Diagnostic Ultrastructure of Non-Neoplastic Diseases

Diagnostic Ultrastructure of Non-Neoplastic Diseases

Edited by

John M. Papadimitriou BA MD PhD FRCPath FRCPA FIBiol

Professor of Ultrastructural Pathology, The University of Western Australia; Consultant in Pathology, Royal Perth Hospital and The Queen Elizabeth II Medical Centre, Perth, Western Australia

Douglas W. Henderson MB BS MRCPath FRCPA

Associate Professor of Pathology, Director of Electron Microscopy and Joint Head of the Department of Histopathology, Flinders Medical Centre, Adelaide; Honorary Consultant in Ultrastructural Pathology, The Queen Elizabeth Hospital, Woodville, South Australia

Dominic V. Spagnolo MB BS FRCPA

Pathologist, Hospital and University Pathology Services, The Queen Elizabeth II Medical Centre, Perth, Western Australia

With the technical assistance of

Peter J. Leppard

Hospital Scientist, Electron Microscopy Unit, Department of Pathology, Flinders Medical Centre, Adelaide, South Australia

Terry A. Robertson

Technologist-in-Charge, Electron Microscopy Unit, Department of Pathology, University of Western Australia, Perth, Western Australia

CHURCHILL LIVINGSTONE
EDINBURGH LONDON MADRID MELBOURNE NEW YORK AND TOKYO 1992

CHURCHILL LIVINGSTONE
Medical Division of Longman Group UK Limited

Distributed in the United States of America by
Churchill Livingstone Inc., 650 Avenue of the Americas, New York,
N.Y. 10011, and by associated companies, branches and
representatives throughout the world.

First published 1992

ISBN 0-443-03464-8

British Library Cataloguing in Publication Data
A catalogue record for this book is available from the British
Library.

Library of Congress Cataloging in Publication Data
Diagnostic ultrastructure of non-neoplastic diseases/edited by John
  M. Papadimitriou, Douglas W. Henderson, Dominic V. Spagnolo;
  with the technical assistance of Peter J. Leppard, Terry A.
  Robertson.
     p. cm.
    Companion v. to: Ultrastructural appearances of tumours/
Douglas W. Henderson, John M. Papadimitriou, Mark Coleman.
1986.
    Includes bibliographical references and index.
    ISBN 0-443-03464-8
    1. Diagnosis, Electron microscopic—Atlases. I. Papadimitriou,
John M. II. Henderson, Douglas W. III. Spagnolo, Dominic V.
IV. Henderson W. Ultrastructural appearances of tumours.
    [DNLM: 1. Microscopy, Electron. 2. Pathology—methods. QZ
25 D536]
RB43.5.D54 1991
616.07'58—dc20
DNLM/DLC
for Library of Congress   90-15129

Printed and bound in Great Britain by
William Clowes Limited, Beccles and London

Preface

This book arose from our perception of the need for a single guidebook to the diagnosis of most non-neoplastic diseases encountered in diagnostic human ultrastructural pathology, as a companion volume to our work, *Ultrastructural Appearances of Tumours*, and this implicit general division between neoplasms versus non-neoplasms seems practical in terms of the workload of most diagnostic electron microscopy (EM) laboratories. Because of their rarity, many of the conditions covered are concentrated in highly specialized laboratories, necessitating a multi-author approach in order to achieve the broadest possible coverage. Nevertheless, it is impossible to discuss and illustrate all of the diagnostic ramifications of EM in a single volume of this size and if more detail is required, the references appended to each chapter should be consulted.

Authorities differ in what they mean by 'diagnostic' in relation to electron microscopy. Some restrict the term to only those disorders in which EM is essential for diagnosis;

by such a yardstick, this would be a slender volume, for there are few diseases in which the diagnosis cannot be made by any other technique. Others are more liberal in their interpretation and would also cover those disorders in which EM can provide useful or contributory information, and even conditions in which the ultrastructure adds much to our understanding of the nature or pathogenesis of the disorder. In conformity with the latter approach, we could equally have chosen the term 'ultrastructural pathology' for the title of this book as an accurate reflection of its scope.

It is our hope that this volume will be useful to ultrastructural pathologists in their everyday practice and that it will further stimulate interest among all pathologists in the ultrastructure of disease processes.

Adelaide and Perth, 1992   J.M.P.
                                            D.W.H.
                                            D.V.S.

Seeing is in some respect an art, which must be learnt. To make a person see with such a power* is nearly the same as if I were to make him play one of Handel's fugues upon the organ.

Sir William Herschel, 18th–19th century astronomer

*The 'power' to which he referred was one of his astronomical telescopes. (In: *The Far Planets*. Time–Life Books, Amsterdam, 1988, p 19)

Seeing does not suffice; it is necessary to learn how to look, how to observe, how to construct a subjective opinion, not one based on a single sense, on seeing, but rather on all available senses, on one's total intellectual capacity . . . Furthermore, it is essential for the microscopist to be free of all sophisticated bias.

Jan Evangelista Purkinje (1787–1869)

(Steiner I, Sajner J, Pollak O J 1988 J E Purkinje memorial lecture. Ultrastructural Pathology 12: 455–459)

For Churchill Livingstone

Publisher: Timothy Horne
Editorial Co-ordination: Editorial Resources Unit
  Copy Editor: Paul Singleton
  Indexer: Nina Boyd
Production Controller: Lesley W Small
Design: Design Resources Unit
Sales Promotion Executive: Hilary Brown

Acknowledgements

Drs Henderson, Papadimitriou and Spagnolo

First and foremost, we are deeply indebted to the multiple authors of this work; its production would have been quite impossible without their willingness to contribute time and talent to the preparation of their various chapters. We also thank them for their forbearance during the long genesis of the book. Any success which this volume achieves will be due largely to their unique contributions, whereas we accept full responsibility for its defects. In addition, completion of this project would have been almost impossible without the continuing support and enthusiasm of Professor M N-I Walters (Perth) and Professor R Whitehead (Adelaide).

We are no less indebted to our families, who have long supported our preoccupation with the world of the very, very small.

We also express our gratitude to Mr P J Leppard (Adelaide), who prepared the illustrations for Chapters 4, 7, 11 and 17, Mr T A Robertson for the figures in Chapters 26 and 29 and to all our technical staff who tirelessly processed tissue for EM and who produced stained ultrathin sections of superlative quality for our scrutiny.

We are especially grateful to Mrs M A Seats, who gallantly and diligently typed the many drafts and final copies of most of the chapters in this book and to Ms Ivonne van Bruggen for checking many of the references.

We thank Drs P W Allen, M Coleman, A E Seymour and J M Skinner for their constructive comments on the manuscript, and Miss L M Smith for secretarial assistance.

In addition, we thank many authors, editors and publishers for permission to reproduce previously published material. Acknowledgements of their contributions can be found below.

Finally, we are most grateful to our publishers, Churchill Livingstone, for their co-operation, enthusiasm and, above all, patience.

Dr Mukherjee

The author wishes to acknowledge the help of Mr K Smith and Mr J G Swift for assistance in compiling this chapter. The permission of SEM Inc Chicago, USA to reproduce Figures 1.1 to 1.4 is also gratefully acknowledged.

Drs Marzella and Trump

We wish to thank Drs Elizabeth McDowell and Thomas Jones and Ms Mary Smith for critical review of this manuscript. We thank the staff of the Publications Division (Wayne J Ivusich, Diane B Dix and Millie M Michalisko), Department of Pathology, University of Maryland School of Medicine for their administrative/secretarial work. We gratefully acknowledge Messrs Robert Pendergrass, Seung Chang, Perry Comegys, Roderick Wierwille and Mrs Janet Folmer of the Electron Microscopy Laboratory in the Department of Pathology for their expert assistance.

Dr Dustin

This review would not have been possible without the collective work of many collaborators. I wish first to thank Professor V J Ferrans, who contributed the material on hyperlipidaemias and Wolman's disease (Figs 6.19 and 6.20) and Professor J J Martin (Fig. 6.18) who sent me an original micrograph. All electron micrographs of conjunctival biopsies are by courtesy of Professor J Libert (Department of Ophthalmology, University of Brussels). My collaborators at the Department of Pathology, University of Brussels, who contributed most of the figures, were Professor J Flament-Durand, Professor A Résibois and Drs M Tondur and J Rutsaert. I wish also to extend my thanks to Mr Jean-Louis Conreur, who did the photographic work for this text and Mrs DeLigne who helped to prepare the Tables.

Figures 6.8, 6.14 and 6.15 are reproduced from J V Johannessen (ed) 1978 Electron microscopy in human medicine, Vol 2, McGraw-Hill Inc, by kind permission of the publishers (copyright date 5.9.90).

Dr Madeley

I am indebted to Dr June Almeida, who originally taught me electron microscopy, Dr Anne Field and my other colleagues on the PHLS EM Advisory Committee for the discussions and occasionally arguments which have helped to shape the opinions outlined in this chapter, and particularly to Mrs Bonnie Cosgrove, Mr Iain Miller, Mr Fred

Laidler and Mr Elliott Wilkinson, with whom I have worked directly.

I am indebted to Churchill Livingstone for permission to reproduce Figures 8.5, 8.8, 8.11, 8.14 and 8.17–8.24; to the Editor, The Lancet for permission to reproduce Figure 8.9.

Dr Wills
The excellent technical assistance of Susan Brammah with this work is gratefully acknowledged. Thanks are also due to those colleagues, named in the appropriate figure legends, who contributed specimens for this chapter.

Drs Corrin and Dewar
We thank all those colleagues, named in the relevant captions, who so readily contributed illustrations. We also thank colleagues and editors who kindly gave permission to reproduce illustrations, again as detailed in the relevant captions.

Drs Kamel, Boyd, Toner, Henderson, Armstrong and Mukherjee
We are indebted to Mr P J Leppard, Electron Microscopy Laboratory, Department of Pathology, Flinders Medical Centre, for technical and photographic assistance in the preparation of this chapter. We also thank Drs G P Davidson and E Cutz for Figure 14.1, and the editor and publisher of *Gastroenterology* — Dr Raj K Goyal and Elsevier Science Publishing Company — for permission to reproduce the figure.

Drs Asa, Horvath and Kovacs
The authors gratefully acknowledge the excellent technical assistance of Mrs G Ilse and Mrs D Lietz and the invaluable secretarial help of Ms M Wong and Mrs W Wlodarski.

Drs Coleman and Seymour
The authors gratefully acknowledge the contribution of Mr P J Leppard who, with meticulous attention to detail, prepared for publication all of the photomicrographs.

Drs Stevens and Boadle
The authors wish to thank Dr John Tyler and Dr David Mortimer for helpful discussion, Carol Robinson for photographic assistance, Celia Tanner for artwork and Dianne Jones for typing the manuscript. Figure 18.4 inset is reproduced by courtesy of the editor of *Pathology*.

Drs Smith and Fenoglio-Preiser
The authors gratefully acknowledge the excellent technical assistance of Mark Boyer.

Dr Sathananthan
The author is indebted to the Royal Children's Hospital, Melbourne, and the National University of Singapore for TEM facilities. Dennis Philipatos and Jean Ho are thanked for technical assistance.

Dr Anton-Lamprecht
I cordially thank all my co-workers, who participated in the ultrastructural investigations over the years and who, with their excellent and dedicated co-operation, contributed significantly to the material that forms the basis of the present chapter. They are: Dr Marie-Luise Arnold, Dr Ingrid Hausser, Barbara Melz-Rothfuss, Inge Werner, Jutta Deimel-Hatzenbühler, Ermelind Schleiermacher, Rita Triebskorn and Dagmar Theiss; their names are indicated in the captions of the respective micrographs taken by them. Anita Lutz prepared the final prints of the light and electron micrographs and Gertrud Lippert and Margot Herold typed the manuscript. I am especially thankful to Margot Herold for her invaluable help in taking care of the final compilation of the entire chapter. I am grateful to colleagues and publishers who agreed to the reproduction of figures from previously published investigations, especially to Professor Ruggero Caputo for his kind permission to include his table on histiocytic disorders (Table 22.3).

Finally, I should like to dedicate this manuscript to my husband. His infinite patience, his appreciation and encouragement throughout all the years have become the firm ground of my past and present work and research.

Dr Vital
The author is very grateful to A Gue, L Huguet, J Rochet and M Turmo for their technical assistance, to S Senon for preparation of the final photographs, to C Bourdillou for her expert secretarial assistance and to R Cooke for linguistic help.

Dr Steiner
The author greatly appreciates the invaluable technical help provided by Lucie Clements in the preparation of the material and illustrations. He also thanks Ms Hilda Castro for typing the manuscript and Drs Bullough and DeCarlo for their help in performing the X-ray microanalysis of the case of tumoural calcinosis (Fig. 27.11) and in taking SEM and performing X-ray analysis of a case of crystal pyrophosphate deposition disease (Figs 28.21 and 28.22). Figure 27.4 is reproduced with the kind permission of the copyright holder; it is from Figure 16 in Bullough P, Davidson D, Lorenzo J C 1981 Morbid anatomy of the skeleton in osteogenesis imperfecta. Clinical Orthopaedics and Related Research 159: 42. Figures 28.1 and 28.18 are reproduced with the kind permission of Dr G Faure, and Figure 28.14 with the kind permission of Dr R Minns.

Drs Spagnolo, Armstrong, Papadimitriou and Henderson
The authors gratefully acknowledge the excellent technical assistance of M Archer and P Caterina (Electron Microscopy Unit, Hospital and University Pathology Services, Queen Elizabeth II Medical Centre), and R Horne, A Lazzaro and S H Wee (Electron Microscopy Unit, Department of Pathology, Royal Perth Hospital). We are also indebted to Drs L R Matz (Royal Perth Hospital) and A Singh (Fremantle Hospital) who made available material for our studies.

Contributors

Ali Ahmed MD
Senior Lecturer in Pathology, Department of Pathology,
University of Manchester, Manchester, UK

Arline Albala MA
Staff Associate, Columbia University College of Physicians
and Surgeons, New York, USA

Ingrun Anton-Lamprecht DSc
Professor and Direktor, Institut für Ultrastrukturforschung
der Haut, Hautklinik der Ruprecht-Karls-Universität,
Heidelberg, Germany

John A. Armstrong DSc FRCPath
Electron Microscopist, Department of Pathology, Royal
Perth Hospital, Perth, Western Australia

Sylvia L. Asa MD PhD
Assistant Professor of Pathology, University of Toronto;
Pathologist, St Michael's Hospital, Toronto, Ontario,
Canada

Ross A. Boadle AAIMLS
Chief Medical Technologist, Electron Microscopy Unit,
Institute of Clinical Pathology and Medical Research,
Westmead Hospital, Westmead, Sydney, New South Wales,
Australia

Sheelagh M. Boyd MB BCh BAO MRCPath
Senior Registrar, Department of Pathology, Royal Victoria
Hospital, Belfast, Northern Ireland

Janine Breton-Gorius PhD
Director of Research, INSERM Unité de Recherche en
Génétique Moléculaire et en Hématologie, Hôpital Henri
Mondor, Creteil, France

Katherine E. Carr BSc PhD MIBiol
Professor of Anatomy and Director of School of Basic
Medical Sciences, Medical Biology Centre, The Queen's
University of Belfast, Belfast, Northern Ireland

Mark Coleman MB BS FRCPA
Senior Staff Specialist and Senior Lecturer in Pathology,
Flinders Medical Centre, Adelaide, South Australia

Bryan Corrin MD FRCPath
Professor of Thoracic Pathology, National Heart and Lung
Institute (London University), Brompton Hospital,
London, UK

Elisabeth Cramer MD PhD
Associate Professor, Service d'Hématologie et INSERM
Unité 91, Hôpital Lariboisière, Paris, France

Ann Dewar MIBiol
Senior Technician in Electron Microscopy, National Heart
and Lung Institute (London University), Brompton
Hospital, London, UK

Pierre Dustin MD
Emeritus Professor of Pathology, Faculty of Medicine,
Université Libre de Bruxelles, Brussels, Belgium

John J. Fenoglio Jr MD (Deceased)
Professor and Vice-Chairman, Department of Pathology,
College of Physicians and Surgeons of Columbia
University, New York, USA

Cecilia M. Fenoglio-Preiser MD
Professor of Pathology, University of New Mexico School
of Medicine; Chief of Laboratory Services, Albuquerque
Veterans Administration Medical Center, Albuquerque,
New Mexico, USA

Jennet M. Harvey MB BS FRCPA
Pathologist, Hospital and University Pathology Services,
The Queen Elizabeth II Medical Centre, Nedlands, Perth,
Western Australia

Douglas W. Henderson MB BS MRCPath FRCPA
Associate Professor of Pathology, Director of Electron
Microscopy and Joint Head of the Department of
Histopathology, Flinders Medical Centre, Adelaide;
Honorary Consultant in Ultrastructural Pathology,
The Queen Elizabeth Hospital, Woodville, South
Australia

Asao Hirano MD
Professor, Department of Pathology and Neuroscience, Albert Einstein College of Medicine, New York; Head of the Division of Neuropathology, Department of Pathology, Montefiore Hospital and Medical Center, New York, USA

Eva Horvath PhD
Associate Professor of Pathology, University of Toronto; Research Associate, St Michael's Hospital, Toronto, Ontario, Canada

Hassan M. H. Kamel MB ChB MSc PhD
Registrar, Department of Pathology, Royal Victoria Hospital, Belfast, Northern Ireland

Gordon K. Klintworth MD PhD
Professor of Ophthalmology and Pathology, Duke University Medical Center, Durham, North Carolina, USA

Kalman Kovacs MD PhD DSc FRCP(C) FCAP FRCPath
Professor of Pathology, University of Toronto; Pathologist, St Michael's Hospital, Toronto, Ontario, Canada

C. Richard Madeley MD FRCPath
Professor of Clinical Virology and Consultant Virologist, University of Newcastle upon Tyne and Royal Victoria Infirmary, Newcastle upon Tyne, UK

Louis Marzella MD PhD
Associate Professor, Division of Hyperbaric Medicine, Maryland Institute for Emergency Medical Services Systems; Associate Professor, Department of Pathology, University of Maryland School of Medicine, Baltimore, Maryland, USA

Tapen M. Mukherjee MD FRCPA
Head of Electron Microscopy, Institute of Medical and Veterinary Science, Adelaide, South Australia

John M. Papadimitriou BA MD PhD FRCPath FRCPA FIBiol
Professor of Ultrastructural Pathology, The University of Western Australia; Consultant in Pathology, Royal Perth Hospital and The Queen Elizabeth II Medical Centre, Perth, Western Australia

Alan D. Proia MD PhD
Assistant Professor of Ophthalmology and Pathology, Duke University Medical Center, Durham, North Carolina, USA

A. Henry Sathananthan PhD
Senior Lecturer, Lincoln School of Health Sciences, Melbourne; Honorary Senior Research Associate, Centre for Early Human Development, Monash Medical Centre, Clayton, Victoria, Australia

Anthony E. Seymour MD FRCPA
Associate Professor of Pathology, Flinders Medical Centre, Adelaide, South Australia; Consultant in Renal Pathology, The Queen Elizabeth Hospital, Woodville; Associate Pathologist, The Adelaide Children's Hospital, North Adelaide, South Australia

Suzanne Meleg Smith MD
Research Assistant Professor, University of New Mexico School of Medicine, Albuquerque, New Mexico, USA

Dominic V. Spagnolo MB BS FRCPA
Pathologist, Hospital and University Pathology Services, The Queen Elizabeth II Medical Centre, Perth, Western Australia

German C. Steiner MD
Director, Department of Pathology and Laboratory Medicine, Hospital for Joint Diseases Orthopaedic Institute; Associate Professor of Surgical Pathology, New York University School of Medicine, New York, USA

Susan M. B. Stevens MD BS PhD DCH(Lond) FRCPA
Senior Staff Specialist, Electron Microscopy Unit, Institute of Clinical Pathology and Medical Research, Westmead Hospital, Westmead, Sydney, New South Wales, Australia

Grant R. Sutherland PhD DSc
Chief Cytogeneticist, Department of Pathology, Adelaide Children's Hospital, North Adelaide, South Australia

Kyuichi Tanikawa MD PhD
Professor and Chairman, The Second Department of Internal Medicine, Kurume University School of Medicine, Kurume, Japan

Peter G. Toner MB ChB DSc FRCPG FRCPath
Musgrave Professor of Pathology, The Queen's University of Belfast, Belfast, Northern Ireland

Benjamin F. Trump MD
Professor and Chairman, Department of Pathology, University of Maryland School of Medicine, Baltimore, Maryland, USA

Claude Vital MD
Professor of Pathology and Neuropathology, Bordeaux II University; Head, Department of Pathology, Pellegrin Hospital, Bordeaux, France

Andrew Warton PhD
Research Fellow, University Department of Pathology, Sir Charles Gairdner Hospital, The Queen Elizabeth II Medical Centre, Nedlands, Perth, Western Australia

Edward J. Wills MD BSc(Med) DCP FRCPA
Senior Staff Specialist and Head, Section of Electron Microscopy, Department of Anatomical Pathology, Royal Prince Alfred Hospital, Sydney, New South Wales, Australia

Contents

1. Introduction

D. W. Henderson   J. M. Papadimitriou   D. V. Spagnolo

The ambit of electron microscopy (EM) in surgical pathology is potentially almost as broad as that of light microscopy (LM), but EM is of diagnostic relevance far less often. It has been estimated that ultrastructural examination can contribute useful information on about 1–5% of the specimens recorded in most teaching hospital–university departments; this applies especially to tumours.[4,8,15,20,31] EM is usually less decisive in the diagnosis of non-neoplastic diseases overall, but it has a well-established role in a broad range of disorders and tissues, notably in virus diagnosis, renal pathology, disorders of skeletal muscle, and certain skin diseases. Although several books on the ultrastructural pathology of tumours have now been published,[3,7,12,15,23,24] there are fewer works dealing with the diagnostic fine structure of non-neoplastic diseases, and these often cover a mixture of both neoplastic and non-neoplastic conditions;[17,29] alternatively, the latter may be dealt with in a specialized text covering a single disease group such as virus infections[5,18] or renal diseases,[28] or a single tissue such as the liver,[22] breast[2] or synovium.[11]

In a general sense, the following roles can be defined for EM in anatomical pathology:[10]

1. *The diagnosis and classification of diseases.* The dysmotile cilia syndrome, microvillous inclusion disease of the intestinal tract, the epidermolysis bullosa group of skin disorders, minimal change nephropathy and other glomerular basement membrane nephropathies are classical examples of disorders in which EM is mandatory for precise diagnosis (see Ch. 13, 14, 17 and 22).

2. *Quality control in diagnostic pathology.* Because of its capacity to detect diagnostic features beyond the resolution of the light microscope, EM can be used on occasions to monitor the accuracy of LM diagnoses, rectifying any tendency to overdiagnosis or underdiagnosis,[10] especially when the LM criteria are vague or highly subjective. In the same way, EM can be used to evaluate the accuracy of immunohistological diagnosis by revealing occasional instances of false-positive or false-negative immunostaining.

3. *A refined appreciation of light microscopy appearances.*

For example, EM has established that the so-called parenthesis bodies seen by LM in *Pneumocystis* cysts represent paired thickenings of the cyst wall.[26]

4. *The delineation of new disease entities.* Once again, ciliary dyskinesia is a classical example.[1,6,19]

5. *Evaluation of the effects of drugs, chemicals and xenobiotics, and of response to therapy.* For example, EM has clarified the nature of amiodarone toxicity in the lung (see Ch. 13), while X-ray microanalysis of xenobiotics is an expanding discipline in its own right and is the subject of a book published recently.[16]

6. *Elucidation of pathogenetic mechanisms.* For example, the identification of the trophozoite form of *Pneumocystis* and the proposed life cycle of the organism, as well as its preferential localization to the surface of type I pneumocytes, has been achieved mainly by EM.[26,30] Similarly, in diffuse alveolar damage the central role of injury to type I pneumocytes has been established by EM (see Ch. 13).

7. *As a fundamental technique in cell biology.* Advances in cell biology are being incorporated into the realm of surgical pathology with increasing frequency, blurring the distinction between 'pure' and 'applied' research.

8. *As a teaching modality at both undergraduate and postgraduate levels.*

Our views[14,15] and those of others[9,22,27] on the principles of diagnostic electron microscopy — whether of tumours or other disease processes — have been stated in detail elsewhere and can be reiterated here quite briefly:

a. Light microscopy examination of tissue or cells is a fundamental prerequisite for diagnostic EM, and the fine-structural findings become most informative when closely correlated with the LM observations, including immunohistology whenever appropriate, and other clinico-pathological data.

b. Clearly, familiarity with normal fine structure is essential if the abnormal is to be recognized and interpreted correctly.

c. As a general consideration, any abnormal ultrastructural finding should preferably fulfil three criteria to be useful in diagnosis:[14] (i) the structure should be sufficiently distinctive to be able to be recognized readily; (ii) the structure should be specific for — or at least characteristic of — a particular cell type or disease process, either in isolation or (more frequently) in combination with other appearances: every finding needs to be evaluated in the light of its cellular or subcellular milieu; and (iii) ideally, the structure should be found with sufficient frequency that it is useful in at least a sizeable proportion of cases.

d. One needs to be aware of the limitations of EM in diagnosis. Overinterpretation of submicroscopic structure should be avoided. For example, we are wary of drawing functional or biochemical conclusions from the static perspective of disordered fine structure, unless these have been well established by experimental data or correlative studies. The lysosomal storage disorders represent one group of diseases in which the nature of the stored material and the underlying enzyme defects have been established by biochemical studies and correlated with the ultrastructural appearances, and a biochemical conclusion can be predicted from the fine structure (see Ch. 6). X-ray microanalysis in the electron microscope[16] is an obvious exception to the general rule stated above, and allows precise chemical analysis of abnormal material (for example, xenobiotics) and many 'normal' substances accumulating in abnormal amounts (for example, iron in siderosomes).

The question of who should perform and interpret diagnostic EM is one issue that arouses passion and argument among electron-microscopists and pathologists alike. Some of our colleagues fervently believe that this should be the exclusive province of the specialist pathologist who can best place the ultrastructural findings into clinical and pathological perspective. Yet we have seen surgical pathologists with little experience of ultrastructure charge into this unfamiliar territory, basing their interpretation on a single subcellular finding, which they have then misinterpreted, thereby reaching a wildly erroneous conclusion.

Historically, diagnostic EM has often been relegated to professional electron-microscopists without formal training in pathology, partly because of the inertia of pathologists and their lack of familiarity with EM procedures, and partly because of the territorial imperatives of some electron-microscopists.[25] Many electron-microscopists are highly competent at ultrastructural diagnosis, and some are outstanding authorities in the field. Regrettably, others lack familiarity with pathological processes; as Rosai[22] has emphasized, the reports originating from their laboratories can be easily spotted, being characterized by lengthy descriptions of almost every organelle in turn — devoid of highlights or correlation with clinical and pathological data, and without a meaningful conclusion; alternatively, a functional aberration may be invoked as opposed to a fine-structural diagnosis. Equally regrettably, some electron-microscopists involved in diagnosis view it as a chore: a tiresome intrusion into their research programmes.

One can long argue about which is less deplorable in diagnostic ultrastructural pathology: wrongful interpretations by a pathologist lacking a detailed knowledge of fine structure, or irrelevant reports by an electron-microscopist without a detailed knowledge or experience of pathology. Our own view is that erroneous reports can spell doom for the credibility of the individual, but that irrelevance can be the death-knell of the discipline. Moreover, it is probably easier for a pathologist to learn fine structure than for an electron-microscopist to acquire a detailed knowledge of pathology, with its clinical implications and priorities.[27] In the final analysis, we believe that the achievement of optimal results is less dependent on the formal qualifications of the professionals concerned than on a detailed knowledge of, and commitment to, diagnosis in surgical pathology and electron microscopy, in roughly equal proportions, together with the capacity for evaluation or correlation of each stage of morphological assessment, from routine light microscopy, to the semithin sections, to actual examination of the ultrathin sections in the electron microscope and finally to the interpretation of the electron micrographs.[22] We do not generate a separate EM report for many of the examinations carried out in our laboratories, notably renal biopsies; instead, a single unified report is issued which correlates the 'routine' light microscopy, immunohistology and electron microscopy. In this setting, the philosophy of diagnostic EM is not that of an isolated discipline but that of a technique integral to surgical pathology, albeit one with its own set of rules and regulations.

REFERENCES

1. Afzelius B A 1976 A human syndrome caused by immotile cilia. Science 193: 317–319
2. Ahmed A 1978 Atlas of the ultrastructure of human breast diseases. Churchill Livingstone, Edinburgh
3. Azar H A (ed) 1988 Pathology of human neoplasms. An atlas of diagnostic electron microscopy and immunohistochemistry. Raven Press, New York
4. Dardick I 1987 The Ottawa course (editorial). Ultrastructural Pathology 11: v–vi
5. Doane F W, Anderson N 1987 Electron microscopy in diagnostic virology: a practical guide and atlas. Cambridge University Press, New York
6. Eliasson R, Mossberg B, Camner P, Afzelius B A 1977 The immotile-cilia syndrome. A congenital ciliary abnormality as an, etiologic factor in chronic airway infections and male sterility. New England Journal of Medicine 297: 1–6
7. Erlandson R A 1981 Diagnostic transmission electron microscopy of human tumors. The interpretation of submicroscopic structures in human neoplastic cells. Masson, New York
8. Erlandson R A 1984 Electron microscopy and human tumor diagnosis. Past, present, and future (editorial). Ultrastructural Pathology 6: iii–v
9. Erlandson R A 1987 Application of transmission electron microscopy to human tumor diagnosis: an historical perspective. Cancer Investigation 5: 487–505
10. Ghadially F N 1981 The role of electron microscopy in the determination of tumour histogenesis. Diagnostic Histopathology 4: 245–262
11. Ghadially F N 1983 Fine structure of synovial joints. A text and atlas of the ultrastructure of normal and pathological articular tissues. Butterworths, London
12. Ghadially F N 1985 Diagnostic electron microscopy of tumours, 2nd edn. Butterworths, London
13. Hammar S P 1986 Editorial: Is electron microscopy dying? Ultrastructural Pathology 10: iii–v
14. Henderson D W 1990 Case for the panel: unusual cytoplasmic inclusions in metastatic tumor cells in retroperitoneal lymph nodes of a man with unknown primary tumor (commentary). Ultrastructural Pathology 14:101–106
15. Henderson D W, Papadimitriou J M, Coleman M 1986 Ultrastructural appearance of tumours. Diagnosis and classification of human neoplasia by electron microscopy, 2nd edn. Churchill Livingstone, Edinburgh
16. Ingram P, Shelburne J D, Roggli V 1989 Microprobe analysis in medicine. Hemisphere Publishing Corporation, New York
17. Johannessen J V (ed) 1978–1983 Electron microscopy in human medicine, vols 1–13a. McGraw-Hill, New York
18. Madeley C R 1972 Virus morphology. Churchill Livingstone, Edinburgh
19. McDowell E M, Beals T F 1986 Biopsy pathology of the bronchi. Chapman and Hall, London, pp 221–241
20. McLay A L C, Toner P G 1981 Diagnostic electron microscopy. In: Anthony PP, MacSween R N M (eds) Recent advances in histopathology, no. 11. Churchill Livingstone, Edinburgh, pp 241–261
21. Phillips M J, Poucell S, Patterson J, Valencia P 1987 The liver. An atlas and text of ultrastructural pathology. Raven Press, New York
22. Rosai J 1981 How not to do diagnostic electron microscopy (editorial). Ultrastructural Pathology 2: iii–iv
23. Russo J, Sommers S C 1986 Tumor diagnosis by electron microscopy, vol 1. Field, Rich and Associates, New York
24. Russo J, Sommers S C 1988 Tumor diagnosis by electron microscopy, vol 2. Field & Wood, Philadelphia
25. Seymour A E, Henderson D W 1981 Electron microscopy in surgical pathology: a selective review. Pathology 13: 111–135
26. Sobonya R E 1988 Pneumocystis infection. In: Dail D H, Hammar S P (eds) Pulmonary pathology. Springer-Verlag, New York, pp 301–313
27. Sobrinho-Simões M, Nesland J M, Johannessen J V 1981 Diagnostic ultrastructural pathology — sub-specialty or special stain? Diagnostic Histopathology 4: 223–236
28. Spargo B H, Seymour A E, Ordóñez N G 1980 Renal biopsy pathology with diagnostic and therapeutic implications. John Wiley & Sons, New York
29. Trump B F, Jones R T 1978–1983 Diagnostic electron microscopy, vols 1–4. John Wiley & Sons, New York
30. Walzer P D 1984 Experimental models of *Pneumocystis carinii* infections. In: Young L S (ed) *Pneumocystis carinii* pneumonia. Pathogenesis. Diagnosis. Treatment. Marcel Dekker, New York, pp 7–76
31. Williams M J 1981 Diagnostic electron microscopy in the US Veterans Administration. Diagnostic Histopathology 4: 279–293

2. Techniques in diagnostic electron microscopy

T. M. Mukherjee

INTRODUCTION

Within the span of a decade, the electron microscope and its ancillary techniques have become invaluable in diagnostic pathology. The early years of electron microscopy (EM) were marked by its extensive use in the submicroscopic investigation of cells and tissues, when it was a mainstay in cell biology and especially in biomedical research. Unfortunately, the limitations associated with electron microscopy at that time — such as prolonged preparatory procedures, and expensive instrumentation which could be handled only by expert technologists — prompted an attitude among many pathologists that EM was an expensive 'tool' not particularly suited to the needs of routine diagnostic pathology, where rapid diagnosis is of the utmost importance.

Developments over the past decade — including modifications to techniques and the application of automation in various preparatory procedures — have made modern-day EM a valuable 'diagnostic tool' and an essential adjunct to other routine methods of laboratory diagnosis.

The formerly complex ancillary procedures such as scanning electron microscopy (SEM), backscattered electron imaging (BEI), analytical electron microscopy (EDX) and, of late, electron energy loss spectrometry (EELS) have now become simplified due to advances in instrument technology and the development of suitable hard- and soft-ware; these advances have brought such sophisticated techniques within the scope of routine pathology laboratories. In addition, modern electron microscopes are user-friendly, various modes of operation being controlled with the flick of a switch.

The purpose of this chapter is to elucidate this growth in the nature of EM techniques and to offer recipes that have proven their worth in routine diagnostic laboratories.

Although surgical biopsies form the majority of specimens requiring diagnostic EM, there are a number of other types of specimen which may yield significant diagnostic information — not only to anatomical pathologists but also to haematologists, virologists and microbiologists. Hence it has been the practice in this laboratory to be prepared to process almost any type of sample for direct transmission electron microscopy (TEM) or any other type of ancillary electron microscopic examination that may be required. These specimens include:

Tissue biopsies
Sputum
Faecal matter
Urinary sediments
Cytology specimens
Cerebrospinal fluid
Bone marrow biopsies
Peripheral blood
Synovial fluid
Calculi
Bronchial lavage fluid

Familiarity with the range of methodologies available for any of these types of material will ensure that the sample is processed by the optimal method for conventional TEM or any of the other ancillary techniques.

The experience of Cleland et al[25] serves as a good example in support of this concept. They reported a 25-year-old man, engaged in the manufacture of fibreglass surf boards, who presented with chronic synovitis in the dorsal exterior sheath of the hand. Synovial fluid aspirates showed unusual needle-shaped particles by phase contrast microscopy. SEM of the particles followed by EDX revealed that the particles consisted of silicon and calcium, indicating their relationship to fibreglass, which was further confirmed by EDX examination of dust from the factory floor. Hence the judicial use of various EM techniques was able to confirm a hitherto unreported diagnosis of fibreglass-induced synovitis. Baker and associates[11] have reviewed the use of microprobe analysis in human pathology, citing many other examples of unusual and unforeseen observations by EDX techniques.

The purpose of this section is to discuss the commonly used methods of tissue preparation which allow specimens to be examined not only by the conventional methods of TEM but also by other ancillary techniques. Also considered are the applications and limitations of various EM techniques in diagnosis — such as SEM (see also Ch. 3), BEI, EDX, EELS, immunocytochemistry and freeze–fracture (FF).

DIFFERENT METHODS OF SPECIMEN PREPARATION

Fixation and processing for conventional thin-section (TEM)

This topic has been extensively covered in the literature,[52,56,58,67,68,105,106,129,171] and these references give a comprehensive account of the problems associated with improper fixation, dehydration and embedding — and how to avoid them.

In our laboratory we have found that 2.5% glutaraldehyde in 0.05 M sodium cacodylate buffer at pH 7.2 is the most suitable fixative. The advantages are many as this fixative can be stored for prolonged periods without compromising its buffering capacity. It can also be used for tissues on which EDX analysis may be required at a later stage. In contrast, phosphate buffer has the disadvantage of possible fungal growth, with alteration of phosphate levels in any material requiring microprobe analysis at a later stage. There is an added advantage of primary fixation in glutaraldehyde in cacodylate buffer in the conventional manner, followed by post- fixation in osmium tetroxide, together with fixation of a concurrent sample in glutaraldehyde in cacodylate buffer alone. Few laboratories realize the benefit of a small tissue sample not postfixed in osmium tetroxide for later use by other ancillary EM techniques: once the tissue has been osmicated, further studies with X-ray microprobe analysis are considerably handicapped due to osmium-related displacement or translocation of various elements or ions of importance. In addition, unosmicated tissues can reveal important details of particulate aggregates within cells and tissues (see Fig. 2.1) since the inner details of such structural entities are otherwise masked by osmium. Further details on this argument are covered in references 50, 51, 110 and 133. Haemosiderin, ferritin particles, other iron-containing inclusions, metallic inclusions with high Z value (high atomic number of the element) can be easily identified by BEI in an unstained unosmicated section because of their electron-scattering properties; this is not true for the tissue itself (see Fig. 2.3). Moreover, osmium and uranyl acetate as pre-embedding staining agents often compete with these metallic components and may translocate them so that their presence in the section is not appropriately represented.

Obviously, the choice of a suitable fixative and embedding material and the subsequent processing procedures are of importance when considered in relation to the varied needs of routine pathology laboratories. These requirements will vary from institution to institution and much has already been written on this aspect;[51,56,58,67,68,105,106,129,171] hence it is natural to expect that each laboratory will have its own recipes to satisfy its individual requirements.

MICROWAVE AS A PREPARATORY PROCEDURE FOR EM

Since the early attempt by Chew et al[23] to use microwave irradiation as an aid to rapid fixation for the study of cell ultrastructure, considerable interest has developed over the years. To hasten primary fixation in aldehydes, numerous workers[73,87,88,89,90,92,93] have used microwave as an adjunct for a brief period such as 26–90 ms[93] to about 90 s.[87] This is then followed by post-fixation in osmium tetroxide, dehydration, and embedding in the usual resin mixtures. Although this method of fixation has merits in reducing the initial fixation time and improving the penetration of aldehydes, it has done little to the time taken for the overall preparatory procedures of dehydration, infiltration in resin mixtures and polymerization. Accordingly, some attempts have been made by Mclay et al[104] to reduce the polymerization time. They observed that uninterrupted exposure of the capsules in a microwave oven for a minute or more produced 'almost explosive polymerization with distortion of the embedding capsule'. They managed to overcome this problem by seven 15-second bursts and two 30-second exposures separated by 30-second cooling intervals, and they found the final results to be quite acceptable. Estrada et al[39] have also used microwave for rapid staining of ultrathin sections: for surgical pathology specimens, 15 seconds in uranyl acetate followed by immersion in lead citrate for a similar time, produced better results than staining them by conventional methods. From their experience it seems that microwave can improve the staining quality of thin sections and can also considerably reduce contamination.

Perhaps the most significant area where microwave fixation has a role is in its future use in EM cytochemistry and immunocytochemistry. Enzyme cytochemistry has a few applications in diagnostic electron microscopy, such as in differentiating acute myeloblastic from acute lymphoblastic leukaemias by localizing myeloperoxidase in the cells belonging to the myeloid series (see Ch. 30). However, the potential for evaluating differences of, for example, membrane-associated enzymes such as alkaline phosphatase, ATPase, and mitochondrial enzymes such as succinic dehydrogenase has been hampered by the problems of prolonged fixation in aldehyde fixatives needed to preserve cell ultrastructure on the one hand, but at the expense of enzyme activity on the other. For this reason, localization of enzymes has been little used for diagnosis. With the aid of this rapid microwave fixation,[88,90,93] the investigation of rapid intracellular physiological processes and preservation of proteins difficult to demonstrate with routine fixation methods (for example, antigens and enzymes, and their qualitative and perhaps quantitative demonstration in health and disease) has come within reach. This technique may also pave the way for an alternative method to cumbersome and demanding quick-freeze and subsequent freeze-drying methods, and low-temperature embedding and cryo-ultramicrotomy techniques.[59,99,155,177,179] Although these methods of tissue preparation have made significant contributions in studies related to non-clinical enzyme cytochemistry and immunocytochemistry by EM, they are as yet far from 'routine' in clinical EM, and rapid microwave fixation and polymerization may represent a method for the future application of enzyme cytochemistry and immunocytochemistry in diagnostic pathology. Preliminary experience appears to indicate that microwave preservation will eventually be important, not only in routine light microscopy but also in routine diagnostic EM, enzyme-cytochemistry and immunocytochemistry.

PREPARATORY TECHNIQUES FOR DIFFERENT SPECIMENS

Standard specimen processing of tissues by fixation in glutaraldehyde, washing in buffer, and postfixation in osmium tetroxide, followed by dehydration through graded ethanols, embedding in a variety of epoxy-based resins and subsequent polymerization in capsules for sectioning and staining, requires no further description: most surgical pathology laboratories are already well versed in the appropriate protocols. Obviously, these methods have many variations. The following discussion centres on the processing of unusual samples:

Effusion fluids and/or bone marrow fragments

1. Centrifuge for 10 min at 1000 r.p.m
2. Remove supernatant
3. Resuspend in 0.5 ml of 8% bovine serum albumin (BSA)
4. Add four drops of 25% glutaraldehyde
5. Mix and immediately centrifuge at 1500 r.p.m for 5 min
6. Remove set BSA with the cell pellet from the centrifuge tube
7. Remove excess BSA
8. Treat as a standard tissue specimen and proceed with the usual postfixation dehydration and embedding

Variations of similar techniques for processing cell suspensions can be found in procedures utilizing agar, fibrin, and albumin cross-linking by glutaraldehyde as has been done in this instance for BSA.[169,176] Burkhardt[19] describes a rapid method for the processing of large numbers of samples of cell suspension for cytochemical and immunocytochemical studies at the ultrastructural level.

Occasionally, one is confronted by cell suspensions with very few 'free-floating' cells. Although the method described above is suitable in most instances, the method used by Kaps & Burkhardt[80] for EM studies of cells in cerebrospinal fluid (CSF) deserves special mention. Their technique involves entrapping CSF cells between two bovine serum albumin cylinders (prepared by the method described by Burkhardt[19]) and linked by glutaraldehyde using microhaematocrit tubes.

The 'sandwiched' specimen can then be processed routinely. It is claimed that this method is rapid and avoids substantial loss of CSF cells — an important consideration when the concentration of cells in a fluid is very low.

Peripheral blood

1. Centrifuge the blood with anticoagulant at 1000 r.p.m for 20 min
2. Remove supernatant
3. Gently add an equal volume of 2.5% glutaraldehyde
4. Allow to fix for 30 min
5. Remove buffy coat and cut into blocks
6. Allow to fix in fresh 2.5% glutaraldehyde in appropriate buffer for 1.5 h
7. Follow standard technique as before, with postosmication, dehydration and embedding in usual resin mixture

Platelet-rich plasma

1. Incubate at 37°C for 1 h
2. Preheat 0.2% glutaraldehyde in appropriate buffer to 37°C
3. Mix equal volumes of both solutions
4. Fix at 37°C for 15 min
5. Discard supernatant
6. Treat pellet as described by the standard technique

Note that glass containers should never be used while preparing platelets since the latter will stick to the surface, leaving the sample devoid of them.

Bone

1. Fix in glutaraldehyde for 2 h
2. Cut bone into small blocks
3. Treat with 'decal', several changes over two days, with stirring
4. Treat by standard technique

Paraffin blocks

1. Select area of block from corresponding H & E section
2. Remove tissue, 1–2 mm^3 or less
3. Deparaffinize with several changes of xylol over 12 h
4. Rehydrate through decreasing alcohol series
5. Treat according to standard technique

Paraffin blocks (urgent)

1. Select corresponding area of block from corresponding H & E section
2. Remove tissue 1–2 mm deep with a scalpel
3. Cut into blocks 1 mm^3
4. Fix in freshly made osmium tetroxide in xylol at 40°C for 15 min and at room temperature for a further 45 min
5. Wash with xylol, dehydrate with propylene oxide and then infiltrate with propylene oxide/resin mixture before embedding in fresh resin and polymerize according to standard procedures

This procedure incorporates the method of rapid deparaffinization as described by Weerman van den Berg & Dingemans.[172]

Tissue for examination from paraffin sections (sometimes termed the 'pop off' method)

1. Locate area of interest and mark on the back of the slide with a diamond pencil
2. Remove cover slip after soaking in xylol
3. Wash in two changes of xylol
4. Rehydrate through decreasing alcohol series
5. Wash in buffer, 2 × 5 min
6. Fix in 2% osmium tetroxide for 1 h
7. Wash in buffer 2 × 5 min
8. Dehydrate through increasing alcohol series; cover the section with resin/propylene oxide 1:1 mixture for 15 mins and then, after draining the mixture, cover the section again with 3:1 mixture for a further 15 min
9. Drain and cover section with final resin mix 2 × 15 min
10. Place a hardened blank block over marked area of section
11. Polymerize at 60°C
12. Chill slide on LN_2-cooled metal block which cracks the slide; 'pop-off' the block with the section on its surface

Yau et al[187] describe an improved method for the reprocessing of paraffin sections for EM, using a 'free-floating technique' in which a paraffin section is deparaffinized and rehydrated, followed by procedures similar to those described above. We prefer the 'pop-off' method, mainly because of its reproducibility.

The methods described here are those followed in this laboratory; they represent a synthesis of the various methods described in the literature. However, it must be admitted that conditions and requirements vary from one laboratory to another. Further reference may therefore be made to papers such as that of Carson et al,[21] where a simple method of handling and orientating small specimens for EM is described, using cyanoacrylic glue (Eastman 910) to affix small pieces of nasal scrapings to lens paper immediately before fixation in glutaraldehyde. In this instance, the lens paper acts as a binding agent and a marker for the presence of the tissue, facilitating its retention during the preparative procedure.

Yasuda & Toida[186] describe a novel pop-off method for the processing of bone marrow and peripheral blood specimens which may be particularly useful where the yield of bone marrow chips or the peripheral blood sample is scanty.

Flat embedding has been a useful method to study cells grown in cultured monolayers. Giamara & Hanker[55] describe an excellent method for the study of cytochemically stained and cultured cells by both light and electron microscopy. This method uses embedding of stained tissue sections, cells, cultured cells or organ cultures in a special polyethylene mould to form epoxy microscope slides in which the cells can be examined, firstly by light microscopy; an appropriate area can then be selected, cut with a scalpel or saw, and glued to the tip of a resin block with cyanoacrylic cement before being sectioned in an ultramicrotome for EM. A similar method of flat embedding was also described by Raymond & Pickett-Heaps;[137] this is a particularly useful method for examining microorganisms.

Another interesting method, described by di Sant'Agnese & Mesy-Jensen,[33] uses a pop-off technique in which small areas of large surgical biopsy specimens of size 10 × 10 × 1 mm — or even as large as 15 × 15 × 2 mm — embedded in Spurr epoxy resin can be selected and sectioned for EM. It is claimed that sampling errors can be avoided by this method.

However, we find that an appropriate semithin section stained with toluidine blue, from all the capsules processed from one specimen, can most often avoid sampling problems. Proper fixation of large surgical biopsy specimens for EM has always been a problem, and will remain so; however, the technique described by di Sant'Agnese & Mesy-Jensen[33] may be very useful if it can be guaranteed that the degree of preservation is optimal.

Other useful fixation and embedding procedures will be discussed with reference to particular EM techniques.

SPECIAL STAINS

Apart from the stains commonly used for enhancing contrast (uranyl acetate and lead citrate) there are now various other stains which demonstrate specific features in biopsy material. Those that we have found to be useful are as follows:

Stains commonly used in this laboratory

1. Myeloperoxidase
2. Alkaline phosphatase
3. Periodic acid–silver
4. Melanin
5. Lanthanum
6. Ruthenium red

Myeloperoxidase

Peroxidase is one of the variety of enzymes intrinsic to polymorphonuclear leukocytes,[10] and as such it represents an important marker for cells of the myeloid series in the discrimination between different forms of leukaemias (see Fig. 2.4).[83] Although the technique described here is useful for this exercise, the method is also applicable for peroxidase associated with eosinophils and other blood constituents.[24] A detailed resumé of the use of ultrastructural peroxidase cytochemistry in routine EM has been given by Dvorak et al.[36] Since then, peroxidase cytochemistry has improved considerably. For further information, the monograph of Hanker[66] gives a comprehensive outline of the various methods available for routine cytochemical localization of various enzymes, using osmiophilic reagents for enzyme cytochemistry. As stated in that monograph,[66] extensive changes in the use of reagents alternative to 3,3'-diaminobenzidine (DAB) have occurred, with the realization that oxidative coupling reactions of aromatic amines in the presence of phenols can provide a suitable substitute for

DAB.[65] Both DAB and *p*-phenylenediamine (PPD) in the presence of pyrocatechol have been proposed by Hanker et al[65] and have also been discussed by Sheibani et al.[144] However, the ease with which Hanker–Yates reagent can be obtained at present through commercial agents (Polysciences, Warrington PA, USA) has led us to use this reagent routinely for the demonstration of myeloperoxidase. The method we adopt is as follows:

1. Fix in 2.5% glutaraldehyde for 1 h. (Refer to Dvorak et al[36] for variations in fixation times relative to peripheral blood or bone marrow samples)
2. Prepare first the Hanker–Yates reagent (Polysciences, Warrington, PA, USA) with H_2O_2 in Tris buffer
3. Incubate at room temperature, in darkness with regular stirring for 1 h
4. Wash thoroughly in cacodylate buffer
5. Fix immediately in 2% osmium tetroxide for 1 h
6. Treat by standard techniques of dehydration and embedding in resin as in conventional methods

Alkaline phosphatase

The method is as follows:

1. Fix in 3% glutaraldehyde for 30 min
2. Wash in buffer for 3 h
3. Prepare medium of lead nitrate, glucose-6-phosphate in Tris-tartrate buffer pH 7.6
4. Incubate tissue in small pieces or else 40-μm cryostat sections at room temperature for 1 h
5. Wash thoroughly
6. Treat by standard technique with osmium tetroxide, dehydration and embedding in resin

Note. In certain circumstances the OsO_4 step can be omitted to demonstrate the localization of the lead precipitates — not only in the TEM mode but also in the BEI mode as well, with enhanced contrast obtained in the SEM, STEM or BEI mode.

Periodic acid–silver

The method is as follows:

1. Process tissue by standard technique
2. Collect ultrathin sections on gold grids
3. Dry thoroughly and float grid, section side down, on 1% periodic acid for 15 min at room temperature
4. Wash in distilled water three times
5. Float on fresh silver methenamine solution for 1 h at 60°C in the dark
6. Wash in distilled water three times
7. Float grid on 3% sodium thiosulphate solution for 5 min at room temperature
8. Wash in distilled water three times; let it dry before viewing in the microscope

Note. Sections treated this way may be seen not only by TEM alone but also by BEI and SEM as well.

Melanin

The method is as follows:

1. Cut ultrathin or semithin sections and collect them onto nickel grids; dry thoroughly
2. Float grid on 1% silver nitrate in acidified water (add sufficient 1% citric acid to water to register a pH of 3.2) and incubate at 43°C for 3 min
3. Float grids in freshly prepared developer (2% silver nitrate ACS grade in acidified water) at 56°C for 20 s
4. Wash in hot or warm running tap water; let the grid dry and examine by TEM, SEM, STEM or BEI. This is especially suited for BEI because silver acts as a useful stain not only for melanosomes but also for nuclear and cytoplasmic morphology

Further information on this method of staining can be found in references 139, 141, 167 and 170.

Apart from the methods described above, silver staining has become a very versatile method in recent years for the visualization of various other cell structures and products. Reduced silver staining techniques have been used extensively in the study of connective and nervous tissue. Furthermore, silver has been used to localize nucleolar organizer regions in interphase cells and in chromosomes, synaptonemal complexes and other components of chromosomes. These techniques have been used in pathology for the visualization of myelin and neurofilament proteins.[49,54,86] Silver staining has therefore brought a new dimension to EM techniques, particularly for the study of tissues, cells and cell organelles, not only by conventional methods of transmission EM but more suitably by BEI.

Lanthanum

The method is as follows:

1. Fix tissue sample in 2.5% glutaraldehyde with 1.3% $LaNO_3$ for 1 h with stirring
2. Wash in buffer three times, 30 min each time
3. Fix in 2% OsO_4 with 1.3% $LaNO_3$ for 1 h with stirring
4. Wash with buffer
5. Follow standard dehydration and embedding procedure

Ruthenium red

The method is as follows:

1. Fix in 2.5% glutaraldehyde with ruthenium red (1.5 mg/ml) for 1 h
2. Wash briefly in buffer
3. Fix in 2% OsO_4 with ruthenium red (1.5 mg/ml) for 3 h
4. Wash with buffer
5. Follow standard dehydration and embedding procedures

These are essentially standard methods that we have followed whenever necessary to demonstrate surface mucopolysaccharides such as the glycocalyx of the cell membranes and, with lanthanum, the sealing properties of various intercellular junctions.

However, many variations to these procedures exist where different staining chemicals have been used 'specifically' to demonstrate the nature of cell membranes or other structures with a view to furthering our knowledge of organelles in health and disease. Ruthenium red staining in borate buffer at pH 9.2 has been used to demonstrate by LM and EM the polyanion-containing structures in thin sections of resin embedded tissues,[60] as well as staining of the cell surface by osmium-low ferrocyanide.[124] Davina et al[29] report an interesting application of 'tannic acid binding' of cell surfaces to differentiate between normal, premalignant and malignant squamous epithelium of the human uterine cervix. In normal epithelium the distinct binding was observed in up to four or five layers of the deep intermediate zone. In premalignant and malignant tissues, however, no binding was noticeable, whereas in moderate dysplasia an intermediate reaction pattern was found. Another variation of tannic acid staining is shown by Buma et al[18] who have used the 'tannic acid ringer incubation (TARI)' method for demonstrating the exocytosis of neural, neuroendocrine and endocrine secretions.

It has also been observed that post-fixation with osmium tetroxide–potassium ferrocyanide (Fe^{II}) imparts high electron density to glycogen and membranes when the tissue is stained en bloc.[30,81] Such methods also improved electron opacity of sarcoplasmic reticulum[46] and endoplasmic reticulum,[47] and the extracellular space[5,78] and cell surface coat.[37,64] Many other references are listed in the article of Neiss[124] regarding the use of osmium and potassium ferrocyanide to contrast selectively different cellular and extracellular material. However, Neiss[124] reports the use of osmium-low ferrocyanide to enhance the staining of the cell surface coat in particular, as opposed to the cell membrane. The modifications as proposed appear to demonstrate the versatility of the osmium-ferrocyanide en bloc staining method and depend on the ferrocyanide concentration: with 40 mM (1%) OsO_4 + 36 mM (1.5%) Fe^{II}, pH 10.4, membranes and glycogen appear to be well stained. However, low ferrocyanide (40 mM (1%) OsO_4 + 2 mM (0.08%) Fe^{II}, pH 7.4) stains the cell surface coat and the basal lamina, but not glycogen.

Elastin is yet another component which has aroused the interest of cytochemists because it is difficult to demonstrate clearly with conventional TEM thin section methods. Elastin is present in many forms of extracellular matrices and is involved in ageing and in several inherited diseases.[3,4,61,144,166] Franc et al[48] describe a useful method for the routine staining of elastin in ordinary ultrathin sections with the use of a 7-minute immersion of the grid in a 7% solution of uranyl acetate in absolute methanol, rinsing several times in absolute methanol and finally counterstaining in Reynold's lead citrate. In contrast, Kageyama et al[79] describe a method of visualizing elastic fibres by staining with a tannate–metal salt. This method appears to be more complex than that of Franc et al[48] and hence should be tested for reproducibility.

Ferritin as a marker

Ferritin has been used for a number of years as a marker of negative charge on cell membranes and in the labelling of antigenic sites following conjugation with a variety of antibodies. This latter aspect has now been replaced by the use of gold or peroxidase labelling procedures which are now well documented in immunocytochemistry. However, ferritin still has an important role in demonstrating the surface charge distribution on cell membranes. Danon et al[27] used cationized ferritin to label negative charges on cell surfaces of old and young erythrocytes and reported significant differences in the charge distribution between the two groups. Greer & Baker[57] also used cationized ferritin at pH 4.4 to demonstrate the distribution of surface charge on erythrocytes. Danon et al[28] studied the surface charges of epithelial cells of urinary bladder with cationized ferritin. Mukherjee[112,113] studied differences in the surface charge of the epithelial cells of mouse jejunum, enunciated various factors affecting iron attachment to the microvilli of the absorptive cells, and proposed a possible mechanism for the regulation of iron absorption.[113]

The significance of these studies with cationized ferritin and of colloidal iron attachment to the cell surface[136] indicates the possible use of these methods in pathological tissues. Indeed, if the studies of Mukherjee[113] can be used as a model one may be able to suggest mechanisms for the regulation of absorption — not only of iron but also of other cations — both normal and abnormal, for example in malabsorptive states.

Having discussed various preparatory procedures relating to fixation, embedding and cytochemical staining we now consider the instrument modalities that are more or less standard accessories with most modern electron microscopes.

INSTRUMENTAL PARAMETERS OF VALUE IN DIAGNOSTIC PATHOLOGY

Dark-field and bright-field imaging

In routine transmission imaging we normally look at the bright-field image of the specimen produced by scattering of electrons due to the presence of heavy metal stains used in the preparatory procedures to produce a shadow of the specimen on the fluorescent screen. By tilting the beam or by placing the objective aperture in the rear focal plane of the objective lens one can achieve an image which is the opposite of the bright field. This is called the dark-field image and is useful in situations where the specimen under bright-field view has little contrast and hence very little capacity to scatter enough electrons to produce an observable shadow. (For theoretical and further information on this technique references 45, 127, 173 and 175 may be consulted.) The use of dark-field imaging to demonstrate the substructure of a variety of electron-translucent crystals and small particles (such as viruses, ferritin and so forth) is well recognized.

In fact, there have been several attempts to overcome the low inherent contrast of biological materials without the use of heavy metals by using dark-field imaging in conventional TEM.[149,173] Sjöstrand[149] used this method to demonstrate the substructure of mitochondrial membranes. Other attempts include mixed signal imaging by scanning transmission or Z contrast (medium to high atomic number of the material) imaging techniques.[20,77,82] We[110] have used the technique to study, by TEM or STEM, material fixed only in glutaraldehyde and embedded in resin mixture to reveal metallic or clay particles in lung tissue, without heavy metal staining. In fact, this is a superior method for the demonstration of such particulate materials because of their high Z value which causes them to stand out distinctly above the background — and studies such as EDX analysis or electron diffraction can be made with ease and without interference from contamination by heavy metal stains. Furthermore, such methods have the inherent advantage of less risk of translocation of metallic ions brought about by preparatory procedures.[50,53]

More recently, Frosch et al,[45] have attempted to improve detail in biological specimens (such as ferritin molecules and muscle) by combining conventional dark-field microscopy with electron spectroscopic imaging to examine extremely thin unstained sections of tissues embedded in a water-soluble melamine resin, nanoplast. This combination has now led to the development of a new Casteing-Ottensmeyer's electrostatic type electron energy loss spectrometer (EELS)-imaging analytical electron microscope, manufactured by Carl Zeiss (model EM 902), for biological use. This system appears to be superior to the conventional magnetic sector type EELS analysing system for biological samples.[107] According to Mizuhara,[107] elastic and inelastic, or dark-field images of unstained ultrathin sections, including frozen sections, can be made with excellent resolution in this microscope fitted with appropriate accessories. This is a new approach to elemental analysis and shows a great deal of promise. The only problem that one can envisage at present is the necessity to cut very thin sections of about 30 nm in thickness, above which the absorption of electrons increases so much that the sensitivity of the instrument diminishes dramatically. For further reading the following references are recommended: 12, 71, 128, 134, 135, 138, 161 and 165.

Although recent, this method of dark-field spectroscopic imaging has much potential for development, so that accurate measurements of cell concentrations of elements from hydrogen to uranium at low atomic energy levels may be obtained with the imaging resolution of the transmission electron microscope. Modern methods of energy dispersive X-ray microanalysis, in spite of significant developments in technology (particularly relating to software for quantifica-tion), unfortunately suffer from a lack of resolution achievable by inelastic dark-field spectroscopy techniques as described before and the commonly used EDX analytical methods utilized in the SEM, BEI, CTEM or STEM modes. When fully developed this instrumentation will hopefully provide an excellent tool for the study of unstained, unfixed tissues in health and disease. Wróblewski and coworkers[182-185] have developed freeze-drying and freeze-substitution methods along with low-temperature embedding, and they have analysed freeze-dried cryosections of human skeletal muscle from normal and diseased states and of different fibre types as well; they reported significant differences in sulphur, magnesium, sodium and potassium contents. Other studies[100-102] similarly examined skeletal muscle after conventional methods of tissue preparation as opposed to cryofixation.[183] It is here that this new method of inelastic dark-field spectroscopy may play a significant role in our understanding of chemical changes, not only in muscle but also in other organs, in health and disease, for it avoids many of the preparatory problems of conventional or cryofixation methods.

Use of specimen tilt to answer some pathological problems

Most electron microscopes of today are equipped with a goniometer stage and in many it is standard equipment, along with a single tilt specimen holder with tilt capability of $\pm 60°$. Yet this accessory is often neglected. In a recent study, Mukherjee et al[111] were able to dispel the notion of Hammerson et al[63] that there are two kinds of intramitochondrial crystalloids by using specimen tilt judiciously, and they were able to define the three-dimensional structure of these intramitochondrial crystalloids as seen in various skeletal muscle disorders known as mitochondrial myopathies.

Mukherjee & Dixon[110] applied the same method of specimen tilt to distinguish a cross-sectioned plate-like inclusion from needle-like inclusions observed in kaolinite-associated interstitial lung disease. The cross-section of a plate-like inclusion cannot be differentiated from a needle-like inclusion in conventionally examined TEM because they both look the same. However, if one studies thick sections of 0.5 μm or more by the STEM mode, and tilts the specimen by 40°, one can easily observe the difference between a plate and a needle (see Fig. 2.1). Dixon et al[34] again used the same method of specimen tilt to identify Auer body precursors in a case of promyelocytic leukaemia.

The purpose of mentioning this facility is to emphasize that specimen tilt can easily resolve the problem of whether a dense structure located between two adjacent cells is a true desmosome (with its typical ultrastructure) or merely a focal density of the adjacent plasma membranes. The same technique can determine whether a secretory granule located close to the membrane is actually fused to the plasma membrane in the process of exocytosis, or merely lying close to the plasma membrane.[117] For a more comprehensive account of the usefulness of specimen tilt, reference may be made to the review by Lange.[85]

Electron diffraction

Perhaps one of the most interesting examples of the application of selected-area diffraction was confirmation of the nature of unknown crystalline inclusions observed in the brain and kidney of patients administered xylitol intravenously. These patients developed a syndrome which led to death in some instances and which was characterized by lactic acidosis and osmotic diuresis.[40,163,164] Many of these cases showed the presence of unusual accumulations of crystals in the brain and kidney. Selected-area diffraction of the crystals in unstained thin sections revealed a crystalline pattern, and after appropriate analysis it was confirmed that the crystals were calcium oxalate dihydrate. This is but one of a large number of applications of electron diffraction facilities which are standard accessories in modern electron microscopes. We have always found that selected-area or micro-beam diffraction can give a rapid answer as to whether an inclusion is crystalline or amorphous (see Fig. 2.2).[110] Electron diffraction is particularly useful nowadays in relation to the growing awareness of the dangers of asbestos fibres and other harmful 'dust' particles as 'lethal agents'. The recent awareness of the diseases that can be associated with exposure to asbestos, silica and non-fibrous silicate minerals published by the Silicosis and Silicate Diseases Committee[35,146,169] emphasizes the value of all modalities in the analysis of such particles. Electron diffraction in association with specimen tilt in one of the conventional TEM, STEM, SEM or BEI modes serves as an excellent adjunct to the instrumental methods available to characterize such materials.

Backscattered electron imaging

Becker & Sagard[13] have discussed the difference between scanning electron microscopy and backscattered electron imaging (BEI). In SEM, due to the interaction of a high-energy electron beam passing through a specimen, many low-energy electrons within the material are produced by electron scattering. The range of these low-energy electrons or secondary electrons is quite short; some close to the surface of the specimen escape and can be collected by a detector to produce an image which we know as the SEM image. In contrast to the SEM image, in BEI the same high-energy electrons which have penetrated the surface of the specimen can collide with electrons belonging to elements with high atomic number (Z) in which case the collision between the two reverses the direction of the electrons without loss of much energy; they then escape from the surface of the specimen and are collected by suitable detectors to demonstrate the backscattered electron image. Therefore, the essential difference between the SEM

image and the BEI image is that the former is useful for visualizing surface detail whereas the latter has the potential to reveal the internal structure of cells and organelles, provided that they either contain a material that has an inherently high Z value or have been stained by high-Z-value materials to reveal their substructure.

The potential of BEI in pathology is immense, and its application was pioneered by Abraham, DeNee & Willard.[1,2,32] Since then, BEI methods have been developed not only for use in conjunction with dedicated scanning electron microscopes but with transmission electron microscopes as well. Many modern transmission electron microscopes now have the capacity for examination by STEM, SEM and BEI, as well as 'routine' examination of thin specimens. This has been achieved by improvements in microelectronic technology and signal and data processing to produce images and spectral data of high quality. In a way, this combination suits the pathologist very well for it gives an opportunity of examining a resin-embedded thin section, a 0.5–1.0-μm resin-embedded thick section, or a 5-μm paraffin section, not only in TEM or STEM modes but also in SEM and BEI modes as well.

In our experience BEI has been highly effective in giving preliminary information of diagnostic significance. One such case concerned a patient presenting with interstitial lung disease of unknown cause. A resin-embedded 0.5 μm thick section of lung tissue was embedded without any osmication. Figure 2.3A shows the SEM image of the section and Fig. 2.3B the BEI image. Note that in both micrographs the same particles are easily visualized but that particles are more numerous in the latter than in the SEM image. This illustration clearly demonstrates the advantage of BEI over SEM since in the BEI mode the electrons penetrate deeply into the section to produce images of particles not observable by conventional SEM means. EDX of these particles showed that they were all stainless steel deposits. The case is fully described in the article by Mukherjee & Dixon.[110]

Figure 2.4 demonstrates yet another example of the usefulness in rapid analysis of a semithin section mounted on a glass slide and viewed in the BEI mode. Figure 2.4A is a comparable image of a thin section TEM image of a specimen of bone marrow taken to ascertain whether this was a case of acute myeloblastic or lymphoblastic leukaemia. The specimens were processed for myeloperoxidase by the DAB/osmium technique. Examination of a semithin section, 0.5 μm thick, placed on a grid or a glass slide without any specific staining in the BEI mode (Fig. 2.4B) gives the definitive answer of myeloperoxidase positivity of the granules and the nuclear membrane. This approach may be used to save time, since semithin are more easily obtained than thin sections.

Figure 2.5(A–C) demonstrates the usefulness of BEI of paraffin sections. It must be emphasized that this 5-μm paraffin section mounted on a glass slide was silver stained by the method of Thiebaut et al[162] and examined by SEM

(Fig. 2.5A) and BEI (Fig. 2.5, B and C). The BEI image clearly displays melanin at low power (Fig. 2.5B) and high power (Fig. 2.5C) and demonstrates the usefulness of BEI in examining paraffin sections both by routine light microscopy and in the higher resolution of EM. The only problem at present is to obtain a common staining method that will include, within the dyes used conventionally for light microscopy, some high-atomic-number elements with specificity in their affinity for tissues, cells and cell organelles. At present we are limited by the requirement of staining by the silver methenamine method of Becker & Sogard,[13] with some modifications or cytochemical methods such as DAB/osmium, which selectively stains certain cell organelles for visualization by BEI.

BEI is also useful in the study of leukocytes, and hence in haematology. Soligo et al[151] used BEI to differentiate between normal and malignant human leukocytes — important in the diagnosis of various leukaemias[14] — by using four different elements with high atomic numbers: iron, silver, lead and osmium. Iron was found to be an excellent marker of phagocytic activity in granulocytes and monocytes. Silver staining was more useful for the staining of the nuclei. Lead was useful for the demonstration of acid phosphatases, and precipitates of DAB/osmium for the demonstration of peroxidase.

Since then de Harven[31] has published an extensive review of the value of BEI in clinical haematology which is recommended to anyone interested in this field. Halter et al[62] also used this method to study cells in effusions.

Scanning transmission imaging (STEM)

This again is a mode of imaging in a transmission electron microscope to obtain information beyond the scope of normal thin-section TEM. The advantage of this technique lies in the fact that specimen contrast does not have to be achieved by heavy metal staining as is essential for routine thin section examination. This method also allows the use of 'thick' (0.5–1.0 μm) sections which cannot be studied by routine TEM. Most microscopes today have this facility as an accessory, and the resolving power in this mode is usually better than 1.5 nm — which is quite sufficient for use in histopathology.

We have extensively used this technique for studying thick sections of unosmicated tissues from patients with interstitial lung disease, illustrated in Fig. 2.5. It should also be emphasized that this technique is a very useful adjunct to analytical EM because with this method an area of approximately 20 nm^2 can be analysed, compared to about 50 nm^2 obtainable in the conventional TEM mode, because of the minimum beam diameter obtainable in the STEM mode. The other advantage of this technique is the possibility of utilizing the usual features of a TEM such as specimen tilt, electron diffraction and other methods used in the conventional TEM for studying 'thick' sections.

ANALYTICAL ELECTRON MICROSCOPY

Analytical electron microscopy has brought a new dimension to the correlation of morphology with chemistry, opening up a new field of pathology never contemplated when the first electron microscope was being constructed, and its relevance to biomedicine was still in the domain of imagination rather than reality. In fact it has been stated that 'the results obtained thus far have been so impressive that many scientists now feel that electron-probe microanalysis may be more valuable to physiology than electron microscopy has been to anatomy'.[50] Ghadially,[50] in his review of electron-probe X-ray microanalysis, covers the limitations of the technique, equipment parameters, methods of specimen preparation and analysis and discusses at length the applications of the technique in solving many unanswered questions in pathology. In the last decade or so analytical electron microscopy has grown enormously — as discussed by Baker et al[11] in their review of the use of microprobe analysis in human pathology.

Roomans & Shelburne,[142] in their anthology compiled from papers relating to biological X-ray microanalysis presented at the SEM Symposia of 1982 and 1983, cover the field of analytical electron microscopy from a variety of perspectives, including the principles of basic instrumentation, methods of biological specimen preparation and a discussion of the limitations of conventional specimen preparatory techniques and cryopreparatory techniques as well. However, much of the advice given in this account is based on optimal preservation of the specimen to be analysed. This is a luxury in pathology practice since such a requirement very often cannot be met in a routine diagnostic laboratory, and in this respect Baker et al[11] give a more practical approach to utilizing analytical electron microscopy in a diagnostic laboratory.

Our experience in this respect, though limited, has revealed certain clear-cut guidelines which are:

1. If a specimen is thought at the time of receipt possibly to require analytical study at a later date, the specimen is divided into two portions; one goes through conventional techniques whereas the other is fixed in 2.5% glutaraldehyde in cacodylate buffer for an average duration of, say, two hours and then is hand processed separately without osmium postfixation or en bloc uranyl acetate staining. Hand processing is important since, if one uses an automated tissue processor, there is always the likelihood of contamination of the specimen from previous operations involving osmium and uranyl acetate procedures. Following dehydration the tissue for analysis is embedded in any epoxy resin.

Thin sections or semithin sections can then be cut, carbon coated, and examined unstained in the routine TEM mode or STEM or BEI mode and chemical analysis of the structure in question can then be made.

2. In many instances it is the material from a paraffin block that requires analysis. In this situation there are two

alternatives, depending on the distribution of the material to be analysed:

(i) If a paraffin block is available, a portion of the block can be enucleated, deparaffinized and subsequently processed for conventional TEM and microprobe analysis on thin sections or semithin sections.

(ii) However, if only a paraffin section is available then, following deparaffinization, the section can be studied in the BEI mode without any staining and the chemical composition of the material in question can be revealed by EDX analysis. It should be remembered that at all stages a layer of carbon should be evaporated on the specimen to prevent problems of charging. This method is useful, as has already been mentioned in the works of Abraham & DeNee,[1,2] but the only problem with this technique is that only materials with high atomic number can be properly analysed, for BEI is mainly dependent upon high Z-contrast of the element in question. Hence, any element that has a low Z value cannot be recognized and thus analysed.

At this stage it is worth discussing the limitations of energy dispersive X-ray analytical systems and how recent progress in instrumentation, development of software and ancillary techniques have improved the usefulness of this technique.

Instrument developments

Every energy-dispersive analytical instrument requires an appropriate Si (Li) detector with resolutions varying from 148 eV to about 162 eV. The limits of resolution are not important in 'routine' diagnosis since few spectral overlap situations arise when looking for unidentified elements. However, when choosing a particular detector notice should be taken of the individual capabilities of the detectors with or without windows, for they can play a significant role in enhancing the sensitivity of EDX analysis. Then again, when one endeavours to quantify the elements observed in any particular intracellular or extracellular inclusion, the problem of resolution of the detector becomes relevant, and the choice between the different makes of analyser now available is best made by the user by matching requirements against the equipment specifications. In addition, a variety of software is available which differentiates one make from the other. Hence, the user needs firstly to define the requirements of the analytical applications, and then to choose the appropriate software for the EDX system installed in the electron microscope.

Common software

Rapid semiquantitative analysis for approximate concentrations

This software is often quite useful for semiquantitative analysis of an inclusion seen while examining a thin section.

It gives some understanding of the variety of elements that can be expected in a pathological specimen. From our perspective this is very useful in instances where nothing was suspected in a biopsy sample and hence no particular precaution was taken for proper quantitative appraisal of the elements present in the inclusion. The next step obviously is proper quantitative appraisal of the elements in a sample, for which one needs appropriate software.

Quantitative analysis package for use with thin biological specimens

This software incorporates spectral analysis with or without any standards and complete absorption and fluoresence corrections useful for biological specimens. To use this software, one must be careful to have the specimen properly prepared, as mentioned before, without postfixation in OsO_4 or staining with either uranyl acetate or lead citrate. Appropriate measures should be taken — such as identical instrument parameters, especially the use of identical beam current for all different samples and, ideally, with analysis of a known standard sample prepared and sectioned in a similar manner to serve as a control. Although the software comes with or without any standards it is always helpful to prepare some known standards so that the element ratios obtained at the time of examination of an unknown sample can be related to a reference 'standard'. Indeed, every laboratory has to develop its own method of standardization and controls for interpretation, for only then do proper quantitative comparisons become a reality.

The use of cryotechniques, along with quantitative analysis, has already been well discussed in the studies of Baker et al,[11] Chandler[22] and Wróblewski et al.[185] Such cryotechniques are far from routine in diagnostic pathology, but advancements in microwave preservation, as discussed earlier, may prove to be of value in making quantitative EDX analysis in routine diagnostic pathology a reality.

Digital imaging

This software provides automatic feature detection and classification according to size, shape and elemental composition of particles. It obviously has many uses — especially in laboratories engaged in environment-related diseases where particle counting is of considerable diagnostic importance.

Electron diffraction pattern analysis programme

This kind of software is of little relevance to pathology at present since its use is essentially limited to the study of thin films of metals and so forth. However, the presence of talc, varieties of clay minerals and many other crystalline particulates that have now been identified in association with human disease,[11] and our own experience with calcium oxalate crystals in patients infused with xylitol,[40] demonstrate the potential usefulness of this kind of software.

Tracking analyser programme

This is an important and excellent programme for biological analytical EM. Normally, while analysing any inclusion or particle specimen, drift is one of the most important hindrances which may reduce the sensitivity of spectral analysis and thus interfere with the calculation of element ratios. This tracking programme has the ability to keep a reference position constant and thus avoid the specimen drift which can often be as much as 2 nm per minute under normal operating conditions.

Stereo measurement package

This is a relatively new application of the image processing capabilities of modern EDX systems. This software allows the automatic measurement and interpretation of topographic information. In this system, a stereo pair of images is obtained directly in the SEM, STEM or any other mode and digitized by using the digital imaging system as mentioned above. TEM images can also be similarly obtained by the use of a TV camera and then the image digitized through the digital imaging system. The pair of digital images can then be compared, one with the other, and the relative heights and so forth can then be computed by the software. The advantage of the system is that, once it has been initiated, measurements of height, depth and any other information can be processed automatically.

In normal microscopy, the determination of a 'stereo pair' requires a high level of skill and the ability of the microscopist to actually see the image in stereo — either by using appropriate stereo instruments or through sheer ability to utilize eyesight in order to calculate the height and depth of a specimen. The use of such software takes the handicap out of such procedures. It is then possible to see the actual shape of an inclusion in a thin section or in a semithin section viewed in the SEM or BEI mode and study the nature of such specimens. Again, in studying white cells or red blood cells in smears in the SEM mode after, say, labelling by immunogold techniques, one may in fact calculate the concentration of gold particles on their surface. These are fields of investigation which have never been applied in pathology before because of the time-consuming nature of such stereo pairing and its interpretation. However, with such software it may now be possible to obtain 'stereo' information rapidly; this may assist in the interpretation of the structural abnormalities in question.

In conclusion, it must be stated that improvements in the field of analytical electron microscopy occur almost daily, and it is impossible to describe all the facilities in a single chapter. The inclusion of a segment on software is essentially to bring to our notice the exceptional progress that has taken place in this field: before ordering such equipment one should take into account all these aspects so that the instrument can be best suited to the use of analytical EM in pathology.

ELECTRON ENERGY LOSS SPECTROMETRY (EELS)

This is a new alternative analytical procedure developed recently, in addition to the energy dispersive X-ray microprobe analysis described above. For an understanding of the physical aspects of EELS one should refer to the papers of Johnson[75,76] and for the advantages in the field of biology to Janguillaume.[74]

In brief, the advantage of EELS lies in its ability to analyse light elements. With the exceptions of hydrogen and helium, all the elements can be analysed by this method — in contrast to EDX systems where, with a standard Si–Li detector, one is limited to analysing elements with atomic number $Z = 11$ or greater, which can be extended with a thin window or windowless detectors to a Z value of 5. However, it is now accepted that EELS typically has a much better resolution than EDX.

In the lung, for example, the detection of beryllium is impossible by routine EDX techniques, and it is here that EELS can become very useful. Another example relates to the ferruginous sheath of iron hydroxide which surrounds asbestos fibres where Fe, O and other pollutants — including Si, O and C — can be easily identified in human biopsies.[74] Janguillaume[74] in fact gives a long list of elements which have been detected through the use of EELS in a variety of biological samples, including human biopsies and surrounding regions of failed joint prostheses as well.

With the development of parallel EELS, whereby element detection can be carried out simultaneously over 1024 channels, thus collating absorption spectra of several elements at one time, the effects of radiation damage due to the electron beam have been further minimized. This is but the first step, but it is significant, for it has now led many biomedical investigators to explore the benefits of this unique analytical tool in new areas of investigative biology and pathology.

IMMUNOLABELLING FOR ELECTRON MICROSCOPY

In their book, Polak & Varndell[132] have covered most of the aspects of immunolabelling for electron microscopy; the topics include choice of markers, choice of resins and a discussion of pre-embedding and post-embedding immunocytochemical techniques. This is a comprehensive textbook which also describes streptavidin–biotin bridging, protein-A-gold techniques for antigen localization, and various other methods — including double immunostaining procedures. These techniques will not be reiterated here, and it is worth emphasizing that immunocytochemistry at the EM level is still not an important adjunct to routine diagnosis. In the great majority of cases immunohistochemistry in surgical pathology can be carried out at the level of light microscopy. Immuno-EM is largely of value in ascertaining the distribution of immunolabelling at the subcellular level, and demonstrating, for example, the polypeptide content within endocrine secretory granules.

In addition, there are difficulties associated with optimum tissue preservation of biopsies, lack of resolution that can be achieved by conventional cryostat and paraffin sections followed by immunocytochemistry, the lack of penetration of gold and ferritin probes into the interior of resin-embedded sections (only antigens exposed at the surface of the sections will be labelled), the large size of the immunoglobulin–colloidal gold probes (which can prevent access of the probe to the epitope), and, finally, the difficulty of using cryo-ultramicrotomy as an alternative to resin-embedded sections. These difficulties have been partially overcome by the use of tissues embedded in polyethylene glycol (PEG) or polymerized polymethyl methacrylate.[7,59,177–179] In this context, the method described by Wolosewick,[179] dealing with hydrated resinless sections produced by a variety of methods, appears to be well suited for post-embedding immunocytochemistry at the EM level.

In summary it appears that, for immunolabelling at the EM level, gentle fixation with a low concentration of glutaraldehyde, the use of relatively small probes, embedding in PEG and increased incubation times allow a more comprehensive labelling of a hydrated thick section and thus enhance the efficacy of the immunotechnique.

More recently, Holm et al[72] have applied a double staining method with colloidal gold conjugates for antigen localization at the ultrastructural level. For demonstrating the distribution of two or more antigens on the same tissue sections, which would be reliable and sensitive indicators of the presence of the different antigens at the ultrastructural level, these authors have compared the following:

1. Indirect double immunogold staining
2. Sequential double protein-A gold staining method
3. Two-face protein-A gold staining method
4. Two-face amplified protein-A gold staining method
5. Formaldehyde blockade protein-A gold staining method
6. Formaldehyde blockade amplified protein-A gold staining method

While reviewing the different methods, these authors[72] were able to conclude that only four of the methods (1, 3, 4 and 5) were reliable and sensitive, whereas 2 and 6 gave cross-reactions between the first and second staining sequences.

Apart from the identification of polypeptide hormones within secretory granules, immunocytochemistry at the EM level has been applied to other intracellular constituents such as alpha actinin, filamin in cultured cells,[84] and tubulin and actin in seminiferous tubule epithelium.[180,181] In addition, modifications of the avidin-biotin complex technique for use in EM[94] appear promising for the localization of different antigens in a variety of cells.

Perhaps the development of appropriate methods of microwave preservation[88–90,93] along with fixation with low concentrations of a mixture of glutaraldehyde and paraformaldehyde, followed by cryosectioning and immunostaining with monoclonal or polyclonal antibodies, will give a rapid and sensitive method of localization of antigens in the near future.

The other area where there has been striking progress is in the field of rapid identification of viruses by immuno-SEM[152] where polystyrene beads were coated with specific monoclonal antibodies — such as those for HIV-1 core, or the HIV-1 envelope antigens gp41 or gp110, or human CMV envelope glycoproteins — and then incubated with cerebrospinal fluid containing the antigen and compared against appropriate controls. After incubation the beads were air-dried, coated with gold, and then examined by SEM; the viral particles were found to be specifically bound to the latex polystyrene beads, thus demonstrating the antigens in the CSF. These results have been similar to those of Andersson et al[6] relating to CMV identification, and they demonstrate that the technique of immuno-SEM is as sensitive as routine serological tests for viral identification. The method described by Sonnerborg et al[152] is in its early stages but it shows a great deal of promise of being able to contribute greatly to the field of rapid virus diagnosis by the use of immuno-SEM.

FREEZE–FRACTURE TECHNIQUE

This technique was first applied to biological materials by Steere,[153] and later developed by Moor, Muhlethaler and coworkers.[108,109] Freeze–fracture[15] is a technique whereby a small sample of tissue (about 0.5 mm³) is snap frozen in liquid freon-22 and then transported to a vacuum evaporator while still under liquid nitrogen at −187°C. The frozen specimen is then fractured by a microtome device which is also cooled to liquid nitrogen temperature. Fracturing occurs along planes of weak bonding. These planes are dictated by the phase differences between the various cells and cell organelles. For example, in the case of the cell membrane the fracture plane may pass through the hydrophobic ends of the lipid bilayer thus splitting the membrane into an inner or outer leaflet. The inner leaflet is apposed to the cytoplasm of the cell and hence is called the P-face, whereas the outer leaflet in contact with the exterior is called the E-face of the plasma membrane. Freeze–fracture technique can also split the membranes which are on the apposed surfaces of adjacent cells. Therefore, this is the only technique that can reveal the intercellular surface of adjoining cells en face; in contrast, thin sections for TEM can demonstrate only the cross-sectional appearance of the intercellular border. Accordingly, freeze–fracture allows one to visualize en face the extent and characteristics of intercellular junctions as opposed to the bidimensional cross-sectional appearances. Thus, any alterations of these intercellular junctions associated with pathological processes can be demonstrated with ease in the replicas, whereas these changes may be inapparent by conventional methods. In summary therefore, the advantage of the freeze–fracture method lies in its capacity to reveal the inner aspects of the plasma membrane or various other cell constituents not readily observable by conventional TEM techniques; hence it represents a valuable alternative method for the ultrastructural study of cells and cell organelles. This is particularly important, because in freeze–fracture the conventional preparatory techniques for TEM can be avoided, thus giving an alternative approach to the investigation of cell structures without the artefactual aberrations that may be associated with chemical procedures. For a more comprehensive review of the freeze–fracture technique and its capabilities the reader is referred to Bullivant[17] and Staehelin.[154]

Freeze–fracture is definitely not a technique for use as a routine diagnostic method in surgical pathology. Its usefulness essentially lies in the future, for at present we are at the beginning of an era of understanding the features exposed in the freeze–fracture replicas. Considerable improvements have also been made in our appreciation of the limitations of the technique and the identification of artefacts.[150]

In considering the relevance of freeze–fracture technique to pathology, two areas of importance standout prominently.

1. The ability to study the distribution of intramembrane particles (IMPs) which represent integral membrane proteins,[16,130,131] thus enabling variations in membrane constituents to be studied morphologically and to relate them to the patho-physiology of a disease process.

2. The capacity to reveal structures on the intercellular surface, especially the various junctions — namely, the tight junctions, gap junctions and desmosomes. The morphological alterations of these structures can be studied with the view that they may be associated with specific physiological or pathological changes in the tissue.

Figure 2.6 shows the capacity of freeze–fracture to display the intercellular border in replicas, thus demonstrating the organization of the tight junction in duodenal epithelial cells where they produce a tight seal between adjacent epithelial cells, so that material in the lumen of the gut is unable to seep into the intercellular space. For a more comprehensive outline of the various physiological functions of the different types of junctions the reader is referred to the review of Staehelin.[154]

Figure 2.7 demonstrates how the FF replicas can show the differences in the organization of gap junctions in cirrhotic liver. In contrast, Fig. 2.8 illustrates the variation in the architecture of the tight junctions between endothelial cells as opposed to those seen between the epithelial cells depicted in Fig. 2.6, thus pointing to their relevance in the physiological differences between the two cell types.

In the light of this knowledge, some of the interesting observations that have already been made by using this technique are now discussed.

The membrane-splitting property of freeze–fracture

It is now well known that the cell membrane consists of a bilayer of lipid interrupted by integral membrane proteins, some of which may lie within the membrane while others traverse its full thickness. In the light of this knowledge, IMP distribution on replicas revealed by FF in normal and pathological erythrocytes has been studied by various authors. From our own experience it was possible to demonstrate translocation of IMPs into discrete aggregates in erythrocytes from patients suffering from paroxysmal nocturnal haemoglobinuria (personal observation) although this was not detected by previous workers.[174] More recently, studies on erythrocytes have been directed towards the demonstration of variation in the IMP density on the membranes in Duchenne muscular dystrophy,[145] and other congenital dystrophies.[8] Other studies include membrane alterations in islet cells produced by diabetogenic drugs;[126] membrane changes associated with mucus production by intestinal goblet cells;[158] and membrane changes associated with muscle fibre damage due to bupivacaine HCl, where regenerating fast twitch fibres revealed alterations similar to those observed in Duchenne muscular dystrophy.[188] Other studies include observations on the membrane structure of the myocardium;[44] decreased IMPs in human dysfunctional corneal endothelial cells;[103] studies of human cochlea;[9] mucus secretion in cystic fibrosis;[125] demonstration of the glycocalyx in colonic epithelial cells;[158] the effect of ovarian hormones on the endometrium;[119,120] alterations in the membrane during pregnancy in the rat;[121,122] and the fluidity of the integral and peripheral membrane components.[123] There are many more studies in the literature which demonstrate the usefulness of freeze–fracture studies in distinguishing changes associated with integral membrane components in various pathophysiological conditions. Indeed, the studies of Madara and coworkers[96,97] on the structural abnormalities of cell membranes of the epithelial cells in patients with coeliac sprue are an excellent example of the usefulness of this technique in understanding the pathological changes in the membrane associated with this disease. These authors observed that the IMP density correlated with the decrease in the specific activity of brush border enzymes, and the tight junctions also showed significant abnormalities.[97]

The demonstration of intercellular junctions

This is perhaps the most important area of investigation that has occupied the interest of many researchers in this field for well over the past decade. There is overwhelming evidence that intercellular junctions are significantly altered in neoplasia;[26,38,51,52,69,70,91,114,116,118,160] all of these studies attempt to enhance our understanding not only of the morphological features of a variety of neoplasms but also histogenesis as well. Mukherjee and coworkers[114,116] have even gone a step further and discussed the value of such morphological markers obtained by freeze–fracture analysis of the junctions in a neoplasm as a means of assisting diagnosis when this has been equivocal by other routine methods. From their experience it appears that cells from different tissues demonstrate distinctive morphological features which are characteristic for a specific tissue under investigation. As well as desmosomes, tight junctions are a constant feature of most epithelia and hence are of diagnostic importance in adenocarcinomas. Mesotheliomas on the other hand have tight junctions, but most importantly gap junctions, which distinguish them from other tumours. Small cell carcinomas demonstrate only poorly developed tight junctions and desmosomes but have no gap junctions. These attempts are only the beginning of more in-depth studies on the application of freeze–fracture technique in the field of tumour pathology.

In non-neoplastic diseases too there have been some attempts made to characterize features associated with certain disease processes. Apart from the disorders mentioned above, junctional abnormalities have also been reported in patients with extrahepatic cholestasis,[140] as well as in microvasculature,[147] and vascular endothelium of arteries and veins.[148]

The demonstration of intracellular detail

Freeze–etching has been of great assistance in the following, for example: in revealing the structural organization of the intramitochondrial crystalloids seen in cases of mitochondrial myopathy;[111] in proving the presence of C and R bodies associated with the epithelial cells of human colon and their alterations seen in ulcerative colitis;[156] revealing the nature of lysosomal inclusions in Crohn's disease;[98] and showing that the core microfilaments of the intestinal microvilli are actin filaments.[115] The recent developments in the field of freeze–fracture cytochemistry have brought FF to heights not even contemplated in its early years. These include the application of filipin- and tomatin-induced membrane deformations;[42] the analysis of cholesterol in the membranes by treating with digitonin to produce tubular complexes which are visible in freeze–fracture replicas;[41] the fracture labelling of thin sections;[95] and the label-fracture of cell surfaces by replica staining developed by Forsman & Pinto da-Silva.[43] Future developments will show whether the addition of these complex procedures will make the freeze–fracture technique any more useful in investigative pathology than it has been in the past. The results of the past surely promise that this technique will have a bright future in its applications.

REFERENCES

1. Abraham J J, DeNee P B 1974 Biomedical applications of backscattered electron imaging. One year's experience with electron histochemistry. Scanning Electron Microscopy III: 252–258
2. Abraham J J, DeNee P B 1973 Scanning electron microscope histochemistry using backscattered electrons and metal stains. Lancet i: 1125
3. Adnet J J, Pinteaux A, Caulet T, Hibon E, Petit J, Pluot M, Roth A 1976 L'elastose dans le cancers du sein. Etude anatome-clinique histochemie et ultrastructurale. Annales de Medicine de Reims 13: 147
4. Adnet J J, Pinteaux A, Pousse G, Caulet T 1976 Caractérisation du tissue élastique et pathologie en microscopié electronique. Pathologie Biologie (Paris) 24: 293
5. Aguas A P 1982 The use of osmium tetroxide–potassium ferrocyanide as an extracellular tracer in electron microscopy. Stain Technology 57: 69–73
6. Andersson J, Nybom R, Larsson P, Andersson U, Britton S, Ehrnst A 1987 Rapid detection of cytomegalovirus using immune scanning electron microscopy. Journal of Virological Methods 16: 55–64
7. Armbruster B L, Carlemalm E, Chiovetti R, Garavito R M, Hobot J A, Kellenberger E, Villiger W 1982 Specimen preparation for electron microscopy using low temperature embedding resins. Journal of Microscopy 126: 77–85
8. Atkinson B G, Nixon B, Atkinson K H 1976 Deformation of the erythrocyte plasma membrane for early identification of congenital muscular dystrophy. Canadian Journal of Genetic Cytology 18: 552
9. Bagger-Sjoback D, Engstrom B, Steinholz L, Hillerdal M 1987 Freeze-fracturing of human stria vascularis. Acta Otolaryngologica (Stockholm) 103: 64–72
10. Bainton D, Farquhar M 1968 Differences in the enzyme content of Azurophil and specific granules of polymorphonuclear leukocytes. II. Cytochemistry and electron microscopy of bone marrow cells. Journal of Cell Biology 39: 299–317
11. Baker B, Kupke K G, Ingram P, Roggli V L, Shelburne J D 1985 Microprobe analysis in human pathology. Scanning Electron Microscopy II: 659–680
12. Bauer R, Hezel U, Kurz D 1987 High resolution imaging of thick biological specimens with an imaging electron energy loss spectrometer. Optik 77: 171–174
13. Becker R P, Sogard M 1979 Visualization of subsurface structures in cells and tissues by backscattered electron imaging. Scanning Electron Microscopy II: 835–870
14. Bennett J M, Catovsky D, Daniel M-T, Flandrin G, Galton D A G, Gralnick H R, Sultan C 1976 Proposals for the classification of the acute leukaemias. British Journal of Haematology 33: 451–458
15. Branton D 1971 Freeze-etching studies of membrane structure. Philosophical Transactions of the Royal Society of London (B) 261: 133–138
16. Bretscher M S, Raff M C 1975 Mammalian plasma membranes. Nature 258: 43–49
17. Bullivant S 1973 Freeze-etching and freeze–fracturing. In: Koehler J (ed) Advanced techniques in biological electron microscopy. Springer, Berlin, pp 67–112
18. Buma P, Roubos E W, Bulis R M 1984 Ultrastructural demonstration of exocytosis of neural neuroendocrine and endocrine secretions with an in vitro tannic acid TARI method. Histochemistry 80: 247–256
19. Burkhardt E 1984 A rapid method for processing large numbers of cell suspension samples for cytochemical and immunocytochemical electron microscopy. Histochemical Journal 16: 1339–1342
20. Carlemalm E, Kellenberger E 1982 The reproducible observation of unstained cellular material in thin sections: visualization of an integral membrane protein by a new mode of imaging for STEM. European Molecular Biology Organisation Journal 1: 63–67
21. Carson J, Lee R M K W, Forrest J B 1982 A simple method for the handling and orientation of small specimens for electron microscopy. Journal of Microscopy 126: 201–203
22. Chandler J A 1985 X-ray microanalysis of biological tissues—an examination of comparative specimen preparation techniques using prostatic tissue as a model. Scanning Electron Microscopy II: 731–744
23. Chew E C, Riches D J, Lam T K, Hou Chan H J 1983 A fine structural study of microwave fixed tissues. Cell Biology International Reports 7: 135–139

24. Chi E Y, Henderson W R 1984 Ultrastructure of mast cell degranulation induced by eosinophil peroxidase: use of diaminobenzidine cytochemistry by scanning electron microscopy. Journal of Histochemistry and Cytochemistry 32: 332–341

25. Cleland L G, Vernon-Roberts B, Smith K 1984 Fibre glass induced synovitis. Annals of Rheumatic Diseases 43: 530–534

26. Coleman M, Henderson D W, Mukherjee T M 1989 The ultrastructural pathology of malignant pleural mesothelioma. Pathology Annual 24: 303–354

27. Danon D, Goldstein L, Marikovsky Y, Skutelsky E 1970 Cationized ferritin used for labelling of negative charges on cell surfaces. Septieme Congres International de Microscopie Electronique, Grenoble, pp 33–34

28. Danon D, Ekblad E B M, Strum J M 1974 Comparative analysis of surface charges on luminal epithelial membranes of urinary bladders from toad frog turtle and tortoise. Anatomical Record 180: 509–520

29. Davina J H M, Laamers G E M, van Haelst U J G M, Kenemans P, Stadhouders A M 1984 Tannic acid binding of cell surfaces in normal premalignant and malignant squamous epithelium of the human uterine cervix. Ultrastructural Pathology 6: 275–284

30. de Bruijn 1968 A modified OsO_4 double fixation procedure which selectively contrasts glycogen. In: Bocciarelli D S (ed) 4th European Regional Conference on Electron Microscopy, Rome, II: pp 65–66

31. de Harven E 1987 Scanning electron microscopy in the backscattered electron imaging BEI mode: applications to clinical haematology. Ultrastructural Pathology 11: 711–721

32. DeNee P B, Abraham J L, Willard P A 1974 Histochemical stains for the scanning electron microscope. Qualitative and semiquantitative aspects of specific silver stains. Scanning Electron Microscopy III: 259–266

33. di Sant'Agnese D E, Mesy-Jensen K L 1984 Diagnostic electron microscopy on re-embedded popped-off areas of large Spur epoxy sections. Ultrastructural Pathology 6: 247–253

34. Dixon B R, Mukherjee T M, Ho J Q K 1984 The ultrastructural identification of Auer body precursors in a case of acute promyelocytic leukemia using high angle specimen tilt. American Journal of Clinical Pathology 81: 132–137

35. Dodson R F, Williams M G, McLarty L G, Hurst G A 1983 Asbestos bodies and particulate matter in sputum from former asbestos workers: an ultrastructural study. Acta Cytologica 27: 635–640

36. Dvorak A M, Monahan R A, Dickerson G R 1981 Diagnostic electron microscopy: 1. Haematology: differential diagnosis of acute lymphoblastic and acute myeloblastic leukemia. Use of ultrastructural peroxidase cytochemistry and routine electron microscopy technology. Pathology Annual 16: 101–137

37. Dvorak A M, Hammond M E, Dvorak H F, Karnovsky M J 1972 Loss of cell surface material from peritoneal exudate cells associated with lymphocyte-mediated inhibition of macrophage migration from capillary tubes. Laboratory Investigation 27: 561–564

38. Erlandson R A 1981 Diagnostic transmission electron microscopy of human tumours. The interpretation of submicroscopic structures in human neoplastic cells. Masson, New York

39. Estrada J C, Brinn N T, Bossen E H 1985 A rapid method of staining ultrathin sections for surgical pathology TEM with the use of the microwave oven. American Journal of Clinical Pathology 83: 639–641

40. Evans G W, Phillips G, Mukherjee T M, Snow M R, Lawrence J R, Thomas D W 1973 Identification of crystals deposited in brain and kidney after xylitol administration by biochemical histochemical and electron diffraction methods. Journal of Clinical Pathology 26: 32–36

41. Fishbeck K H, Bonilla E, Schotland D L 1983 Freeze–fracture analysis of plasma membrane cholesterol in Duchenne muscle. Annals of Neurology 13: 532–535

42. Forsman C A 1985 Freeze–fracture cytochemistry of sympathetic ganglia: distribution of filipin and tomatin induced membrane deformations in neurons and satellite cells. Histochemistry 82: 209–218

43. Forsman C A, Pinto da-Silva P 1988 Label fracture of cell surfaces by replica staining. Journal of Histochemistry and Cytochemistry 36: 1413–1418

44. Frank J S, Beydler S, Mottino G 1987 Membrane structure in ultrarapidly frozen, unpretreated, freeze–fractured myocardium. Circulation Research 61: 141–147

45. Frosch D, Westphal C, Bauer R 1987 Dark-field electron microscopy of unstained biological materials embedded in nanoplast. Journal of Microscopy 147: 313–321

46. Forbes M S, Planholt B A, Sperelakis N 1977 Cytochemical staining procedures selective for sarcotubular systems of muscle: modifications and applications. Journal of Ultrastructure Research 60: 306–327

47. Forbes M S, Sperelakis N 1980 Membrane system in skeletal system of the lizard *Anolis carolinensis*. Journal of Ultrastructure Research 73: 245–261

48. Franc S, Garrone R, Bosch A, Franc J M 1984 A routine method for contrasting elastin at the ultrastructural level. Journal of Histochemistry and Cytochemistry 32: 251–258

49. Gallyas F 1979 Silver staining of myelin by means of physical development. Neurology Research 1: 203–209

50. Ghadially F N 1979 The technique and scope of electron-probe X-ray microanalysis in pathology. Pathology 11: 95–110

51. Ghadially F N 1982 Ultrastructural pathology of the cell and matrix, 2nd edition. Butterworths, London, p 7

52. Ghadially F N 1985 Diagnostic electron microscopy of tumours. Butterworths, London

53. Ghadially F N, Lalonde J M A, Mukherjee T M 1979 Electron-probe X-ray analysis of intramitochondrial iron deposits in sideroblastic anaemia. Journal of Submicroscopic Cytology 11: 503–510

54. Gambetti P, Autilio-Gambetti L, Papasozomenos S Ch 1981 Bodian's silver method stains neurofilament peptides. Science 213: 1521–1522

55. Giamara B L, Hanker J S 1986 Epoxy slide embedment of cytochemically stained tissues and cultured cells for light and electron microscopy. Stain Technology 61: 51–58

56. Glauert A M 1974 Practical methods of electron microscopy, vol 3. North-Holland, Elsevier, Amsterdam, New York

57. Greer M H, Baker R F 1970 The distribution of surface charges on the human erythrocyte as shown by ferritin labelling. Septieme Congres International de Microscopie Electronique, Grenoble, pp 31–32

58. Griffin R L 1972 Ultramicrotomy. Williams & Wilkins, Baltimore

59. Griffiths G, McDowall A, Back R, Dubochet J 1984 On the preparation of cryosections for immunocytochemistry. Journal of Ultrastructure Research 89: 65–78

60. Gutierrez-Gonzalvez M G, Stockert J C, Ferrer J M, Tato A 1984 Ruthenium red staining of polyanion containing structures in sections from epoxy-resin embedded tissues. Acta Histochemica 74: 115–120

61. Guay M, Lamy F 1980 Élastine une protéine fibreuse impliquée dans pleusieurs processus pathologiques. Union Medicale (Paris) 109: 1

62. Halter S, Hunt L S, Roche B, Reidel R D 1984 Backscattered electron imaging of cells from effusions. Scanning Electron Microscopy IV: 1883–1892

63. Hammerson F, Gidlof A, Larsson J, Lewis D H 1980 The occurrence of paracrystalline inclusions in normal skeletal muscle. Acta Neuropathologica 49: 41–47

64. Hammond M E, Roblin R O, Dvorak A M, Selvaggio S S, Black P H, Dvorak H F 1974 MIF-like activity in simian virus 40-transformed 3T3 fibroblast cultures. Science 185: 955–957

65. Hanker J S, Yates P E, Metz C B, Rustioni A 1977 A new specific sensitive and non-carcinogenic reagent for the demonstration of horseradish peroxidase. Histochemical Journal 9: 789–792

66. Hanker J S 1979 Osmiophilic reagents in electron microscopic histochemistry. Gustav Fisher Verlag, Stuttgart, New York

67. Hayat M A 1970 Principles and techniques in Electron Microscopy: Biological Applications, vol 1. Van Nostrand Reinhold Company, New York

68. Hayat M A 1972 Basic Electron Microscopy Techniques. Van Nostrand Reinhold Company, New York

69. Henderson D W, Leppard P J, Brennan J S, Mukherjee T M, Swift J G 1989 Primitive neuroepithelial tumours of soft tissues and of bone: further ultrastructural and immunocytochemical clarification of 'Ewings sarcoma', including freeze–fracture analysis. Journal of Submicroscopic Cytology and Pathology 21: 35–57

70. Henderson D W, Papadimitriou J M, Coleman M 1986 Ultrastructural appearances of tumours: diagnosis and classification of human neoplasia by electron microscopy, 2nd edition. Churchill Livingstone, Edinburgh

71. Hezel U B, Bauer R, Zellman E, Miller W I 1986 Proceedings of the 44th Annual Meeting of Electron Microscopy Society of America. San Francisco, pp 68–69

72. Holm R, Nesland J M, Attramadal A, Johannessen J V 1988 Double staining methods at the ultrastructural level applying colloidal gold conjugates. Ultrastructural Pathology 12: 279–290

73. Hopgood D, Coghill G, Ramsey J, Milne G, Kerr M 1984 Microwave fixation: its potential for routine techniques, histochemistry, immunocytochemistry and electron microscopy. Histochemical Journal 16: 1171–1191

74. Janguillaume C 1987 Electron energy loss spectroscopy and biology. Scanning Microscopy I: 437–450

75. Johnson D E 1979 Energy loss spectrometry for biological research. In: Hren J J, Joy D C (eds) Introduction to analytical electron microscopy. Plenum, New York, London, pp 245–258

76. Johnson D E 1979 Electron energy loss microanalysis of biological material. In: Lechene C P, Warner R R (eds) Microbeam analysis in biology. Academic Press, pp 99–109

77. Jones A V, Leonard K R 1978 Scanning transmission electron microscopy of unstained biological sections. Nature 271: 659–660

78. Kaissling B 1980 Ultrastructural organization of the transition from the distal nephron to the collecting duct in the desert rodent *Psammomys obesus*. Cell and Tissue Research 212: 475–495

79. Kageyama M, Takagi M, Parmley R T, Toda M, Hirayama H, Toda Y 1985 Ultrastructural visualization of elastic fibres with a tannate–metal salt method. Histochemical Journal 17: 93–103

80. Kaps M, Burkhardt E 1985 An improved method for electron microscopic observation of cerebrospinal fluid cells. Acta Cytologica 29: 484–486

81. Karnovsky M J 1971 Use of ferrocyanide-reduced osmium in electron microscopy. Proceedings of the 14th Annual Meeting of the American Society of Cell Biology, p 146

82. Kellenberger E, Carlemalm E, Villiger W, Wurtz M, Mory C, Colliex C 1986 Z contrast in biology. A comparison with other imaging modes. Annals of the New York Academy of Science 483: 202–228

83. Koike T 1984 Megakaryoblastic leukemia: the characterisation and identification of megakaryocytes. Blood 64: 683–692

84. Langanger G, DeMay J, Moeremans M, DeBrabander M, Small J V 1984 Ultrastructural localization of α-actinin and filamin in cultured cells with the immunogold IGS method. Journal of Cell Biology 49: 1324–1334

85. Lange R H 1976 Tilting experiments in the electron microscope. In: Hayat M A (ed) Principles and techniques of electron microscopy, vol 6. pp 241–270

86. LaVelle A 1985 Some introductory comments on silver staining. Stain Technology 60: 271–273

87. Leong A S-Y 1985 Microwave irradiation as a form of fixation for light and electron microscopy. Journal of Pathology 146: 313–321

88. Leong A S-Y, Milios J 1986 Rapid immunoperoxidase staining of lymphocyte antigens using microwave irradiation. Journal of Pathology 148: 183–187

89. Leong A S-Y 1988 Microwave irradiation in histopathology. Pathology Annual Part 2: 213–234

90. Leong A S-Y, Milios J, Duncis C G 1988 Antigen preservation in microwave irradiated tissues: a comparison with formaldehyde fixation. Journal of Pathology 156: 275–282

91. Loewenstein W R 1979 Junctional intercellular communication and the control of growth. Biochemica et Biophysica Acta 560: 1–65

92. Login G R, Dvorak A M 1985 Microwave energy fixation for electron microscopy. American Journal of Pathology 120: 230–243

93. Login G R, Stavinoha W B, Dvorak A M 1986 Ultrafast microwave energy fixation for electron microscopy. Journal of Histochemistry and Cytochemistry 34: 381–387

94. Lombardi L, Della Torre G, Giardini R, Delia D, Rilke F 1986 Light and electron-microscopic immunocytochemical study of cytoplasmic immunoglobulins in non-Hodgkin's lymphomas. In: Fenoglio-Preiser C, Wolff M, Rilke F (eds) Progress in surgical pathology. Field & Wood, Philadelphia, pp 17–32

95. Lotti L V, Pavan A, Mancini P, Frati L, Torrisi M R 1988 Wheat germ agglutinin fracture label of Golgi apparatus membranes in proliferating cells. Cell Biology International Reports 12: 597–605

96. Madara J L, Trier J S, Neutra M R 1980 Structural changes in the plasma membrane accompanying differentiation of epithelial cells in human and monkey small intestine. Gastroenterology 78: 963–975

97. Madara J L, Trier J S 1980 Structural abnormalities of jejunal epithelial cell membranes in coeliac sprue. Laboratory Investigation 43: 254–261

98. Marin M L, Greenstein A J, Geller S A, Gordon R E, Aufse, A H Jr 1984 Freeze–fracture analysis of epithelial cell lysosomal inclusions in Crohn's disease. Ultrastructural Pathology 6: 39–44

99. Marshall A T 1980 Freeze substitution as a preparatory technique for biological X-ray microanalysis. Scanning Electron Microscopy II: 395–408

100. Maunder C A, Yarom R, Dubowitz V 1977 Electron microscopic X-ray microanalysis of normal and diseased human skeletal muscle. Journal of Neurological Science 33: 323–334

101. Maunder-Sewry C A, Dubowitz V 1979 Myonuclear calcium in carriers of Duchenne muscular dystrophy. An X-ray microanalysis study. Journal of Neurological Science 42: 337–347

102. Maunder-Sewry C A, Dubowitz V 1980 X-ray microanalysis of elemental changes in muscle nuclei of carriers of Duchenne muscular dystrophy. Electron Microscopy 3: 82–83

103. McCartney M D, Wood T O, McLaughlin B J 1987 Freeze–fracture label of functional and dysfunctional human corneal endothelium. Current Eye Research 6: 589–597

104. McLay A L C, Anderson J D, McMeekin W 1987 Microwave polymerisation of epoxy resin: rapid processing technique in ultrastructural pathology. Journal of Clinical Pathology 40: 350–352

105. Meek G A 1970 Practical electron microscopy for biologists. Wiley-Interscience, New York

106. Mercer E H, Birbeck M S C 1972 Electron microscopy: a handbook for biologists, 3rd edition. Blackwell Scientific, Oxford

107. Mizuhira V 1989 Recent advances in biomedical microbeam analysis — from EDX to EELS. Imaging analysis of biomedical specimens with respect to calcifying tissue. Journal of Electron Microscopy 285: 5142–5146

108. Moor H, Muhlethaler K, Waldner H, Frey-Wyssling A 1961 A new freezing ultramicrotome. Journal of Biophysical Biochemical Cytology 10: 1–13

109. Moor H, Muhlethaler K 1963 Fine structure in frozen–etched yeast cells. Journal of Cell Biology 17: 609–628

110. Mukherjee T M, Dixon B 1983 The role of electron microscopy and microanalytical techniques in the understanding of the pathophysiology of environmental dusts associated with lung disease. Scanning Electron Microscopy II: 663–679

111. Mukherjee T M, Dixon B R, Blumbergs P C, Swift J G, Hallpike J F 1986 The fine structure of intramitochondrial crystalloids in mitochondrial myopathy. Journal of Submicroscopic Cytology 18: 595–604

112. Mukherjee T M 1972 Surface charge on human colonic epithelial cells. Proceedings of the Electron Microscopy Society of America and First Pacific Regional Conference on Electron Microscopy. XXXth Annual Meeting, pp 266–267

113. Mukherjee T M 1972 Factors affecting iron attachment to microvilli. Medical Journal of Australia 2: 378–381

114. Mukherjee T M 1982 The role of electron microscopy in the diagnosis of neoplastic cells in effusion fluids. Journal of Submicroscopic Cytology 14: 776–784

115. Mukherjee T M, Staehelin L A 1971 The fine structural organization of the brush border of the intestinal epithelial cells. Journal of Cell Science 8: 573–599

116. Mukherjee T M, Smith K, Swift J G 1983 Scope of scanning electron microscopy, transmission electron microscopy and freeze-fracture technique in diagnostic cytology of effusions. Scanning Electron Microscopy III: 1317–1327

117. Mukherjee T M, Swift J G, Smith K, Smith L A 1983 Exocytosis of neurosecretory granules in small cell undifferentiated carcinoma. Ultrastructural Pathology 4: 187–195

118. Mukherjee T M, Swift J G, Henderson D W 1988 Freeze–fracture study of intercellular junctions in benign and malignant mesothelial

cells in effusions and a comparison with those seen in pleural mesotheliomas (solid tumour). Journal of Submicroscopic Cytology and Pathology 20: 195–208

119. Murphy C R, Swift J G, Mukherjee T M, Rogers A W 1979 Effects of ovarian hormones in the rat uterus. I. Freeze–fracture studies of the apical membrane of the luminal epithelium. Cell Biophysics 1: 181–193

120. Murphy C R, Swift J G, Mukherjee T M, Rogers A W 1981 Effects of ovarian hormones on cell membranes in the rat uterus. II. Freeze–fracture of tight junctions of the lateral plasma membrane of the luminal epithelium. Cell Biophysics 3: 57–69

121. Murphy C R, Swift J G, Mukherjee T M, Rogers A W 1982 The structure of tight junctions between uterine luminal epithelial cells at different stages of pregnancy in the rat. Cell and Tissue Research 223: 281–286

122. Murphy C R, Swift J G, Mukherjee T M, Rogers A W 1982 Changes in the fine structure in the apical plasma membrane of the endometrial epithelial cells during implantation in the rat. Journal of Cell Science 55: 1–12

123. Murphy C R, Swift J G, Mukherjee T M, Rogers A W 1982 Fluidity of integral and peripheral membrane components in uterine epithelial cells. Acta Anatomica 114: 361–366

124. Neiss W F 1984 Electron staining of the cell surface coat by osmium-low ferrocyanide. Histochemistry 80: 231–242

125. Neutra M R 1978 Intestinal mucus secretion in cystic fibrosis: autoradiographic and freeze–fracture studies. Acta Paediatrica Belgica 31: 103–104

126. Orci L, Amherdt M, Malaisse-Lagae F, Ravazzola M, Malaisse W J, Perrelet A, Renold A E 1976 Islet cell membrane alteration by diabetogenic drugs. Laboratory Investigation 34: 451–454

127. Parsons D F 1970 Some biological techniques in: electron microscopy. Academic Press, New York, London

128. Peachey L D, Heath J P, Lamprecht G 1986 Proceedings of the 44th Annual Meeting of the Electron Microscopy Society of America. San Francisco Press, pp 88–91

129. Pease D C 1964 Histological techniques for elecron microscopy, 2nd edition. Academic Press, New York

130. Pinto da Silva P, Nicholson G L 1974 Freeze-etch localization of concanavalin A receptors to the membrane intercalated particles of human erythrocyte ghost membranes. Biochimica Biophysica Acta 363: 311–319

131. Pinto da Silva P, Moss P S, Fudenberg H H 1973 Anionic sites on the membrane intercalated particles of human erythrocyte ghost membranes: freeze–etch localization. Experimental Cell Research 81: 127–138

132. Polak J M, Varndell I 1984 Immunolabelling for electron microscopy. Elsevier, New York

133. Pounder D J, Ghadially F N, Mukherjee T M, Hecker R, Rowland R, Dixon B, Lalonde J-M A 1982 Ultrastructure and electron probe X-ray analysis of the pigment in melanosis duodeni. Journal of Submicroscopic Cytology 14: 389–400

134. Probst W 1986 Ultrastructural localization of calcium in the CNS of vertebrates. Histochemistry 85: 231–239

135. Probst W, Seiler H 1986 Microanalytical methods and identification of calcium in vertebrate nervous tissue. Proceedings of the XIth International Congress on Electron Microscopy, Kyoto, pp 579–580

136. Rao S N, Mukherjee T M, Wynn Williams A 1972 Quantitative variation in the disposition of the enteric surface coat in mouse jejunum. Gut 13: 33–37

137. Raymond O L, Pickett-Heaps J D 1983 A routine flat embedding method for electron microscopy of microorganisms allowing selection and precisely orientated sectioning of single cells by light microscopy. Journal of Microscopy 130: 79–84

138. Reimer L, Ross-Messemer R 1987 Top-bottom effect in energy-selecting transmission electron microscopy. Ultramicroscopy 21: 385–388

139. Rennison A, Duff C, McPhie J L 1987 Electron microscopic identification of aberrant melanosomes using a combined DOPA/ Warthin-Starry technique. Journal of Pathology 152: 333–336

140. Robenek H, Herwig J, Themann H 1980 The morphologic characteristics of intercellular junctions between normal human liver cells and cells from patients with extrahepatic cholestasis. American Journal of Pathology 100: 93–104

141. Rodriguez H A, McGavran M H 1969 A modified DOPA reaction for the diagnosis and investigation of pigment cells. American Journal of Clinical Pathology 52: 219–227

142. Roomans G M, Shelburne J D 1983 Basic methods in biological X-ray microanalysis. Scanning Electron Microscopy. AMF O'Hare, Illinois, USA

143. Sandberg L B, Soskel N T, Leslie J G 1981 Elastin structure biosynthesis and relation to disease states. New England Journal of Medicine 304: 566

144. Sheibani K, Lucas F V, Tubbs R R, Savage R A, Hoeltge G A 1981 Alternate chromogens as substitutes for benzidine for myeloperoxidase cytochemistry. American Journal of Clinical Pathology 75: 367–370

145. Shivers R R, Atkinson B G 1979 Freeze–fracture analysis of intramembrane particles of erythrocytes from normal, dystrophic, and carrier mice: a possible diagnostic tool for detection of carriers of human muscular dystrophy. American Journal of Pathology 94: 97–102

146. Silicosis and Silicate Diseases Committee, National Institute for Occupational Safety and Health: special article 1988. Diseases associated with exposure to silica and non-fibrous silicate minerals. Archives of Pathology and Laboratory Medicine 112: 673–723

147. Simionescu M, Simionescu N, Palade G E 1975 Segmental differentiations of cell junctions in the vascular endothelium: the microvasculature. Journal of Cell Biology 67: 863–885

148. Simionescu M, Simionescu N, Palade G E 1976 Segmental differentiations of cell junctions in the vascular endothelium: arteries and veins. Journal of Cell Biology 68: 705–723

149. Sjöstrand F S 1978 The structure of mitochondrial membranes: a new concept. Journal of Ultrastructure Research 64: 217–245

150. Sleytr U B, Robards A W 1982 Understanding the artefact problem in freeze–fracture replication. Journal of Microscopy 126: 101–122

151. Soligo D, Lampen N, de Harven E 1981 Backscattered electron imaging of human leukocytes. Scanning Electron Microscopy II: 95–103

152. Sonnerborg A, Nybom R, Britton S, Ehrnst A, Forsgren M, Larsson P H, Stranegord O, Andersson J (unpublished information)

153. Steere R L 1957 Electron microscopy of ultrastructural detail in frozen biological specimens. Journal of Biophysical and Biochemical Cytology 3: 45–69

154. Staehelin L A 1974 Structure and function of intercellular junctions. International Review Cytology 39: 191–283

155. Stewart M, Vigers G 1986 Electron microscopy of frozen–hydrated biological material. Nature 231: 631–636

156. Stone J, Mukherjee T M, Hecker R 1977 C bodies and R bodies in the epithelial cells of normal and diseased human rectum. Archives of Pathology and Laboratory Medicine 101: 437–441

157. Swift J, Mukherjee T M, Rowland R 1983 Intercellular junctions in hepatocellular carcinoma. Journal of Submicroscopic Cytology 15: 799–810

158. Swift J G, Mukherjee T M 1978 Membrane changes associated with mucus production by intestinal goblet cells. Journal of Cell Science 33: 301–316

159. Swift J G, Mukherjee T M 1976 Demonstration of the fuzzy surface coat of rat intestinal microvilli. Journal of Cell Biology 69: 491–494

160. Swift J G, Mukherjee T M, Meredith D J, Henderson D W, Smith K 1989 Freeze–fracture study of the intercellular junctions in bronchioloalveolar carcinoma (Clara cell type). Journal of Submicroscopic Cytology and Pathology 21: 239–247

161. Theveny B, Bailly A, Rauch C, Rauch M, Delain E, Milgrom E 1987 Association of DNA-bound progesterone receptors. Nature 329: 79–81

162. Thiebaut F, Rigaut J P, Rectan J, Reith A 1986 Spatial visualization of junctional complexes by backscattered electron imaging and silver staining. Ultrastructural Pathology 10: 265–273

163. Thomas D W, Edwards J B, Gilligan J E, Lawrence J R, Edwards R G 1972 Complications following intravenous administration of solutions containing xylitol. Medical Journal of Australia 24: 1238–1246

164. Thomas D W, Gilligan J E, Edwards J B, Edwards R G 1972 Lactic acidosis and osmotic diuresis produced by xylitol infusion. Medical Journal of Australia 24: 1246–1248
165. Trinik J, Berriman J 1987 Zero-loss electron microscopy with the Zeiss EM902. Ultramicroscopy 21: 393–398
166. Uitto L 1979 Biochemistry of the elastic fibers in normal connective tissues and its alterations in diseases. Journal of Investigative Dermatology 72: 1–10
167. Van Duinen S G, Ruiter D J, Schefer E 1983 A staining procedure for melanin in semithin and ultrathin epoxy sections. Histopathology 7: 35–48
168. Valyathan V, Shi X, Dalala N S, Irr W, Castranova V 1988 Generation of free radicals from freshly fractured silica dust: potential role in acute silica-induced lung injury. American Review of Respiratory Diseases 138: 1213–1219
169. Walker M H, Roberts E M 1982 A thin film albumin method for encapsulating single cells for ultramicrotomy. Histochemistry Journal 14: 999–1001
170. Warkel R L, Luna L G, Helwig H B 1980 A modified Warthin-Starry procedure at low pH for melanin. American Journal of Clinical Pathology 73: 812–815
171. Weakley B S 1972 A beginners handbook in biological electron microscopy. Churchill Livingstone, Edinburgh, London
172. Weerman van den Berg M A, Dingemans K P 1984 Rapid deparaffinization for electron microscopy. Ultrastructural Pathology 7: 55–57
173. Weibull C 1974 Dark-field electron microscopy of thin sections of Trichosporon cutaneum. Journal of Bacteriology 120: 527–531
174. Weinstein R S, Williams R A 1967 Freeze–cleaving of red cell membranes in paroxysmal nocturnal hemoglobinurea. Blood 30: 785
175. Westfall C, Frosch D 1984 Electron-phase-contrast imaging of unstained biological materials embedded in melamine resin. Journal of Ultrastructure Research 88: 282–286
176. Wilks P N 1979 Sample preparation of cytological cell suspensions for electron microscopy: a routine method. Medical Laboratory Sciences 36: 95–97
177. Wolosewick J J 1984 Cell fine structure and protein antigenicity after polyethylene glycol processing. In: Revel J-P, Barnard T, Haggis G H (eds) The science of biological specimen preparation. Scanning Electron Microscopy Inc. AMF O'Hare, Chicago, Illinois, pp 83–95
178. Wolosewick J J 1985 To resin or not to resin in immunocytochemistry. In: Muller M, Becker R T, Boyde A, Wolosewick J J (eds) The proceedings of the fourth Pefferkorn conference on the science of biological specimen preparation. Scanning Electron Microscopy Inc. AMF O'Hare, Chicago, Illinois, pp 229–234
179. Wolosewick J J 1986 Polyethylene glycol embedding protocol for immunofluorescence microscopy. Methods in Enzymology 134: 580–591
180. Wolosewick J J, DeMay J 1982 Localization of tubulin and actin in polyethylene glycol embedded rat seminiferous epithelium. Biology of the Cell 44: 85–88
181. Wolosewick J J, DeMay J, Meininger V 1983 Ultrastructural localization of tubulin and actin in polyethylene glycol embedded rat seminiferous epithelium by immunogold staining. Biology of the Cell 49: 219–226
182. Wróblewski J, Wróblewski R 1986 Why low temperature embedding for X-ray microanalytical investigations? A comparison of recently used preparation methods. Journal of Microscopy 142: 351–362
183. Wróblewski R 1982 Healthy and diseased striated muscle studied by analytical scanning electron microscopy with special reference to fibre type. Scanning Electron Microscopy III: 1173–1189
184. Wróblewskl R, Wróblewski J 1984 Freeze–drying and freeze substitution with low temperature embedding. Preparation techniques for microprobe analysis of biological soft tissues. Histochemistry 81: 469–475
185. Wróblewski R, Wróblewski J, Anniko M, Edstrom L 1985 Freeze drying and related preparation techniques for biological X-ray microanalysis. Scanning Electron Microscopy I: 447–454
186. Yasuda H, Toida S 1986 Application of pop-off method to bone marrow and peripheral blood specimens for purposes of electron microscopy. Ultrastructural Pathology 10: 577–582
187. Yau W L, Or S B, Ngai H K 1985 A 'free floating' technique for reprocessing paraffin sections for electron microscopy. Medical Laboratory Sciences 42: 26–29
188. Yoshimura T, Schotland D L 1987 Freeze–fracture analysis of muscle plasma membrane in bupivacaine HCl-induced degeneration and regeneration. Journal of Neuropathology and Experimental Neurology 46: 522–532

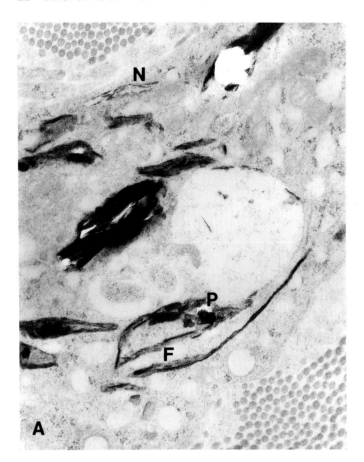

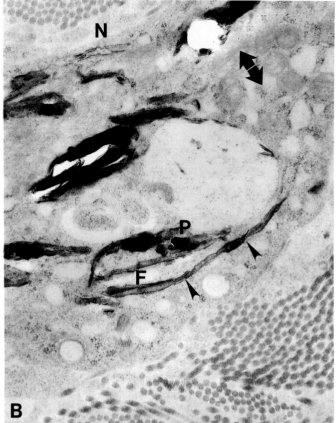

Fig. 2.1   Specimen tilt: kaolinite crystals. Lung biopsy specimen of kaolinite-associated interstitial disease, fixed only in glutaraldehyde and thin sections examined by TEM. Light microscopy showed the presence of variably-sized nodules, interstitial fibrosis and the presence of birefringent crystalline material in the nodules. Interstitial macrophages showed a variety of inclusions. The inclusions have been tilted from 0°, in **A**, to 35° of tilt in the direction of the double headed arrow (**B**). Some needle-like inclusions maintain their appearance with tilting (N), whereas others (F) take on a flake-like appearance. Regions of flake which overlap are indicated by the arrowheads. The flakes are more electron-lucent than the inclusions classified as plates (P). Sections unosmicated but stained. (× 42 000)

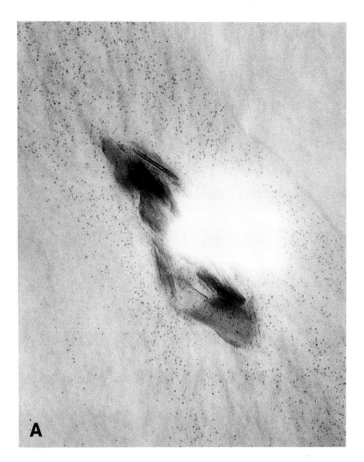

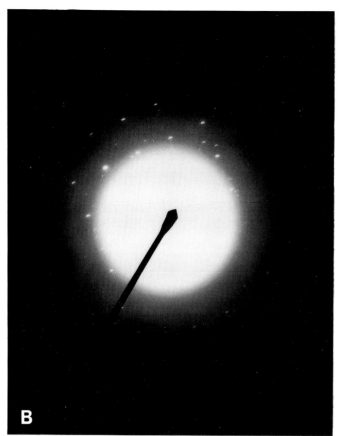

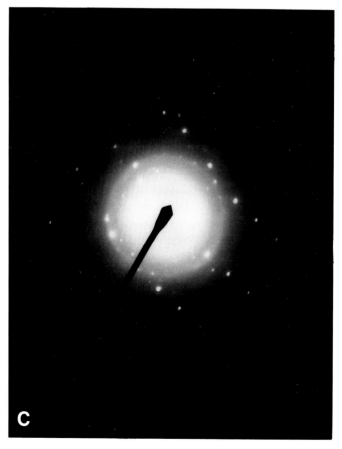

Fig. 2.2 Electron diffraction: kaolinite crystals. A small phagosome with needle-like inclusions from the same case as shown in Fig. 2.1. **A** The clear area in the centre is the size of the microbeam used for diffraction, shown here by double exposure, before and after the diffraction patterns were obtained. ($\times$ 180 000). **B** Microbeam diffraction from the area double-exposed in A. **C** Microbeam diffraction pattern from a hexagonal plate.

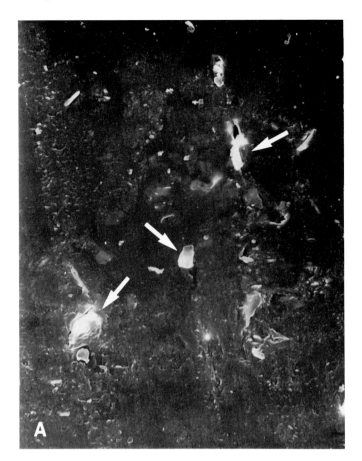
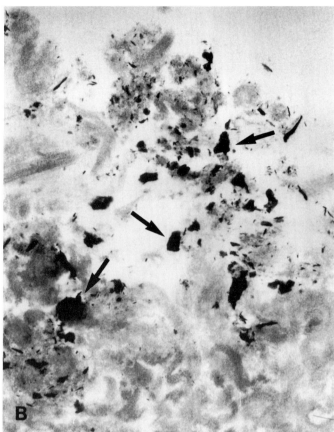

Fig. 2.3 Backscattered electron imaging (BEI): stainless steel-associated interstitial lung disease. One-micrometre epoxy resin sections of lung tissue mounted on copper grids were examined after staining with uranyl acetate. EDX examination of this tissue showed the presence of stainless steel.[110] **A** Scanning electron microscopy (SEM) shows the presence of possible particles on the surface of the section (arrows). (× 2400) **B** BEI of the same field shows the same particles to be electron-dense (arrows). The value of this technique is illustrated by the detection of particles of greater electron-density than the surrounding tissue (arrowheads) which are within the thickness of the section. The number of backscattered (elastically scattered) electrons is greater from areas with higher density or elements of higher atomic number. (× 2400)

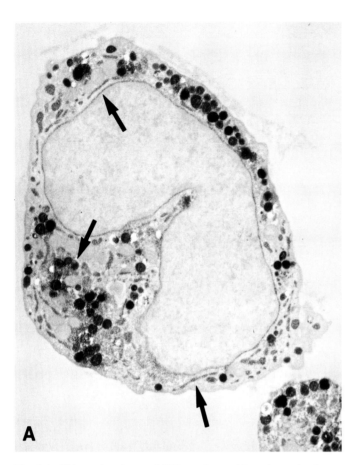
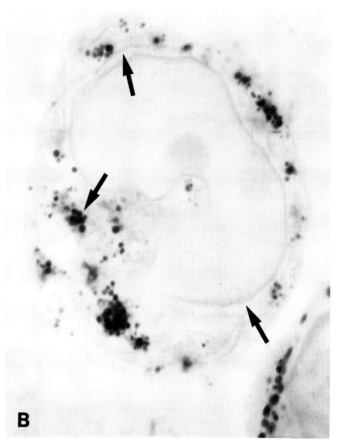

Fig. 2.4 EM cytochemistry and BEI: myeloperoxidase. A sample of bone marrow was stained by the DAB/osmic acid method for myeloperoxidase reaction. This method is especially useful in distinguishing cases of poorly differentiated acute myeloid leukaemia (AML) from acute lymphocytic leukaemia (ALL).[14] **A** An ultrathin section stained with lead citrate and uranyl acetate and examined by transmission electron microscopy (TEM) shows dense myeloperoxidase reaction product (arrows) on the nuclear membrane, endoplasmic reticulum cisternae and granules of the myeloid series. This reaction, together with morphological features, were used to make the diagnosis of AML. (× 8300) **B** A half-micrometre section from the same block was examined by BEI with no extra staining. The resolution of the morphology and enzyme reaction deposits are good enough to make a diagnosis by this simpler method. (× 7200)

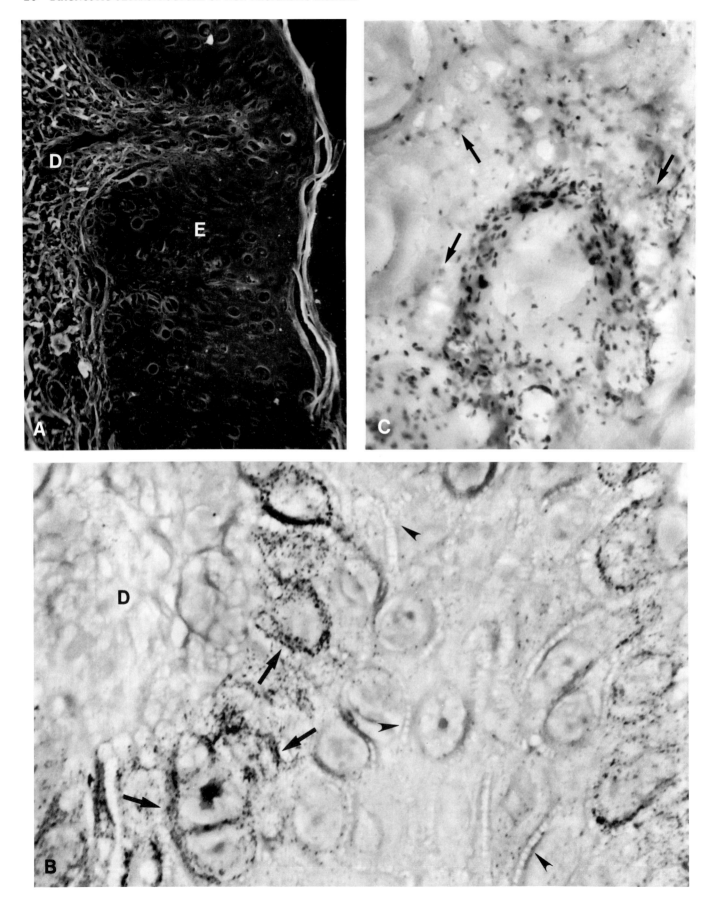

Fig. 2.5 The use of BEI in paraffin sections: demonstration of melanin. Paraffin sections (5 μm) of skin placed on glass were stained for the presence of melanin by a silver deposition method.[163] **A** SEM examination of the section surface shows the arrangement of the layers of the skin from the dermis (D) to the outermost layer of the epidermis (E). SEM will not show the silver stain as it uses only the low energy (inelastically scattered) electrons emitted by the sample. (× 360) **B** BEI, on the other hand, clearly images the distribution of the staining reaction (arrowheads). Details of the cell morphology, such as intercellular bridges (arrows) can also be easily identified. The dermis (D) is totally free of reaction products. (× 1800) **C** Higher magnification of an area of the same field reveals more detail of the distribution of melanin in the tissue and even the shape of the silver grains. Fainter images of silver grains (arrows) show the distribution of melanin within the thickness of the section. (× 6000)

Fig. 2.6 Freeze–fracture: tight junction I. Freeze–fracture replica of a tight junction (TJ) on a villus epithelial cell of mouse duodenum. Loosely-organized strands (arrows) extend basally down the lateral plasma membrane below the tight junction network. M = microvilli; P = protoplasmic fracture face of membrane; E = exoplasmic fracture face of membrane. (× 58 000)

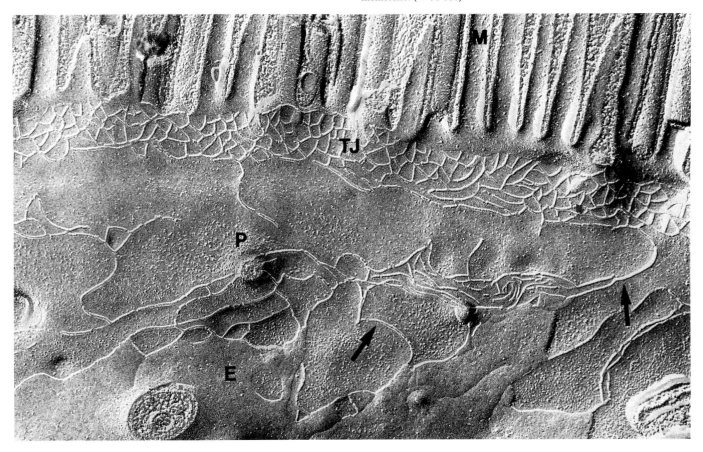

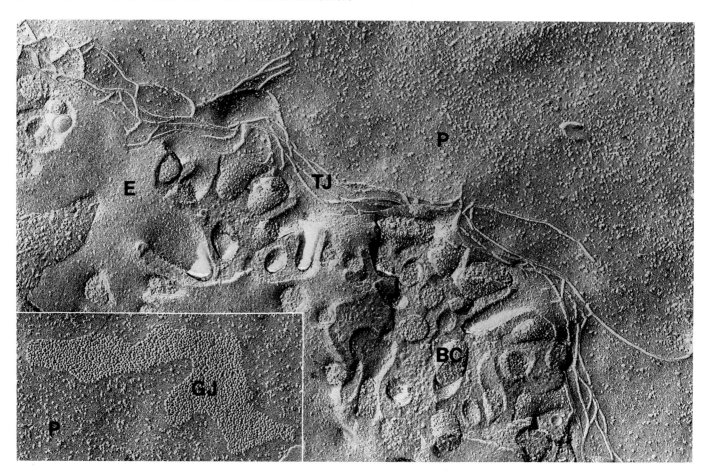

Fig. 2.7   Freeze–fracture: tight junction II. Freeze–fracture replica of a
tight junction (TJ) in cirrhotic human liver. Normal liver cells have small
gap junctions within the tight junction network. Gap junctions were
absent from the tight junction networks in this cirrhotic liver, but large
gap junctions (GJ, inset) were present on the lateral plasma membranes.
BC = bile canaliculus. ($\times$ 66 000)

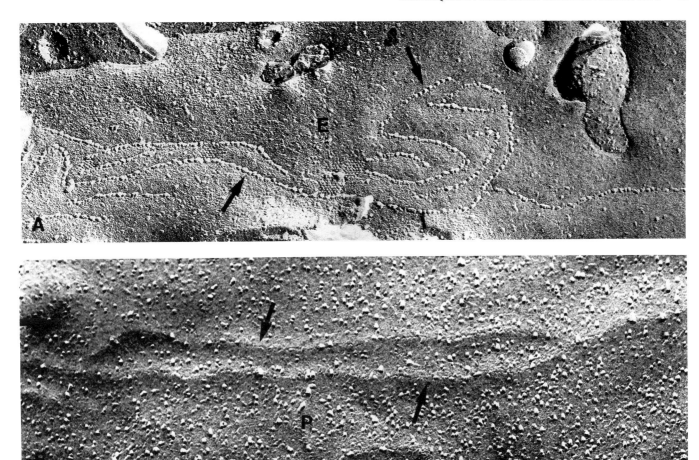

Fig. 2.8 Freeze–fracture: tight junction III. In freeze-fracture replicas, most tight junctions appear as ridges or rows of particles on the P-face and as particle-free grooves on the E-face. However, the tight junctions of some endothelial cells show a different appearance in replicas: on the E-face the tight junction grooves are occupied by rows of particles (A, arrows), whereas on the P-face the junction is represented by low profile ridges without organized rows of particles (B, arrows). Endothelial cell of kitten retina. (× 103 000)

3. Diagnostic applications of scanning electron microscopy

H. M. H. Kamel   Katherine E. Carr   P. G. Toner

INTRODUCTION

Although the scanning electron microscope (SEM) is capable of operating in several distinct modes, each offering unique new information, it is the familiar secondary electron image which is the usual starting point for beginners in the technique. When operated in this mode, the SEM provides information on the surface structure or topography of the specimen. This information is conceptually similar to that offered by the familiar binocular dissecting light microscope, but in the case of the SEM there is a much wider range of instrument magnification: the available resolution extends far beyond the capability of the light microscope, and the depth of field is much greater at any given level of resolution than in a corresponding light optical image. In addition to this, through the other available imaging modes, the modern SEM can add a wide range of further information to the purely structural data of the secondary electron image.

When the scanning electron microscope became commercially available in the 1960s there were understandable reasons for optimism regarding the potential of this technique in the study of disease.[3,41,96,104,107,157,165,167,188,189,190] The enthusiastic investigative work which followed soon identified specific contributions. The new three-dimensional images, which often provided new structural insights, could not be obtained by other methods. Scanning microscopy proved invaluable in visualizing certain effects of disease and in obtaining a better understanding of a variety of pathological processes.[12,30,38,39,42] The SEM quickly established itself as an essential research tool in various areas of anatomy and experimental pathology, being used routinely alongside other familiar techniques such as transmission electron microscopy and immunocytochemistry.

Despite the rapid development of the technique during the last 20 years, the parallel discipline of routine diagnostic pathology has been much slower to bring the SEM into general use, even in its most straightforward secondary electron mode. This cannot simply be attributed to any general mistrust of new methods, since both immunocytochemistry and transmission electron microscopy were accepted over the same period of time and already have an established role in pathological diagnosis.

There are probably several reasons behind this relative failure of SEM to make a major impact in diagnosis. Firstly, although the SEM is in many ways more simple in its routine operation than the TEM, the technique has always tended to be seen as 'specialized'. Secondly, specimen limitations have confined the range of SEM, largely restricting its effective use to the study of naturally occurring tissue surfaces, such as epidermal, mucosal and serosal surfaces, or, at higher magnification, the surfaces of individual cells in cytological specimens. Pathologists in general, however, have continued to mistrust the 'skin deep' quality of the secondary electron image, being more convinced by the demonstration in tissue sections of the underlying pathological process, than by what are seen as no more than its superficial manifestations.

In summary, there remain uncertainties amongst pathologists as to the practical advantages of such 'topographical' data over the more immediately familiar 'transmission' data provided by routine histology and TEM, at least in relation to diagnostic evaluations. In the future there may well be a practical role for SEM in diagnosis, but before this will be widely accepted, the potentially interested histopathologist must become more familiar with the technique, the information it can provide, and the applications in which it has been used to date. Some of these topics are considered in this chapter (see also Chapter 2).

TECHNICAL ASPECTS

Specimens suitable for SEM examination

Almost any type of specimen can be examined in the SEM, including individual cells or groups of cells; discrete tissue structures such as individual renal glomeruli; particulate material from specific locations such as renal casts or calculi and gallstones; specimens of hair; needle or endoscopic biopsies; surgical biopsies, autopsy material, and so forth. Table 3.1 summarizes different types of specimens that can be examined in the SEM.

Table 3.1 Principal categories of pathological specimens studied by SEM

1. Subcellular structures: mitochondria, chromosomes, cytoskeleton, nucleus and nuclear matrix, intracellular antigens — refs 8, 75, 90, 126, 184 and 187
2. Individual cells or groups of cells: glomeruli, blood cells, spheroids, renal casts, cytology specimens, seminal fluid — refs 1, 4, 9, 12–14, 153, 160, 168 and 188
3. Biopsy material: needle biopsy, endometrial curettage, endoscopic biopsies, postoperative biopsies — refs 3, 15, 30, 37–39, 42, 60, 61, 82, 83, 91, 101, 143 and 174
4. Autopsy material (provided it is rapidly fixed) — ref. 173
5. Hard tissues and structures: cartilage, bone, teeth, nails, renal and pancreatic calculi (either directly or by the replica technique) — refs 10, 19, 44, 45, 52, 58, 70, 91, 113, 118, 139, 157 and 179
6. Prosthetic and synthetic structures (either directly or by the replica technique):
   (a) Intravenous catheters — ref. 31
   (b) Endocardial electrodes — ref. 47
   (c) Peritoneal dialysis catheters — ref. 53
   (d) Contact lenses — ref. 73
   (e) Intrauterine contraceptive devices — refs 112, 129 and 176
   (f) Urine droppers — ref. 130
   (g) Bioprosthetic heart valves — refs 142, 158, 159 and 163
7. Corrosion resin casts (mainly for blood vessels of different tissues) — refs 79, 98 and 119
8. Replicas of resected, *in vivo* or prosthetic structures: nails, tooth surfaces — refs 24, 40, 66, 118, 164 and 191
9. Paraffin or resin blocks and sections — refs 33, 34, 59, 80, 121, 147 and 180

Methods of specimen preparation for SEM

In general, most SEM preparation methods are simple and easy to learn and are neither expensive nor time consuming. Routine specimens must be dry and conductive to electrons.[21,202] The two most common methods of specimen drying are critical point drying[6,22,48,123,168] and freeze drying.[20,22,168] The results are similar after both procedures, although variations in the types of tissue under examination and in the technical details of specimen preparation between different laboratories might be factors contributing to the variable quality of the reported final results.[22,144,168,202]

The specimen must also be conductive to electrons. The two most common methods of achieving conductivity are conductive staining of fixed tissue prior to critical point drying[134,135] and sputter coating of the specimen surface to achieve a thin metallic film, using metals such as gold, palladium or a mixture of the two.[20,65,100] Certain materials, such as kidney stones, can be examined without prior conductive staining or metal coating using low voltage SEM.[45]

The recent availability of low-temperature specimen chambers for the SEM makes possible the examination of fresh unfixed frozen hydrated specimens, hence avoiding the steps of fixation, drying and coating.[34,35,46,74,133] The main advantage of this method is that it preserves the fine structural details of tissues from any artefactual alterations induced by the process of fixation and drying. This technique, which is used mainly for X-ray microanalysis studies in the SEM, is at present still too tedious and time consuming for routine use.

Specimens processed for SEM examination can subsequently be reprocessed for further correlative light and transmission microscopy.[36,175] Preservation of the ultrastructural details in the reprocessed tissue is dependent to a considerable extent on the quality of the original preservation and fixation of the fresh material.

Several techniques have been described for the examination of paraffin or plastic sections in the SEM.[33,34,136,147] Examples include heavy metal staining and subsequent examination in the backscattered electron mode (Fig. 3.1).[59] Plasma-etched resin sections produce images comparable to those of light microscopy or low magnification transmission electron micrographs (Fig. 3.2).[33,34,136,180] Colloidal gold-immunolabelled surfaces and sections can also be examined in the SEM (Fig. 3.3).[17,95,97,125,132,140,141] Autoradiography (Fig. 3.4) and morphometric analysis are also applicable to SEM.[43,78,99,149,200] Table 3.2 summarizes the wide range of techniques by which specimens can be examined by SEM.

Imaging modalities in the SEM

Secondary electron imaging

The major advantage of the SEM, although one which is still under-utilized, is the diversity of imaging modalities which it offers and the variety of forms and states of materials which it can examine (see also Chapter 2). As referred to above, the most commonly used modality is surface scanning, as imaged by the secondary electron detector. The images produced by this detector can be referred to as the conventional or standard SEM images, whereas the other modalities, referred to below, are sometimes referred to as 'non-conventional' or 'non-standard' imaging methods. In the surface scanning modality the images obtained are the topographical features of the specimen surface; natural surfaces have been most widely studied. These images are representative of any existing surface pathology, such as alterations of tissue contours, cell surface irregularities, abnormal cell shedding, or ulceration.

Backscattered electron imaging (BEI)

The backscattered electron detector takes advantage of the differential backscattering produced by elements of

Table 3.2 Various techniques applicable to pathological specimens studied by SEM

1. Secondary electron imaging and backscattered electron imaging of natural surfaces — refs 3, 5, 15, 30, 32, 37–39, 42, 169 and 177
2. Secondary electron imaging and backscattered electron imaging of cut or fractured surfaces — refs 23, 33, 34, 59, 64, 71, 90, 95, 117, 121 and 192
3. STEM — refs 49, 54, 55, 67, 124 and 145
4. X-ray elemental microanalysis — refs 2, 72, 74, 111, 112, 127, 133 and 162
5. Correlative light and transmission electron microscopy — refs 16, 29, 36, 116, 137, 147, 156, 175 and 183
6. Immunolabelling and surface marker techniques — refs 17, 95, 97, 132, 140, 141 and 193
7. Plasma etched sections — refs 33, 34 and 180
8. Backscattered electron imaging of heavy-metal-stained paraffin and semithin plastic sections — refs 36, 59 and 136
9. Autoradiography — refs 43, 99 and 149
10. Morphometric analysis, cell volume and surface area determination — refs 56, 78 and 115
11. Mass mapping and determination — refs 124, 181 and 198
12. Replicas — refs 25, 40 and 66
13. Corrosion casts — refs 79, 98, 106 and 119
14. Cytochemistry — refs 177 and 178
15. Simultaneous light and scanning electron microscopy — refs 204 and 205
16. High-resolution SEM imaging of macromolecular structure — refs 145, 151 and 187

different atomic numbers.[59,116,124,136,141,169] The potential usefulness of this modality has been documented in a wide range of fields such as biochemical analysis, immunocytochemistry, cytochemistry and mass determination.[23,95,115,124,141,177,178,181,192,193] Images similar to those of conventionally stained histological sections can also be produced by backscattered imaging, using sections stained by histological metallic impregnation techniques (Fig. 3.1).[36,59]

Transmitted electron detectors in the SEM

The transmitted electron detector fitted in the SEM provides a scanning transmission (STEM) image of a thin specimen, such as a tissue section, equivalent to that obtained by the conventional TEM,[54,55,67] although the best available resolution on most commercial instruments currently falls short of the performance of the average TEM. Unconventional modes such as backscattered electron imaging can also be used by the STEM.[49]

X-ray microanalysis in the SEM

The use of X-ray detectors in the SEM provides for elemental analysis both of sections and of bulky specimens of either fixed or unfixed frozen hydrated tissues.[74,127,131,133,162] X-ray detector and analyser systems are currently obtainable for most commercially available scanning microscopes.

Other detectors and developments in SEM technology

SEM technology is advancing very rapidly, with technical advances steadily improving the performance of established modalities and allowing the development of others. Computerized digital image processing,[93,105] cryoscanning electron microscopy,[138] scanning tunnelling,[5] and scanning auger spectroscopy,[84] photoelectron microscopes,[88] and high magnification scanning microscopy,[150,151] are some current examples reflecting the growing diversity of SEM techniques. Recently, a new instrument combining simultaneous light and scanning electron microscopy has been described[204,205] which, through allowing accurate correlative studies, would maximize information retrieval.

SEM IN PATHOLOGY: GENERAL CONSIDERATIONS

The slow development of SEM in clinical practice is partly due to pathologists' unfamiliarity with the technique. This should be remedied by the wider use of correlative studies.[29,32,36,37,42,116,117,137,147,175,183] Cut or fractured surfaces of various tissues,[64,71,75,121,126,137] although sometimes informative, often produce unsatisfactory or uninterpretable images. In general, therefore, body systems which have wide natural surfaces are more suitable for SEM than solid organs. Even in an ideal anatomical site, the potential contribution of SEM depends heavily on the nature of the underlying pathology.

It must be appreciated that much of the interest to date in the pathological applications of SEM has centred on the study of dysplastic and neoplastic lesions, particularly of epithelial surfaces. There has also been great interest in the applications of the technique in forensic medicine.[11,108,152] In the following review, however, attention is concentrated specifically on the application in non-neoplastic human disease. The extent of the relevant literature makes detailed discussion difficult, so that for the most part this chapter attempts only to highlight areas of interest rather than to explore the results of such studies in any detail.

APPLICATIONS IN SYSTEMATIC PATHOLOGY

Digestive system

The gastrointestinal tract, with its varied and highly differentiated luminal morphology, offers ideal opportunities for SEM. Pathologists not infrequently use the dissecting light microscope to observe surface mucosal changes in the small intestine. SEM provides a similar service, but with much better resolution over a wide range of magnification, from the level of the hand lens to the threshold of macromolecular structure.[94,150,151,187] Pathological conditions represented by changes in mucosal topography are sometimes more readily appreciated and more easily understood through SEM than through the study of single, or even serial histological sections. Examples include lesions throughout the gastrointestinal tract, referred to individually below.[15,16,33,34,36,88,154,172,174] The technique of SEM also has an established role in dental and oral pathology, particularly with the use of the replica technique.[10,19,60,61,70,139,206]

In the human oesophageal mucosa, significant differences in the surface microridge patterns were observed between cases with no identified pathology and those with oesophagitis (Fig. 3.5) or dysplasia.[82,160,174] Irregularity and desquamation of the epithelial cells, with diminution of their microridges and an abundant acute inflammatory infiltrate, were seen by SEM in cases of oesophagitis.[174] The SEM, in conjunction with other techniques, is described as a useful tool for identifying and recognizing the nature of masses of foreign material occasionally encountered in the stomach (bezoars).[122] A recent study[16] used colloidal gold/silver labelling techniques for human gastric mucosal biopsies, examined in the backscattered electron mode, to detect intracellular mucin. The SEM observations, in conjunction with immunocytochemical studies, suggested that impaired mucus secretion may play a role in the pathogenesis of gastric ulcer. In cases of duodenal peptic ulceration, marked alterations in the surface architecture of the mucosa surrounding the ulcers, such as partial villus atrophy, villus spacing, distortion and swelling, are identified by SEM. It is suggested that the monitoring of enterocyte alterations by SEM could facilitate the identification of patients who may be prone to recurrence of ulceration.[15]

In coeliac disease the importance of SEM studies has been repeatedly emphasized.[3,15,91,94,154] In untreated cases, the 'flat' mucosa, characterized by the absence of villi and the presence of irregular crypt openings, is easily distinguished (Fig. 3.6). Three numerical stages of architectural disturbance are described, stage three being the most severe.[154] The recovery process and the early assessment of dietary response can be reliably monitored by SEM.[15,91] In cases of giardiasis, well preserved parasites can be clearly seen trapped between, and attached to, the surfaces of the villi (Fig. 3.7). Bacterial organisms,[88] such as Campylobacter/Helicobacter pylori (Fig. 3.8), have a characteristic undulant morphology. Rectal and appendiceal spirochaetes are also easily distinguished by SEM (Fig. 3.9) although their clinical significance is much less clear (see also Ch. 14). In acute appendicitis, SEM can provide information about the extent of the inflammatory process (Fig. 3.10).

There are several other gastrointestinal diseases in which the SEM has been reported to contribute to diagnosis and prognostic evaluation. The list includes milk protein and soy protein intolerance, cystic fibrosis, ulcerative colitis, Crohn's disease (Fig. 3.11) and drug induced colitis.[15,154,172]

The examination of liver biopsies in the SEM has attracted several studies.[101,143,195,196,197,207] These emphasized the value of this technique in recognizing pathological features which would be hard to appreciate by other methods. Vascular changes in different liver diseases, such as sinusoidal stenosis, are described as easily detectable and more readily appreciated by SEM than by histology. Unrecognized morphological and functional aspects of the perisinusoidal cells during mesenchymal reaction can also be revealed. The list of liver diseases in which SEM can offer a significant contribution includes intrahepatic and extrahepatic cholestasis, polycystic disease, veno-occlusive disease and Budd–Chiari syndrome.[196] Although methods for the SEM study of needle and wedge biopsies of human liver have been reported, and their significance has been emphasized, paucity of material and unfamiliarity with technique still confine the usage of SEM mainly to experimental studies of the liver.

Integumentary system

The hair and skin are ideal specimens for SEM. Several reports have documented and reviewed the undoubted significance of the SEM findings in many skin diseases.[72] Distinctive features have been recognized in different skin lesions, including warts, seborrhoeic keratosis,[203] moles and melanomas,[62,128] psoriasis, ichthyosis and bullous and non-bullous ichthyosiform erythroderma. Useful diagnostic information can be obtained through qualitative and quantitative elemental analysis in different skin conditions using the X-ray microanalysis technique in the SEM.[2,72,166] So far, however, the SEM does not yet have an established place in the routine dermatopathology service. The pathology of the hair is in a different situation. The SEM is said to be the most frequently used instrument for assessing hair damage of all types, especially with regard to cosmetic science.[26,27] The value of SEM in the study of the hair pathology associated with many inherited and acquired conditions has been reviewed.[28,42,81,155,186] Several hair diseases have diagnostic morphological features when studied by SEM. Examples include 'uncombable hair', or 'spun glass' hair,[81] Menke's disease, or 'kinky hair syndrome' showing pili torti (twisted hair) appearance (Fig. 3.12),[186] brittle hair and abuse of hair dyes[26] (see also Ch. 22). Examination of nails,[52,146] or their in vivo replicas, demonstrated distinctive changes in the surface structure of diseased nails such as clubbed nails, nails with onychogryphosis and the 'yellow nail syndrome'. X-ray microanalysis in the SEM is also of value in detecting and quantifying the uptake of various elements in certain pathological conditions of the hair and nails.[72]

Renal system

In glomerulopathies the information contributed by SEM is described as difficult or impossible to achieve by other techniques.[12,103] SEM has increased our knowledge of the normal morphology of intact glomeruli, and in particular the appearance of their podocyte foot processes. The technique has revealed unrecognized three-dimensional patterns of pathological changes which are inaccessible to other techniques. The complementary role of SEM in renal pathological diagnosis has been reported in a number of diseases, including glomerular disease, hypertensive kidney disease and tubular disease such as medullary cystic disease, adult polycystic disease and acute tubular necrosis.[103]

In recent years, the use of cell extraction techniques prior to SEM examination,[13,14,199] has allowed more accurate interpretation of structural changes in the glomerular basement membrane. This new technique permits the three-dimensional visualization of the naked glomerular basement membrane and of any structural alterations arising as a result of immune complex deposition. SEM studies of different types of glomerulonephritis using this technique revealed three-dimensional patterns of pathological change which were previously unrecognized. The types of glomerulopathy studied include lupus nephritis,[199] idiopathic membranous glomerulopathy[199] and minimal change disease.[13,14,103]

SEM techniques, especially when associated with X-ray microanalysis, have recently been used in the diagnosis of different types of urinary tract calculi. The elemental composition of different calculi has been accurately assessed by these techniques.[44,45,58,110,111,113,179]

Reproductive system

The female genital tract in health and disease has been widely investigated by SEM.[51,69,77,148,182,208] In the vagina, age-associated changes and pathological conditions such as vaginal adenosis and tampon-associated vaginal ulceration have been described. The surface of the endometrium shows interesting cyclical changes in its lining ciliated and glandular cell components. These SEM changes have been correlated with those seen in the endometrial glands by light microscopy. An increased ratio of ciliated to glandular epithelial cells is observed in the lining endometrium in cases of endometrial hyperplasia,[68] while in cases of endometrial carcinoma these ciliated cells are often depleted or absent (Fig. 3.13).

In the fallopian tube the morphological effects of both clinical and experimentally induced specific infection were studied. A decreased percentage of ciliated cells was reported in cases of hydrosalpinx and tuberculous pyosalpinx.[51,109,148,208]

Intrauterine contraceptive devices have been repeatedly examined by SEM in studies aimed at improving their design and manufacturing quality and identifying the constituents of the coating deposited on the surface of the device in the form of crusts.[112,129,176] The effects of the devices on the endometrium and the endometrial blood vessels have also been studied. Other general areas of the female genital system where SEM might offer a diagnostic contribution include pathological lesions of the placenta and the examination of cervical and ascites cytology.[109] SEM has a potential diagnostic role in human sperm pathology (see Ch. 18). Different abnormalities in human sperm morphology contributing to infertility, such as straight tailed, short tailed, round-headed and double spermatozoa have distinct and easily recognizable features.[4,109]

Cardiovascular system

Most of the SEM studies of the cardiovascular system to date are of experimental work, with few exceptions. The SEM appearances of normal human myocardium and the myocardium of hypertensive patients have been reported.[173] SEM studies have shown the presence of para-arterial fibrosis in the myocardium of hypertensive patients in the stages of decompensation. Differences in vascularity between normal and hypertensive myocardium can also be observed. Surgically resected human myocardium in cases of rheumatic valvulitis has been studied by SEM.[171] Abnormalities in the pulmonary artery endothelium in patients with congenital heart diseases and pulmonary hypertension have been studied by correlative light, scanning and transmission electron microscopy.[156] The SEM has been used to study different types of prosthetic heart valve.[142,158,159,163] Adhesion of various types of leukocytes to the surface of the leaflets, deposition of platelet aggregates and microthrombi on the leaflet surface and destruction of collagen fibres are seen in degenerating porcine bioprosthetic valves.[159] Useful clinical information has also been gained through SEM studies of other different prosthetic materials such as intravenous catheters,[31] and endocardial electrodes for cardiac pacemakers.[47] The contribution of SEM and SEM microanalysis to the study of atherosclerotic diseases has recently been reviewed.[120]

Respiratory system

In the lung, SEM in conjunction with X-ray microanalysis is often used for the detection and study of particulate-induced lung diseases, especially those due to asbestos.[24,57,170] Asbestos fibres are easily identified in the SEM where elemental quantitative analysis can also be performed to identify the fibre type (see also Ch.13).

Ophthalmic and central nervous system (CNS)

SEM has been widely used in eye and retinal research.[7,18,63,76,80,85,86,102,114,161,194] Diseases of the retina and iris which have been described include retrolental fibroplasia, fundal flavimaculatus, retina in trisomy 18, rubeosis iridis and juvenile diabetic retinopathy. Diseases of the cornea and conjunctiva include Fuch's endoepithelial dystrophy of the cornea, adenovirus follicular conjunctivitis, hay fever conjunctivitis and kerato-conjunctivitis sicca (see also Ch. 24). Contact lenses and contact lens wearing problems can also be examined in the SEM.[87,194] In the CNS the bulk of the SEM work remains confined to experimental situations.[82]

CONCLUSIONS

There is an ever-increasing literature describing the basic topographical features in a wide variety of pathological conditions. In many instances this information — while interesting and often visually arresting — still falls short of the level of critical diagnostic utility attained routinely by conventional histological techniques. Only recently has SEM started to reveal pathological aspects of certain diseases which would be unrecognizable by any other available technique. Therefore, it is not yet possible, in routine diagnostic practice, to point to certain clearly defined categories of disease which can be securely claimed both to be of clinical importance and to require the use of SEM for their recognition. Such conditions may well exist, but their identity has not yet been firmly established.

In general, the most that can now be said is that SEM is a useful confirmatory method of investigation in certain pathological conditions, adding significantly to the understanding and morphological evaluation of the underlying pathological process. Certain materials, such as hair and nails, are ideal specimens for SEM study, while other specimens such as prosthetic heart valves and IUDs are difficult to study effectively by any other technique — but these are far from routine problems in diagnostic pathology.

It is not surprising, or even particularly disappointing, that this should be so. Diagnostic pathology is essentially a practical problem-solving discipline, and is increasingly constrained by economic considerations which place a heavy emphasis on reaching an adequate diagnosis by the most cost-effective route. A new technique, such as SEM, will quickly displace existing methods only if it is self-evidently the best, the only, or the cheapest way to reach an adequate diagnosis.

Diagnostic pathology is a captive of its own history. The current primacy of routine histological methods simply reflects the long experience of many practitioners in the application of these methods; this has permitted the evolution of a reliable consensus on most practical diagnostic problems. It will take a considerable period of time before the diagnostic applications of SEM have been tried and tested to anything approaching the same level of confidence. Until then, the mainstream practitioner will correctly remain satisfied with the more familiar — and cheaper — routine techniques. As with other earlier developments in the technology of diagnostic pathology, the processes of evaluation and exploration will continue in academic centres and can be expected to diffuse only slowly into the general professional environment of service pathology.

However, the SEM, with its many accessories and operating modalities, is already fully established as a major research instrument, gathering data from three dimensional structure through to elemental composition and immuno-cytochemical reactivity. In time, a defined role in diagnostic pathology will certainly emerge, initially in the more highly specialized areas of practice, and perhaps extending from there into more routine applications, as familiarity with topographical images increases amongst diagnostic service pathologists.

REFERENCES

1. Albrecht R M, Jasdan C, Hong R 1978 Identification of monocytes and lymphocytes: correlation of histological, histochemical and functional properties with surface structure as viewed by scanning electron microscopy. Scanning Electron Microscopy II: 511–524
2. Andres T L, Vallayathan N V, Madison J F 1980 Electron probe microanalysis. Aid in the study of skin granulomas. Archives of Dermatology 116: 1272–1274
3. Asquith P, Johnson A G, Cook W T 1970 Scanning electron microscopy of normal and coeliac jejunal mucosa. American Journal of Digestive Diseases 15: 511–521
4. Bacetti B, Renieri T, Soldlini P 1981 Scanning electron microscopy and human sperm pathology. Scanning Electron Microscopy IV: 151–156
5. Baro A M, Miranda R, Alaman J, Garcia N, Binnig G, Rohrer H, Gerber C, Carrascosa J L 1985 Determination of surface topography of biological specimens at high resolution by scanning tunnelling microscopy. Nature 315: 253–254
6. Barlett A A, Burstyn H P 1975 A review of the physics of critical point drying. Scanning Electron Microscopy 1975: 305–316
7. Basu P K 1983 Application of scanning electron microscopy in ophthalmic research. Indian Journal of Ophthalmology 31: 476–485
8. Bell P B Jr 1981 The application of scanning electron microscopy to the study of the cytoskeleton of cells in culture. Scanning Electron Microscopy II: 139–157
9. Berga L, Vives-Corrons J L, Ferran M J, Rozman C, Aguilar I, Bascompte J L, Jou J, Feliu E, Ester A, Dolz J 1982 Contribution of scanning electron microscopy (SEM) to the study of erythrocyte morphology and to the diagnosis of haemolytic syndromes. Sangre (Barcellona) 27: 445–460
10. Blumershine R V 1982 A bibliography of scanning electron microscopy in dentistry. Part II. Scanning Electron Microscopy IV: 1809–1815
11. Bohm E, Bohm I 1983 Bibliography of scanning electron microscopy application in forensic medicine. Scanning Electron Microscopy I: 305–309
12. Bonsib S M 1984 Scanning electron microscopy of acellular glomeruli in human glomerulonephritis: application of a technique. Ultrastructural Pathology 7: 215–217
13. Bonsib S M 1985 Scanning electron microscopy of acellular glomeruli in nephrotic syndrome. Kidney International 27: 678
14. Bonsib S M 1985 Segmental subepithelial deposits in primary glomerulonephritis: scanning electron microscopic examination of acellular glomeruli. Human Pathology 16: 1115–1121

15. Bonvicini F, Zoli G, Maltarello M C, Bianchi D, Pasquinelli G, Versura P, Gasbarrini G, Laschi R 1985 Clinical applications of scanning electron microscopy in gastrointestinal diseases. Scanning Electron Microscopy III: 1279–1294

16. Bonvicini F, Zoli G, Maltarello M C, Versura P, Bianchi D, Gasbarrini G, Laschi R 1986 Correlative scanning electron microscopy in the study of human gastric mucosa. Scanning Electron Microscopy II : 687–702

17. Borg M 1985 Comparison of various immune surface labelling methods for scanning electron microscopy with the example of a surface antigen protein in the yeast *Candida albicans*. Zeitschrift fur Naturforschung Section C 40: 539–550

18. Borwein B 1985 Scanning electron microscopy in retinal research. Scanning Electron Microscopy I: 279–301

19. Bowen R L 1985 Bonding of restorative materials to dentine: the present status in the United States. International Dental Journal 35: 154–155

20. Boyde A 1974 Freezing, freeze–fracturing and freeze drying in biological specimen preparation for the SEM. Scanning Electron Microscopy 1043–1046

21. Boyde A 1976 Do's and don'ts in biological specimen preparation for the SEM. Scanning Electron Microscopy I: 683–690

22. Boyde A 1978 Pro's and Con's of critical point drying and freeze drying for SEM. Scanning Electron Microscopy I: 303–314

23. Boyde A, Jones S F 1983–84 Back-scattered electron imaging of skeletal tissues. Metabolic Bone Diseases and Related Research 5: 145– 150

24. Brody A R 1984 The early pathogenesis of asbestos-induced lung disease. Scanning Electron Microscopy I: 167–171

25. Bromage T G 1985 Systematic inquiry in tests of negative/positive replica combinations for SEM. Journal of Microscopy 137: 209–216

26. Brown A C, Broyles J A 1980 Accumulative scarring of the scalp due to hair dye. In: Brown A C and Croune R G (eds) Hair, trace elements, and human illness. Praeger Publishers, New York, pp 348–360

27. Brown A C, Swift J A 1975 Hair breakage: the scanning electron microscope as a diagnostic tool. Journal of Cosmetic Chemistry 26: 289–297

28. Brown A C 1978 The integumentary system. In: Hayat M A (ed) Introduction to biological scanning electron microscopy. University Park Press, Baltimore/London, pp 65–125

29. Brummer M E G, Lowrie P M, Tyler W S 1975 A technique for sequential examination of specific areas of large tissue blocks using SEM, LM and TEM. Scanning Electron Microscopy: 333–340

30. Buss H, Hollweg H G 1980 Application of scanning electron microscopy to diagnostic pathology. A critical review. Scanning Electron Microscopy II: 139–153

31. Bylock A, Hultman E, Gustavsson B, Linder L E, Curelaru I 1986 Surface morphology of unused and used hydromer-coated intravenous catheters. Scanning Electron Microscopy I: 157–164

32. Carr K E, Chung P, McLay A L, Toner P G, Wong A L 1981 The role of scanning electron microscopy in diagnostic pathology. Diagnostic Histopathology 4: 237–244

33. Carr K E, Hayes T L, Hume S P, Kamel H M H 1983 Qualitative and quantitative SEM of gastrointestinal tract. Proceedings of the 41st Annual Meeting of the Electron Microscopy Society of America, San Francisco Press, USA, pp 496–499

34. Carr K E, Hayes T L, McKoon M, Bastacky S J, Kamel H M H 1984 Etched surfaces of plastic embedded and frozen hydrated gastrointestinal tissue. Journal of Submicroscopic Cytology 16: 216–226

35. Carr K E, Hayes T L, McKoon M, Sprague M, Bastacky S J 1983 Low temperature scanning electron microscope studies of mouse small intestine. Journal of Microscopy 132: 209–217

36. Carr K E, Kamel H M H, Toner P G, McGadey J 1984 Correlative scanning electron microscopy in gastrointestinal pathology. Scanning Electron Microscopy II: 761–772

37. Carr K E, McLay A L, Toner P G, Chung P, Wong A 1980 SEM in service pathology: a review of its potential role. Scanning Electron Microscopy III: 121–138

38. Carr K E, Toner P G 1981 Scanning electron microscopy in biomedical research and routine pathology. Journal of Microscopy 123: 147–159

39. Carr K E, Toner P G, Saleh K. M 1982 Scanning electron microscopy. Histopathology 6: 3–14

40. Carrassi A, Abati S 1984 Replication technique in scanning electron microscopy: possibilities for use in the field of biology. Comparative study of various materials and methods. Mondo Odontostomatalogico 26: 11–23

41. Carteaud A J P 1969 Scanning electron microscope in dermatology. British Medical Journal 3: 239–240

42. Carter H W 1980 Clinical applications of scanning electron microscopy (SEM) in North America with emphasis on SEM's role in comparative microscopy. Scanning Electron Microscopy III: 115–120

43. Cheng G, Hodges G M, Trejdosiewicz L K 1985 A methodological basis for SEM autoradiography: biosynthesis and radioligand binding. Journal of Microscopy 137: 9–16

44. Cheng P T, Reid A D, Pritzker K P H 1985 Ultrastructural studies of crystal–organic matrix relations in renal stones. Scanning Electron Microscopy I: 201–207

45. Cheng P T, Reid A D 1985 Low voltage scanning electron microscopy of uncoated kidney stones. Scanning Electron Microscopy I: 1551–1554

46. Chiu W 1986 Electron microscopy of frozen hydrated biological specimens. Annual Review of Biophysical Chemistry 15: 237–257

47. Clawson C C, Parins D J, White J G, MacCarter D J 1980 Interactions of blood with solid and porous endocardial electrodes for cardiac pacemakers. Scanning Electron Microscopy III: 211–218

48. Cohen A L 1979 Critical point drying — principles and procedures. Scanning Electron Microscopy II: 303–323

49. Colliex C, Jeanguillaume C, Mary C 1984 Unconventional modes for STEM imaging of biological structures. Journal of Ultrastructure Research 88: 177–206

50. Cooper M D, Jeffrey C 1985 Scanning and transmission electron microscopy of bacterial attachment to mucosal surfaces with particular reference to the human fallopian tube. Scanning Electron Microscopy III: 1183–1190

51. Cooper M D, Jeffrey C, Dever C A 1984 Electron microscope studies of attachment to human fallopian tube mucosa by a gonococcal IgA1 protease deficient mutant and wild type parent. Scanning Electron Microscopy IV: 1925–1930

52. Cotton D W K, Inman C B E 1986 Quantitative evaluation of SEM morphology of nail surfaces. Journal of Pathology 148: 595A (synopsis)

53. Cregory D W, Youngsons G G, Marshall D 1985 Implantation failure of peritoneal dialysis catheters. A scanning electron microscopic study. Scanning Electron Microscopy III: 1223–1229

54. Crewe R V 1983 High-resolution scanning transmission electron microscopy. Science 221: 325–330

55. Crewe R V 1984 An introduction to the STEM. Journal of Ultrastructure Research 88: 94–104

56. Dadoune J P, Fain-Maurel M A, Guillaumin M, Guillaumin D 1980 Scanning electron microscopic morphometry of a discriminated population of elongated human spermatozoa. International Journal of Fertility 25: 18–27

57. Davis M L, Dodson R F 1985 A scanning electronmicroscopic study of the early response of the lung tissue to amosite asbestos exposure. Cytobios 44: 169–182

58. Deganello S, Chou S 1985 The uric acid whewellite association in human kidney stones. Scanning Electron Microscopy IV: 1545–1550.

59. Dichiara J F, Rowley P P, Ogilvie R W 1980 Backscatter electron imaging (BEI) of paraffin sections stained with heavy metal histopathologic stains, with observation on some variables encountered in BEI. Scanning Electron Microscopy III: 181–188

60. Dourov N 1980 Scanning electron microscopy in the study of tongue pathology. Acta Otorhinolaryngealogica Belgica 34: 627–629

61. Dourov N 1984 Scanning electron microscopy contribution in oral pathology. Scanning Electron Microscopy I: 243–248

62. Drzewieck K T 1977 The surface morphology of the melanoma cell. A scanning electron microscope study on the primary cutaneous melanoma. Scandinavian Journal of Reconstructive Surgery 11: 9–16

63. Eagle R C Jr, Lucier A C, Bernardino V B Jr, Yanoff M 1980 Retinal pigment epithelial abnormalities in fundus flavimaculatus. Ophthalmology 87: 1189–1200

64. Eakin R M, Brandenburger J L 1980 Method for observing the

interior of biological specimen by scanning electron microscopy. Mikroskopic 36: 33–34

65. Echlin P 1978 Coating techniques for scanning electron microscopy and X-ray microanalysis. Scanning Electron Microscopy I: 109–132

66. Ekfeldt A, Fli Oystrand F, Oilo G 1985 Replica techniques for in vivo studies of tooth surfaces and prosthetic materials. Scandinavian Journal of Dental Research 93: 560–565

67. Engel A, Reichelt R 1984 Imaging of biological structures with the scanning transmission electron microscope. Journal of Ultrastructure Research 88: 105–120

68. Farzadegan H, Roth I L 1975 Scanning electron microscopy and freeze-etching of gonorrhoeal urethral exudate. British Journal of Venereal Diseases 51: 83–91

69. Ferenczy A 1980 The female reproductive system. In: Hodges G M, Hallowes R C (eds) Biomedical Research Application of Scanning Electron Microscopy, vol 2, Academic Press, London, pp 127–165

70. Fischlschweiger W, Antonson D E 1983 Scanning electron microscopy in clinical dental research. Methodology for clinical and laboratory studies. Florida Dental Journal 54: 17–19, 37–38

71. Flood P R 1975 Dry fracturing techniques for the study of soft-internal biological tissues in the scanning electron microscope. Scanning Electron Microscopy : 287–294

72. Forslind B 1984 Clinical applications of scanning electron microscopy and X-ray microanalysis in dermatology. Scanning Electron Microscopy I: 183–206

73. Fowler S A, Allansmith M R 1981 The effect of cleaning soft contact lenses. A scanning electron microscopic study. Archives of Ophthalmology 99: 1382–1386

74. Fuchs H, Fuchs W 1980 The use of frozen-hydrated bulk specimens for X-ray microanalysis. Scanning Electron Microscopy II: 371–382

75. Fukudome H, Tanaka K 1986 A method for observing intracellular structures of free cells by scanning electronmicroscopy. Journal of Microscopy 141: 171–178

76. Fulton A B, Craft J L, Zakov Z N, Howard R O, Albert D M 1980 Retinal anomalies in trisomy 18. Albrecht von Graefes Archiven für Klinische und Experimentelle Ophthalmologie 213: 195–205

77. Garcia Tamayo, J, Castillo G, Martinez A J 1982 Human genital candidiasis: histochemistry, scanning and transmission electron microscopy. Acta Cytologica (Baltimore) 26: 7–14

78. Gattone V H, Fineberg N S, Evan A P 1985 A proposed technique for the morphometric analysis of arteriolar smooth muscle cells from scanning electron microscopic preparations. Journal of Submicroscopic Cytology 17: 551–554

79. Gaudio E, Pannarole L, Marrinozzi G 1985 A SEM corrosion cast study on pericyte localization in microcirculation of skeletal muscle. Angiology 36: 458–464

80. Giereck A, Sosnierz M, Bialas B 1974 A slide of a retinal surface viewed under a scanning electron microscope and associated histopathological process observed after operation for detached retina in a human eye. Ophthalmology 168: 52–57

81. Goerz G, Busch P 1981 Das Glasswall-Haar. 'Spun-glass Hair'. Archives of Dermatological Research 270: 353–359

82. Goran D A, Shields H M, Bates M L, Zuckerman G R, De Schryuer–Kecskemeti K 1984 Oesophageal dysplasia. Assessment by light microscopy and scanning electron microscopy. Gastroenterology 86: 39–50

83. Gok G, Molenaar I 1983 Some applications of scanning electron microscopy on the study of biopsies in central nervous system pathology. Scanning Electron Microscopy I: 143–150

84. Goto K 1984 Aspects of quantitative auger electron spectroscopy. Scanning Electron Microscopy I: 103–110

85. Gattinger W 1981 Formation of basement membranes and collagenous fibrils on peripheral cystoid degeneration and retinoschisis. Developmental Ophthalmology 2: 362–368

86. Greiner J V, Covington H J, Allansmith MR 1978 Surface morphology of giant papillary conjunctivitis in contact lens wearers. American Journal of Ophthalmology 85: 242–252

87. Greiner J V, Covington H I, Korb D R, Allansmith M R 1978 Conjunctiva in asymptomatic contact lens wearers. American Journal of Ophthalmology 86: 403–413

88. Griffith O H, Rempfer G F, Lesch G H 1981 A high vacuum photoelectron microscopy for the study of biological specimens. Scanning Electron Microscopy II: 123–130

89. Guentzel M N 1983 Application of scanning electron microscopy to the study of microorganisms in gastrointestinal pathology. Scanning Electron Microscopy II: 279–292

90. Haggis G H, Schweitzer I, Hall R, Bladon T 1983 Freeze fracture through the cytoskeleton, nucleus and nuclear matrix of lymphocytes studied by scanning electron microscopy. Journal of Microscopy 132: 185–194

91. Halter S A, Green H L, Helink G 1982 Gluten sensitive enteropathology: sequence of villous regrowth as viewed by scanning electron microscopy. Human Pathology 13: 811–818

92. Harada H, Takeda M, Tanaka J, Miki H, Ochi K, Kimura I 1983 The fine structure of pancreatic stones as shown by scanning electron microscopy and X-ray probe microanalyser. Gastroenterologia Japonica 18: 530–537

93. Hardy W, Vance J, Jones K, Kokubo Y 1982 Digital image processing: a path to better pictures. Scanning Electron Microscopy II: 485–494

94. Hardoff D, Levanon D, Gitay H, Nir I 1986 Evaluation of microvilli in gluten-sensitive enteropathology by means of scanning and transmission electron microscopy. Journal of Pediatric Gastroenterology and Nutrition (New York) 5: 560–564

95. Hartman A L, Nakane P K 1981 Intracellular localization of antigens with backscatter mode of SEM using peroxidase labelled antibodies. Scanning Electron Microscopy II: 33–44

96. Heinze J, Carroll N 1969 The scanning electron microscope in external eye disease. Transactions of the Australian College of Ophthalmologists 1: 122–126

97. Hisano S, Adachi T, Maegawa M, Daikoku S 1986 Some improvement in tissue preparation and colloidal gold immunolabelling for electron microscopy. American Journal of Anatomy 175: 245–266

98. Hodde K C, Nowell J A 1980 SEM of micro-corrosion casts. Scanning Electron Microscopy II: 89–106

99. Hodges G M, Muir M D 1974 Autoradiography of biological tissues in the scanning electron microscope. Nature 247: 383–385

100. Ingram P, Morosoff N, Pope L, Allen F, Tisher C 1976 Some comparisons of the techniques of sputter (coating) and evaporative coating for scanning electron microscopy. Scanning Electron Microscopy I: 75–81

101. Itoshima T, Yoshino K, Yamamoto K, Munetomo F, Murakami T 1978 Scanning electron microscopy of puncture perfused human liver biopsy samples. Observation of bile ductules and bile canaliculi. Scanning Electron Microscopy II: 169–174

102. John T, Sassani J W, Eagle R C Jr 1982 Scanning electron microscopy of rubeosis iridis. Transactions of the Pennsylvania Academy of Ophthalmology and Otolaryngology 35: 119–121

103. Jones D B 1983 The complementary role of scanning electron microscopy in renal pathological diagnosis. Scanning Electron Microscopy I: 323–332

104. Kanagawa H, Hafez E S, Baechler C A, Pitchford W C, Barnhart M E 1972 Improved methodology for scanning electron microscopy of the female reproductive tract. International Journal of Fertility 17: 75–80

105. Kanaya K, Baba N, Shino M K, Kai M, Oho E, Muranaka Y 1982 Digital processing methods using scanning densitometer and microcomputer for the structural analysis of a scanning electron micrograph. Scanning Electron Microscopy I: 61–72

106. Karaganov I A L, Mironov A A, Mironov V A 1982 Scanning electron microscopy with corrosive preparations in pathology. Arkhiv Patologii (Moskva) 44: 63–69

107. Kavin H, Hamilton D G, Greasley R E, Eckert J D, Zuidema G 1970 Scanning electron microscopy. A new method in the study of rectal mucosa. Gastroenterology 59: 426–432

108. Keeley R 1984 The forensic scanning electron microscope. Medico-Legal Journal 52: 211–226

109. Kenemans P, Hafez S E L 1984 Clinical application of scanning electron microscopy in human reproduction. Scanning Electron Microscopy I: 215–242

110. Khan S R, Hackett R L 1986 Calcium oxalate urolithiasis in the rat: is it a model for human stone disease? A review of recent literature. Scanning Electron Microscopy III: 1247–1251

111. Khan S R, Hackett R L 1986 Identification of urinary stone and sediment crystals by scanning electron microscopy and X-ray microanalysis. Journal of Urology 135: 818–825

112. Khan S R, Wilkinson E J 1985 Scanning electron microscopy as analytical tool for the study of calcified intrauterine contraceptive devices. Scanning Electron Microscopy III: 1247–1251

113. Kim K M, Resau J, Chung J 1984 Scanning electron microscopy of urinary stones as a diagnostic tool. Scanning Electron Microscopy I: 1819–1831

114. Kretzer F L, Hiltner H M, Johnson A T, Mehta R S, Godio L B 1982 Vitamin E and retrolental fibroplasia: ultrastructural support of clinical efficacy. Annals of New York Academy of Science 393: 145–166

115. Kristensen S E, Papadimitriou J M 1981 The measurement of cell volume and surface area by SEM photogrammetry. Journal of Microscopy 124: 155–161

116. Kushida H, Kushida T 1982 An improved method for both light and electron microscopy of identical sites in semi-thin tissue sections embedded in epoxy resin 'quentol 651'. Journal of Electron Microscopy (Tokyo) 2: 202–205

117. Kushida H, Kushida T, Nagato Y, Ogura K 1982 An improved method for both light and scanning electron microscopy in back-scattered electron mode of identical sites in semi-thin tissue sections embedded in GMA and Quetal 523. Journal of Electron Microscopy 31: 202–205

118. Lambrecht P, Vanherle G, Davidson C 1981 A universal and accurate replica technique for scanning electron microscope study in clinical dentistry. Microscopica Acta 85: 45–58

119. Lametschwandtner A, Lametschwandtner U, Weiger T 1984 Scanning electron microscopy of vascular corrosion casts. Techniques and applications. Scanning Electron Microscopy II: 663–695

120. Laschi R 1985 Contribution of scanning electron microscopy and associated analytical techniques to the study of atherosclerotic disease. Scanning Electron Microscopy III: 1215–1222

121. Leighton S B 1981 SEM images of block faces cut by a miniature microtome within the SEM. Scanning Electron Microscopy III: 73–76

122. Levison D A, Crocker P R, Baxall T A, Randall K J 1986 coconut matting bezoar identified by a combined analytical approach. Journal of Clinical Pathology 39: 172–175

123. Lewis E R, Jackson L, Scott T 1975 Comparison of miscibilities and critical point drying properties of various intermediate and transitional fluids. Scanning Electron Microscopy: 317–324

124. Linders P W, Hagemann P 1983 Mass determination of thin biological specimens using back-scattered electrons. Application in quantitative X-ray microanalysis on an automated STEM system. Ultramicroscopy 11: 13–19

125. Linke A, Rose H J, Frick G 1983 Demonstration of immune complexes on erythrocytes by scanning electron microscopy. Folia Haematologica (Leipzig) 110: 852–857

126. Makita T, Sandborn E B 1971 Identification of intracellular components by scanning electron microscopy. Experimental Cell Research 67: 211–214

127. Makita T, Ueda H, Hirose H, Idegomori T 1982 X-ray microanalysis of hydrated biological specimens. Scanning Electron Microscopy III: 1215–1220

128. Marks R, Dawber R P R 1971 Skin surface biopsy. An improved technique for the examination of the horny layer. British Journal of Dermatology 84: 117–123

129. Marrie T J, Costerton J W 1983 A scanning and transmission electron microscopic study of the surfaces of intrauterine contraceptive devices. American Journal of Obstetrics and Gynaecology 146: 384–394

130. Marrie T J, Costerton J W 1983 A scanning electron microscopic study of urine droppers and urine collecting systems. Archives of Internal Medicine 143: 1135–1141

131. Marshall A T 1980 Quantitative X-ray microanalysis of frozen hydrated bulk biological specimens. Scanning Electron Microscopy II: 335–348

132. Molday R S, Maher P 1980 A review of cell surface markers and labelling techniques for scanning electron microscopy. Histochemical Journal 12: 273–315

133. Moreton R B, Echlin P, Gupta B L 1974 Preparation of frozen hydrated tissue sections for X-ray microanalysis in the scanning electron microscope. Nature 247: 113–115

134. Murakami T, Iida N, Taquchi T, Ohtani O, Kikuta A, Ohtsuka A, Itoshima T 1983 Conductive staining of biological specimen for scanning electron microscopy with special reference to ligand-mediated osmium impregnation. Scanning Electron Microscopy I: 235–246

135. Murphy J A 1980 Non-coating techniques to render biological specimens conductive: 1980 update. Scanning Electron Microscopy: 209–220

136. Nagato Y, Kushida T, Kushida H, Ogura K 1983 Observation on back-scattered electron image (BEI) on a scanning electron microscope (SEM) in semi-thin sections prepared for light microscopy. Tokai Journal of Experimental and Clinical Medicine 8: 167–174

137. Nagele R G, Doane K J, Lee H, Wilson F J, Roisen F J 1984 A method for exposing the internal anatomy of small and delicate tissues for correlated SEM/TEM studies using polyethylene glycol embedding. Journal of Microscopy 133: 177–183

138. Naguro T, Saito M, Natatani T 1980 A simple method for observing soft biological tissue with the cryo-scanning electron microscope. Journal of Electron Microscopy (Tokyo) 29: 195–196

139. Nakabayashi N 1985 Bonding of restorative materials to dentine: the present status in Japan. International Dental Journal 35: 145–154

140. Nakane P K, Hartman A L 1980 Immunocytochemical localization of intracellular antigens with SEM. Histochemical Journal 12: 435–447

141. Nava M T, Soligo D, Pozzoli E, Lambertenghi-Deliliers G 1984 Back-scattered electron imaging for immunogold viewing by scanning electron microscope. Journal of Immunological Methods 70: 269–271

142. Nelson A C, Schoen F J, Levy R J 1985 Scanning electron microscopy for study of the pathophysiology of calcification in bioprosthetic heart valves. Scanning Electron Microscopy I: 209–213

143. Nopanitaya W, Grisham J W, Lesense H R 1977 A preliminary assessment of the use of scanning electron microscopy for diagnostive evaluation of liver biopsies. Scanning Electron Microscopy II: 159–169

144. Nordestgaard B G, Rostgaard J 1985 Critical-point drying versus freeze drying for scanning electron microscopy: a quantitative and qualitative study on isolated hepatocytes. Journal of Microscopy 137: 189–207

145. Ohtsuk M 1980 Observation of unstained biological macromolecules with the STEM. Ultramicroscopy 5: 317–323

146. Pfister T H C, Neukirchner A 1980 Raster elektronenmikroskopische Untersuchungen an kranken Nagel mittles Abdruck-Verfahren. Fortschritte der Medizin (Leipzig) 98: 1465–1470

147. Pasquinelli G, Scala C, Borsetti G P, Martegani F, Laschi R 1985 A new approach for studying semi-thin sections of human pathological material: intermicroscopic correlation between light microscopy and scanning electron microscopy. Scanning Electron Microscopy III: 1133–1142

148. Patek E, Nilsson L 1977 Hydrosalphinx simplex as seen by the scanning electron microscope. Fertility and Sterility 28: 962–971

149. Paul D, Hecker E 1970 Autoradiography in the scanning electron microscope. Nature 227: 488–489

150. Peters K-R 1979 Scanning electron microscopy at macromolecular resolution in low energy mode on biological specimens coated with ultrathin metal films. Scanning Electron Microscopy II: 133–148

151. Peters K-R 1985 Working at higher magnification in scanning electron microscopy with secondary and back-scattered electrons on metal coated biological specimens and imaging macromolecular cell membrane structures. Scanning Electron Microscopy IV: 1519–1544

152. Plister R I982 The use of scanning electron microscopy and associated techniques in forensic sciences (a bibliographic update). Scanning Electron Microscopy III: 1037–1042

153. Polak B, Daunter B 1983 Scanning electron microscopy and histological examination of human seminal coagulum. Andrologia 15: 542–562

154. Poley J R 1983 The small bowel mucosa in disease states characterized by chronic diarrhoea. Observations by scanning electron microscopy. Scanning Electron Microscopy III: 1293–1306
155. Price V H, Odom R B, Ward W H, Jones F T 1980 Trichothio-dystrophy. Sulphur deficiency brittle hair as a marker for a neuroectodermal symptom complex. Dermatology 116: 1375–1384
156. Rabinovitch M, Bothwell T, Hayakawa B N, Williams W G, Trusler G A, Rowe R D, Olley P M, Cutz E 1986 Pulmonary artery endothelial abnormalities in patients with congenital heart defects and pulmonary hypertension: a correlation of light with scanning electron microscopy and transmission electron microscopy. Laboratory Investigation 55: 632–653
157. Redler I, Zimny M L 1970 Scanning electron microscopy of normal and abnormal articular cartilage and synovium. Journal of Bone and Joint Surgery 52: 1395–1404
158. Reece I J, Anderson J D, Wain W H, Carr K, Toner P G, Tindale W, Black M M, Wheatley D J 1985 A new porcine bioprosthesis: *in vivo* and *in vitro* evaluation. Life Support Systems 3: 207–227
159. Riddle J M, Jenning J J, Stein P D, Magilligan D J Jr 1984 A morphological overview of the porcine bioprosthetic valve — before and after its degeneration. Scanning Electron Microscopy I: 207–214
160. Robinson K M, Maistry L, Evers P 1981 Surface features of normal and neoplastic human oesophageal cells *in vivo* and *in vitro*. Scanning Electron Microscopy II: 213–222
161. Rodrigues M M, Leurier C A 1983 Histopathology of argon laser photocoagulation in juvenile diabetic retinopathy. Ophthalmology 90: 1023–1027
162. Roomans G M 1981 Quantitative electron probe X-ray microanalysis of biological specimens. Scanning Electron Microscopy II: 345–356
163. Rosenbauer K A, Herzer J A 1980 Further scanning electron microscopic studies of different types of prosthetic heart valves which were in place between two and more than ten years. Scanning Electron Microscopy III: 219–226
164. Ryan R L, Hing S A, Theiler R F 1983 A replica technique for the evaluation of human skin by scanning electron microscopy. Journal of Cutaneous Pathology 10: 262–276
165. Sakagushi H 1973 Scanning electron microscopy in the field of pathology. Journal of Electron Microscopy 22: 1–3
166. Sato S, Murphy G F, Bernhard J D, Mihm M C Jr, Fitzpatrick T B 1981 Ultrastructural and X-ray microanalytical observations of minocycline-related hyperpigmentation of the skin. Journal of Investigative Dermatology 77: 264–271
167. Schaff Z, Lapis K, Irene K B 1974 The role and possibilities of use of scanning electron microscope as a new morphologic examination method in medicine. Orvosi Hetilap (Budapest) 1I5: 1263–1267
168. Schneider G B, Pockwinse S M, Brillings-Gagllardi S 1978 Morphological changes in isolated lymphocytes during preparation for SEM. A comparative TEM/SEM study of freeze drying and critical point drying. Scanning Electron Microscopy : 305–316
169. Sedar A W, Silver M J, Ingerman-Wojenski C M 1983 Back-scattered electron imaging to visualise arterial endothelial detachment in the scanning electron microscope. Scanning Electron Microscopy II: 969–974
170. Siegesmund K A, Funahashi A, Pintar K, Dragen R, Schlueter D P 1980 Elemental content in alveolar septa in various pneumoconioses. Scanning Electron Microscopy II: 485–491
171. Siew S 1978 Scanning electron microscopy of acute rheumatic valvulitis. Scanning Electron Microscopy II: 234, 341–348
172. Siew S 1983 The application of scanning electron microscopy in the clinical investigation of the human colon. Scanning Electron Microscopy IV: 1911–1929
173. Siew S 1985 Scanning electron microscopy of the human myocardium. Scanning Electron Microscopy IV: 1295–1304
174. Siew S, Goldstein M L 1981 Scanning electron microscopy of mucosal biopsies of the human upper gastrointestinal tract. Scanning Electron Microscopy IV: 178–181
175. Siklos L, Rozsa M, Zombori J 1986 A simple method for correlative light, scanning electron microscope and X-ray microanalytical examination of the same section. Journal of Microscopy 142: 107–110
176. Sheppard B L, Bonnar J 1980 Scanning and transmission electron microscopy of material adherent to intrauterine contraceptive devices. British Journal of Obstetrics and Gynaecology 87: 155–162
177. Soligo D, de Harven E 1981 Ultrastructural cytochemical localizations by back-scattered electron imaging of white blood cells. Journal of Histochemistry and Cytochemistry 29: 1071–1079
178. Soligo D, de Harven E, Pozzoli E, Nava M T, Polli N, Lambertenchi-Deliliers G 1985 Scanning electron microscope cytochemistry of blood cells. Scanning Electron Microscopy II: 817–825
179. Stacholy J, Goldberg E P 1985 Microstructural matrix–crystal interactions in calcium oxalate monohydrate kidney stones. Scanning Electron Microscopy II: 781–787
180. Steflik D E, McKinney R V Jr, Singh B B 1983 Retrieval of plastic embedded light microscopy specimens for plasma etched scanning electron microscope analysis. Stain Technology 58: 59–61
181. Stols A L, Standhouders A M, Linders P W, van de Vorstenbosch R A 1986 The use of back-scattered electrons in analytical electron microscopy for the measurement of the mass of the individual rat blood platelets. Histochemistry 84: 379–382
182. Sundstrom P, Nilsson O, Liedholm P 1983 Scanning electron microscopy of human preimplantation endometrium in normal and clomiphene/human chorionic gonadotrophin-stimulated cycles. Fertility and Sterility 40: 642–647
183. Sweney L R, Shapiro B L 1981 One to one correlation of histological and histochemical light microscopy with scanning electron microscopy. Scanning Electron Microscopy II: 63–72
184. Tanaka K 1981 Medical use of scanning electron microscope and recent morphological findings on organelles. Nippon Rinsho 39: 3570–3578
185. Tanaka K, Mitsushima A 1984 A preparation method for observing intracellular structures by scanning electron microscopy. Journal of Microscropy 133: 213–222
186. Taylor C J, Green S H 1981 Menke's syndrome (Trichopaliodystrophy): use of scanning electron microscope in diagnosis and carrier identification. Developmental Medicine and Child Neurology 23: 361–368
187. Tichelaar W, Oostergetel G T, Haker J, van Heel M G, van Bruggen E F 1980 Scanning transmission electron microscopy of biological macromolecules. Ultramicroscopy 5: 27–33
188. Tokunaga J, Fujita T, Hattori A 1969 Scanning electron microscopy of normal and pathological human erythrocytes. Archivum Histolologicum Japonicum 31: 21–35
189. Toner P G, Carr K E 1969 The use of scanning electron microscopy in the study of the intestinal villi. Journal of Pathology 97: 611–617
190. Tyler W S, Dungworth D L, Nowell J A 1973 The potential of SEM in studies of experimental and spontaneous diseases. Scanning Electron Microscopy: 403–410
191. Ureina F, Azofeifa A, Akahari H 1985 An improved method for the surface replica. Journal of Electron Microscopy (Tokyo) 34: 144–145
192. Ushiki T, Fujita T 1986 Back-scattered electron imaging. Its applications to biological specimens stained with heavy metals. Archivum Histolologicum Japonicum 49: 139–154
193. Ushiki T, Yonehara K, Iwanaga T, Fujita T 1984 Application of a back-scattered electron image to immunocytochemistry in freeze-cracked tissues. Archivum Histolologicum Japonicum 47: 553–557
194. Versura P, Bonvincini F, Caramazza R, Laschi R 1985 Scanning electron microscopy study of human cornea and conjunctiva in normal and various pathological conditions. Scanning Electron Microscopy IV: 1695–1708
195. Vonnahme F J 1980 An improved method for transparenchymal fixation of human liver biopsies for scanning electron microscopy. Scanning Electron Microscopy III: 177–180
196. Vonnahme F J 1984 The scanning electron microscope as a diagnostic tool in liver pathology. Scanning Electron Microscopy I: 173–182
197. Vonnahme F J, Brolsch C H 1981 Ultrastructural observations of the hepatic vascular system in Budd-Chiari's syndrome. Bibliotheca Anatomica 20: 98–101

198. Wall J S, Hainfeld J F 1986 Mass mapping with the scanning transmission electron microscope. Annual Reviews of Biophysical Chemistry 15: 355–376

199. Weidner N, Lorentz W B Jr 1986 Scanning electron microscopy of the acellular glomerular basement membranes in idiopathic membraneous glomerulopathy. Laboratory Investigation 54: 84–92

200. Weiss R L 1980 Scanning electron microscope autoradiography of critical point dried biological samples. Scanning Electron Microscopy IV: 124–130

201. Weiss R L 1984 Improved coating and fixation methods for scanning electron microscope autoradiography. Biology of the Cell 50: 157–161

202. Wenzel M, Wenzel J, Klausch D, Slems W, Stracke R, Weise H 1984 Methods of preparing various tissues for scanning electron microscopy. Zeitschrift fur Mikroskopisch — Anatomische Forschung 98: 705–720

203. Wilborn W H, Dismukes D E, Montes L F 1978 Seborrhoeic keratoses. Journal of Cutaneous Pathology 5: 373–375

204. Wouters C H, Koerten H K, Bonnet J, Daems W T, Ploem J S 1986 Quantitative DNA measurement in an instrument combining scanning microscopy and light microscopy. Journal of Microscopy 141: 41–53

205. Wouters C H, Ploem J S 1985 A new instrument combining simultaneous light and scanning electron microscopy. Progress in Clinical and Biological Research 196: 115–133

206. Yamashita S, Sugihara K, Nagata M, Kawashima K, Hamazaki E 1980 Observation of various diseases in the oral area by scanning electron microscopy. Shikai Tenbo 3: 385–396

207. Yoshino K 1979 Scanning electron microscopy of the liver of primary biliary cirrhosis. Scanning Electron Microscopy III: 697–704

208. Zamberletti D, Fedele L, Verecellini P, Candiani G D 1981 Scanning electron microscopy of the tubercular fallopian tube. Acta Europea Fertilatis 12: 213–221

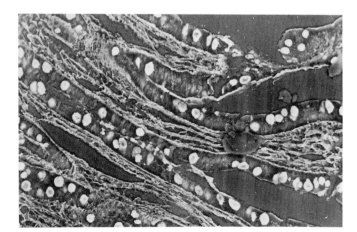

Fig. 3.1 Small intestine. A plastic-embedded small intestinal tissue section stained with a silver impregnation method and examined in the scanning electron microscope by the backscattered electron mode. Goblet cells and reticulin framework are clearly seen. (× 275)

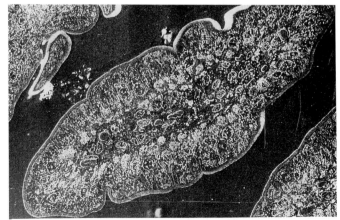

Fig. 3.2 Small intestine. Plasma-etched semi-thin plastic section of the mouse small intestine examined in the backscattered electron mode. Subcellular structures such as the microvillous border, nuclei and mitochondria are identifiable by this technique. (× 476)

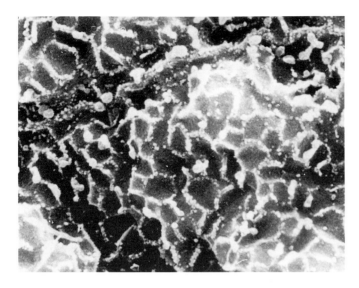

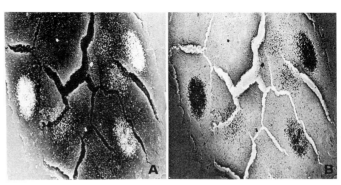

Fig. 3.4 Urothelial carcinoma. SEM autoradiography of human bladder carcinoma-derived epithelial (RT4) cells (3HTdr labelled carbon and L4 emulsion-coated; 10 min trypsin degelatination treatment) showing secondary (A) and backscattered (B) electron images of silver grain concentrations localized over cell nuclei. Differences in labelling intensity are in evidence. (× 530) (Courtesy of Dr G M Hodges, Imperial Cancer Research Fund)

Fig. 3.3 Urothelium. Luminal surface distribution of concanavalin A receptor sites marked by indirect labelling with 30 nm gold particles on the superficial terminally differentiated urothelial cells of mouse urinary bladder. (× 18 600) (Courtesy of Dr G M Hodges, Imperial Cancer Research Fund)

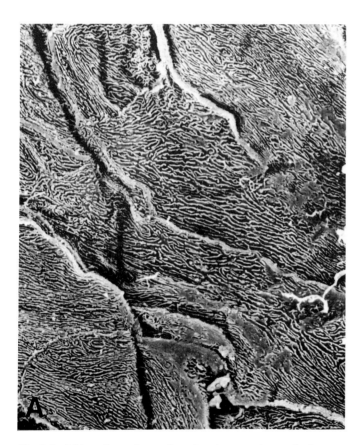

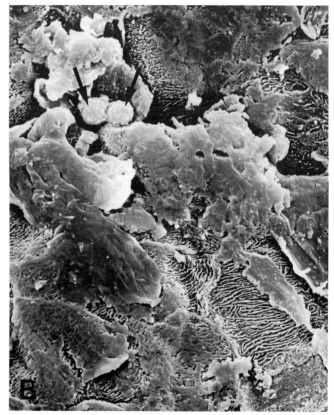

Fig. 3.5 A Normal oesophagus. Scanning electron micrograph of normal oesophageal biopsy showing characteristic microridge pattern on the surface of the superficial stratified squamous epithelial cells. Cell boundaries are clearly demarcated. Dewaxed paraffin block. (× 2200)
B Oesophagitis. Surface debris obscuring the characteristic microridge pattern in a case of oesophagitis. Two round cells (arrows), presumably inflammatory cells, can be seen. Dewaxed paraffin block. (× 2200)

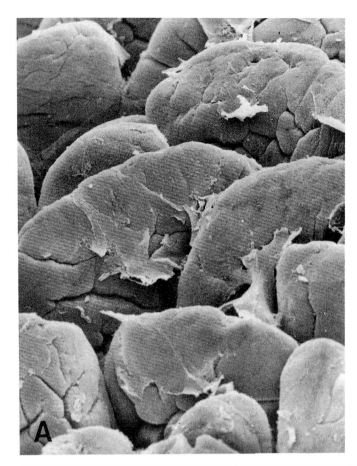
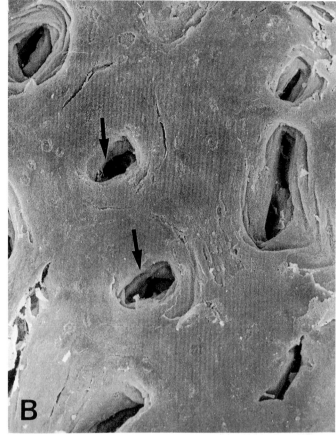
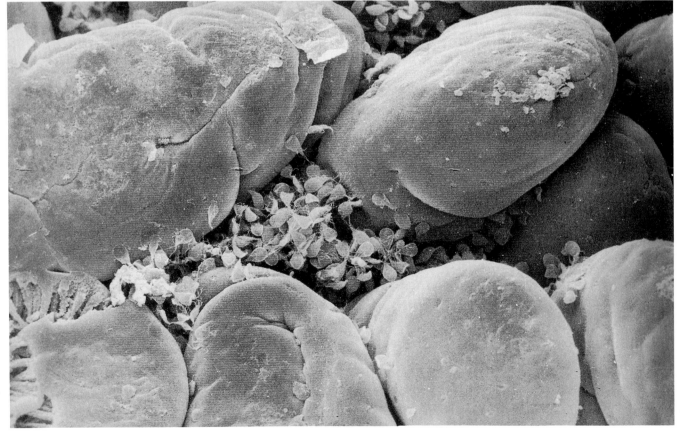

Fig. 3.6 **A** Normal small intestine. Scanning electron micrograph of normal leaf-shaped human intestinal villi. Dewaxed paraffin block. (× 250). **B** Coeliac disease. The small intestinal mucosa in a case of coeliac disease. The absence of the villi, the flat mucosa and the irregularly shaped crypt openings (arrows) contrast with the normal morphology seen in **A**. Dewaxed paraffin block. (× 250)

Fig. 3.7 Giardiasis. *Giardia lamblia* on the surface of apparently normal human duodenal villi. Dewaxed paraffin block. (× 550)

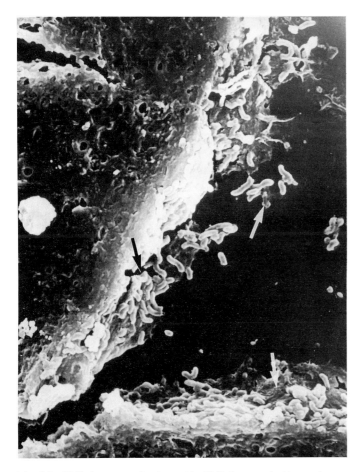

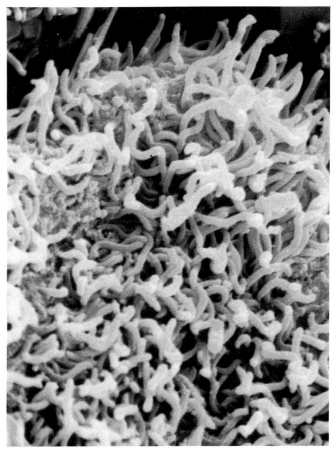

Fig. 3.8 *Helicobacter*-associated gastritis. *Helicobacter pylori* (arrows) on the surface of the gastric mucosa in a case of gastritis. The characteristic, slightly twisted organisms are easily identifiable by SEM. Dewaxed paraffin section. (× 2940)

Fig. 3.9 Spirochaetosis. Co-existing appendiceal spirochaetosis found by chance during the examination of a case of acute appendicitis. The elongated twisted spirochaetes cover the mucosal surface of the appendix, obscuring the underlying microvilli. Dewaxed paraffin block. (× 8770)

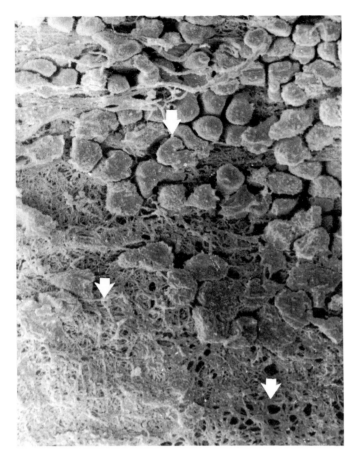

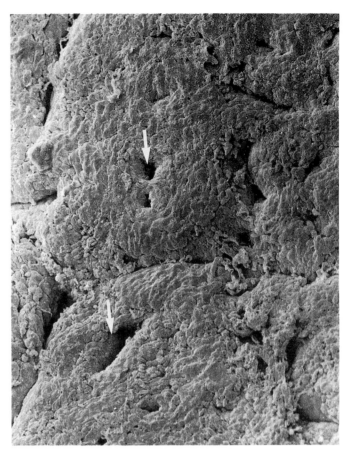

Fig. 3.10 Acute appendicitis with peritonitis. The serosal surface of the appendix is covered with acute inflammatory cells (arrows) and a fibrin network (short arrows). Dewaxed paraffin block. (× 1350)

Fig. 3.11 Crohn's disease. Scanning electron micrograph of the small intestinal mucosal surface showing non-specific mucosal changes in a case of Crohn's disease. The mucosa is flattened, and no villi are seen in this micrograph. The crypt openings (arrows) are of irregular sizes and shapes. Dewaxed paraffin block. (× 200)

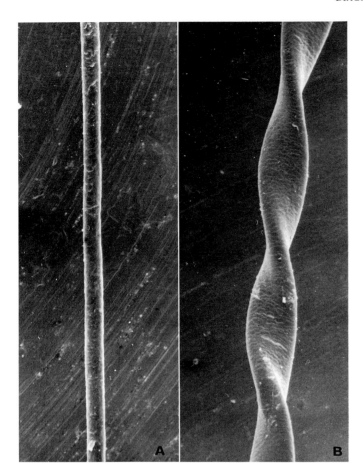

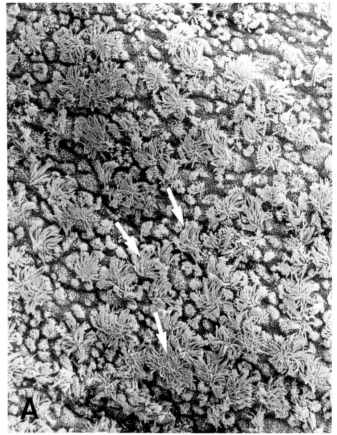

Fig. 3.12 Normal and twisted hair. **A** Scanning electron micrograph of normal hair showing straight hair shafts with the characteristic cylindrical structure. (× 135) (Courtesy of Dr C. H. S. Cameron, Queen's University Department of Pathology, Royal Victoria Hospital, Belfast.) **B** Scanning electron micrograph of pili torti (twisted hair). The hair is flattened and twisted around its long axis (see also Fig. 22.45). In cross-section the hair is ellipsoidal or triangular. (× 145) (Courtesy of Dr M Y Walsh and Dr C H S Cameron, Queen's University Department of Pathology, Royal Victoria Hospital, Belfast)

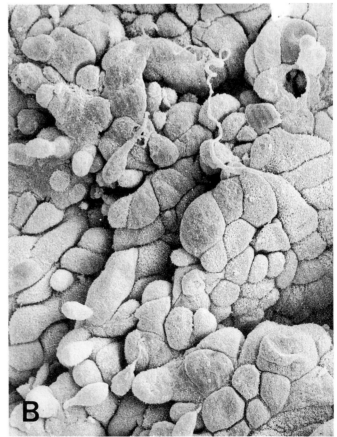

Fig. 3.13 **A** Endometrial hyperplasia. Scanning electron micrograph of the endometrial surface in a case of endometrial hyperplasia. Ciliated cells (arrows) are prominent amongst non-ciliated cells, but the overall appearances are of a relatively ordered epithelial sheet. (× 1000) **B** Endometrial adenocarcinoma. Scanning electron micrograph appearance of endometrial adenocarcinoma. Note the pleomorphism and irregular arrangement of cells. No ciliated cells are present. Dewaxed paraffin block. (× 1000)

4. Pathology of the cell: ultrastructural features

L. Marzella   B. F. Trump

INTRODUCTION

The purpose of this chapter is to describe some of the common ultrastructural alterations induced by acute cell injury. Particular emphasis will be given to alterations of subcellular organelles. The functional significance of the morphological alterations will be described, as it is currently understood. The relationship between the ultrastructural alterations and the severity of the cell injury state will be indicated. In this chapter we shall use the normal ultrastructure of the hepatocyte as a reference point for the description of the ultrastructural alterations induced by cell injury. Examples from other tissues will be used to illustrate the commonality of these changes.

DEFINITION OF CELL INJURY

Cellular injury is defined as a state of pathologically altered cellular function. Under physiological conditions normal cells are in homeostasis. When an injurious stimulus is applied cells expend metabolic energy to maintain homeostasis. If the stimulus is severe enough, or lasts sufficiently long, the ability of the cells to adapt may be exceeded and cellular functions become altered; the cell is said to be injured. If the injury is sublethal, the cell survives even though it may function abnormally. A chronically injured state induces cells to undergo stable, structural and functional alterations that may restore homeostasis.[20] Sublethally injured cells may also continue to deteriorate structurally and functionally to reach a point from which recovery is no longer possible. The so-called 'point-of-no-return' is not yet precisely defined, either ultrastructurally or functionally. However, it has been possible to define the point-of-no-return empirically. Tissues are, for example, subjected to injury of reproducible severity for progressively longer periods of time. In this manner, the duration of injury (for example, anoxia) needed to induce cell death in a particular tissue is established. It therefore becomes possible to study the cells to determine what distinctive structural or functional alterations have taken place at or near the point-of-no-return.[5] These alterations are likely to be important determinants of the death of cells.

SUSCEPTIBILITY TO INJURY

It is clear that cells differ in their susceptibility to injury. Many structural factors influence this susceptibility — for example, organelle composition, histological organization and relationship to extracellular matrix. Other physical, mechanical and environmental factors such as nutrition, ionic composition of extracellular milieu, diffusion of gases, nutrients and waste products, blood flow and contractility of adjacent tissues also contribute to susceptibility to injury. Even within the same tissue, some cells may be more susceptible to injury than others because of differences in the stage of the cell cycle, differences in metabolic rates and inability to dissociate metabolic rates from availability of high energy compounds. Despite these sources of variability, it is remarkable that, at the ultrastructural level, quite diverse types of insults — such as ischaemic, toxic, immunological and infectious injuries — all induce similar ultrastructural alterations in cells. At the biochemical level, these insults induce more distinct alterations by virtue of modification of specific biochemical pathways or by modification of a specific organelle. However, with time, the initial biochemical alteration inevitably affects integrated diverse cellular functions. As a consequence, despite differences in the initial insult, injured cells manifest common structural and functional alterations. These common functional alterations reflect a loss of homeostasis.

Cells that pass the point-of-no-return are irreversibly injured: they are committed to cell death. Dead cells lose structural integrity due to osmotic and other physical factors and to the degradative action of intracellular and extracellular enzymes (the process of necrosis). Factors such as blood flow (which allows the influx of inflammatory cells), adjacent tissue cells and extracellular matrices influence the rapidity of necrosis. At the light microscopy level, dead cells are morphologically indistinguishable from living cells until the process of necrosis begins to induce changes. However, at the ultrastructural level readily identifiable alterations permit the identification of irreversibly injured cells several hours before the necrotic process begins and even more hours before histological alterations become apparent in the tissue by light microscopy. Cell death, due to changes in hormonal levels, occurs in endocrine-dependent tissues. It has been proposed that, mechanistically and morphologically, this type of cell death represents a distinct entity called apoptosis.[36] However, little is known about the mechanisms which govern this process.

STAGES OF CELL INJURY

The ultrastructural criteria of cell injury are useful markers for staging the level of tissue injury and have been validated for many tissues. Deviations from normal physiological temperature and in vitro conditions can alter the evolution and the characteristics of these ultrastructural alterations.[34,35] For classification and for didactic purposes, it is helpful to divide the ultrastructural alterations of injured cells into stages.[56] However, this does not imply that sharp transition points exist in the evolution of the ultrastructural alterations or that all organelles within a cell move synchronously through the various stages. Intracellular and histological micro-environments respond to injury at different rates, and consequently various stages of cell injury may be occurring simultaneously in different cells or even within the same cell.

Parallel biochemical and ultrastructural analyses can be used to elucidate the functional significance of ultrastructural alterations of injured cells. For example, simultaneous morphological and spectrofluorometric studies have been performed to understand the functional significance of blebbing.[21] Correlations of observations made by TEM with other ultrastructural techniques have established the importance of ion shifts in the swelling of injured cells. For example, analytic techniques such as X-ray microanalysis permit the quantification of ion shifts within specific organelles of injured cells. Scanning microscopy is particularly suited to studying the surface features of injured cells. These features may not be adequately preserved by the vigorous processing techniques required for TEM. In addition, structures such as surface blebs are not adequately visualized in thin sections. Immunocytochemistry can assist in the study of cellular structures that are too altered by cell injury to be identified reliably by ultrastructural criteria alone.

These various analytical and morphological techniques have identified characteristic biochemical and physical alterations that parallel the ultrastructural stages of injury. The presence of these common biochemical and morphological alterations indicates that cell injury ultimately interferes with basic integrative cellular functions. There is a general agreement that key cellular functions, if interfered with sufficiently, will cause cell death.

MECHANISMS OF CELL INJURY

Maintenance of structural and functional integrity of the cell surface membrane and of specialized intracellular membrane compartments is critical to maintain ionic equilibrium. The integrity of intracellular membranes is also essential to separate the subcellular compartments with their specialized functions. These membrane-bound micro-environments facilitate enzymatic reactions for biosynthesis and oxidative phosphorylation, regulate availability of ions and substrates, and segregate lytic reactions. The ability to generate ATP needed to drive chemical reactions and maintain chemical equilibrium is another key function whose loss may lead to irreversible injury. The earliest and most important consequence of dysfunction of energy metabolism is thought to be the loss of homeostasis of ions such as Na^+, Ca^{2+}, K^+ and H^+.

Loss of ionic regulation, energy loss and altered membrane permeability enhance each other in a deleterious way. Thus, after a specific initiating event, cell injury may evolve into a vicious cycle sustained by cellular biochemical pathways. However, in the early stages of injury, some of these functional alterations may be adaptive responses. For example, in ischaemia of cardiac muscle, loss of Ca^{2+} regulation by the sarcoplasmic reticulum is a very early event and may be caused by inactivation of a key regulatory protein.[49] Yet this inactivation causes immediate loss of contractility of the injured myocyte, with consequent preservation of metabolic energy. Similarly, inactivation of transcriptional and/or translocational activity may be beneficial initially as it decreases ATP consumption. Acidification of the cell due to anaerobic metabolism during ischaemia or hypoxia may also enhance the resistance of the cell to injury.[39] During injury states, active repair and detoxification processes are also activated to restore homeostasis. Excision and repair of macromolecules, proteolytic degradation of denatured proteins, re-acylation of lysophosphatides, endocytosis, and lysosomal degradation of cell surface membranes bearing complement lesions are some examples. In some instances, however, active metabolic and detoxication processes are responsible for biotransformation of compounds into chemically reactive toxic species.

Other functions are also affected by cell injury but are less likely to cause cell death because the alterations are often reversible. These functions are: (1) cytoskeletal organization required to maintain cell shape, integrity of the plasma membrane, and locomotion of cell and subcellular organelles; (2) transcription of DNA, translation of mRNA transcripts, and translocation and export of macromolecules; (3) intermediary metabolism of fuels; (4) intercellular communication and adherence to other cells and to the extracellular matrix; and (5) uptake, processing and degradation of macromolecules derived from outside or inside cells. Interference with any one of these processes may induce characteristic ultrastructural alterations that will be illustrated.

INFLUENCE OF FIXATION AND SPECIMEN PROCESSING ON APPEARANCE OF CELLS

Alterations induced by cell injury will be discussed by reference to changes of subcellular organelles. Therefore, detailed knowledge of the normal ultrastructural features of organelles in the tissue of interest is essential. Changes in shape, size, texture, electron density, orientation and numbers of organelles are the main criteria used to assess cell injury. Some of these features can be profoundly affected by the chemical composition and physical characteristics of the fixative employed to preserve the tissue. In addition, the manner of application of the fixative, dehydration, embedding and sectioning of the specimen also may affect, in specific ways, the appearance of the organelles. Proper fixation is undoubtedly the most important preparative step. The volume of cells, tissue and vascular spaces are affected by the fixative and by the mode of application of the fixative. The fixative may be applied by vascular perfusion, by immersion or, topically, by dripping the fixative onto the surface of the organ. In injured tissue, perfusion may be rendered difficult by swelling and by microvascular occlusion. Slow penetration of fixative causes poor fixation. Poor penetration of the fixative creates a state of in vitro autolysis often difficult or impossible to distinguish from *in vivo* injury and/or autolysis. Optimal fixation should stop cellular biochemical reactions quickly in order to preserve the morphology of the cell in a condition as close as possible to that which it was in in the living state. Poor fixation can also be due to inappropriate osmolality, chemical composition or pH of the buffer in which the fixative is made up. Mechanical damage to the tissue during sectioning and handling is also an important source of distortion of histological as well as subcellular structure.[23]

The type of fixative used has a profound influence on the appearance of the cells and on the amount of cellular components retained in the cell. Marked losses of water-soluble components and some extraction and redistribution of proteins and lipids normally occurs during fixation. Fixatives used for electron microscopy stabilize cellular proteins and lipids by cross-linking to specific residues on adjacent molecules. These reactions stop the biological activity of cellular molecules and can induce oxidative breakdown of the molecules if prolonged. By changing the concentration, temperature and duration of application of the fixative, these reactions can be controlled to suit the specific needs of the pathologist. The traditional procedure for TEM fixation involves the sequential use of two fixatives, namely glutaraldehyde followed by osmium tetroxide. Glutaraldehyde fixes tissue by cross-linking proteins. However, it penetrates very slowly, and in large tissue blocks cells in the centre of the block may undergo anoxic injury before fixation is complete. To enhance the rapidity of fixation, mixtures of formaldehyde and glutaraldehyde may be employed.[23] Formaldehyde penetrates faster and reaches greater depths within tissue blocks because of its lower molecular weight. During aldehyde fixation, cellular swelling or contraction is induced if the osmolality of the fixative vehicle is unsuitable. After glutaraldehyde fixation, osmium tetroxide fixation is routinely used. Osmium cross-links lipids and enhances the electron-density of membranes. Even with this double fixation procedure, some cell components are not preserved. However, despite the extraction and redistribution of certain cellular components, a standard ultrastructural appearance of the cell is produced. The following criteria are considered the norm for well-fixed tissue: the presence of unbroken membranes and uniform electron density of cytosol and mitochondrial matrix; the preservation of structural continuity and the topological organization of cellular organelles.

To diminish extraction and redistribution of cell constituents that occur during chemical fixation, physical fixation by quick freezing may be employed. The frozen tissue is fixed anhydrously with osmium and is freeze–substituted over several days. After infiltration with Lowicryl resin, polymerization can be carried out at $-20\,^\circ$C with ultraviolet light. The ultrastructural appearance of this type of preparation is illustrated in Fig. 4.1. Chromatin and (in general) organelles and cytosol, appear electron-dense. Glycogen, triglyceride droplets and lipoproteins appear electron-lucent. Linear densities appear in intermembranous spaces. Abundant electron-dense granules are often present in the matrix of mitochondria. The composition and functional significance of these granules is uncertain. Figure 4.2 illustrates the increased electron-lucency of cytosol and nucleus induced by prolonged primary fixation in osmium tetroxide in s-collidine buffer. Notice the electron density of membranes and of lipids in lysosomes and secretory granules. Some vesiculation of membranes is apparent. The fixation of this cell is poor because a substantial amount of protein is lost.

ULTRASTRUCTURAL MANIFESTATIONS OF CELL INJURY IN SUBCELLULAR ORGANELLES

Nuclei

The interphase nucleus is surrounded by an envelope consisting of two separate membranes (Fig. 4.3). The two membranes converge at the site of nuclear pores, where transport between nucleus and cytoplasm occurs. The outer nuclear membrane is structurally continuous with the RER cisternae, contains typical ER marker enzymes and bears ribosomes on the cytosolic face. The inner membrane of the nuclear envelope is associated with a dense lamina and with dense clusters of (hetero)-chromatin that extend into the nuclear matrix. The lamina and nuclear matrix are made up of polypeptides which are structurally continuous and function as a karyoskeleton and which contract in response to changes in Ca^{2+} and Mg^{2+} concentrations.[6] The appearance of the chromatin is very variable and reflects the biosynthetic activity of the cell. Inhibition of transcription induces condensation of chromatin (Fig. 4.3) and may increase the electron-lucency of the nuclear matrix because of decreases in ribonuclear and other soluble proteins. Structurally, the chromatin consists of 2–3-nm strands of DNA coiled into dense fibres (20–30 nm in diameter) or dispersed fibres (12 nm in diameter). In conventional thin sections the chromatin rarely appears fibrillar; most commonly it has a granular appearance.[44,66] The appearance of the chromatin can be altered by changes in the tonicity, pH and ionic composition of fixative and its vehicle.[66] The nucleolus is round or oval and contains granular components, dense fibrillar components and fibrillar centres (Fig. 4.3). Functionally, the nucleolus consists of regions of DNA containing genes for ribosomal RNA undergoing transcription. Ribosomal particles at various stages of processing, biosynthetic enzymes and associated proteins complete the nucleolus. Transcription of DNA in the fibrillar centres generates fibrillar components, which are the precursors of the granular components.[14] Nucleoli increase in numbers and size in transcriptionally active cells. Acute cell injury causes the nucleoli to decrease in size and become more compact. Granular components may disappear and the nucleolus may become a small spherical aggregate containing only fibrillar components. Fragmentation and segregation of the nucleolar components into distinct regions is induced by toxins that inhibit protein synthesis.[9]

Chromatin condensation is an early reversible manifestation of cell injury. More severe injury induces marked condensation of the chromatin (Figs 4.4, C and D). Changes in pH and ionic and water shifts are thought to be responsible for these alterations. In dead cells, a gradual disappearance of chromatin and associated proteins occurs (Fig. 4.5) due to the activity of nucleases and proteases. Rupturing of the nuclear envelope and fragmentation of the nucleus (karyolysis) is a late event in the necrotic process. Figure 4.6 summarizes the ultrastructural changes of the nucleus induced by acute cell injury.

Endoplasmic reticulum and Golgi apparatus

We shall next consider alterations induced by acute cell injury in the endoplasmic reticulum (ER). This organelle is made up of an intracellular (endoplasmic) reticulum (network) of membrane sheets and tubules. The sheets are closely apposed and form flattened sacs (cisternae) with a lumen of 25 nm average diameter. The cytosolic side of the membranes is rough because it is studded with ribosomes. In conventional ultrathin sections, the rough ER cisternae are arranged in parallel rows, oriented towards the smooth ER and Golgi apparatus. An early subtle manifestation of cell injury is a loss of this polarity. As the severity of cell injury increases the rough ER becomes more disorganized and rounded concentric whorls may form (Fig. 4.7). The rough ER is structurally continuous with a tortuous network of

smooth-surfaced tubules — the smooth endoplasmic reticulum (SER). In acute cell injury due to certain toxins, the tubular structures of the SER may become compacted (Fig. 4.8) and large aggregates of ER may form. These aggregates are thought to be due to redistribution of ER since no increases in ER marker enzymes can be detected.[19] In injury induced by microtubular disruption, fluorescence microscopy has confirmed the occurrence of retraction of the ER into clusters located near the centre of the cells.[54]

The ER functions in: (1) the biosynthesis of protein, phospholipid, cholesterol and oligosaccharide moieties; (2) the integration of these biosynthetic products into membrane bilayers or translocation into the lumen of the saccules; and (3) translocation of membranes and luminal contents to other intracellular compartments or to the extracellular space. These functions are very prominent in secretory cells. In addition, the ER functions in the regulation of cytosolic Ca^{2+} and in the detoxification of toxins. The synthesis of proteins destined for the ER begins with the translation of mRNA in the cytosol by the ribosomes. The amino-terminal oligopeptide (signal or leader peptide) of the nascent protein binds to a cytosolic signal-recognition particle (SRP). The SRP associates with a receptor (docking protein, DP) on the ER. Thus, the ribosome comes into contact with ribophorins, which function as ribosome receptors in association with other membrane proteins which are localized exclusively in the RER. The ribophorins, and other yet to be characterized proteins, are required for the translocation of the nascent protein through the membrane of ER.[60] The amount of ribophorin mRNA increases in rat liver after partial hepatectomy — reflecting the synthesis of RER in the proliferating liver cells. Ribophorin mRNA is also present in proliferating neoplastic cells which have a well developed secretory apparatus.[15] Moreover, regions of homology exist between the amino acid sequence of ribophorin and that of cytoskeletal proteins such as lamin C and keratin. This suggests that ribophorins alone, or in association with cytoskeletal proteins, may maintain the ultrastructural appearance of the flattened sacs which are typical of RER.[15]

An early and universal alteration induced by cell injury is dilatation of the ER (Fig. 4.9). The precise mechanism is unknown. It is thought that disorganization of cytoskeletal and integral proteins on ER membrane and the accumulation of iso-osmotic fluid in the cells as they swell, play a role. In severe states of acute cell injury vesiculation of the reticulum occurs. The identity of the Golgi apparatus is lost; however, vesicles derived from the RER retain some ribosomes (Fig. 4.10). The Golgi apparatus is particularly susceptible to disruption as can be demonstrated with the use of antimicrotubular drugs.[47] Break up of ER and Golgi apparatus membranes into sealed membrane vesicles also occurs during cell division and can be readily induced by homogenization of tissue.

The ER adjoins the Golgi apparatus in a transition zone

containing many smooth vesicles. The Golgi apparatus consists of a stack of small flattened sacs (saccules). Each sac has club-like dilatations at each end. The Golgi stack is polarized, with a cis region related to SER, a medial region, and a trans region. At the trans region, numerous coated and smooth vesicles are present. There is no structural continuity between ER and the Golgi apparatus; transport between the two compartments occurs by means of smooth vesicles. Both ultrastructurally and biochemically these transport vesicles remain uncharacterized. The Golgi stacks appear to lack structural continuity. It has been suggested that oligomerization of protein subunits and acquisition of stable tertiary or quaternary structure are essential for transport of proteins to the Golgi apparatus. Errors in assembly, folding or glycosylation of proteins, induced by toxins or mutations, cause the accumulation of proteins in the RER.[63] Accumulation of lipid in the ER can also result from inhibition of transport to the Golgi apparatus. Figure 4.11 illustrates accumulation of triglyceride caused by inhibition of protein synthesis. Transport vesicles are thought to function in vectorial transport of proteins across the Golgi stack.[40] In the trans region of the Golgi apparatus secretory storage granules form with a partial clathrin coat. A non-clathrin-coated vesicle seems to participate in constitutive secretion. Uncoating of the clathrin coat is an energy-requiring process and is necessary to allow fusion of transport vesicles with other cellular organelles such as lysosomes or plasma membranes.

Enzymes for the biosynthesis of phospholipids are located on the cytoplasmic side of the ER. Rapid translocation of phospholipid to the luminal side of the membrane bilayer is facilitated by transporter proteins. These membranes are essential for maintenance and growth of the Golgi apparatus, secretory granules, lysosomes and plasma membranes. The ER is an important regulator of cytosolic Ca^{2+} homeostasis. Inositol 1,4,5-triphosphate, generated by the signal transduction pathway, causes rapid release of calcium from the lumen of the ER.[43] The ER transport system has a high affinity for Ca^{2+} and can quickly take up Ca^{2+} and restore normal cytosolic Ca^{2+} levels by activation of ATP-dependent pumps. ATP-dependent pumps in the plasma membrane are also activated, leading to extrusion of calcium from the cells.[1] Loss of ATP can permit sustained elevation of cytosolic Ca^{2+}. In the presence of ATP, a massive influx of calcium into the cell can saturate the ER transport. At this point the lower affinity — but higher capacity — mitochondrial Ca^{2+} transport system is activated.

The SER is active in the biotransformation of non-polar drugs via the cytochrome P-450 mixed-function oxidase system. In the first stage of drug biotransformation, reactive drug intermediates are created by oxidation through cytochrome P-450. Reactive drug intermediates induce cell injury by covalent binding to proteins, nucleic acids and lipids. In the second stage of biotransformation, conjugation reactions add residues such as sulphates or glucuronides that render the drug water soluble and therefore exportable to the bloodstream for eventual excretion. It is clear, however, that these drug conjugates, such as glutathione, may be toxic or may undergo transformation to reactive intermediates that can induce tissue damage.[2]

Mixed-function oxidase enzymes are highly enriched in the liver and are present in different quantitites in different regions of the hepatic lobule. Marked oxygen gradients also exist across the liver lobules. These factors, along with nutritional status and availability of cofactors, explain the marked heterogeneity to toxic and ischaemic injury manifested by hepatocytes in different regions of the liver lobule.[10] In addition, free radicals such as superoxide anion can be generated from the dissociation of cytochrome P-450–oxygen complexes which chemically interact with cellular components. An example of cell injury mediated by drug biotransformation reaction is the damage seen after carbon tetrachloride intoxication. Carbon tetrachloride is converted to a trichloromethyl free radical by the ER. Hypoxia and a reducing environment favour this activation.[4,27] Figure 4.12 illustrates the marked ER dilatation that may be induced in the hepatocytes by carbon tetrachloride. Impaired sequestration of calcium by the ER has been demonstrated in the presence of this toxin.[22] Figure 4.13 summarizes the ultrastructural alterations induced by cell injury on the ER.

Plasma membrane

The ionic composition of cells is markedly different from that of the extracellular space; in addition, cells contain large amounts of negatively charged proteins. In the case of calcium, for example, the extracellular concentration is in the millimolar range, whereas the cytosolic concentration of free calcium is four orders of magnitude smaller. The plasma membrane of cells maintains these ionic gradients. In epithelial cells the plasma membrane is polarized into an apical and baso-lateral domain. These domains are bounded by junctional structures that anchor cells to each other, to the extracellular matrix and to cytoskeletal components. Membrane proteins are exchanged in both directions between cell surface membrane and intracellular organelles through vesicular transport mechanisms which involve endocytic and exocytic pathways. In addition, soluble proteins and other molecules also enter cells through endocytic processes that are morphologically well defined and functionally well understood. The plasma membrane of cells is therefore important for the maintenance of cellular shape, homeostasis, and for traffic between the cellular organelles, the cell surface and the extracellular space.

The plasma membrane constitutes a permeability barrier that restricts the free movement of ions and metabolites between the cellular interior and the extracellular space. Metabolic energy is expended to maintain the concentration of ions and metabolites in the two compartments at different levels. Na^+ and Ca^{2+} are extruded from the cells by energy-dependent pumps and exchanger systems. Efflux of potassium occurs from concentration gradients and may be increased during vigorous exercise leading to 'physiological hyperkalaemia'; these fluxes are influenced by catecholamine levels.[62] Physiologically altered fluxes of Na^+, K^+ and H^+, due to changes in the activity of the Na^+/H^+ exchanger and of the Na^+/K^+ ATPase, can directly or through changes in intracellular Ca^{2+}, induce differentiation of cells as well as promote cell proliferation. Loss of ability to regulate ionic homeostasis is thought to be an important event in cell injury. In cell injury loss of ATP (needed to drive Na^+/K^+ ATPase) may cause a rise in cytosolic Na^+ levels. The presence of Na^+/K^+ ATPase inhibitors such as digitalis or ouabain will have an analogous effect. Increased Na^+ levels block efflux of Ca^{2+}, dependent on the Na^+/Ca^{2+} exchanger; the exchanger normally functions to regulate intracellular Ca^{2+} by utilizing the downhill movement of Na^+ to provide energy for the uphill extrusion of Ca^{2+}. Membrane depolymerization may occur due to the influx of sodium. The change in membrane potential can cause voltage-dependent calcium channels to open, increasing the influx of Ca^{2+}. The ability to extrude protons from the cells in exchange for the uptake of Na^+ is also impaired in injured cells. Since protons are generated continuously from cellular metabolism the intracellular pH declines as the intracellular buffering capacity is exceeded. Loss of ATP also prevents Ca^{2+} extrusions by the Ca^{2+} ATPase. This enzyme is one of the major plasma membrane systems for ejecting Ca^{2+} in non-excitable cells.[8] Loss of ion homeostasis in cell injury can be aggravated if the permeability of the surface membrane is perturbed by the detergent-like activity of Ca^{2+}-dependent phospholipases in the plasma membrane. Toxins such as heavy metals, which oxidize thiol groups, alter the permeability of the plasma membrane. This permits influx of Na^+ and Ca^{2+} which may accelerate cell death.[50] Biological toxins such as complement can create channels through the plasma membrane bilayer. In these conditions, because of functioning mitochondria, massive intramitochondrial accumulations of calcium may occur.

In summary, dysfunction of the plasma membrane may cause loss of ion homeostasis and induce sustained elevations of cytosolic calcium. Increased cytosolic calcium levels function as a second messenger system that modulates a great variety of cellular activities. By virtue of the great importance of calcium in the integration of cell functions, it has been hypothesized that calcium deregulation is a common mechanism in the evolution of cell injury towards cell death.[11,56] Increased intracellular calcium can cause profound cellular alterations by modulation of enzyme activity. Nucleases, lipases, proteases and protein kinases can be activated. Increased expression of oncogenes may occur, with far-reaching effects on regulation of cellular metabolism.

Transport and fusion of membrane vesicles can be affected by changes in cytosolic calcium levels.[31] The cytoskeleton is modified, increased Ca^{2+} depolymerizes microtubules and enhances cross-linking of keratins. Calcium levels also have a profound influence on cell junction structures, namely the desmosomes and the zonula adherens.[37] Elevation of calcium can close gap junctions, but only at very high levels, such as may be achieved during cell injury. Decreases in pH of various amplitudes are also effective blockers of junctional conductance.[51] Generation of free radicals by cytochrome P-450-dependent metabolism can also close gap junctions.[48] The uncoupling of injured cells from normal cells induced by acidosis or oxidative stress may be an example of adaptive cellular response designed to prevent further amplification of injury.

In addition to causing altered ion regulation, loss of plasma membrane permeability causes an influx of water and other solutes. The cell undergoes osmotic swelling. In conditions where blood flow is interrupted the intracellular environment may become hypertonic due to the accumulation of low-molecular-weight metabolites. Upon blood reflow, osmotic swelling may occur. Epithelial cells can respond to osmotic stress by increasing the number of ionic channels or transport proteins in the plasma membrane. This increased capacity for ion transport is associated with fusion of cytoplasmic vesicles and tubular structures with the plasma membrane. Decreases in ionic transport correlated with decreased surface areas of plasma membrane are also known to occur.[45,53] In so far as it is possible, cells may also alter their shape and the organization of the plasma membrane to adapt to severe increases in cell volume. The movement of water across biological membranes is sufficiently rapid not to play any role in determining cellular volume. Even in polarized cells with water-impermeable domains of plasma membrane it is primarily the solute load that determines cellular volume. Cells swell rapidly in response to an increased osmotic load until the influx of water abolishes the differences in colloid osmotic pressure across the plasma membrane. Loss of intracellular water activates the uptake of solute from the extracellular space. Rapid adjustments occur to restore cellular volume. In addition, the intracellular generation of low-molecular-weight substances tends to restore osmolality to normal and to normalize cell volume.

Shifts in ions such as Na^+, K^+ and Ca^{2+} and in small molecules such as amino acids and other organic components are primarily responsible for cell swelling.[12,16] The volume of cells is regulated by the plasma membrane by actively extruding sodium to balance the colloid osmotic pressure of large molecules. At the ultrastructural level, swelling is evident from increased electron-lucency of the cytosol. As swelling continues, and the cell volume increases, the plasma membrane begins to lose its surface microvilli. An early manifestation of cell injury is the formation of rounded sacs of surface membrane and cytosol which protrude in the extracellular space (Fig. 4.14). These blebs may seal at the base and detach from the cell in a non-leaky fashion, or they may persist unaltered, be resorbed or burst. In many types of injury, clusters of vacuoles form at the apex of epithelial cells. Occasionally, as in the case of hypoxia, these vacuoles can become very large and be seen to arise from invaginations on the plasma membrane (Fig. 4.15). If cellular swelling is not halted, rupture of the plasma membrane occurs. Cellular proteins are extruded, and plasma proteins may enter cells (Fig. 4.16). Swelling and cell bursting may occur explosively during conditions of reflow following ischaemia (see Fig. 4.32). Figure 4.17 summarizes the ultrastructural alterations characteristic of the plasma membranes of injured cells.

Cytoskeleton

The plasma membrane is linked to cytoskeletal components through spectrin and ankyrin-like proteins. Disruption of these links can be induced by toxins and by ionic shifts, and may enhance the susceptibility of the plasma membrane to deformations. Disruption of the cytoskeleton in myocytes seems to be responsible for increased osmotic fragility of irreversibly injured cells.[13] Marked changes in numbers and cellular distribution of cytoskeletal filaments occur in acute and chronically injured cells (Fig. 4.18). For example, it is known that increases in calcium concentration to a micro-molar level cause solubilization of actin filaments and vesiculation of membranes.[7,61]

In contractile tissues, ultrastructural alterations of actin and myosin filaments are readily seen in response to both acute and chronic cell injury.[26] The myofibrils may become split, branched or misaligned in many pathological conditions. Fragmentation of Z bands may occur in zonal lesions such as occur in shock.[46] Contracture of filaments is readily seen in necrotic myocytes.

In most cells the actin and myosin filaments and other cytoskeletal components are inadequately visualized in the thin sections used in conventional TEM. As a result, in cell injury, cytoskeletal alterations are not assessed directly. Rather, it is inferred that they occur from observations of other cellular structures. For example, blebs are readily seen on the plasma membrane. However, the underlying cytoskeletal disorganization can be visualized only by immuno-cytochemistry.

Mitochondria

Ultrastructural alterations of mitochondria are a reliable means of assessing the severity of cell injury. Small electron-dense granules are present in the matrix of mitochondria (Fig. 4.19); their loss is one of the earliest manifestations of cell injury. Less commonly seen — but also an early indication of cell damage — is the presence of electron-dense deposits between the inner and outer membranes and

between the cristae of mitochondria (Fig. 4.20). The functional significance of these ultrastructural alterations is not known. It is likely that loss of ability to carry out oxidative phosphorylation is an important mechanism which contributes to cell death. Whereas mitochondrial respiration is very resistant to injury, the ability of mitochondria to phosphorylate ADP is very sensitive and is lost relatively early following ischaemic injury.[25,32] Decreases in cellular levels of ATP render cells more susceptible to certain types of injury. In chronic hypoxic or hypermetabolic states characterized by lowered cellular ATP levels, protection against cell necrosis is achieved by reducing cellular metabolism.[38,55] Recently, interest has been focused on the role of altered regulation of mitochondrial Ca^{2+} in the evolution of cell injury. Inhibition of mitochondrial respiration by anoxia or by toxins causes a loss of mitochondrial membrane potential. This potential is used to generate ATP and to achieve Ca^{2+} uptake. The condensed appearance of the mitochondria is thought to be the ultrastructural manifestation of a state of low ATP levels in the cell (Fig. 4.21). In various cells, release of calcium from mitochondria can be induced by agents such as t-butyl hydroperoxide[3] or cysteine conjugates.[59] Oxidation or other covalent modifications of mitochondrial membrane proteins that regulate proton permeability may be responsible for the loss of mitochondria membrane potential. This early mitochondrial injury leads to elevation of cytosolic calcium even in the absence of Ca^{2+} influx from the extracellular environment.[50,52] In normal conditions, efflux of Ca^{2+} from the cell would ensue as the systems for calcium translocation are activated in the plasma membrane.

In healthy cells, mitochondria play no role in the physiological regulation of cytosolic calcium levels, because the ER has an active transport system with high affinity for Ca^{2+}.[49] However, in types of cell injury which affect primarily the permeability of the plasma membrane, and where blood flow is maintained, influx of calcium will cause elevations of cytosolic calcium which overwhelm the low capacity system of the ER. As a consequence, massive uptake of calcium by the mitochondria occurs. This is seen during reflow after ischaemia and in mercury nephrotoxicity *in vitro*. The uptake of calcium by the mitochrondria of injured cells is paralleled by progressive mitochondrial swelling. Mild degrees of swelling (low amplitude) are seen in reversibly injured cells. Marked increases in swelling (high amplitude) are commonly seen in cells near the point of no return. In dead cells, the outer mitochondrial membrane may be disrupted (Fig. 4.22) and the inner membrane may unfold and balloon out. Massive Ca^{2+} uptake may lead to the formation of calcium precipitates seen in the matrix of the mitochondria.[58] A reliable indicator of cell death is the appearance of amorphous densities in the matrix of mitochondria (Fig. 4.23). These densities are termed 'flocculent', and they appear to consist of denatured proteins and degraded lipid components. In Fig. 4.23 cell death was due to anoxia without blood reflow. The ultrastructural alterations are relatively mild. Subacute and chronic cell injury frequently induces non-specific alterations in the shape and size of mitochondria. An example of mitochondrial enlargement is shown in Fig. 4.24. The ultrastructural alterations of mitochondria induced by cell injury are summarized in Fig. 4.25.

Lysosomes

The lysosomes are acidic vacuoles active in the degradation of intracellular (autophagy) and extracellular (heterophagy) materials. The lysosomes display a marked heterogeneity in shape, size and contents. The heterogeneity is due to the presence of different types and amounts of cytoplasmic organelles in various stages of degradation inside the lysosomes. Various stages in the segregation and degradation of organelles by lysosomes are recognized ultrastucturally. Figure 4.26 illustrates various stages in the formation and maturation of autophagic vacuoles and the heterogeneity in their appearance. Autophagic degradation is a physiological mechanism for the turnover of intracellular organelles and can be identified morphologically (Fig. 4.27A). Autophagy is energy-dependent and can be stimulated in some cell types during starvation to generate amino acids for protein synthesis and to maintain blood amino acid and glucose homeostasis.[28] Ultrastructurally the increased catabolism of stressed cells is reflected by an increase in the size and numbers of lysosomes. Hormonal signals and amino acid levels are important regulators of protein degradation and thus also of the size of the lysosomal compartment. An expansion of the lysosomal compartment can also occur if the degradation inside the lysosomes is blocked by decreases in the ATP needed to acidify the vacuoles. The numbers and size of lysosomes often increase in injured cells (compare B with A in Fig. 4.27). In many cases, both a stimulation in the segregation of organelles and a retardation in their degradation may be occurring. In any case, it seems that ionic deregulation and cytoskeletal disorganization of injured cells are not sufficient conditions for the generation of autophagic vacuoles.[64]

The numbers and size of the lysosomes can also increase in cell injury due to heterophagy of necrotic debris. While this change is most prominent in macrophages (Fig. 4.28), other cell types, both mesenchymal and epithelial, may show evidence of increased phagocytic uptake of cellular debris. Cell injury may also disturb other endocytic pathways to the lysosomes as well as vesicular traffic between the various organelles. In subacute or chronic types of cell injury, non-degradable material — such as lipids and lipid peroxides, haemoproteins and metals — may accumulate in the lysosomes.[18,65]

The lysosomal milieu is acidic due to the presence of a proton pump. The acidic pH facilitates degradation of intralysosomal materials by the hydrolases, all of which have acid pH optima. Weak bases such as chloroquine accumulate in the lysosomes[42] and can cause their enlargement by osmotic effects and by inhibiting lysosomal degradation (Fig. 4.29). Weak bases can also induce errors in the translocation of lysosomal enzymes and induce their secretion, rather than translocation to primary lysosomes (see Fig. 4.30). It is thought that rupture of lysosomes and leakage of hydrolases occur after cell death. The pH optima of the lysosomal hydrolases mitigate against cellular damage, were leakage of lysosomal contents to occur before death — the pH of the cytosol is higher than the pH optimum of lysosomal hydrolases. In addition, lysosomal enzyme inhibitors are present inside the cell. The pathways for lysosomal degradation of organelles and extracellular material, and the route in the biogenesis of lysosomal enzymes are summarized schematically in Fig. 4.30.

ULTRASTRUCTURAL ALTERATIONS OF VASCULATURE

In this chapter we have emphasized the role of injury to parenchymal cells in the evolution of tissue necrosis. As a guide in the evaluation of the injury we have focussed on ultrastructural alterations of cellular organelles and have described criteria for staging the severity of the injury. Assessment of the status of the blood vessels, and the microvasculature in particular, is also necessary to evaluate the status of the tissue. Vascular structures are generally more resistant to injury than are parenchymal cells. The microvasculature is the conduit through which recruitment of neutrophils and macrophages to sites of injury occurs and initiates the process of necrosis, namely the clearing of dead tissue (Fig. 4.31). Release of lysosomal enzymes through active secretion or through lysis of neutrophils may, in some conditions,[33] amplify the initial injury. Figure 4.32 illustrates the appearance of ultrastructurally equivalent degrees of injury in microvasculature and in parenchymal cells. The usefulness of alterations of subcellular organelles in staging the severity of the injury in parenchymal cells is illustrated. In the case of endothelium the paucity of subcellular organelles makes the assessment difficult. Damage to the microvasculature may be the primary event which ultimately leads to cessation of blood flow and causes necrosis of parenchymal cells. Frostbite (Fig. 4.33) is an example of this type of injury.[29]

EVOLUTION OF CELL INJURY IN VITRO

The evolution of cellular injury in isolated perfused organs *in vitro* and in isolated cells in culture and suspension differs from that observed *in vivo*. Several obvious pathogenetic mechanisms such as inflammatory mediators, inflammatory cells and platelets, metabolic and mechanical stresses may be absent *in vitro*. In addition, cultured cells are exposed to a buffered medium with stable concentrations of substrates and metabolites. Accumulation of metabolites does not occur, but, on the other hand, a virtually unlimited reservoir of various ions and substrates is present in the media. As a consequence, damage, particularly at the ultrastructural level, may develop later and possibly differ in characteristic from injury induced in *vivo*.[17] However, in general, the type of ultrastructural alterations seen in injured cells parallel those seen *in vivo* (Fig. 4.34).

OVERVIEW OF EVOLUTION OF CELL INJURY

The characterization of the functional disturbances associated with morphological alterations in injured cells has shown the common occurrence of increased level of calcium in the cytosol. This elevation occurs early on and may induce an unregulated stimulation of calcium-dependent phenomena in the cell. Some of these events, such as the activation of proteases and lipases, can induce alterations of the cytoskeleton and of membrane permeability and create a vicious cycle of further disruption of ionic homeostasis and ATP depletion.

Other functional disturbances, such as enzyme inactivation, lipid peroxidation, thiol depletion, loss of substrates and cofactors, covalent binding, inhibition of biosynthesis, and DNA damage have been identified in injured cells. However, disrupted ion homeostasis, in particular Ca^{2+}, is the currently favoured biochemical mechanism proposed to lead to cell death. The diagram in Fig. 4.35 emphasizes the role of increased membrane permeability and loss of regulatory function by mitochondria, ER and plasma membranes in the initiation of cell injury and in the evolution of cell injury towards cell death.

REFERENCES

1. Alkon D L, Rasmussen H 1988 A spatial-temporal model of cell activation. Science 239: 998–1005
2. Anders M W, Lash L H, Elfarra A A 1986 Nephrotoxic amino acid and glutathione s-conjugates: formation and renal activation. Advances in Experimental Medicine and Biology 197: 443–445
3. Bellomo G, Thor H, Orrenius S 1984 Increase in cytosolic Ca^{2+} concentration during t-butyl hydroperoxide metabolism in hepatocytes involves NADPH oxidation and mobilization of intracellular Ca^{2+} stores. FEBS Letters 168: 38–42
4. Bernacchi A, Myers R A M, Trump B F, Marzella L 1984 Protection of hepatocytes with hyperbaric oxygen against carbon tetrachloride-induced injury. Toxicologic Pathology 12: 315–323
5. Borgers M, Shu L G, Xhonneux R, Thone F, Van Overloop P 1986 Changes in ultrastructure and Ca^{2+} distribution in the isolated working rabbit heart after ischemia. A time-related study. American Journal of Pathology 126: 92–102
6. Brasch K 1982 Fine structure and localization of the nuclear matrix *in situ*. Experimental Cell Research 140: 161–171
7. Burgess D R, Prum B E 1982 Reevaluation of brush border motility: calcium induces core filament isolation and microvillar vesiculation. Journal of Cell Biology 94: 97–107
8. Carafoli E 1984 Calmodulin-sensitive calcium-pumping ATPase of plasma membranes: isolation, reconstitution, and regulation. Federation Proceedings 43: 3005–3010
9. Cole K E, Jones T W, Lipsky M M, Trump B F, Hsu I C 1989 Comparative effect of three carcinogens on human, rat and mouse hepatocytes. Carcinogenesis 10: 139–143
10. de Groot H, Noll T 1987 Oxygen gradients: the problem of hypoxia. Biochemical Society Transactions 15: 363–365
11. Farber J L 1982 Membrane injury and calcium homeostasis in the pathogenesis of coagulative necrosis. Laboratory Investigation 47: 114–123
12. Foskett J K, Spring K R 1985 Possible role for calcium and cytoskeleton in epithelial volume regulation. American Journal of Physiology 248: C27–C36
13. Ganote C E, Van der Heide R S 1987 Cytoskeletal lesions in anoxic myocardial injury. A conventional and high-voltage electron-microscopic and immunofluorescence study. American Journal of Pathology 129: 327–344
14. Goessens G 1984 Nucleolar structure. International Review of Cytology 87: 107–158
15. Harnick-Ort V, Prakash K, Marcantonio E, Colman D R, Rosenfeld M G, Adesnik M, Sabatini D D, Kreibich G 1987 Isolation and characterization of cDNA clones for rat ribophorin. I: Complete coding sequence and *in vitro* synthesis and insertion of the encoded product into endoplasmic reticulum membranes. Journal of Cell Biology 104: 855–863
16. Hoffman E K, Lambert I H 1983 Amino acid transport and cell volume regulation in Ehrlich ascites tumor cells. Journal of Physiology (London) 338: 613–625
17. Jennings R B, Reimer K A, Steenbergen C 1986 Myocardial ischemia revisited. The osmolar load membrane damage and reperfusion. Journal of Molecular and Cellular Cardiology 18: 769–780
18. Jerome W G, Lewis J C 1987 Early atherogenesis in White Carneau pigeon. III. Lipid accumulation in nascent foam cell. American Journal of Pathology 128: 253–264
19. Jones T W, Chopra S, Kaufman, J S, Flamenbaum W, Trump B F 1985 Cis-diamminedichloroplatinum (II)-induced acute renal failure in the rat. Correlation of structural and functional alterations. Laboratory Investigation 52: 363–374
20. Keenan K P, McDowell E M 1986 Injury and regeneration of the respiratory epithelium. In: Ruben R W et al (eds) The biology of change in otolaryngology. Elsevier, Amsterdam, pp 373–382
21. Lemasters J J, Diguiseppi J, Nieminen A L, Herman B 1987 Blebbing, free calcium and mitochondrial membrane potential preceding cell death in hepatocytes. Nature 325: 78–81
22. Long R M, Moore L 1986 Elevated cytosolic calcium in rat hepatocytes exposed to carbon tetrachloride. Journal of Pharmacology and Experimental Therapeutics 238: 186–191
23. McDowell E, Trump B F 1976 Histologic fixatives suitable for diagnostic light and electron microscopy. Archives of Pathology and Laboratory Medicine 100: 405–411
24. Majerus P W, Connolly T M, Deckmyn H, Ross T S, Bross T E, Ishii H, Bansal V S, Wilson D B 1986 The metabolism of phosphoinositide-derived messenger molecules. Science 234: 1519–1526
25. Malis C D, Bonventre J V 1986 Mechanism of calcium potentiation of oxygen free radical injury to renal mitochondria. A model for post-ischemic and toxic mitochondrial damage. Journal of Biological Chemistry 261: 14 201–14 208
26. Marzella L, Trump B F 1986 Microfilament alterations induced by cell injury. Pathology, Research and Practice 181: 612–614
27. Marzella L, Muhvich K, Myers R A M 1986 Effects of hyperoxia on liver necrosis induced by hepatotoxins. Virchows Archiv, Cell Pathology 51: 497–507
28. Marzella L, Glaumann H 1987 Autophagy, microautophagy and crinophagy as mechanisms for protein degradation. In: Glaumann H, Ballard J (eds) Lysosomes, their role in protein breakdown. Academic Press, London, pp 319–370
29. Marzella L, Jesudass R, Manson P N, Myers R A M, Bulkley G B 1989 Morphological characterization of acute injury to vascular endothelium of skin after frostbite. Plastic Reconstructive Surgery 83: 65–75

30. Matsumura T, Thurman R G 1983 Measuring rates of O_2 uptake in periportal and pericentral regions of liver lobule: stop-flow experiments with perfused liver. American Journal of Physiology 244: G656–G659

31. Mellgren R L 1987 Calcium-dependent proteases: an enzyme system active at cellular membranes. FASEB Journal 1: 110–115

32. Mergner W J, Marzella L, Mergner C , Kahng M W, Smith M W, Trump B F 1977 Studies on the pathogenesis of ischemic cell injury. VII. Proton gradient and respiration of renal tissue cubes, renal mitochondrial and submitochondrial particles following ischemic cell injury. Beitrage zur Pathologische 161: 230–243

33. Movat H Z, Cybulsky M I, Colditz I G, Chan M K W, Dinarello C A 1987 Acute inflammation in gram-negative infection: endotoxin, interleukin 1, tumor necrosis factor, and neutrophils. Federation Proceedings 46: 97–104

34. Myagkaya G, van Veen H, James J 1984 Ultrastructural changes in rat liver sinusoids during prolonged normothermic and hypothermic ischemia in vitro. Virchows Archiv, Cell Pathology 47: 361–373

35. Myagkaya G, van Veen H, James J 1987 Ultrastructural changes in rat liver during Euro-Collins storage, compared with hypothermic in vitro ischemia. Virchows Archiv B 53: 176–182

36. Nawaz S, Lynch M P, Galand P, Gerschenson L E 1987 Hormonal regulation of cell death in rabbit uterine epithelium. American Journal of Pathology 127: 51–59

37. O'Keefe E J, Briggman R A, Herman B 1987 Calcium-induced assembly of adherens junctions in keratinocytes. Journal of Cell Biology 105: 807–817

38. Orrego H, Blake J E, Blendis L M, Compton K V, Israel Y 1987 Long-term treatment of alcoholic liver disease with propylthiouracil. New England Journal of Medicine 317: 1421–1427

39. Pentilla A, Trump B F 1974 Extracellular acidosis protects Ehrlich ascites tumor cells and rat renal cortex against anoxic injury. Science 185: 277–278

40. Pfeffer S R, Rothman J E 1987 Biosynthetic protein transport and sorting by the endoplasmic reticulum and Golgi. Annual Review of Biochemistry 56: 829–852

41. Phillips T E, Boyne A F 1984 Liquid nitrogen-based quick freezing: experiences with bounce-free delivery of cholinergic nerve terminals to a metal surface. Journal of Electron Microscopy Technique 1: 9–29

42. Poole B, Ohkuma S 1981 Effect of weak bases on the intralysosomal pH in mouse peritoneal macrophages. Journal of Cell Biology 90: 665–669

43. Prentki M, Biden T J, Janjic D, Irvine R F, Berridge M J, Wollheim C B 1984 Rapid mobilization of calcium from rat insulinoma microsomes by inositol-1,4,5-triphosphate. Nature 309: 562–564

44. Puvion-Dutilleul F 1983 Morphology of transcription at cellular and molecular levels. International Review of Cytology 84: 57–101

45. Rastegar A, Biemesderfer D, Kashgarian M, Hayslett J P 1980 Changes in membrane surfaces of collecting duct cells in potassium adaptation. Kidney International 18: 293–301

46. Ratcliffe N B, Kopelman R I, Goldner R D, Gruz P T, Kackel D B 1975 Formation of myocardial zonal lesions. American Journal of Pathology 79: 321–328

47. Rogalski A A, Singer S J 1984 Association of elements of the Golgi apparatus with microtubules. Journal of Cell Biology 99: 1092–1100

48. Saez J C, Bennett M V L, Spray D C 1987 Carbon tetrachloride at hepatotoxic levels blocks reversibly gap junctions between rat hepatocytes. Science 236: 967–969

49. Shamoo A E, Ambudkar I S 1984 Regulation of calcium transport in cardiac cells. Canadian Journal of Physiology and Pharmacology 62: 4–22

50. Smith M W, Ambudkar I S, Phelps P C, Regec A L, Trump B F 1987 $HgCl_2$-induced changes in cytosolic Ca^{2+} of cultured rabbit renal tubular cells. Biochimica et Biophysica Acta 931: 130–142

51. Spray D C, Ginzberg R D, Morales E A, Gatmaitan Z, Arias I M 1986 Electrophysiological properties of gap junctions between dissociated pairs of rat hepatocytes. Journal of Cell Biology 103: 135–144

52. Snowdowne K W, Freudenrich C C, Borle A B 1985 The effects of anoxia on cytosolic free calcium fluxes and cellular ATP levels in cultured kidney cells. Journal of Biological Chemistry 260: 11 619–11 626

53. Stanton B A, Biemesderfer D, Wade J B, Giebish G 1981 Structural and functional study of the rat distal nephron: effects of potassium adaptation and depletion. Kidney International 19: 36–48

54. Terasaki M, Chen L B, Fujiwara K 1986 Microtubules and the endoplasmic reticulum are highly interdependent structures. Journal of Cell Biology 103: 1557–1568

55. Thurman R G, Matsumura T, Lemasters J J 1984 Is hypoxia involved in the mechanism of alcohol-induced liver injury? Fundamental and Applied Toxicology 4: 125–133

56. Trump B F, Berezesky I K 1984 The role of sodium and calcium regulation in toxic cell injury. In: Mitchell J R, Horning M G ; (eds) Drug metabolism and drug toxicity. Raven Press, New York, pp 261–300

57. Trump B F, Berezesky I K 1987 Cell injury, ion regulation and tumor promotion. In: Butterworth B E, Slaga T J (eds) Banbury report 25. Non-genotoxic mechanisms in carcinogenesis. Cold Spring Harbor Laboratory, New York, pp 69–79

58. Trump B F, Croker B P, Mergner W J 1971 The role of energy metabolism, ion, and water shifts in the pathogenesis of cell injury. In: Richter G W, Scarpelli D G (eds) Cell membranes: biological and pathological apects. Williams & Wilkins, Baltimore, pp 84–128

59. Wallin A, Jones T W, Vercesi A E, Cotgreave I, Ormstad K, Orrenius S 1987 Toxicity of s-pentachlorobutadienyl-L-cysteine studied with isolated rat renal cortical mitochondria. Archives of Biochemistry and Biophysics 258: 365–372

60. Walter P, Gilmore R, Blobel G 1984 Protein translocation across the endoplasmic reticulum. Cell 38: 5–8

61. White J R, Naccache P H, Sha' afi R I 1983 Stimulation by chemotactic factor of actin association with the cytoskeleton in rabbit neutrophils. Effects of calcium and cytochalasin B. Journal of Biological Chemistry 258: 14 041–14 047

62. Williams M E, Gervino E V, Rosa R M, Landsberg L, Young J B, Silva P, Epstein F H 1985 Catecholamine modulation of rapid potassium shifts during exercise. New England Journal of Medicine 312: 823–827

63. Yamamoto T, Bishop R W, Brown M S, Goldstein J L, Russell D W 1986 Deletion in cysteine-rich region of LDL receptor impairs transmission to cell surface in WHHL rabbit. Science 232: 1230–1237

64. Yu Q-C, Marzella L 1988 Response of autophagic protein degradation to physiologic and pathologic, stimuli in rat hepatocyte monolayers. Laboratory Investigation 58: 643–652

65. Yu Q-C, Lipsky M, Trump B F, Marzella L 1988 Response of human hepatocyte lysosomes to postmortem anoxia. Human Pathology 19: 1174–1180

66. Yunis E J, Agostini R M, Devine W A 1984 Studies on the nature of fibrillar nuclei. Distinction from viral nucleocapsid. American Journal of Pathology 115: 84–91

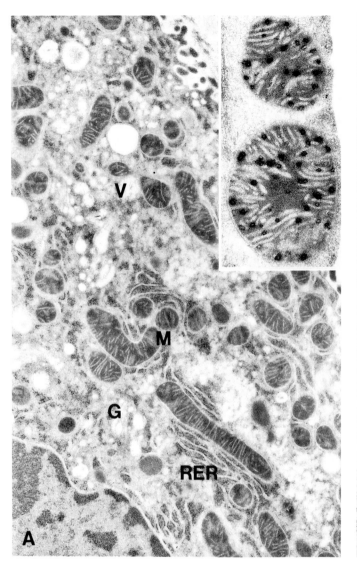

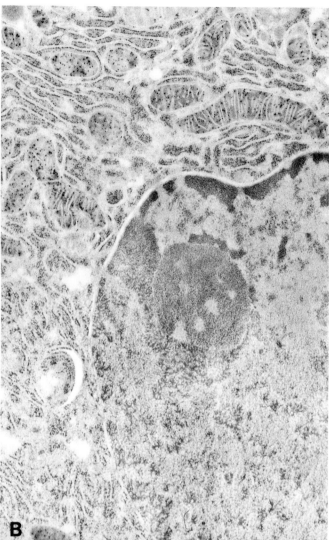

Fig. 4.1 Physical fixation. A tissue sample was rapidly obtained from a mouse liver. The sample was quick-frozen with the freezing device designed by Boyne.[41] The frozen specimen was postfixed and freeze–substituted in a mixture of tetrahydrofuran and osmium tetroxide, embedded in Lowicryl 4KM and double-stained with uranyl acetate and lead citrate. **A** The ultrastructure of the hepatocytes immediately below Glisson's capsule is well preserved. Many of the structures such as lipoproteins in secretory vacuoles (V) and membranes appear as negative images in the micrograph. M = mitochondria; RER = rough endoplasmic reticulum; G = Golgi complex. ($\times$ 18 000) **Inset** Electron-dense deposits in the mitochondrial matrix are present in mesenchymal cells at the surface of the tissue block. ($\times$ 36 000) **B** Artefacts induced by physical fixation. This micrograph was taken from an improperly frozen area of the sample. Mitochondrial cristae are poorly preserved. At a depth of approximately 10 μm from the surface of the liver, ice crystal damage becomes evident (compare ultrastructure at top of micrograph with bottom). ($\times$ 23 000)

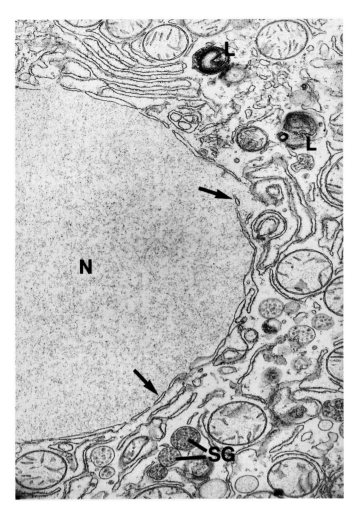

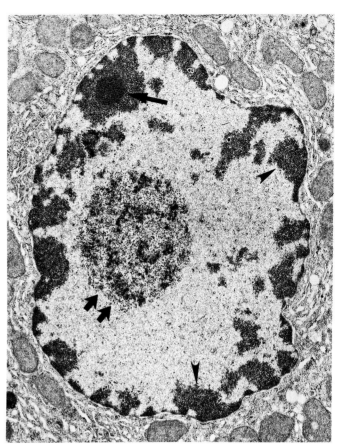

Fig. 4.2 Artefacts induced by chemical fixation. Loss of ions and of small molecules, as well as some extraction and redistribution of cellular proteins and lipids, occur during routine fixation and processing for transmission electron microscopy. These changes are not detectable by TEM and usually do not affect what is considered the standard ultrastructural appearance of tissues. More drastic changes, such as the ones illustrated in this micrograph, are considered artefactual — namely, fragmentation and vesiculation of membranes (arrows) as well as swelling and extraction of cytosol and matrix of organelles. The ultrastructural alterations induced by poor penetration of fixative, unsuitable osmolality and pH of fixative vehicle or improper processing are similar to alterations caused by in vitro autolysis and by cell injury. N = nucleus; L = lysosomes; SG = secretory granules. (× 14 000)

Fig. 4.3 Ultrastructural alterations of nucleus: margination of chromatin and of nucleolus. The clustering of condensed nuclear chromatin at the nuclear envelope (arrowhead) is an early and uniform manifestation of cell injury. Toxins which alter cellular protein synthesis frequently also induce margination of nucleoli (arrow). The fibrillar, granular and amorphous components of this nucleolus are not interspersed as in the more centrally located nucleolus (double arrow). Note the abundance of perichromatin granules. (× 14 000)

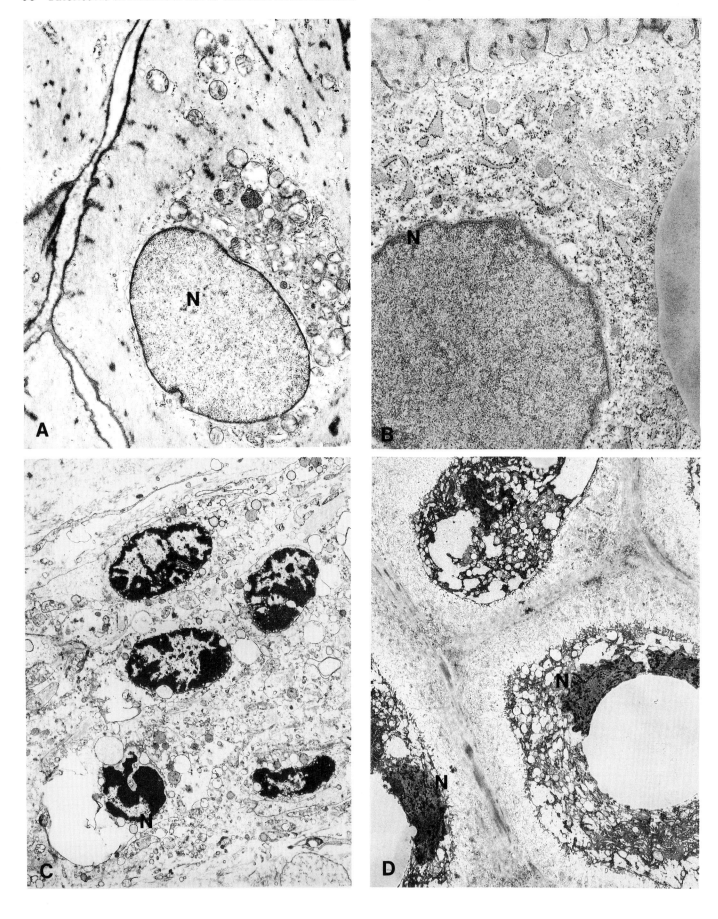

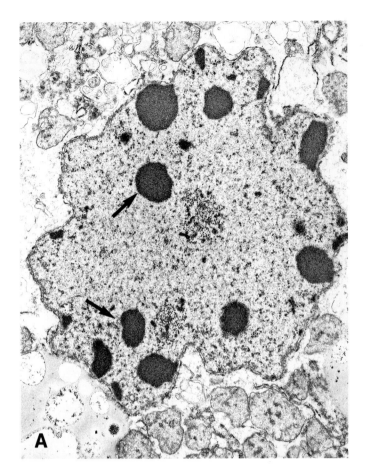

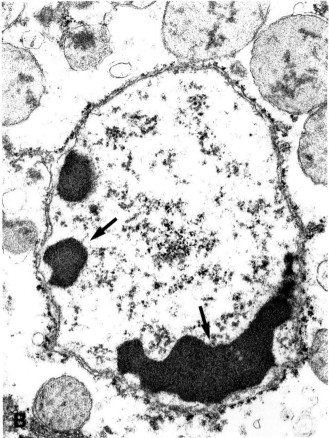

Fig. 4.5 A and **B** Ultrastructural alterations of nucleus: clumping and lysis of chromatin in necrotic cells. The chromatin of dead cells is very electron-dense and homogeneous (arrows). During necrosis, electron-lucent areas appear in the nucleus, presumably because of degradation of the DNA and RNA by nucleases of intracellular and extracellular origin. From rat liver, 24 h after administration of carbon tetrachloride (A, × 16 000; B, × 24 000)

Fig. 4.4 (Facing page) Ultrastructural alterations of nucleus: condensation of chromatin. The chromatin of biosynthetically active cells is finely dispersed. The typical euchromatin pattern is illustrated in a smooth muscle cell (**A**) and in a chondrocyte (**B**). Cell injury initially causes margination of chromatin, followed by progressively more severe condensation of chromatin and shrinkage of the nucleus (**C** and **D**). Swelling and/or condensation of these irreversibly injured cells can be seen. **C** From arteriole in rat skin subjected to 12 h of ischaemia and 1 h of reflow. **D** From rabbit ear cartilage 6 h after frostbite injury. N = nucleus. (A, 13 000; B, × 10 500; C, × 3500; D, × 4000)

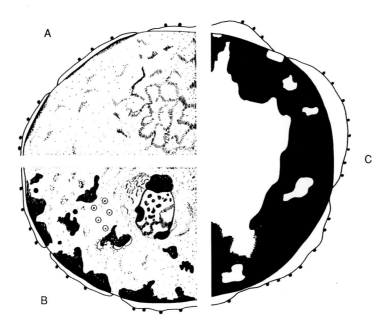

Fig. 4.6 Schematic overview of ultrastructural alterations of the nucleus. The nuclear shape, size and chromatin distribution vary in different cells and are influenced by the stages of the cell cycle and by protein biosynthetic activity. **A** Nucleus in cell with high DNA transcription shows evenly dispersed chromatin and interchromatin granules; the nucleolus contains interspersed filamentous structures, chromatin fibrils and dense granules. **B** In the early stages of cell injury, condensation of the chromatin occurs particularly near the nuclear envelope (margination). Agents known to interrupt protein synthesis may induce nucleolar segregation, namely separation of nucleolar components into distinct regions. **C** More severe injury causes clumping of the chromatin. The appearance of electron-lucent spaces occurs after cell death (karyolysis) due to degradative activity of DNAses. Swelling of nuclear envelope is also depicted.

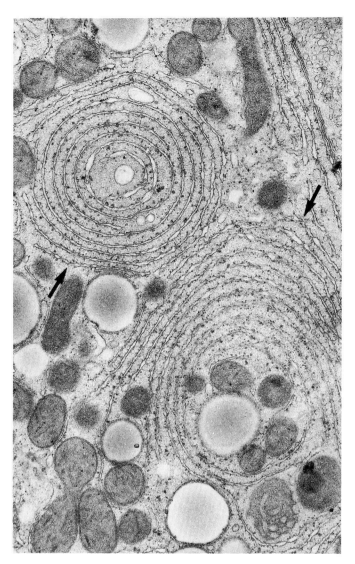

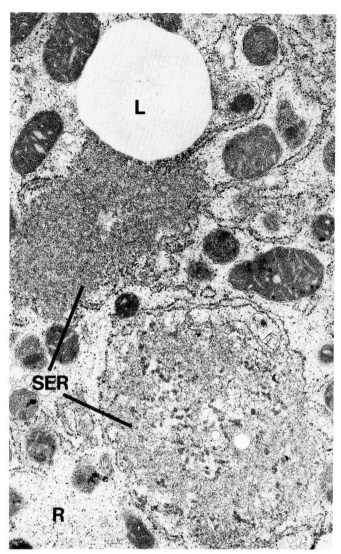

Fig. 4.7 Ultrastructural alterations of endoplasmic reticulum (ER): loss of polarity. In the secretory cells, the rough ER is well developed and the ER cisternae are arranged in parallel arrays. In various types of cell injury, several cisternae may form concentric whorls (arrows). These structures often become segregated into autophagic vacuoles. (× 18 000)

Fig. 4.8 Ultrastructural alterations of endoplasmic reticulum (ER): aggregation of smooth ER, decreased numbers of polysomes. Toxic cell injury in the acute stages or during recovery induces the formation of compact aggregates of smooth ER. These aggregates can, on occasion, be seen sequestered inside autophagic vacuoles where they are degraded. Toxins often inhibit protein synthesis and consequently decrease the number of ribosomes (R) in polysomal configurations in the cytosol and in the RER. L = lipid. (× 22 000)

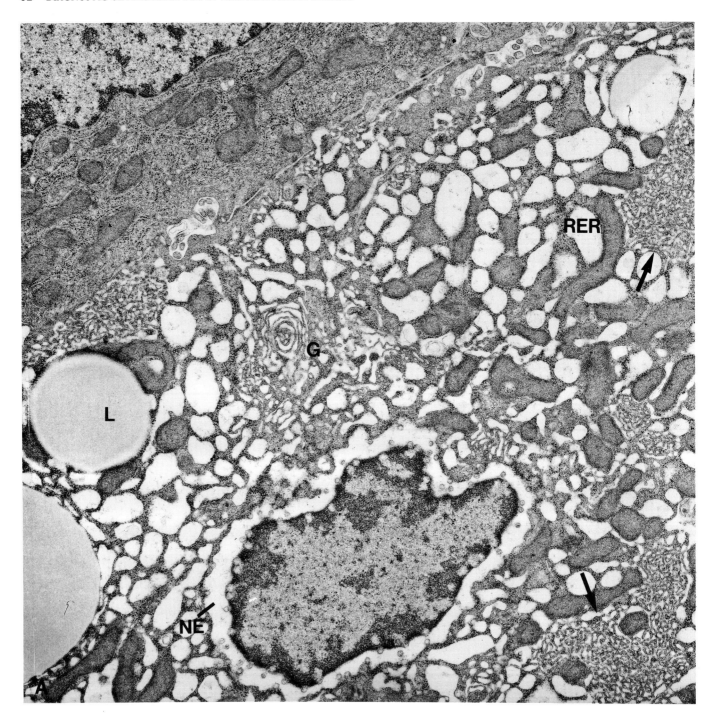

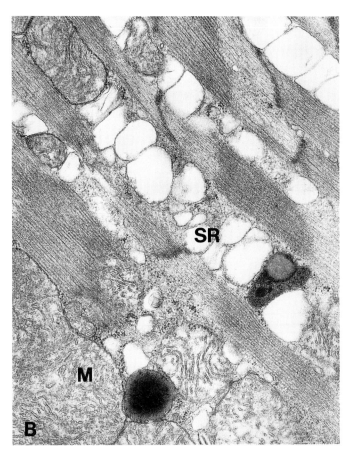

Fig. 4.9 Ultrastructural alterations of endoplasmic reticulum (ER) and Golgi apparatus. **A** (Facing page) Dilatation of the ER is frequently the first ultrastructural manifestation of cellular injury. In more severe states of injury, the nuclear envelope (NE) also becomes dilated. The Golgi (G) apparatus dilates, usually in parallel with the ER; it often fragments and becomes morphologically non-identifiable. In some types of cell injury, clustering of smooth ER (arrows) may develop. Lipid (L) accumulation in the form of triglyceride is a characteristic feature of injury in many cell types. All the changes illustrated in this micrograph are thought to be reversible. The presence of a structurally normal contiguous hepatocyte illustrates the focal nature of the injury. Differences in metabolic activity, blood flow, oxygenation and enzyme composition between the hepatocytes may account for the difference in susceptibility to the injury. From a rat liver 4 h after exposure to carbon tetrachloride. (× 14 000) **B** It is hypothesized that loss of ion regulation is responsible for the swelling of the ER. This myocyte is from a mouse diaphragm incubated in the presence of a calcium ionophore (A23l87). Dilatation of the sarcoplasmic reticulum (SR) is induced by the presence of the toxin. (× 22 000)

Fig. 4.10 Ultrastructural alterations of endoplasmic reticulum (ER): vesiculation. In this hepatocyte the rough ER (RER) cisternae have broken up into multiple vesicles. The number of peroxisomes (P) is increased. Proliferation of peroxisomes may be induced by substrates such as ethanol and long chain fatty acids which are oxidized by this organelle with concomitant generation of H_2O_2. From the liver of a patient who died in irreversible shock. (× 20 000)

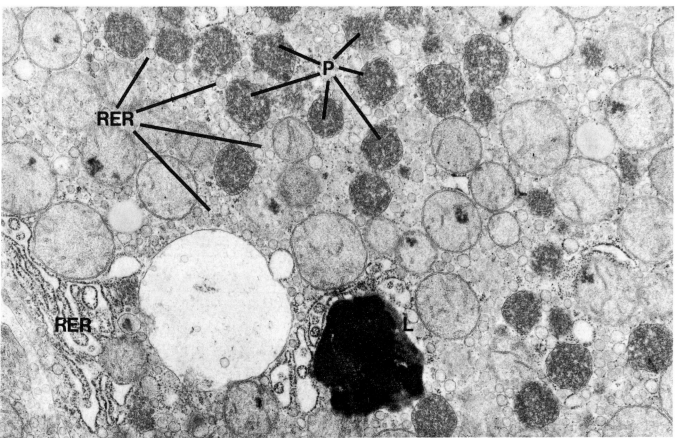

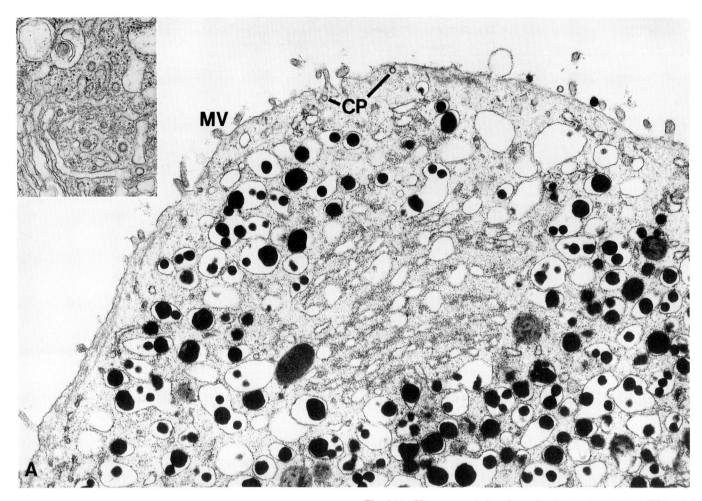

Fig. 4.11 Ultrastructural alterations of endoplasmic reticulum (ER) and Golgi apparatus: lipid accumulation. **A** Increase in VLDL lipid in dilated smooth ER in a cultured hepatocyte. Normal structural features of the plasma membrane, namely microvilli (MV) and coated pits (CP), are also illustrated. (× 19 000) ***Inset*** Several coated pits and vesicles in the trans region of a dilated Golgi apparatus. (× 25 000) **B** (Facing page) Imbalances between the transport into cells, export, or oxidation of fatty acids occur in sepsis, ischaemia and toxic cell injury. The fatty acids are re-esterified into triglycerides. Triglyceride lipid (L) appears as droplets in the cytosol. Inhibition of triglyceride export in hepatocytes may be caused by inhibition of protein synthesis and failure to synthesize the apoprotein moiety of VLDL. In this case, the lipid accumulates in smooth ER (arrows). From a rat liver 24 h after carbon tetrachloride exposure. (× 35 000)

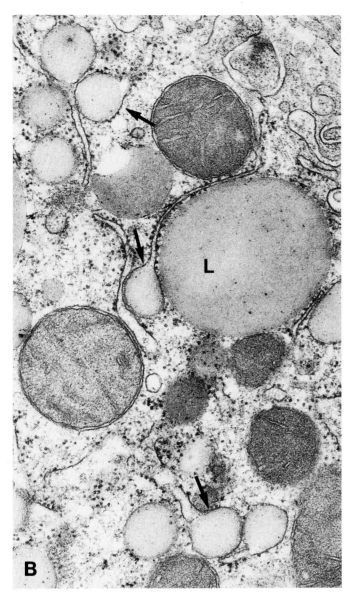

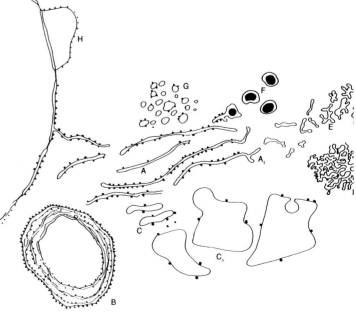

Fig. 4.12 Ultrastructural alterations of endoplasmic reticulum (ER): massive dilatation. The pathological change called 'ballooning degeneration' is illustrated in this micrograph. The ER is markedly dilated. The nucleus appears normal; the mitochondria are slightly condensed. From a rat liver 24 h after exposure to carbon tetrachloride. (× 7000)

Fig. 4.13 Schematic overview of ultrastructural alterations of endoplasmic reticulum (ER). **A** Normal ultrastructural appearance of rough ER; narrow parallel cisternae with ribosomes attached to cytoplasmic surface. **A1** Normal appearance of smooth ER; highly convoluted smooth cisternae structurally continuous with rough ER. **B** Loss of polarity of rough ER: cisternae lose orientation towards the Golgi apparatus and plasma membrane, and form concentric whorls. **C** Dilatation of ER is a frequent early response to sublethal injury. **C1** Massive dilatation of ER occurs in CCl$_4$ intoxication. **D** Aggregates of smooth ER are found in many types of toxic cell injury. **E** Proliferation of smooth ER is induced by compounds metabolized by the cytochrome P-450 system. **F** Lipid droplets accumulate in smooth ER when blocks occur in protein synthesis or phospholipid synthesis and transport. **G** Break-up of rough and smooth ER results when the cisternae pinch off into sealed vesicles that retain their luminal contents. Detachment of ribosomes can be seen — indicating interference with protein synthesis. **H** The outer membrane of the nuclear envelope is continuous with the rough ER and can undergo dilatation during cell injury.

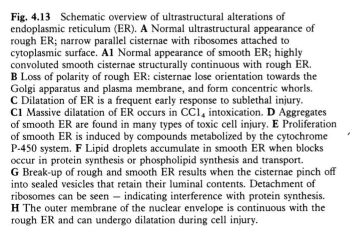

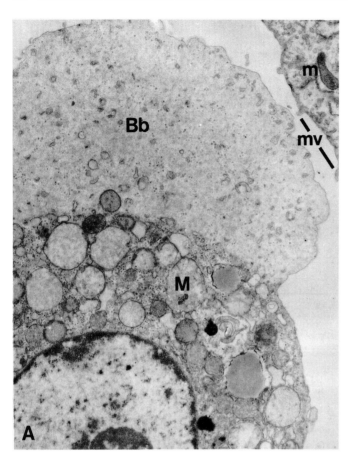

Fig. 4.14 Ultrastructural alterations of plasma membrane: blebbing. During reversible stages of injury, blebs develop on the surface of the cell, grow to various sizes, and may pinch off at the base and detach from the cell. It is thought that cytoskeletal filaments at the base of the blebs prevent the entry of large organelles and cause the apposition and fusion of the plasma membrane at the base of the bleb. **A** Human hepatocytes in suspension after isolation from a liver removed at autopsy and perfused with collagenase. (× 8000) **B** Human renal tubular epithelium. B = bleb; mv = microvilli; M = swollen mitochondria; m = normal mitochondria. (× 14 000)

Fig. 4.15 Ultrastructural alterations of plasma membrane: apical vacuolization. During severe cellular injury, pitting of the cell surface occurs. These pits are best visualized by scanning EM. The pits extend into the interior of the cell by infolding of the plasma membrane. The pits may seal at the surface and lose their continuity with the surface of the cell. Large apical vacuoles are commonly induced by hypoxia and artefactually by poor perfusion fixation. **A** Vacuolization (V) in an irreversibly injured human hepatocyte. Note the increased size of the lysosomes (L). (× 13 000) **B** (Facing page) Vacuoles (V) in reversibly injured hepatocytes from an anaesthetized dog subjected to hypovolaemic shock. Note the concomitant blebbing (B) in the space of Disse (SD). The mitochondria (M) are swollen. The endothelial cell lining the sinusoid (S) is intact. (× 11 000)

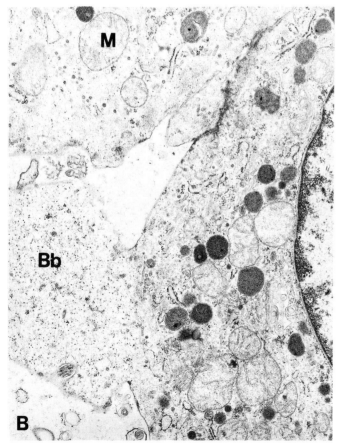

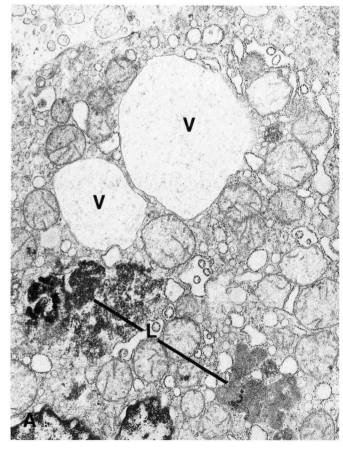

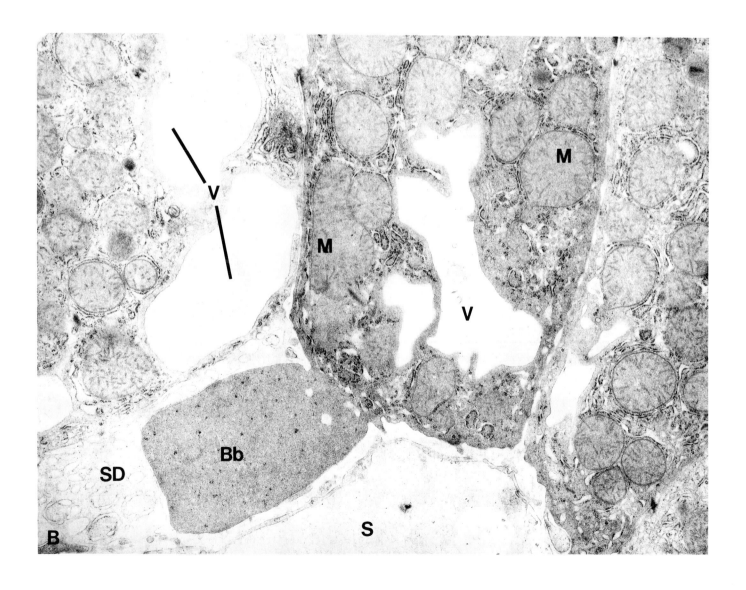

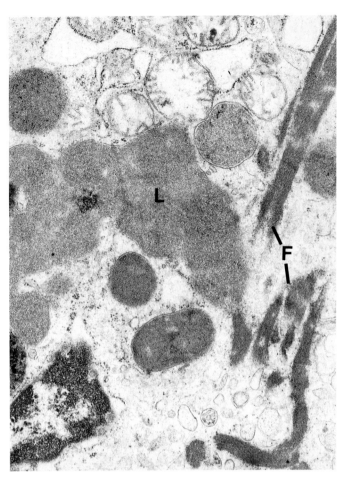

Fig. 4.16 Ultrastructural alterations of plasma membane: entry of plasma proteins into dead cells. After cell death, breaks in the continuity of the plasma membrane occur. These breaks hasten the release of cytosolic proteins such as enzymes into the blood stream. Plasma proteins such as fibrinogen can enter the cell and may, on occasion, be seen polymerized in the dead cells. F = fibrin; L = lysosomes. (× 19 000)

Fig. 4.18 (Facing page) Ultrastructural alterations of cytoskeleton. The cytoskeleton is responsible for cell shape, locomotion and division as well as organelle distribution and movement in the cell. Changes in the number and organization of cytoskeletal components are commonly seen in injured cells and may be responsible for the plasma membrane changes illustrated in previous figures. **A** In this normal cell, microtubules seen on longitudinal (arrow) or cross-section, radiate from the centrioles (C). N = nucleus. (× 15 000) **B** As an adaptation to culture conditions, intermediate filament bundles (IFB) develop near the surface of the plasma membrane. Note the presence of several vesicles, some of which are coated (arrows). Similar filament bundles may develop in cells that are terminally differentiated, as well as in injured cells. From human umbilical vein endothelial cells in culture. MT = microtubules. (× 25 000)

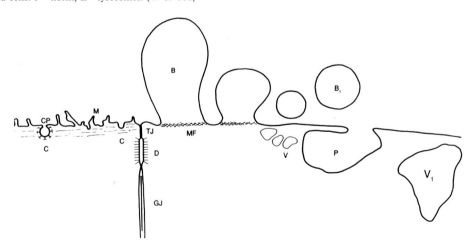

Fig. 4.17 Schematic overview of ultrastructural alterations of plasma membrane induced by cell injury. Structural features such as microvilli (M), caveolae (C), and coated pits (CP) tend to disappear from the surface of severely injured cells. The plasma membrane becomes smoother and rounded, and blebs (B) protrude into the extracellular space. Blebs vary in size and shape and can be observed in cultured cells to pinch off and detach (B1). The microfilament network (MF) allows only cytosolic components to enter the bleb. Intense vacuolization (V) of apical cytoplasm can be seen in many types of cell injury. Large pits (P) and large apical vacuoles (V1) may be seen in some hypoxic cells. The large vacuoles may represent complex involutions of plasma membrane. The junctional complexes of epithelial cells separate. Gap junctions (GJ) become non-functional early on. Desmosomes (D) and tight junctions (TJ) separate at later stages of injury.

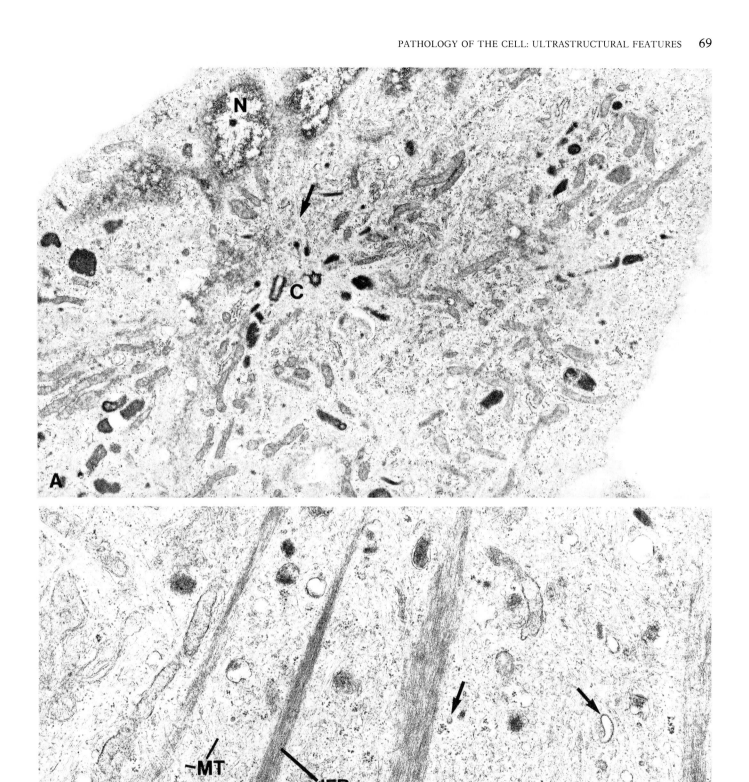

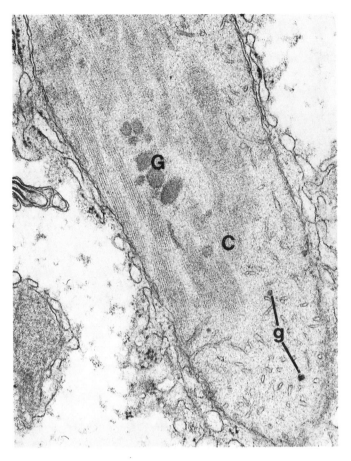

Fig. 4.20 (Facing page) Ultrastructural alterations of mitochondria: increased electron-density of mitochondrial membranes. Electron-dense linear deposits (arrows) may be seen in the cristae and between inner and outer membranes of mitochondria in cells such as ischaemic myocytes. This alteration is thought to be reversible. (× 28 000) *Inset* Dense deposits in a mitochondrion from a mouse diaphragm incubated for 60 min in the presence of a calcium ionophore. (× 49 000)

Fig. 4.19 Ultrastructural alterations of mitochondria: mitochondrial granules and crystals. Dense granules of various shapes and sizes are found in the matrix of the mitochrondria. The granules tend to be larger, more dense and/or more abundant in quick-frozen tissues (see Fig. 4.1); it is not clear whether these granules are preserved by this technique or artificially induced by it. In conventionally fixed, plastic-embedded tissues, the larger granules (G) are more commonly seen in pathologically altered cells. The chemical composition of the granules is not known with certainty. The loss of the small matrix granules (g) is one of the earliest manifestations of cell injury. Crystalline (C) deposits of undetermined composition have also been described in cells chronically exposed to various agents. From a dog hepatocyte. (× 35 000)

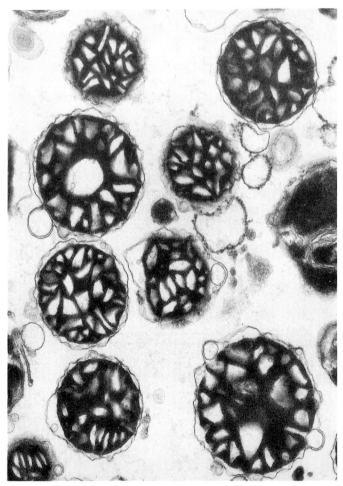

Fig. 4.21 Ultrastructural alterations of mitochondria: condensation of matrix. A subcellular fraction from rat liver is shown. The extreme condensation of the mitochondrial matrix is associated with expansion of the space between inner and outer membranes, as well as expansion of the cristae. The condensation is caused by cessation of mitochondrial respiration as well as by the use of a slightly hypertonic isolation medium in the isolation procedure. This morphological appearance is compatible with the proposal that the condensation of mitochondria seen in cell injury is caused by shifts in ions and water from mitochondrial compartments. (× 32 000)

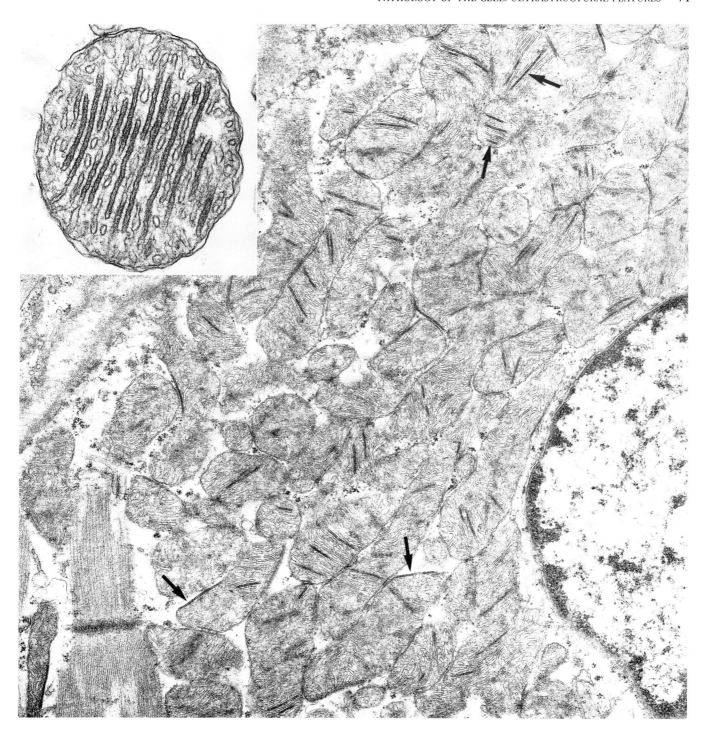

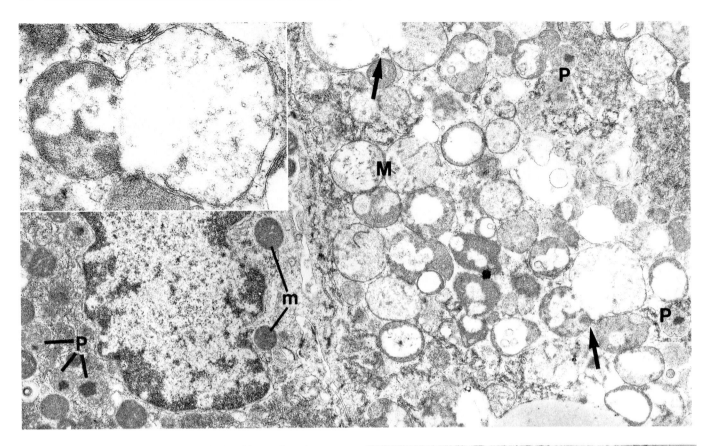

Fig. 4.22 Ultrastructural alterations of mitochondria: condensation, swelling and disruption, and extraction. Two hepatocytes are shown — one reversibly, the other irreversibly injured. Condensed mitochondria (m) are seen in both hepatocytes and are characterized by dense matrices and dilated cristae. The necrotic hepatocyte also shows swollen mitochondria (M) characterized by electron-lucent matrices and apparent loss of cristae. Rupture of the mitochondrial outer membrane (arrows) causes unfolding of the cristae and ballooning out of the inner membrane (inset). Note the electron-lucent zones in several mitochondria due to extraction of matrix components. It is also interesting to note that the peroxisomes (P) of the necrotic cell are not swollen. From rat liver 24 h after administration of carbon tetrachloride. (× 17 000; inset, × 39 000)

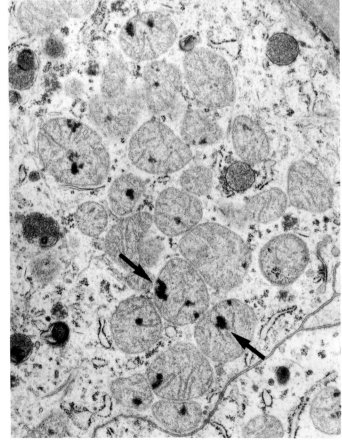

Fig. 4.23 Ultrastructural alterations of mitochondria: flocculent densities. Amorphous electron dense deposits (arrows) are present in the matrix of the mitochondria. These deposits have been designated 'flocculent densities' and are typically seen in mitochondria of irreversibly injured cells. Human renal epithelium. (× 18 000)

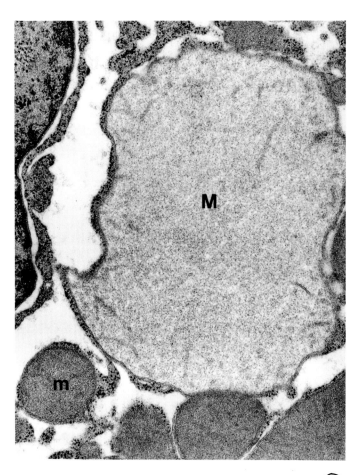

Fig. 4.24 Ultrastructural alterations of mitochondria: enlargement. Increase in the number and/or size of organelles is a comman manifestation of subacute cell injury. With regard to mitochondria, increased size of isolated organelles can be seen in chronically injured cells. This micrograph illustrates the presence of enlargement due to hypertrophy in a mitochondrion (M) from the liver of a rat after acetaminophen intoxication. Compare to the size of a normal mitochondrion (m). (× 22 000)

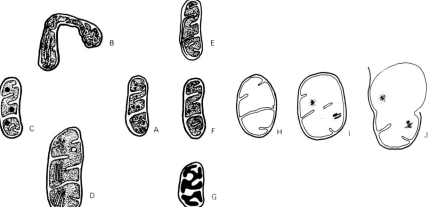

Fig. 4.25 Schematic overview of ultrastructural alterations of mitochondria. **A** Normal appearance of a mitochondrion. Typically, the mitochondria are uniform in shape and size and are surrounded by two membranes; the inner membrane forms several infoldings. The matrix contains granules variable in numbers and shape. **B** In some chronically injured cells, the shape and size of the mitochondria and the orientation of the cristae become variable. **C** The size and numbers of matrix granules vary depending upon tissue type and fixation procedure. **D** Very large mitochondria can be induced by chronic toxic injury; crystalline structures in the mitochondrial matrix can be induced by ethanol and by oestrogens. **E–G** Electron-dense linear deposits in the intermembranous space, loss of matrix granules and condensation of matrix, are early reversible alterations. **H** Mitochondrial swelling is an indication of more severe injury. **I** Appearance of flocculent densities is pathognomonic of cell death. **J** As swelling progresses, the outer mitochondrial membrane ruptures and membrane ghosts are formed.

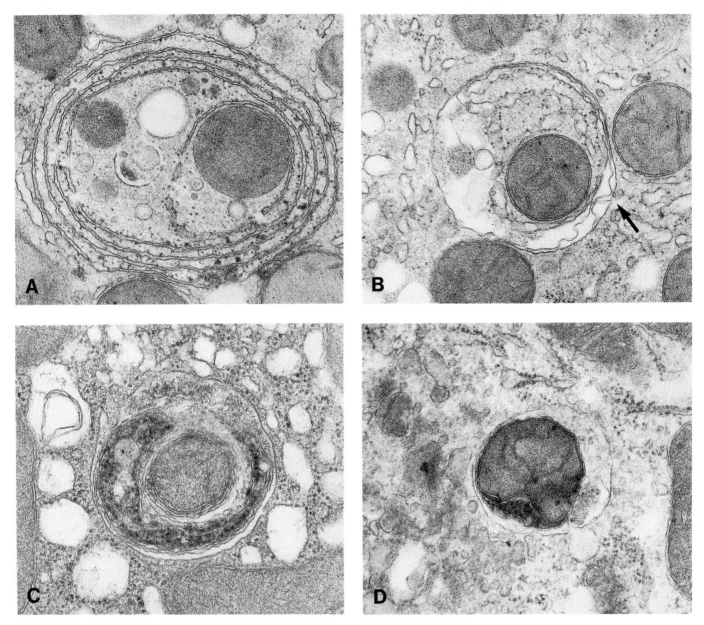

Fig. 4.26 Ultrastructural alterations of lysosomes: stages in the formation of autophagic vacuoles. The lysosomes are responsible, in part, for the physiological degradation of cellular organelles. Cell injury may enhance or inhibit lysosomal degradation with consequent alterations in the numbers, shapes, sizes and contents of the lysosomes. Lysosomal autophagic degradation occurs through sequential steps that can be recognized ultrastructurally. **A** and **B** The first step, sequestration, occurs with the formation of an autophagic vacuole bounded typically by two membranes morphologically similar to endoplasmic reticulum (arrow). **C** and **D** The autophagic vacuole acquires digestive enzymes by fusing with a lysosome and the inner bounding membrane is degraded. The sequestered organelles are broken down and become progressively amorphous. Degradation of the sequestered organelles proceeds to the level of molecular constituents which re-enter the cytosol for re-utilization. **A** and **B** are from cultured rat hepatocyte. **C** and **D** are from rat liver. (A, × 32 000; B, × 32 000; C, × 40 000; D, × 40 000)

Fig. 4.27 Ultrastructural alterations of lysosomes: expansion of the lysosomal compartment through autophagy. In some types of cell injury, the lysosomes increase in numbers and size due to the presence of many partially degraded organelles apparently taken up by autophagic sequestration. **A** This micrograph illustrates the typical appearance and presumed maturation of autophagic vacuoles (AV1, AV2) into lysosomal dense bodies (DB). From a cultured human umbilical vein endothelial cell. (× 14 500) **B** This micrograph illustrates the massive accumulation of lysosomes that can occur in cell injury. Because of rapid degradation of autophagic vacuole contents (t½ approximately 10 min), the cellular volume occupied by lysosomes of epithelial cells is typically 1–3%. This explant from hamster pancreas was cultured in the presence of a carcinogen. Close to 50% of acinar cell volume is occupied by lysosomes (L). The following mechanisms, acting separately or in concert, may be responsible for this alteration: sequestration of large areas of cytoplasm into autophagic vacuoles, fusion of several autophagic vacuoles and/or block in maturation of autophagic vacuoles. Direct biochemical measurements of protein degradation coupled with morphometry of lysosomal volume are used to identify the precise mechanism of the expansion. The appearances of the nucleus (N) and mitochondria (M) indicate that the acinar cells are viable. (× 17 000)

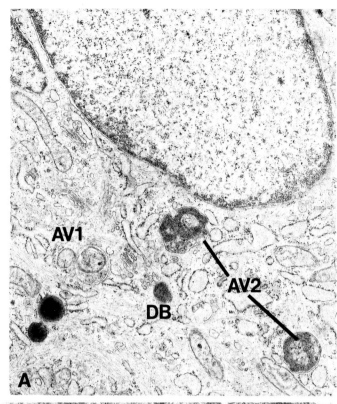

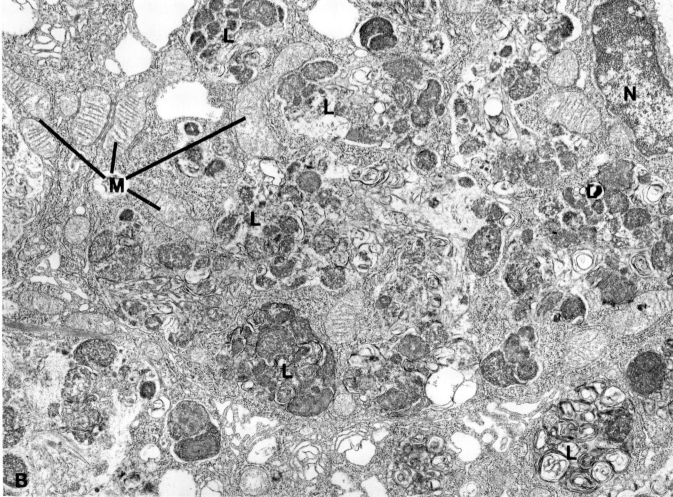

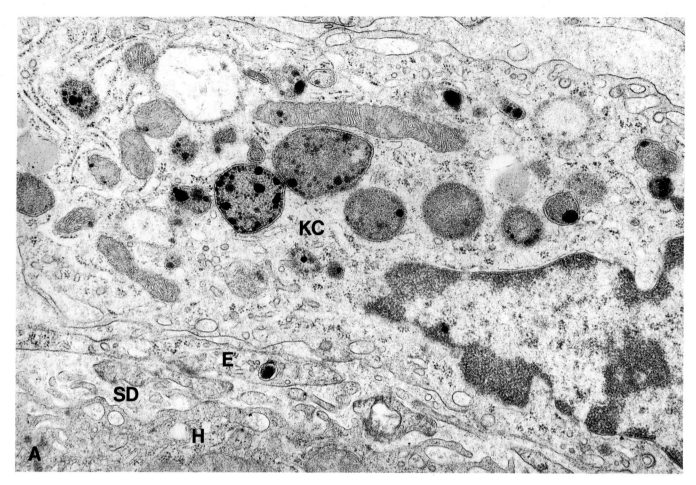

Fig. 4.28 Ultrastructural alterations of lysosomes: expansion of the lysosomal compartment through heterophagy. Tissue macrophages are responsible for phagocytosis and degradation of necrotic cells. Some other mesenchymal and epithelial cells also manifest limited capacity for heterophagic uptake of necrotic debris. **A** Kupffer cell (KC) from rat liver. The lysosomal compartment occupies approximately 15% of cell volume in this cell type. (× 21 000) **B** (Facing page) From human liver following shock. Note the enlargement of the lysosomes (arrows) in a Kupffer cell (KC). Amorphous material of variable electron density is present in the lysosomes. Note the swelling and disruption of endothelial cells (E).
SD = space of Disse; H = hepatocyte. (× 11 000)

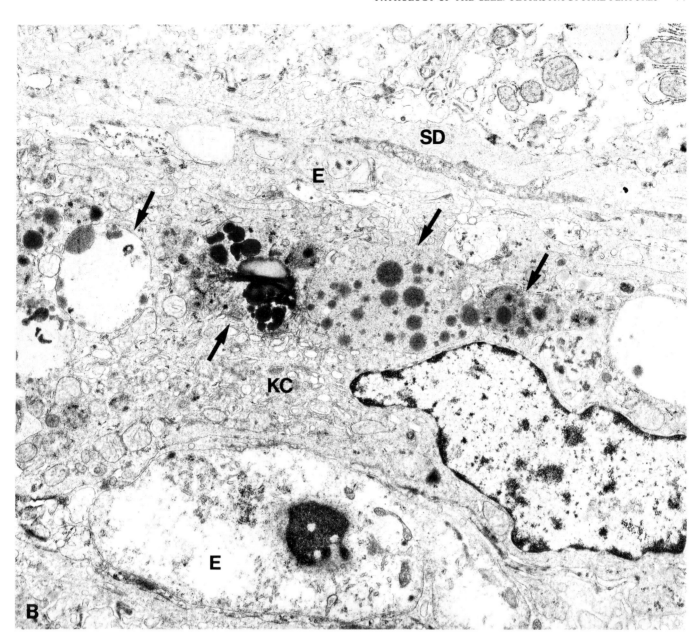

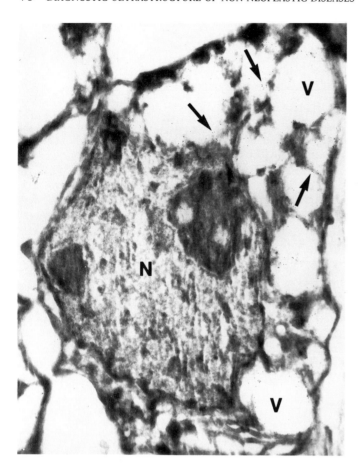

Fig. 4.29 Ultrastructural alterations of lysosomes: expansion of the lysosomal compartment by swelling. The lysosomal milieu is acidic because of the activity of an ATP-dependent proton pump. Weak bases such as chloroquine enter the lysosomes by free diffusion and are protonated and trapped inside the lysosomes. The accumulation of the drugs and osmotic effects cause swelling of the lysosomes and vacuolization (v) of cells. The lysosomes in the micrograph are identified by colloidal gold (arrows) immunolabelling with an antibody to an integral protein of the lysosomal membrane. U-937 cells were fixed with 2% paraformaldehyde and ultrathin frozen sections were prepared. After immunolabelling, the sections were stained with uranyl acetate and embedded in methylcellulose. N = nucleus. (× 10 000)

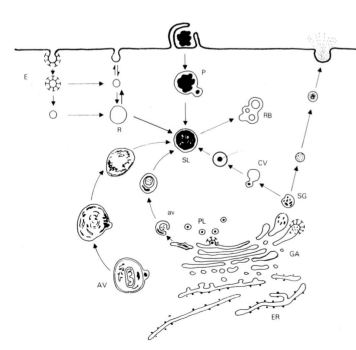

Fig. 4.30 Schematic overview of ultrastructural alterations of lysosomes. The vacuolar structures participating in lysosomal degradation pathways are illustrated, namely, (macro) autophagic vacuoles (AV), microautophagic vacuoles (av), crinophagic vacuoles (CV), (hetero) phagosomes (P), and smooth or coated endocytic (E) vesicles. The size, numbers and contents of these vacuoles and vesicles are altered during acute cell injury. Rates of formation and/or degradation of these vacuoles can be affected. Typically, the lysosomes (L) are increased in numbers and size in injured cells. Accumulations of myelin figures and lipofuscin in lysosomal residual bodies (RB) are often seen. ER = endoplasmic reticulum; GA = Golgi apparatus; SG = secretory granule; R = receptosome; PM = plasma membrane.

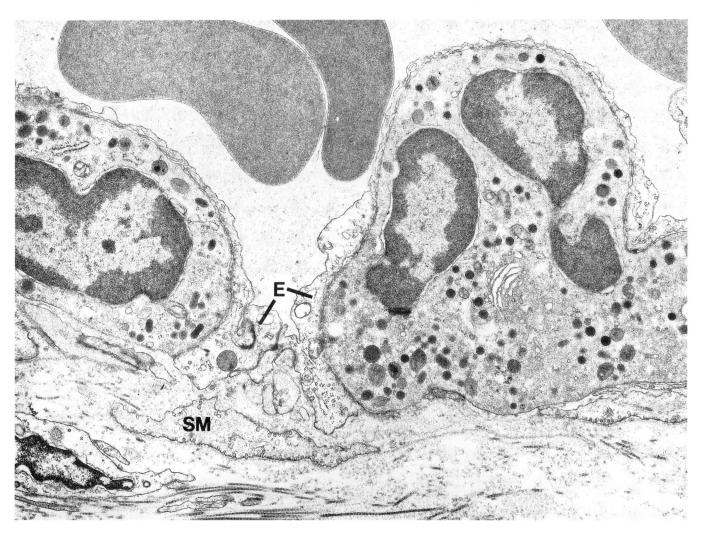

Fig. 4.31 Ultrastructural alterations of vasculature. The micrograph is from the epigastric vein of a skin flap in rat dermis. The skin was subjected to 7 h of ischaemia. Diapedesis of neutrophils through the wall of the viable vessel can be seen. In this injury model, the viability of the microvasculature determines the ultimate survival of the skin.
E = endothelium; SM = smooth muscle cell. (× 17 000)

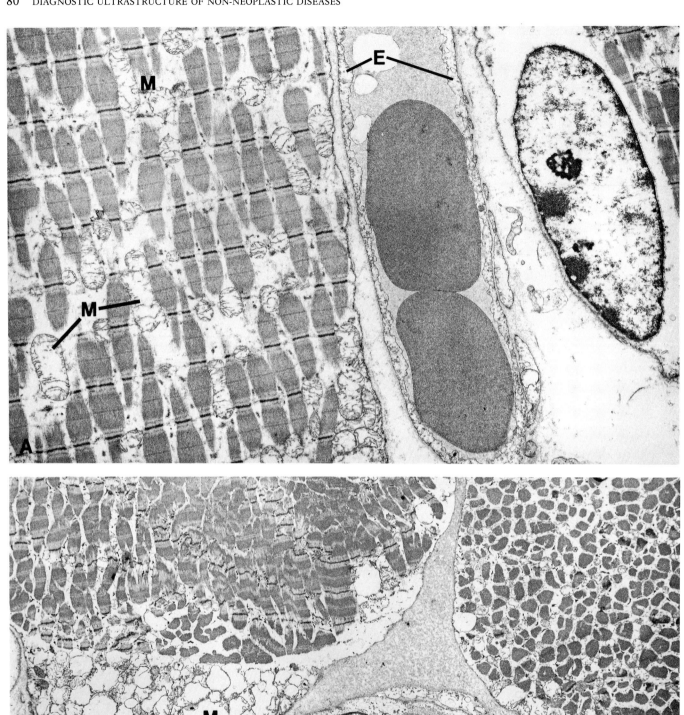

Fig. 4.32 Ultrastructural alterations of vasculature. In tissues containing parenchymal cells that are relatively resistant to injury, damage to the microvasculature may be seen in parallel with damage to parenchyma. These micrographs are from the tibialis anterior (TA) or gastrocnemius muscle from rabbit limb, subjected to 7 h of ischaemia and to re-perfusion ranging from 5 to 60 min. The time of evolution of the injury in the muscle is variable. Micrographs of TA myocytes were selected to illustrate the appearance of areas demonstrating progressively increasing injury. **A** (Facing page) TA muscle, 5 min reflow. Swelling of mitochondria (M) and cytosol. E = endothelium. (× 7000) **B** (Facing page) TA muscle, 15 min reflow. High-amplitude swelling of mitochondria (M) and cytosol. Endothelial (E) swelling is also seen. (× 4000) **C** TA muscle, 1 h reflow. Blebbing and rupture (arrows) of the plasma membrane (PM) are seen. Stasis of red blood cells (RBC) contributes to the injury. (× 6000) **D** Illustrates injury to gastrocnemius (7 h ischaemia, 60 min reflow). Swelling of mitochondria (M), as well as dilatation and vesiculation of sarcoplasmic reticulum (arrows) are evident. Injury to gastrocnemius is, in general, less severe because of lack of increased compartment pressures in this muscle. (× 14 000)

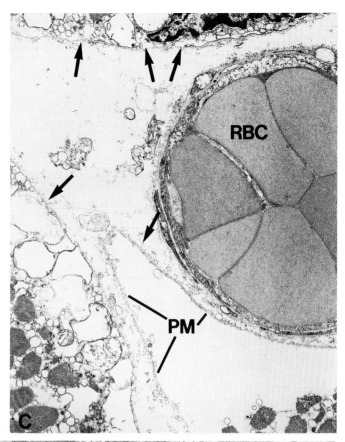

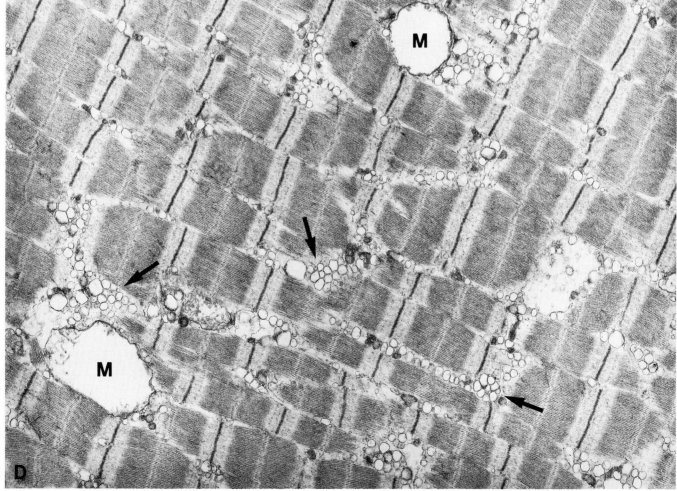

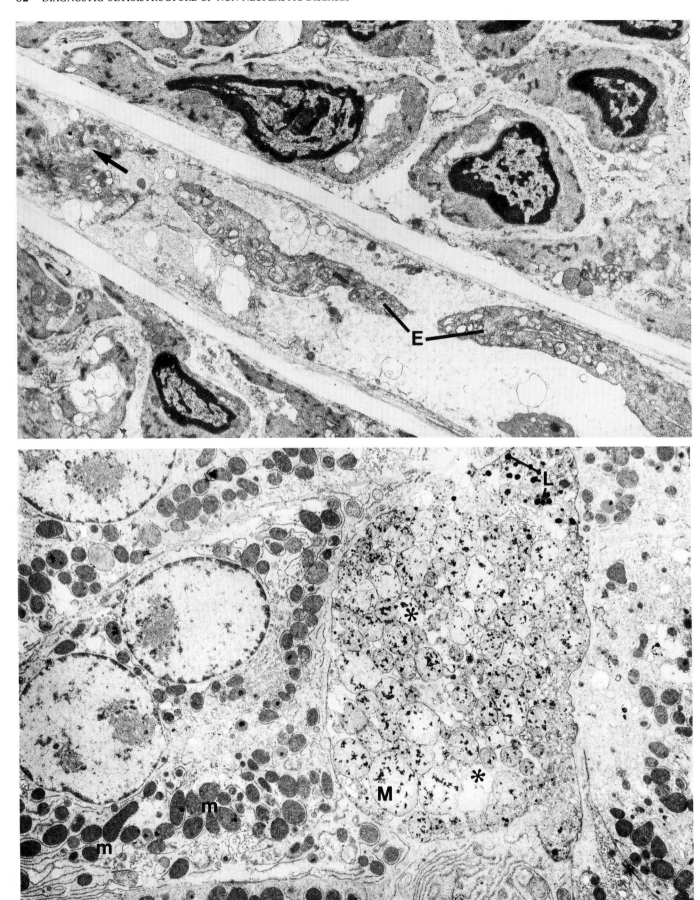

Fig. 4.33 (Facing page) Ultrastructural alterations of vasculature. In some types of injury, selective damage to the vasculature may be induced. This micrograph is from the ear of an anaesthetized rabbit subjected to frostbite. The ear was quick-frozen and thawed. A skin sample was taken 10 min after freezing. Note separation of endothelial cells (E) from the basal lamina of arteriole and vacuolization of smooth muscle cells. Platelet deposition can also be seen (arrow). (× 12 000)

Fig. 4.34 (Facing page) Ultrastructural alterations induced by cell injury in cultured cells. The ultrastructural manifestations of cell injury and necrosis in vitro are similar to those seen in vivo. In these cultured hepatocytes, the viable cells show very mild vacuolization; the mitochondria (m) are normal. The necrotic hepatocyte (asterisks) shows marked vacuolization and vesiculation. Some lipid (L) deposits are present. The mitochondria (M) are massively swollen. The electron-dense deposits in the normal mitochondria may be an artefact of culture. (× 5000)

Fig. 4.35 Schematic overview of key functional cellular alterations induced by acute cell injury. In this overview, the roles of plasma membrane, mitochondria and endoplasmic reticulum in the maintenance of ionic homeostasis are emphasized. It is hypothesized that loss of regulation of intracellular ion levels (particulary calcium) is a key event which leads to irreversible cell injury and cell death. Reproduction from Trump & Berezesky[56] with permission. For further discussion of the role of calcium in cell differentiation and gene expression see Trump & Berezesky.[57]

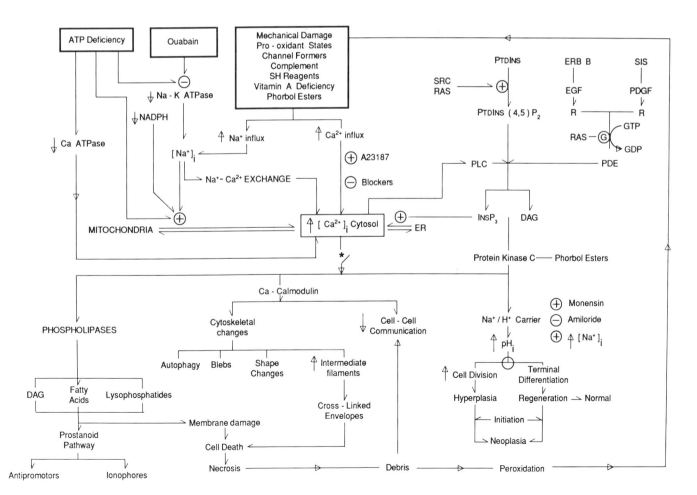

5. Stromal aberrations

Jennet M. Harvey   Ingrun Anton-Lamprecht

PART 1
GENERAL REMARKS
Jennet M. Harvey

INTRODUCTION

With its complex architecture of cellular elements, fibrous components and extracellular matrix, connective tissue serves a multitude of functions of which the following are some of the most important: mechanical properties such as tensile strength and elasticity, extensibility, flexibility and protection for the enclosed and underlying microvasculature, nerves, and resident cells; maintenance of the fluid and electrolyte balance; nutritional, and immunological control functions.[124,254] Most of these functions are related to the biochemical composition and molecular structure and constitution of the fibrous proteins that contribute to collagen[29], microfilaments, elastic microtubules (oxytalan fibrils), and elastin,[77,223] and of the glycoproteins and mucopolysaccharides such as proteoglycans and glycosaminoglycans[39,246] constituting the non-fibrous extracellular matrix. In addition, basement membranes separate cells from the underlying or surrounding connective tissue; they form specialized thin extracellular matrices of special collagens (types IV and V), proteoglycans (heparan sulphate) and glycoproteins (laminin, fibronectin, nidogen), most of which are probably synthesized by the respective cells themselves.[35,129]

A variety of ultrastructural abnormalities may be observed in the stroma in non-neoplastic diseases — including changes in the vasculature and the presence of a cellular exudate — but in general these changes lack precise diagnostic significance. This chapter focuses primarily on the two main extracellular components of the stroma, namely: (1) the fibrous component — collagen and the elastic system; and (2) the extracellular matrix. Several, mostly non-specific, ultrastructural abnormalities in these components will be listed, followed by a description of some of the disease states in which they occur.

COLLAGEN

The term 'collagens' is used to refer to a heterogeneous group of macromolecular proteins with the capacity to aggregate and form extracellular supporting elements. The amino acid composition of the collagens is characterized by a high content of glycine, alanine, proline and hydroxyproline, an absence of tryptophan and usually cysteine, a low tyrosine content and the presence of a rare hydroxylated amino acid, hydroxylysine.[207] The most distinctive feature of the component chains of the various molecular species of collagen is the presence of lengthy sequences of repetitive triplets; these tripeptide units are an absolute requirement for the triple helical structure of the tropocollagen molecule and are therefore the fundamental structural feature of the group.

At least 10 different types of collagens have been identified so far in various locations (Table 5.1). Each type of collagen contains three polypeptide chains that may be identical to, or different from, each other, forming the triple helical collagen molecule. At least 16 different collagen chains are known so far. Each of the chains is coded for by separate genes.[35] These collagen genes are not clustered but are widely distributed throughout the human genome. Collagen genes have been identified on chromosomes 2 (type III α 1 chain; type V α 2 chain), 7 (type I α 2 chain), 12 (type II α 1 chain), 13 (type IV α 1 chain), and 17 (type I α 1 chain); collagen-like sequences are localized on chromosomes 1, 5, 7, 13, 14 and 15.[85] Mutations may affect any of these gene loci and DNA sequences. In only a few cases have exact phenotype–genotype correlates been defined.[35] Moreover, collagen molecules and collagen fibrils interact in a complex manner with macromolecules in the surrounding matrix. This may explain why morphological changes of collagen are not only found in those genetic disorders that are due to mutations of collagen genes, but in

Table 5.1 Collagen types

A. Interstitial collagens (form broad-banded fibrils)		
Type I fibrils	Diameter 45–180 nm	Widely distributed in most connective tissues except cartilage: major component of bone, tendon, skin, dentin
Type II fibrils	Diameter 10–80 nm	Found almost exclusively in cartilage
Type III fibrils 'reticulin'	Diameter 5–40 nm	Found with type I; relatively high concentration in distensible connective tissue (skin, blood vessels, gut, uterus, etc)
B. Minor collagens (do not form broad-banded fibrils)		
Type IV	Basement membranes	Main component of basal laminae: postulated to form two-dimensional lattice-like network
Type V	Fibril forms unknown	Pericellular and interstitial location in most tissues except cartilage
Type VI	? 100 nm periodic filaments and fibrils[27]	Aortic intima[81] and a wide variety of other tissues
Type VII	Fibril form; the major anchoring fibril protein	Skin, amniotic membrane; possibly associated with all stratified epithelia
Type VIII 'EC collagen'	Fibril form undetermined	Broad distribution in vertebrate tissues; first isolated from aortic endothelial cells[226]
Type IX	Fibril form unknown	Cartilaginous tissue
Type X 'G collagen'	Fibril form unknown	Cartilage growth plate

many other genetic conditions and non-heritable disturbances.

There are several ways of classifying the various types of collagen. To the electron microscopist there are two main categories: those that form periodically banded fibres and those that do not.[275] Some of the collagens in the latter group have been identified as specific fibrous or lamellar form but there are others whose structure is unknown and some which require special techniques such as electron immunohistochemistry for their identification.[83,84,113]

There are probably no structural abnormalities of collagen fibrils which are entirely specific, although certain ultrastructural alterations or patterns of alteration may be predictive of a certain disease. In some instances overall architectural derangements may be detected using scanning electron microscopy (SEM), and this technique has been employed in the investigation of many diseases of connective tissue, both hereditary[128] and acquired.[5,131,155,156,158,168,173,186,206,210,271,273,301]

Interstitial collagens

These appear as a characteristic banded fibril, usually of fairly uniform diameter, which depends on the site, for example, approximately 100 nm in the reticular dermis of the skin but up to 160 nm in the semilunar cartilage of the knee. Special techniques show the fibrils to be composed of filaments 3–5 nm in diameter, each made up of five rows of approximately quarter-staggered tropocollagen molecules.[253] It is this quarter-staggered arrangement which gives the collagen fibril its characteristic axial periodicity; this varies from 64 to 70 nm in fresh wet tissue, to 52 to 62 nm in most ultrathin sections. Table 5.1 summarizes the ultrastructural characteristics (where known) and the distribution of presently known collagen types. In some instances the formation of collagen not normally

present in that site, or the presence of abnormal proportions of the various types of collagen may be an integral part of the disease,[125,143,145] and biochemical or other specialized techniques may be necessary to detect the change. Fibrils with abnormally small or large diameters, or with an abnormal variation in diameter, may also be a feature of certain diseases, particularly the inherited connective tissue disorders[76,125,126,143,196,282] (Table 5.2 and Part 2).

Anchoring fibrils

Anchoring fibrils are collagenous in nature, and related to type VII collagen.[275] They are present in normal human skin,[21,22,37,101,106,161,267,297] as well as in other normal tissues and in certain disease states.[98,149,167,191,235,261,266,268,298] The term is used to describe fibrils measuring 400–600 nm in length and 20–60 nm in diameter which present as U- or J-shaped structures linking the basal lamina of epithelial cells to the underlying collagen. Anchoring fibrils have been shown to bind IgA in the skin of patients with dermatitis herpetiformis,[297] but may be absent or hypoplastic in the skin of patients with some types of epidermolysis bullosa dystrophica[23] (see Ch. 22).

Fibrous long-spacing collagen

The fibrils of so called 'fibrous long-spacing' (FLS) collagen demonstrate a periodicity markedly greater than the approximately 64 nm periodicity of usual collagen fibrils. In vivo the periodicity varies between 100 and 150 nm, and there is some doubt as to whether this material is exactly the same as the fibrous long-spacing collagen first produced in vitro[114,115] with a periodicity of 200–260 nm. It is probable that both the in vitro and in vivo fibrous

Table 5.2 Ultrastructural alteration of collagen in inherited connective tissue diseases*

Disease	Collagen alteration	References
Buschke–Ollendorff	Collagen flowers	276, 277
Cutis laxa (dominant and recessive)	Collagen unaltered;	94, 150, 170
	variable diameter;	104
	collagen flowers;	180
	diminished collagen,	126
	small fibres	
(X-linked)	Large fibrils, densely packed, excessive matrix	32
Elastosis perforans serpiginosa	Collagen flowers; mingling of collagen and elastic fibres	286
Ehlers–Danlos type I		
Adult	Increased fibril diameter,	121
	collagen flowers,	283
	excess matrix;	240
	small fibrils variable	14
	diameter; disorganized bundles on SEM	
Infant	Bizarre flowers, poorly integrated bundles	126
Ehlers–Danlos type II	Large-diameter fibrils,	121
	collagen flowers, serrated	240
	fibrils;	
	variable fibril diameter,	126
	collagen flowers;	
	small-diameter fibrils,	14
	small bundles	190
Ehlers–Danlos type III	Large-diameter fibrils, collagen flowers, serrated fibrils	240
Ehlers–Danlos type IV	Small variable-diameter fibrils, excessive matrix, dilated	125
	rough endoplasmic reticulum of dermal fibroblasts	
Ehlers–Danlos type V	Small diameters, collagen	14, 240
	flowers, serrated collagen	
Ehlers–Danlos type VI	Large-diameter fibrils,	121
	collagen flowers; small-diameter fibrils	263
Ehlers–Danlos type VII	Fibrils irregularly shaped	284
	or variable in diameter,	294
	collagen degeneration	
Ehlers–Danlos type VIII	Variable-diameter	126
	dissociated bundles,	
	excessive diffuse matrix;	
	small-diameter fibrils,	
	excessive diffuse material	
Ehlers–Danlos type IX	Large-diameter collagen	34, 35, 126
	fibrils, collagen flowers,	
	excessive density of collagen fibre bundles	
Ehlers–Danlos type X	Collagen flowers,	34, 35, 126
	altered packing of	
	collagen fibrils into fibre bundles	
Marfan's syndrome	Dense angular fibrils	33, 71, 82, 126
	dissociated bundles, excessive diffuse matrix;	
	small-diameter fibrils, excessive diffuse material	
Osteogenesis imperfecta	Small-diameter fibrils	143
Pseudoxanthoma elasticum	Diminished amount of collagen,	80, 102, 224, 227
	collagen flowers or unaltered	

*Table modified from Holbrook & Byers.[126] See also Ch. 5, part 2, and Table 5.5

long-spacing collagens are composed of a combination of proteoglycans or glycoproteins and collagen, and that FLS collagen is likely to develop in the presence of excess glycosaminoglycans in tissue,[87] although it is uncertain whether FLS collagen results from the breakdown or the abnormal development of connective tissue. FLS collagen was first described in vivo in Descemet's membrane of the cornea,[141] and it is frequently seen in a variety of normal tissues[9,48,130,172,183,256,280] and pathological conditions, both neoplastic[111] and non-neoplastic (Table 5.3). It has recently been suggested that FLS collagen fibrils are, at least in some instances, type VI collagen.[27]

Amianthoid fibres

Amianthoid fibres are composed of collections of giant collagen fibrils up to 6–10 times thicker than normal (up to 1 μm or more in diameter). The reported periodicity varies according to the preparative techniques but is comparable to that of native collagen.[87] It has been suggested that giant collagen fibrils may represent an age-related or degenerative process in native collagen. 'Amianthoid change' has been reported in numerous light microscopic studies on ageing cartilage since the initial observations of Bohmig,[16] and ultrastructural descriptions have also been provided of amianthoid fibres in human costal

Table 5.3 FLS collagen in non-neoplastic conditions

Skin	Scleroderma[162]
	Hereditary haemorrhagic telangiectasia[109]
	Tuberous sclerosis[12]
	Lepromatous leprosy[63]
	Blue naevus[11]
	Raynaud's syndrome[279]
Heart	Rheumatic carditis[9]
Lung	Sarcoidosis[111]
Nervous system	Cauda equina in compression[234]
	Experimentally constricted nerve[211]
	Traumatic neuroma, acoustic nerve[116]
Eye	Type VI mucopolysaccharidosis (Maroteaux–Laury syndrome) (Henderson, unpublished observation)
	Cornea guttata[142]
	Kayser–Fleischer rings[142]
	Exfoliation syndrome[220]
	Glaucoma[138,221,222]
Ear	Menieres disease[78]
Kidney	Experimental amyloidosis[154]
	Multiple myeloma[236]
Lymphohaemopoietic system	Sarcoidosis[264,265]
	Reaction to Freund's adjuvant[10]
	Lymphadenitis[185]
	Reactive lymphadenopathy[193]
	Angio-immunoblastic lymphadenopathy[66,153,159,182,198]
	Myeloproliferative disorder[147]
Tumour-like proliferations	Pigmented villonodular synovitis[4]
	Proliferative fasciitis[42]
	Fibromatosis hyalinica multiplex juvenilis[291,296]

cartilage,[132,133] osteoarthritic human articular cartilage,[88] the fascia of a patient with congenital fascial dystrophy,[139] De Quervain's disease,[137] muscle tissue associated with temporo-mandibular joint ankylosis[65] as well as in various neoplasms.[111]

Composite collagen fibrils/collagen flowers

These fibrils, which have been observed in a variety of inherited[126] (Table 5.2 and Fig. 5.1) and acquired disorders,[55,56,105,163,168,184,199,203,209,218,257,259] (Fig. 5.2) are referred to by several different terms. Lengthwise, they appear as loosely aggregated thick bundles wound in a shallow spiral (collagen 'ropes' or 'wires') while in transverse section they may appear serrated, lobulated or fused and are referred to as collagen 'flowers', 'aggregates' or 'composites'. It is not known whether composite fibrils represent an abnormality in the process of fibrillogenesis or a degenerative change. Elevated levels of proteoglycans in the vicinity of the developing fibrils have been suggested as a possible mechanism and may explain why in many instances there are simultaneous alterations in both collagen fibrils and elastic fibres.[275] Alternatively, the action of hydrolytic enzymes might be responsible for the abnormality which would thus represent a degenerative phenomenon.

Unravelled collagen fibrils

An apparent unravelling of collagen fibrils may occur in tissues, often associated with other abnormalities, such as composite morphology, variation in fibril diameter etc. In some instances this unravelling takes the form of separation of fibrils into parallel banded units approximately 20 nm in diameter (so called 'microfibrils') whereas in other instances fibrils dissociate into even finer filaments with no obvious banding ('microfilaments'). Again it is not known whether this change in collagen represents an abnormality in synthesis or a degradative phenomenon. Unravelled fibrils have been described in Marfan's syndrome,[229] spondyloepiphyseal dysplasia,[31] hyalinosis cutis et mucosae,[105] amyloidosis,[56,103] tuberous sclerosis,[163] solar elastosis,[171] ocular pterygia and pinguecula,[6] Ehlers Danlos type I,[126] arthritis,[59] sclerema neonatorum[205] and a variety of experimental situations.[157,229]

Hieroglyphic fibrils

Like composite fibrils, these are composed of loosely aggregated, spiralled subunits, but they differ on transverse section, appearing as small twisted ribbons. These fibrils have been described in dermatosparactic sheep, cattle, cats and dogs,[51,75,99,123,127,200] and represent the structural consequence of a molecular defect in these animals, namely, a deficiency of the procollagen peptidase enzyme which is responsible for cleaving the amino terminal propeptide of type I collagen (see Table 5.5).

Spiny collagen

The term 'spiny collagen' was used by Banfield et al,[9] to refer to collagen fibrils in myocardium with electron-dense granules regularly attached to the periodic bands producing a beaded appearance. This change has also been observed in vitro in numerous experimental animals and in human neoplasms,[49,72,87,97,208,217,232,262,303] but the nature of the electron-dense granules and the significance of this change are obscure.

ELASTIN

To the electron microscopist, normal mature elastic fibres have two distinct components representing two different proteins. The main component, elastin, appears as an amorphous material of variable electron density, possibly dependent upon the age of the elastic tissue. Since mature elastic tissue is relatively electron-lucent, various techniques have been suggested to enhance the contrast of elastin — including fixation in solutions containing tannic acid,[50] or staining with silver tetraphenylporphine sulphonate.[1] Special techniques using SEM and negative contrast are said to show a fibrillary substructure with filaments about 2.5 nm in diameter not visible in routine TEM.[96] Within and around this material are aggregates of electron-dense fibrils, of the order of 11–14 nm in diameter. Morphologically similar fibrils unassociated with amorphous material occur in skin at the dermo-epidermal junction as well as in ligaments, tendons and other sites and are referred to as oxytalan fibrils. Another group of structurally similar fibrils associated with a small amount of elastin are seen in the skin, connecting oxytalan fibrils to the elastic fibres of the reticular dermis, and are referred to as elaunin fibrils. It has been postulated that the three groups of fibrils represent different stages in the development of elastic tissue, the amorphous component being progressively laid down around the fibrillar template; however, it has not been definitely established that the three different fibril types are identical, and, indeed, their exact chemical composition is unknown. When examined by SEM, elastic fibres appear as smooth-surfaced cords or ribbons assembled into a continuous network. In the skin, this mesh-like arrangement can be easily demonstrated by SEM studies after autoclaving. The process destroys collagen and other tissues and enables the elastic tissue architecture to be examined.[274]

In some diseases involving elastic tissue, the molecular defect is well delineated, but in most instances the exact biochemical abnormality is not known and the group of disorders is categorized according to quantitative or qualitative changes in the elastic content. Very often that change can be demonstrated on light microscopic examination, and the ultrastructural abnormalities, while providing supportive morphological evidence, are not diagnostic in themselves. Electron microscopic abnormalities seen in elastic tissue in various hereditary and acquired conditions are summarized in Table 5.4 (see also Figs 5.4 & 5.5).

OTHER CONNECTIVE TISSUE COMPONENTS

Numerous filamentous structures, other than those readily identifiable as collagenous or elastic, occur in the extracellular matrix. They vary in size from 2–3 nm to 20 nm and some can be related to intrinsic matrix components including proteoglycans, fibronectin,[68–70,216,247,270] or non-striated interstitial collagen fibrils. Other fibrillar or tubular structures have been associated with various pathological circumstances[36,164,176] including amyloidosis. In addition to all these, however, there are many filamentous structures occurring in tissues whose identity cannot be established on ultrastructural features alone.

Proteoglycan molecules

Proteoglycans are complex macromolecules consisting of a core of protein to which is bound a variety of complex carbohydrate structures (glycosaminoglycans). They appear to play a role in cell–cell and cell–matrix interactions and in salt and water distribution. By TEM proteoglycans are extremely variable in shape and morphology (Figs 5.1 to 5.3), presumably undergoing distortion during preparation procedures. Special techniques including ruthenium red staining[64] have been employed to facilitate their demonstration. They appear as round, oval or stellate non-membrane-bound structures measuring 25–60 nm in maximum extent in most connective tissues, but are most abundant in the matrix of hyaline articular cartilage. They may be seen in a variety of neoplasms, notably chondrosarcoma.[87]

Spherical microparticles

This term is used to describe extracellular 40–100 nm diameter particles and membrane-bound vesicles, of variable electron density, found in or adjacent to the basement membrane. They are likely to be derived by budding from the cell membrane or as a degenerative change in cells or cell processes and hence are of cellular rather than stromal origin. First described in tissue culture fluids, they have since been seen in a variety of circumstances, sometimes in association with virus particles.[53,189] There have been several reports of spherical microparticles in the kidney (see Ch. 17)[10,28,30,42,43,58,117,118,135,179,202,225,241,255,302] as well as in the heart, arteries and other tissues.[74,120,175]

Ferrans et al[74] have suggested that the shedding of spherical microparticles is part of the process of cell surface remodelling but that the process may be greatly exaggerated with increasing age and in various pathological circumstances.

Matrix vesicles and calcifying bodies

Structures similar in morphology and probably also in origin to spherical microparticles are found in the matrix

Table 5.4 Ultrastructural alterations in elastic tissue*

Disease	Elastic tissue alteration	References
A. Inherited connective tissue diseases[126]		
Buschke–Ollendorff	Branched elastic fibres,	277
	clumps of electron-dense	47
	material with fibrillar coating	
Cutis laxa (dominant	Thick elastic fibres,	94
and recessive)	increased electron density;	
	irregular globular fibres;	180
	deficient elastin adjacent to	231
	amorphous electron-dense	26
	material; thin bundles of	104
	fibres; separation of micro-	
	fibrillar and elastin	170
	components	
(X-linked)	Unaltered	32
Ehlers–Danlos type I		
Adult	Fragmented or unaltered	126
		240
		284
Infant	Excessive microfibrils	126
Ehlers–Danlos type II	Fragmented variably stained, excessive amount or	240
	unaltered	126
Ehlers–Danlos type III	Unaltered	240
Ehlers–Danlos type IV	Excessive relative amount;	125
	fragmented, with inclusions	126
Ehlers–Danlos type V	Fragmented or irregular	240
		77
Ehlers–Danlos type VI	Electron-dense elastin or unaltered	126
Ehlers–Danlos type VII	Small irregular unevenly stained fibres or large and	294
	unaltered	284
Ehlers–Danlos type IX	Elastic fibres unaltered	34, 35, 125, 126, personal observations (Anton-Lamprecht)
Elastosis perforans serpiginosa	Large branched fibres, excessive microfibrils and other smaller filaments	286
Marfan's syndrome	Frayed fibres containing	269
	cystic areas, increased osmiophilia	230
Pseudoxanthoma	Large irregular fibres,	80
elasticum	granular elastin containing	224
	electron-dense inclusions,	77
	focal calcification	102
B. Acquired conditions affecting elastic tissue		
Actinic and senile elastosis	Irregular electron-dense	169
	inclusions in elastin;	272
	initially increased numbers	18
	of enlarged microfibrils, later diminished microfibrillar	275
	component, cystic spaces and fragmentation	
Anetoderma	Fragmented thin irregular	201
	fibres, paucity of elastin	281
Diabetes mellitus	Disruption, splitting and granular degeneration	19
Diverticular disease	Elastic tissue deposits between muscle of taeniae coli	293
Elastoderma	Electron-dense material associated with elastic fibres	275
Elastofibroma	Granular aggregates	8
	of electron-dense material	288
		295
		192
Myxoedema	Variable fibre diameter and diminished microfibrils	181
Ocular pterygia and pinguecula	Electron-dense inclusions, degeneration	6
Pancreatitis	Fragmentation of fibres in elastic lamina	110
Raynaud's syndrome	Elastin of variable density associated with granulofibrillar material; randomly arranged microfibrils	279
Relapsing polychondritis	Fragmentation of fibres	60
Penicillamine therapy	Diminished or increased, abnormal coating	107
PUVA therapy	Fragmentation of fibres	300

*Part A has been modified from Holbrook & Byers.[126]

of cartilage of various types, and from differing sites, in man and various animals. They may appear as vesicular structures bounded by a trilaminar membrane but more usually have a solid appearance. Their lipid nature has resulted in terms such as 'matrical lipidic debris', 'osmiophilic bodies' and 'extracellular lipid'. Since crystals of calcium particles are sometimes found near these structures, alternative terms ('calcifying globules', 'crystal bodies' or 'calcifying bodies') have also been used. These bodies are believed to represent at least one way in which calcification occurs, for example, in the cartilaginous growth plate,[2,3] the mineralization of dentine[148] and in various pathological lesions.[79,151,152,178,219,228,238] Calcium salts can also be seen in other situations, both intracellularly and in the stroma where they appear as electron-dense fine particles, needles or sheets between collagen fibrils. In the dermis, mineralization of collagen fibrils may occur in hyalin,[105] and amyloid[56] accumulations. In other circumstances calcium salts may be deposited in elastic fibres, notably in the genetic disorder pseudoxanthoma elasticum (Fig. 5.5). In this disease, electron-dense deposits of calcium crystals appear within the elastin component, around the elastic fibre or related to collagen fibrils.[67,203,224] Identical deposits can also be seen in saltpetre-induced cutaneous lesions, following calcium chloride contact and in some examples of atherosclerosis and metastatic calcification.[140,203,278,299]

PART 2
SPECIFIC DISORDERS OF CONNECTIVE TISSUE
Ingrun Anton-Lamprecht

Connective tissue disorders such as Ehlers–Danlos syndrome, osteogenesis imperfecta, Marfan's syndrome, cutis laxa, or pseudoxanthoma elasticum are due to mutations of genes involved in the synthesis or post-translational modification of collagen proteins, microfibrils, or elastin, or in the synthesis and/or regulation of matrix constituents. In only a few of the disorders is the underlying basic abnormality known.

Ehlers–Danlos syndrome (EDS)

Skin hyperextensibility and fragility, easy bruising with formation of cigarette paper scars, joint hypermobility, and muscle weakness are common features to the various types of this heterogeneous syndrome. At present, 10 genetic types can be differentiated (Table 5.5). They share ultrastructural changes of collagen fibrils (Fig. 5.1), partly associated with disturbances of regular bundle formation and thus tissue architecture, and partly with changes and abnormalities in the extrafibrillar matrix constituents (Fig. 5.1F). Changes of elastic fibres are found in some types only[126,129] and are probably signs of secondary effects from interaction with matrix components. Thus, in general, Ehlers–Danlos syndrome (EDS) genotypes seem to be expressions of mutations affecting the primary protein structure of collagen chains or their post-translational processing to the final collagen fibrils.[34,35,212]

Biochemical defects have been identified, or are assumed,

for EDS types IV, V, VI, VII, IX and X (Table 5.5); in type X the defect is not directly related to collagen and its biosynthesis but is the result of interaction with one of the matrix glycoproteins, fibronectin. Chromosome 8 bears a gene (FNZ) responsible for fibronectin binding; a structural gene for fibronectin (gene locus FN1) is mapped to chromosome 2. EDS types II and IV may be linked to chromosome 2 (gene locus COL3A1), and type VII (like one type of Marfan's syndrome and type IV osteogenesis imperfecta) to chromosome 7 (gene locus COL1A2).[85] Types V and IX are linked to the X-chromosome, though the significance of defective lysyl oxidase in both types is still questioned.[35,212]

Holbrook & Byers[126,129] have stressed that collagen changes — such as composite collagen fibrils (flowers) and ropes of unravelled collagen; variable (larger and smaller than normal) diameters; serrated and irregular contours — are non-specific and are not suited to identify single types of EDS. They may also occur in other types of connective tissue disorders of genetic and non-genetic origin (compare Figs 5.1 and 5.2). However, Holbrook & Byers[129] agree that different *patterns* in the presence and combination of these ultrastructural abnormalities exist in different types of EDS and may be helpful in identifying a given type. In our personal experience this is especially true for the three most frequent dominant types, I–III, for which the underlying biochemical abnormalities are still unknown. Differentiation of EDS types I and II at the ultrastructural level is shown in Fig. 5.1. The most important criteria are outlined in the legends and in Table 5.5.

Possibilities for prenatal diagnosis of EDS have been discussed by Byers & Wenstrup[34] and Byers et al.[35]

Scleroedema adultorum Buschke

Collagen changes resembling those found in EDS (Fig. 5.1) occur under circumstances of connective tissue disturbances of non-genetic origin as well. Abnormalities of matrix substances, such as proteoglycans and glycosaminoglycans (GAG), predominate in these instances and are of greater diagnostic significance.

The classical Buschke type of scleroedema may occur in children (29%), adolescents (22%) and adults (49%), often following viral or bacterial infections, with a good prognosis for remission. The diabetes-associated type, with a poor prognosis, is related to chronic insulin-resistant diabetes. Both are clinically similar, with tight oedema of the neck and shoulders. Histologically, the dermis is thickened and sclerotic, with tight collagen bundles and an increase of intervening alcian blue-positive material.[108]

Ultrastructurally, collagen flowers and broad twisted ropes (Fig. 5.2, B and C) are found in sclerotic areas with tight collagen bundles. Within the oedematous areas ('fenestrations') collagen fibrils show flexures and bending (Fig. 5.2, A and D), possibly because of disturbed or incomplete cross-linking. These oedematous spaces are filled with tiny networks of matrix constituents, most probably GAG, with fine strands branching at right angles (Fig. 5.2A). During dehydration and tissue processing, water bound to proteoglycans and glycosaminoglycans is largely removed, whereas the protein and sugar moieties of these substances are nicely retained.

The matrix filaments are distinctly different in EDS type II (Fig. 5.1F), scleroedema (Fig. 5.2A), and scleromyxoedema (Fig. 5.3, A and B) indicating different biochemical molecules. Similar branching strands, probably proteoglycans, are also found in pretibial myxoedema (occurring in association with LATS-hyperthyroidism) (see Ref. 108, Fig. 28).

Scleromyxoedema Arndt–Gottron

This is another non-hereditary, acquired connective tissue disorder, often associated with monoclonal gammopathies or multiple myeloma, with pathological deposition of immunoglobulins (Fig. 5.3D), and with sclerotic skin, pachydermia and lichenoid papules. Increased cell proliferation in the dermis (macrophages) and deposition of alcian blue-positive substances (hyaluronic acid) are the most significant changes (Fig. 5.3, A and B). Phagocytosis of connective tissue elements such as elastic fibres (Fig. 5.3A) and the specific morphology of GAG in the intercellular spaces with bulky nodes of filamentous dark-staining material (Fig. 5.3, A and B) are diagnostically significant and demonstrated in all cases investigated by us so far.[100,260]

Cutis laxa

Cutis laxa is a descriptive term for a variety of non-related hereditary or acquired disorders of different aetiology. Skin laxity is often described as cutis laxa; it may be a predominating feature in other connective tissue disorders such as EDS (see type IX EDS, X-linked 'cutis laxa'; Table 5.5 and Ref. 35), pseudoxanthoma elasticum, or leprechaunism.[52]

In inherited and acquired cases of cutis laxa, severe disturbances of the elastic fibres are the most pronounced changes, in contrast to EDS where disturbances of collagens predominate. Dominant and recessive types of inherited cutis laxa exist, with different types of disturbances of normal elastogenesis and ultrastructure.[126,129,276] Separation of elastotubules (oxytalan fibrils)[77] and elastin, and excessive amounts of elastotubules (Fig. 5.4) are typical findings in inherited cases of cutis laxa.

Collagen changes may also be found in these cases occasionally; they reflect the delicate interactions of the various connective tissue constituents with each other and are probably less specific.[129]

Acquired cutis laxa is frequently secondary to immunopathies with Bence–Jones paraproteinemia due to plasmacytomas.[57,104,195,285] The pattern of disturbances is much more complex, including destruction and phagocyto-

sis of elastic (and collagen) fibres, and systemic (AL) amyloidosis (see Fig. 5.6 C–E).

Pseudoxanthoma elasticum (PXE)

Although by LM this abnormality seems to be restricted to the elastic fibres, PXE is a systemic connective tissue disorder of heterogeneous origin that involves not only elastic fibres but also collagen and ground substance of the skin and the vasculature of all inner organs. Skin lesions often give the diagnostic clue to severe internal disturbances (heart, kidneys, CNS).

The first skin manifestations are yellowish xanthomatous plaques appearing during childhood or adolescence on the neck and axillae, on the elbows (flexures), and in the groins. Angioid streaks in the fundus oculi often develop before or with the first skin manifestation and generally lead to impairment of vision in the second to third decade of life, with the risk of blindness.[54,57]

PXE is heterogeneous. At least four genetic types have been identified in England:[213,214] two dominant and two recessive traits. Because severe internal manifestations (vascular abnormalities, cerebral, renal and gastrointestinal haemorrhages) mostly develop later than at reproductive age, genetic counselling of at-risk persons and affected patients is important. Early detection of affected individuals is possible from skin biopsy samples (sites of predilection) by EM before clinical and histopathological changes become evident (ref. 224; personal unpublished data). In a child with unexplained renovascular hypertension, periodic headaches and nausea, the first xanthomatous papules were recorded at the age of 7.5 years; ultrastructural examination confirmed the diagnosis of PXE, possibly of the severe, recessive type.[233]

Different degrees of elastic fibre abnormalities[54,224] are revealed in the central and peripheral parts of the lesions (Fig. 5.5, A and B). Control of various parts of tissue samples is therefore required to verify the diagnosis. The degree of calcification of the fibres (Fig. 5.5, A and C) varies largely, probably due to heterogeneity, severity, age of the patient and of the lesion, and site of the sample. Occasionally, the von Kossa stain may fail to show calcium deposition. At the EM level the following permit identification of PXE: the typical abnormalities of elastic fibres with small focal calcium deposits that are inapparent by LM; surrounding oedema of the matrix; and the changes of collagen fibrils close to abnormal elastic fibres.[57,233]

The aetiology and pathogenesis of PXE are still unclear.[54,276] Molecular defects of the elastin molecule might underlie dominant PXE types, whereas enzymes participating in its synthesis, processing, and degradation might be defective in the recessive PXE types.[276] It has been shown that PXE elastic fibres contain high amounts of abnormal proteoglycans. Secretion of excessive amounts of a serine proteinase, as demonstrated for cultured PXE fibro-

Table 5.5   Differential diagnosis of Ehlers–Danlos syndrome (EDS)

Type	Name	Inheritance	Frequency (%)	Clinical features	Biochemical defect[a]	Ultrastructural abnormalities[b]
EDS I	Gravis	AD	40	Marked skin hyperextensibility, bruising, and fragility; poor wound healing; cigarette-paper scars, molluscoid pseudotumours; hernia; joint hypermobility and frequent dislocations; risk of miscarriage	Unknown	Thickened dermis; pronounced variation in shape and diameter of collagen fibrils, irregular sizes and contours, extensive dense aggregations, bizarre flowers and broad irregular ropes of unravelled collagen, most pronounced in central reticular dermis; disorganized bundles, collagen-free matrix
EDS II	Mitis (chromosome 2?)	AD	30	Moderate skin hyperextensibility and bruising; moderate joint hypermobility, milder than in type I	Unknown; excessive matrix production?	Flower-like collagen fibrils and large fragmented ropes of unravelled collagen with normal banding periodicity among normal collagen fibrils; increase of matrix substances (proteoglycans? glycosaminoglycans?) in form of deep-staining irregular strands and filaments in a branched network
EDS III	Benign hypermobility type	AD	~12	Marked large and small joint hypermobility, mild skin extensibility, soft skin, often hypotonic musculature	Unknown	Isolated collagen flowers; smaller ropes of incompletely cross-linked unravelled collagen; excessive flocculent or fuzzy material
EDS IV	Ecchymotic type (chromosome 2?)	AD AR	~6	Thin and translucent skin, easy bruising, marked ecchymosis with minimal trauma; not hyperextensible except acral joints; bowel and arterial ruptures frequent; risk of uterine rupture in late pregnancy	Defective structure or synthesis of type III collagen or defective secretion	Thinned dermis overall; small collagen fibril diameters, variable diameter fibrils with irregular contours; excessive diffuse matrix; excessive amounts of branched or fragmented elastic fibres; fibroblasts with distended ER cisternae filled with type III collagen

EDS V	X-linked type (X-chromosome)	XR	~4	Hyper-elastic, easily bruising skin (similar to type II); heart valve prolapse	Lysyl oxidase deficiency in some patients	Variable collagen fibril diameters, flowers and serrated cross sections
EDS VI	Ocular type	AR	~2	Hyperextensibility of skin, cigarette-paper scars; haematomas; hypermobile joints and bone deformities (kyphoscoliosis), muscular weakness and hypotonus; ocular fragility, ruptures of sclerae and cornea, keratoconus, microcornea, glaucoma	Lysyl hydroxylase deficiency, lack of hydroxylysine	Large-diameter collagen fibrils; collagen flowers; poorly organized and small bundles; excessive diffuse matrix
EDS VII	Arthrochalasis multiplex congenita (chromosome 7)	AD	~3	Marked joint hypermobility and dislocations (congenital hip dislocation)	Defective cleavage of procollagen: amino acid substitution near NH_2 terminal cleavage site of proα2(1)	Irregularly shaped collagen fibrils, variable diameters
	Dermatosparaxis in animals	AR		Easily bruising skin in animals	NH_2 terminal protease deficiency; accumulation of procollagen	Hieroglyphic-shaped fibrils, poorly organized, in dermatosparactic animals
EDS VIII	Periodontitis type	AD	?	Extensive periodontal destruction, early loss of teeth; skin fragility marked, minimal skin extensibility; cigarette-paper scars	Unknown	Variable diameters of collagen fibrils; elastic fibres unaltered
EDS IX	X-linked cutis laxa (X-chromosome)	XR	?	Soft skin, mild laxity, long thin facies, abnormalities of bones, obstructive uropathy (bladder rupture)	Decreased lysyl oxidase activity due to abnormal copper utilization with multiple enzyme abnormalities	Large-diameter collagen fibrils, collagen flowers, excessive density of collagen fibre bundles; elastic fibres unaltered
EDS X	Platelet dysfunction type (chromosome 8?)	AR	?	Thin skin, easily bruising, mild joint hypermobility; defective platelet aggregation	Defective ability of fibronectin to bind to platelets; fibronectin defect	Collagen flowers, altered packing of collagen fibrils into fibre bundles

[a]Summarized according to Byers & Wenstrup,[34] Byers et al.[35] and Pinnell.[212]
[b]Summarized according to Holbrook & Byers[126,129] and personal data.
AD = Autosomal Dominant
AR = Autosomal Recessive
XR = Sex-linked

blasts, is thought to be responsible for degradation of high-molecular-weight proteoglycans; their products, like abnormal polyanionic molecules bound to elastic fibres, could trigger calcification via binding of inorganic phosphate to elastin and subsequent precipitation of calcium in the form of apatite crystals (Fig. 5.5, A and C).[77,276,289] Abnormalities of the matrix composition and presence of abnormal proteoglycans would also explain the regular presence of lesional collagen abnormalities.

Amyloidosis

Amyloidosis is characterized by the extracellular accumulation of fibrillar proteins with characteristic tinctorial properties including congophilia with green birefringence on polarization microscopy. In most types of amyloid the protein fibrils are characterized by having a serum precursor,[45] a high degree of anti-parallel beta-sheet conformation on X-ray diffraction analysis,[17,62,89] and a distinctive ultrastructure. Under the electron microscope the fibrils are composed of a generally haphazard arrangement of rigid non-branching filaments ('fibrils') of indeterminate length but measuring 7–10 nm in diameter.[46,242,292] In some instances the filaments aggregate laterally to form fibrils of up to 40 nm in diameter. Special techniques reveal the filaments to consist of two or more protofilaments 3–4 nm in diameter, not visualized in routine plastic-embedded sections.[87]

In addition to the characteristic protein fibrils, a minor second component is always present in amyloid, known as the 'amyloid P component' (AP). This appears ultrastructurally as a pentagonal, doughnut-shaped body measuring 8 nm in diameter,[15,40,244] and is composed of the normal serum alpha-1 glycoprotein.[13,20] Other mucopolysaccharide and glycosaminoglycan residues, as well as lipids, fibrinogen and complement may also be associated with some types of amyloid.

Amyloid deposits can occur in a great variety of pathological circumstances in a localized or systemic distribution. The pathological typing of amyloid is related to the clinical setting and an identification of the component protein; amyloids are now classified according to the various precursor proteins from which they originate[119] (Table 5.6). Immuno-electron microscopy has contributed significantly to the identification and classification of amyloid.[177]

Primary and secondary amyloidoses differ in the mode of amyloid distribution, the kind of deposition, and in organ involvement. In primary systemic amyloidosis, amyloid is formed by immunoglobulin light chains,[92] most often due to multiple myeloma, and occasionally to other gammopathies, plasmacytoma, or Waldenström's macroglobulinaemia (light chain or AL amyloidosis). Light chains may be of the kappa[285] or of the lambda type (Fig. 5.6, C–E).

Secondary systemic amyloidoses most often follow chronic inflammatory disorders (e.g. rheumatoid diseases) or chronic infections (lepromatous leprosy; tuberculosis) and are caused by the deposition of protein AA, derived from a serum precursor SAA which is a normal serum alphaglobulin. Chronic inflammation increases the amount of this serum component. Biochemically, amyloid A is completely different from immunoglobulins. The distribution of its deposition also differs from that of AL amyloidosis involving multiple organs, particularly kidney, liver, spleen, adrenals, pancreas and lymph nodes. The skin is often clinically unremarkable though amyloid may be demonstrable in biopsies (see ref. 108 for a review). Cutaneous nodular amyloidosis with systemic involvement[93a] probably belongs to secondary systemic or protein AA amyloidosis (Fig. 5.6F).

The cutaneous forms, lichen amyloidosis and macular amyloidosis, differ clinically, though they are said to be identical by LM and EM. In these conditions the amyloid filaments (amyloid K)[119] are assumed to originate from keratin filaments of epidermal keratinocytes (Fig. 5.6B) in a sequence of degenerative and transforming steps;[165] immunoglobulins may be trapped in this sponge-like material. In skin disorders with inflammatory reactions or with a ten-

Table 5.6 Stromal amyloid in disease

Nomenclature	Clinical disorder	Chemical composition	References
Systemic amyloidosis			
AL	Primary; myeloma-associated amyloid	Kappa or lambda immunoglobulin light chains	90,91,197,248
AA	Secondary amyloid; familial Mediterranean fever	Unique 18 500 dalton protein 'amyloid A'	95,112,134,174 249,250,287
AF	Familial amyloid, e.g. AF$_p$ (Portuguese) etc	Normal and variant pre-albumins in some types	61,194,215,290
AH (AβM)	Haemodialysis-associated amyloid	β2-Microglobulin	38,86,146,166,243
Localized amyloidosis			
AE	Endocrine-tissue-related amyloid, e.g. medullary carcinoma of thyroid*	Calcitonin or precalcitonin	251
	Pancreatic islets in type II diabetes mellitus	Protein unidentified	44
	Pituitary adenoma	Growth hormone	188
AS	Senile amyloid: heart, ASc$_1$	Pre-albumin	237.252
	brain ASb$_1$	?Pre-albumin, ?other	93,136,239,245
AD (AK)	Cutaneous (dermal) amyloid	Keratin-related	160,165

*Amyloid deposits may occasionally also be seen in association with a variety of other neoplasms.[111]

dency to lichenification, amyloid may be demonstrable in the papillary dermis (Fig. 5.6A). It has been stressed until now[108] that the various forms of amyloid are ultrastructurally identical. However, by comparing parts A, B, C–E and F of Fig. 5.6 it is evident that the heterogeneity of the various amyloids is also reflected in ultrastructural differences of their microfilaments.

REFERENCES

1. Albert E N, Fleischer E 1970 A new electron dense stain for elastic tissue. Journal of Histochemistry and Cytochemistry 18: 697–708
2. Ali S Y, Sajdera S W, Anderson H C 1970 Isolation and characterization of calcifying matrix vesicles from epiphyseal cartilage. Proceedings of the National Academy of Sciences of the USA 67: 1513–1520
3. Anderson H C 1969 Vesicles associated with calcification in the matrix of epiphyseal cartilage. Journal of Cell Biology 41: 59–72
4. Archer-Harvey J M, Henderson D W, Papadimitriou J M, Rozenbilds, M A M 1984 Pigmented villonodular synovitis associated with psoriatic polyarthropathy: an electron microscopic and immunocytochemical study. Journal of Pathology 144: 57–68
5. Arem A J, Kischer C W 1980 Analysis of striae. Plastic and Reconstructive Surgery 65: 22–29
6. Austin P, Jakobiec F A, Iwamoto T 1983 Elastodysplasia and elastodystrophy as the basis of ocular pterygia and pinguecula. Ophthalmology 90: 96–109
7. Bairati A, Petruccioli M G, Pernis B 1967 Ultrastruttura e natura del tessuto fibroso ialino postumo al granuloma da adiuvante di Freund II. Indagini al microscopio elettronico. Bolletino-Società, Italiana Biologia Sperimentale 43: 1443–1444
8. Banfield W G, Lee C K 1968 Elastofibroma. An electron microscopic study. Journal of the National Cancer Institute 40: 1067–1077
9. Banfield W G, Lee C K, Lee C W 1973 Myocardial collagen of the fibrous long spacing type. Archives of Pathology 95: 262–266
10. Bariety J, Callard P 1975 Striated membranous structures in renal glomerular tufts: an electron microscopy study of 340 human renal biopsies. Laboratory Investigation 32: 636–641
11. Bhawan J, Edelstein L M 1976 Banded structure in cellular blue naevus. Archives of Dermatology 112: 1176–1177
12. Bhawan I, Edelstein L M 1977 Angiofibromas in tuberous sclerosis: a light and electron microscopic study. Journal of Cutaneous Pathology 4: 300–307
13. Binette P, Binette M, Calkins E 1974 The isolation and identification of the P-component of normal human plasma proteins. Biochemical Journal 143: 253–254
14. Black C M, Cathercole L J, Bailey A J, Beighton P 1980 The Ehlers–Danlos syndrome: an analysis of the structure of the collagen fibres of the skin. British Journal of Dermatology 102: 85–96
15. Bladen H A, Nylen M U, Glenner G G 1966 The ultrastructure of human amyloid as revealed by the negative staining technique. Journal of Ultrastructure Research 14: 449–459
16. Bohmig R 1928 Uber die kataplastischen Veranderungen im menschlichen Rippenknorpel. Beitrage zur pathologischen Anatomie und zur allgemeinen Pathologie 81: 172–210
17. Bonar L C, Cohen A S, Skinner M 1969 Characterization of the amyloid fibril as a cross-beta protein. Proceedings of the Society for Experimental Biology and Medicine 131: 1373–1375
18. Braverman I M, Fonferko E 1982 Studies in cutaneous aging. I. The elastic fibre network. Journal of Investigative Dermatology 78: 434–443
19. Braverman I M Keh-Yen A 1984 Ultrastructural abnormalities of the microvasculature and elastic fibres in the skin of juvenile diabetics. Journal of Investigative Dermatology 82: 270–274
20. Breathnach S M, Bhogal B, Dyck R F, DeBeer F C, Black M M, Pepys M B 1981 Immunohistochemical demonstration of amyloid P component in skin of normal subjects and patients with cutaneous amyloidosis. British Journal of Dermatology 105: 115–124
21. Briggaman R A, Dalldorf F G, Wheeler C E 1971 Formation and origin of basal lamina and anchoring fibrils in adult human skin. Journal of Cell Biology 51: 384–395
22. Briggaman R A, Wheeler C E 1968 Epidermal–dermal interactions in adult human skin: role of dermis in epidermal maintenance. Journal of Investigative Dermatology 51: 454–465
23. Briggaman R A, Wheeler C E 1975 Epidermolysis bullosa dystrophica-recessive: a possible role of anchoring fibrils in the pathogenesis. Journal of Investigative Dermatology 65: 203–211
24. Briggaman R A, Wheeler C E 1975 The epidermal–dermal junction. Journal of Investigative Dermatology 65: 71–84
25. Brody I 1960 The ultrastructure of the tonofibrils in the keratinization process of normal human epidermis. Journal of Ultrastructure Research 4: 264–297
26. Brown F R III, Holbrook K A, Byers P H, Stewart D, Dean J, Pyeritz R E 1982 Cutis laxa. Johns Hopkins Medical Journal 150: 148–153
27. Bruns R R, Press W, Engvall R, Gross J 1986 Type VI collagen in extracellular, 100 nm periodic filaments and fibrils: identification by immuno electron microscopy. Journal of Cell Biology 103: 393–404
28. Busch G J, Galvanek E G, Reynolds E S Jr 1971 Human renal allografts: analysis of lesions in long term survivors. Human Pathology 2: 253–298
29. Burgeson R E 1987 The collagens of skin. Current Problems in Dermatology 17: 61–75
30. Burkholder P M, Hyman L R, Barber T A 1973 Extracellular clusters of spherical microparticles in glomeruli in human renal glomerular disease. Laboratory Investigation 28: 415–425
31. Byers P H, Holbrook K A, Chandler J W, Bornstein P, Hall J G 1978 Electron microscopy as an aid to diagnosis of the extracellular matrix: a new type of spondyloepiphyseal dysplasia. Birth Defects Original Article Series 14 (6B): 221–232
32. Byers P H, Siegel R C, Holbrook K A, Narayanan A S, Bornstein P, Hall J G 1980 X-linked cutis laxa. Defective cross-link formation in collagen due to decreased lysyl oxidase activity. New England Journal of Medicine 303: 61–65
33. Byers P H, Siegel R C, Peterson K E, Rowe D W, Holbrook K A, Smith L T, Change Y H, Fu J C 1981 Marfan syndrome: abnormal alpha 2 chain in Type 1 collagen. Proceedings of the National Academy of Sciences 78: 7745–7749
34. Byers P H, Wenstrup R J 1984 Prenatal diagnosis of inherited connective tissue disorders. Seminars in Dermatology 3: 257–264
35. Byers P H, Wenstrup R J, Bonadio J F, Starman B, Cohn D H 1987 Molecular basis of inherited disorders of collagen biosynthesis: implications for prenatal diagnosis. Current Problems in Dermatology 16: 158–174
36. Camilleri J-P, Phat V N, Bruneval P, Tricottet V, Balaton A, Fiessinger J-N, Cormier J-M 1985 Surface healing and histologic maturation of patent polytetrafluoroethylene grafts implanted in patients for up to 60 months. Archives of Pathology and Laboratory Medicine 109: 833–837
37. Caputo R, Peluchetti D 1977 The junctions of normal human epidermis: a freeze–fracture study. Journal of Ultrastructure Research 61: 44–61
38. Casey T T, Stone W J, Di Raimondo C R, Brantley B D, Di Raimondo C V, Gorevic P D, Page D L 1986 Tumoral amyloidosis of bone of beta-2-microglobulin origin in association with long-term haemodialysis: a new type of amyloid disease. Human Pathology 17: 731–738
39. Caterson B, Baker J R, Christens J E, Couchman J R 1982 Immunologic methods for the detection and determination of connective tissue proteoglycans. Journal of Investigative Dermatology 79 (suppl 1): 45s–50s
40. Cathcart E S, Comerford F R, Cohen A S 1965 Immunologic studies on a protein extracted from human secondary amyloid. New England Journal of Medicine 273: 143–146
41. Chiricosta A, Jindal S L, Metuzals J, Koch B 1970 Hereditary nephropathy with haematuria (Alport's syndrome). Canadian Medical Association Journal 102: 396–340

42. Chung E B, Enzinger F M 1975 Proliferative fasciitis. Cancer 36: 1450–1458
43. Churg J, Sherman R L 1973 Pathologic characteristics of hereditary nephritis. Archives of Pathology 95: 374–379
44. Clark A, Holman R P, Matthews D R, Hockaday T D R, Turner R C 1984 Non-uniform distribution of islet amyloid in the pancreas of 'maturity onset' diabetic patients. Diabetologia 27: 527–528
45. Cohen A S, Connors L H 1987 The pathogenesis and biochemistry of amyloidosis. Journal of Pathology 151: 1–10
46. Cohen A S, Shirahama T 1973 Electron microscopic analysis of isolated amyloid fibrils from patients with primary, secondary and myeloma-associated disease. A study utilizing shadowing and negative staining techniques. Israel Journal of Medical Sciences 9: 849–856
47. Cole G W, Barr R J 1982 An elastic tissue defect in dermatofibrosis lenticularis disseminata. Buschke–Ollendorff syndrome. Archives of Dermatology 118: 44–46
48. Cornah M S, Meachim G, Parry E W 1970 Banded structures in the matrix of human and rabbit nucleus pulposus. Journal of Anatomy 107: 351–362
49. Cornell R 1969 Spontaneous neoplastic transformation in vitro. Ultrastructure of transformed cell strains and tumours produced by injection of cell strains. Journal of the National Cancer Institute 43: 891–906
50. Cotta-Periera G, Guerra Rodrigo F, Bittencourt-Sampaio S 1976 Oxytalan, elaunin and elastic fibres in the human skin. Journal of Investigative Dermatology 66: 143–148
51. Counts D F, Byers P H, Holbrook K A, Hegreberg G A 1980 Dermatosparaxis in a Himalayan cat: I. Biochemical studies of dermal collagen. Journal of Investigative Dermatology 74: 96–99
52. Dallaire L, Cantin M, Melançon S B, Perreault G, Potier M 1976 A syndrome of generalized elastic fiber deficiency with leprechaunoid features: a distinct genetic disease with an autosomal recessive mode of inheritance. Clinical Genetics 10: 1–11
53. Dalton A J 1975 Microvesicles and vesicles of the multivesicular bodies versus 'virus-like' particles. Journal of the National Cancer Institute 54: 1137–1148
54. Danielsen L 1979 Morphological changes in pseudoxanthoma elasticum and senile skin. Acta Dermato-venereologica Supplement 83
55. Danielsen L, Kobayasi T 1972 Degeneration of dermal elastic fibres in relation to age and light exposure. Preliminary report on electron microscopic studies. Acta Dermato-venereologica 52: 1–10
56. Danielsen L, Kobayasi T 1973 An ultrastructural study of cutaneous amyloidosis. Acta Dermato-venereologica 53: 13–21
57. Daróczy J, Rácz I 1987 Diagnostic electron microscopy in practical dermatology. Adademiai Kiado, Budapest
58. Deodhar S D, McCormack L J, Osborne D, Gifford R W 1973 Unusual ultrastructural and immunologic findings in a case of membranous glomerular disease with renal vein thrombosis. Proceedings of the 31st Annual Electron Microscopic Society of America Meeting, pp 418
59. Dorwart B B, Schumacher H R 1981 Arthritis in β thalassaemia trait: clinical and pathological features. Annals of the Rheumatic Diseases 40: 185–189
60. Dryle A, Lansaman J, Meyer O, Bardin T, Ryckewaert A 1981 Relapsing polychondritis. An ultrastructural study of elastic and collagen fibres degradation revealed by tannic acid. Virchows Archiv A, Pathological Anatomy Histopathology 390: 109–119
61. Dwulet F E, Benson M D 1983 Polymorphism of human plasma thyroxine binding prealbumin. Biochemical and Biophysical Research Communications 114: 657–662
62. Eanes E D, Glenner G G 1968 X-ray diffraction studies on amyloid filaments. Journal of Histochemistry and Cytochemistry 16: 673–677
63. Edwards R P 1975 Long spacing collagen in skin biopsies of patients with lepromatous leprosy. British Journal of Dermatology 93: 175–182
64. Eisenstein R, Sorgente N, Kuettner K E 1971 Organization of extracellular matrix in epiphyseal growth plate. Americal Journal of Pathology 65: 515–534
65. El-Labban N G, Harris M, Hopper C, Barber P 1986 Amianthoid fibres in muscle tissue associated with temporomandibular joint ankylosis. Ultrastructural Pathology 10: 571–576
66. Emura I, Yanagisawa S, Ohnishi Y 1977 FLS-like fibril in two autopsy cases of so called immunoblastic lymphadenopathy. Igaku No Ayumi 101: 644–645
67. Eng A M, Bryant J 1975 Clinical pathological observations in pseudoxanthoma elasticum. International Journal of Dermatology 14: 586–605
68. Engel J, Odermatt E, Engel A, Madri J A, Furthmayr H, Rohde H, Timpl R 1981 Shapes, domain organizations and flexibility of laminin and fibronectin, two multifunctional proteins of the extra cellular matrix. Journal of Molecular Biology 150: 97–120
69. Erickson H P, Carrell N, McDonagh J 1981 Fibronectin molecule visualized in electron microscopy: a long thin flexible strand. Journal of Cell Biology 91: 673–678
70. Erickson H P, Carrell N A 1983 Fibronectin in extended and compact conformations. Electron microscopy and sedimentation analysis. Journal of Biological Chemistry 258: 14 539–14 544
71. Fabre M-Th, Duret J Cl, Brousset A, Buisson H 1968 Ultrastructure du derme dans le syndrome de Marfan. Presse Medicale 76: 419–423
72. Favara B E, Johnson W, Ito J 1968 Renal tumours in the neonatal period. Cancer 22: 845–855
73. Faust E C, Beaver P C, Jung R C 1975 Animals, agents and vectors of human disease, 4th edn. Lea and Febiger, Philadelphia, pp 118–121
74. Ferrans V J, Thiedemann K-U, Jones M, Robert W C 1976 Spherical microparticles in human myocardium. An ultrastructural study. Laboratory Investigation 35: 349–368
75. Fjølstad M, Helle O 1974 A hereditary dysplasia of collagen tissues in sheep. Journal of Pathology 112: 183–188
76. Fleischmajer R, Krieg T, Dziadek M, Altchek D, Timpl R 1984 Ultrastructure and composition of connective tissue in hyalinosis cutis et mucosae of skin. Journal of Investigative Dermatology 82: 252–258
77. Frances C, Robert L 1984 Elastin and elastic fibres in normal and pathologic skin. International Journal of Dermatology 23: 166–179
78. Friedman I, Cawthorne T, Bird E S 1965 The laminated cytoplasmic inclusions in the sensory epithelium of the human macula. Journal of Ultrastructure Research 12: 92–103
79. Friedmann I, Galey F R 1980 Initiation and stages of mineralization in tympano-sclerosis. Journal of Laryngology and Otology 94: 1215–1229
80. Fukushiro R, Fukui Y, Hirone T, Konishi Y 1972 Alterations of dermal elastic fibres in senile elastosis and pseudoxanthoma elasticum. Japanese Journal of Dermatology (A) 82: 661–666
81. Furthmayr H, Wiedemann H, Timpl R, Odermatt E, Engel J 1983 Electron-microscopical approach to a structural model of intima collagen. Biochemical Journal 211: 303–311
82. Gauthier Y, Surleve-Bazielle J-E, Gauthier O, Texier L 1973 Etude comparative ultrastructurale au comportemente du tissue collagene et du tissu elastique au cours de trois états pathologique (maladie de Marfan, sclerodermie apres vitamin K, effet lathyrogene de la penicillamine). Annales de Dermatologie et de Syphiligraphie 100: 525–529
83. Gay S, Martinez-Hernandez A, Rhodes R K, Miller E J 1981 The collagenous exocytoskeleton of smooth muscle cells. Collagen and Related Research 1: 377–384
84. Gay S, Miller E J 1983 What is collagen, what is not? Ultrastructural Pathology 4: 365–377
85. Gedde-Dahl T Jr 1987 The human gene map and genes expressed in the skin. Current Problems in Dermatology 16: 45–64
86. Gejyo F, Yamada T, Odani S, Nakagawa Y, Arakawa M, Kunitomo T, Kataoka H, Susuki M, Hirasawa Y, Shirahama T, Cohen A S, Schmid K 1985 A new form of amyloid protein associated with chronic haemodialysis was identified as beta-2-microglobulin. Biochemical and Biophysical Research Communications 129: 701–706
87. Ghadially F N 1982 Ultrastructural pathology of the cell and matrix, 2nd edition. Butterworths, London, pp 881–947
88. Ghadially F N, Lalonde J-M A, Yong N K 1979 Ultrastructure of amianthoid fibres in osteoarthritic cartilage. Virchows Archiv Abreilung B, Cell Pathology 31: 81–86
89. Glenner G G 1980 Amyloid deposits and amyloidosis: the beta fibrilloses. New England Journal of Medicine 302: 1283–1292, 1333–1343

90. Glenner G G, Ein D, Eanes E D, Bladen H A, Terry W, Page D L 1971 Creation of 'amyloid' fibrils from Bence–Jones protein in vitro. Science 174: 712–714

91. Glenner G G, Terry W, Harada M, Isersky C, Page D 1971 Amyloid fibril proteins: proof of homology with immunoglobulin light chains by sequence analysis. Science 172: 1150–1151

92. Glenner G G, Terry W D, Isersky C 1973 Amyloidosis: its nature and pathogenesis. Seminars in Hematology 10: 65–86

93. Glenner G G, Wong C W 1984 Alzheimer's disease: initial report of the purification and characterization of a novel cerebrovascular amyloid protein. Biochemical and Biophysical Research Communications 120: 885–890

93a. Goerttler E, Anton-Lamprecht I, Kotzur B 1976 Amyloidosis cutis nodularis. Klinische, histopathologische und ultra strukturelle Befunde. Hautarzt 27: 16–25

94. Goltz R W, Hult A-M, Goldfarb M, Gorlin R J 1965 Cutis laxa. Archives of Dermatology 92: 373–387

95. Gorevic P D, Greenwald M, Frangrove B, Pras M, Franklin E C 1977 The amino acid sequence of duck amyloid A (AA) protein. Journal of Immunology 118: 1113–1118

96. Gotte L, Serafini-Fracassini A 1963 Electron microscope observations on the structure of elastin. Journal of Atherosclerosis Research 3: 247–251

97. Grimley P M, Deftos L J, Weeks J R, Rabson A S 1969 Growth in vitro and ultrastructure of cells from a medullary carcinoma of the human thyroid glands transformation by Simian Virus 40 and evidence of thyrocalcitonin and prostaglandins. Journal of the National Cancer Institute 42: 663–680

98. Hackemann M, Grubb C, Hill K R 1968 The ultrastructure of normal squamous epithelium of the human cervix uteri. Journal of Ultrastructure Research 22: 443–457

99. Hanset R, Ansay M 1967 Dermatosparaxie (peau dechieree) Chez le veau: un defaut general du tissu conjonctif, de nature hereditaire. Annales de Medecine Veterinaire 111: 451–470

100. Hardmeier T, Vogel A 1970 Electron microscopic lesions in scleromyxedema Arndt-Gottron. Archiv für klinische und experimentelle Dermatologie 237: 722–736

101. Hashimoto K 1970 The ultrastructure of the skin of human embryos V. The hair germ and perifollicular mesenchymal cells. Hair germ — mesenchyme interaction. British Journal of Dermatology 83: 167–176

102. Hashimoto K, Di Bella R J 1967 Electron microscopic studies of normal and abnormal elastic fibres of the skin. Journal of Investigative Dermatology 48: 405–423

103. Hashimoto K, Gross B G, Lever W F 1965 Lichen amyloidosus. Histochemical and electron microscopic studies. Journal of Investigative Dermatology 45: 204–219

104. Hashimoto K, Kanzaki T 1975 Cutis laxa. Ultrastructural and biochemical studies. Archives of Dermatology 111: 861–873

105. Hashimoto K, Klingmuller G, Rodermund O E 1972 Hyalinosis cutis et mucosae. An electron microscopic study. Acta Dermato-venereologica 52: 179–195

106. Hashimoto K, Lever W F 1969 Histogenesis of skin appendage tumours. Archives of Dermatology 100: 356–369

107. Hashimoto K, McEvoy B, Belcher R 1981 Ultrastructure of penicillamine induced skin lesions. Journal of the American Academy of Dermatology 4: 300–315

108. Hashimoto K, Niizuma K 1983 Skin pathology by light and electron microscopy. Igaku-Shoin, New York

109. Hashimoto K, Ohyama H 1974 Cross-banded filamentous aggregation in the human dermis. Journal of Investigative Dermatology 62: 106–112

110. Helin H, Mero M, Helin M, Markkula H 1981 Elastic tissue injury in human acute pancreatitis. Pathology Research and Practice 172: 170–175

111. Henderson D W, Papadimitriou J M, Coleman M 1986 Ultrastructural appearance of tumours, 2nd edn. Churchill Livingstone, Edinburgh, London, Melbourne, New York, pp 57–72

112. Hermodson M A, Kuhn R W, Walsh K A, Neurath H, Eriksen N, Benditt E P 1972 Amino-acid sequence of monkey amyloid-protein A. Biochemistry 11: 2934–2938

113. Hessle H, Engvall E 1984 Type VI Collagen. Studies on its localization, structure, and biosynthetic form with monoclonal antibodies. Journal of Biological Chemistry 259: 3955–3961

114. Highberger J H, Gross I, Schmitt F O 1950 Electron microscopic observations of certain fibrous structures obtained from connective tissue extracts. Journal of the American Chemical Society 72: 3321–3322

115. Highberger J H, Gross J, Schmitt F O 1951 The interaction of mucoprotein with soluble collagen: an electron microscope study. Proceedings of the National Academy of Sciences of the USA 37: 286–291

116. Hilding D A, House W F 1965 Acoustic neuroma: comparison of traumatic and neoplastic. Journal of Ultrastructure Research 12: 611–623

117. Hill J S, Jenis E H, Goodloe S Jr 1974 The non-specificity of the ultrastructural alterations in hereditary nephritis, with additional observations on benign familial haematuria. Laboratory Investigation 31: 516–531

118. Hinglais N, Grunfeld J P, Bois E 1972 Characteristic ultrastructural lesion of the glomerular basement membrane in progressive hereditary nephritis (Alport's syndrome). Laboratory Investigation 27: 473–487

119. Hintner H, Stoessl H, Hoepfl R, Grubauer G, Fritsch P 1988 Amyloid K. Hautarzt 39: 419–425

120. Hoff H H 1972 Human intracranial atherosclerosis: a histochemical and ultrastructural study of gross fatty lesions. American Journal of Pathology 69: 421–438

121. Holbrook K A, Byers P H 1978 Ultrastructural characterization of several varieties of the Ehlers–Danlos syndrome (EDS). Clinical Research 27: 570Aa

122. Holbrook K A, Odland G F 1980 Regional development of human epidermis in the first trimester embryo and the second trimester fetus. Journal of Investigative Dermatology 74: 161–168

123. Holbrook K A, Byers P H, Counts D F, Hegreberg G A 1980 Dermatosparaxis in a Himalayan cat. II. Ultrastructural studies of dermal collagen. Journal of Investigative Dermatology 74: 100–104

124. Holbrook K A, Smith L T 1981 Ultrastructural aspects of human skin during the embryonic, fetal, premature, neonatal, and adult periods of life. Birth defects original article series vol 17, no 2. March of Dimes Birth Defects Foundation. Alan R Liss, New York, pp 9–13

125. Holbrook K A, Byers P H 1981 Ultrastructural characteristics of the skin in a form of the Ehlers–Danlos syndrome Type IV. Storage in the rough endoplasmic reticulum. Laboratory Investigation 44: 342–350

126. Holbrook K A, Byers P H 1982 Structural abnormalities in the dermal collagen and elastic matrix from the skin of patients with inherited connective tissue disorders. Journal of Investigative Dermatology 79 (suppl 1): 7s–16s

127. Holbrook K A, Byers P H 1982 Structural abnormalities in the dermal collagen and elastic matrix from the skin of patients with inherited connective tissue disorders. Journal of Investigative Dermatology 79: 7s–16s

128. Holbrook K A, Byers P H, Pinnell S R 1982 The structure and function of dermal connective tissue in normal individuals and patients with inherited connective tissue disorders. Scanning Electron Microscopy (part 4): 1731–1744

129. Holbrook K A, Byers P H 1989 Skin is a window on heritable disorders of connective tissue. American Journal of Medical Genetics 34: 105–121

130. Holmberg A S 1965 Schlemm's canal and the trabecular meshwork. An electron microscopic study of the normal structure in man and monkey (Cercopithecus aethiops). Documenta Ophthalmologica (Den Haag) 19: 339–373

131. Hoshino K, Ohashi M 1981 Scanning electron microscopic studies of dermal skin and connective tissue disorders. Journal of Investigative Dermatology (Tokyo) 8: 97–107

132. Hough A J, Mottram F C, Sokoloff L 1973 The collagenous nature of amianthoid degeneration in human costal cartilage. American Journal of Pathology 73: 201–216

133. Hukins D W L, Knight D P, Woodhead-Galloway J 1976 Amianthoid change: orientation of normal collagen fibrils during aging. Science 194: 622–624

134. Husby G, Natvig J B, Sletten K, Nordstoga K, Anders R F 1975 An experimental model in mink for studying the relation between amyloid fibril protein AA and the related serum protein SAA. Scandinavian Journal of Immunology 4: 811–816

135. Hyman L R, Burkholder P M, Joo P A, Segar W E 1973 Malignant lymphoma and nephrotic syndrome. A clinico-pathologic analysis with light immunofluorescence and electron microscopy of the renal lesions. Journal of Pediatrics 82: 207–212

136. Igbal K, Zaid T, Thompson C H, Merz P A, Wisniewski H M 1984 Alzheimer paired helical filaments: bulk isolation, solubility and protein composition. Acta Neuropathologica 62: 167–177

137. Ippolito E, Postacchini F, Scola E, Bellocci M, De Martino C 1985 De Quervain's disease. An ultrastructural study. International Orthopaedics 9: 41–47

138. Iwamoto T, Witmer R, Landolt E 1971 Light and electron microscopy in absolute glaucoma with pigment dispersion phenomena and contusion angle deformity. American Journal of Ophthalmology 72: 420–434

139. Jablonska S, Groniowski J, Krieg T, Nerlich A, Peltonen L, Oikarinen A, Dabrowski J, Pietrow D 1984 Congenital fascial dystrophy — a non-inflammatory disease of fascia: the stiff skin syndrome. Paediatric Dermatology 2: 87–97

140. Jacotot B, Beaumont J L, Monnier G, Szigeti M, Robert B, Robert L 1973 The role of elastic tissue in cholesterol deposition in the arterial wall. Nutrition and Metabolism 15: 46–58

141. Jakus M A 1956 Studies on the cornea: II. The fine structure of Descemet's membrane. Journal of Biophysical and Biochemical Cytology 2: 243–252

142. Jakus M A 1962 Further observations of the fine structure of the cornea. Investigative Ophthalmology 1: 202–225

143. Jones C J, Cummings C, Ball J, Beighton P 1984 Collagen defect of bone in osteogenesis imperfecta (Type I). An electron microscopic study. Clinical Orthopaedics and Related Research 183: 208–214

144. Jones C J, Cummings C, Ball J, Beighton P 1984 Collagen defect of bone in osteogenesis imperfecta (Type I). An electron microscopic study. Clinical Orthopaedics and Related Research 183: 208–214

145. Jozsa L, Reffy A, Balint J B 1984 Polarization and electron microscopic studies on the collagen of intact and ruptured human tendons. Acta Histochemica 74: 209–215

146. Kachel H G, Altmeyer P, Baldamus C A, Koch K M 1983 Deposition of an amyloid-like substance as a possible complication of regular dialysis treatment. Contributions to Nephrology 36: 127–132

147. Kamiyama R 1982 Fibrous long-spacing-like fibres in the bone marrow of myeloproliferative disorder. Virchows Archiv B, Cell Pathology 39: 285–291

148. Katchburian E 1973 Membrane-bound bodies as initiators of mineralization of dentine. Journal of Anatomy 116: 285–302

149. Kawanami O, Ferrans V J, Roberts W C, Crystal R G, Fulmer J D 1978 Anchoring fibrils. A new connective tissue structure in fibrotic lung disease. American Journal of Pathology 92: 389–410

150. Kaye C I, Esterly N, Booth C W 1976 Cutis laxa and lamellar ichthyosis in siblings. Clinical Genetics 9: 508–512

151. Kim K M 1976 Calcification of matrix vesicles in human aortic valve and aortic media. Federation Proceedings 35: 156–162

152. Kim K M, Trump B F 1975 Amorphous calcium precipitations in human aortic valve. Calcified Tissue Research 18: 155–160

153. Kimoto M, Morinaga S, Yamagushi H, Asai I, Tsukada T, Nozawa Y, Hara M, Kamiyama R 1979 Five cases of (angio) immunoblastic lymphadenopathy. Japanese Journal of Clinical Haematology 20: 933–942

154. Kimura K, Koizumi F, Kihara I, Kitamura S 1975 Fibrous long spacing type collagen fibrils in the glomeruli of experimental amyloidosis in rabbit. Laboratory Investigation 32: 279–285

155. Kischer C W 1984 Comparative ultrastructure of hypertrophic scars and keloids. Scanning Electron Microscopy (part 1): 423–431

156. Kischer C W, Brody G S 1981 Structure of the collagen nodule from hypertrophic scars and keloids. Scanning Electron Microscopy (part 3): 371–376

157. Kischer C W, Droegemueller W, Shetlar M, Schvapil M, Vining J 1980 Ultrastructural changes in the architecture of collagen in the human cervix treated with urea. American Journal of Pathology 99: 525–538

158. Kischer C W, Shetlar M R, Chvapil M 1981 Hypertrophic scars and keloids: a review and new concept concerning their origin. Scanning Electron Microscopy (part 4): 1699–1713

159. Knecht H, Lennert K 1981 Ultrastructural findings in lymphogranulomatosis X ([angio] immunoblastic lymphadenopathy). Virchows Archiv B, Cell Pathology 37: 29–47

160. Kobayashi H, Hashimoto K 1981 Antigenic identity of amyloid in localized cutaneous amyloidosis with keratin. Journal of Investigative Dermatology 76: 320

161. Kobayasi T 1968 Electron microscopy of the elastic fibres and the dermal membrane in normal human skin. Acta Dermato-venereologica (Stockholm) 48: 303–312

162. Kobayasi T, Asboe-Hansen G 1972 Ultrastructure of generalized scleroderma. Acta Dermato-venereologica (Stockholm) 52: 81–93

163. Kobayasi T, Wolf-Jurgensen P, Danielsen L 1973 Ultrastructure of shagreen patch. Acta Dermato-venereologica 53: 275–278

164. Korbet S M, Schwartz M M, Rosenberg B F, Sibley R K, Lewis E J 1985 Immunotactoid glomerulopathy. Medicine 64: 228–243.

165. Kumakiri M, Hashimoto K 1979 Histogenesis of primary localized cutaneous amyloidosis: sequential change of epidermal keratinocytes to amyloid via filamentous degeneration. Journal of Investigative Dermatology 73: 150–162

166. Kuntz D, Bardin T, Voisin M C, Zingraff J 1984 Amyloidosis in patients on long term haemodialysis. Arthritis and Rheumatism 27: S27

167. Laguens R 1972 Subepithelial fibrils associated with the basement membrane of human cervical epithelium. Journal of Ultrastructure Research 41: 202–208

168. Laschi R 1985 Contribution of scanning electron microscopy and associated analytical techniques to the study of atherosclerotic disease. Scanning Electron Microscopy (part 3): 1215–1222

169. Lavker R M 1979 Structural alterations in exposed and unexposed aged skin. Journal of Investigative Dermatology 73: 59–66

170. Ledoux-Corbusier M 1983 Cutis laxa, congenital form with pulmonary emphysema: an ultrastructural study. Journal of Cutaneous Pathology 10: 340–349

171. Ledoux-Corbusier M, Achten G 1974 Elastosis in chronic radiodermatitis. An ultrastructural study. British Journal of Dermatology 91: 287–295

172. Leeson T S, Speakman J S 1961 The fine structure of extracellular material in the pectinate ligament (trabecular meshwork) of the human iris. Acta Anatomica (Basel) 46: 363–379

173. Legge J W, Finlay J B, McFarlane R M 1981 A study of Dupuytren's tissue with the scanning electron microscope. Journal of Hand Surgery 6: 482–492

174. Levin M, Pras M, Franklin E C 1973 Immunologic studies of the major non-immunoglobulin protein of amyloid. I. Identification and partial characterization of a related serum component. Journal of Experimental Medicine 138: 373–380

175. Liebhart M, Janczewska E 1973 Ultrastructural changes in the placenta of a newborn with diabetes mellitus. Pathologia Europaea 8: 127–134

176. Liftin A, Schwarz R, Jagirdar J 1985 Fibronectin-containing hyaline globules in malignant melanoma. American Journal of Dermatopathology 7 (suppl): 17–21

177. Linke R P, Nathrath W B J, Wilson P D 1983 Immuno-electron microscopic identification and classification of amyloid in tissue sections by post-embedding protein-A gold method. Ultrastructural Pathology 4: 1–7

178. Lipper S, Dalzell J C, Watkins P J 1979 Ultrastructure of psammoma bodies of meningioma in tissue culture. Archives of Pathology and Laboratory Medicine 103: 670–675

179. Mandal A K, Mask D R, Nordquist J, Chrysant K S, Lindeman R D 1974 Membranous glomerulonephritis: virus-like inclusions in glomerular basement membrane. Annals of Internal Medicine 80: 554–555

180. Marchase P, Holbrook K, Pinnell S R 1975 A familial cutis laxa syndrome with ultrastructural abnormalities of collagen and elastin. Journal of Investigative Dermatology 75: 399–403

181. Matsuoko L Y, Wortsman J, Uitto J, Hashimoto K, Kupchella C E, Eng A M, Dietrich J E 1985 Altered skin elastic fibres in hypothyroid myxoedema and pretibial myxoedema. Archives of Internal Medicine 145: 117–121

182. Matz L R, Papadimitriou J M, Carroll J R, Barr A L, Dawkins R L, Jackson J M, Hermann R P, Armstrong B K 1977 Angioimmunoblastic lymphadenopathy with dysproteinaemia. Cancer 40: 2152–2160

183. Meachim G, Cornah M S 1970 Fine structure of juvenile human nucleus pulposus. Journal of Anatomy 107: 337–350

184. Mensing H, Schaeg G 1984 Composites — an aberrant structure of the collagen fibril. Dermatologica 168: 1–9

185. Mollo F, Monga G 1971 Banded structures in the connective tissue of lymphomas, lymphadenitis and thymomas. Virchows Archiv Abteilung B, Zellpathologie 7: 356–366

186. Montagna W, Carlisle K 1979 Structural changes in ageing human skin. Journal of Investigative Dermatology 73: 47–53

187. Morita T, Suzuki M, Kamimura A, Hirasawa Y 1985 Amyloidosis of a possible new type in patients receiving long term haemodialysis. Archives of Pathology and Laboratory Medicine 109: 1029–1032

188. Mori H, Mori S, Saitoh Y, Moriwaki K, Ida S, Matsumoto K 1985 Growth hormone-producing pituitary adenoma with crystal-like amyloid immunohistochemically positive for growth hormone. Cancer 55: 96–102

189. Moses H L, Glade P R, Kasel J A, Rosenthal A S, Hirshant Y, Chessin L N 1968 Infectious mononucleosis: detection of herpes-like virus and reticular aggregates of small cytoplasmic particles in continuous lymphoid cell lines derived from peripheral blood. Proceedings of the National Academy of Sciences of the USA 60: 489–496

190. Masutani M, Unno T 1984 Structural abnormalities in the mitis form (Type II) of Ehlers–Danlos syndrome. Journal of Dermatology (Tokyo) 11: 433–437

191. Nakai H, Rose G G, Cattoni M 1971 Electron microscopic study of chronic desquamative gingivitis. Journal of Periodontal Research 6 (suppl): 7–30

192. Nakamura Y, Okamoto K, Tanimura A, Masahiro K, Morimatsu M 1986 Elastase digestion and biochemical analysis of the elastin from an elastofibroma. Cancer 58: 1070–1075

193. Nakanishi I, Masuda S, Kitamura T, Morizumi I, Kajikawa K 1981 Distribution of fibrous long spacing fibres in normal and pathological lymph nodes. Acta Pathologica Japonica 31: 733–745

194. Nakazato M, Kangano K, Minamino N, Tawara S, Matsuo H, Araki S 1984 Revised analysis of amino acid replacement in a prealbumin variant (SKO-III) associated with familial amyloidotic polyneuropathy of Jewish origin. Biochemical and Biophysical Research Communications 123: 921–928

195. Nanko H, Voss Jepsen L, Zachariae H, Soegaard H 1979 Acquired cutis laxa (generalized elastolysis): light and electron microscopic studies. Acta Dermato-venereologica 59: 315–324

196. Nanto-Salonen K, Pelliniemi L J, Autio S, Kivimaki T, Rapola J, Penttinen R 1984 Abnormal collagen fibrils in aspartylglycosaminuria. Altered dermal ultrastructure in a glycoprotein storage disorder. Laboratory Investigation 51: 464–468

197. Natvig J B, Westermark P, Sletten K, Husby G, Michaelson T 1981 Further structural and antigenic studies of light chain amyloid proteins. Scandinavian Journal of Immunology 14: 89–94

198. Neiman R S, Dervan P, Handenschild C, Jaffe R 1978 Angioimmunoblastic lymphadenopathy. An ultrastructural and immunologic study with review of the literature. Cancer 41: 507–518

199. Nemetschek Th, Meinel A, Nemetschek-Gansler H, Reill P, Riedl H 1976 Zur Ätiologie der Kontraktur beim Morbus Dupuytren. Virchows Archiv A, Pathological Anatomy and Histopathology 372: 57–74

200. O'Hara P J, Read W K, Romane W M, Bridges C H 1970 A collagenous tissue dysplasia of calves. Laboratory Investigation 23: 307–314

201. Oikarinen A I, Palatzi R, Adomian G E, Oikarinen H, Clark J G, Uitto J 1984 Anetoderma: biochemical and ultrastructural demonstration of an elastin defect in the skin of three patients. Journal of the American Academy of Dermatology 11: 64–72

202. Olsen S, Bohman S-O, Petersen V P 1974 Ultrastructure of the glomerular basement membrane in long term renal allografts with transplant glomerular disease. Laboratory Investigation 30: 176–189

203. Otkjaer-Nielsen A, Christiansen O B, Hentzer B, Johnson E, Kobayasi T 1978 Saltpeter-induced dermal changes electron-microscopically indistinguishable from pseudoxanthoma elasticum. Acta Dermato-venereologica 58: 323–327

204. Otkjaer-Nielsen A, Johnson E, Hentzer B, Danielsen L, Carlsen F 1977 Apatite crystals in pseudoxanthoma elasticum: a combined study using electron microscopy and selected area diffraction analysis. Journal of Investigative Dermatology 69: 376–378

205. Pasyk K 1980 Sclerema neonatorum. Virchows Archiv A, Pathological Anatomy and Histology 388: 87–103

206. Perejda A J, Abraham P A, Carnes W H, Coulson W F, Uitto J 1985 Marfan's syndrome: structural, biochemical and mechanical studies of the aortic media. Journal of Laboratory and Clinical Medicine 106: 376–383

207. Perez-Tamayo R 1978 Pathology of collagen degradation. A review. American Journal of Pathology 92: 508–566

208. Perk K, Hod I, Nobel T A 1971 Pulmonary adenomatosis of sheep (jagsiekta) I. Ultrastructure of the tumour. Journal of the National Cancer Institute 46: 525–537

209. Peyrol S, Grimaud J A, Borojevic R 1976 Pathologie ultrastructurale. Les septa fibreux actifs et passifs dans les fibroses hépatiques sévères chez l'homme: mise en évidence d'hyperfibres de collagéne en microscopie électronique. Comptes Rendus Hebdomadaires des Sénces de L'Académie des Sciénces (D) 282: 333–336

210. Pieraggi M T, Julian M, Delmas M, Bouissou H 1982 Striae: morphological aspects of connective tissue. Virchows Archiv A, Pathological Anatomy and Histopathology 396: 279–289

211. Pillai P A 1964 A banded structure in the connective tissue of nerve. Journal of Ultrastructure Research 11: 455–468

212. Pinnell S R 1982 Molecular defects in Ehlers-Danlos syndrome. Journal of Investigative Dermatology 79 (suppl 1): 90s–92s

213. Pope F M 1974 Two types of autosomal recessive pseudoxanthoma elasticum. Archives of Dermatology 110: 209–212

214. Pope F M 1975 Historical evidence for the genetic heterogeneity of pseudoxanthoma elasticum. British Journal of Dermatology 92: 493–509

215. Pras M, Prelli F, Franklin E C, Frangione B 1983 Primary structure of an amyloid prealbumin variant in familial polyneuropathy of Jewish origin. Proceedings of the National Academy of Sciences of the USA 80: 539–542

216. Price T M, Rudec M L, Pierschbacher M, Ruoslahti 1982 Structure of fibronectin and its fragments in electron microscopy. European Journal of Biochemistry 129: 359–363

217. Renteria V G, Ferrans V J, Roberts W C 1976 The heart in the Hurler syndrome: gross histological and ultrastructural observations in five necropsy cases. American Journal of Cardiology 38: 487–501

218. Reymond J L, Stoebner P, Zambelli P, Beani J C, Amblard P 1982 Penicillamine induced elastosis perforans serpiginosa: an ultrastructural study of two cases. Journal of Cutaneous Pathology 9: 352–357

219. Rice N S C, Jones B R, Ashton N 1968 Punctate keratopathy of West Indians. British Journal of Ophthalmology 52: 865–875

220. Ringvold A, Vegge T 1971 Electron microscopy of the trabecular meshwork in eyes with exfoliation syndrome (pseudoexfoliation of the lens capsule). Virchows Archiv Abteilung A, Pathologische Anatomie 353: 110–127

221. Rohen J W, Linner E, Witmer R 1973 Electron microscopic studies on the trabecular meshwork in two cases of corticosteroid glaucoma. Experimental Eye Research 17: 19–31

222. Rohen J W, Witmer R 1972 Electron microscopic studies on the trabecular meshwork in glaucoma simplex. Albrecht von Graefes Archiv für Klinische und Experimentelle Ophthalmologie 183: 251–266

223. Ross R 1973 The elastic fiber: a review. Journal of Histochemistry and Cytochemistry 21: 199–208

224. Ross R, Fialkow P, Altman L K 1978 Fine structure alterations of elastic fibres in pseudoxanthoma elasticum. Clinical Genetics 13: 213–223

225. Rowlands D T Jr, Burkholder P M, Bossen E H, Lin H H 1970 Renal allografts in HL-A matched recipients: light immunofluorescence and electron microscopic studies. American Journal of Pathology 61: 177–210

226. Sage H, Pritzl P, Bornstein P 1980 A unique pepsin-sensitive collagen synthesized by aortic endothelial cells in culture. Biochemistry 19: 5747–5755

227. Saito Y, Klingmuller G 1977 Elektronenmikroskopische Untersuchungen zur Morphogenese elastischer Fasern bei der senilen Elastose und dem Pseudoxanthoma elasticum. Archives of Dermatological Research 260: 179–191

228. Sarkar K, Uhthoff H K 1978 Ultrastructural localization of calcium in calcifying tendinitis. Archives of Pathology and Laboratory Medicine 102: 266–269

229. Saruk M, Eisenstein R 1977 Aortic lesions in Marfan syndrome: the ultrastructure of cystic medial degeneration. Archives of Pathology and Laboratory Medicine 101: 74–77

230. Sayers C P, Goltz R W, Mottaz J 1975 Pulmonary elastic tissue in generalized elastolysis (cutis laxa) and Marfan's syndrome. A light and electron microscopic study. Journal of Investigative Dermatology 65: 451–457

231. Sayers C P, Goltz R W, Mottaz J 1975 Pulmonary elastic tissue in generalized elastolysis (cutis laxa) and Marfan's syndrome. A light and electron microscopic study. Journal of Investigative Dermatology 65: 451–457

232. Schafer I A, Silverman L, Sullivan J C, Robertson W van B 1967 Ascorbic acid deficiency in cultured human fibroblasts. Journal of Cell Biology 34: 83–95

233. Schärer K, Hausser I, Anton-Lamprecht I, Tilgen W 1990 Clinical quiz (pseudoxanthoma elasticum). Pediatric Nephrology 4: 97–99

234. Scholtz C L 1975 Banded structures in cauda equina. Pathology 7: 129–132

235. Schroeder H E, Theilade J 1966 Electron microscopy of normal human gingival epithelium. Journal of Periodontal Research 1: 95–119

236. Schubert G E, Adam A 1974 Glomerular nodules and long spacing collagen in kidneys of patients with multiple myeloma. Journal of Clinical Pathology 27: 800–805

237. Schwarz P 1965 Senile cerebral, pancreatic insular and cardiac amyloidosis. Transactions of the New York Academy of Sciences 27: 393–413

238. Sela J, Boyde A 1977 Further observations on the relationship between the matrix and the calcifying fronts in osteosarcoma. Case report. Virchows Archiv A, Pathological Anatomy and Histopathology 376: 175–180

239. Selkoe D J, Abraham C R, Podlisny M B, Duffy L K 1986 Isolation of low molecular weight proteins from amyloid plaque fibres in Alzheimer's disease. Journal of Neurochemistry 46: 1820–1834

240. Sevenich M, Schultz-Ehrenburg V, Orfanos C E 1980 Ehlers–Danlos syndrome: a disease of fibroblasts and collagen fibrils. Archives of Dermatological Research 267: 237–252

241. Sherman R L, Churg J, Yudis M 1974 Hereditary nephritis with a characteristic renal lesion. American Journal of Medicine 56: 44–51

242. Shirahama T, Cohen A S 1967 High-resolution electron microscopic analysis of the amyloid fibril. Journal of Cell Biology 33: 679–708

243. Shirahama T, Skinner M, Cohen A S, Gejyo F, Arakawa M, Susuki M, Hirasawa Y 1985 Histochemical and immunohistochemical characterization of amyloid associated with chronic haemodialysis as β_2-microglobulin. Laboratory Investigation 53: 705–709

244. Shirahama T, Skinner M, Sipe J D, Cohen A S 1985 Widespread occurrence of AP in amyloidotic tissues. An immunohistochemical observation. Virchows Archiv B, Cell Pathology 48: 197–206

245. Shirahama T, Skinner M, Westermark P, Rubinow A, Cohen A S, Brun A, Kemper T L 1982 Senile cerebral amyloid: prealbumin as a common constituent in the neuritic plaque, in the neurofibrillary tangle and in the microangiopathic lesion. American Journal of Pathology 107: 41–50

246. Silbert J E 1982 Structure and metabolism of proteoglycans and glycosaminoglycans. Journal of Investigative Dermatology 79 (suppl 1): 31s–37s

247. Singer I I, Kawka D W, Kazazis D M, Clark R A 1984 *In vivo* codistribution of fibronectin and actin fibres in granulation tissue: immunofluorescence and electron microscope studies of the fibronexus at the myofibroblast surface. Journal of Cell Biology 98: 2091–2106

248. Skinner M, Benson M D, Cohen A S 1975 Amyloid fibril protein related to immunoglobulin chains. Journal of Immunology 14: 89–94

249. Skinner M, Cathcart E S, Cohen A S, Benson M D 1974 Isolation and identification by sequence analysis of experimentally induced guinea pig amyloid fibrils. Journal of Experimental Medicine 140: 871–876

250. Skinner M, Shirahamo T, Benson M D, Cohen A S 1977 Murine amyloid protein AA in casein-induced experimental amyloidosis. Laboratory Investigation 36: 420–427

251. Sletten K, Westermark P, Natvig J B 1976 Characterization of amyloid fibril proteins from medullary carcinoma of the thyroid. Journal of Experimental Medicine 143: 993–997

252. Sletten K, Westermark P, Natvig J B 1980 Senile cardiac amyloid is related to prealbumin. Scandinavian Journal of Immunology 12: 503–506

253. Smith J W 1968 Molecular pattern in native collagen. Nature 219: 157–158

254. Smith L T, Holbrook K A, Byers P H 1982 Structure of the dermal matrix during development and in the adult. Journal of Investigative Dermatology 79 (suppl 1): 93s–104s

255. Spear G S, Slusser R J 1972 Alport's syndrome: emphasizing electron microscopic studies of the glomerulus. American Journal of Pathology 69: 231–242

256. Spelsberg W W, Chapman G B 1962 Fine structure of human trabeculae. Archives of Ophthalmology 67: 773–784

257. Staubesand J 1977 Matrix Vesikel und Mediadysplasie. Ein neues Konzept zur formalen Pathogenese der Varikose (Kurzbericht) Medizinische Welt 28: 1943–1946

258. Staubesand J, Fischer N 1979 Collagen dysplasia and matrix vesicles. Researches with the electron microscope into the problem of so-called 'weakness of the vessel wall'. Pathology, Research and Practice 165: 374–391

259. Staubesand J, Fischer N 1980 The ultrastructural characteristics of abnormal collagen fibrils in various organs. Connective Tissue Research 7: 213–217

260. Stiefel A, Hausser I 1988 Skleromyxödem Arndt-Gottron. Hautarzt 39: 478–479

261. Stern I B 1965 Electron microscopic observations of oral epithelium 1. Basal cells and the basement membrane. Periodontics 3: 224–238

262. Stiller D, Katenkamp D 1978 Intercellular substances in Hodgkin's lymphomas. Ultrastructural observations. Virchows Archiv A, Pathological Anatomy and Histopathology 380: 81–90

263. Sulica V I, Cooper P H, Pope F M, Hambrick G W, Gerson B M, McKusick V A 1979 Cutaneous histologic features in Ehlers–Danlos syndrome. Archives of Dermatology 115: 40–42

264. Sun C N, White H J 1973 A study of banded structures, 'long-spaced collagen' in the connective tissue. Journal of Cell Biology 59: 340a

265. Sun C N, White H J 1975 Extracellular cross-striated banded structures in human connective tissue. Tissue and Cell 7: 419–432

266. Susi F R, Belt W D, Kelly J W 1967 Fine structure of fibrillar complexes associated with the basement membrane of human oral mucosa. Journal of Cell Biology 34: 686–690

267. Swanson J L, Helwig E B 1968 Special fibrils of human dermis. Journal of Investigative Dermatology 50: 195–199

268. Takarada H, Cattoni M, Sugumoto A, Rose G G 1974 Ultrastructural studies of human gingiva. IV. Anchoring fibrils and perforations of the basal lamina in chronic periodontitis. Journal of Periodontology 45: 809–814

269. Takebayashi S, Kubota I, Takagi A 1973 Ultrastructural and histochemical studies of vascular lesions in Marfan's syndrome with report of 4 autopsy cases. Acta Pathologica Japonica 23: 847–866

270. Tooney N M, Mosesson M W, Amrani D L, Hainfield J F, Wall J S 1983 Solution and surface effects on plasma fibronectin structure. Journal of Cell Biology 97: 1686–1692

271. Tsuji T 1980 Scanning electron microscope studies of solar elastosis. British Journal of Dermatology 102: 307–312

272. Tsuji T 1981 Ultrastructural studies of elastotic material and elastic fibres in aged skin before and after autoclaving. Journal of

Investigative Dermatology 77: 452–457

273. Tsuji T 1984 The surface structural alterations of elastic fibres and elastotic material in solar elastosis: a scanning electron microscopic study. Journal of Cutaneous Pathology 11: 300–308

274. Tsuji T, Lavker R M, Kligman A M 1978 A new method for scanning electron microscopic visualization of dermal elastic fibres. Journal of Microscopy (Oxford) 115: 165–173

275. Uitto J, Perejda A 1987 Connective tissue disease. In: Littlo J, Perejda A (eds) The biochemistry of disease, vol 12. Marcel Dekker, New York, pp 3–28, 101–140, 399–422

276. Uitto J, Ryhänen L, Abraham P A, Perejda A J 1982 Elastin in diseases. Journal of Investigative Dermatology 79 (suppl 1): 160s–168s

277. Uitto J, Santa Cruz D J, Starcher B, Whyte M, Murphy M A 1981 Biochemical and ultrastructural demonstration of elastin accumulation in skin lesions of the Buschke–Ollendorff syndrome. Journal of Investigative Dermatology 76: 284–287

278. Urry D W 1975 Molecular aspects of the elastic fibre as a site of vascular pathology. Alabama Journal of Medical Sciences 12: 361–368

279. Vajda K, Kadar A, Kali A, Urai L 1982 Ultrastructural investigations of finger pulp biopsies: a study of 31 patients with Raynaud's syndrome. Ultrastructural Pathology 3: 175–186

280. Vegge T, Ringvold A 1971 The ultrastructure of the extracellular components of the trabecular meshwork in the human eye. Zeitschrift für Zellforschung und Mikroskopische Anatomie 115: 361–376

281. Venencie P Y, Winkelmann R K, Moore B A 1984 Ultrastructural findings in the skin lesions of patients with anetoderma. Acta Dermato-venereologica 64: 112–120

282. Vitellaro-Zuccarello L, Garino Canina G, De Biasi S, Cocchini F, Vitellaro-Zuccarello P 1984 Ultrastructural study on the stapes and skin in a case of type I osteogenesis imperfecta. Journal of Submicroscopic Cytology 16: 779–786

283. Vogel A, Holbrook K A, Steinmann B, Gitzelmann R, Byers P H 1979 Abnormal collagen fibril structure in the gravis form (Type I) of Ehlers–Danlos syndrome. Laboratory Investigation 40: 201–206

284. Vogel A, Steinmann B 1980 Ultrastructural studies of skin from a patient with a new type of Ehlers–Danlos syndrome (EDS) characterized by a structural mutation of procollagen. Journal of Cutaneous Pathology 6: 177

285. Voigtländer V, Arnold M-L, Neu P, Anton-Lamprecht I, Jung E G 1985 Cutis laxa acquise avec amyloidose cutanée et paraprotéinemie (IgG kappa). Annales de Dermatologie et Vénéréologie 112: 779–780

286. Volpin D, Pasquali-Ronchetti I, Castellani M G, Peserico A, Mori G 1978 Ultrastructural and biochemical studies on a case of elastosis perforans serpiginosa. Dermatologica 156: 209–223

287. Waalen K, Sletten K, Husby G, Nordstoga K 1980 The primary structure of amyloid fibril protein AA in endotoxin-induced amyloidosis of the mink. European Journal of Biochemistry 104: 407–412

288. Waisman J, Smith D W 1968 Fine structure of an elastofibroma. Cancer 22: 671–677

289. Walker E R, Frederickson R G, Mayes M D 1989 The mineralization of elastic fibers and alterations of extracellular matrix in pseudoxanthoma elasticum. Archives of Dermatology 125: 70–76

290. Wallace M R, Dwulet F E, Conneally P M, Benson M D 1986 Biochemical and molecular genetic characterization of a new variant pre-albumin associated with hereditary amyloidosis. Journal of Clinical Investigation 78: 6–12

291. Wang N-S, Knaack J 1982 Fibromatosis hyalinica multiplex juvenilis. Ultrastructural Pathology 3: 153–160

292. Westermark P 1977 Amyloid of human islets of Langerhans. II. Electron microscopic analysis of isolated amyloid. Virchows Archiv A, Pathological Anatomy and Histopathology 373: 161–166

293. Whiteway J, Morson B C 1985 Elastosis in diverticular disease of the sigmoid colon. Gut 26: 258–266

294. Williams B, Cranley R, Doty S, Lichtenstein T 1973 Morphological observations on connective tissue from individuals with pro-collagen peptidase deficiency (Ehlers–Danlos Type VII Syndrome). American Journal of Human Genetics 25: 86A

295. Winkelmann R K, Sams W M 1969 Elastofibroma: report of a case with special histochemical and electron microscopic studies. Cancer 23: 406–415

296. Woyke S, Domagala W, Olszewski W 1970 Ultrastructure of fibromatosis hyalinica multiplex juvenilis. Cancer 26: 1157–1168

297. Yaoita H, Katz S I 1976 Immunoelectromicroscopic localization of IgA in skin of patients with dermatitis herpetiformis. Journal of Investigative Dermatology 67: 502–506

298. Younes M S, Steele H D, Robertson E M, Benscosme S A 1965 Correlative light and electronmicroscope study of the basement membrane of the human ectocervix. American Journal of Obstetrics and Gynaecology 92: 163–171

299. Yu S Y, Blumenthal H T 1963 The calcification of elastic fibres. II. Ultramicroscopic characteristics. Journal of Gerentology 18: 127–134

300. Zelickson A S, Mottaz J H, Zelickson B D, Muller S A 1980 Elastic tissue changes in skin following PUVA therapy. Journal of the American Academy of Dermatology 3: 186–192

301. Zheng P, Lavker R M, Kligman A M 1985 Anatomy of striae. British Journal of Dermatology 112: 185–193

302. Zollinger H U, Moppert J, Thiel G, Rohr H P 1973 Morphology and pathogenesis of glomerulopathy in cadaver kidney allografts treated with antilymphocyte globulin. Current Topics in Pathology 57: 1–48

303. Zwillenberg H H L, Zwillenberg L O, Laszt L 1972 Ultrastructural changes in organ cultures of bovine veins. Symposia Angiologica Santoriana. Fourth International Symposium, Fribourg-Nyon. Angiologica 9: 292–300

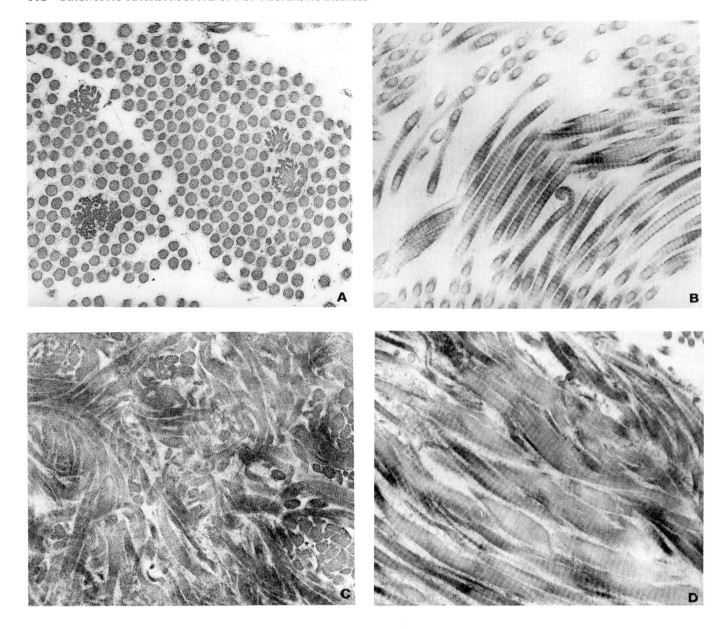

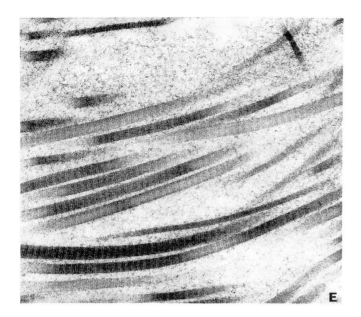

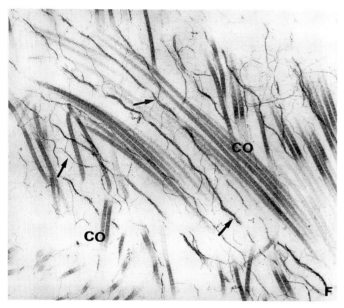

Fig. 5.1 Ehlers–Danlos syndrome (EDS). **A** and **B** Principal abnormalities concern the collagen fibrils. Due to incomplete cross-linking of individual polypeptide chains, loosely aggregated fibrils large in diameter produce flower-like arrangements in cross-section (**A**) whereas in longitudinal section they appear as loose, fragmented ropes with twisted helical subfibrils, but showing the normal periodic cross-banding (**B**). EDS type II (mitis type); tissue samples from elbow. **A** adult female, 29 years old, middle part of reticular dermis. (× 41 600); **B** adult male, 39 years old, lower part of reticular dermis. (× 25 300) **C** and **D** In EDS type I (gravis type) changes may be somewhat similar. A clear distinction of both dominant types is, however, possible by the much more severe disturbance (in EDS type I) of collagen fibrils in the central parts of the reticular dermis, resulting in a tangled disorderly pattern of densely packed fibrils of highly variable diameters and with irregular circumference in cross-sections (**C**). Broad fragmented collagen ropes have the normal banding pattern in longitudinal sections (**D**). Adult male, 27 years old, tissue sample from right elbow. (C, × 41 600; D, × 31 200) **E** Increase of finely flocculent material between the collagen fibrils and among loose collagen fibres that possibly represents non-fibrillar collagen precursors or aberrant partly degraded collagen. This fuzzy material is ultrastructurally different from serum proteins. Adult male, clinically EDS type II, 25 years old; tissue sample from left elbow. (× 32 500) **F** In addition to changes of collagen fibrils, EDS type II is characterized by an increase in proteoglycans and glycosaminoglycans (GAG) in the papillary and reticular dermis. These are seen as irregular deeply dark-staining strands and filaments (arrows) running in parallel with mostly small collagen fibrils; they are connected to them with fine branches and form a tiny network as a result of their interconnections. The deep staining is due to binding of uranyl acetate by the aldehyde residues of the sugar moieties of proteoglycans and GAG. Female patient, 29 years old; same case as in Fig. 22.37A; papillary dermis. (× 16 800) Electron micrographs A, E and F: I Werner; B: J Deimel-Hatzenbühler.

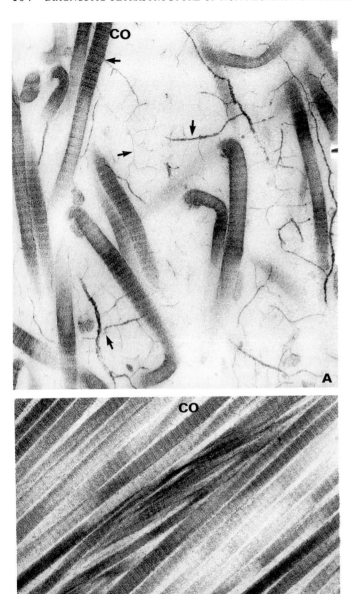

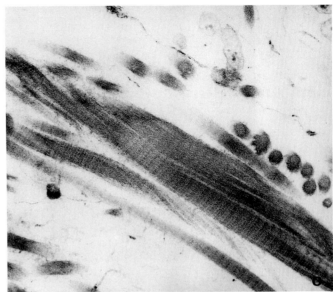

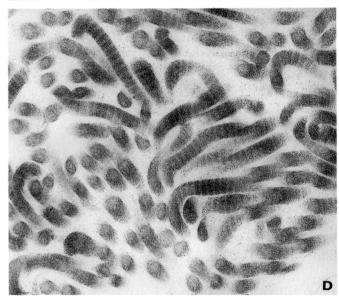

Fig. 5.2 Scleroedema adultorum Buschke. **A–D** Changes of the collagen fibrils such as collagen flowers and collagen ropes are not highly specific from the diagnostic point of view and occur not only in the various types of EDS (see Fig. 5.1A and B) but also in many other conditions with disturbances of the delicate balance between fibrous elements and ground substance of the connective tissue. Scleroedema adultorum Buschke is assumed to lead to an enormous increase in components of the ground substance, such as GAG (**A**, arrows), seen as a network of finely branching strands, the appearance of which is significantly different from the GAG strands in EDS type II (compare with Fig. 5.1F). Collagen flowers (not shown) and long and broad collagen fibrils, twisted in appearance like ropes (**B**, **C**), are intermingled with more normal-appearing collagen (**B**). Normal cross-banding is present in normal and in enlarged, twisted collagen fibrils (**B**, **C**). Isolated collagen fibrils show conspicuous bending (**A**, **D**), especially when surrounded by masses of ground substance (**A**). These flexures and the high amount of GAG in the dermal connective tissue are of special diagnostic significance. **A** and **D** Adult female, neck. **B** and **C** Adult male, shoulder. (A, × 55 000; B, × 36 400; C, × 51 700; D, × 35 700) Electron micrographs B–E: I. Werner.

Fig. 5.3 (Facing page) Scleromyxoedema Arndt–Gottron. Increased cellularity with predominance of fibroblasts and macrophages, high amounts of GAG, low amounts of collagen, and destruction of elastic tissue in the connective tissue of affected skin areas are the main features of scleromyxoedema Arndt–Gottron. **A** and **B** Phagocytosis of abnormal elastic fibres (with elastotic changes resembling those in solar or actinic elastosis) by macrophages reflects the progressive loss of normal tissue architecture. GAG of the ground substance fill wide spaces of the dermal connective tissue with a network of extremely fine strands interconnected by bulky, clumped nodes of dark-staining material (arrows), probably hyaluronic acid (**A** and **B**; compare with GAG networks in Fig. 5.1F and 5.2A). They correspond to alcian blue-positive mucosubstances, mainly hyaluronic acid, in routine histopathology sections. **C** and **D** A different network of fine filaments (fibronectin?) span between the collagen fibrils. Collagen is present only in small groups, forming loose bundles and incomplete fibres. Most fibrils have a regular banding pattern (**C**) and a smooth outer surface (**D**); small-diameter fibrils predominate. Coarse granular material (*), probably immunoglobulins, is intermingled with the collagen fibrils in the deep reticular dermis. **A**, **C** and **D** Adult female, 73 years old. (A, × 21 800; C, × 70 400; D, × 71 700) **B** Adult male, 56 years old . (× 41 600) Electron micrograph B: Dr I Hausser.

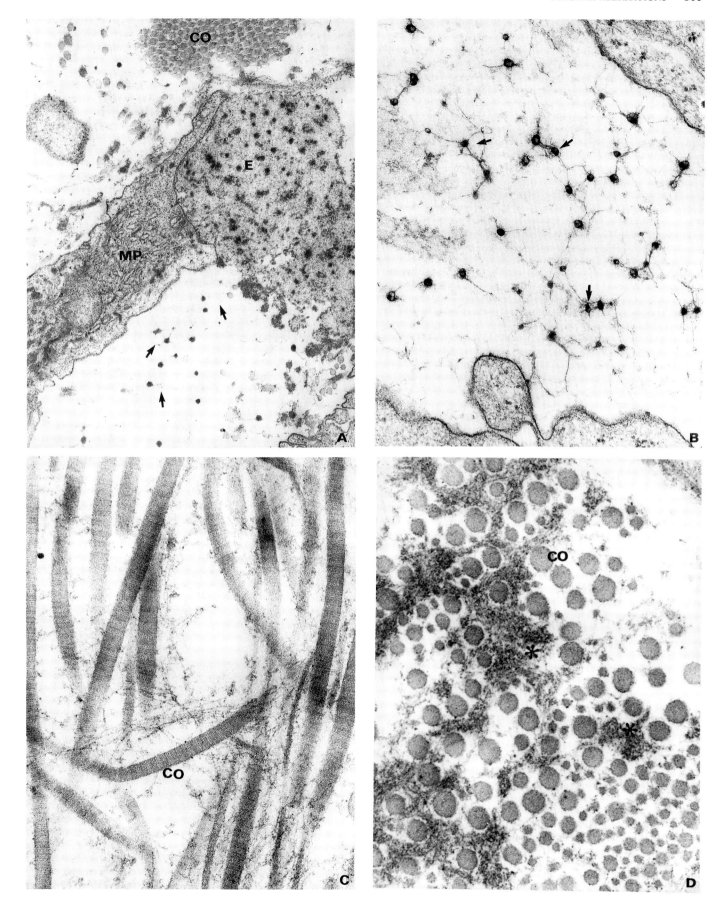

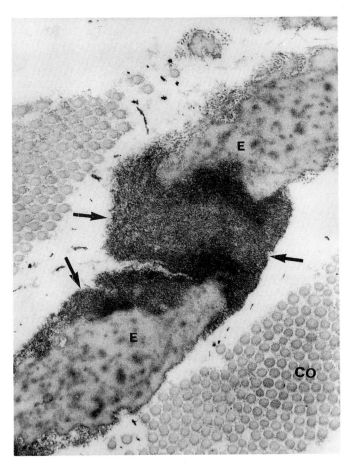

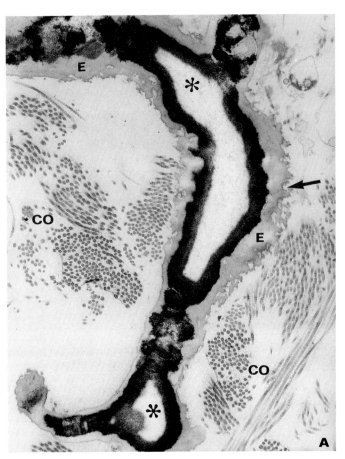

Fig. 5.4 Cutis laxa with autosomal dominant inheritance. Elastic fibres show varying degrees of dissociation of elastotubules from the elastic moieties: excessive amounts of tangled elastotubules (arrows), reduced elastin deposition and clumped, disorderly shaped fibres. Collagen appears unaltered. Female, 32 years old from a kindred with a dominant transmission of cutis laxa (clinical observation: Professor Dr V. Voigtländer, Mannheim). (× 41 700) Electron micrograph: Dr M-L Arnold.

Fig. 5.5 Pseudoxanthoma elasticum (PXE). A The classic appearance of PXE is exemplified by this clumped, swollen, branching degenerated elastic fibre with severe central mineralization (*) (deposition of calcium and phosphorus). In the periphery of the fibre, elastin and a small margin of unmineralized elastotubules (arrows) are recognizable. Collagen fibrils in the neighbourhood show slight changes. Sample from the centre of a xanthomatous papular lesion. B Malformed elastic fibre close to a fibroblast, with four areas of lateral branching protuberances (arrows), and with dark-staining granular precipitates (*) parallel to the longitudinal axis of the fibre (calcium deposition). Irregular groups of elastotubules (curved arrows) surround the fibre. Sample from the margin of a xanthomatous lesion. A and B Adult female, aged 45 years, with dominantly inherited PXE and severe CNS involvement. (A, × 9000; B, × 21 300) C Ultrastructural detail of central mineralization (*) with a concentric arrangement of partly extracted granular core, a reticulated mantle with radial arrangement of needle-like calcium apatite crystals (arrows) and irregularly deposited mineral substances (*); elastin is dislocated to the fibre periphery. Curved arrows indicate marginal elastotubules. Oedema of ground substance, collagen fibrils with collagen flowers and longitudinal ropes of broad unravelled, twisted fibrils are most pronounced in close proximity to degenerate, mineralized elastic fibres. C Adult female, 29 years old. (× 51 700)

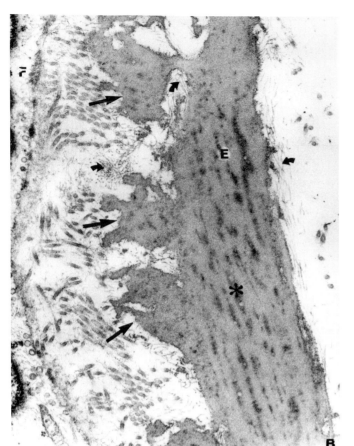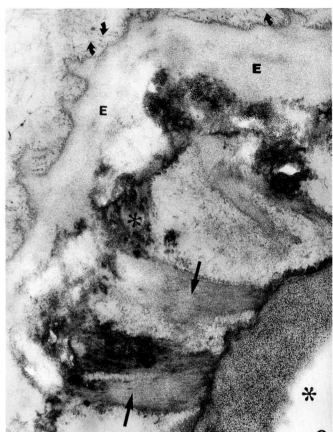

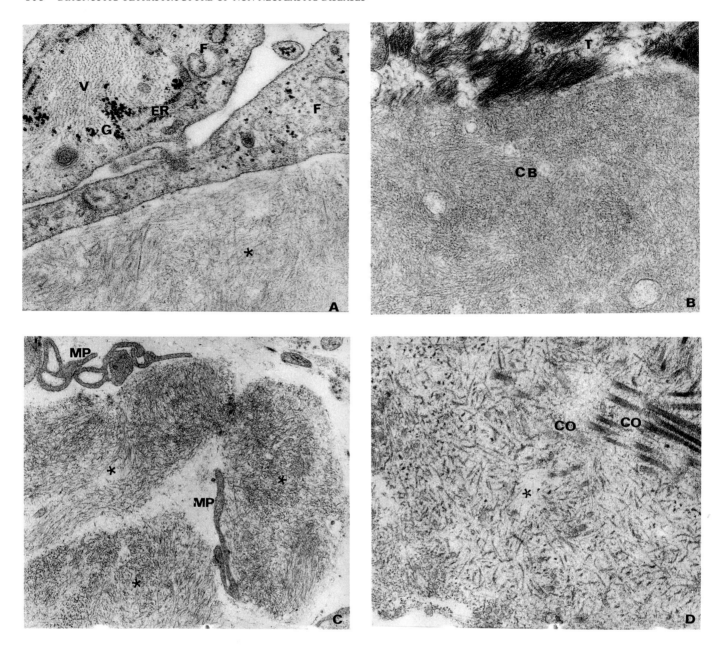

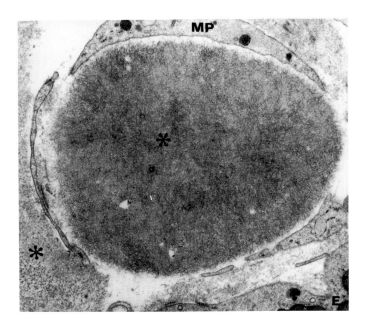

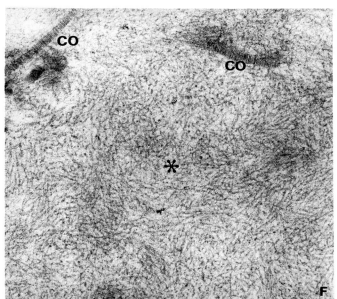

Fig. 5.6 Amyloidoses. **A** Localized cutaneous amyloidosis associated with congenital reticular ichthyosiform erythroderma (see Figs 22.13 and 22.14). Amyloid islands (*) in the papillary dermis appear as a tangled texture of very thin, straight filaments intermingled with few collagen fibrils underneath the dermo-epidermal junction with basal lamina, normal hemidesmosomes and anchoring fibrils. There is no sign of degeneration of basal or suprabasal epidermal cells, and there are no intra-epidermal amyloid precursors. Amyloid microfilaments (*) are clearly different from the cytofilaments, for example the vimentin filaments (v) seen in a fibroblast. Adult female, 57 years old; no signs of systemic involvement and immunoglobulins normal. (× 43 000) **B** Intra-epidermal fibrillar or Civatte body (see also Fig. 22.20B) composed of keratin filaments in a curving array (adjacent to a bundle of tonofilaments of higher density and diameter). According to some authors, fibrillar bodies originating from degenerating epidermal cells ('hyaline degeneration'; apoptosis) give rise to amyloid in cases of lichen amyloidosis and macular amyloidosis (i.e. localized amyloidoses of the skin). Blister edge, newborn female, 10 days old, with epidermolysis bullosa herpetiformis Dowling–Meara. (× 41 600) **C–E** Primary systemic amyloidosis, light-chain or AL amyloidosis. Amyloid islands (*) fill the interstitium of the entire connective tissue and are present as ovoid (**C**) or globular (**E**) masses of straight filaments of varying thickness and appearance. These include loose aggregates of short, straight, partly needle-like filaments (**C, D**), and tightly packed globular aggregations (**E**) of straight filaments that are smaller in size than those in (**D**). Male patient, 75 years old, with pronounced acquired cutis laxa due to amyloid AL (monoclonal gammopathy, kappa type) deposition throughout the entire dermal connective tissue with destruction of collagen and elastic fibrous matrix components.[228] Note the distinctive differences in the amyloid fibril ultrastructure of this case.
(**C**, × 12 100; **D**, × 28 100; **E**, × 9600). **F** Nodular amyloidosis of the skin with systemic involvement (secondary systemic or protein AA amyloidosis). Amyloid islands filling the connective tissue of the nodular lesions are composed of straight filaments that are distinctly different from those in the localized cutaneous amyloidoses (compare with **A**) and from those in kappa-type light-chain amyloidosis (compare with **C–E**). They are intermingled with some few isolated thin collagen fibrils. Adult female, 45 years old, with nodular amyloidosis of the face and amyloid deposition in rectum[93a]. At that time, determination of the type of amyloid was not performed, and a possible origin from immunoglobulins was not considered. (× 41 600) Electron micrographs C–E: Dr M-L Arnold; F: B Melz-Rothfuss.

6. Storage diseases

P. Dustin

INTRODUCTION

Many hereditary defects of catabolic pathways lead to the intracellular accumulation of various metabolites. Similar cellular changes may also result from the administration of several drugs, and others have no definite biochemical explanation as yet. Different mechanisms may be involved, but the role of lysosomes is central and many forms of storage result from deficiencies of their enzymes.

This field has grown in complexity in recent years as the result of the thorough investigation of the biochemistry of most metabolic diseases.[89] Contrary to early ideas, it has become evident that the accumulation of metabolites does not result simply from the absence of an enzyme involved in the catabolism of complex molecules, but also from abnormalities of enzyme activity resulting from mutations of their genes, or the absence of activating or protective factors. The polymorphism of most human storage disorders is an indication of the variety of enzyme defects.

Not all storage disorders are hereditary, and genocopies may result from the administration of drugs which penetrate into the lysosomes, disturbing their pH and the transport and functioning of their enzymes. The resulting morphological changes may resemble closely those secondary to hereditary defects.

While advances in the biochemical evaluation of missing enzymes and accumulated metabolites may appear to have overtaken ultrastructural observations, the latter remain indispensable — particularly in diseases where the biochemical defect has not been defined. Moreover, they also provide a rapid method of diagnosis.[22] Advances in biopsy techniques[46,47] and of tissue processing make possible rapid demonstration of the cellular changes. Morphology and biochemistry are complementary since, in some conditions, similar ultrastructural appearances may result from quite different biochemical defects — for instance the mucopolysaccharidoses and I-cell disease. Lastly, extracellular accumulations of abnormal metabolites, such as amyloid, calcium oxalate or phytanic acid will not be considered in this chapter.

DEFECTS OF LIPID TRANSPORT AND STORAGE

Tables 6.1 and 6.2 cover a large number of hereditary conditions — some quite frequent, such as familial hyperlipidaemia,[9,32,61] and some exceptional, such as Tangier disease.[15,36] Hyperlipidaemia leading to similar increases of intracellular lipids may also be secondary to other conditions such as the nephrotic syndrome, hypothyroidism, alcoholism, glycogenosis type I, diabetes and so forth.

The morphology and the intracellular location of lipids is similar in most of these conditions. Lipid droplets are found either in endocytotic vacuoles or in the ground cytoplasm. They may be birefringent (cholesterol esters) or not (triglycerides). Intracellular cholesterides may appear as elongated prismatic crystals — as observed extracellularly in xanthomas and atheromatous deposits — while chylomicrons may be observed in cell vacuoles. Lipids may also be located in lysosomes, in particular in Wolman's disease (see below). Generally the lipids captured by the LDL receptors at the cell surface are transported eventually into lysosomes to be digested.[56] Lastly, excessive intralysosomal ceroid-lipofuscin pigment may be associated with some forms of hyperlipidaemia.[24,31]

By electron microscopy (EM), the lipid droplets appear structureless and without a definite limiting membrane. No enzymes, such as acid phosphatase, can be detected in the pseudovacuoles visible after embedding. Ceroid and lipofuscin are dense lamellated inclusions located in lysosomes which show only slight enzyme activity (telolysosomes). None of these features are pathognomonic, and the diagnosis relies mainly on the composition of the blood lipids and their apoproteins.[78]

INTRALYSOSOMAL STORAGE: GENERAL MECHANISMS

Lysosomes play a central role in the catabolism of endogenous and exogenous metabolites. Since the early studies of their role in various storage diseases (reviewed by Résibois et al[68] and Hers & van Hoof[38]), a large number of publications

Table 6.1 Familial lipoprotein and lipid metabolic disorders I

Disease	Frequency and genetics	Age of onset and evolution	Deficiency	Pathology	Principal clinical signs
Alpha-beta lipoproteinaemia[36]	Rare autosomal recessive	Neonatal, progressive	Apolipoprotein B	Lipids in intestinal cells, hepatic steatosis, ceroid in fibroblasts and macrophages, acanthocytosis	Ataxic neuropathy, retinitis pigmentosa, fat malabsorption
Hypo-beta-lipoproteinaemia[36]	Rare, autosomal recessive heterozygous	Childhood, adults	Apolipoprotein B	Lipid in intestinal epithelium, hepatic steatosis (in homozygotes only)	Similar to a-beta-lipo-proteinaemia
Tangier disease[15,36]	Rare, autosomal recessive	Childhood, progressive	Apolipoprotein A	Cholesteryl esters in most organs (in cytoplasm and lysosomes): endothelia, liver, bone marrow, leukocytes; intestine unaffected	Hyperplastic yellow tonsils, neuromuscular dysfunction
Familial lipoprotein-lipase deficiency (type I hyperlipoproteinaemia[24,61])	Rare, autosomal recessive	Childhood	Lipoprotein lipase	Xanthomas, hepatosplenomegaly with chylomicron fat in macrophages	Abdominal pain, pancreatitis
Familial C-II deficiency[61]	Rare, autosomal recessive	Young adults	C-II deficiency (co-factor for lipoprotein lipase)	Eruptive xanthomas	

Table 6.2 Familial lipoprotein and lipid metabolic disorders II

Disease	Frequency and genetics	Age of onset and evolution	Deficiency	Pathology	Principal clinical signs
Familial type 5 hyperlipoproteinaemia[61]	Uncommon, autosomal dominant?	20–50 years	Unknown	Eruptive xanthomas, atherosclerosis	Elevated VLDL, fasting chylomicronaemia, decreased glucose tolerance
Lecithin-cholesterol acyltransferase deficiency[31]	Rare, autosomal recessive	Adults	Lecithin-cholesterol acyltransferase	Foam cells in bone marrow and renal glomeruli; sea-blue histiocytes in spleen	Corneal opacities, anaemia with target-cells, early atherosclerosis
Dys-beta-lipo proteinaemia (type 3 hyperlipoproteinaemia)[9]	Rare; homozygous for Ed allele + other factor	Adults (after 20 years)	Apoprotein E	Foam cells and ceroid in spleen; palmar, tuberous xanthomas	Elevated cholesterol and triglycerides
Hypercholesterolaemia (type 2 hyperlipoproteinaemia)[32]	Autosomal dominant, frequent	At birth; clinical manifestation in adults	Receptor for plasma LDL	Tuberous xanthomas, foam cells and ceroid in spleen	Premature atherosclerosis
Cerebro-tendinous xanthomatosis[75]	Rare, autosomal recessive	Adults	Liver enzyme hydroxylating cholestanesterol	Cholesterol and cholestanol xanthomas; pigment (ceroid?) in liver cells	Dementia, cerebellar ataxia, cataracts, premature atherosclerosis
Sitosterolaemia[75]	Rare, autosomal recessive	Adults	Metabolic defect affecting plant sterols	Cholesterol and sitosterol xanthomas	Tendon xanthomas

have dealt with this subject. Apart from the series published by Dingle et al[18] and the chapter on storage diseases in the volumes edited by Johannessen,[22] two important relatively recent monographs have helped in the preparation of this chapter — those of Callahan & Lowden[11] and Barranger & Brady.[3]

The principal mechanisms which lead to excessive intra-lysosomal storage are summarized in Table 6.3. Complete absence of one of the dozens of lysosomal enzymes is more the exception than the rule, while some lysosomal changes have as yet no biochemical definition, such as those of the ceroid–lipofuscinoses. Lysosomal storage may also result from an excessive amount of substances in the blood, or defects of transport, as in the case of iron and copper accumulation. Deficiency of activators or protectors of lysosomal enzymes is also a cause of excessive storage, while in cystinosis the accumulation results from defective transport from the lysosomal compartment to the cytoplasm. In so-called I-cell disease (or mucolipidosis II) on the other hand, there is excessive leaking of enzymes from the lysosomes into the extracellular compartment. The clinical variability of these disorders — some deficiencies being rapidly lethal while others are compatible with survival to adulthood — is an indication of the diversity of the genetic defect.

THE GLYCOGENOSES

Glycogen storage occurs in several genetic disorders (Table 6.4), but excessive amounts are mainly found in glycogenoses I and II. Type IV (Andersen's disease) will be mentioned in relation to local deposits of amylopectins in some other conditions.

In glycogeneosis type I, normal glycogen rosettes are stored in the cytoplasm, without any preferential organellar location. The liver and kidney cells in particular contain large amounts of glycogen.[41] The enzymatic defect explains the frequent hypoglycaemic episodes. On the other hand,

the mechanism of the hyperuricaemia and the hyperlipid-aemia are imperfectly understood.

Pompe's disease (glycogenosis II), although infrequent, was the first hereditary recessive metabolic defect in which the role of lysosomes was demonstrated.[37] While it is known that glycogen may be present in lysosomes ('glycogeno-somes') in infancy and in animals injected with glucagon, the role of lysosomes in glycogen metabolism had not been considered before the studies of Hers[37] and Hers & van Hoof.[38] In type II glycogenosis the tissues mainly affected are the heart, striated muscle, liver and various other cells, such as brain and spinal neurons. Large amounts of glycogen are found in the cytoplasm, and the lysosomes are considerably swollen by the accumulation of normal-appearing glycogen rosettes (Figs 6.1 and 7.3).

While cytoplasmic glycogen is normally degraded by glucose-6-phosphatase after starvation or adrenalin injection, the lysosomes, lacking acid maltase, remain loaded with glycogen. The alpha-glucosidase (acid maltase) deficiency may, however, result from several other mechanisms: an impairment of the conversion of a precursor molecule; the absence of its phosphorylation; or too rapid degradation of the precursor before it reaches the lysosomes.[95]

Several problems, however, remain. Large glycogen particles cannot be assembled in the lysosomes, and must aggregate into these by autophagy.[33] In striated muscle, large amounts of extralysosomal glycogen may be observed, and also deposits of strongly metachromatic material. It has been proposed that another enzymatic defect leading to the accumulation of acid mucopolysaccharides may be involved. In a study of muscle biopsies, Griffin[33] has shown that the enlarged lysosomes rupture and that the glycogen is progressively digested, leaving empty zones of sarcoplasm. The metachromatic material is located in zones of undigested extralysosomal glycogen where the glycogen granules stain deeply with silver periodate and become large and irregular. This ultrastructural study of the metachromatic deposits concludes that they may consist of partly digested glycogen

Table 6.3 Some mechanisms of pathological lysosomal storage*

Total or partial absence of lysosomal enzymes (proenzymes, absence of mRNA)	Pompe's disease
Absence of mannose–phosphate receptor	I-cell disease
Instability; rapid degradation	Gaucher type I
	Fucosidosis
Absence of protective factors	Galactosialidosis
Absence of activators or helping factors	Gaucher's disease
	AB variant of Tay–Sachs disease
	Aryl sulphatase-positive sulphatidosis
	Niemann–Pick disease type C
	Morquio's disease
Abnormal egress from lysosomes	Cystinosis
Intoxication of enzymes by undigestible metabolites	Ceroid–lipofuscinosis
Weakening of lysosomal membranes	Haemochromatosis
Drug-induced change	Chloroquine, amiodarone

*References: 1, 7, 10, 42, 45, 49, 64, 65, 67, 76, 87, 95 and 96.

Table 6.4 The glycogenoses*

Type	Eponym	Age	Enzyme deficiency	Main organs affected	Other consequences
I	von Gierke	Congenital	Glucose-6-phosphatase	Liver, kidney	Xanthomas, hyperlipidaemia hyperuricaemia, fasting hypoglycaemia, amino-aciduria (Fanconi), liver adonomas,
II	Pompe	Infantile	Alpha-1,4-glucosidase (acid maltase)	Heart, muscle, motor neurons of spinal cord	Cardio-respiratory failure
		Childhood		Muscle	
		Adult		Muscle	Muscle weakness
III	Cori (six different forms)		Amylo-1-6-glucosidase (debrancher enzyme)	Muscle, liver	Hypoglycaemia
IV	Andersen (amylopectinosis)		Alpha-1,4-glucan-glucosyl transferase (brancher enzyme)	Liver, heart	Neurological dysfunction
V	McArdle	Adult	Muscle phosphorylase	Muscle	
VI	Hers		Hepatic phosphorylase	Liver	
VII	Hers		Muscle phosphofructokinase	Muscle	
VIII	Hers		Liver phosphorylase-kinase	Liver	

*References: 37,41,78 and 82.

with their electron-negative groups closer together than is normal; this would explain the metachromasia.

While the infantile forms of Pompe's disease progress rapidly to death from myocardial failure, other patients may survive into adulthood with only minor problems — notwithstanding a strongly depressed lysosomal maltase. This indicates that the lysosomal catabolism of glycogen is only an accessory pathway. It is also possible that, besides the glycogen-loaded lysosomes deficient in maltase, normally functioning lysosomes may be present and may degrade the glycogen. In fact, heterogeneity of lysosomes has been demonstrated in many pathological conditions.[3,69]

Besides rare cases of generalized amylopectinosis[82] (Andersen's disease) in which insufficiently branched glycogen accumulates mainly in the heart muscle, amylopectins are found in two conditions which are not hereditary. In the central nervous system, amylaceous bodies (corpora amylacea) are frequently found in relation to ageing, tumours, or circulatory disturbances. They are formed in glial cells and later accumulate in the Virchow–Robin perivascular spaces. The mechanism underlying their formation remains unknown. Ultrastructurally (Fig. 23.18), they appear as filamentous structures composed of polyglucosans, probably linked to proteins.[80,82,88]

In one rare disease — the myoclonic form of epilepsy described by Unverricht — similar amylopectin bodies are found in neurons. These Lafora bodies (see also Ch. 23) are weakly metachromatic, have the same fibrous structure as amylaceous bodies and, like them, are destroyed by amylase.[74,94] No enzymatic defect has been demonstrated in these patients. Both amylaceous bodies and Lafora bodies have no particular relation to cytoplasmic organelles.

LYSOSOMAL STORAGE OF COMPLEX LIPIDS

This is a most important group of storage diseases, (Tables 6.5 to 6.8), since pathognomonic lysosomal change may often help to establish their diagnosis. The lipids involved are ceramide, or esters of ceramide (N-acylsphingosine), sphingosine being linked to a long-chain fatty acid with 14–26 carbon atoms. From this molecule, various anabolic pathways lead to the formation of gangliosides, sulphatides and sphingomyelin.

These molecules play an important role in a variety of cell functions, in particular those associated with membranes and myelin. Their synthesis involves many enzymes, and the same is true for their catabolism, where lysosomes are involved through the action of several of their acid hydrolases. These inherited conditions are all autosomal recessive, with the exception of Fabry's disease, which is sex-linked. The anomalies of the lysosomal enzymes or the absence of their activators, often have serious consequences, leading to early death — although some forms are compatible with survival to adulthood. Some evidence of enzyme deficiencies without clinical signs has also been described, and this is perhaps explicable by a possible compensatory mechanism involving the action of extralysosomal enzymes with similar activity.

The most frequent of these conditions is Tay–Sachs disease, a gangliosidosis. In some population groups, principally Jews originating from Poland, it affects up to 100 children born each year (1970 estimate in the United States).[63] Other conditions are quite exceptional, only a few cases having been reported, and still fewer with ultrastructural studies. However, these experiments of nature are

Table 6.5 Lysosomal storage disorders of ceramide and ceramide esters I

Eponym	Type	Age evolution	Missing enzyme	Stored metabolites	Ultrastructure of lysosomes	Main organs affected and clinical aspects
Sulphatidosis[25,43]	1	Late infantile	Arylsulphatase A, no precursor formed	Sulphatides (ceramide gal–SO$_4$)	Herring-bone pattern discs	Severe brain lesions (metachromatic leukodystrophy), gallbladder involvement
	2	Juvenile variant	Sulphatase activator	Sulphatides (ceramide gal–SO$_4$)	Herring-bone pattern discs	Gallbladder involvement
	3	Adult (under 16 years)	Arylsulphatase A (rapidly degraded in lysosomes)	Sulphatides (ceramide gal–SO$_4$)	Herring-bone pattern discs	Gallbladder involvement
	4	4–6 years	Multiple sulphatase deficiency (arylsulphatase A,B,C steroid and mucopolysaccharide sulphatases (deficiency of a stabilizing factor for sulphatase?)	Sulphatides + mucopolysaccharides	Herring-bone pattern discs; Adler–Reilly granules in leukocytes	Bone involvement, excess mucopolysaccharides in tissues and urine
Fabry[16]		Mean death about 40 years	Alpha-galactosidase A, (sex-linked)	Ceramide trihexosides and dihexosides (ceramide glu–gal–gal, ceramide–gal–gal)	Concentric and parallel lamellae	Endothelial cells, glomeruli (renal failure), smooth muscle, connective tissue, skin (angiokeratoma)

Table 6.6 Lysosomal storage disorders of ceramide and ceramide esters II

Eponym	Type	Age evolution	Missing enzyme	Stored metabolites	Ultrastructure of lysosomes	Main organs affected
Gaucher[8]	1	Adult, chronic	Acid beta-glucosidase (decreased stability)	Glucosylceramide	Tubular	Splenomegaly, liver, blood-forming organs
	2	Infancy (fatal before 2 years)	Impaired maturation	Glucosylceramide	Tubular	Neuropathy, acute hepatosplenomegaly
	3	Juvenile (lethal)	Impaired maturation	Glucosylceramide	Tubular	Neuropathy, monocytes, blood-forming organs, nervous system (dementia)
Krabbe[92]	1	Infantile (1 year)	Galactocerebroside-beta-galactosidase	Galactosylceramide	Tubular	Globoid-cell leukodystrophy (macrophages) globoid cells
	2	Late onset				
	3	Adult (2–10 years)				Mental deterioration

Table 6.7 Lysosomal storage disorders of ceramide and ceramide esters III

Eponym	Type	Age	Missing enzyme	Stored metabolites	Ultrastructure of lysosomes	Main organs affected
Farber[55]	–	Infancy, fatal	Acid ceramidase	Ceramide	Curved bilamellar leaflets	Connective tissues, joints; nodular, granulomatous lesions
Niemann–Pick[7,10]	A	Infancy, acute	Sphingomyelinase	Sphingomyelin (ceramide-phosphorylcholine)	Irregular, dense lamellae	Blood-forming tissues, central nervous system
	B	Infancy or childhood (chronic)	Sphingomyelinase	Sphingomyelin	Irregular, dense lamellae	Visceral (no neural involvement)
	C	Fatal before 20 years (chronic)	Sphingomyelinase activator	Sphingomyelin	Irregular, dense lamellae	Spleen

Table 6.8 The gangliosidoses*

Eponym	Type	Age at death	Missing enzyme	Stored metabolites and evolution	Ultrastructure of lysosomes	Main organs affected
Generalized GM$_1$ gangliosidoses	1	Infantile, under 2 years	Beta-galactosidase A	GM$_1$ gangliosides (more than 30 different ones)	Enlarged, fine fibrillary content	Nervous system, liver, kidney, bone
	2	Juvenile (3–10 years)	Beta-galactosidase A	GM$_1$ gangliosides		Nervous system, no visceral storage
	3	Adult (above 20 years)	Beta-galactosidase A	GM$_1$ gangliosides	?	Progressive cerebellar dysarthria
Tay–Sachs		2–5 years	Beta-hexosaminidase A	GM$_2$ gangliosides + asialo derivatives	Concentric, lamellar	Brain, early blindness
Sandhoff	1	2–5 years	Beta-hexosaminidase A and B (beta-subunit)	GM$_2$ gangliosides + asialo derivatives + N-acetylglucosaminyl oligosaccharides	Polymorphic	Brain, blindness, bone deformities
Tay–Sachs	2	Juvenile (5–15 years)	Hexosaminidase A	GM$_2$ gangliosides		
	3	Adult	Hexosaminidase A (like Tay–Sachs + other allele mutation)			Late blindness
Tay–Sachs AB(+) variant	4		Glycoprotein activator of GM$_2$ hydrolysis	GM$_2$ gangliosides		Brain

*References: 12, 44, 45, 58 and 63.

interesting for the study of the morphological aspects of intralysosomal storage in relation to the enzyme deficiencies. Their description will be given in order of increasing complexity of the stored lipids. Comprehensive descriptions of the biochemical and clinical characteristics of these conditions are to be found in the textbook of Stanbury et al.[89]

Farber's disease

No more than 30 cases of this exceptional condition have been reported, and few have been studied by EM.[22,55] It affects infants and is characterized by accumulation of ceramide resulting from the absence of ceramidase, a lysosomal enzyme. Ceramide is found in enlarged macrophages, some of which fuse and contribute to the formation of nodular granulomatous lesions, which may calcify. The most obvious are located close to limb joints. Similar granulomas are found in other tissues, in particular the lungs and the mucosa of the small intestine.

The stored ceramide appears as multiple curved double leaflets (Fig. 6.2). This differs from other diseases of this group but has some resemblance to the inclusions found in ceroid–lipofuscinosis (see below). Overloading *in vitro* cultures of macrophages from a case of Farber's disease with ceramide containing non-hydroxylated fatty acids reproduces these structures.[72]

Niemann–Pick disease

The accumulation of sphingomyelin in lysosomes, mainly in macrophages, is the consequence of deficient sphingomyelinase activity in both the acute and chronic forms (A and B). In the chronic form, however, sphingomyelinase is present and the disease results from absence of an enzyme activator.[3,7,10]

Two forms — the infantile and type C — are accompanied by serious central nervous system damage, while in type B only macrophages (in the blood-forming tissues and the liver) are loaded with excessive amounts of sphingomyelin. These differences are difficult to explain as sphingomyelin is an important component of the central nervous system. The relationship to blood-forming tissues may be similar to that in Gaucher's disease where the lipids originate from the normal destruction of white and red blood cells.

The different forms have similar ultrastructural features, whether the patients die in infancy or survive for several years. The morphology of the lysosomes is characteristic: they are enlarged, and the cells have a foamy appearance by LM. EM shows dense irregular lamellar inclusions, with some clear zones (Figs 6.3 and 6.4). This appearance differs from that of other lipid storage diseases, such as Tay–Sachs and Fabry's diseases, where the lamellae are more regular.

Gaucher's disease

This is also a polymorphic disorder, although the same gene is affected in the three main clinical forms.[4,96] It affects mainly the blood-forming tissues, although in the infantile form it seriously involves the nervous system. The chronic forms are compatible with life into adulthood, with considerable hepatosplenomegaly. While the infantile form is rare, the adult type — resulting from a decreased stability of beta-glucosidase — is frequent, mainly in persons of Ashkenazi Jewish origin (more than 4000 cases in the United States[8]).

A helping factor or cohydrolase — a small acidic protein — has been found in significantly increased amounts in the spleen of Gaucher patients, and the disease possibly results from insufficient binding of this factor to beta-glucosidase. This cohydrolase may also be required for the activation of enzymes involved in other forms of lipid storage disorders (galactocerebrosidase, sphingomyelinase).[65,76]

The accumulation of glucosylceramide is apparent in macrophages of various tissues, particularly the spleen and blood-forming organs. The light-microscopy appearances of these cells are typical, with a striated cytoplasm as observed in bone-marrow smears. This results from enlargement of the lysosomes which become elongated, in contrast to other storage disorders. They contain long tubular inclusions with a diameter of about 50 nm (Figs 6.5 and 15.20), similar to those which form when cerebrosides associate *in vitro*. These appearances are similar to those seen in Krabbe's disease, but the tubules of Gaucher's disease, however, stain strongly with aqueous phosphotungstic acid, suggesting the presence of other components (possibly proteins).[23,68]

Gaucher-like cells have been described in various conditions.[17] Their ultrastructure is not always similar to that of true Gaucher cells, and the lysosomal inclusions may be lamellar, not tubular. Some of these cells contain ceroid-like autofluorescent pigments. They resemble the so-called sea-blue histiocytes observed in haemopoietic tissue in several conditions, often associated with excessive destruction of blood cells. They have been observed also in various metabolic disorders such as dyslipidoses, ceroid–lipofuscinoses and lecithin–cholesterol acyl transferase deficiency.[22,26]

Krabbe's disease

This rare condition (about 50 cases have been published world-wide) results from the intralysosomal accumulation of lactosyl-ceramide.[92] There are several forms — infantile, juvenile and adult — indicating polymorphism of the enzyme deficiency. Severe mental deterioration is present in all cases. The nervous system is infiltrated by large mononuclear cells (globoid leukodystrophy) where ultrastructure is similar to that of Gaucher's disease, with intralysosomal tubular lipids. Globoid cells are also found in the connective tissue of most organs.

The sulphatidoses

Sulphatides — sulphuric esters of ceramide–galactose — are components of myelin. Disturbances of their metabolism lead to extensive destruction of white matter (metachromatic leukodystrophy or Greenfield's disease) but sulphatase esters of cerebrosides and steroids may accumulate in other tissues.[43] The polymorphism of this group of diseases results not only from the deficiency of sulphatase, but also from that of a sulphatase activator. There are several sulphatases (A, B and C) and all three may be deficient in the form called multiple sulphatase deficiency. Less than 100 cases of sulphatidosis have been published.[43]

In the most typical forms — infantile and adult — extensive destruction of the brain myelin leads to the accumulation of phagocytes staining brownish-red (by toluidine blue) in the white matter. These sulphatide-laden cells are also found in other tissues — in particular the gallbladder, where they accumulate in the thickened submucosa. The ultrastructure is quite characteristic: the sulphatides form short leaflets which pile into more or less cylindrical structures, with a herring-bone configuration (Figs 6.6 and 6.7). This differs from other dyslipidoses and is of diagnostic value. Similar features have been reproduced experimentally by overloading macrophages cultured from cases of the disease with sulphatides.[71] The cause of the myelin breakdown, however, is not well understood.

In the juvenile form arylsulphatases are present and the disease results from the absence of a specific activator (pseudoarylsulphatase deficiency).[25] In multiple sulphatase deficiency an increase of dermatan and heparan sulphates, and also cholesteryl-sulphate, is reported. Sulphatases are deficient in cultured fibroblasts from these patients, although A, B and C sulphatases may be detectable but at lower levels than normal. They appear qualitatively normal but their synthesis or their activity is decreased.

Fabry's disease

This sex-linked deficiency of lysosomal alpha-galactosidase A leads, in hemizygous males, to deposits of globotriosylceramide (Cer–gal–gal–glu) and to a lesser extent of galbiosylceramide (Cer–gal–gal), in most tissues, and particularly in endothelial cells. Heterozygous females have a decreased level of alpha-galactosidase, with or without clinical symptoms.[16]

Fabry's disease is manifested by peculiar cutaneous lesions resulting from vascular dilatations (angiokeratomas), severe painful crises affecting the extremities, and eventually renal failure secondary to the deposition of large quantities of lipids in the glomeruli. The frequency is low, the disease affecting about 2 in 40 000 people, but more than 350 cases have been reported in various countries. As alpha-galactosidase is involved in the catabolism of several types of glycoliplds, multiple metabolites are stored, in particular B blood group substances. Increased quantities of glycosphingolipids may also be found in the urine.

The typical lysosomal inclusions are most frequent in endothelial cells; they have a dense lamellar, regular, structure (Figs 6.8, 6.9 and 22.40) and become quite large. The parallel lamellae differ from the irregular ones found in Niemann–Pick's disease. Similar lipid deposits have also been observed in the kidney of hemizygous females. The endothelial location of the lipids explains the cutaneous, nervous and some of the renal complications. However, the disease may run a relatively slow course, sometimes becoming apparent only in adulthood. The lysosomal changes are specific in their distribution and intensity, but resemble some inclusions induced by drugs such as chloroquine.

The gangliosidoses

Gangliosides (Table 6.8) are components of cell membranes, and the human brain contains about ten different types. The lysosomal enzyme deficiencies affecting these lipids are quantitatively the most important, as one form (Tay–Sachs disease or gangliosidosis GM_2), affects many children. It appears that the gene required for the catabolism of GM_2 gangliosides is frequently affected, particularly in subjects of Ashkenazi Jewish origin.[63]

Gangliosides are complex, and their metabolism follows many pathways. The genetic diversity of the gangliosidoses is shown by the various clinical forms resulting from abnormalities of the enzymes required for the catabolism of these large molecules. Activator proteins may also play a role in one form of Tay–Sachs disease.

Biochemically, two main groups of gangliosides may be stored: GM_1 and GM_2, which differ by the presence or absence of a terminal galactose. The catabolic pathways, involving enzymes such as galactosidase, sialidase and mannosidase, are related to those implicated in other lysosome storage diseases affecting glycoproteins and mucopolysaccharides.

GM_1 gangliosidosis is uncommon (less than 200 cases have been reported), the most frequent being the infantile form. It results from the absence of lysosomal beta-galactosidase A.[44,45] Gangliosides accumulate in many tissues, and the ultrastructure is mainly that of large lysosomes with a fluffy, finely granular content with some lipid lamellae. This appearance is not specific and resembles that of mucopolysaccharidoses (in particular Morquio's disease where there is also a galactosidase deficiency, apparently resulting from absence of an activator protein).[44,45]

Tay–Sachs disease is by far the most frequent gangliosidosis. The accumulation of GM_2 gangliosides in the lysosomes of many tissues, and in particular the nervous system, leads to the condition earlier described as amaurotic familial idiocy.[63] The missing enzyme is hexosaminidase A. This is

Table 6.9   The mucopolysaccharidoses I

Age	Eponym	Enzyme deficiency	Urinary mucopolysaccharides	Gross pathology	Ultrastructural pathology
MPS 1H	Hurler	Alpha-L-iduronidase	Dermatan and heparan sulphates	Dwarfing, clouding of cornea, skeletal abnormalities, hepatosplenomegaly, pseudo-atheromatosis	Clear vacuoles, 'zebra-bodies' in neurons
MPS 1S	Scheie	Alpha-L-iduronidase	Dermatan and heparan sulphates	As in Hurler's disease	Vacuolation, without neuronal changes (except slight increase in lipofuscin)
MPS 1H/S	Hurler–Sheie	Alpha-L-iduronidase	Dermatan and heparan sulphates	As in Hurler's disease	Vacuoles, concentric lamellar inclusions in spinal cord neurons, less frequent in brain neurons
MPS II XR	Hunter (two clinical forms: mild, severe)	Iduronate sulphatase (X-linked)	Dermatan sulphate	Dwarfism, stiff joints, heart lesions, retinitis pigmentosa	Metachromatic vacuoles in fibrocytes, membranous bodies in neural ganglion cells
MPS IIIA	Sanfilippo A	Heparan-N-sulphatase (= sulphamidase)	Heparan sulphate	Mental retardation	Extensive vacuolation of most tissue cells, and neurons
MPS IIIB	Sanfilippo B	N-acetyl-alpha-D-glucosaminidase	Heparan sulphate	Mental retardation	Vacuolation

Table 6.10:   The mucopolysaccharidoses II*

Age	Eponym	Enzyme deficiency	Urinary mucopolysaccharides	Gross pathology	Ultrastructural pathology
MPS IIIC	Sanfilippo C	Acetyl coA: alpha-glucosaminide-N-acetyltransferase	Heparan sulphate	Mental retardation	Vacuolation
MPS IIID	Sanfilippo D	N-acetyl-alpha-D-glucosaminide-6-sulphatase	Heparan sulphate	Mental retardation	Vacuolation
MPS IVA	Morquio A	Galactosamine-6-sulphatase	Keratan sulphate	Skeletal and joint deformities	Cell vacuolation (not in neurons)
MPS IVB	Morquio B	Beta-galactosidase	Keratan sulphate	Skeletal and joint deformities	Cell vacuolation (not in neurons)
MPS VI	Marotaux–Lamy	N-acetylgalactosamine-4-sulphatase (arylsulphatase B)	Dermatan sulphate	Growth retardation, skeletal deformities, corneal clouding	Cytoplasmic vacuolation (metachromatic)
MPS VII	Sly	Beta-glucuronidase	Dermatan and heparan sulphates	Hepatosplenomegaly	Metachromatic granules in granulocytes

*References: 28 and 50.

formed by the assembly of two polypeptide chains, alpha and beta, whose genes are respectively located on chromosomes 15q and 5q. The mechanisms leading to hexosaminidase deficiency are multiple, and even in the classic form (in which death results before the age of five), several types have been identified. The enzyme may be abnormal in the absence of translation of the alpha subunit, in an unusual molecular configuration, in its excessive lability or in a defective alpha–beta association.[58] The accumulation of GM_2 gangliosides and of some of their asialo derivatives leads to the formation of pathognomonic concentric lamellar deposits in lysosomes of all neurons (Figs 6.10 and 6.11), with demyelination and gliosis of the central nervous system.

Sandhoff's disease is a polymorphic group of lysosomal lesions with complex deficiencies of both hexosaminidases A and B, resulting from a defect of the beta subunit or a defective association between alpha and beta subunits.[63] In the forms leading to early death, the nervous system is mainly affected, as in Tay–Sachs disease. The lysosomes show polymorphic inclusions, resembling those of GM_1 gangliosidosis (Fig. 6.12). In the juvenile form there may also be an increase of neuronal lipofuscin, resembling that of Batten–Spielmeyer's disease. Chemically, GM_2 gangliosides, asialo derivatives, globosides and oligosaccharides accumulate as the consequence of the enzyme deficiency.

The so-called AB variant of Tay–Sachs disease results from the absence of an activator protein.[12,58] Its ultrastructural pathology does not appear to have been described.

THE MUCOPOLYSACCHARIDOSES

This large group of diseases affecting skeletal growth (Tables 6.9 and 6.10) is important to the paediatrician,[50] and results from various deficiencies of the lysosomal enzymes involved in the catabolism of glycosaminoglycans (mucopolysaccharides). The ultrastructural appearances are rather uniform. Mucopolysaccharides are large molecules comprising various acetylated or sulphated sugars forming long chains attached to protein substrates. Their degradation involves the successive action of several enzymes. In most of these conditions there is excretion of large amounts of undegraded heparan and/or dermatan sulphates in the urine. The skeleton and joints, the connective tissue, the eyes (corneal clouding) and — in the most severe forms — the nervous system, are involved. Dwarfism is common. The bone abnormalities are usually apparent in the early years of life, but some forms are compatible with survival into adulthood and even old age. There is a considerable polymorphism, with many subtypes.

The frequency of these conditions varies from country to country, and some (such as Sly's disease) are known only from a few observations. The most frequent are the various forms of Sanfilippo's disease, which affect about 1 in 25 000 births, but which may often go undiagnosed. The Hurler and Hunter diseases affect about one in 100 000 births. All

are autosomic and recessive except Hunter's disease, which is sex-linked.

The typical ultrastructure is a vacuolar change of the lysosomes, apparent in various cells, mainly of the connective tissue. These vacuoles may stain metachromatically, indicating the presence of negatively-charged polymers. The ultrastructure is without diagnostic value: the lysosomes contain a finely granular fluffy poorly stained material, sometimes with a few lipid leaflets (Figs 6.13 and 15.21). There is one exception: the neurons of Hurler's disease (and the Hurler–Scheie variant) contain large lamellar structures known as zebra bodies (Fig. 6.14), because of the grouping of bundles of more or less parallel lipid leaflets. This appearance resembles that of lipidoses, and it has been suggested that it may result from the accumulation of gangliosides, although this has not been demonstrated chemically. It could be explained by the fact that several enzymes involved in glycosaminoglycan catabolism also play a role in ganglioside degradation.

DISTURBANCES OF GLYCOPROTEIN CATABOLISM

Multiple types of glycoproteins are degraded in the lysosomes by the action of several enzymes — absence or deficiency of which leads to accumulation of proteins with mannose, fructose or aspartylglucosamine residues.[5,21,90] These diseases (Tables 6.11 and 6.12) are related to the gangliosidoses and the mucolipidoses — sialidosis, for example, was previously known as mucolipidosis type I.[19]

The importance of glycoproteins in many tissues explains the severe clinical consequences of these enzyme deficiencies, which affect the skeleton (as in the mucopolysaccharidoses), the eyes and the central nervous system. The bone changes resemble those of some mucopolysaccharidoses, while the neural disturbances are similar to those of the lipidoses. Eye lesions are frequent and may resemble those of the fundus in Tay–Sachs disease (cherry-red spot). In contrast to the mucopolysaccharidoses, the urinary excretion of heparan or dermatan sulphate is not excessive.

As in other storage diseases, multiple clinical forms have been described, although these conditions are infrequent. The ultrastructure, with clear, vacuolated lysosomes containing some lipid droplets or leaflets is not specific and has no diagnostic value.

Mannosidosis

About 50 cases had been reported by 1983. In both clinical forms skeletal and neural lesions predominate. The urine contains the trisaccharide mannose–mannose–N–acetylglucose and other oligosaccharides. Apart from the vacuolation of lymphocytes, few microscopic studies have been reported. The swollen lysosomes may contain some lipid droplets (Fig. 6.15).[22]

Table 6.11 Disturbances of glycoprotein catabolism I

Name	Age of onset	Missing enzyme	Accumulated metabolites	Clinical manifestations					Ultrastructure
				Skeleton	Liver, spleen	Blood cells, lymphocytes	Eye	Nervous system	
Mannosidosis type I	3–12 months	Alpha-D-mannosidase	Mannose-containing oligosaccharides	Coarse facies dysostosis	Enlarged	Vacuoles	Corneal opacities, cataracts	Mental retardation, hearing loss	Clear vacuoles
type II	1–4 years	Alpha-D-mannosidase	Mannose-containing oligosaccharides	Coarse facies dysostosis	Enlarged	Vacuoles	Corneal opacities, cataracts	Mental retardation, hearing loss	Clear vacuoles
Fucosidosis type I	3–18 months	Alpha-L-fucosidase	Several fucose-containing oligosaccharides	Mild changes, dysostosis	Enlarged	Vacuoles	–	Mental retardation	Lamellar inclusions, clear vacuoles, angiokeratoma
type II	1–2 years	Alpha-L-fucosidase	Several fucose-containing oligosaccharides	Mild changes	Enlarged	Vacuoles	Abnormal conjunctival vessels	Mental retardation	Lamellar inclusions, clear vacuoles, angiokeratoma

*References: 1, 5, 19–21, 48, 62 and 90.

Table 6.12 Disturbances of glycoprotein catabolism II*

Name	Age of onset	Missing enzyme	Accumulated metabolites	Clinical manifestations					Ultrastructure
				Skeleton	Liver, spleen	Blood cells, lymphocytes	Eye	Nervous system	
Sialidosis type I (normomorphic)	8–25 years	Sialidase	Sialido-oligosaccharides	Normal	Normal	Rare vacuoles	Blindness,	Myoclonic seizures	Clear vacuoles and lamellar inclusions
type II juvenile (dysmorphic)	2–20 years	Sialidase	Sialido-oligosaccharides	Dysostosis	Normal	Vacuoles	Reduced acuity	Mental retardation	Vacuoles and lamellae, angiokeratoma
infantile	0–12 months	Sialidase	Sialido-oligosaccharides	Dysostosis, coarse facies	Slightly enlarged	Vacuoles	Cherry-red spots	Mental retardation	?
congenital		Sialidase	Sialido-oligosaccharides	Dysostosis, coarse facies	Enlarged	Vacuoles	?	Mental retardation	
Aspartylglycosaminuria	1–5 years	Aspartylglycosamine amidohydrolase	Glyco-asparagine	Mild changes	Normal	Vacuoles	Lens opacities	Mental retardation	Vacuoles photosensitivity

*References: 1, 5, 19–21, 48, 62 and 90.

Table 6.13 The ceroid-lipofuscinoses*

Type	Eponyms	Age of onset	Duration, course	Clinical manifestations	
				Nervous system	Eye
Infantile	Hagberg–Santavuoni	First year	Rapidly progressive	Psychomotor retardation	Optic atrophy, pigmentary degeneration of retina
Late	Jansky–Bielchowski	2–4 years	From 1 to 6 years	Psychic retardation, dementia	Optic atrophy, pigmentary degeneration of retina
Juvenile	Batten–Spielmeyer–Vogt	4–8 years	Slowly progressive	Psychomotor retardation, late onset dementia	Retinitis pigmentosa
Adult	Kufs	After 20 years	Slowly progressive	Variable, slight retardation	No retinal changes

*References: 38, 98, 100 and 101.

Fucosidosis

This is also a rare condition and about 50 cases are known.[5] The angiokeratoma is similar to that of Fabry's disease, while skeletal and neurological lesions are constantly present, although milder than in mannosidosis. Many fucose-containing glycolipids have been identified in the liver and are excreted in the urine, and they result from faulty degradation of gangliosides and polysaccharides. Glycoasparagines are also present in the urine. A few ultrastructural descriptions have been published: polymorphic lysosomal inclusions, sometimes clear, sometimes lamellated, have been observed in biopsy samples of liver and brain.

Sialidosis

This is a rare condition which has been recognized only recently.[19] Various forms have already been reported, differing mainly in the age of onset[20,45,48,62] while angiokeratomas are present in some patients. The lymphocytes are vacuolated, and lysosomal vacuoles are visible in Kupffer cells, fibroblasts and neurons, with pleomorphic clear or lamellar inclusions (Fig. 6.16). In some patients not only sialidase is deficient but also the lysosomal enzyme beta-galactosidase.[27,28]

Aspartylglycosaminuria

This disease has been mainly observed in Finland, where nearly 100 cases have been reported.[5] Aspartylglycosamine is present in the urine of all patients, as well as various other glycoasparagines, resulting from the degradation of glycoproteins. EM of most tissues show mainly vacuolated lysosomes, except in the brain where dense granular bodies have been observed.

I-CELL DISEASE AND PSEUDO-HURLER POLYDYSTROPHY

These conditions — previously known as mucolipidoses II and III (mucolipidosis I is sialidosis) — have contributed important information on the mechanisms of transportation and fixation of enzymes into lysosomes.[57,59,60] These rare conditions were first considered to belong to the mucopolysaccharidoses since the cells showed similar large vacuolated lysosomes — hence the name inclusion cell disease proposed in 1967.[52,53] The clinical evolution, with severe skeletal changes, joint contractures, and mental retardation (leading to early death at about five years), is similar to that of neonatal Hurler's disease and some cases may have been described under this name. The term 'mucolipidosis' was proposed since these patients appeared to have coexistent symptoms of mucopolysaccharidoses and lipidoses, although urinary excretion of heparan or dermatan was not excessive.

The main ultrastructural change, very apparent in cultured fibroblasts, consists of large swollen clear lysosomes (Fig. 6.17) demonstrated by their positive acid phosphatase reaction. In pseudo-Hurler polydystrophy, the cell changes are similar, but the clinical signs appear later in life, with joint stiffness and corneal clouding. This is compatible with survival into adulthood. In fact, these are two forms of the same autosomal recessive enzyme deficiency.[59]

In these conditions lysosomes lack multiple hydrolases (glycosidases, cathepsins, sulphatases), and an excessive amount of these enzymes leaks into the plasma and body fluids.[54] This suggests that the cells are unable to fix the enzymes into their lysosomes properly. As mentioned above,[40,60] biochemical studies have indicated that enzymes can only pass into lysosomes provided that they are conjugated to appropriate factors such as phosphorylated mannose residues. I-cell disease demonstrates the importance of this phosphorylation. The missing enzyme is the phosphotransferase required to phosphorylate the mannose residues.[34,67] However, there is evidence that mannose-phosphate is not required for the passage of all enzymes into lysosomes, since those of I-cell disease contain acid phosphatase, which must have been transferred by another mechanism.[26] In I-cell disease there may also be other abnormalities of lysosomal enzymes, as their molecular weight is often higher than normal.

It is also evident that not all cells are similarly affected: hepatocytes, neurons and granulocytes are normal.[26,59] The biochemical diagnosis relies on the considerable amount of enzymes such as beta-hexosaminidase, arylsulphatase A and iduronate sulphatase being found in body fluids. The ultrastructure resembles that of the mucopolysaccharidoses, with large clear lysosomes (Fig. 6.18). These may also contain some lamellar inclusions indicating a possible deficiency of lipid catabolic enzymes.[53]

WOLMAN'S DISEASE AND CHOLESTERYL ESTER STORAGE DISEASE

Lysosomes contain an acid lipase, deficiency of which leads to early death in Wolman's disease, or which can be tolerated into adulthood in the more benign cholesteryl ester storage disease.[2] Wolman's disease is characterized by vacuolation of lymphocytes, and foam cells in the bone–marrow. The liver and spleen are enlarged and the adrenal glands become calcified. In addition, there is a progressive mental deterioration. Cholesteryl ester storage disease is characterized by slow evolution, hepatomegaly, malnutrition, and large foam cells in the bone marrow. Calcification of the adrenals is exceptional. Both conditions are quite rare.

Absence of lysosomal lipase explains the accumulation of triglycerides and cholesterides in the lysosomes, these often appearing as elongated crystals (Figs 6.19 and 6.20). The total cholesterol content of the liver is increased about ten-fold. The plasma cholesterides are elevated and premature atherosclerosis was present in an autopsied case.

CYSTINOSIS

This autosomal recessive disease leads to the accumulation of rectangular birefringent cystine crystals in the conjunctiva, the bone-marrow, the lymph-nodes, the leucocytes and other organs (but not muscle and brain).[79] The crystals are located in large acid-phosphatase positive vacuoles (Fig. 6.21). Fatal renal failure is a possible consequence. Three forms are described: infantile (6–18 months), with impaired growth, retinopathy and Fanconi's renal syndrome; late onset (1–17 years) with less typical features and nephropathy; and a benign form with crystalline deposits in cornea and conjunctiva without renal failure. The frequency, probably variable from country to country, is about 1 per 300 000 in France.

The presence of acid phosphatase demonstrates the lysosomal nature of the inclusions. The biochemical defect is related to the relative absence of transport of cystine from the lysosomes towards the cytoplasm. This results from failure of an ATPase-dependent mechanism, which appears specific for cystine, as the exodus of lysine remains normal. This mechanism has been studied in cultured fibroblasts from cases of cystinosis.[42,64]

THE CEROID-LIPOFUSCINOSES

This group of hereditary recessive diseases (Table 6.13), affecting the lysosomes, with severe disturbances of the central nervous system, was earlier grouped with the gangliosidoses, and was delineated only in 1970.[100,101] The lesions result from the accumulation in neurons and other cells of brown autofluorescent pigments of two types: lipofuscin and ceroid.[98] While lipofuscin is known mainly as an age pigment, present in neurons, liver, myocardium and other non-dividing cells in old age,[86,97] ceroid was first described in experimental vitamin E deficiency. Both pigments are insoluble polymers differing mainly by their inorganic contents: more zinc in lipofuscin, and more calcium, copper and iron in ceroid.

Ultrastructurally, lipofuscin shows two components: a clear lipid region, and a dense granular material (Fig. 6.22). It is formed in old lysosomes (telolysosomes) often without any active enzymes except sometimes acid phosphatase. By light microscopy, the difference between lipofuscin and ceroid is slight: both are acid-fast, autofluorescent, and coloured by fat stains.

The typical ultrastructure (Figs 6.23 and 6.24) is that of lysosomes containing curvilinear or finger-print structures.[98] Denser, granular inclusions, with irregular contours, more closely resembling the lipofuscins of old age, may also be observed. EM is particularly important in the diagnosis of these conditions, as the enzymatic defects remain poorly understood.

The chemical nature of purified curvilinear granules from Batten's disease has been studied by Wolfe et al;[98] in this study, chromatography indicated the presence of polyisoprenols and dolichols — which are alcohols with long-chain isoprene units (up to more than 100 carbon units). It appears that cells may have lost the ability to recycle these derivatives (deficiency in polyprenol esterases?). On the other hand, the autofluorescent material may derive from oxygenated retinoic acid, a metabolite of vitamin A. Ceroid pigments are also involved in the formation of the sea-blue histiocytes described above in the lipid storage diseases.[73]

The clinical forms of ceroid-lipofuscinoses vary between rapidly evolving brain atrophy with blindness, and chronic conditions present in adulthood and manifesting slight mental retardation and some disturbances of retinal pigmentation; transitions between these various forms are also reported.

STORAGE OF METALS AND METALLOPROTEINS

In all conditions where the amount of iron is excessive, the metalloprotein ferritin, formed in the cytoplasm, is captured by lysosomes (siderosomes) — probably by autophagy. The main disease of iron metabolism is haemochromatosis; it is autosomal and recessive, linked to the HLA locus, and relatively frequent.[6] Although well tolerated in its heterozygous form, in homozygotes there is an accumulation of iron in nearly all tissues, except the central nervous system, where only the choroid plexus is affected.

Some of the clinical complications of haemochromatosis result from the weakening of the lysosomal membranes secondary to their iron overloading, with an excessive leakage of their enzymes. In the lysosomes, the protein component of ferritin (apoferritin) may be digested, the iron then remaining in the form of larger granules or haemosiderin (see Fig. 15.19).[66,99]

The causal mechanism remains unknown, as iron transport in the blood is normal, while transferrin is increased and nearly saturated with iron, and blood ferritin is also increased. The tissues appear to have an excessive affinity for iron which could induce the synthesis of ferritin.

The main complications are cardiac failure and cirrhosis of the liver, often complicated by the development of hepatocellular carcinoma. Iron infiltration of the endocrine tissues is one cause of the associated diabetes and the increased secretion of melanocyte stimulating hormone leading to the bronze colour of the skin.

Similar ultrastructural features may result from excessive iron absorption in various conditions: these include multiple blood transfusions in bone marrow aplasia; an iron-rich diet; the thalassaemia syndromes (mainly beta-thalassaemia major); and the sideroblastic anaemias, where iron-loaded lysosomes are seen in immature blood cells.[81] If the iron overload is severe the same complications observed in haemochromatosis may result: cirrhosis of the liver, diabetes and endocrine disturbances.[77]

Excessive storage of copper is found in Wilson's disease,

which is much less frequent than haemochromatosis.[14] The symptoms appear at an early age or in adulthood. The most typical is the Kayser–Fleischer corneal ring. Renal tubular injury, arthropathy and severe neuronal damage result from the excessive copper load. The intestinal absorption of this metal is normal, while there is decreased incorporation in caeruloplasmin — the copper-containing protein of the blood — whose exact function remains poorly understood. Cultured fibroblasts from patients with Wilson's disease capture more copper than normal ones. Ultrastructurally, copper accumulates as dense granules in the liver lysosomes (Fig. 15.18).

In experimental conditions, many other heavy metals may be stored in lysosomes: uranium, lead, silver, mercury and thorium.[91] Gold salts, used in anti-rheumatic therapy lead to the formation of dense intralysosomal inclusions ('aurisomes'). Their structure is quite different from that of siderosomes, since gold (or gold–protein compounds) forms elongated dense bodies with a distinctly spiculated substructure (see Fig. 17.22).[29]

DRUG-INDUCED LYSOSOMAL STORAGE

Experimentally, a large number of drugs can modify lysosomes and lead to accumulation of dense lipid leaflets or to the formation of clear vacuoles. All these are amphiphilic bases which enter rapidly into the lysosomes (see also Ch. 12). Ammonium chloride, long known to vacuolate cells, induces a swelling of the lysosomes and inactivates their enzymes through an increased pH of their contents.[39,57,85] The dissociation rate of enzymes from the mannose–

phosphate receptors may also be decreased.[87] Other drugs may have more complex actions, for example by combining with lipids and rendering them undigestible by the lysosomal enzymes.[84] Some of these changes resemble those described in hereditary diseases.

The number of active drugs in human pathology is limited. The most important is the antimalarial chloroquine,[87] which induces vacuoles and lamellar inclusions in leukocytes, the cornea and striated muscle (Fig. 6.25); these lesions are thought to be reversible. A drug finding wide use in cardiology as anti-arrhythmic is amiodarone, which is an iodine-containing benzofurane derivative.[35,83] It forms lamellated lysosomal inclusions in the endothelium of conjunctival capillaries, in the conjunctival epithelial cells, and in the lung where it may lead to fibrosis (see also Ch.13). Two other drugs used in the treatment of angina pectoris may induce similar changes: they are 4,4-diethylamino-ethoxyhexestrol and perhexilline.

The list of drugs active in experimental conditions is far longer and is thoroughly discussed in the extensive review by Lüllman-Rauch.[49] While these drug-induced lesions appear to be well tolerated and probably reversible, they may depress the activity of the lysosomal enzymes. They are important, since the ultrastructural changes may closely mimic those of some lipid storage diseases.

Finally, the ultrastructure of several cytoplasmic inclusions in various storage disorders is schematically depicted in Fig. 6.26. Although not drawn to exact scale, the diagram highlights the major structural features of the stored products as they appear by electron microscopy.

REFERENCES

1. Alhadeff J A 1981 Human α-L-fucosidases and fucosidosis. In: Callahan J W, Lowden J A (eds) Lysosomes and lysosome storage diseases. Raven Press, New York, pp 299–314

2. Assmann G, Fredrickson D S 1983 Acid lipase deficiency: Wolman's disease and cholesteryl ester storage disease. In: Stanbury J B, Wyngaarden J B, Goldstein J L, Brown M S (eds) The metabolic basis of inherited disease, 5th edition. McGraw-Hill, New York, pp 803–819

3. Barranger J A, Brady R O (eds) 1984 Molecular basis of lysosomal storage disorders. Academic Press, Orlando, Florida

4. Barranger J A, Murray G J, Ginns E I 1984 Genetic heterogeneity of Gaucher's disease. In: Barranger J A, Brady R O (eds) Molecular basis of lysosomal storage disorders. Academic Press, Orlando, Florida, pp 311–323

5. Beaudet A L 1983 Disorders of glycoprotein degradation: mannosidosis, fucosidosis, sialidosis, and aspartylglycosaminuria. In: Stanbury J B, Wyngaarden J B, Goldstein J L, Brown M S (eds) The metabolic basis of inherited disease, 5th edition. McGraw-Hill, New York, pp 788–802

6. Botwell T H, Charlton R W, Motulsky A G 1983 Idiopathic hemochromatosis. In: Stanbury J B, Wyngaarden J B, Goldstein J L, Brown M S (eds) The metabolic basis of inherited disease, 5th edition. McGraw-Hill, New York, pp 1269–1300

7. Brady R O 1983 Sphingomyelin lipidosis: Niemann–Pick disease. In: Stanbury J B, Wyngaarden J B, Goldstein J L, Brown M S (eds) The metabolic basis of inherited disease, 5th edition. McGraw-Hill, New York, pp 831–841

8. Brady R O, Barranger J A 1983 Glucosylceramide lipidosis: Gaucher's diseases. In: Stanbury J B, Wyngaarden J B, Goldstein J L, Brown M S (eds) The metabolic basis of inherited disease, 5th edition. McGraw-Hill, New York, pp 842–856

9. Brown M S, Goldstein J L, Fredrickson D S 1983 Familial type 3 hyperlipoproteinemia (dysbeta-lipoproteinemia) In: Stanbury J B, Wyngaarden J B, Goldstein J L, Brown M S (eds) The metabolic basis of inherited disease, 5th edition. McGraw-Hill, New York, pp 655–671

10. Callahan J W, Jones C S, Shankaran P, Gerrie J 1981 Sphingomyelinases and Niemann–Pick disease type C. In: Callahan J W, Lowden J A (eds) Lysosomes and lysosome storage diseases. Raven Press, New York, pp 205–218

11. Callahan J W, Lowden J A (eds) 1981 Lysosomes and lysosome storage diseases. Raven Press, New York

12. Conzelmann E, Sandhoff K 1978 AB variant of infantile GM_2 gangliosidosis: deficiency of a factor necessary for stimulation of hexosaminidase A-catalyzed degradation of ganglioside GM_2 and glycolipid GA_2. Proceedings of the National Academic of Science of the USA 75: 3979–3983

13. Creek K E, Sly W S 1984 The role of the phosphomannosyl receptor in the transport of acid hydrolases to lysosomes. In: Dingle J T, Dean R T, Sly W (eds) Lysosomes in biology and pathology. Elsevier, Amsterdam, vol. 7, pp 63–82

14. Danks D M 1983 Hereditary disorders of copper metabolism in Wilson's disease and Menkes' disease. In: The metabolic basis of inherited disease, 5th edition. McGraw-Hill, New York, pp 1251–1269

15. Dechelotte P, Kantelip B, De la Guillaumie B V, Labbe A, Meyer M 1985 Tangier disease — a histological and ultrastructural study. Pathology, Research and Practice 180: 424–430

16. Desnick R J, Sweeley C C 1983 Fabry's disease: α–galactosidase deficiency. In: The metabolic basis of inherited disease, 5th edition. McGraw-Hill, New York, pp 906–944

17. Dingemans K P, Mooi W J, van den Bergh Weerman M A 1983 Angulate lysosomes. Ultrastructural Pathology 5: 113–122

18. Dingle J T, Dean R T, Sly W 1969–1984 Lysosomes in biology and pathology, vols 1–7. Elsevier, North-Holland, Amsterdam

19. Durand P, Gatti R, Cavalieri S, Borrone C, Tondeur M, Michalski J C, Strecker G 1977 Sialidosis (mucolipidosis I). Helvetica Paediatrica Acta 32: 391–400

20. Durand P, Gatti R, Borrone C, Siliato F 1982 Sialidosis: a newly recognized inherited storage disease due to neuroaminidase deficiency. In: Francois F, Maione M (eds) Paediatric Ophthalmology. John Wiley, Chichester, pp 217–218

21. Durand P, O'Brien J S (eds) 1982 Genetic errors of glycoprotein metabolism. Edi-ermes, Milano, and Springer-Verlag, Berlin

22. Dustin P, Tondeur M, Libert J 1978 Metabolic and storage diseases. In: Johannessen J V (ed) Electron microscopy in human medicine. McGraw Hill, New York, vol. 2, pp 149–245

23. Elleder M, Šmid F 1977 Lysosomal non-lipid component of Gaucher's cells. Virchows Archiv B, Cell Pathology 26: 133–138

24. Ferrans V J, Buja L M, Roberts W C, Fredrickson D S 1971 The spleen in type I hyperlipoproteinemia: histochemical, biochemical, microfluorometric and electron microscopic observations. American Journal of Pathology 64: 67–84

25. Fluharty A L, Kihara H 1984 Cerebroside sulfatase activator deficiency. In: Calahan J W, Lowden J A (eds) Lysosomes and lysosome storage diseases. Raven Press, New York, pp 51–60

26. Gabel C A, Goldberg D E, Kornfeld S 1984 Evidence of a mannose-6-phosphate-independent pathway for lysosomal enzyme targeting. In: Calahan J W, Lowden J A (eds) Lysosomes and lysosome storage diseases. Raven Press, New York, pp 175–193

27. Galjaard H, d'Azzo A, Hoogeveen A, Verheijen F 1984 Combined beta galactosidase-sialidase deficiency in man: genetic defect of a 'protective factor'. In: Calahan J W, Lowden J A (eds) Lysosomes and lysosome storage diseases. Raven Press, New York, pp 175–193

28. Galjaard H, Heuser A J J 1984 Genetic aspects of lysosomal storage diseases. In: Dingle J T, Dean R T, Sly W (eds) Lysosomes in Biology and Pathology. North-Holland, Amsterdam, vol 7, pp 315–345

29. Ghadially F N 1982 Ultrastructural pathology of the cell and matrix, 2nd edition. Butterworths, London

30. Glew R H, Basu A, Prench E M, Remaley A T 1985 Lysosomal storage diseases. Laboratory Investigation 53: 250–269

31. Glomset J A, Norum K R, Gjona E 1983 Familial lecithin-cholesterol acyltransferase deficiency. In: Stanbury J B, Wyngaarden J B, Goldstein J L, Brown M S (eds). The metabolic basis of inherited disease, 5th edition. McGraw-Hill, New York, pp 643–654

32. Goldstein J L, Brown M S 1983 Familial hypercholesterolemia. In: Stanbury J B, Wyngaarden J B, Goldstein J L, Brown M S (eds) The metabolic basis of inherited disease, 5th edition. McGraw Hill, New York, pp 672–712

33. Griffin J L 1984 Infantile acid maltase deficiency. Virchows Archiv B, Cell Pathology 45: 23–63

34. Hasilik A, Waheed A, von Figura K 1981 Enzymatic phosphorylation of lysosomal enzymes in the presence of UDP-N-acetyl-glucosamine; absence of the activity in I-cell fibroblasts. Biochemical and Biophysical Research Communications 98: 761–767

35. Heath M F, Costa-Jussa F R, Jacobs J M, Jacobson W 1985 The induction of pulmonary phospholipidosis and the inhibition of lysosomal phospholipases by amiodarone. British Journal of Experimental Pathology 66: 391–397

36. Herbert P N, Assmann G, Gotto A M, Fredrickson D S 1983 Familial lipoprotein deficiency: a-beta-lipoproteinemia, hypobetalipoproteinemia, and Tangier disease. In: Stanbury J B, Wyngaarden J B, Goldstein J L, Brown M S (eds) The metabolic basis of inherited disease, 5th edition. McGraw-Hill, New York, pp 589–621

37. Hers H G 1963 α–glucosidase deficiency in generalized glycogen storage disease (Pompe's disease). Biochemical Journal 86: 1–16

38. Hers H G, van Hoof F 1973 Lysosomes and storage diseases. Academic Press, New York

39. Heyworth C M, Wynn C H 1985 Heterogeneity of lysosomal enzymes in cultured normal and sialidosis type II human fibroblasts and the effects of ammonium chloride on this heterogeneity. Molecular Cell Biochemistry 67: 25–30

40. Hickman S, Neufeld E F 1972 A hypothesis for I-cell disease: defective hydrolases do not enter lysosomes. Biochemical and Biophysical Research Communications 49: 992–999

41. Howell R R, Williams J C 1983 The glycogen storage diseases. In: Stanbury J B, Wyngaarden J B, Goldstein J L, Brown M S (eds) The metabolic basis of inherited disease, 5th edition. McGraw-Hill, New York, pp 141–166

42. Jonas A J, Smith M L, Schneider J A 1982 ATP-dependent lysosomal cystin efflux is defective in cystinosis. Journal of Biological Chemistry 257: 13 185–13 188

43. Kolodny E H, Moser A W 1983 Sulfatide lipidosis: metachromatic leukodystrophy. In: Stanbury J B, Wyngaarden J B, Goldstein J L, Brown M S (eds) The metabolic basis of inherited disease, 5th edition. McGraw Hill, New York, pp 881–905

44. Li Y T, Li S C 1984 The occurrence and physiological significance of activator proteins essential for the enzymic hydrolysis of GM_1 and GM_2 gangliosides. In: Barranger J A, Brady R O (eds) Molecular basis of lysosomal storage disorders. Academic Press, Orlando, Florida pp 79–91

45. Li Y T, Li S C 1984 Activator proteins related to the hydrolysis of glycosphingolipids catalyzed by lysosomal glycosidases. In: Dingle J T, Read R T, Sly W (eds) Lysosomes in Biology and Pathology. Elsevier, Amsterdam, vol 7, pp 99–118

46. Libert J, D'Amico D, Kenyon K 1985 Diagnosis of lysosomal storage disease by the ultrastructural study of conjunctival biopsies. Prceedings of the VIIth Congress of the European Society of Ophthalmology, Helsinki, pp 239–241

47. Libert J, Kenyon K R 1986 Clinicopathologic correlations in inborn lysosomal storage diseases. In: Goldberg M F (ed) Genetic and metabolic eye diseases. Little Brown, Boston, pp 111–138

48. Lowden J A, O'Brien J S Sialidosis: a review of human neuraminidase deficiency. American Journal of Human Genetics 31: 1–18

49. Lüllman-Rauch R 1979 Drug-induced lysosomal storage disorders. In: Dingle T T, Jacques P J, Shaw I H (eds) Lysosomes in applied biology and therapeutics. North-Holland, Amsterdam, vol 6, pp 49–130

50. McKusick V A, Neufeld E F 1983 The mucopolysaccharide storage diseases. In: Stanbury J B, Wyngaarden J B, Goldstein J L, Brown M S (eds) The metabolic basis of inherited disease, 5th edition. McGraw-Hill, New York, pp 751–777

51. Marzella L, Glaumann H 1983 Biogenesis, translocation, and function of lysosomal enzymes. International Review of Experimental Pathology 25: 239–278

52. Martin J J, Leroy J G, Farriaux J P, Fontaine G, Desnick R J 1975 I-cell disease (mucolipidosis II). A report on its pathology. Acta Neuropathologica (Berlin) 33: 285–305

53. Martin J J, Leroy J G, van Eygen M, Ceuterick C 1984 I-cell disease. A further report on its pathology. Acta Neuropathologica (Berlin) 64: 234–243

54. Miller A L, Freeze H H, Kress B C 1981 I-cell disease. In: Callahan J W, Lowden J A (eds) Lysosomes and lysosome storage diseases. Raven Press, New York, pp 271–287

55. Moser H W, Chen W A 1983 Ceramidase deficiency: Farber's disease. In: Callahan J W, Lowden J A (eds) Lysosomes and lysosome storage diseases. Raven Press, New York, pp 271–287

56. Myant N B 1984 The catabolism of low-density lipoprotein by the LDL-receptor lysosomal system. In: Dingle J T, Dean R T, Sly W

(eds) Lysosomes in biology and pathology. Elsevier, Amsterdam, vol. 7, pp 261–296

57. Neufeld E F 1981 Recognition and processing of lysosomal enzymes in cultured fibroblasts. In: Callahan J W, Lowden J A (eds) Lysosomes and lysosome storage diseases. Raven Press, New York, pp 115–129

58. Neufeld E F, d'Azzo A, Proia R L 1984 Defective synthesis or maturation of the alpha-chain of beta-hexosaminidase in classic and variant forms of Tay–Sachs disease. In: Barranger J A, Brady R O (eds) Molecular basis of lysosomal storage disorders. Academic Press, Orlando, Florida, pp 251–256

59. Neufeld E F, McKusick V A 1983 Disorders of lysosomal enzyme synthesis and localization: I-cell disease and pseudo-Hurler polydystrophy. In: Stanbury J B, Wyngaarden J B, Goldstein J L, Brown M S (eds) The metabolic basis of inherited disease, 5th edition. McGraw-Hill, New York, pp 778–787

60. Neufeld E F, Sando G N, Garvin A J, Rome L H 1977 The transport of lysosomal enzymes. Journal of Supramolecular Structure 6: 95–101

61. Nikkilä E A 1983 Familial lipoprotein–lipase deficiency and related disorders of chylomicron metabolism. In: Stanbury J B, Wyngaarden J B, Goldstein J L, Brown M S (eds) The metabolic basis of inherited disease, 5th edition. McGraw-Hill, New York, pp 622–642

62. O'Brien J S 1981 Enzymology of the sialidoses. In: Callahan J W, Lowden J A (eds) Lysosomes and lysosome storage diseases. Raven Press, New York, pp 263–269

63. O'Brien J S 1983 The gangliosidoses. In: Stanbury J B, Wyngaarden J B, Goldstein J L, Brown M S (eds) The metabolic basis of inherited disease, 5th edition. McGraw-Hill, New York, pp 945–972

64. Pisoni R L, Thoene J G, Christensen H N 1985 Detection and characterization of carrier-mediated cationic amino acid transport in lysosomes of normal and cystinotic human fibroblasts. Role in therapeutic cystine removal? Journal of Biological Chemistry 260: 4791–4798

65. Radin N S 1984 The cohydrolases for cerebroside β glucosidase. In: Barranger J A, Brady R O (eds) Molecular basis of lysosomal storage disorders. Academic Press, Orlando, Florida, pp 93–112

66. Richter G W 1984 Studies of iron overload. Rat liver siderosome ferritin. Laboratory Investigation 50: 26–35

67. Reitman M L, Varki A, Kornfeld S 1981 Fibroblasts from patients with I-cell disease and pseudo-Hurler polydystrophy are deficient in uridine-5'-diphosphate-N-acetylglucosamine:glycoprotein N-acetyl glucosaminyl-phosphotransferase activity. Journal of Clinical Investigation 67: 1574–1579

68. Résibois A, Tondeur M, Mockel M, Dustin P 1970 Lysosomes and storage diseases. International Review of Experimental Pathology 9: 93–149

69. Reuser A J J 1984 Genetic heterogeneity in lysosomal storage diseases studied by somatic cell hybridization. In: Barranger J A, Brady R O (eds) Molecular basis of lysosomal storage disorders. Academic Press, Orlando, Florida, pp 287–309

70. Rothman J E 1985 The compartmental organization of the Golgi apparatus. Scientific American 253: 84–93

71. Rutsaert J, Menu R, Résibois A 1973 Ultrastructure of sulfatide storage in normal and sulfatase-deficient fibroblasts in vitro. Laboratory Investigation 29: 527–535

72. Rutsaert J, Tondeur M, Vamos-Hurwiz E, Dustin P 1977 The cellular lesions of Farber's disease and their experimental reproduction in tissue culture. Laboratory Investigation 36: 474–480

73. Rywlin A M, Lopez-Gomez A, Tachmes P, Pardo V 1971 Ceroid histiocytosis of the spleen in hyperlipemia relationship to the syndrome of the sea-blue histiocyte. American Journal of Clinical Pathology 56: 572–579

74. Sakai M, Austin J, Witmer F, Trube L 1970 Studies in myoclonus epilepsy (Lafora body form). Polyglycosans in the systemic deposits of myoclonus epilepsy and corpora amylacea. Neurology (Minneapolis) 20: 160–176

75. Salen G, Shefer S, Berginer V M 1983 Familial disease with storage of sterols other than cholesterol:cerebrotendinous xanthomatosis and sitosterolemia with xanthomatosis. In: Stanbury J B, Wyngaarden J B, Goldstein J L, Brown M S (eds) The metabolic basis of inherited disease, 5th edition. McGraw-Hill, New York, pp 713–730

76. Sandhoff K 1984 Function and relevance of activator proteins for glycolipid degradation. In: Barranger J A, Brady R O (eds) Molecular basis of lysosomal storage disorders. Academic Press, Orlando, Florida, pp 19–49

77. Schafer A I, Cheron R G, Dluhy R, Cooper B, Gleason R E, Soeldner J S, Bunn H F 1981 Clinical consequences of acquired transfusional iron overload in adults. New England Journal of Medicine 304: 319–324

78. Schiaffino S, Hanzlikova V 1972 Autophagic degradation of glycogen in skeletal muscles of the newborn rat. Journal of Cell Biology 52: 41– 51

79. Schneider J A, Schulman J D 1983 Cystinosis. In: Stanbury J B, Wyngaarden J B, Goldstein J L, Brown M S (eds) The metabolic basis of inherited disease, 5th edition. McGraw-Hill, New York, pp 1844–1866

80. Schwalbe H P, Quadbeck G 1975 Die corpora amylacea in menschlichen Gehirn. Virchows Archiv A, Pathological Anatomy and Histopathology 366: 305–311

81. Selden C, Owen M, Hopkins J M P, Peters T J 1980 Studies on the concentration and intracellular localization of iron proteins in liver biopsy specimens from patients with iron overload with special reference to their role in lysosomal disruption. British Journal of Haematology 44: 593–603

82. Schochet S S Jr, McCormick W F, Zellweger H 1970 Type IV glycogenosis (amylopectinosis). Light and electron microscopic observations. Archives of Pathology 90: 354–363

83. Simon J B, Manley P N, Brien J F, Armstrong P W 1984 Amiodarone hepatotoxicity simulating alcoholic liver disease. New England Journal of Medicine 311: 167–172

84. Sly W S, Matowicz M, Gonsalez-Noriega A 1981 The role of mannose-6-phosphate recognition marker and its receptor in the uptake and intracellular transport of lysosomal enzymes. In: Callahan J W, Lowden J A (eds) Lysosomes and lysosome storage diseases. Raven Press, New York, pp 131–146

85. Sly W S, Grubb J H 1984 The role of acidification in transport of acid hydrolases to lysosomes. In: Barranger J A, Brady R O (eds) Molecular basis of lysosomal storage disorders. Academic Press, Orlando, Florida, pp 163–174

86. Sohal R S (ed) 1981 Age pigments. Elsevier, Amsterdam

87. Sosa M A, Bertini F 1985 The effect of the lysosomotropic drug chloroquine on the binding of N-acyl-beta-D-glucosaminidase to mannose-6-phosphate-recognizing receptors of liver. Biochemical and Biophysical Research Communications 131: 634–639

88. Stam F C, Roukema P A 1973 Histochemical and biochemical aspects of corpora amylacea. Acta Neuropathologica (Berlin) 25: 95–102

89. Stanbury J B, Wyngaarden J B, Goldstein J L, Brown M S (eds) 1983 The metabolic basis of inherited disease (5th edition). McGraw-Hill, New York

90. Strecker G 1981 Oligosaccharides in lysosomal storage diseases. In: Callahan J W, Lowden J A (eds) Lysosomes and lysosome storage diseases. Raven Press, New York, pp 95–113

91. Sternlibe I, Goldfischer S 1976 Heavy metals and lysosomes. In: Dingle J T, Dean R T (eds) Lysosomes in Biology and Pathology. North-Holland, Amsterdam, vol 5, pp 185–200

92. Susuki K, Susuki Y 1983 Galactosylceramide lipidosis: globoid cell leukodystrophy (Krabbe's disease). In: Stanbury J B, Wyngaarden J B, Goldstein J L, Brown M S (eds) The metabolic basis of inherited disease, 5th edn. McGraw-Hill, New York, pp 857–880

93. Tager J M 1985 Biosynthesis and deficiency of lysosomal enzymes. Trends in Biochemical Science 10: 324–326

94. Vanderhaeghen J J 1971 Correlation between ultrastructure and histochemistry of Lafora bodies. Acta Neuropathologica (Berlin) 17: 24–36

95. von Figura K, Hasilik A, Steckel F 1984 Lysosomal storage disorders caused by instability of the missing enzyme. In: Barranger J A, Brady R O (eds) Molecular basis of lysosomal storage disorders. Academic Press, Orlando, Florida, pp 133–146

96. Wenger D A, Olson G C 1981 Heterogeneity in Gaucher's disease. In: Callahan J W, Lowden J A (eds) Lysosomes and lysosome storage diseases. Raven Press, New York, pp 157–171

97. Wharton S A, Riley P A 1984 Lysosomes and ageing. In: Dingle J T, Dean R T, Sly W (eds) Lysosomes in biology and pathology. Elsevier, Amsterdam, vol. 7, pp 401–420

98. Wolfe L S, Ng Ying Kin N M K, Baker R R 1981 Batten's disease and related disorders: new findings on the chemistry of the storage material. In: Callahan J W, Lowden J A (eds) Lysosomes and lysosome storage diseases. Raven Press, New York, pp 325–330

99. Wixon R L, Prutkin L, Munro H N 1980 Hemosiderin: nature, formation and significance. International Review of Experimental Pathology 22: 193–227

100. Zeman W, Siakotos A N 1973 The neuronal ceroid–lipofuscinoses. In: Hers H G, van Hoof F (eds) Lysosomes and storage diseases. Academic Press, New York, pp 519–553

101. Zeman W 1974 Studies in the neuronal ceroid–lipofuscinoses. Journal of Neuropathology and Experimental Neurology 33: 1–12

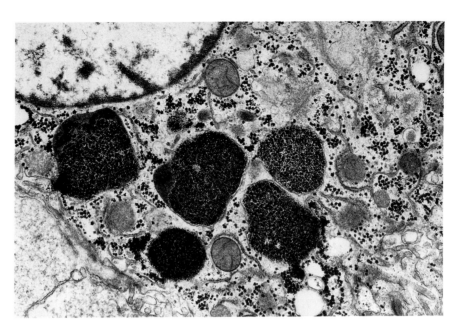

Fig. 6.1 Pompe's disease: liver. Large lysosomes containing glycogen granules are present. (× 13 900) (Courtesy of J M Papadimitriou) (see also Fig. 7.3)

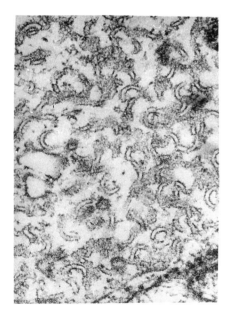

Fig. 6.2 Farber's disease: lung. High magnification of parallel curved leaflets of ceramide in an enlarged lysosome. (× 47 500)

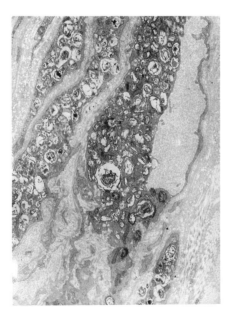

Fig. 6.3 Niemann–Pick disease: conjunctival biopsy. Numerous lysosomes with dense irregular inclusions in pericytes and endothelial cells are present. (× 7 300)

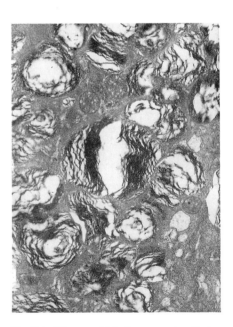

Fig. 6.4 Niemann-Pick disease: conjunctival biopsy. High magnification of the lamellar lysosomal accumulations of sphingolipids. (× 22 000)

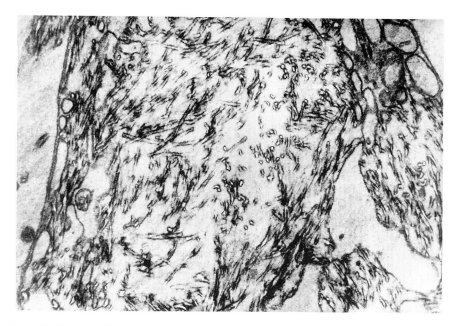

Fig. 6.5 Gaucher's disease: spleen. Phosphotungstic acid staining at low pH reveals large elongated lysosomes with tubular structures whose walls are strongly stained. (× 25 100) (From Résibois et al[68])

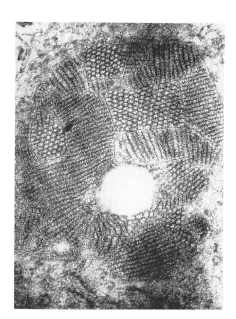

Fig. 6.6 Sulphatidosis (metachromatic leukodystrophy): brain biopsy. A large lysosome with prisms of parallel or herring-bone patterns. (× 48 900) (From Résibois et al[68])

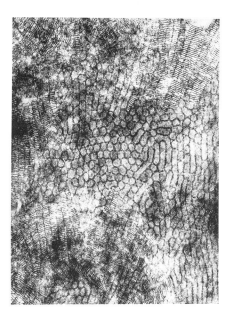

Fig. 6.7 Sulphatidosis: large lysosome loaded with sulphatides. Piles of small leaflets limited by a darker zone are present. The honeycomb pattern becomes apparent when sectioned parallel to the leaflets. (× 48 900) (From Résibois *et al.*[68])

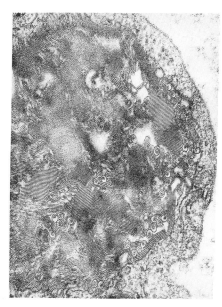

Fig. 6.8 Fabry's disease: conjunctiva. The contents of an enlarged lysosome display parallel lipid leaflets, some of which are curled. (× 41 000)

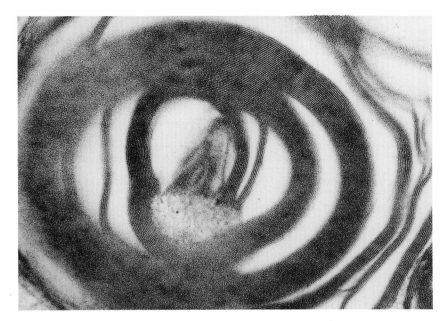

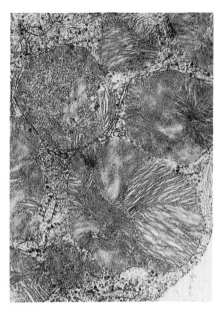

Fig. 6.9 Fabry's disease: kidney. Detail of a concentric myelinoid lysosomal inclusion showing the lamellar configuration, the lamellae being spaced at intervals of about 4 nm. (× 125 000) (Courtesy of M Coleman)

Fig. 6.10 Tay–Sachs disease: conjunctival biopsy. Large lysosomes with parallel lipid leaflets sectioned in various planes are present. (× 8300)

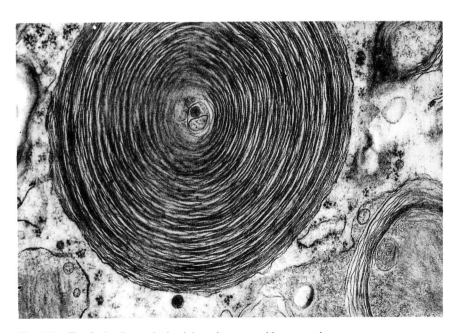

Fig. 6.11 Tay–Sachs disease: brain. A large lysosome with concentric parallel lipid leaflets is depicted. (× 26 400)

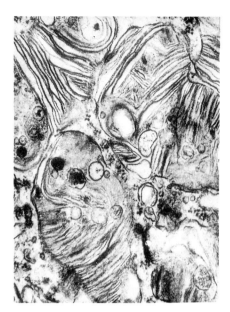

Fig. 6.12 Sandhoff's disease: neurone with pleomorphic inclusions. Lipid leaflets and clear granular zones. (× 17 800) (Courtesy of G Fontaine in Dustin et al[22])

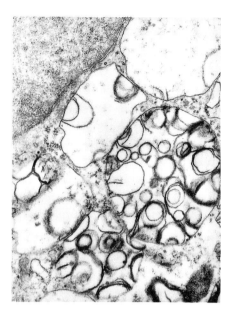

Fig. 6.13 Sanfilippo's disease: kidney biopsy. Enlarged lysosomes with curved lamellar lipid leaflets and/or fluffy material similar to that seen in Hunter's and Hurler's diseases can be discerned. (× 24 800)

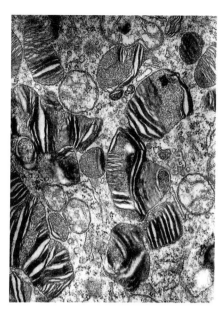

Fig. 6.14 Hurler's disease: brain biopsy. Typical large lysosomes with alternating parallel lipid membranes and granular material ('zebra bodies') are present. (× 17 800)

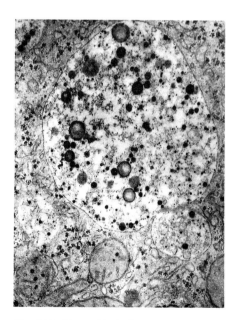

Fig. 6.15 Mannosidosis: liver biopsy. Large pleomorphic lysosomes with dark lipid droplets and a granular background can be seen. (× 16 500)

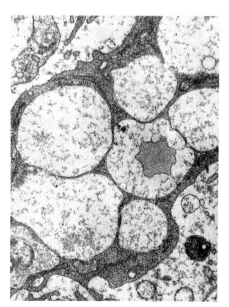

Fig. 6.16 Sialidosis (mucolipidosis I): endothelial cell. Large swollen clear granular lysosomes similar to those of the mucopolysaccharidoses are present. (× 13 200)

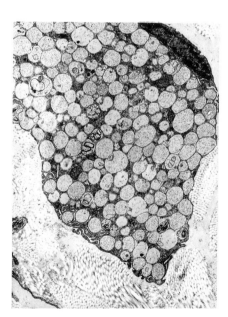

Fig. 6.17 I-cell disease: conjunctival biopsy. Typical appearance of a connective tissue cell with numerous swollen, clear, lysosomes. (× 4600)

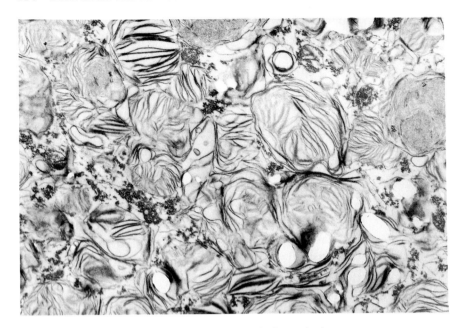

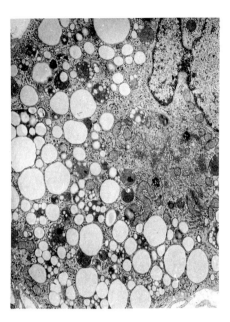

Fig. 6.18 I-cell disease: spinal cord. The lysosomes of this anterior horn neurone show an accumulation of leaflets similar to the zebra bodies of Hurler's disease (compare with Fig. 6.14). (× 21 300) (Courtesy of J J Martin et al[52])

Fig. 6.19 Wolman's disease: bone-marrow. Foam cell with numerous lipid vacuoles is present; note the large Golgi zone. (× 7300) (Courtesy of V J Ferrans in Dustin et al[22])

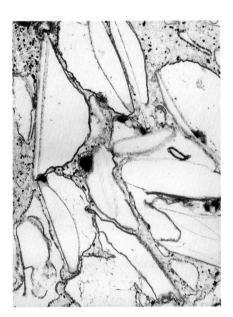

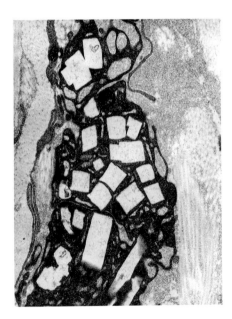

Fig. 6.20 Cholesterol ester storage disease: bone marrow. Clear lipid vacuoles and several needle-like inclusions of cholesterides are seen. (× 12 200) (Courtesy of V J Ferrans in Dustin et al[22])

Fig. 6.21 Cystinosis: conjunctival biopsy. Intracellular accumulation of polygonal, mainly rectangular, clear crystals of cystine. (× 21 100)

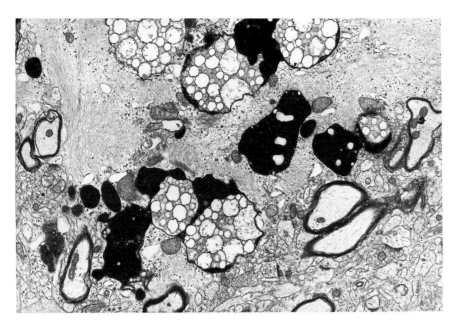

Fig. 6.22 Alzheimer's disease: brain biopsy. Accumulation of lipofuscin granules showing dark and clear zones. (× 9000)

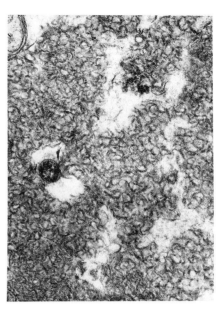

Fig. 6.23 Ceroid–lipofuscinosis (Jansky–Bielchowski's disease): conjunctival biopsy. A large lysosome in an endothelial cell contains many curved lipid lamellae (compare with Fig. 6.11). (× 27 700) (Courtesy of J M Papadimitriou)

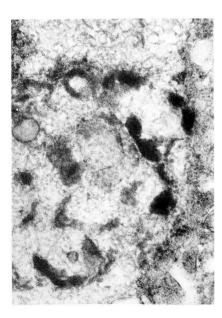

Fig. 6.24 Ceroid–lipofuscinosis (juvenile or Spielmyer–Sjögren type): neuronal inclusion. A fingerprint-like substructure is seen in the inclusion. (× 24 900) (Courtesy of J M Papadimitriou)

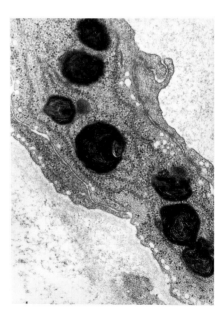

Fig. 6.25 Chloroquine-related injury: conjunctival biopsy. An endothelial cell with dark lamellar lysosomes is shown. (× 43 600)

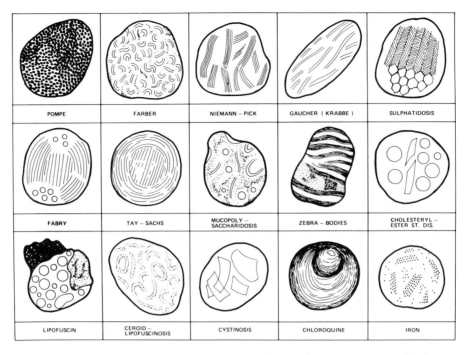

Fig. 6.26   Diagram illustrating the major ultrastructural features of several storage materials in a variety of storage disorders.

7. Prenatal diagnosis of genetic disease by electron microscopy

G. R. Sutherland   D. W. Henderson

INTRODUCTION

Prenatal diagnosis usually refers to the diagnosis of birth defects early enough in pregnancy for termination of gestation if it can be shown that the fetus does have a serious birth defect.[12,36] Prenatal diagnosis is now standard in many genetic counselling situations. Virtually all inborn errors of metabolism have a 25% recurrence risk and most couples will avoid this risk of a seriously handicapped child. The only alternatives to prenatal diagnosis for such couples wishing to have children are artificial insemination (not applicable for X-linked disorders), or ovum donation, or adoption (not a realistic alternative in most western countries because of the paucity of infants available). In general, dominant disorders, where the recurrence risk is 50%, are not amenable to prenatal diagnosis using standard biochemical studies.

There are several approaches to prenatal diagnosis. The most common is amniocentesis to collect a sample of amniotic fluid at 15–18 weeks' gestation. The amniotic fluid contains cells which can be studied either directly or after tissue culture. Cultured cells are used primarily for the diagnosis of fetal chromosome abnormalities but they can also be studied biochemically for the detection of many inborn errors of metabolism. Components of the amniotic fluid itself can be assayed, and the principal group of disorders for which this approach is used are the neural tube defects, diagnosable by measurement of α-fetoprotein and secretory acetylcholinesterase.

There are other approaches to prenatal diagnosis. Chorionic villus biopsy now complements amniocentesis for the prenatal diagnosis of chromosome disorders and many inborn errors of metabolism (see below). It can also provide a source of DNA for the increasing number of disorders which can either be unequivocally diagnosed prenatally by recombinant DNA technology, or can be suspected or excluded with a high degree of probability as a result of genetic linkage studies using the same technology. Fetal blood sampling via the fetoscope or by puncture of the sinus venosus under ultrasound guidance provides another source of material which has been used mainly for detection of haematological disorders, many of which are now diagnosable from chorionic villus biopsy using DNA technology.

The rapid development of high quality ultrasound in recent years has added a very useful technique for the detection of birth defects associated with morphological changes in the fetus. The use of electron microscopy (EM) in prenatal diagnosis has been confined largely to the detection of skin disorders and a few inborn errors of metabolism. Potentially, other disorders could be diagnosed prenatally by EM if tissue samples could be obtained.

TISSUE FOR ELECTRON MICROSCOPY

Several tissues are potentially available for prenatal diagnosis by EM:

1. Uncultured amniotic fluid cells. These have been studied in normal amniotic fluids by Hoyes[22] and have been reported to be a suitable tissue for the prenatal diagnosis of infantile Pompe disease.[23]

2. Cultured amniotic fluid cells. In some ways these resemble cultured skin fibroblasts, although the variation in cell morphology, even at the light microscopy level, is much greater than in skin fibroblasts.[17,41] Studies on the fine structure of normal cultured amniotic fluid cells have been reported by Bartman[8] and Nieland et al.[32]

3. Chorionic villi. Prenatal diagnosis using amniotic fluid cells or samples of fetal skin, liver or blood can be accomplished only during the second trimester (usually at 15–18 weeks' gestation). However, chorionic villi can be biopsied from either the implantation site or the extraplacental chorion during the first trimester (for example, at 8–11 weeks' gestation).[12,34] This procedure has a number of advantages over second-trimester biopsy techniques, including minimal maternal hazards and seemingly low fetal mortality in excess of the 'normally' high fetal wastage due to spontaneous abortion in the first trimester.[34] In addition, termination of an abnormal fetus during the first trimester is safer than second-trimester abortion, and can avoid the

emotional problems resulting from termination after the onset of fetal movements.[34] This procedure has been developed only recently but its application in the diagnosis of genetic disorders is evolving rapidly. Such chorionic tissue has been used for chromosome studies and enzyme or DNA analyses for approximately 100 different single gene disorders.[13]

There are few reports on the fine structure of normal human chorionic tissue secured by this technique[15,39] (see Figs 7.1 and 7.2). It has yet to be determined whether genetic disorders amenable to diagnosis by EM later in life — notably some of the storage disorders — are generally expressed in direct chorionic biopsies in ultrastructural terms as early as the first trimester. There is some evidence that mucolipidosis type IV (MLIV) is not. Ornoy and associates[32a] reported a single case of MLIV in which the fine structure of a direct chorionic villus biopsy did not differ significantly from control samples, and the diagnosis was established by electron microscopy of cultured chorionic cells and, later, in cultured amniotic fluid cells. They suggested that inability to make the diagnosis on direct chorionic biopsy may be related to a paucity of blood vessels in early chorionic villi and that this limitation may extend to other storage disorders in which the diagnosis is dependent on ultrastructural changes in endothelial or other mesenchymal cells.

4. Fetal skin. Fetal skin biopsy is possible either directly through the fetoscope[37] or by fine-needle biopsy under ultrasound guidance.[28]

5. Fetal liver. Fetal liver biopsy has been successfully accomplished to provide tissue for enzyme assay,[38] and is appropriate for the prenatal diagnosis of certain enzyme deficiences which cannot be detected by examination of amniotic fluid — for example ornithine carbamyltransferase (OCT) deficiency[38] or phenylketonuria.[34] These disorders can, however, be diagnosed prenatally using DNA techniques.

6. Fetal blood. Fetal blood sampling has been used largely for the diagnosis of the thalassaemias and other haematological disorders, and for rapid or specialized chromosome studies.[1] Successful prenatal ultrastructural diagnosis of type IIa glycogenosis can also be accomplished by the detection of intralysosomal glycogen in circulating lymphocytes obtained by fetal venepuncture (Fig. 7.3).

DIAGNOSIS BY ELECTRON MICROSCOPY

Inborn errors of metabolism

There are a number of inborn errors of metabolism, particularly lysosomal storage disorders, in which there are characteristic ultrastructural features in fibroblast culture,[42] which suggest that diagnosis using cultured amniotic fluid cells may be possible. However, in the majority of these diseases the biochemical defect is known, and prenatal

diagnosis normally uses this approach. The exception is mucolipidosis IV, in which the biochemical defect has not been delineated and where prenatal diagnosis is by EM of cultured amniotic fluid cells, which show characteristic membrane-bound cytoplasmic lamellar bodies.[25,26,32a]

If uncultured amniotic fluid cells could be used for prenatal diagnosis this would be a major advantage over the use of cultured cells, since several weeks in tissue culture is usually necessary to produce sufficient cells for enzyme assays or other studies. This tissue is, however, highly variable: many of the cells in amniotic fluid are dead or anucleate, and the absolute numbers per volume of fluid vary widely. However, this approach has been documented by Hug et al[23] to be successful for the prenatal diagnosis of glycogen-storage disease type IIa (infantile Pompe disease). They monitored 26 at-risk pregnancies and diagnosed six as being affected within 3–6 days of amniocentesis, compared with 3–6 weeks required for an enzymatic diagnosis on cultured cells. The prenatal diagnoses were all confirmed as correct. The same group[24] has shown that this approach is not successful for the prenatal diagnosis of mucopolysaccharidosis type I (Hurler disease).

MacLeod et al[30] reported finding lysosomal curvilinear deposits in the uncultured amniotic fluid cells of a pregnancy at risk for the late infantile Jansky–Bielschowsky variant of neuronal ceroid lipofuscinosis. They stated that these findings were pathognomonic for this disease, thus establishing a prenatal diagnosis. The pregnancy was not terminated, and studies on the infant at the age of three months confirmed the prenatal diagnosis.[31]

Genetic skin diseases (see also Ch. 22)

There are a number of genetic diseases of the skin and its appendages which are lethal, handicapping or severely disfiguring, for which prenatal diagnosis is appropriate[2,9] — notably the epidermolysis bullosa (EB) and ichthyosis congenita groups (see Table 7.1). An underlying biochemical defect has been identified in only a few of these disorders: defects in DNA repair in xeroderma pigmentosum; steroid sulphatase and arylsulphatase C deficiency in the X-linked recessive ichthyosis of Wells–Kerr;[2] phytanic acid accumulation due to its impaired oxidation in Refsum disease;[40] production of an abnormal collagenase by dermal fibroblasts leading to dermolytic blister formation in the Hallopeau–Siemens type of EB dystrophica;[2] and abnormalities of keratins and filaggrins in bullous ichthyosiform erythroderma.[3,21] Even so, positive prenatal diagnosis of most genetic skin disorders is primarily dependent on ultrastructural examination of fetal skin. By the same token, EM is of value in excluding these disorders in at-risk pregnancies, hence avoiding unnecessary abortion of healthy fetuses.[2]

The clumped tonofibrils characteristic of bullous congenital ichthyosiform erythroderma (CIE; see Figs 22.9–22.11) have been reported in a 'significant proportion' of amniotic

Table 7.1 Genetic skin disorders which have been studied prenatally

Disease	Inheritance	Prenatal diagnosis made	Characteristics
Epidermolysis bullosa:			
Hallopeau–Siemens type	AR	Yes[4]	Lysis of anchoring fibrils and collagen fibres, with sublaminal cleavage
Herlitz type	AR	Yes[29,37]	Hypoplasia of hemidesmosomes
Atrophicans inversa	AR	Exclusion[2]	Hypoplasia of hemidesmosomes
Bullous ichthyosiform erythroderma	AD	Yes[14]	Intracellular epidermal oedema and large globular keratohyaline granules
Non-bullous ichthyosiform erythroderma	AR	Yes[28,33]	Epidermal acanthosis, premature and excessive keratinization
Harlequin ichthyosis	AR	Yes[11]	Premature hyperkeratosis, plugs of hyperkeratotic debris
Sjögren–Larsson syndrome	AR	Yes[2,27]	LM used only, but potential for EM
Anhydrotic ectodermal dysplasia	XL	Yes[7]	Absence of all skin appendages
Oculocutaneous albinism	AR	Yes[10]	Arrest in melanosome development

fluid cells in this disorder, and Holbrook et al[21] suggest that prenatal diagnosis should be possible on cells obtained by amniocentesis. This may be a useful first line of ultrastructural investigation for suspected bullous CIE, and a positive result seems to obviate the need for fetal skin biopsy. However Arnold & Anton-Lamprecht[6] caution that failure to detect the tonofibril abnormalities in amniotic fluid cells does not exclude the diagnosis: cultured amniotic fluid cells in their case appeared normal, clumping of tonofibrils being pronounced only in severely hyperkeratotic plantar and palmar epidermis.[3] In such circumstances and in the other forms of ichthyosis congenita and the EB group, fetal skin biopsy is mandatory for prenatal diagnosis. The ultrastructural abnormalities in these disorders are described and illustrated in Chapter 22 and will not be reiterated here.

Although prenatal diagnosis of the EB group by electron microscopy is relatively straightforward, the ichthyosis congenita group poses considerable problems — especially in relation to false-positive diagnosis on the one hand, and confident exclusion of the suspected disorder on the other. These difficulties relate largely to the stage of development of the fetal epidermis and its regional variations at the time of biopsy.[6] In the past, 'precocious' keratinization has been used as the criterion for identification of scaling disorders such as bullous CIE,[6] but it is still uncertain whether the mutant gene is expressed before or after the normal onset of keratinization (precocious versus excessive keratinization).[6] Interpretation of fetal skin biopsies in these disorders requires a background knowledge of the normal development and keratinization of fetal epidermis — which have been documented in detail by Holbrook & Odland.[18–20]

At 17–19 weeks' gestation age, keratinization is restricted to developing hair follicles in the scalp, and differentiation and keratinization of hair follicles then pro-

ceed cephalocaudally.[19] (Gestational age is usually calculated from the date of first day of the last menstrual period, i.e. menstrual age. Some authors, particularly those publishing in the fields of embryology and teratology frequently refer to the postconceptual age or estimated gestation age, EGA, which is approximately 14 days less than the menstrual age. This use of two methods of timing fetal development can cause confusion. Throughout this account we refer to the menstrual age.) By 23 weeks, hair follicles are present in all areas of the body.[19] At this stage, the hair canals pursue a protracted oblique course through the epidermis; the diameter of the canals exceeds that of the interfollicular epidermis and they possess a lining of two to five layers of keratinized cells.[19] Hair shafts are exposed on the head, but they are only partly exposed on the trunk and upper limbs, and on the lower limbs they are completely enclosed within intraepidermal hair canals.[19] The openings of the hair canals sometimes run parallel to the surface of the epidermis, potentially creating a false impression of precocious keratinization.[6] Chance sampling of such an area can lead to a false-positive diagnosis of ichthyosis congenita.[6] Therefore, multiple biopsies which include the interfollicular epidermis should be taken.

Keratinization of the interfollicular epidermis on most areas of the body does not begin until 24–26 weeks' gestation.[5,6] At this time, keratinization is complete only on the scalp, face and plantar region.[19] Holbrook & Odland[20] report that the interfollicular epidermis over most of the body is roughly uniform in development. Nevertheless, regional variation is recorded, and Arnold & Anton-Lamprecht[6] observed interfollicular keratinization in two skin biopises taken at 20–22 weeks' gestation from fetuses who did not have ichthyosis congenita (Figs 7.4 and 7.5); in both instances the biopsies appeared to be derived from nipple.

For these reasons, and from the diagnostic problems discussed in detail by Arnold & Anton-Lamprecht,[6] the following conclusions can be drawn concerning fetal skin biopsy when ichthyosis congenita is suspected:

1. Ideally, biopsies should not be performed before 24 weeks' gestation since precocious-excessive inter follicular keratinization may not be present.[6] However, legislative or sociomedical attitudes towards potential fetal viability at about this time may either necessitate biopsy earlier or preclude prenatal diagnosis of this group of disorders.

2. In biopsies taken before 24 weeks' gestation, less definite signs — for example, irregularities of horn cell contents — may have to suffice as evidence of the disorder.[6] Bullous ichthyosiform erythroderma is recognisable by markers other than keratinization (abnormal clumping of tonofibrils)[5,21] while some disorders — such as harlequin ichthyosis and the Sjögren-Larsson syndrome — can be identified by truly precocious keratinization,[5] but the situation is less clear for other disorders of keratinization. Anton-Lamprecht et al[5] recommend performance of prenatal skin biopsies for keratinization disorders 'after week 20 and until week 22'.

3. Confident exclusion of ichthyosis may be impossible from biopsies taken before 22 weeks' gestation.[6]

4. Multiple biopsies are mandatory, and the anatomical sites from which they are derived should be known.

5. Since apparently precocious or excessive keratinization may be found rarely in fetuses not at risk for ichthyosis, other ultrastructural markers — such as frequent lipid droplets, cholesterol clefts or membrane structures — should ideally be present before an unequivocal diagnosis of ichthyosis is made.[6]

Fortunately, skin biopsies from fetuses at risk for epidermolysis bullosa can be taken a little earlier since the components of the epidermal–dermal interface region (desmosomes, hemidesmosomes, basal lamina and anchoring fibrils) develop as early as 12 weeks' gestation and are well constructed by 22 weeks.[3] Successful diagnosis of EB letalis (Herlitz) and EB dystrophica (Hallopeau–Siemens) is well documented with biopsies taken at 18–22 weeks' gestation.[2,4,29,37]

REFERENCES

1. Alter B P 1981 Prenatal diagnosis of haemoglobinopathies: a status report. Lancet 2: 1152–1155
2. Anton-Lamprecht I 1981 Prenatal diagnosis of genetic disorders of the skin by means of electron microscopy. Human Genetics 59: 392–405
3. Anton-Lamprecht I 1983 Genetically induced abnormalities of epidermal differentiation and ultrastructure in ichthyoses and epidermolysis: pathogenesis, heterogeneity, fetal manifestation, and prenatal diagnoses. Journal of Investigative Dermatology 81: 149s–156s
4. Anton-Lamprecht I, Rauskolb R, Jovanovic V, Kern B, Arnold M L, Schenck W 1981 Prenatal Diagnosis of epidermolysis bullosa dystrophica Hallopeau–Siemens with electron microscopy of fetal skin. Lancet ii: 1077–1079
5. Anton-Lamprecht I, Arnold M-L, Holbrook K A 1984 Methodology of sampling fetal skin and pitfalls in the interpretation of fetal skin biopsy specimens. Seminars in Dermatology 5: 203–215
6. Arnold M-L, Anton-Lamprecht I 1985 Problems in prenatal diagnosis of the ichthyosis congenita group. Human Genetics 71: 301–311
7. Arnold M-L, Rauskolb R, Anton-Lamprecht I, Schinzel A, Schmid W 1984 Prenatal diagnosis of anhidrotic ectodermal dysplasia. Prenatal Diagnosis 4: 85–98
8. Bartman J 1971 Ultrastructure of cultivated amniotic fluid cells. Obstetrics and Gynecology 38: 838–840
9. Eady R A J, Rodeck C H 1984 Prenatal diagnosis of disorders of the skin. In: Rodeck C H and Nicolaides K H (eds) Prenatal diagnosis. Proceedings of the Eleventh Study Group RCOG. RCOG, London, pp 147–158
10. Eady R A, Gunner D B, Garner A, Rodeck C H 1983 Prenatal diagnosis of oculocutaneous albinism by electron microscopy of fetal skin. Journal of Investigative Dermatology 80: 210–212
11. Elias S, Mazur M, Sabbagha R, Esterly N B, Simpson J L 1980 Prenatal diagnosis of harlequin ichthyosis. Clinical Genetics 17: 275–280
12. Fraccaro M, Simoni G, Brambati B 1985 First trimester fetal diagnosis. Springer-Verlag, Berlin
13. Galjaard H 1986 Survey of fetal diagnosis of genetic disease using DNA analysis and (enzyme) protein assays of chorionic villi. Proceedings of the Seventh International Congress of Human Genetics, Berlin
14. Golbus M S, Sagebiel R W, Filly R A, Gindhart T D, Hall J G 1980 Prenatal diagnosis of congenital bullous ichthyosiform erythroderma (epidermolytic hyperkeratosis) by fetal skin biopsy. New England Journal of Medicine 302: 93–95
15. Gosden J R, Mitchell A R, Gosden C M, Rodeck C H, Morsman J M 1982 Direct vision chorion biopsy and chromosome-specific DNA probes for determination of fetal sex in first trimester prenatal diagnosis. Lancet ii: 1416–1419
16. Hähnel R, Stratton C J, Wysocki S J, Hockey A 1981 Prenatal detection of Pompe's disease by induction of alkaline phosphatase in cultured amniotic fluid cells. Australian and New Zealand Journal of Obstetrics and Gynaecology 21: 43–46
17. Hoehn H, Bryant E M, Karp L E, Martin G M 1974 Cultivated cells from diagnostic amniocentesis in second-trimester pregnancies. I. Clonal morphology and growth potential. Pediatric Research 8: 746–754
18. Holbrook K A, Odland G F 1975 The fine structure of developing human epidermis: light, scanning, and transmission electron microscopy of the periderm. Journal of Investigative Dermatology 65: 16–38
19. Holbrook K A, Odland G F 1978 Structure of the human fetal hair canal and initial hair eruption. Journal of Investigative Dermatology 71: 385–390
20. Holbrook K A, Odland G F 1980 Regional development of the human epidermis in the first-trimester embryo and the second-trimester fetus (ages related to the timing of amniocentesis and fetal biopsy). Journal of Investigative Dermatology 74: 161–168
21. Holbrook K A, Dale B A, Sybert V P, Sagebiel R W 1983 Epidermolytic hyperkeratosis: ultrastructure and biochemistry of skin and amniotic fluid cells from two affected fetuses and a newborn infant. Journal of Investigative Dermatology 80: 222–227
22. Hoyes A D 1968 Ultrastructure of the cells of the amniotic fluid. Journal of Obstetrics and Gynecology of the British Commonwealth 75: 164–171

23. Hug G, Soukup S, Ryan M, Chuck G 1984 Rapid prenatal diagnosis of glycogen-storage disease type II by electron microscopy of uncultured amniotic fluid cells. New England Journal of Medicine 310: 1018–1022
24. Hug G, Soukup S, Chuck G, Ryan M 1984 Antenatal diagnosis of mucopolysaccharidosis type I (Hurler's disease) is not possible by electron microscopy of uncultured amniotic fluid cells. Journal of Medical Genetics 21: 359–363
25. Kohn G, Livni N, Ornoy A, Sekeles E, Beyth Y, Legum C, Bach G, Cohen M M 1977 Prenatal diagnosis of mucolipidosis IV by electron microscopy. Journal of Pediatrics 90: 62–66
26. Kohn G, Sekeles E, Arnon J, Ornoy A 1982 Mucolipidosis IV. Prenatal diagnosis by electron microscopy. Prenatal Diagnosis 2: 301–307
27. Kousseff B G, Matsuoka L Y, Stenn K S, Hobbins J C, Mahoney M J, Hashimoto K 1982 Prenatal diagnosis of Sjogren–Larsson syndrome. Journal of Pediatrics 101: 998–1001
28. Langlois S Le P, Henderson D W, Chen C, Sutherland G R 1985 Antenatal diagnosis of lamellar ichthyosis by ultrasonically guided needle biopsy of foetal skin. Fourth Meeting of the World Federation of Ultrasound in Medicine and Biology, Sydney, Pergamon, p 305
29. Löfberg L, Anton-Lamprecht I, Michaëlsson G, Gustavii B 1983 Prenatal exclusion of Herlitz syndrome by electron microscopy of fetal skin biopsies obtained at fetoscopy. Acta Dermatovener (Stockholm) 63: 185–189
30. MacLeod P M, Dolman C L, Nickel R E, Chang E, Zonana J, Silvey K 1984 Prenatal diagnosis of neuronal ceroid lipofuscinosis. New England Journal of Medicine 310: 595
31. MacLeod P M, Dolman C L, Nickel R E, Chang E, Nag S, Zonana J, Silvey K 1985 Prenatal diagnosis of neuronal ceroid-lipofuscinoses. American Journal of Medical Genetics 22: 781–789
32. Nieland M L, Parmley T H, Woodruff J D 1970 Ultrastructural observations on amniotic fluid cells. American Journal of Obstetrics and Gynecology 108: 1030–1042
32a. Ornoy A, Arnon J, Grebner E E, Jackson L G, Bach G 1987 Early prenatal diagnosis of mucolipidosis IV (letter). American Journal of Medical Genetics 27: 983–985
33. Perry T B, Holbrook K A, Hoff M S, Hamilton E F, Senikas V, Fisher C 1987 Prenatal diagnosis of congenital non-bullous ichthyosiform erythroderma (lamellar ichthyosis). Prenatal Diagnosis 7: 145–155
34. Rodeck C H, Morsman J M 1983 First-trimester chorion biopsy. British Medical Bulletin 39: 338–342
35. Rodeck C H, Nicolaides K H 1983 Fetoscopy and fetal tissue sampling. British Medical Bulletin 39: 332–337
36. Rodeck C H, Nicolaides K H (eds) 1984 Prenatal Diagnosis. Proceedings of the Eleventh Study Group RCOG. RCOG, London
37. Rodeck C H, Eady R A, Gosden C M 1980 Prenatal diagnosis of epidermolysis bullosa letalis. Lancet ii: 949–952
38. Rodeck C H, Patrick A D, Pembrey M E, Tzannatos C, Whitfield A E 1982 Fetal liver biopsy for prenatal diagnosis of ornithine carbamyl transferase deficiency. Lancet ii: 297–300
39. Rodeck C H, Morsman J M, Gosden C M, Gosden J R 1983 Development of an improved technique for first-trimester microsampling of chorion. British Journal of Obstetrics and Gynaecology 90: 1113–1118
40. Steinberg D, Vroom F Q, Engel W K, Cammermeyer J, Mize C E, Avigan J 1967 Refsum's disease — a recently characterized lipidosis involving the nervous system. Annals of Internal Medicine 66: 365–395
41. Sutherland G R, Bauld R, Bain A D 1974 Observations on human amniotic fluid cell strains in serial culture. Journal of Medical Genetics 11: 190–195
42. Wyatt P R, Cox D M 1977 Utilization of electron microscopy in the prenatal diagnosis of genetic disease. Human Heredity 27: 22–37

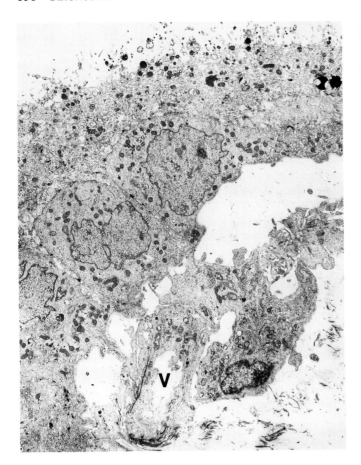

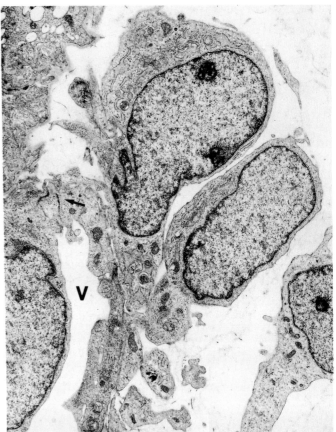

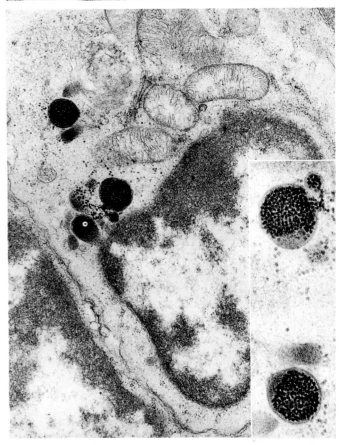

Fig. 7.1 Normal human chorionic villus: first-trimester villus biopsy I. The surface layer of syncytiotrophoblast is not well preserved in this field, but the microvillous free surface of the cells is evident. In other areas these cells had elaborate villiform processes, abundant dilated RER and multiple irregular nuclear profiles. The cytotrophoblast layer is well maintained and the cells rest on a continuous basal lamina. Fetal mesenchyme containing a small vessel (V) and an adjacent fibroblastoid cell is also present. (× 3600) References: 15 and 39.

Fig. 7.2 Normal human chorionic villus: first trimester villus biopsy II. Fetal mesenchyme within the villus is depicted. The basal lamina at the base of the cytotrophoblast is evident at top left. A developing blood vessel (V) is apparent, and junctions can be seen between adjoining endothelial plasma membranes (arrow). Luminal erythrocytes were found in other areas. Adjacent fibroblastoid cells are also present. The abundant extracellular matrix contains only a few collagen fibres, but these may be abundant.[15] (× 6400)

Fig. 7.3 Type IIa glycogenosis (infantile Pompe's disease): intralysosomal glycogen in circulating fetal lymphocytes. Lymphocytes from fetal blood obtained by umbilical cord puncture at 16 weeks' gestation. A few glycogen particles are present within the background cytoplasm, but most are concentrated within the clustered lysosomes. **Inset** Detail of glycogen-rich lysosomes. (× 20 500; *Inset* × 38 000) (Case contributed by Professor J M Papadimitriou; further details on this case have been published elsewhere.[16]) References: 16 and 23.

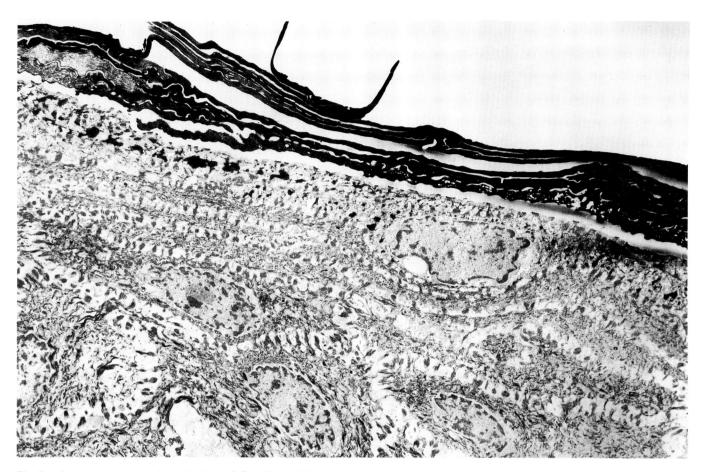

Fig. 7.4 Ichthyosis congenita: fetal skin biopsy I. Figs. 7.4 and 7.5 are from the same case. Second trimester transuterine needle biopsy of skin from a fetus at risk from lamellar ichthyosis. The parents were non-consanguineous and had previously had a daughter with lamellar ichthyosis; at birth, the infant had had the appearance of a 'collodion' baby, and she died aged 2 days. The mother presented at the age of 39; two separate sets of biopsies were performed at 20 and 22 weeks' gestation, and on each occasion, four separate biopsies were taken from the fetal buttock.

At the first examination, two fragments of skin were obtained. Keratinization was evident, and a diagnosis of ichthyosis was indicated with a high index of probability, but because of doubt concerning chance sampling of a hair follicle region, a repeat biopsy was performed. Again, the appearances of the skin biopsies by light and electron microscopy suggested a diagnosis of ichthyosis. The pregnancy was terminated and a fetus of 23 weeks' gestation was delivered. There was both gross and microscopic evidence of ichthyosis; the fetus had a 'pinched' expression, with a taut mouth, and white areas were seen around the mouth and forehead region. Light microscopy revealed epidermal acanthosis, premature-excessive keratinization, and marked keratotic plugging of hair follicles, the changes being most severe in the facial and scalp regions.

The second skin biopsy, taken at 22 weeks' gestation, is depicted. Glycogen-rich and periderm cells are not present in this field. The keratinocytes forming the stratum spinosum are characterized by numerous cell processes with desmosome-tonofilament complexes. Tonofibrils appear to be over-abundant in comparison to the gestational age. Keratohyaline granules can be seen in the stratum granulosum. Up to nine layers of heavily keratinized cells are evident on the surface, but these are consistent with a 'flat' hair follicle extending along the surface of the epidermis.

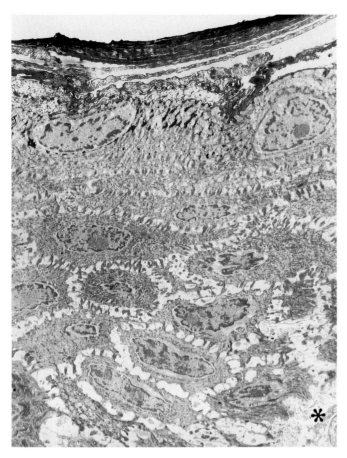

Fig. 7.5 Ichthyosis congenita: fetal skin biopsy II. The second skin biopsy (22 weeks' gestation) is again shown here. A small amount of dermal connective tissue occupies the lower right corner (*). The epidermis is acanthotic, lacking evidence of immaturity, and several layers of keratinized cells are present on the surface, the latter being consistent with a hair follicle lying parallel to the surface. (× 3600) Details of this case, including the biopsy procedure, have been published elsewhere,[28] and it appears to resemble quite closely the case reported by Perry et al.[33] We are grateful to Professor I Anton-Lamprecht for confirmation of the diagnosis of ichthyosis in this case.

8. The search for viruses by negative contrast

C. R. Madeley

INTRODUCTION

This chapter deals with finding and identifying viruses directly in diagnostic specimens — specifically human specimens — but the principles discussed can be applied to veterinary virology and, to some extent, plant and insect virology as well. The underlying intention is to concentrate as many viruses onto the microscope grid as possible, free of most contaminating debris and with their surface or internal details efficiently displayed. This is important at any time, but becomes still more important when the virus concerned is one not hitherto recognized: certainty of recognition grows rapidly with the numbers of particles seen.

Not surprisingly, the finding of viruses depends on good techniques — preparation, examination and microphotography. Each stage is important, and what follows is a guide for the inexperienced. It does not provide a comprehensive atlas of the viruses which may be found — the reader is referred to other textbooks for this, although it is most unlikely that all viruses are already known. There are still many cases of disease of probable viral origin from which no virus has been recovered, and the challenge to find something 'new' remains.

At present the electron microscope is still the only catch-all system of virus detection — no prior decision as to which virus may be present is required. In its simplest terms, it is a matter of making a suitable preparation and examining it. Nonetheless, these preparations must be properly executed, and this begins long before the actual microscopy.

The methods outlined below form the basis of techniques which have been found to be suitable, but they should not be considered the last word on specimen preparation. Indeed, the reader is challenged to make them only a starting point. Seemingly, everything is rediscovered every 25 years, and any trained microscopist may find a new highly sensitive method and, with it, hitherto undiscovered viruses.

PREPARATION

This section is not intended to provide methods of preparation but to discuss the principles involved. Because the steps of preparation of different specimens and different examples of the same specimen (for example, faeces) require judgement rather than the rigid application of a recipe, it is better for the microscopist to understand what he is trying to achieve and to modify his handling of the specimen according to circumstances.

Aims of preparation

Simply stated, these are to concentrate as many undamaged viruses from the specimen as possible onto the grid, and with as little contaminating material as possible. It must be remembered that the electron microscope is an insensitive tool for detecting viruses, due to the small amount of material that can be put on a 3 mm grid, and the need to remove at least some of the contaminating biological debris which will have similar physical characteristics to the viruses. This inevitably involves the loss of some of the viruses and may amount to 99% or more.

It seems that it is generally difficult physically to damage viruses; they survive high speed centrifugation at forces up to 100 000 g with no obvious damage. All EM preparations are artefacts, but in the case of viruses examined by negative contrast they are very constant, different preparations of the same virus being indistinguishable from each other.

Chemical damage on the other hand is easily done. The use of stains, buffers, enzymes, detergents, disinfectants and so forth, can all result in effects which, at their worst, will make the virus unrecognizable either by changing surface detail or disintegrating the particles. The use of some chemicals is unavoidable in preparation, but this concept should always be at the back of the microscopist's mind, and the objects seen subsequently in the microscope interpreted accordingly. Some specific examples are discussed later.

Viruses grow in cells, usually killing them in the process. Release from the cell may occur by budding over a period of time, by immediate lysis, or sometimes after release of the whole cell from its place in the body. In any case, viruses are later found in regions of the body (secretions, faeces, serum and so forth) where they will be well mixed with other material with characteristics (size, density, appearance) very similar to their own. Removal of contaminants may be only at the expense of losing a substantial proportion of the viruses present. At first sight the loss of 99% is unacceptable, but where the original concentration of viruses in faeces, for example, may reach 10^{11}/g of the original stool, losses of even this magnitude will reduce the concentration only to about 10^9/ml of extract — which lies well above the probable threshold of detection of 10^6/ml.

The best naturally occurring specimen for routine detection of viruses is the fluid in the vesicles of chickenpox or herpes simplex. This vesicle fluid (VF) contains high levels of viruses in a medium relatively free of particulate contaminants. The intention of the approaches to preparing various specimens which are discussed below is to make an extract which is as close to natural VF as possible. Such high-titre fluids are then finally prepared for the microscope in much the same way, regardless of source.

With most specimens the microscopist will want to concentrate any virus present and this will usually mean centrifugation. Before considering the preparation of various types of specimen it is necessary to understand what centrifugation in a bench centrifuge or an ultracentrifuge can and cannot achieve.

To centrifuge or not to centrifuge

In any gravitational field, large dense particles will sediment more quickly than their lighter and smaller companions. If the field is strong enough and acts for a sufficiently long time all particles suspended in a fluid of lesser density will reach the bottom. The speed with which they do so depends on their size and density and on the size of the force. However, in a fluid of increasing density (a density gradient) these particles will eventually reach an equilibrium where the fluid density is the same as their own, and the sedimenting force is balanced by a buoyant one.

These parameters limit what can be achieved by centrifugation:

1. Low-speed centrifugation (LSC)

Bench centrifuges can only provide up to about 5000 g. This is enough to sediment cells, bacteria (most) and larger debris after 20 minutes. It is not enough to sediment most viruses as individual particles but a considerable amount may finish in the pellet either as aggregates (some of this may be antibody-mediated) or carried down in, or by, contaminating debris.

Whether this makes the difference between finding a virus or not is debatable. With a high titre virus, detectable amounts are usually left in the supernatant, mostly as individual particles or small aggregates. Where diagnosis alone is the intention, this may not be important but assessing what proportion of the virus is aggregated may

require examination of uncentrifuged material as well, while accepting the difficulties provided by too much irrelevant debris on the grid. By itself low-speed centrifugation cannot concentrate virus.

2. High-speed centrifugation (HSC)

This is done with the intention of sedimenting viral particles to the bottom of the centrifuge tube. Hence the speed (force) and time combination is chosen to make sure of this. Rarely it is chosen to sediment a particular virus — more often it is an excess to make sure any virus present does reach the bottom. This is usually acceptable because viruses survive such clumsy treatment very well.

The parameters used will vary from one laboratory to another but a good round figure is 100 000 g for one hour. This is an average figure and takes no account, for example, of differences between the top and bottom of the tube. It is so much greater than that necessary to bring down even the smallest viruses that such distinctions are unimportant.

What is not so clearly understood, however, is what is achieved by this. Although usually undertaken to concentrate viruses, the concentration achieved in practice may not be substantial or even significant. The volume in the centrifuge tube is often about 5 ml and, with many stool extracts for example, this produces a substantial pellet after an hour's centrifugation. Diluting this to a level where the grid is not overloaded will reverse the concentrating effect and the effective final concentration may not even reach ten-fold.

What high speed centrifugation does achieve, however, is removal of soluble protein and salt. Both are enemies of good microscopy and are discarded from the preparation as the supernatant is poured off. This is an important, and generally unrecognized, achievement and applies equally to specimens producing only small pellets, where the above argument about concentration applies less clearly.

Either angle or swing-out rotors may be used but there are two reasons for preferring the latter if they are available; the pellet will always be at the bottom of the tube, and the filling and capping of angle rotor tubes is much more tedious and time-consuming — an increasingly important factor if many specimens are handled.

3. Medium-speed centrifugation

This has been used as an additional cleaning-up step in preparation. Forces such as 11 000 g for an hour have been used. Because its introduction may achieve the worst of both worlds — in losing some virus into the pellet while leaving much of the debris of similar size and density to the virus in the supernatant — this should not be used without proving its value first.

4. Gradients

Centrifugation to equilibrium in a suitable density gradient (such as caesium chloride) will provide valuable information about the density of a virus — but usually at the expense of characteristic surface morphology. The trouble and expense of preparing, loading, running, fractionating and examining the various fractions individually make this a technique for obtaining further evidence about a virus already found, rather than for routine diagnosis. It is easier to do when there is enough virus in the specimen to produce a visible band on the gradient. This is not always so, and in its absence some guesswork is needed or too many grids will require examination for this to be practicable, except as part of a research project.

These arguments apply even more to velocity gradients (such as sucrose, tartrate) in which the virus is not sedimented to equilibrium, and its position on the gradient is even more a matter of guesswork.

Preparation of different types of specimen

The preparation of a variety of specimens is outlined below. In all, it is axiomatic that if an extract is being made for isolation in cell culture in addition to microscopy, it will have to be made in saline (usually buffered with non-volatile salts), while distilled or deionised water (DW) is preferable for EM alone. Routine diluents typically consist of DW containing a small polypeptide such as bacitracin (0.1%) as a wetting agent. Types of specimen are listed in Table 8.1 and further aspects of their preparation are discussed below.

1. Vesicle fluid (VF)

This can be collected most conveniently with a small syringe and a fine (25 gauge) needle. The quantity needed is very small and is rinsed out of the syringe (or even out of the needle alone) with a small amount of EM diluent. Because phosphotungstate can lyse envelopes, allowing the stain-virus mixture to stand in the syringe for up to 20 minutes can improve the apparent level of virus present — enough to convert negative results to positive in some cases.

2. Cerebrospinal fluid

It is rarely possible to get more than about 1 ml of what will be largely EM-compatible fluid. Levels of protein will be fairly low, as will particulate debris. Salt may be a problem, but the dilution necessary for HSC may be thought too risky (some losses are inevitable). Minimal dilution in EM diluent may be the only practical solution.

3. Faeces

An approximately 10% extract is made, from the whole stool if available; from the solid part if from a napkin. In the latter case, particularly with a very fluid stool, much may be lost. After brisk shaking, the extract is clarified by LSC (approx-

imately 3000 r.p.m for 20 min) and the supernatant removed carefully. This can be difficult with a fatty stool and it is better not to be too ambitious over quantities. The supernatant is removed and ultracentrifuged (HSC) while the pellet is discarded. This second supernatant is poured off, the tube plugged with a tissue while inverted, and then allowed to drain for several minutes. The pellet is gently resuspended in a few drops of EM diluent to provide the equivalent of VF. With some specimens considerable dilution is needed to reduce the concentration of background debris so that any viruses present will be visible. The optimal dilution must be learnt by trial and error but more is generally preferable to less, despite the apparent dangers of overdilution. The vast numbers of virus particles in many stools protect against this, but the number present in successive specimens from one patient diminishes with time, and some judgement is necessary to achieve the right dilution. Experience will help here but, occasionally, two or more grids may need to be prepared.

4. Urine

The quantity of specimen is not usually a problem with children and adults, but difficulties in securing an adequate volume is a problem with infants and uncooperative subjects. The concentration of virus is likely to be low, and minute quantities of 0.5 ml or less give the microscopist little chance.

The percentage of urines positive for viruses by culture is low and reflects low concentrations of viruses. They should be examined by EM as soon as possible after micturition. With fresh urines there is little to be gained by LSC, but HSC will allow protein and salt to be discarded. The pellet is often too small to be seen (an argument for using a swing-out rotor) but a surprising and adequate amount of formed debris will be found in it. Nonetheless, viruses will be difficult to find by any technique, and the yield by EM will also be low — both in the number of positive cases and the amount of virus in each.

5. Serum

Quantity is not usually a problem. The two viruses listed in Table 8.1 are not the only ones to be found in blood but the others are present in the cellular fractions and do not achieve levels in the serum that are detectable by EM. Electron microscopy is not used routinely to diagnose infections with hepatitis B — for which other antibody-based assays are more appropriate — but it is the only widely available technique which can detect with certainty the presence of infectious viruses (Dane particles).

The amounts of protein and salt in serum makes HSC essential. The amount of other debris is small but includes spherical lipoprotein-like material which can mimic the appearance of hepatitis B surface antigen closely.

The parvovirus B18 associated with 'fifth disease' (erythema infectiosum or 'slapped-cheek' syndrome) appears to be present only transiently after onset of the disease and has often disappeared by the time the specimen is taken.

6. Pharyngeal washes

These should not be confused with nasopharyngeal aspirates but are the products of gargling a saline solution. They can be obtained only with the active co-operation of the patient, but this defines the suitable patient as one not seriously ill and in whom the need to make a definite diagnosis of a respiratory tract infection is not going to be life-saving. Bronchial lavage may be done on unconscious patients and is now more widely used; viruses may be found by EM after HSC. Prior LSC is necessary if the specimen contains much particulate debris visible to the naked eye. This technique has not been widely used hitherto but may become so with the increasing numbers of older children and adults who are immunosuppressed for whatever reason.

7. Biopsies

Table 8.1 lists three types of biopsy and the viruses which may be found in them. However, viruses of any kind may be sought in any piece of tissue suspected of containing them.

Because the ratio of cells containing morphologically intact virions to those without them is small it is never easy to find viruses in biopsies except from common warts early in their existence. In genital warts and herpes encephalitis the level is usually close to undetectable.

To break up the tissue, biopsies are ground with clean (or sterile) sharp sand in a small amount of DW in a pestle and mortar which should have been chilled to $-20°C$ beforehand. The objective is to disrupt (osmotically by DW and through ice-crystal formation by freezing) the cells and release any viruses present. Grinding with sand is probably better than using all-glass homogenizers because most biopsies contain fibro-elastic tissue and collagen which is too rubbery and hardened by the freezing to disrupt easily without sand.

The resultant slurry is allowed to thaw, put in a conical glass centrifuge tube and left for a few minutes to separate. The usually milky supernatant can be treated as VF but, if necessary, it can be diluted in more DW and purified by LSC and HSC. It should be remembered that some enveloped viruses, for example, do not exist as complete virions inside cells and that only incomplete viral particles may be present in a biopsy extract.

8. Other specimens

These can include any specimen (fluid or solid) obtained

Table 8.1 Viruses which may be found in specimens

Specimen	Possible viruses	Morphology	Quantity in average specimens
Vesicle fluid	Herpesvirus	Herpesvirus	+ +
	Poxvirus	Poxvirus	+ +
	Parapoxvirus	Parapoxvirus	+ + +
Cerebrospinal fluid	Mumps	Paramyxovirus/RNP helix	+
	Enterovirus	SRV	+
Faeces	Rotavirus	Rotavirus	+ + + +
	Adenovirus	Adenovirus	+ + + +
	Astrovirus	Astrovirus	+ + + +
	Calicivirus	Calicivirus	+ +
	Norwalk	SRSV	+
	Coronavirus	Coronavirus	+
	SRV	SRV	+ +
	SRSV	SRSV	+ +
	Breda-like	Coronavirus	+
	Parvovirus	Parvovirus	+ + + +
	Bacteriophage	Tailed 'phage	+ + +
		SRV	?
Urine	Cytomegalovirus	Herpesvirus	+
	Papovavirus	Papovavirus	+ +
Serum	Hepatitis B	Dane particles	+
		HB surface antigen	+ +
	B18	Parvovirus	+ +
Pharyngeal washes	Influenza A or B	Myxovirus	+
	Parainfluenza	Paramyxovirus	+
	Adenovirus	Adenovirus	+
Biopsies: brain	Herpesvirus hominis (simplex)	Herpesvirus	+
skin	Wart: common	Papillomavirus	+ + +
	genital	Papillomavirus	+
	Molluscum contagiosum	Poxvirus	+ + +

from a patient, with extraction of any viruses present according to the principles discussed above. In novel circumstances it may be justifiable to extract the material with fluorocarbon and/or proteolytic or other enzymes. When looking at the resultant preparations in the EM the possibilities that the viruses are present only in altered or damaged forms must be kept in mind. If anything is present which might be a virus, the preparation should be repeated with or without alterations in the method to clarify the situation.

MICROSCOPY

The use of the electron microscope itself is central to the business of finding viruses in diagnostic specimens. In this section some aspects crucial to success are discussed, but it is assumed that the reader knows how to operate his microscope and that most of the technical terms used are familiar to him.

A suitable electron microscope properly aligned, good technique in finding viruses, good technique in taking high-resolution micrographs, and standardization of the magnification(s) used are unlikely to be thought controversial. Nevertheless, insufficient attention is paid to them if the published results are a fair guide. Table 8.2 lists features which are particularly important in a microscope to be used for routine diagnosis.

Stains, buffers and grids

Viruses are biological structures and might best be expected to survive intact at physiological osmolarities and pH values. This is generally true, but most viruses survive as morphological entities surprisingly well in DW and EM diluent, and both salt and phosphates will precipitate out as visible crystals on the grid and provide unwanted background 'noise'. Volatile buffers which do not precipitate out in drying have not been a serious requirement for routine use, provided the pH of the negative stain is controlled.

However, different stains and pH values can alter the appearance of virus particles considerably; for example, the architecture of enveloped viruses is best preserved and revealed by ammonium molybdate at the high pH of 9. Nevertheless, a high-contrast stain at a neutral pH probably provides the best routine stain, although most microscopists will want to have other stains available and at a variety of pH values.

The stain which has been used most widely and remains first choice for most microscopists is phosphotungstic acid, prepared as a 2–3% solution in distilled water and adjusted from its very acid pH to neutrality with 1 M potassium hydroxide. This stain both preserves virus structure well and helps the particles to stand out from the background.

High-quality micrographs are essential for virus recognition. These depend on the technique of the microscopist and the mechanical stability of the specimen on the microscope grid. For this purpose, fine mesh grids are vital. At the magnifications normally used to find and examine viruses a mesh wider than 16 squares/mm (400 squares/inch) is unnecessary. The grids should be coated with a thin film such as formvar and stabilized with evaporated carbon.

Disinfection

The theme of virological safety is outside the scope of this chapter but the consequences of attempting to disinfect grid preparations before putting them in the microscope is not. The use of ultraviolet irradiation has no effect on morphology, but all forms of liquid disinfectant (such as formaldehyde, glutaraldehyde or hypochlorite) either do, or are liable to, alter the morphology of virus particles so that they may be poorly recognizable or not recognizable at all with certainty.

Finding viruses and standardization of magnification

These two aspects of diagnostic work are closely related. Finding a virus is essentially an act of recognition. With a well-known virus it is seeing at least one particle which is indistinguishable from those seen before; with an unknown one it is seeing something consistent with the memory's concept of a virus. Most material in a diagnostic specimen has no conveniently recognizable size so that we have to provide our own context, and the easiest way to do so is to use the same magnification all the time. This allows a build-up of memory and experience which cannot happen if the magnification used for searching for viruses is varied from specimen to specimen.

Table 8.2 Requirements for an electron microscope for virus diagnosis

1. A magnification step of about $50\,000\times$ ($>40\,000\times$, $<60\,000\times$)
2. Stability, i.e. lens currents do not fluctuate significantly, magnification does not vary, no electronic drift
3. Fine-grain viewing screens
4. High resolution (0.2 nm)
5. Good illumination at the working magnification
6. Large viewing screen
7. Good object contrast (from a small objective aperture — 30 nm)

Table 8.3 Standard magnifications for diagnostic virology of the Philips EM 300 (Department of Virology, Newcastle upon Tyne)

	Magnification	
	Nominal	Calibrated
Scanning and taking micrographs	50 000 ×	51 700 ×
Printing		200 000 ×

If this argument is accepted it follows that the magnification at which the resultant micrographs are taken and printed should also be standardized. Those used in the author's laboratory are shown in Table 8.3. The true magnification on the focussing screen is less than 50 000 ×, and with 8 × binoculars the apparent magnification is similar to the 200 000 × used in printing micrographs. The printed pictures and the images seen in the microscope consequently reinforce each other, and the operator will be able to estimate whether dimensions of the object seen are appropriate.

Finding a virus is, therefore, a matter of looking for particles at the standard magnification. However, it will not take a new microscopist long to discover that all grid squares are not equally likely to contain either any viruses at all or the same number of viruses. Hence it becomes necessary to assess the quality of the preparation on the grid before searching seriously. This means examining the grid at a low enough magnification to see most of it at once. The grid so visualized can then be assessed for quality of preparation. A substantial proportion of the grid squares should have an intact formvar film over them. Of these there should be several with neither too much material (nearly black all over) nor too little (no debris visible). Practice will soon allow these promising half-tone areas to be identified and these should be scanned at high magnification first. If there are no such grid squares (usually because they are all overloaded), it is better to prepare another grid. If the half-tone areas yield no viruses the darker squares may be explored, but the formvar on most will tear rapidly when heated by the electrons in the beam.

Taking good-quality high-resolution micrographs

High-quality micrographs provide the only conclusive evidence of viral presence. Micrographs taken at 50 000 × ruthlessly expose flaws in technique which do not show at 10 000–15 000 ×.

There are three enemies of micrography, and all need attention if the microscopist is to be able to make a case for his virus.

1. Focus

Technically this is the point of least contrast but this is difficult to see in virus preparations, and most microscopists prefer a slight degree of under-focus, which produces an apparently sharper image with greater contrast in the detail. This is, it must be admitted, much easier said than done but is a matter of practice allied to a careful and systematic assessment of each negative. This should be done using a 20 × magnifier, most conveniently provided by a dissecting microscope, focussing on the background carbon grain of the specimen (not on the silver grains of the negative). At this enlargement the carbon grains should be pin-point in size. Negatives with a grain size larger than this should be ruthlessly discarded.

2. Astigmatism

Only those who habitually operate at high magnification will be acutely aware of objective astigmatism as a problem. It is partly inherent (from the objective pole pieces and the objective aperture holder) and partly acquired (from contamination build-up on the objective aperture). The latter is kept to a minimum with thin-foil apertures, but whatever residual astigmatism exists must be removed by adjusting the objective stigmators or the object will appear blurred on the micrograph. Careful inspection will show the blurring to be due to a directional distortion of the background grain. Correction may be done either on a holey carbon film or on the background grain of the specimen (preferably the latter).

3. Drift

Drift is movement in the specimen due to local overheating, or, more rarely, movement of the grid in the specimen holder. In some microscopes it may be due to electronic instability but this is unlikely in modern instruments. Drift cannot be overcome and it, too, will produce a directional grain in the micrograph. It can largely be prevented by an adequate coating of evaporated carbon on the formvar covering the grid. This conducts the impinging electrons away and prevents the local accumulation of their energy on parts of the grid. This uneven heating may produce distortion and hence movement in the specimen.

Drift may occur with any specimen and quite unpredictably. If the microscopist is patient, stability will develop with time but waiting for this to happen allows carbon contamination and radiation damage to build up on the specimen — with the consequent deterioration showing as a loss of fine detail.

IDENTIFICATION OF VIRAL PARTICLES

Diagnostic specimens always contain a considerable amount of debris as well as any viruses, and the microscopist must beware of seeing a virus where none is present or spending too long examining objects of no significance. Newcomers always want to look in more detail at objects that the more experienced eye will instantly dismiss as 'not virus'. Experience, then, is vital, and any would-be diagnostic virologist should spend time examining: (a) known positive specimens and (b) cell-culture viruses grown specifically for the purpose; he should also browse through any micrographs available. Looking at known positive specimens and cell-culture viruses is more important than browsing through available micrographs. Time spent at the instrument building up memory of the ways in which standard viruses vary is valuable, but should be organized — mere man-hours at the console are not enough. In acquiring this experience a number of guidelines should be borne in mind:

1. Keep an open mind

Table 8.1 lists the probable viruses to be found in various diagnostic specimens. However, the unexpected may occur, and it is unwise to decide what will be found before starting to look. It is important to have the full clinical details but these should not become a straitjacket. Finding papovaviruses in vesicle fluid is very unexpected (and rare) but it would be very unprofessional to miss them because the microscopist was convinced that only herpes viruses were likely to be present.

As an extension of this, one should be prepared for second, third or even fourth viruses in the specimen. This applies particularly, but not only, to stool extracts from children. It is an argument against pooling specimens, even from the same patient, for different stools can (and frequently do) contain different viruses even when they are consecutive. Similarly, different skin biopsies from a single patient may contain wart and molluscum contagiosum viruses.

2. Remember that the specimen is an artefact

A few years ago a scientist wrote an article in one of the popular science journals reminding microscopists of this factor, and it was widely interpreted as discrediting electron microscopy as a biological technique. This conclusion failed to understand the nature of microscopy — there is no claim that what is seen is the material *au naturel*; all is altered to some extent, but the artefacts produced are remarkably constant if the preparative technique is also constant, and it is usually not a major problem to recognize instantly and with certainty many of the common viruses.

Nevertheless, routine methods of preparation involve extraction from cells, centrifugation, staining and, possibly, disinfection followed by exposure to a high vacuum and bombardment with electrons and carbon atoms (contamination). Not surprisingly, these processes may do considerable damage to virus particles and prevent their appearing in the classic form seen in the micrographs published in journal papers on their detailed structure. Complete herpesvirus capsids with clearly visible ring-like capsomers in ordered rows are rarities in vesicle fluid; more often they show considerable damage, much of it probably due to decay occurring between production inside cells and removal of the specimen for diagnosis. Relating these ruined remains to the original virus requires familiarity with the appearance and understanding of the construction of the complete virion.

3. Certainty increases with numbers

It is possible to recognize with complete certainty one particle of a virus with a highly characteristic morphology, provided it is sufficiently intact. Other less characteristic viruses are more difficult, and this point is well illustrated by the enteroviruses. From cell cultures these appear as featureless circular objects 25 nm in diameter, and are frequently isolated from the stools of children. Rarely, if ever, do they reach EM-detectable levels but their possible presence in a stool extract puts pressure on the microscopist to identify compatible objects as enteroviruses. This point is discussed in more detail below, but the microscopist's certainty will increase rapidly as the number of such objects in the preparation rises. It would not be difficult to convince anyone that the particles shown in Fig. 8.1 are likely to be viruses, but the single particle in Fig. 8.2 from a stool extract may or may not be a virus. A specimen in which no virus is seen may still contain up to 100 000 particles/ml but this does not make it possible to recognize one particle with certainty. However, one possible particle is a challenge to search for more, and certainty rises with each additional sighting. If none is found, the microscopist will have to assess his certainty before deciding what to report, but it is wise to under-report rather than over-diagnose.

4. It must be the right size

The size of spherical viruses varies little, and some form of measuring device (other than taking a micrograph and measuring it later) is valuable. This may take the form of a scale (or a circle of known size) on the main screen (provided it is horizontal when in use), or a graticule in one of the binocular eyepieces, or even a television attachment with a scale drawn on the monitor's screen. Variations in size will become immediately apparent as will inappropriate sizes (for example, spherical viruses >30 nm in diameter are too large to be enteroviruses). In such estimations the unaided eye is not reliable enough, although experience helps.

Spherical viruses up to 25–30 nm in diameter may have no visible surface subunit structure — no visible capsomers

— but particles larger than this always do. Hence larger spheres are not viruses if they are plain.

5. *The image is two-dimensional*

On the screen all objects are two-dimensional, even though the original has thickness as well. This third dimension can be inferred by the width and density of the 'collar' of stain around the particle. An actual estimate of this third dimension may be made by shadowing with evaporated carbon but this is too tedious and unreliable to be used routinely.

6. *Contamination builds up with time*

Carbon is continually being deposited on the specimen and this will finally obscure fine detail. The rate of build-up can be greatly reduced by using a 'cold finger' as a contamination trap, but many diagnostic microscopists do not employ one because it delays brisk scanning and microscopy. Well over 90% of the contamination is deposited on the area being scanned so that other areas of the specimen are relatively unharmed. Bombardment with electrons will also induce damage in the specimen — destroying the fine detail at rates which vary with the specimen. This also puts a premium on working without delay.

The points made above indicate that the image observed on the screen (or the micrograph) must be interpreted. To do so requires imagination from the microscopist but it is also all too easy to see 'viruses' which are not there; therefore, imagination needs to be disciplined, with the discipline deriving from experience.

There is a further way in which the disciplined imagination is important. We must not assume that all viruses have been identified and their morphology recognized. Further viruses presumably remain to be discovered, but any candidate is likely to be constructed along the same general lines as those already identified. Any 'new' virus should then be seen in this context, and an understanding of virus architecture is part of the microscopist's background study.

Is it a virus?

This section offers some help in answering this question with some viruses. Because the damage to particles is both variable and unpredictable, this advice cannot be comprehensive. Some aspects of these problems are discussed under general headings below.

Small round (structured) viruses

There is a considerable number of small cubic viruses with sizes of 20–40 nm the identification of which poses problems to the microscopist. Some, such as astroviruses and caliciviruses, possess surface structure which, if visible, allows their specific identification. In neither case will all the particles present show the pathognomonic morphology but careful searching will usually yield some with the necessary features. Whether the other atypical particles are also regarded as astroviruses or caliciviruses will depend on their appearance and their distribution on the microscope grid. Nevertheless, the recognition of astroviruses and caliciviruses is more a challenge to the microscopist's patience than to his imagination.

These apart, there remains a considerable number of spherical virus-like particles, particularly in stool specimens, which might be viruses and which require a decision about this likelihood. They can be divided into two morphological types (Figs 8.3 and 8.4) according to whether they appear to be featureless spheres (SRVs; Fig. 8.3) or whether they appear to have some surface structure (SRSVs; Fig. 8.4). This SRSV surface structure is not well enough defined on the particles to give clear recognition features — it gives the particle a hairy appearance. Some, which have been identified antigenically, are Norwalk, Montgomery County and Hawaii viruses, but the identity of most is unknown. The recognition of both SRVs and SRSVs as viruses (and of what kind) is not easy. They differ in whether some surface structure is present, but even their identity as viruses may be called into question. Some points to consider in coming to a conclusion are:

a. Are they three-dimensional? By the negative contrast technique, objects are delineated by the stain forming a collar round the object. It also fills the sulcus, if any, between the particle and the supporting membrane (for example, formvar) covering the grid. As shown in Fig. 8.5A, a spherical object provides a good-sized sulcus and a correspondingly dense collar of stain, while a flat coin-shaped object provides no equivalent sulcus and a much less dense collar (Fig. 8.5B). This means that the enterovirus particles in Fig. 8.6 stand out rather better than the other debris, something that is even more apparent on the viewing screen. For this reason particles with a sufficient thickness to provide the necessary sulcus will attract the microscopist's attention more readily, and the best example of such three-dimensional structures is a sphere. If a particle, then, appears to demand attention it is likely to do so because it has thickness. It is not surprising that such particles can cast a shadow while enveloped viruses do not (Fig. 8.7).

b. Are they consistent in size? Figure 8.8 depicts five objects in a group but, because they vary substantially in size, are not convincingly virus-like, regardless of their average size. Cubic viruses with icosahedral symmetry are constructed of a finite number of similar or identical subunits (32, 60 or 180). No matter what detailed differences exist between one virus family or another, the construction of each member of a family remains the same and hence any differences will be minimal. In practice, the scatter is very narrow, as Fig. 8.9 indicates. Because the subunits are too small to be resolved in the microscope, it is not surprising that an assembly using the same finite number of them produces fine manufacturing tolerances.

In a number of cases the genome-sized piece of nucleic acid (DNA or RNA) provides a template round which the coat assembles. Nonetheless, in its absence (in stain-penetrated apparently 'empty' particles) the size mostly remains the same, but in the case of the small 20 nm spheres and 20 nm wide bacillary forms of self-assembled hepatitis B surface antigen (HBsAg) there is more variation than in other small particles (Fig. 8. 10).

c. Are they round (spherical)? The third dimension has to be inferred from the collar of stain but any icosahedral virus will appear round or regularly hexagonal. The lowest particle in Fig. 8.8 possesses a well-defined collar but is clearly not round. Unlikely to be a virus, it may nonetheless appear round when seen through the viewing port. Scrutiny through the binoculars will show its true nature.

Despite this comment, viruses are biological objects and can be distorted. How much is within acceptable limits is open to debate, but Fig. 8.11 illustrates the problem, in which x and y are the short and long dimensions. Norwalk is the only virus of this type specifically thought to be oval, but inspection of the published pictures suggests that this is probably an artefact. Other virus particles may also appear oval but these distorted ones are clearly a minority. Nevertheless, some probably non-viral objects seen in the microscope appear oval, and a good working rule is that y should not be more than 10% longer than x, and a virus that is naturally oval has yet to be described.

d. Are SRSVs merely SRVs covered with antibody? It is not easy to answer this with certainty but it seems unlikely. Attempted removal of antibody by treatment with a low-pH buffer requires a return to neutrality before staining and leaves the appearance of at least one SRSV essentially unaltered (Fig. 8.12, A and B). A true antibody coating is finer than the surface structure of SRSVs on which there is a hint of an ordered network, although the details cannot be discerned. For example, enterovirus coated with antibody (Fig. 8.13A) does not really resemble an SRSV (Fig. 8.13B). The distinction is fine and not conclusive but during the course of an infection SRVs have not been reported to convert to SRSVs nor have SRSVs been reported to become more densely hairy. If not antibody, then what? Because no virus with SRSV morphology has been grown in cell culture or in an experimental animal, no experimental work on them has been done. As spherical viruses, they are likely to have icosahedral symmetry but this requires proof before any further conclusions can be drawn. Treatment with enzymes to digest any surface antibody is also liable to remove some virion structure. This may give some information about how it is put together without indicating the nature of the surface threads.

e. How many are needed to make the diagnosis? Only the operator can decide, and the numbers required will be inversely proportional to the degree of certainty about each particle. The more present the better, for this allows them to be measured, but this in turn means micrographs, and small numbers well scattered will be expensive to record. Anything, even one particle, *may* be a virus, but recording and analysis of small numbers will often be thought to be more effort than is warranted. Nevertheless, more information may be present on a micrograph than is visible on the viewing screen, and the micrograph provides a permanent record for future comparison.

Many microscopists do not take SRVs and SRSVs very seriously, partly because they are difficult to find (a challenge to technique) and partly because finding takes interpretation little further. They are important epidemiologically because they are often the only apparent culprits in common source outbreaks of food poisoning, and finding similar objects in endemic stools is (a) good practice and (b) the background against which to see positive stools in the next outbreak. It is not an aspect of diagnostic electron microscopy from which firm conclusions can be drawn, but it provides a challenge to the microscopist (and encourages the operator to keep an open mind).

Herpesviruses

These are large viruses, with a 100-nm capsid made up of 162 capsomers which are apparently tubular and 9 nm in diameter, with the whole surrounded by a double envelope derived from host cell membranes. Identifying such a well-characterized group of viruses might be thought to present few problems but this is not so.

Fluid from a fresh vesicle will often contain a considerable number of easily identified enveloped particles showing typical capsids, and some of the best particles to be found will come from such a source (Fig. 8.14). Other preparations will contain only occasional particles, most of which are severely damaged and in which the presence of an envelope is not a conclusive feature. Features to look for in such damaged particles are:

a. Size. The capsid of a herpesvirus is very close to 100 nm in diameter, and surprisingly few other circular objects approximate this size. The large viewing screen of a number of Philips microscopes has a 5 mm-diameter circle marked on it. At a magnification of 50 000 × this is equivalent to 100 nm and is very convenient for measuring possible capsids.

b. Capsomers. In plan, capsomers are 9 nm in diameter and appear organized in a geometric way even when the whole capsid is not clearly visible. Both size and organization must be present before a confident identification can be made (Fig. 8.15). At the capsid periphery they may be seen as castellations, particularly on stain-penetrated particles (Fig. 8.16). Such castellations may extend round the entire periphery, but diagnosis is possible if they are resolved clearly on only one sixth of the periphery. Individual castellations will be seen to be formed from two short parallel 'lines' about 8–10 nm long (Fig. 8.16) and may be the only feature clearly visible on the capsid. These are not found on other debris and are a good recognition feature. The outline of the capsid should be hexagonal, but damage or distortion may round this off.

c. Nucleoids. Ill-defined concentric nucleoids may be seen inside the capsids. Figure 8.17 shows examples in cytomegalovirus virions grown in culture. The nucleoids appear to have an empty centre, about 25 nm in diameter, and the outer surface is about 30–35 nm. They are not an invariable feature, but they add certainty if present.

The first particles seen may have no clearly identifiable features other than approximately correct size. However, suspicion should stimulate the microscopist to find other particles, even to making a second preparation from the original specimen. It is not uncommon to find that the particles in this second preparation are better stained or more characteristic although the reason is not clear. A considerable number of particles 100 nm in diameter, which are easily seen by the observer, are likely to be herpesvirus particles, and at least one should have one of the features listed above. The only doubt will be *which* herpesvirus is present for they are not distinguishable in the EM. The only correct report to the clinician, therefore, is 'Herpesvirus particles seen' — further typing must depend on other information, such as direct immunofluorescence or culture.

Membranes or envelopes

Any preparation containing cellular debris is likely to contain membranous material that may be the remains of virus envelopes. With three exceptions discussed below, they lack any clearly distinguishable features so that any virological nature is impossible to recognize. This lack of certainty is particularly marked with paramyxoviruses (parainfluenza, measles, mumps, Newcastle disease, SV5, and so forth), where even complete virions may be difficult to identify (Fig. 8.18), but their completeness gives a clue. They do not have a standard size; however, two features may help in their identification:

a. The virus contains a helical nucleocapsid which is invariably present and recognizable as herringbone or zipper forms separate from the virions (Fig. 8.19). It is virtually unknown for such pieces of ribonucleocapsid (RNP) *not* to be present in a paramyxovirus preparation. They are unmistakable and, in some preparations, are the only visible form. The ultrastructural appearances of these pieces of ribonucleo-capsid are morphologically indistinguishable among the paramyoxoviruses, but they are a unique characteristic of the family.

b. Stain-penetrated particles may show the RNP in situ but, even if the helical structure is not clearly visible, the stain may occasionally penetrate only the central canal of the RNP, outlining its length (Fig. 8.20)

The envelope of paramyxoviruses has a specific fringe on it which is constant in length at about 10 nm (Fig. 8.18) but it lacks any clearly distinguishing features so that recognition of virus on this feature alone is not possible. Three viruses, however, do have clearly recognizable envelopes. These are:

a. Influenza A and B (Orthomyxoviruses). These viruses, not distinguishable from each other, have an envelope bearing a very regular and recognizable palisade of surface spikes (Fig. 8.21). These are very constant in length at 9 nm and are absolutely characteristic. They may also be visible on the presenting surface as well, but this is uncommon. It used to be thought that ammonium molybdate at a pH of 9.0 displayed the surface fringe even more clearly. However, for unknown reasons, this is no longer the case. It appears to be due to the stain itself but no one knows what has changed. Rarely, stain penetrates into influenza virions revealing the contained RNP (Fig. 8.22). The characteristic bobbin appearance is unmistakable, but to rely on finding it (in contrast to paramyxoviruses) is a mistake.

b. Coronaviruses. Coronavirus-like particles may be found in faeces. Their identity as true viruses (and as pathogens) is still open to debate, but their surface fringe of pin-like projections is their only constant feature, with the particles themselves being very pleomorphic (Fig. 8.23). The fringe may sometimes appear to be a two-tiered one, but the more elaborate the fringe the less likely is the particle to be truly a virus.

c. Rhabdoviruses. These bullet-shaped viruses are unlikely to be found in diagnostic specimens, but their unmistakable envelope could hardly be missed (Fig. 8.24).

These exceptions apart, most of the membranous debris in diagnostic material must be ignored. Only if virus-specific features are present can they contribute to the diagnosis; otherwise, the temptation to linger on them should be resisted.

Contaminants

A proportion of diagnostic specimens will contain viruses which are not thought to contribute to the disease. The best example is provided by tailed bacteriophages which may be present in stool extracts in large numbers. Their lollipop shape is unique (Fig. 8.25) and their contribution to any diarrhoea is obscure. They vary in morphology from stool to stool but more than one type in any one stool is uncommon, though by no means unknown.

Cell cultures may carry contaminating animal viruses whose presence may be unknown to the isolation part of the diagnostic laboratory. The main source of these is simian tissue and they are usually simian viruses SV40 (polyomavirus) or SV5 (paramyxovirus). They do not appear to interfere greatly with the isolation of viruses, but SV5 in particular can spread into all cell types, primary or continuous, and widespread isolation of paramyxovirus identified by EM should be accepted with great caution.

CONCLUSIONS

For all the foregoing, many of the specimens offered to the microscopist will be negative. This has led some to argue that EM is only an interim technique, acceptable only until a better test is available. This is to deny the catch-all nature of EM and to disregard the pleasure and certainty of finding an unmistakable virion — which is enough to make the diagnosis in a specimen.

In the end, electron microscopy provides the best — and often the fastest — evidence for a virus in diagnostic material; the results have an elegance not provided by many other techniques, and good EM should be an integral part of any diagnostic laboratory with ambitions to offer an effective service.

REFERENCES

1. Almeida J D, Waterson A P 1980 Viruses. In: Johannessen J V (ed) Electron microscopy in human medicine, vol 3, Infectious agents. McGraw-Hill, New York, pp 3–45
2. Doane F W, Anderson N 1987 Electron microscopy in diagnostic virology: a practical guide and atlas. Cambridge University Press, New York
3. Grimley P M, Henson D E 1983 Electron microscopy in virus infections. In: Trump B F, Jones R T (eds) Diagnostic electron microscopy, vol. 4. John Wiley and Sons, New York, pp 1–73
4. Madeley C R, Field A M 1988 Virus morphology 2nd ed. Churchill Livingstone, Edinburgh.
5. Nermut M V, Steven A C 1987 Animal virus structure. Elsevier, Amsterdam

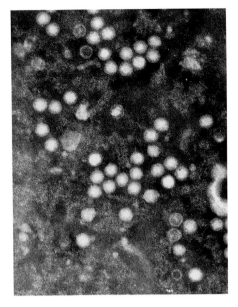

Fig. 8.1 Group of viruses in faecal extract. It is not only the morphology of the individual particles, but also their numbers in particular which establishes these as viral in character. (× 132 000)

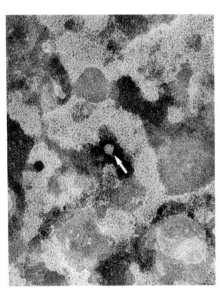

Fig. 8.2 Single virus-like particle in a faecal extract. There are no diagnostic features, and no other particles for comparison; it may be a virus (arrow) but one can never be sure. (× 132 000)

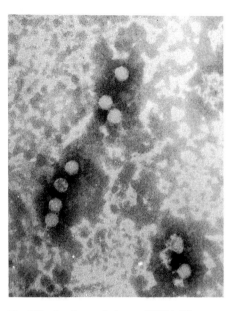

Fig. 8.3 Small round viruses (SRVs). These are featureless spheres, with an occasional 'empty' particle. (× 132 000)

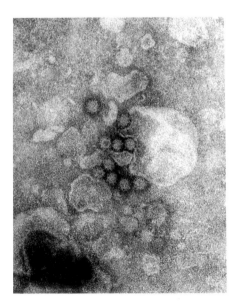

Fig. 8.4 Small round structured viruses (SRSVs). Particles with an ill-defined feathery edge and a suggestion of surface structure. (× 132 000)

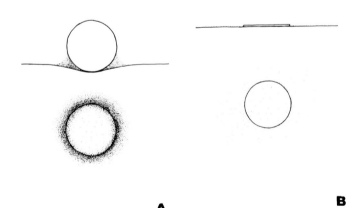

Fig. 8.5 **A** Elevation and plan view of spherical 'virus', showing accumulation of stain in the sulcus between the particle and the supporting membrane. **B** Elevation and plan view of coin-shaped flat object showing the absence of a collar of stain.

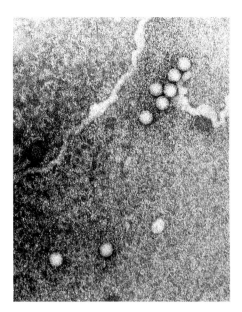

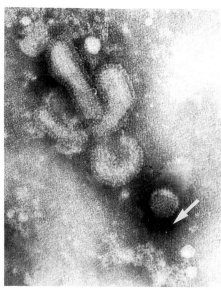

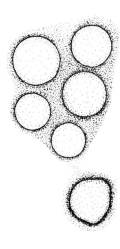

Fig. 8.6 Enteroviruses. Group of enterovirus particles (Coxsackie B) showing how they stand out from the background. (× 132 000)

Fig. 8.7 Adenovirus and influenza virus. Adenovirus (lower right) and influenza virus (upper left) particles, shadowed with evaporated carbon from the lower left. Note the shadow cast by the adenovirus (arrow) and the absence of shadow downstream from the influenza virus, suggesting that the latter is almost totally flat after dehydration. (× 132 000)

Fig. 8.8 Diagram of six 'particles'. The upper five are approximately circular in outline but vary too much in size to be convincingly SRVs. The lowest particle has a good collar of 'stain' but is clearly not circular and it, too, is not convincing.

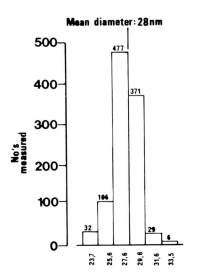

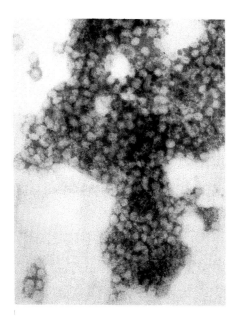

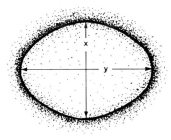

Fig. 8.9 Histogram of astrovirus particle sizes measured on EM negatives. Over 1000 particles were measured but the scatter is small, about a mean of 28 nm.

Fig. 8.10 Hepatitis B surface antigen. These particles consist of virus coat protein only, which has self-assembled into spheres and bacillary forms. The former are about 20 nm in diameter and the latter are about the same width. Note that there is more variation than with the astroviruses due, perhaps, to the absence of a template function provided by nucleic acid. (× 132 000) See also Chapters 9 and 15.

Fig. 8.11 Diagram to illustrate the problem posed by distortion of spherical particles. See text for details.

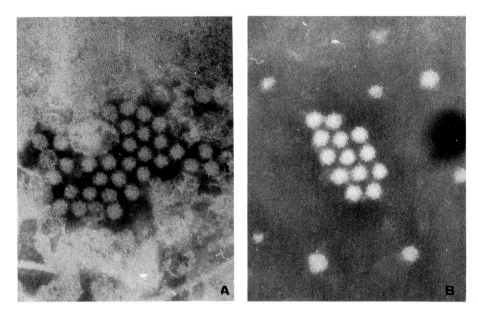

Fig. 8.12   SRSVs from faecal extracts before (**A**) and after (**B**) treatment at pH 3 to dissociate any antibody combined with the surface. Note that the surface has not altered appreciably and, in particular, that an SRSV has not been converted to an SRV. (× 132 000)

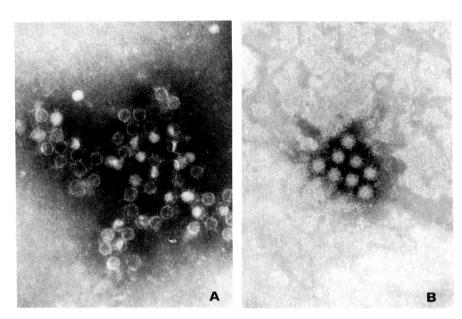

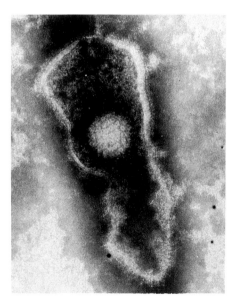

Fig. 8.13   Comparison of enterovirus (echovirus type 11) coated with antibody (**A**) and an SRSV (**B**). Thread-like structures join the particles in **A** but are absent in **B** where the surface is merely ill-defined. (× 132 000)

Fig. 8.14   Enveloped complete herpesvirus particle (herpes simplex). Note both surface ring-like capsomers and irregular fringed envelope. (× 132 000)

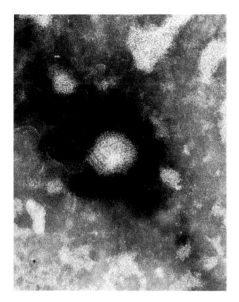

Fig. 8.15 Solitary herpesvirus capsid (herpes simplex). No envelope is present but the capsomers are unmistakable. (× 132 000)

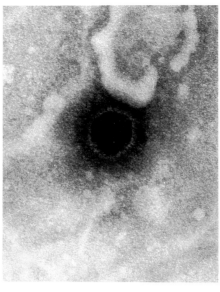

Fig. 8.16 Stain-penetrated herpesvirus capsid (herpes simplex). No ring-like capsomers but only peripheral castellations, seen as short parallel rods in pairs. (× 132 000)

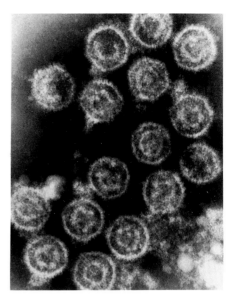

Fig. 8.17 Group of herpes virus capsids (cytomegalovirus) showing internal 'nucleoids'. (× 132 000)

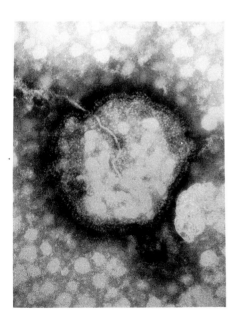

Fig. 8.18 Paramyxovirus virion. Particle with an ill-defined surface fringe and no other distinguishing features. (× 132 000)

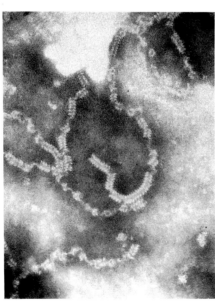

Fig. 8.19 Separate nucleoprotein helix from paramyxovirus. Note characteristic herringbone or zipper appearance. Paramyxovirus helix is unmistakable but is indistinguishable regardless of which virus it comes from. (× 132 000)

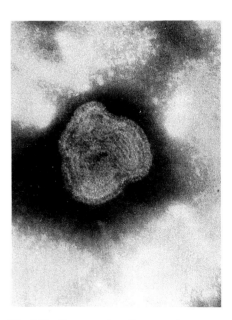

Fig. 8.20 Paramyxovirus. Paramyxovirus particle in which the stain appears to have penetrated down the central canal of the nucleoprotein. (× 132 000)

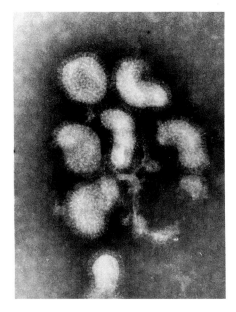 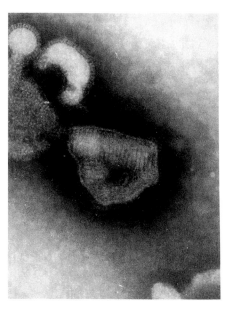 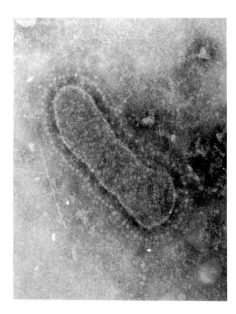

Fig. 8.21 Orthomyxovirus (influenza A) virions. Note better-defined and regular surface fringe compared with paramyxovirus (Fig. 8.18). It is very regular in length (about 10 nm). Note also the absence of leaking nucleoprotein. (× 132 000)

Fig. 8.22 Orthomyxovirus. Rare micrograph of a stain-penetrated orthomyxovirus particle showing nucleoprotein helix in situ. Note that it is quite different from that of paramyxoviruses and is rarely, if ever, seen outside the virions. (× 132 000)

Fig. 8.23 Faecal coronavirus. Note pin-like surface projections (peplomers). The fringe made up from these projections is regular but the stalks of the pins cannot be discerned. (× 132 000)

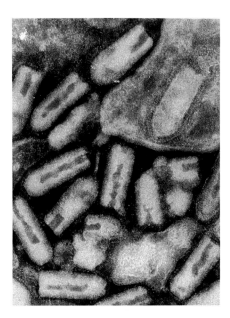 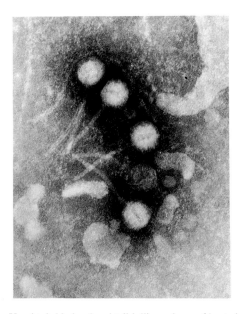

Fig. 8.24 A specialized envelope seen on vesicular stomatitis virus (a rhabdovirus). Unlike most enveloped viruses, this has a regular size and shape which gives this group of viruses their characteristic bullet-shaped appearance. (× 132 000)

Fig. 8.25 Unmistakable head and tail lollipop-shape of bacteriophages. No animal or human virus of this shape has yet been described, but they may be present in high concentration in faecal extracts. (× 132 000)

9. Infectious agents: fungi, bacteria and viruses

E. J. Wills

INTRODUCTION

Most infectious diseases have been traditionally diagnosed in the laboratory by cultural identification. More recently, the introduction of techniques such as enzyme-linked or radio-immunoassays have made same-day diagnosis a practical proposition. However, there will be occasions when such methods are inapplicable — for example, when there is no established method for growing the organism, or because only a fixed-tissue specimen is available. In such circumstances light microscopy may be diagnostic, or at least arouse a level of suspicion which may be resolved in a limited number of cases by immunohistochemical or nucleic acid probing techniques. However, many of these procedures rely on the detection of individual microbial antigens and will answer only specific questions. The 'open ended' approach of electron microscopy (EM) offers a useful alternative measure — provided that the examiner is conversant not only with the morphology of mature organisms, but also with their developmental stages and their effects on cells and tissues, and that he can distinguish them from the many degenerate cell products that are often present. This chapter will be restricted to transmission microscopy of sectioned material, a method available in any laboratory where diagnostic EM is practised. Negative staining techniques, which frequently offer the speediest diagnosis in viral infections, are discussed in Chapter 8. Scanning and high-voltage microscopy, freeze–fracture and electron cytochemistry, whilst of considerable research interest, have not shown diagnostic merit, and the future of immuno-electron microscopy of ultrathin sections remains to be established. There is a voluminous literature on the ultrastructural appearances of infectious agents in vitro and on host–parasite relationships in experimental animals. These studies have contributed to an understanding of the structure and life cycle of many agents, together with the pathogenesis and pathology of the diseases they cause (and they still are, as witnessed by current AIDS research); however, an attempt has been made to limit the references cited to those concerning human material, with selected review articles providing access to the wider literature.

No special preparative methods are required for tissue specimens. Although optimum preservation is to be preferred, the fixation requirements of most infectious agents are less stringent than human tissues, and diagnosis may be feasible on inappropriately fixed material, reprocessed paraffin blocks or postmortem specimens that would ordinarily be deemed unsuitable for EM. Screening by light microscopy of semithin sections is essential for the selection of appropriate tissue for ultrathin sectioning; where lesions are very focal, the reprocessing of selected areas in paraffin blocks or sections may be worth consideration as a means of increasing the diagnostic yield. Reprocessing of cytology smears is also possible, particularly for virus diagnosis.

PROTOZOA

Phylum Protozoa includes many parasites of medical importance,[1,3–68] particularly the following:

1. Parasitic amoebae (including *Entamoeba histolytica*[6,7,9,10,14,34,43,50] and amoebae belonging to the genera *Naegleria* and *Acanthamoeba*[4,6,9,10,18,21,33,56])
2. Coccidial protozoa (including *Toxoplasma gondii*,[3,5–7,9,10,27,32,36,49,51,55,60] *Cryptosporidium*,[17,22,31,42] and other members of the suborder Eimerina,[5,7,9,27,44,52,55,62] *Babesia*,[5,7] and *Plasmodium*[5,6,9,11–13,24,54,61]).
3. Flagellate protozoa (including the trypanosomatid flagellates,[5–10,25,26,29,64] the trichomonad flagellates,[7,29,30,39,47,48] and the diplomonad flagellate *Giardia lambla*[8,10,19,28,40,41,45,46,59])
4. Ciliate protozoa (for example, *Balantidium coli*[9,10,68])
5. Parasites of uncertain taxonomic classification (*Pneumocystis carinii*[1,4,16,20,35,37,57,58,63,65]).

Most of these protozoa are discussed and illustrated in Chapter 10, while *P. carinii* is dealt with in Chapters 10 and 13; accordingly, they are not considered here any further.

FUNGI

Fungi[1,69,71-75] exist in yeast and mould forms (Figs 9.1–9.12). Yeasts (Figs 9.2–9.12) are spherical or ovoid single cells with a rigid cell wall, and they reproduce by budding (blastospore formation). Separation of the daughter cell normally leaves a 'bud scar' on the parent cell surface, but persistent terminal attachment may generate chains of cells (pseudohyphae). Yeasts multiply to a lesser extent by binary fission like bacteria or by sporulation like moulds. Moulds are filamentous and multicellular, with vegetative hyphae and reproductive spores. Hyphae are relatively thick-walled branched tubular structures (Figs 9.1, 9.2 and 9.4) that are generally divided by septa into compartments, each with its cytoplasm and one or more nuclei. Moulds reproduce asexually by spores, which vary greatly in their organization and manner of development and may be borne on specialized structures, or by fusion of hyphae or modified hyphae endowed with male and female characteristics. Such diversity facilitates the identification of fungi in clinical specimens or culture by morphological characteristics apparent to the naked eye or light microscope. Although many deep mycoses occur in yeast form, the organisms involved are mostly dimorphic and identification is possible after culture on media that stimulate sporulation and conversion to moulds. For these reasons, EM does not play a significant role in the diagnosis of fungal infections, although there is a considerable literature on the ultrastructure of fungi in vitro,[69,71,73-75] and on the effects of antifungal drugs.[70,71,75] Nuances of species differences that are inapparent by transmission EM may be demonstrable by scanning techniques, which may have some application to taxonomy.[72]

The cell wall is the most distinctive feature of fungi. The composition of the outer layers affects antigenicity and virulence, whilst changes in the spatial arrangement of its components influence dimorphic transition. Ultrathin sections usually show a moderately opaque outer zone of amorphous matrix material and a paler inner zone of fibrils embedded in the matrix. Special methods of fixation or staining may reveal more elaborate stratification, particularly in thick-walled yeasts. The chemistry and synthesis of cell walls is imperfectly understood but, in general, crystalline polysaccharides (chitin and glucans) make up the skeletal portion and polysaccharide/protein complexes (particularly mannans) the matrix. Hyphal septa are formed of invaginations from the inner aspect of the cell wall and may contain pores allowing the free passage of cell constituents (Fig. 9.2). Some fungi, notably *Cryptococcus neoformans* (Figs 9.9–9.12), have an outermost capsule that can be regarded as a separate cell constituent affording protection and affecting pathogenicity. The plasma membrane is closely applied to the inner aspect of the cell wall except where lomasomes, spherical or ovoid bodies of variable density and uncertain function, lie between the

two. There are the usual components of eukaryotic cells, namely a nucleus (sometimes multiple) enclosed in an envelope with pores, along with cytoplasmic organelles such as ribosomes, rather scanty endoplasmic reticulum of both rough and smooth surfaced varieties, mitochondria that may contain ribosomes or DNA fibrils, lysosomes, lipid droplets, glycogen and a variety of vacuoles that increase with ageing and may coalesce to occupy much of the cytoplasm. At the hyphal growing tip the only organelles are specialized vesicles that migrate from a Golgi-like vesicle-generating system to fuse with the plasmalemma, contributing to its surface area as well as transporting cell wall material for further growth.

ULTRASTRUCTURE OF FUNGAL INFECTIONS

Dermatomycoses

Electron microscopy is not required for diagnosis, direct microscopic examination of infected hairs or skin scrapings and culture sufficing. Saprobic infections of human hair have been ultrastructurally studied in vitro but may differ from those occurring under natural conditions.[75] Some species of *Trichophyton*[77] and *Microsporum*[88,89] develop perforating organs from eroding mycelia that invade and digest the hair cortex in vitro, but keratinolysis in vivo is difficult to prove; in tinea capitis, *Microsporum gypseum* seems to gain nutrients by growing within hair cells.[91] The hair nodules of black piedra consist of a mixture of broken strands of cuticle with fungal hyphae and ascospores that do not seem to penetrate beyond the cuticle.[79]

Non-keratinolytic fungi have been investigated to a lesser degree, but *Malassezia furfur* has been found both between and within keratinized cells of the stratum corneum in tinea versicolor.[90]

Deep and systemic mycoses

The host defences[75] to fungal invasion of deep tissues include cells of the mononuclear phagocyte system, which may form granulomas with or without giant cells (Figs 9.7, 9.9 and 9.12), and granulocytes, which may form small abscesses. Phagocytosis of the organisms does not always lead to their death, and intracellular multiplication can produce swelling of the nucleus, mitochondria and endoplasmic reticulum, or vacuolation in the host cell. The presence of a perifungal organelle-free zone, not to be confused with an electron-lucent capsule or shrinkage artefact, may indicate a local effect of fungal toxins. Phagocytic killing of fungi is in fact less apparent than extracellular destruction by surrounding host cells.

Fungal ultrastructure in vivo reflects the combined effects of host defences and the less-than-ideal growth conditions.[75] Hyphae generally appear larger and more convoluted than in culture, especially where pursuing a tortuous course between epithelial cells or within vessel walls. In immune hosts the few surviving fungal elements may be blown up into grotesque shapes that are identifiable with difficulty, or else are completely empty save for their resistant cell wall. In chronic mycoses excess antigenic cell wall material may be produced and antigen–antibody complexes may create an indented dense outer coat, the asteroid body of light microscopy.

BACTERIA

The bacterial cell is a simple prokaryotic structure.[1,103,108,110] There is no envelope around the nuclear material, and cytoplasmic organelles such as mitochondria, endoplasmic reticulum and Golgi areas are lacking. However, the few structures present are capable of complex biochemical activities — the plasma membrane, for instance, fulfilling mitochondrial as well as the more obvious barrier and transport functions. The copious literature on bacterial ultrastructure is derived largely from the study of pure cultures in vitro.

Differences between Gram-positive and Gram-negative organisms are to be seen in the cell wall:[103,105,110]

a. Gram-positive bacteria (Fig. 9.13) have a broad (20–30 nm), rather featureless layer of peptidoglycan (also known as mucopeptide or murein) whose thickness may increase with age. This layer maintains bacterial shape and accounts for 40–60% of cell wall dry weight.
b. The wall of most Gram-negative bacteria (Fig. 9.14) is multilayered. There is an outer membrane with specific receptor, barrier, transport and antigenic properties, that differs in chemical composition from the plasma membrane and includes lipopolysaccharide endotoxin. A relatively electron-transparent zone of varying thickness separates the outer membrane from the underlying 3–5 nm peptidoglycan layer that forms only 5–15% of the cell wall.

However, any correlation between Gram-staining and cell wall ultrastructure falls short in organisms whose peptidoglycan layer is either very thick or very thin.[103] For this reason, Gram-positivity or negativity is better attributed to permeability differences not necessarily visible by electron microscopy. Bacterial L-forms and mycoplasmas (Fig. 9.26) have no cell wall. The plasma membrane is in close contact with the cell wall, and any apparent periplasmic space separating the two is probably a fixation artefact.[106] The plasma membrane is 7–8 nm in width and may appear asymmetric, with the outer layer thicker and denser than the inner. The inner face of the plasma membrane is enzymatically very active. Mesosomes are invaginations of the plasma membrane filled with membranous whorls and are most conspicuous in Gram-positive organisms (Fig. 9.13). Their function is still unsettled but the prior belief that they represent bacterial mitochondria seems refuted; some even

regard them as fixation artefacts and as non-existent in living organisms. The interior of the bacterial cell (protoplast) is very simple (Figs 9.13 and 9.14). Although fibrillar DNA is evident in ultrathin sections, and a supercoiled chromosome is demonstrable by isolation and spreading techniques, freeze–etching rarely provides evidence of chromatin at all, making it likely that nuclear material is dispersed in the living state.[103] The protoplast often contains little else than 10-nm diameter ribosomes, but there may be occasional vesicles, lipid droplets and small polyphosphate (volutin) granules.

External prokaryotic specializations may be evident.[103,107,109,110] Bacterial flagella (Figs 9.14 and 9.22) are organelles of motility bearing no morphological resemblance to the flagella of eukaryotes. Bacterial flagella are long thread-like processes of uniform diameter (12–19 nm unsheathed, up to 55 nm when sheathed) that are attached to a hook-like body that is itself attached to a basal structure in the cell wall and plasma membrane. The flagella consist of helical fibres formed from flagellin subunits. Flagellar localization is useful in taxonomy. Fimbriae or pili are hair-like appendages 3–14 nm in diameter and 0.2–2.0 μm in length that are not seen in conventional ultrathin sections, but may be visualized by ruthenium red or negative staining. They are notably present on enterobacteria and are concerned with adhesion to surfaces. Gonococcal fimbrial variation is related to alteration in pathogenicity. Sex pili, which are involved in DNA transfer between bacteria, are thicker and less numerous than fimbriae.

A glycocalyx (capsule or slime layer) composed of fibrous polysaccharides or globular proteins covers the surface of many bacteria in vivo (Fig. 9.15), but is lost on subculture in vitro. Often invisible after conventional processing, the layer can be revealed after stabilization by cross-linking lectins or specific antibody and by freeze–etching.[104] Some bacterial groups form endospores with a DNA and protein core surrounded by multiple layers of modified cell wall material, spore coats and exosporium.

Mycoplasmas

Mycoplasmas (Fig. 9.26) are amongst the smallest known free-living bacteria capable of replication on artificial growth media without the necessity for other living cells. Their principal morphological characteristic is their extreme pleomorphism due to the absence of a cell wall;[108,111,112,117,128,130,135] variations in processing technique can also have a profound influence on morphology.[117] There have been few ultrastructural studies on human material[123,165] and the organisms are of considerably more importance in veterinary than human medicine.

Rickettsiae and chlamydiae

These small bacteria are obligate intracellular parasites. Rickettsiae include human pathogens of the genera *Rickett-*

sia, *Rochalimaea* and *Coxiella*, highly pleomorphic small bacilli or coccobacilli with Gram-negative structure. Some species have a capsular slime layer. The range of cells infected in humans is restricted; endothelial cells of small vessels are parasitized by *Rickettsia*, macrophages by *Coxiella*. Most ultrastructural investigations[108,114,156,176] have been performed on cell systems in vitro or on insect vectors. Depending on the organism, multiplication occurs within cytoplasmic vacuoles or ground substance, rarely the nucleoplasm.

Chlamydiae are unable to synthesize ATP and have evolved a unique growth cycle with two functionally and morphologically distinct forms, the elementary and the reticulate bodies (Fig. 9.27).[108,114,125,133,169,173,178]

ULTRASTRUCTURE OF BACTERIAL INFECTIONS

Bacterial surface glycocalyx may be quite profuse in infected tissues (Fig. 9.15).[104] The organisms often appear degenerate, particularly when phagocytozed, and — although it is an exaggeration that all bacteria look alike under these circumstances — ultrastructural identification beyond a basic level is difficult. EM can detect bacteria whose small size or staining properties impede their visualization by light microscopy, but the main value of the technique has been in the investigation of diseases of suspected bacterial origin in which the organisms have proved difficult to culture or classify (Figs 9.16–9.18).

VIRUSES

The value of EM in infectious diseases is about inversely proportional to the size of the organism, and it is in the diagnosis of viral infections that this technique has proved to be of greatest practical assistance.[1,183,184,186,193,195] Viruses are the smallest known infectious agents (ranging from 20 to 300 nm in diameter) and replicate only in living cells.[181,183,184,186,192] The complete particle (virion) contains only one kind of nucleic acid — often visible as an electron-dense nucleoid or core — that is protected by a protein shell (capsid) composed of repeating polypeptide subunits (capsomers). The whole may be surrounded by a host-derived lipoprotein envelope containing additional inserted viral glycoprotein antigens. Morphology plays an important part in viral classification, with size, naked or enveloped state, capsid symmetry (icosahedral, helical or complex) and the number of capsomers being utilized. All but the last of these can be applied to diagnosis in ultrathin sections, although it should be realized that, with few exceptions, it is impossible to subclassify viruses of a particular family by EM; Herpes simplex, varicella-zoster, cytomegalovirus and EB virus particles, for example, are morphologically identical to each other.

STAGES OF VIRAL REPLICATION

Distinct phases, most with morphological expression, have been defined in tissue culture systems.[181,183–185,190–192] Little is known of the equivalent early steps in natural infections, but familiarity with the later stages not only allows recognition of the particular agent concerned but may also permit diagnosis in infections in which no replicative virus is formed (Figs 9.49 and 9.50).

1. Adsorption involves the attachment of virus to the plasma membrane of the host cell through specific receptors that partly determine viral tissue tropism.

2. Penetration is traditionally considered to occur by endocytosis (viropexis) but some organisms may penetrate directly into the cell, which, in the case of enveloped viruses, is preceded by fusion of viral envelope and host plasma membrane.

3. Uncoating releases viral nucleic acid. Host cell lysosomes are involved with at least some viruses.

4. Synthesis. There is little visual evidence other than nucleolar alterations during early shut-down of host protein and nucleic acid synthesis, transcription, or the formation of early proteins (proteins necessary for replication but not forming part of the mature virus). Late viral components are often visible, sometimes as virus factories, and nuclear inclusion bodies or altered cytomembrane systems may appear at this stage.

5. Assembly (morphogenesis) involves the formation of progeny virus from its components. Apart from exceptions such as pox viruses (Figs 9.28–9.31), most DNA viruses replicate in the nucleus (Figs 9.32, 9.33, 9.38–9.41, 9.44 and 9.45) and most RNA viruses replicate in the cytoplasm (Figs 9.47, 9.51–9.54). The process is often inefficient, with the production of particles that are both morphologically and functionally defective, or the accumulation of one or more components synthesized in excess of requirements. Rapid assembly of particles in a single locus at a rate exceeding the rate of release may lead to the formation of crystalline arrays of virus in the nucleus or cytoplasm (Figs 9.33, 9.44 and 9.51).

6. Release may occur by liberation through host cell lysis or else as a process of continuous leakage by budding from the cell surface (Fig. 9.53).

ULTRASTRUCTURE OF VIRAL INFECTIONS

Because viruses are obligate intracellular parasites, the changes induced are mostly intracellular. Toxins are unimportant and the inflammatory response consists of lymphocytes and mononuclear phagocytes. The effects of viruses on cells can be considered as follows:[1,181,182,184,189,190,192]

1. Abortive infection is more common than productive infection. One or more of the early replication stages may occur so that — even though the cell may not support viral

growth — it may still be damaged in the course of an infection.

2. Degeneration is the most important as well as the most obvious consequence, and many viruses have characteristic cytopathic effects. Cell swelling, often seen as vacuolar degeneration of organelles, is a fundamental expression of virus-induced injury, and autophagic activity is frequently enhanced. Nuclear changes are common (Figs 9.32, 9.34–9.37, 9.44, 9.45 and 9.49). The production of inclusion bodies has long been recognized as a histological feature of viral infection (for example, Negri bodies in rabies, Guarnieri bodies in smallpox, cytomegalic inclusions in cytomegalovirus infection), and their recognition by light microscopy in semithin sections can reduce the time spent examining ultrathin sections. Inclusions may be nuclear or cytoplasmic and consist of replicative virus (Figs 9.28, 9.32, 9.33 and 9.44), viral components that are produced in excess (Fig. 9.46), or which accumulate because of a later rate-limiting step, as well as non-viral bodies such as macronucleoli and pseudo-inclusions of cytoplasm in nuclei, or large autophagic vacuoles.

3. Fusion. Some viruses induce fusion of plasma membranes. Migration of the nucleus of the merger cells to the nuclear region of the 'host' cell produces multinucleated syncytial cells (Fig. 9.34).

4. Persistent infections. These are characterized by a steady state with a protracted low turnover of infected cells and may take several forms:

a. Chronic infections in which the effects remain subclinical for a considerable period (e.g. congenital rubella, the hepatitis B carrier state [Figs 9.46–9.48 and 16.7–16.8], subacute sclerosing panencephalitis (Figs 9.49 and 9.50).

b. Latent infections in which the virus persists in an occult or non-replicant state until reactivated (e.g. herpes cold sores, shingles, warts in immunosuppressed patients).

c. Slow infections in which a very long incubation period is followed by progressive tissue destruction in the central nervous system (e.g. subacute spongioform encephalopathies).

5. Transformation. Many viruses have long been recognized as oncogenic in animals, but only in recent years have similar human parallels been found. Viral nucleic acid is generally integrated with the tumour cell genome, and in the case of DNA viruses the infection is non-productive, although virus particle formation may be induced after culture of the tumour cells in vitro. Retroviruses (RNA viruses) still produce mature viruses in vivo.

'VIRUS-LIKE' AND 'VIRUS-ASSOCIATED' PARTICLES

Finally, mention should be made of structures which, from time to time, are misinterpreted as viruses (Figs 9.55–9.68), often with the unfortunate term 'virus-like particles' attached to them, or are claimed to be specific markers of infections. Apart from demonstrating ignorance of various normal cell components or non-specific pathological alterations, the repeated publication of such examples underlines the need for strict criteria for the identification of virus particles, particularly with regard to uniformity of size, structure and staining.[184,193,195,301,304,306]

REFERENCES

Infectious agents: general

1. Burns W A 1980 Microorganisms. In: Trump B F, Jones R T (eds) Diagnostic electron microscopy, vol. 3. Wiley, New York, pp 1–35
2. Fejerskov O, Andersen L, Philipsen H P 1980 Oral mucous membrane. In: Johannessen J V (ed) Electron microscopy in human medicine, vol. 7, Digestive system. McGraw-Hill, New York, pp 25–58
3. Font R L, Jakobiec F A 1979 The role of electron microscopy in ophthalmic pathology. In: Trump B F, Jones R T (eds) Diagnostic electron microscopy, vol. 2. Wiley, New York, pp 163–219
4. Myerowitz R L 1983 Ultrastructural characteristics of some opportunistic infections. In: Myerowitz R L (ed) The pathology of opportunistic infections. With pathogenetic, diagnostic and clinical correlations. Raven Press, New York, pp 51–64

Protozoa: general

5. Aikawa M, Sterling C R 1974 Intracellular parasitic protozoa. Academic Press, New York
6. Jadin J-M, Jadin J-B 1980 Protozoa. In: Johannessen J V (ed) Electron microscopy in human medicine, vol 3, Infectious agents. McGraw-Hill, New York, pp 281–332

7. Scholtyseck E 1979 Fine structure of parasitic protozoa. An atlas of micrographs, drawings and diagrams. Springer-Verlag, Berlin
8. Vickerman K 1982 Parasitic protozoa: aspects of the host–parasite interface. In: Mettrich D F, Desser S S (eds) Parasites — their world and ours. Elsevier Biomedical Press, Amsterdam, pp 43–52
9. Zaman V 1978 Atlas of medical parasitology. An atlas of important protozoa, helminths and arthropods, mostly in colour. Adis Press, New York
10. Zaman V 1983 Scanning electron microscopy of medically important parasites. Adis Health Science Press, Sydney

Protozoa: specific organisms

11. Aikawa M 1977 Variations in structure and function during the life cycles of malarial parasites. Bulletin of the World Health Organization 55: 139–156
12. Aikawa M, Miller L H 1983 Structural alteration of the erythrocyte membrane during malarial parasite invasion and intraerythrocytic development. In: Evered D, Whelan J (eds) Malaria and the red cell. CIBA Foundation Symposium 94. Pitman, London, pp 45–63
13. Aikawa M, Seed T M 1980 Morphology of plasmodia. In: Kreier J P (ed) Malaria, vol 1, Epidemiology, chemotherapy, morphology and metabolism. Academic Press, New York, pp 285–344

14. Albach R A, Booden T 1978 Amoebae. In: Kreier J P (ed) Parasitic protozoa, vol 2. Academic Press, New York, pp 455–506

15. Askin F B, Katzenstein A-L A 1981 Pneumocystis infection masquerading as diffuse alveolar damage. A potential source of diagnostic error. Chest 79: 420–422

16. Barton E G, Campbell W G 1967 Further observations on the ultrastructure of *Pneumocystis*. Archives of Pathology 83: 527–534

17. Bird R G, Smith M D 1980 Cryptosporidiosis in man: parasite life cycle and fine structural pathology. Journal of Pathology 132: 217–233

18. Bowers B, Korn E D 1968 The fine structure of *Acanthamoeba castellani*. I. The trophozoite. Journal of Cell Biology 39: 95–111

19. Brooks S E H, Audretsch J, Miller C G, Sparke B 1970 Electron microscopy of *Giardia lamblia* in human jejunal biopsies. Journal of Medical Microbiology 3: 196–199

20. Campbell W G 1972 Ultrastructure of *Pneumocystis* in human lung. Life cycle in human pneumocystosis. Archives of Pathology 93: 312–324

21. Carter R F 1970 Description of a *Naegleria* sp. isolated from two cases of primary amoebic meningoencephalitis, and of the experimental pathological changes induced by it. Journal of Pathology 100: 217–244

22. Casemore D P, Sands R L, Curry A 1985 *Cryptosporidium* species a 'new' human pathogen. Journal of Clinical Pathology 38: 1321–1336

23. Daneshbod K 1978 Localized lymphadenitis due to leishmania simulating toxoplasmosis. Value of electron microscopy for differentiation. American Journal of Clinical Pathology 69: 462–467

24. De Brito T, Barone A A, Faria R M 1969 Human liver biopsy in *P. falciparum* and *P. vivax* malaria. A light and electron microscopy study. Virchows Archiv A, Pathology Pathologische Anatomie 348: 220–229

25. De Souza W 1984 Cell biology of *Trypanosoma cruzi*. International Review of Cytology 86: 197–283

26. De Souza W, Benchimol M 1984 High voltage electron microscopy of critical point dried trypanosomatids. Journal of Submicroscopic Cytology 16: 237–242

27. Dubey J P 1977 *Toxoplasma, Hammondia, Besnoitia, Sarcocystis* and other tissue cyst-forming coccidia of man and animals. In: Kreier J P (ed) Parasitic protozoa, vol 3. Academic Press, New York, pp 101–237

28. Erlandsen S L, Chase D G 1974 Morphological alterations in the microvillous border of villous epithelial cells produced by intestinal microorganisms. American Journal of Clinical Nutrition 27: 1277–1286

29. Eyden B P 1976 Fibrous structures in zooflagellate protozoa. In: Fuller R, Lovelock D W (eds) Microbial ultrastructure. The use of the electron microscope. Academic Press, London, pp 305–320

30. Garcia-Tamayo J, Nunez-Montiel J T, de Garcia H P 1978 An electron microscopic investigation on the pathogenesis of human vaginal Trichomoniasis. Acta Cytologica 22: 447–455

31. Garda L A, Stein S A, Cleary K A, Ordonez N G 1983 Human cryptosporidiosis in the acquired immune deficiency syndrome. Archives of Pathology and Laboratory Medicine 107: 562–566

32. Ghatak N R, Zimmerman H M 1973 Fine structure of Toxoplasma in the human brain. Archives of Pathology 95: 276–283

33. Gonzalez M M, Gould E, Dickinson G, Martinez A J, Visvesvara G, Cleary T J, Hensley G T 1986 Acquired immunodeficiency syndrome associated with *Acanthamoeba* infection and other opportunistic organisms. Archives of Pathology and Laboratory Medicine 110: 749–751

34. Griffin J L, Juniper K 1971 Ultrastructure of *Entamoeba histolytica* from human amebic dysentery. Archives of Pathology 91: 271–280

35. Ham E K, Greenberg S D, Reynolds R C, Singer D B 1971 Ultrastructure of *Pneumocystis carinii*. Experimental and Molecular Pathology 14: 362–372

36. Hammond D M 1973 Life cycles and development of coccidia. In: Hammond D M, Long P L (eds) The coccidia. *Eimeria, Isospora, Toxoplasma* and related genera. University Park Press, Baltimore, pp 45–79

37. Haque A u, Plattner S B, Cook R T, Hart M N 1987 *Pneumocystis carinii*. Taxonomy as viewed by electron microscopy. American Journal of Clinical Pathology 87: 504–510

38. Hasleton P S, Curry A, Rankin E M 1981 *Pneumocystis carinii* pneumonia: a light microscopical and ultrastructural study. Journal of Clinical Pathology 34: 1138–1146

39. Honigberg B M 1978 Trichomonads of importance in human medicine. In: Kreier J P (ed) Parasitic protozoa, vol 2. Academic Press, New York, pp 275–454

40. Klima M, Gyorkey P, Min K-W, Gyorkey F 1977 Electron microscopy in the diagnosis of giardiasis. Archives of Pathology and Laboratory Medicine 101: 133–135

41. Kulda J, Nohýnková E 1978 Flagellates of the human intestine and of intestines of other species. In: Kreier J P (ed) Parasitic protozoa, vol. 2. Academic Press, New York, pp 1–138

42. Lefkowitch J H, Krumholz S, Feng-Chen K-C, Griffin P, Despommier D, Brasitus T A 1984 Cryptosporidiosis of the human small intestine: a light and electron microscopic study. Human Pathology 15: 746–752

43. Ludvik J, Shipstone A C 1970 The ultrastructure of *Entamoeba histolytica*. Bulletin of the World Health Organisation 43: 301–308

44. Mehlhorn H, Heydorn A O 1978 The sarcosporidia (Protozoa, Sporozoa): life cycle and fine structure. In: Lumsden W H R, Muller R, Baker J R (eds) Advances in Parasitology, vol 16. Academic Press, London, pp 43–91

45. Meyer E A, Radulescu S 1979 Giardia and giardiasis. In: Lumsden W H R, Muller R, Baker J R (eds) Advances in Parasitology, vol 17. Academic Press, London, pp 1–47

46. Morecki R, Parker J G 1967 Ultrastructural studies of the human *Giardia lamblia* and subjacent jejunal mucosa in a subject with steatorrhoea. Gastroenterology 52: 151–184

47. Nielsen M H, Nielsen R 1975 Electron microscopy of *Trichomonas vaginalis Donné*: interaction with vaginal epithelium in human trichomoniasis. Acta Pathologica et Microbiologica Scandinavica Section B Microbiology 83: 305–320

48. Nielsen M H, Ludvik J, Nielsen R 1966 On the ultrastructure of *Trichomonas vaginalis* Donné. Journal de Microscopie 5: 229–250

49. Nistal M, Santana A, Paniaqua R, Palacios J 1986 Testicular toxoplasmosis in two men with the acquired immunodeficiency syndrome (AIDS). Archives of Pathology and Laboratory Medicine 110: 744–746

50. Pittman F E, El-Hashimi W K, Pittman J C 1973 Studies of human amebiasis II. Light and electron-microscopic observations of colonic mucosa and exudate in acute amebic colitis. Gastroenterology 65: 588–603

51. Powell H C, Gibbs C J, Lorenzo A M, Lampert P W, Gajdusek D C 1978 Toxoplasmosis of the central nervous system in the adult. Electron microscopic observations. Acta Neuropathologica 41: 211–216

52. Restrepo C, Macher A M, Radany E H 1987 Disseminated extraintestinal isosporiasis in a patient with acquired immune deficiency syndrome. American Journal of Clinical Pathology 87: 536–542

53. Ridley M J, Wells C W 1986 Macrophage-parasite interactions in the lesions of cutaneous leishmaniasis. An ultrastructural study. American Journal of Pathology 123: 79–85

54. Rosen S, Hano J E, Inman M M, Gilliland P F, Barry K G 1968 The kidney in blackwater fever. Light and electron microscopic observations. American Journal of Clinical Pathology 49: 358–370

55. Scholtyseck E 1973 Ultrastructure. In: Hammond D M, Long P L (eds) The coccidia. *Eimeria, Isospora, Toxoplasma* and related genera. University Park Press, Baltimore, pp 81–144

56. Schuster F L 1975 Ultrastructure of cysts of *Naegleria* spp: a comparative study. Journal of Protozoology 22: 352–359

57. Seed T M, Aikawa M 1977 Pneumocystis. In: Kreier J P (ed) Parasitic protozoa, vol 4. Academic Press, New York, pp 329–357

58. Sueishi K, Hisano S, Sumiyoshi A, Tanaka K 1977 Scanning and transmission electron microscopic study of human pulmonary pneumocystosis. Chest 72: 213–216

59. Takano J, Yardley J H 1965 Jejunal lesions in patients with giardiasis and malabsorption. An electron microscopic study. Bulletin of the Johns Hopkins Hospital 116: 413–429

60. Tang T T, Harb J M, Dunne M, Wells R G, Meyer G A, Chusid M J, Casper J T, Camitta B M 1986 Cerebral toxoplasmosis in an immunocompromised host. A precise and rapid diagnosis by electron microscopy. American Journal of Clinical Pathology 85: 104–110

61. Trager W, Rudzinska M A, Bradbury P C 1966 The fine structure of

Plasmodium falciparum and its host erythrocytes in natural malarial infections in man. Bulletin of the World Health Organisation 35: 883–885

62. Trier J S, Moxey P C, Schimmel E M, Robles E 1974 Chronic intestinal coccidiosis in man: intestinal morphology and response to treatment. Gastroenterology 66: 923–935

63. Vavra J, Kučera K 1970 *Pneumocystis carinii* Delanoë, its ultrastructure and ultrastructural affinities. Journal of Protozoology 17: 463–483

64. Vickerman K 1974 The ultrastructure of pathogenic flagellates. In: Trypanosomiasis and leishmaniasis with special reference to Chagas' disease. CIBA Foundation Symposium 20 (new series). Associated Scientific Publishers, Amsterdam, pp 171–198

65. Walzer P D 1986 Attachment of microbes to host cells: relevance of *Pneumocystis carinii* (editorial). Laboratory Investigation 54: 589–592

66. Wang N-S, Huang S-N, Thurlbeck W M 1970 Combined *Pneumocystis carinii* and cytomegalovirus infection. Archives of Pathology 90: 529–535

67. Wickramasinghe S N, Abdalla S H, Kasili E G 1987 Ultrastructure of bone marrow in patients with visceral leishmaniasis. Journal of Clinical Pathology 40: 267–275

68. Zaman V 1978 *Balantidium coli*. In: Kreier J P (ed) Parasitic protozoa, vol 2. Academic Press, New York, pp 633–653

Fungi: general

69. Beckett A, Heath I B, McLaughlin D J 1974 An atlas of fungal ultrastructure. Longman, London

70. Borgers M 1980 Mechanism of action of antifungal drugs, with special reference to the imidazole derivatives. Reviews of Infectious Disease 2: 520–534

71. Carbonell L M 1971 Ultrastructure of human pathogenic fungi and their mycoses. In: Baker R D (ed) Handbuch der speziellen pathologischen anatomie und histologie Section 3, Vol. 5 The pathologic anatomy of mycoses. Springer-Verlag, Berlin, pp 38–66

72. Davenport R R, Bole B, McLeod B, Parsons E 1976 Microfungi, yeasts and yeast-like organisms. In: Fuller R, Lovelock D W (eds) Microbial ultrastructure. The use of the electron microscope. Academic Press, London, pp 265–270

73. Emmons C W, Binford C H, Utz J P, Kwon–Chung K J 1977 Medical Mycology, 3rd edn. Lea and Febiger, Philadelphia

74. Moore R T 1965 The ultrastructure of fungal cells. In: Ainsworth G C, Susman A S (eds) The fungi. An advanced treatise, vol I, The fungal cell. Academic Press, New York, pp 95–118

75. Müller J 1980 Fungi. In: Johannessen J V (ed) Electron microscopy in human medicine, vol 3, Infectious agents. McGraw-Hill, New York, pp 335–390

Fungi: specific organisms

76. Al-Doory Y, Baker C A 1971 Comparative observations of ultrastructure of five species of *Candida*. Mycopathologia et Mycologia Applicata 44: 355–367

77. Baxter M, Mann P R 1969 Electron microscopic studies of the invasion of human hair *in vitro* by three keratinophilic fungi. Sabouraudia 7: 33–37

78. Cawson R A, Rajasingham K C 1972 Ultrastructural features of the invasive phase of *Candida albicans*. British Journal of Dermatology 87: 435–443

79. Chong K C, Adam B A, Soo-Hoo T S 1975 Morphology of *Piedra hortai*. Sabouraudia 9: 157–160

80. Collins D N, Oppenheim I A, Edwards M R 1971 Cryptococcosis associated with systemic lupus eythematosus. Light and electron microscopic observations on a morphological variant. Archives of Pathology 91: 78–88

81. Cruickshank J G, Cavill R, Jelbert M 1973 *Cryptococcus neoformans* of unusual morphology. Applied Microbiology 25: 309–312

82. Djaczenko W, Cassone A 1971 Visualization of new ultrastructural components in the cell wall of *Candida albicans* with fixatives containing TAPO. Journal of Cell Biology 52: 186–190

83. Dumont A, Piché C 1969 Electron microscopic studies of human histoplasmosis. Archives of Pathology 87: 168–178

84. Garcia-Tamayo T, Castillo G, Martinez A J 1982 Human genital candidiasis. Histochemistry, scanning and transmission electron microscopy. Acta Cytologica 26: 7–14

85. Gutierrez F, Fu Y S, Lurie H I 1975 Cryptococcosis histologically resembling histoplasmosis. A light and electron microscopical study. Archives of Pathology 99: 347–352

86. Hino H, Takizawa K, Asboe-Hansen G 1982 Ultrastructure of *Cryptococcus neoformans*. Acta Dermato-Venereologica 62: 113–117

87. Hiruma M, Kagawa S 1985 Ultrastructure of *Cryptococcus neoformans* in the cerebrospinal fluid of a patient with cryptococcal meningitis. Mycopathologia 89: 5–12

88. Kanbe T, Tanaka K 1982 Ultrastructure of the invasion of human hair *in vitro* by the keratinophilic fungus *Microsporum gypseum*. Infection and Immunity 38: 706–715

89. Kanbe T, Suzuki S, Tanaka K 1986 Structural differentiation in the frond and boring hypha of the dermatophyte *Microsporum canis* invading human hair *in vitro*. Journal of Electron Microscopy 35: 38–46

90. Keddie F M 1966 Electron microscopy of *Malassezia furfur* in tinea versicolor. Sabouraudia 5: 134–137

91. Keddie F M 1967 Further investigations of the electron microscopic examination of human hair naturally infected by *Microsporum gypseum*. Sabouraudia 6: 1–4

92. Marrie T J, Costerton J W 1981 The ultrastructure of *Candida albicans* infections. Canadian Journal of Microbiology 27: 1156–1164

93. Marrie T J, Cooper J H, Costerton J W 1984 Ultrastructure of *Candida parapsilosis* endocarditis. Infection and Immunity 45: 390–398

94. Mirra S S, Trombley I K, Miles M L 1980 Ultrastructural study of a cerebral toruloma. Acta Neuropathologica 50: 153–157

95. Montes L F, Wilborn W H 1968 Ultrastructural features of host-parasite relationship in oral candidiasis. Journal of Bacteriology 96: 1349–1356

96. Montes L F, Wilborn W H 1985 Fungus–host relationship in candidiasis. A brief review. Archives of Dermatology 121: 119–124

97. Myerowitz R L 1978 Ultrastructural observations in disseminated candidiasis. Archives of Pathology and Laboratory Medicine 102: 506–511

98. Odds F C 1979 Candida and candidosis. Leicester University Press, Leicester

99. Poulain D, Tronchin G, Dubremetz J F, Biguet J 1978 Ultrastructure of the cell wall of *Candida albicans* blastospores: study of its constitutive layers by the use of a cytochemical technique revealing polysaccharides. Annales de Microbiologie (L'Institut Pasteur) 129A: 141–153

100. Rajasingham K C, Cawson R A 1984 Plasmalemmasomes and lomasomes in *Candida albicans*. Cytobios 40: 21–25

101. Scherwitz C 1982 Ultrastructure of human cutaneous candidosis. Journal of Investigative Dermatology 78: 200–205

102. Williams A O, Lawson E A, Lucas A O 1971 African histoplasmosis due to *Histoplasma duboisii*. Archives of Pathology 92: 306–318

Bacteria: general

103. Costerton J W 1979 The role of electron microscopy in the elucidation of bacterial structure and function. Annual Review of Microbiology 33: 459–479

104. Costerton J W, Irvin R T 1981 The bacterial glycocalyx in nature and disease. Annual Review of Microbiology 35: 299–324

105. Glauert A M, Thornley M J, Thorne K J I, Sleytr U B 1976 The surface structure of bacteria. In: Fuller R, Lovelock D W (eds) Microbial ultrastructure. The use of the electron microscope. Academic Press, London, pp 31–47

106. Hobot J A, Carlemalm E, Villiger W, Kellenberger E 1984 Periplasmic gel: new concept resulting from the reinvestigation of bacterial cell envelope ultrastructure by new methods. Journal of Bacteriology 160: 143–152

107. Hodgkiss W, Short J A, Walker P D 1976 Bacterial surface structures. In: Fuller R, Lovelock D W (eds) Microbial

ultrastructure. The use of the electron microscope. Academic Press, London, pp 49–71
108. Holt S C 1980 Bacteria. In: Johannessen J V (ed) Electron microscopy in human medicine, vol 3, Infectious agents. McGraw-Hill, New York, pp 91–278
109. Lawn A M 1976 Sex pili of enterobacteria. In: Fuller R, Lovelock D W (eds) Microbial ultrastructure. The use of the electron microscope. Academic Press, London, pp 73–86
110. Rogers H J 1983 Bacterial morphology. In: Wilson G, Dick H M (eds) Topley and Wilson's principles of bacteriology, virology and immunity, vol 1, 7th edn. Arnold, London, pp 16–38

Bacteria: specific organisms

111. Anderson D R 1965 Subcellular particles associated with human leukemia as seen with the electron microscope. Wistar Institute Symposium Monographs 4: 113–141
112. Anderson D R 1969 Ultrastructural studies of mycoplasmas and the L-phase of bacteria. In: Hayflick L (ed) The mycoplasmatales and the L-phase of bacteria. North-Holland, Amsterdam, pp 365–402
113. Ashworth C T, Douglas F C, Reynolds R C, Thomas P J 1964 Bacillus-like bodies in Whipple's disease; disappearance with clinical remission after antibiotic therapy. American Journal of Medicine 37: 481–490
114. Avakyan A A, Popov V L 1984 Rickettsiaceae and Chlamydiaceae: comparative electron microscopic studies. Acta Virologica 28: 159–173
115. Azar H A, Pham T D, Kurban A K 1970 An electron microscopic study of a syphilitic chancre. Engulfment of Treponema pallidum by plasma cells. Archives of Pathology 90: 143–150
116. Blackmon J A, Chandler F W, Cherry W B, England A C, Feeley J C, Hicklin M D, McKinney R M, Wilkinson H W 1981 Legionellosis. American Journal of Pathology 103: 429–465
117. Boatman E S 1979 Morphology and ultrastructure of the mycoplasmatales. In: Barile M F, Razin S (eds) The mycoplasmas, vol 1, Cell biology. Academic Press, New York, pp 63–102
118. Boddingius J 1974 The occurrence of Mycobacterium leprae within axons of peripheral nerves. Acta Neuropathologica 27: 257–270
119. Burchard G-D, Bierther 1985 An electron microscopic study on macrophages and lymphocytes in lepromatous and borderline leprosy. International Journal of Leprosy 53: 64–69
120. Chandler F W, Blackmon J A, Hicklin M D, Cole R M, Calloway C S 1979 Ultrastructure of the agent of legionnaires' disease in the human lung. American Journal of Clinical Pathology 71: 43–50
121. Chears W C, Ashworth C T 1961 Electron microscopic study of the intestinal mucosa in Whipple's disease. Demonstration of encapsulated bacilliform bodies in the lesion. Gastroenterology 41: 129–138
122. Chen X G, Correa P, Offerhaus J, Rodriguez E, Janney F, Hoffmann E, Fox J, Hunter F, Diavolitsis S 1986 Ultrastructure of the gastric mucosa harboring Campylobacter-like organisms. American Journal of Clinical Pathology 86: 575–582
123. Collier A M, Clyde W A 1971 Relationships between Mycoplasma pneumoniae and human respiratory epithelium. Infection and Immunity 3: 694–701
124. Collier A M, Clyde W A 1974 Appearance of Mycoplasma pneumoniae in lungs of experimentally infected hamsters and sputum from patients with natural disease. American Review of Respiratory Diseases 110: 765–773
125. De la Maza L M, Peterson E M 1982 Scanning electron microscopy of McCoy cells infected with Chlamydia trachomatis. Experimental and Molecular Pathology 36: 217–226
126. Denholm R B, Mills P R, More I A R 1981 Electron microscopy in the long term follow-up of Whipple's disease. Effect of antibiotics. American Journal of Surgical Pathology 5: 507–516
127. Dharkar D, Kraft J R, Bjornsson L, Gould V E 1984 Tumorlike proliferation of 'granular histiocytes' in a lymph node. Ultrastructural Pathology 7: 339–343
128. Dmochowski L, Dreyer D A, Grey C E, Hales R, Langford P L, Pipes F, Recher L, Seman G, Shively J A, Shullenberger C C, Sinkovics J G, Taylor H G, Tessmer C F, Yumoto T 1967 Studies on the submicroscopic morphology of structures resembling

129. Dobbins W O, Ruffin J M 1967 A light- and electron-microscopic study of bacterial invasion in Whipple's disease. American Journal of Pathology 51: 225–242
130. Domermuth C H, Nielsen M H, Freundt E A, Birch-Andersen A 1964 Ultrastructure of Mycoplasma species. Journal of Bacteriology 88: 727–744
131. Draper P 1982 The anatomy of mycobacteria. In: Ratledge C, Stanford J (eds) The biology of the mycobacteria, vol 1, Physiology, identification and classification. Academic Press, London, pp 9–52
132. Editorial 1984 Intestinal spirochaetes. Lancet i: 720
133. Evans B A 1982 Chlamydial infection of the human cervix — an ultrastructural study. Journal of Infection 4: 225–228
134. Finlayson M H, Bilbao J M, Lough J O 1974 The pathogenesis of the neuropathy in dimorphous leprosy: electron microscopic and cytochemical studies. Journal of Neuropathology and Experimental Neurology 33: 446–455
135. Freundt E A, Vinther O 1980 Mycoplasmas. In: Johannessen J V (ed) Electron microscopy in human medicine, vol 3, Infectious agents. McGraw-Hill, New York, pp 69–87
136. Ghillin J S, Urmacher C, West R, Shike M 1983 Disseminated Mycobacterium avium-intracellulare infection in acquired immunodeficiency syndrome mimicking Whipple's disease. Gastroenterology 85: 1187–1191
137. Giesbrecht P, Wecke J, Reinicke B 1976 On the morphogenesis of the cell wall of staphylococci. International Review of Cytology 44: 225–318
138. Glavin F L, Winn C, Craighead J E 1979 Ultrastructure of the lung in legionnaires' disease. Observations of three biopsies done during the Vermont epidemic. Annals of Internal Medicine 90: 555–559
139. Goodwin C S, Armstrong J A, Marshall B J 1986 Campylobacter pyloridis, gastritis and peptic ulceration. Journal of Clinical Pathology 39: 353–365
140. Goodwin C S, McCulloch R K, Armstrong J A, Wee S H 1985 Unusual cellular fatty acids and distinctive ultrastructure in a new spiral bacterium (Campylobacter pyloridis) from the human gastric mucosa. Journal of Medical Microbiology 19: 257–267
141. Gress F M, Myerowitz R L, Pasculle A W, Rinaldo C R, Dowling J N 1980 The ultrastructural morphologic features of Pittsburgh pneumonia agent. American Journal of Pathology 101: 63–78
142. Harland W A, Lee F D 1967 Intestinal spirochaetosis. British Medical Journal 3: 718–719
143. Hasegawa T 1969 Electron microscopic observations on the lesions of condyloma latum. British Journal of Dermatology 81: 367–374
144. Henrik-Nielsen R, Lundbeck F A, Teglbjaerg P S, Ginnerup P, Hovind-Hougen K 1985 Intestinal spirochetosis of the vermiform appendix. Gastroenterology 88: 971–977
145. Holt S C 1978 Anatomy and chemistry of spirochetes. Microbiological Reviews 42: 114–160
146. Hovind-Hougen K 1983 Morphology. In: Schell R F, Musher D M (eds) Pathogenesis and immunology of Treponemal infection. Dekker, New York, pp 3–28
147. Hovind-Hougen K, Birch-Andersen A, Henrik-Nielsen R, Orholm M, Pedersen J O, Teglbjaerg P S, Thaysen E H 1982 Intestinal spirochetosis: morphological characterization and cultivation of the spirochete Brachyspira aalborgi gen. nov., sp. nov. Journal of Clinical Microbiology 16: 1127–1136
148. Imaeda T, Convit J 1962 Electron microscope study of Mycobacterium leprae and its environment in a vesicular leprous lesion. Journal of Bacteriology 83: 43–52
149. Job C K 1970 Mycobacterium leprae in nerve lesions in lepromatous leprosy. An electron microscopic study. Archives of Pathology 89: 195–207
150. Kahn P, Scott T 1974 The pathology of a radial nerve biopsy in leprosy: light and electron microscopy. Journal of Pathology 114: 97–100
151. Katz S M, Hashemi S, Brown K R, Habib W A, Hammel J M 1984 Pleomorphism of Legionella pneumophila. Ultrastructural Pathology 6: 117–129
152. Klainer A S, Pollack J D 1973 Scanning electron microscopy techniques in the study of the surface structure of mycoplasmas. Annals of the New York Academy of Sciences 225: 236–245

153. Knutton S, Lloyd D R, Candy D C A, McNeish A S 1984 Ultrastructural study of adhesion of enterotoxigenic *Escherichia coli* to erythrocytes and human intestinal epithelial cells. Infection and Immunity 44: 519–529

154. Kölbel H K 1984 Electron microscopy. In: Kubica G P, Wayne L G (eds) The mycobacteria. A sourcebook, Part A. Dekker, New York, pp249–300

155. Lie J T, Davis J S 1976 Pancarditis in Whipple's disease. Electron microscopic demonstration of intracardiac bacillary bodies. American Journal of Clinical Pathology 66: 22–30

156. McCaul T F, Williams J C 1981 Development cycle of *Coxiella burnetii*: structure and morphogenesis of vegetative and sporogenic differentiation. Journal of Bacteriology 147: 1063–1076

157. Morioka H, Hara K, Suganuma A 1981 Cell envelope of staphylococci as revealed by electron microscopy. Zentralblatt für Bakteriologie, Mikrobiologie und Hygiene 1 Abteilung (supplement 10, Staphylococci and staphylococcal infections) pp 449–454

158. Nishiura M 1960 The electron microscopic basis of the pathology of leprosy. International Journal of Leprosy 28: 357–400

159. Okada S, Fukunishi Y, Mukherjee A, Ramu G, Desikan K V 1980 An improved embedding method for electron microscopy of lepromata. International Journal of Leprosy 48: 408–413

160. Pasculle A W, Myerowitz R L, Rinaldo C R 1979 New bacterial agent of pneumonia isolated from renal-transplant recipients. Lancet ii: 58–61

161. Phillips A D, Hine K R, Holmes G K T, Woodings D F 1984 Gastric spiral bacteria. Lancet ii: 100–101

162. Phillips D M 1978 Detection of mycoplasma contamination of cell cultures by electron microscopy. In: McGarrity G J, Murphy D G, Nichols W W (eds) Mycoplasma infection of cell cultures. Plenum Press, New York, pp 105–118

163. Roberts D M, Themann H, Knust F-J, Preston F E, Donaldson J R 1970 An electron-microscope study of bacteria in two cases of Whipple's disease. Journal of Pathology 100: 249–255

164. Rodgers F G 1979 Ultrastructure of *Legionella pneumophilia*. Journal of Clinical Pathology 32: 1195–1202

165. Rollins S, Colby T, Clayton F 1986 Open lung biopsy in *Mycoplasma pneumoniae* pneumonia. Archives of Pathology and Laboratory Medicine 110: 34–41

166. Rothbaum R J, Partin J C, Saalfield K, McAdams A J 1983 An ultrastructural study of enteropathogenic *Escherichia coli* infection in human infants. Ultrastructural Pathology 4: 291–304

167. Silva M T, Macedo P M 1983 The interpretation of the ultrastructure of mycobacterial cells in transmission electron microscopy of ultrathin sections. International Journal of Leprosy 51: 225–234

168. Suganuma A 1965 Fine structure of *Staphylococcus aureus*. Annals of the New York Academy of Sciences 128 Article 1: 26–44

169. Swanson J, Eschenbach D A, Alexander E R, Holmes K K 1975 Light and electron microscopic study of *Chlamydia trachomatis* infection of the uterine cervix. Journal of Infectious Diseases 131: 678–687

170. Sykes J A, Kalan J 1975 Intracellular *Treponema pallidum* in cells of a syphilitic lesion of the uterine cervix. American Journal of Obstetrics and Gynecology 122: 361–367

171. Sykes J A, Miller J N, Kalan A J 1974 *Treponema pallidum* within cells of a primary chancre from a human female. British Journal of Venereal Diseases 50: 40–44

172. Takeuchi A, Jervis H R, Nakazawa H, Robinson D M 1974 Spiral-shaped organisms on the surface colonic epithelium of the monkey and man. American Journal of Clinical Nutrition 27: 1287–1296

173. Todd W J, Caldwell H D 1985 The interaction of *Chlamydia trachomatis* with host cells: ultrastructural studies of the mechanism of release of a biovar II strain from HeLa 229 cells. Journal of Infectious Diseases 151: 1037–1044

174. Tricottet V, Bruneval P, Vire O, Camilleri J P, Bloch F, Bonte N, Roge J 1986 Campylobacter-like organisms and surface epithelium abnormalities in active, chronic gastritis in humans: an ultrastructural study. Ultrastructural Pathology 10: 113–122

175. Trier J S, Phelps P C, Eidelman S, Rubin C E 1965 Whipple's disease: light and electron microscope correlation of jejunal mucosal histology with antibiotic treatment and clinical status. Gastroenterology 48: 684–707

176. Turck W P G, Howitt G, Turnberg L A, Fox H, Longson M, Matthews M B, Das Gupta R 1976 Chronic Q fever. Quarterly Journal of Medicine 45: 193–217

177. Van Spreeuwel J P, Duursma G C, Meijer C J L M, Bax R, Rosekrans P C M, Lindeman J 1985 Campylobacter colitis: histological immunohistochemical and ultrastructural findings. Gut 26: 945–951

178. Ward M E 1983 Chlamydial classification, development and structure. British Medical Bulletin 39 (2): 109–115

179. Wiegand S E, Strobel P L, Glassman L H 1972 Electron microscopic anatomy of pathogenic *Treponema pallidum*. Journal of Investigative Dermatology 58: 186–204

180. Yardley J H, Hendrix T R 1961 Combined electron and light microscopy in Whipple's disease. Bulletin of the Johns Hopkins Hospital 109: 80–98

Viruses: general

181. Boyd R F, Hoerl B G 1986 Viruses. In: Boyd R F, Hoerl B G (eds) Basic medical microbiology, 3rd edn. Little, Brown, Boston, pp 653–706

182. Cheville N F 1975 Cytopathology in viral diseases. In: Melnick J L (ed) Monographs in virology, vol 10. Karger, Basel

183. Fisher H W 1981 Use of electron microscopy in virology. In: Fraenkel-Conrat H, Wagner R W (eds) Comprehensive virology, vol 17, Methods used in the study of viruses. Plenum Press, New York, pp 83–127

184. Grimley P M, Henson D E 1983 Electron microscopy in virus infections. In: Trump B F, Jones R T (eds) Diagnostic electron microscopy, vol 4. Wiley, New York, pp 1–73

185. Howe C, Coward J E, Fenger T W 1980 Viral invasion: morphological, biochemical and biophysical aspects. In: Fraenkel-Conrat H, Wagner R W (eds) Comprehensive virology, vol 16, Virus–host interactions. Viral invasion, persistence and disease. Plenum Press, New York, pp 1–71

186. Hsiung G-D, Fong C Y, August M J 1979 The use of electron microscopy for diagnosis of virus infections: an overview. Progress in Medical Virology 25: 133–159

187. Lutzner M A 1967 Virus diseases. In: Zelickson A S (ed) Ultrastructure of normal and abnormal skin. Kimpton, London, pp 365–387

188. Lutzner M A 1985 Virus diseases of the skin and mucosa. In: Johannessen J V, Hashimoto K (eds) Electron microscopy in human medicine, vol 11a, The skin. McGraw-Hill, New York, pp 277–308

189. Nasemann T 1977 Viral diseases of the skin, mucous membranes and genitals. Clinical features, differential diagnosis and therapy, with basic principles of virology. Thieme, Stuttgart

190. Rabin E R, Jenson A B 1967 Electron microscopic studies of animal viruses with emphasis on *in vivo* infections. Progress in Medical Virology 9: 392–450

191. Russell W C, Winters W D 1975 Assembly of viruses. Progress in Medical Virology 19: 1–39

192. White D O, Fenner F J 1986 Medical virology, 3rd edn. Academic Press, Orlando

193. Wills E J 1983 Ultrathin section electron microscopy in the diagnosis of viral infections. In: Sommers S C, Rosen P P (eds) Pathology annual. Appleton–Century–Crofts, Norwalk 18 (part 1), pp 139–180

194. Wolinsky J S 1979 Viral diseases. In: Johannessen J V (ed) Electron microscopy in human medicine, vol 6, Nervous system, sensory organs and respiratory tract. McGraw-Hill, New York, pp 54–84

195. Yunis E J, Hashida Y, Haas J E 1977 The role of electron microscopy in the identification of viruses in human disease. In: Sommers S C, Rosen P P (eds) Pathology annual. Appleton–Century–Crofts, New York 12 (part 1), pp 311–330

Viruses: specific organisms

196. Almeida J D, Howatson A F, Williams M G 1962 Electron microscope study of human warts; sites of virus production and nature of the inclusion bodies. Journal of Investigative Dermatology 38: 337–345

197. Armstrong J A, Horne R 1984 Follicular dendritic cells and virus-like particles in AIDS-related lymphadenopathy. Lancet ii: 370–372

198. Balázs M 1984 Electron microscopic examination of congenital cytomegalovirus hepatitis. Virchows Archiv A, Pathology Pathologische Anatomie 405: 119–129

199. Beneck D, Greco M A, Feiner H D 1986 Glomerulonephritis in congenital cytomegalic inclusion disease. Human Pathology 17: 1054–1059

200. Bernhard W 1960 The detection and study of tumor viruses with the electron microscope. Cancer Research 20: 712–727

201. Bianchi L, Gudat F 1976 Sanded nuclei in hepatitis B. Eosinophilic inclusions in liver cell nuclei due to excess in hepatitis B core antigen formation. Laboratory Investigation 35: 1–5

202. Bouteille M, Fontaine C, Vedrenne Cl, Delarue J 1965 Sur un cas d'encéphalite subaiguë à inclusions. Étude anatomo-clinique et ultrastructurale. Revue Neurologique 113: 454–458

203. Boyle W F, Riggs J L, Oshiro L S, Lennette E H 1973 Electron microscopic identification of papova virus in laryngeal papilloma. Laryngoscope 83: 1102–1108

204. Breitfeld V, Hashida Y, Sherman F E, Odagiri K, Yunis E J 1973 Fatal measles infection in children with leukemia. Laboratory Investigation 28: 279–291

205. Casas-Cordero M, Morin C, Roy M, Fortier M, Meisels A 1981 Origin of the koilocyte in condylomata of the human cervix. Ultrastructural study. Acta Cytologica 25: 383–392

206. Chou S M, Cherry J D 1967 Ultrastructure of Cowdry type A inclusions. I. In herpes simplex encephalitis. Neurology 17: 575–586

207. Chou S M, Roos R, Burrell R, Gutmann L, Harley J B 1973 Subacute focal adenovirus encephalitis. Journal of Neuropathology and Experimental Neurology 32: 34–50

208. Coleman D V, Russell W J I, Hodgson J, Pe T, Mowbray J F 1977 Human papovavirus in Papanicolaou smears of urinary sediment detected by transmission microscopy. Journal of Clinical Pathology 30: 1015–1020

209. Crawford D H, Achong B G, Teich N M, Finerty S, Thompson J L, Epstein M A, Giovanella B C 1979 Identification of murine endogenous xenotropic retrovirus in cultured multicellular tumour spheroids from nude mouse-passaged nasopharyngeal carcinoma. International Journal of Cancer 23: 1–7

210. Dalton A J 1972 Further analysis of the detailed structure of Type B and C particles. Journal of the National Cancer Institute 48: 1095–1099

211. De Vos R, Ray M B, Desmet V J 1979 Electron microscopy of hepatitis B virus components in chronic active liver disease. Journal of Clinical Pathology 32: 590–600

212. Diebold J, Marche C, Audoin J, Aubert J P, Le Tourneau A, Bouton C, Reynes M, Wizniak J, Capron F, Tricottet V 1985 Lymph node modification in patients with the acquired immunodeficiency syndrome (AIDS) or with AIDS related complex (ARC). A histological, immuno-histopathological and ultrastructural study of 45 cases. Pathology Research and Practice 180: 590–611

213. Donnellan W L, Chantra-Umporn S, Kidd J M 1966 The cytomegalic inclusion cell. An electron microscopic study. Archives of Pathology 82: 336–348

214. Dunn A E G, Ogilvie M M 1968 Intranuclear virus particles in human genital wart tissue: observations on the ultrastructure of the epidermal layer. Journal of Ultrastructure Research 22: 282–295

215. Epstein W L, Fukuyama K 1973 Maturation of molluscum contagiosum virus (MCV) in vivo: quantitative electron microscopic autoradiography. Journal of Investigative Dermatology 60: 73–79

216. Epstein W L, Fukuyama K 1975 Human wart virus proliferation and its influence on keratinization in epidermal cells. In: Prunieras M (ed) Biomedical aspects of human wart virus infection. Fondation Mérieux, Lyon, pp 7–30

217. Esiri M M, Tomlinson A H 1972 Herpes zoster. Demonstration of virus in trigeminal nerve and ganglion by immunofluorescence and electron microscopy. Journal of the Neurological Sciences 15: 35–48

218. Ferenczy A, Braun L, Shah K V 1981 Human papillomavirus (HPV) in condylomatous lesions of cervix. A comparative ultrastructural and immunohistochemical study. American Journal of Surgical Pathology 5: 661–670

219. Fine D, Schochetman G 1978 Type D primate retroviruses: a review. Cancer Research 38: 3123–3139

220. Font R L, Jenis E H, Tuck K D 1973 Measles maculopathy associated with subacute sclerosing panencephalitis. Immunofluorescent and immuno-ultrastructural studies. Archives of Pathology 96: 168–174

221. Foucar E, Mukai K, Foucar K, Sutherland D E R, Van Buren C T 1981 Colon ulceration in lethal cytomegalovirus infection. American Journal of Clinical Pathology 76: 788–801

222. Gardner S D, Field A M, Coleman D V, Hulme B 1971 New human papovavirus (BK) isolated from urine after renal transplantation. Lancet i: 1253–1257

223. Gerber M A, Thung S N 1979 The localization of hepatitis viruses in tissues. International Review of Experimental Pathology 20: 49–76

224. Godman G C 1973 Picornaviruses. In: Dalton A J, Haguenau F (eds) Ultrastructure of animal viruses and bacteriophages: an atlas. Academic Press, New York, pp 133–153

225. Gonda M A, Wong-Staal F, Gallo R C, Clements J E, Narayan O, Gilden R V 1985 Sequence homology and morphologic similarity of HTLV-III and visna virus, a pathogenic lentivirus. Science 227: 173–177

226. Gray F, Gherardi R, Baudrimont M, Gaulard P, Meyrignac C, Vedrenne C, Poirier J 1987 Leucoencephalopathy with multinucleated giant cells containing human immune deficiency virus-like particles in one patient with AIDS. Acta Neuropathologica 73: 99–104

227. Gudat F, Bianchi L, Sonnabend W, Thiel G, Aenishaenslin W, Stalder G A 1975 Pattern of core and surface expression in liver tissue reflects state of specific immune response in hepatitis B. Laboratory Investigation 32: 1–9

228. Gyorkey F, Cabral G A, Gyorkey P K, Uribe-Botero G, Dreesman G R, Melnick J L 1978 Coxsackievirus aggregates in muscle cells of a polymyositis patient. Intervirology 10: 69–77

229. Gyorkey F, Melnick J L, Sinkovics J G, Gyorkey P 1985 Retrovirus resembling HTLV in macrophages of patients with AIDS. Lancet i: 106

230. Haas J E, Yunis E J 1970 Viral crystalline arrays in human coxsackie myocarditis. Laboratory Investigation 23: 442–446

231. Hasegawa T 1971 Further electron microscopic observations of herpes zoster virus. Archives of Dermatology 103: 45–49

232. Hashida Y, Yunis E J 1970 Re-examination of encephalitic brains known to contain intranuclear inclusion bodies: electron-microscopic observations following prolonged fixation in formalin. American Journal of Clinical Pathology 53: 537–543

233. Huang S-N 1971 Hepatitis-associated antigen hepatitis. An electron microscopic study of virus-like particles in liver cells. American Journal of Pathology 64: 483–500

234. Huang S-N, Groh V, Beaudoin J G, Dauphinee W D, Guttmann R D, Morehouse D D, Aronoff A, Gault H 1974 A study of the relationship of virus-like particles and Australia antigen in liver. Human Pathology 5: 209–222

235. Iwasaki Y, Koprowski H 1974 Cell to cell transmission of virus in the central nervous system. I. Subacute sclerosing panencephalitis. Laboratory Investigation 31: 187–196

236. Kasnic G, Sayeed A, Azar H A 1982 Nuclear and cytoplasmic inclusions in disseminated human cytomegalovirus infection. Ultrastructural Pathology 3: 229–235

237. Kimura A, Tosaka K, Nakao T 1972 An electron microscopic study of varicella skin lesions. Archiv für die gesamte Virusforschung 36: 1–12

238. Kovi J, Tillman L, Lee S M 1974 Malignant transformation of condyloma acuminatum. A light microscopic and ultrastructural study. American Journal of Clinical Pathology 61: 702–710

239. Lapis K 1979 Chronic hepatitis. In: Johannessen J V (ed) Electron microscopy in human medicine, vol 8, The liver, gallbladder and biliary ducts. McGraw-Hill, New York, pp 137–157

240. Laurent R, Agache P, Coume-Marquet J 1975 Ultrastructure of clear cells in human viral warts. Journal of Cutaneous Pathology 2: 140–148

241. Laverty C R, Russell P, Hills E, Booth N 1978 The significance of non condylomatous wart virus infection of the cervical transformation zone. A review with discussion of two illustrative

cases. Acta Cytologica 22: 195–201

242. Le Tourneau A, Audoin J, Diebold J, Marche C, Tricottet V, Reynes M 1986 LAV-like viral particles in lymph node germinal centers in patients with persistent lymphadenopathy syndrome and the acquired immunodeficiency syndrome-related complex: an ultrastructural study of 30 cases. Human Pathology 17: 1047–1053

243. Lutzner M A 1962 Fine structure of the zoster virus in human skin. Journal of Ultrastructure Research 7: 409–417

244. Martin A M, Kurtz S M 1966 Cytomegalic inclusion disease. An electron microscopic histochemical study of the virus at necropsy. Archives of Pathology 82: 27–34

245. Martinez-Palomo A, Le Buis J, Bernhard W 1967 Electron microscopy of adenovirus 12 replication. 1. Fine structural changes in the nucleus of infected KB cells. Journal of Virology 1: 817–829

246. Munn R J, Marx P A, Yamamoto J K, Gardner M B 1985 Ultrastructural comparison of the retroviruses associated with human and simian acquired immunodeficiency syndromes. Laboratory Investigation 53: 194–199

247. Muñoz D G, Perl D P, Pendlebury W W 1987 Comparison of cytomegalovirus infection of brain and lung in a patient with subacute encephalopathy of acquired immunodeficiency syndrome. Archives of Pathology and Laboratory Medicine 111: 234–237

248. Nahmias A J, Griffith D, Snitzer J 1967 Fatal pneumonia associated with adenovirus type 7. American Journal of Diseases of Children 114: 36–41

249. Nowoslawski A, Brzosko W J, Madalinski K, Krawczynski K 1970 Cellular localisation of Australia antigen in the liver of patients with lymphoproliferative disorders. Lancet i: 494–498

250. O'Callaghan D J, Randall C C 1976 Molecular anatomy of herpesviruses: recent studies. Progress in Medical Virology 22: 152–210

251. Oriel J D, Almeida J D 1970 Demonstration of virus particles in human genital warts. British Journal of Venereal Diseases 46: 37–42

252. Oyanagi S, Rorke L B, Katz M, Koprowski H 1971 Histopathology and electron microscopy of three cases of subacute sclerosing panencephalitis (SSPE). Acta Neuropathologica 18: 58–73

253. Patrizi G, Middlecamp J N, Reed C A 1968 Fine structure of herpes simplex virus hepatoadrenal necrosis in the newborn. American Journal of Clinical Pathology 49: 325–341

254. Pilotti S, Rilke F, De Palo G, Della Torre G, Alasio L 1981 Condylomata of the uterine cervix and koilocytosis of cervical intraepithelial neoplasia. Journal of Clinical Pathology 34: 532–541

255. Pinkerton H, Carroll S 1971 Fatal adenovirus pneumonia in infants. Correlation of histologic and electron microscopic observations. American Journal of Pathology 65: 543–548

256. Press M F, Riddell R H, Ringus J 1980 Cytomegalovirus inclusion disease. Its occurrence in the myenteric plexus of a renal transplant patient. Archives of Pathology and Laboratory Medicine 104: 580–583

257. Price P J, Arnstein P, Suk W A, Vernon M L, Huebner R J 1975 Type-C RNA viruses of the NIH nude mouse. Journal of the National Cancer Institute 55: 1231–1232

258. Prunieras M 1975 Ultrastructure of the epidermis in epidermodysplasia verruciformis. In: Prunieras M (ed) Biomedical aspects of human wart virus infection. Fondation Mérieux, Lyon, pp 165–170

259. Roizman B, Spear P G 1973 Herpesviruses. In: Dalton A J, Haguenau F (eds) Ultrastructure of animal viruses and bacteriophages: an atlas. Academic Press, New York, pp 83–107

260. Rosen S, Harmon W, Krensky A M, Edelson P J, Padgett B L, Grinnell B W, Rubino M J, Walker D L 1983 Tubulo-interstitial nephritis associated with polyomavirus (BK type) infection. New England Journal of Medicine 308: 1192–1196

261. Sakamoto Y, Yamada G, Mizuno M, Nishihara T, Kinoyama S, Kobayashi T, Takahashi T, Nagashima H 1983 Full and empty particles of hepatitis B virus in hepatocytes from patients with HBsAg-positive chronic active hepatitis. Laboratory Investigation 48: 678–682

262. Schweitzer I L, Dunn A E G, Peters R L, Spears R L 1973 Viral hepatitis B in neonates and infants. American Journal of Medicine 55: 762–771

263. Scotto J, Stralin H, Caroli J 1970 Amas de particules viriformes dans les noyaux d'hépatocytes chez un sujet atteint d'hépatite virale

mortelle et porteur de l'antigène Australia dans le sérum. Comptes Rendus de l'Académie des Sciences, Paris 271 (series D): 1603–1604

264. Sharer L R, Epstein L G, Cho E-S, Joshi V V, Meyenhofer M F, Rankin L F, Petito C K 1986 Pathologic features of AIDS encephalopathy in children: evidence for LAV/HTLV–III infection of brain. Human Pathology 17: 271–284

265. Sobonya R E, Hiller F C, Pingleton W, Watanabe I 1978 Fatal measles (rubeola) pneumonia in adults. Archives of Pathology and Laboratory Medicine 102: 366–371

266. Stanbridge C M, Mather J, Curry A, Butler E B 1981 Demonstration of papilloma virus particles in cervical and vaginal scrape material: a report of 10 cases. Journal of Clinical Pathology 34: 524–531

267. Stein O, Fainaru M, Stein Y 1972 Visualization of virus-like particles in endoplasmic reticulum of hepatocytes of Australia antigen carriers. Laboratory Investigation 26: 262–269

268. Sun S-C, Anderson K E, Hsu C-P, Kau S-L 1974 Hepatocellular ultrastructure in asymptomatic hepatitis B antigenemia. Archives of Pathology 97: 373–379

269. Suringa D W R, Bank L J, Ackerman A B 1970 Role of measles virus in skin lesions and Koplik's spots. New England Journal of Medicine 283: 1139–1142

270. Sutton J S, Burnett J W 1969 Ultrastructural changes in dermal and epidermal cells of skin infected with molluscum contagiosum virus. Journal of Ultrastructure Research 26: 177–196

271. Swanson J L, Craighead J E, Reynolds E S 1966 Electron microscopic observations on *Herpesvirus hominis* (herpes simplex virus) encephalitis in man. Laboratory Investigation 15: 1966–1981

272. Tang T T, Sedmak G V, Siegesmund K A, McCreadie S R 1975 Chronic myopathy associated with coxsackievirus type A9. A combined electron microscopical and viral isolation study. New England Journal of Medicine 292: 608–611

273. Teich N 1982 Taxonomy of retroviruses. In: Weiss R, Teich N, Varmus H, Coffin J (eds) RNA tumor viruses. Molecular biology of tumor viruses, 2nd edn 1/text. Cold Spring Harbor Laboratory, pp 25–207

274. Tenner-Racz K, Racz P, Dietrich M, Kern P 1985 Altered follicular dendritic cells and virus-like particles in AIDS and AIDS-related lymphadenopathy. Lancet i: 105–106

275. Tralka T S, Yee C L, Rabson A B, Wivel N A, Stromberg K J, Rabson A S, Costa J C 1983 Murine type C retroviruses and intracisternal A-particles in human tumors serially passaged in nude mice. Journal of the National Cancer Institute 71: 591–599

276. Watanabe I, Preskorn S H 1976 Virus-cell interaction in oligodendroglia, astroglia and phagocyte in progressive multifocal leukoencephalopathy. An electron microscopic study. Acta Neuropathologica 36: 101–115

277. Weiss R 1982 The search for human RNA tumor viruses. In: Weiss R, Teich N, Varmus H, Coffin J (eds) RNA tumor viruses. Molecular biology of tumor viruses, 2nd edn 1/text. Cold Spring Harbor Laboratory, pp 1205–1281

278. Weiss R 1985 Human T-cell retroviruses. In: Weiss R, Teich N, Varmus H, Coffin J (eds) RNA tumor viruses, 2nd edn 2/ supplements and appendices. Cold Spring Harbor Laboratory, pp 405–485

279. Whitelaw A, Davies H, Parry J 1977 Electron microscopy of fatal adenovirus gastroenteritis. Lancet i: 361

280. Williams M G, Howatson A F, Almeida J D 1961 Morphological characterization of the virus of the human common wart (verruca vulgaris). Nature 189: 895–897

281. Yabe Y, Sadakane H 1975 The virus of epidermodysplasia verruciformis: electron microscopic and fluorescent antibody studies. Journal of Investigative Dermatology 65: 324–330

282. Yamada G, Nakane P K 1977 Hepatitis B core and surface antigens in liver tissue. Light and electron microscopic localization by the peroxidase-labeled antibody method. Laboratory Investigation 36: 649–659

283. Yamada G, Sakamoto Y, Mizuno M, Nishihara T, Kobayashi T, Takahashi T, Nagashima H 1982 Electron and immunoelectron microscopic study of Dane particle formation in chronic hepatitis B virus infection. Gastroenterology 83: 348–356

284. Yeh H-P, Soltani K 1974 Ultrastructural studies in human orf. Archives of Dermatology 109: 390–392
285. Yunis E J, Atchison R W, Michaels R H, De Cicco F A 1975 Adenovirus and ileocecal intussusception. Laboratory Investigation 33: 347–351
286. Zu Rhein G M 1969 Association of papova-virions with a human demyelinating disease (progressive multifocal leukoencephalopathy). Progress in Medical Virology, 11: 185–247

'Virus-like' and 'Virus-associated' structures

287. Afzelius B A 1984 Glycocalyx and glycocalyceal bodies in the respiratory epithelium of nose and bronchi. Ultrastructural Pathology 7: 1–8
288. Anderson M G, Key P, Tovey G, Murray-Lyon I M, Lawrence A, Byrom N, Dixey J, Ellis D S, McCaul T F, Gazzard B, Evans B, Zuckerman A J 1984 Persistent lymphadenopathy in homosexual men: a clinical and ultrastructural study. Lancet i: 880–882
289. Bariéty J, Callard P 1972 Round 'virus-like' extracellular particles in glomerular tufts. An electron microscopic study of 190 human renal biopsies. Virchows Archiv A, Pathology Pathologische Anatomie 357: 125–135
290. Bariéty J, Richer D, Appoy M D, Grossetete J, Callard P 1973 Frequency of intraendothelial 'virus-like' particles: an electron microscopic study of 376 human renal biopsies. Journal of Clinical Pathology 26: 21–24
291. Basset F, Escaig J, Le Crom M 1972 A cytoplasmic membranous complex in histiocytosis X. Cancer 29: 1380–1386
292. Chandra S 1968 Undulating tubules associated with endoplasmic reticulum in pathologic tissues. Laboratory Investigation 18: 422–428
293. Collins D N, Gilbert E F 1977 Glycogen complexes in muscle in Reye's syndrome simulating virus-like particles. Laboratory Investigation 36: 91–99
294. Dalton A J 1975 Microvesicles and vesicles of multivesicular bodies versus 'virus-like' bodies. Journal of the National Cancer Institute 54: 1137–1148
295. De Vos R, Vanstapel M J, Desmyter J, De Wolf-Peeters C, De Groote G, Colaert J, Mortelmans J, De Groote J, Fevery J, Desmet V 1983 Are nuclear particles specific for non-A, non-B hepatitis? Hepatology 3: 532–544
296. Ericsson J L E, Biberfeld P 1967 Studies on aldehyde fixation. Fixation rates and their relation to fine structure and some histochemical reactions in liver. Laboratory Investigation 17: 281–298
297. Ewing E P, Spira T J, Chandler F W, Callaway C S, Brynes R K, Chan W C 1983 Unusual cytoplasmic body in lymphoid cells of homosexual men with unexplained lymphadenopathy. A preliminary report. New England Journal of Medicine 308: 819–822
298. Fawcett D W 1966 An atlas of fine structure. The cell. Its organelles and inclusions. Saunders, Philadelphia
299. Ferrans V J, Thiedemann K-U, Maron B J, Jones M, Roberts W C 1976 Spherical microparticles in human myocardium. An ultrastructural study. Laboratory Investigation 35: 349–368
300. Gardiner T, Kirk J, Dermott E 1983 'Virus-like particles' in lymphocytes in AIDS are normal organelles, not viruses. Lancet ii: 963–964
301. Ghadially F N 1982 Ultrastructural pathology of the cell and matrix, 2nd edn. Butterworths, London
302. Grimley P M, Davis G L, Kang Y-H, Dooley J S, Strohmaier J, Hoofnagle J H 1985 Tubuloreticular inclusions in peripheral blood mononuclear cells related to systemic therapy with α-interferon. Laboratory Investigation 52: 638–649
303. Gyorkey F, Gyorkey P, Sinkovics J G 1980 Origin and significance of intranuclear tubular inclusions in type II pulmonary alveolar epithelial cells of patients with bleomycin and busulfan toxicity. Ultrastructural Pathology 1: 211–221
304. Haguenau F 1973 'Virus like' particles as observed with the electron microscope. In: Dalton A J, Haguenau F (eds) Ultrastructure of animal viruses and bacteriophages: an atlas. Academic Press, New York, pp 391–397
305. Hammar S P, Bockus D, Remington F, Friedman S 1984 More on ultrastructure of AIDS lymph nodes. New England Journal of Medicine 310: 924
306. Henderson D W, Papadimitriou J M, Coleman M 1986 Ultrastructural appearances of tumours. Diagnosis and classification of human neoplasia by electron microscopy, 2nd edn. Churchill Livingstone, Edinburgh
307. Katsuragi S, Miyayama H, Takeuchi T 1981 Picornavirus-like inclusions in polymyositis — aggregation of glycogen particles of the same size. Neurology 31: 1476–1480
308. Kessel R G 1983 The structure and function of annulate lamellae: porous cytoplasmic and intranuclear membranes. International Review of Cytology 82: 180–303
309. Kostianovsky M, Orenstein J M, Schaff Z, Grimley P M 1987 Cytomembranous inclusions observed in acquired immunodeficiency syndrome. Clinical and experimental review. Archives of Pathology and Laboratory Medicine 111: 218–223
310. Kuhn C 1972 Fine structure of bronchiolo-alveolar cell carcinoma. Cancer 30: 1107–1118
311. Lampert F, Lampert P 1975 Multiple sclerosis. Morphologic evidence of intranuclear paramyxovirus or altered chromatin fibers? Archives of Neurology 32: 425–427
312. Marcus P B 1981 Glycocalyceal bodies and their role in tumor typing. Journal of Submicroscopic Cytology 13: 483–500
313. Marquart K-H 1984 An unusual form of endoplasmic reticulum in mononuclear cells of a giant cell tumor of bone. Ultrastructural Pathology 7: 161–165
314. Murray A B, Becke H, Marquart K-H 1984 Vermicellar bodies in osteosarcoma cell nuclei. Ultrastructural Pathology 6: 363
315. Onerheim R M, Wang N-S, Gilmore N, Jothy S 1984 Ultrastructural markers of lymph nodes in patients with acquired immune deficiency syndrome and in homosexual males with unexplained persistent lymphadenopathy. A quantitative study. American Journal of Clinical Pathology 82: 280–288
316. Orenstein J M, Simon G L, Kessler C M, Schulof R S 1985 Ultrastructural markers in circulating lymphocytes of subjects at risk for AIDS. American Journal of Clinical Pathology 84: 603–609
317. Rich S A 1981 Human lupus inclusions and interferon. Science 213: 772–775
318. Schaff Z, Heine U, Dalton A J 1972 Ultramorphological and ultracytochemical studies on tubuloreticular structures in lymphoid cells. Cancer Research 32: 2696–2706
319. Shaw C-M, Sumi S M 1975 Non viral intranuclear filamentous inclusions. Archives of Neurology 32: 428–432
320. Sidhu G S, Stahl R E, El-Sadr W, Cassai N D, Forrester E M, Zolla-Pazner S 1985 The acquired immunodeficiency syndrome. An ultrastructural study. Human Pathology 16: 377–386
321. Singh G, Katyal S L, Torikata C 1981 Carcinoma of type II pneumocytes. Immunodiagnosis of a subtype of 'bronchioloalveolar carcinomas'. American Journal of Pathology 102: 195–208
322. Tralka T S, Yee C, Triche T J, Costa J 1982 Unusual intranuclear inclusions in malignant fibrous histiocytoma: presence in primary tumor, metastases and xenografts. Ultrastructural Pathology 3: 161–167
323. Uzman B G, Saito H, Kasac M 1971 Tubular arrays in the endoplasmic reticulum in human tumor cells. Laboratory Investigation 24: 492–498
324. Yunis E J, Agostini R M, Devine W A 1984 Studies on the nature of fibrillar nuclei. Distinction from viral nucleocapsid. American Journal of Pathology 115: 84–91
325. Zucker-Franklin D 1983 'Looking' for the cause of AIDS. (Editorial) New England Journal of Medicine 308: 837–838

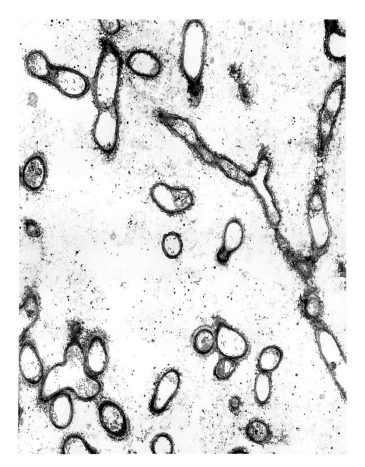

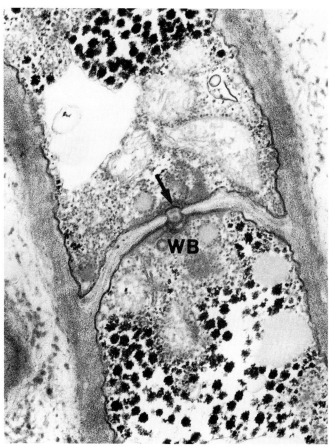

Fig. 9.1 *Aspergillus fumigatus* in lung I: fungal hyphae. Post-mortem specimen. Septate hyphae with dichotomous branching at 45 degrees can be recognized but, as is common in specimens from the contents of lung cavities, many are swollen and ghost-like. Fungal elements in the cavity wall are usually better preserved. (× 22 000)

Fig. 9.2 *Aspergillus fumigatus* in lung II: hypha and hyphal septum. The cell wall invaginates to form the septal plate whose centre is occupied by the pore apparatus (arrow). The wavy plasma membrane is applied to the cell wall and the cytoplasm contains glycogen, mitochondria, ribosomes, lipid droplets and lucent vacuoles. Adjacent to the septal pore are Woronin bodies (WB), whose apparent function is to plug the pore of damaged or degenerating hyphae. (× 37 000)

The specimen was from a fungus ball (aspergilloma) within an old lung cavity in a patient who had a long history of chronic obstructive airway disease. Aspergillus does not usually spread from these lesions or the bronchial plugs of allergic aspergillosis. Invasive aspergillosis can develop as an opportunistic infection in immunosuppressed patients by hyphal outgrowth from lung cavities or other sites, to produce acute necrotizing or suppurative lesions. Vascular involvement may be followed by thrombosis and local infarction or distant dissemination. Conidiophores bearing fruiting bodies, though uncommon in clinical specimens, allow the fungus to be positively identified as *Aspergillus* sp. References: 1, 4 and 73.

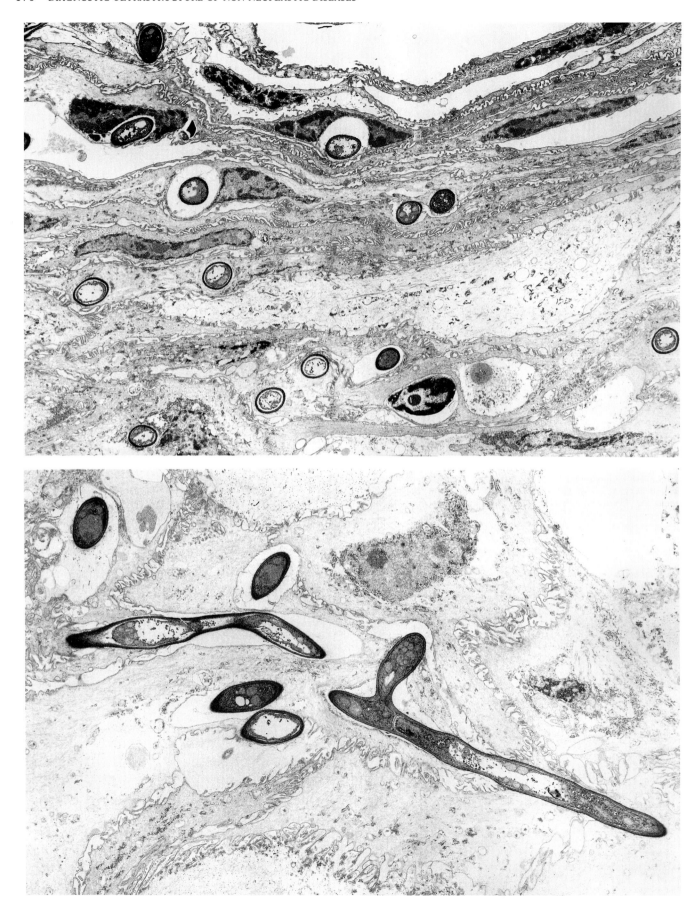

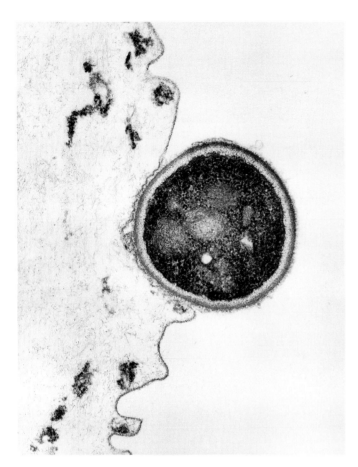

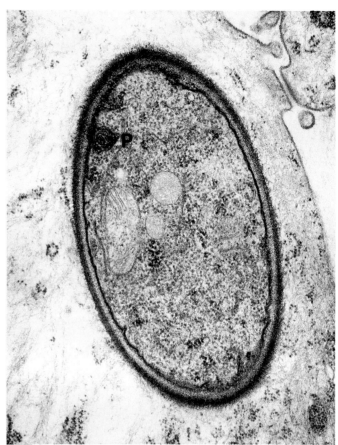

Fig. 9.5 Oesophageal candidosis III: attachment of *Candida* to surface squame. Selective adherence to epithelial cells is a property of pathogenic *Candida* species and is probably a prerequisite for invasion. Loose adherence by an additional surface layer of the fungal cell wall (stainable with ruthenium red) is apparent here; tight adherence also occurs. The nature and function of cell surface receptors in fungal infections is poorly understood. (× 34 000)

Fig. 9.3 (Facing page, top)   Candidal ulceration of the oesophagus I: extra and intracellular blastospores. Post-mortem specimen. Multiple yeast forms (blastospores) lie between and within superficial squamous epithelial cells at the edge of an oesophageal ulcer. Cytoplasmic vacuolation, probably related to ageing, is apparent in some organisms. (× 4000)

Fig. 9.4 (Facing page, bottom)   Oesophageal candidosis II: blastospores, pseudohypha and true hypha. The combination of blastospores, pseudohyphae and true hyphae identifies the organism as *Candida* sp. Despite minor cultural differences, the various species appear similar in vivo. The nucleus and nucleolus are prominent in the two blastospores towards the top left of the field. Below them lies a pseudohypha formed by yeasts that have failed to separate after budding. For comparison, the cells of the true branched hypha (bottom right) are separated by a septum. Both the pseudohypha and true hypha are invading epithelial cells. (× 5000)

Fig. 9.6 Oesophageal candidosis IV: intracellular *Candida*. Conventional aldehyde fixation demonstrates pale inner and layered dense outer zones of the blastospore cell wall; five layers are seen with acrolein/TAPO fixation whilst a further three may be revealed by the Thiéry polysaccharide stain. The plasma membrane shows occasional intracytoplasmic indentations and a mesosome-like plasmalemmasome (P) that is probably formed by fusion of cytoplasmic vesicles with the plasma membrane. Cytoplasmic organelles include ribosomes, endoplasmic reticulum, a mitochondrion with shelf-like cristae, glycogen and vacuoles. The nucleus has not been included in this section. Lomasomes may sometimes also be seen. (× 34 000)

Candida is a classic opportunistic pathogen responsible for infections with protean manifestations. In candidosis of the skin and mucous membranes the organism generally penetrates no deeper than the stratum corneum but oesophageal or bronchial ulceration may develop in terminal illnesses, as in the case illustrated. Systemic candidosis may produce multiple abscesses in sites such as the brain and kidney, along with endocarditis in which exuberant vegetations contain numerous fungal elements that may penetrate the underlying valve tissue. References: 1, 2, 73, 75, 76, 78, 82, 84, 92, 93 and 95–101.

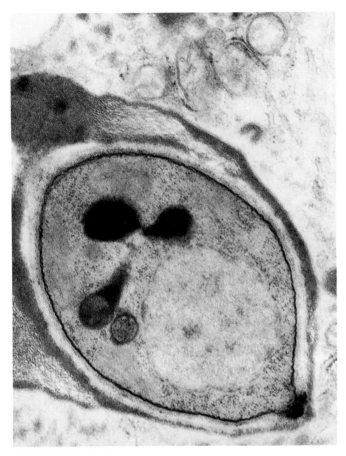

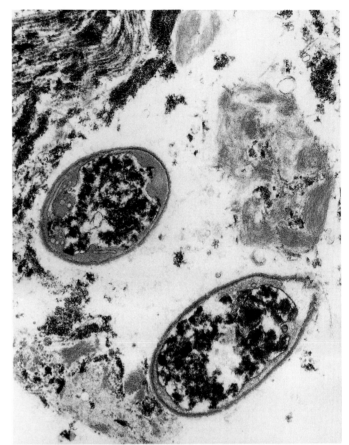

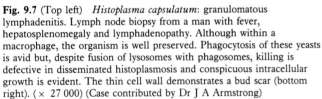

Fig. 9.7 (Top left)   *Histoplasma capsulatum*: granulomatous lymphadenitis. Lymph node biopsy from a man with fever, hepatosplenomegaly and lymphadenopathy. Although within a macrophage, the organism is well preserved. Phagocytosis of these yeasts is avid but, despite fusion of lysosomes with phagosomes, killing is defective in disseminated histoplasmosis and conspicuous intracellular growth is evident. The thin cell wall demonstrates a bud scar (bottom right). (× 27 000) (Case contributed by Dr J A Armstrong)

As the name *Histoplasma* implies, the organism is an intracellular parasite of the mononuclear phagocyte system; *capsulatum*, however, is a misnomer that reflects shrinkage artefact simulating a capsule in histological sections. *Histoplasma capsulatum* occurs as small (American form) and large (African form, var. *duboisii*) yeasts that are ultrastructurally similar, apart from their disparity in size. Mould forms are seen in culture only.

Fig. 9.8 (Top right)   *Histoplasma capulatum*: solitary pulmonary histoplasmoma. From a specimen excised after detection by routine chest X-ray in a woman previously resident in Central America. Two degenerate yeasts lie amongst cell debris and fibrin. (× 16 000)

Most primary histoplasma infections produce a pulmonary lesion resembling a tuberculous Ghon complex. Histoplasmomas develop after slow healing with excessive concentric fibrosis. Fungi in the central zone are typically extracellular and dead. References: 1, 73, 83 and 102.

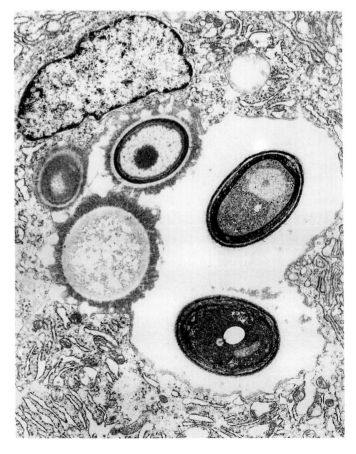

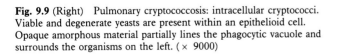

Fig. 9.9 (Right)   Pulmonary cryptococcosis: intracellular cryptococci. Viable and degenerate yeasts are present within an epithelioid cell. Opaque amorphous material partially lines the phagocytic vacuole and surrounds the organisms on the left. (× 9000)

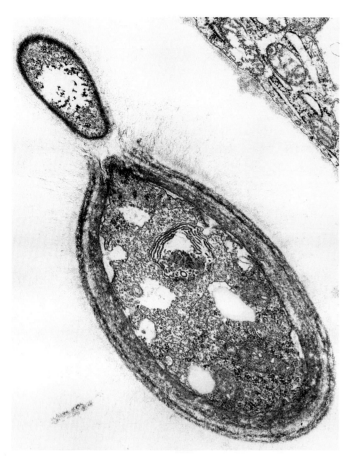

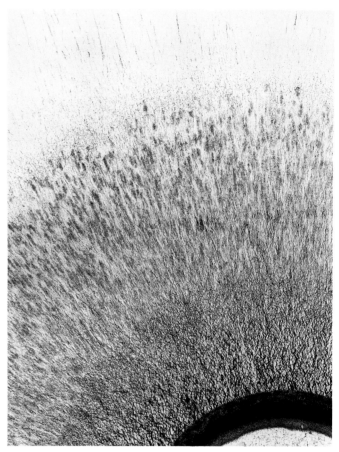

Fig. 9.10 (Top left) *Cryptococcus neoformans*: bud formation. This and the preceding figure come from a lung biopsy specimen of a diabetic cane farmer whose clinical state suggested allergic hypersensitivity pneumonitis. Budding yeasts, found in active lesions, develop from a capsule-covered outgrowth of cytoplasm, plasma membrane and inner cell wall layer through a defect in the outer cell wall. Separation of the daughter cell after the transfer of nuclear and cytoplasmic components leaves a bud scar on the mother cell. The young daughter cell wall is thinner than that of the parent. (× 22 000)

Fig. 9.11 (Top right) *Cryptococcus neoformans*: envelope. At bottom right, the plasma membrane is applied to the inner layer of the lamellated cell wall. The radial coiled and intertwining fibrils of the capsule are enhanced by printing at increased density. The clumping and shedding of the outer capsule are probably age-related degenerative changes. (× 12 000)

The distinctive capsule is usually more abundant in tissues than in culture and is responsible for the gelatinous appearance of cryptococcal lesions. Variations in capsule thickness may produce giant cryptococci up to 40 μm in diameter (normal range 2–8 μm) or small forms histologically resembling histoplasma, with a capsule that is thin or absent.

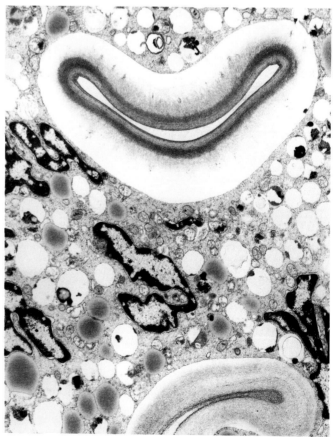

Fig. 9.12 (Right) Pulmonary cryptococcosis: residual cryptococci in a muitinucleated giant cell. From an asymptomatic lung nodule. Disintegration of nuclei and cytoplasm has left only collapsed envelopes that are nevertheless still diagnostic. (× 7000) References: 1, 73, 80, 81, 85–87 and 94.

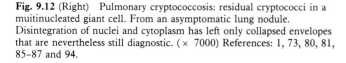

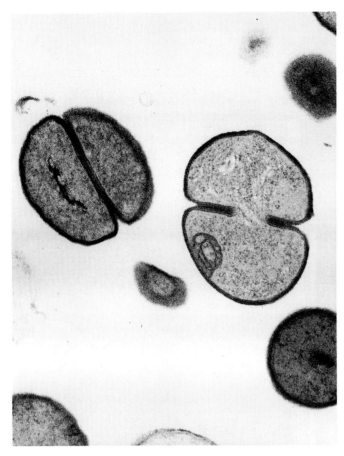

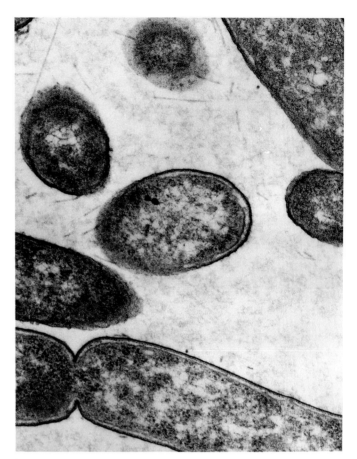

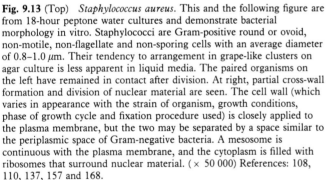

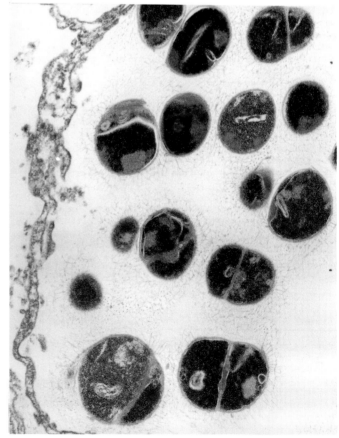

Fig. 9.13 (Top) *Staphylococcus aureus*. This and the following figure are from 18-hour peptone water cultures and demonstrate bacterial morphology in vitro. Staphylococci are Gram-positive round or ovoid, non-motile, non-flagellate and non-sporing cells with an average diameter of 0.8–1.0 μm. Their tendency to arrangement in grape-like clusters on agar culture is less apparent in liquid media. The paired organisms on the left have remained in contact after division. At right, partial cross-wall formation and division of nuclear material are seen. The cell wall (which varies in appearance with the strain of organism, growth conditions, phase of growth cycle and fixation procedure used) is closely applied to the plasma membrane, but the two may be separated by a space similar to the periplasmic space of Gram-negative bacteria. A mesosome is continuous with the plasma membrane, and the cytoplasm is filled with ribosomes that surround nuclear material. ($\times$ 50 000) References: 108, 110, 137, 157 and 168.

Fig. 9.14 (Top right) *Salmonella typhimurium*. Enterobacteria do not differ materially from one another in shape, size and structure. The complex cell wall is typical of Gram-negative bacteria. A very thin peptidoglycan layer is enclosed by a dense outer membrane and separated from the plasma membrane by a periplasmic space. The occasional globular extrusions of the cell wall are common in glutaraldehyde–osmium-fixed Gram-negative bacteria. Flagella (top left) arise from the entire cell surface (peritrichous arrangement). Early division septum formation is apparent at bottom left. ($\times$ 50 000) References: 106, 108 and 110.

Fig. 9.15 (Right) Bacterial glycocalyx. This group of unidentified cocci lies at the edge of an oesophageal ulcer. Each organism is surrounded by a filamentous glycocalyx or slime layer that serves as a means of attachment to the surface squame on the left, provides a fabric for microcolonial growth, and offers protection against antibacterial agents. ($\times$ 18 000) Reference: 104.

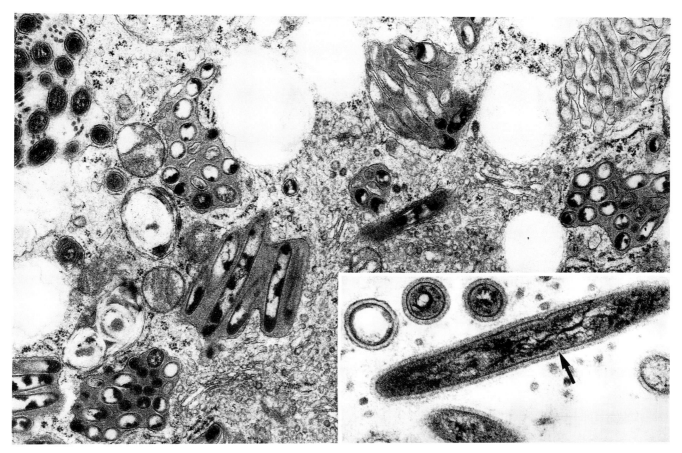

Fig. 9.16 Whipple's disease: intracellular bacteria. A macrophage in the intestinal lamina propria contains membrane-bound clusters of bacilli separated by amorphous material. Compared with the intact extracellular organisms at top left, most of those within the cell are degenerate, with little other than bacterial cell walls remaining at top right. (× 25 000) *Inset* Extracellular bacilli, one of which has commenced division (arrow). (× 61 000) (See also Figs 14.6–14.12)

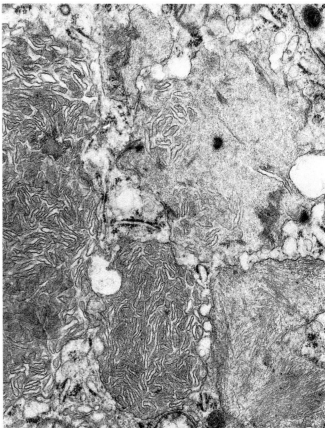

Fig. 9.17 Whipple's disease: late inclusions in Whipple cell. In this macrophage from the deep lamina propria the bacteria have been reduced to membranous and granulofibrillary remnants within phagolysosomes. These forms predominate in specimens obtained during remission. (× 25 000)

Although Whipple conjectured at the significance of the bacilli he observed in intestinal lipodystrophy in 1907, the disorder was generally regarded as some form of storage disease until its aetiology and pathogenesis were demonstrated by electron microscopy over half a century later. To date, the agent has defied attempts at isolation or identification, so that ultrastructural examination has a role both in diagnosis and monitoring of the disease; antibiotic therapy is associated with loss of the organisms within days and their reappearance heralds relapse. The cell wall residues, rendered indigestible by some intrinsic property or host enzyme defect, produce the characteristic PAS-positive cells; however, such PAS-positive macrophages can no longer be considered pathognomonic, even in the small intestine (see caption to Fig. 9.20). The organisms are also found within neutrophils and epithelial cells infected from the lamina propria rather than via the lumen. Absorptive cell injury, reversible by therapy, includes shortened irregularly distributed microvilli, increased numbers of lysosomes, dilated endoplasmic reticulum and prominent lipid. References: 113, 121, 126, 129, 155, 163, 175 and 180.

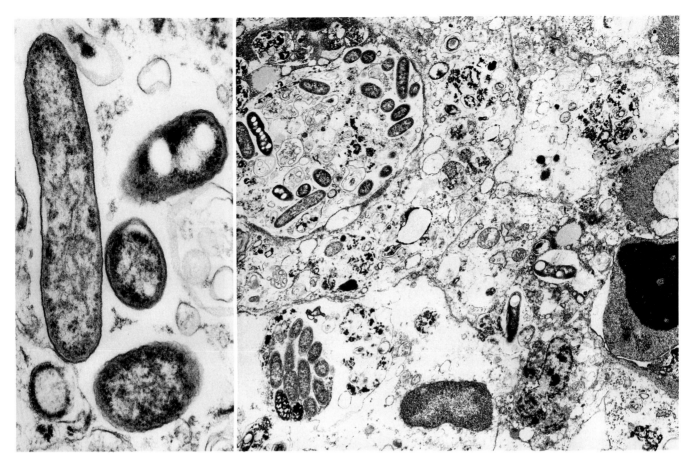

Fig. 9.18 Legionnaires' disease: *Legionella pneumophila*. Well preserved organisms may be hard to find in tissue sections and often lie amongst extracellular debris and fibrin. When present within cells (left) they are typically clustered in phagocytic vacuoles of macrophages and neutrophils, which are often themselves degenerate (× 8000) *Inset Legionella pneumoophila* has the appearance of a Gram-negative bacillus measuring 0.5 × 2.0 μm (up to 5.00 in culture). The wrinkling of the outer membrane and cytoplasmic vacuolation may be artefacts of glutaraldehyde fixation. There has been contention over the presence of a peptidoglycan layer in the periplasmic space; in the Pittsburgh pneumonia agent, *Legionella micdadei*, this layer is usually obvious in clinical tissue specimens but appears to vary with growth conditions in vitro. (× 46 000)

Legionnaires' disease is an acute fibrinopurulent pneumonia of small air spaces in which macrophages may be the predominant cells. When this apparently new disease appeared in 1976 the nature of the infective agent was difficult to determine. EM helped to demonstrate that the infection was indeed bacterial, and eventually the fastidious cultural requirements of this new family were defined. Legionellae in tissue sections are best detected by the Dieterle silver stain but interpretation is not always easy and EM has been suggested as an alternative. Direct immunofluorescent antibody staining is the only morphological method that is specific. References: 116, 120, 138, 141, 151, 160 and 164.

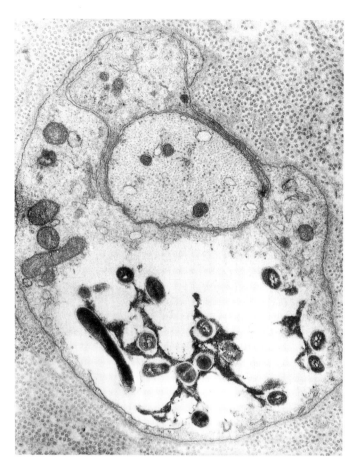

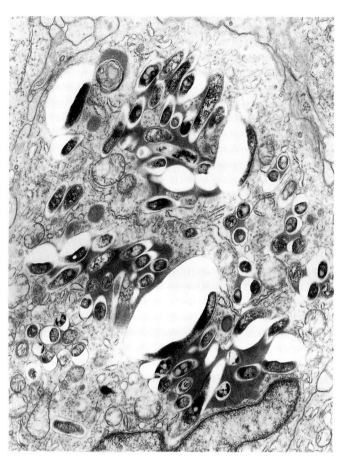

Fig. 9.19 Sural nerve biopsy: *Mycobacterium leprae*. Bacilli with their long axis parallel to the nerve fibre lie in a region of cytoplasmic clearing in a Schwann cell. The axon is undamaged. (× 19 000) (Case contributed by Professor J G McLeod.)

Although all mycobacteria appear similar in ultrathin sections, *M. leprae* is the only bacterium known to invade nerves. Schwann cells are the main target, the organisms multiplying within the cytoplasmic matrix and causing cell degeneration, consequent focal demyelination with axon loss, and dense replacement fibrosis that prevents nerve regeneration. The bacilli infect axons only rarely, but they may also be found in nerve macrophages, perineurial cells and endothelial cells of the vasa nervorum; angiopathy probably contributes to the fibrosis. Lepra cells contain multiple bacilli in cigar bundles (globi) or more random arrays within phagolysosomes and scattered in the cytoplasmic matrix. The accumulation of degenerate organisms, their electron-transparent substance, fat vacuoles and myelin figures produce the foamy macrophages visible in histological sections. Similar material is present in the foamy Schwann cells that sometimes develop in lepromatous leprosy. References: 108, 118, 119, 131, 134, 148–149, 150, 154, 158, 159 and 167.

Fig. 9.20 *Mycobacterium avium–intracellulare*: intracellular mycobacteria in macrophage. Cervical lymph node biopsy from an AIDS patient demonstrating multiple bacilli within phagolysosomes. The tearing of the section by the electron beam is due to uneven infiltration with epoxy resin [159] and is characteristic of intracellular mycobacteria. (× 9000) (Case contributed by Dr J A Armstrong)

The *Mycobacterium avium–intracellulare* complex includes the avian tubercle bacillus and closely related *M. intracellulare*. These ubiquitous atypical acid-fast bacilli are saprophytes that occasionally cause lymphadenitis or chronic lung disease resembling tuberculosis. AIDS patients may develop disseminated disease with Whipple's-like macrophages filled by bacteria in bone marrow, lymph nodes, intestine and liver. Apart from the ultrastructural differences, the distinction from Whipple's disease is facilitated by the clinico-pathological background and the demonstration of acid-fast bacilli by a Ziehl–Neelsen stain at the light microscopy level.

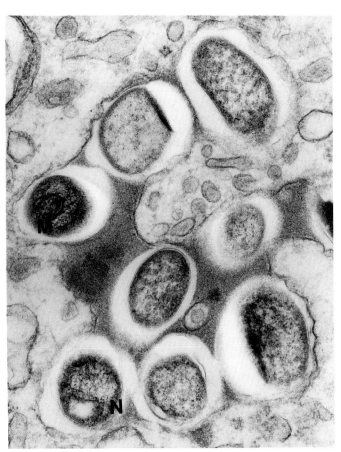

Fig. 9.21 (Left) *Mycobacterium avium-intracellulare*: details. The electron-lucent layer around each organism is characteristic of intracellular mycobacteria and is thought to ensure survival and growth. Mycobacterial nuclear material (N) is more organized than it is in other bacteria, and it is seen better in longitudinally sectioned organisms. An intracellular membrane system (M) is also visible. (× 46 000) (Case contributed by Dr J. A. Armstrong.)

The distinctive lipid-rich envelope of mycobacteria is immunogenic and responsible for resistance to the bacteriocidal action of many physical, chemical and cellular agents. A rigid inner peptidoglycan layer resembling that of other Gram-positive bacteria is linked to an intermediate layer of complex lipopolysaccharides that may appear rope-like when freeze–etched. In some species the outermost glycolipid and peptidoglycolipid (mycoside) layer, transparent in ultrathin sections, is revealed by freeze–etching or negative staining as ribbon-like fibrils wrapped around the organism. References: 108, 127, 131, 136, 154, 159 and 167.

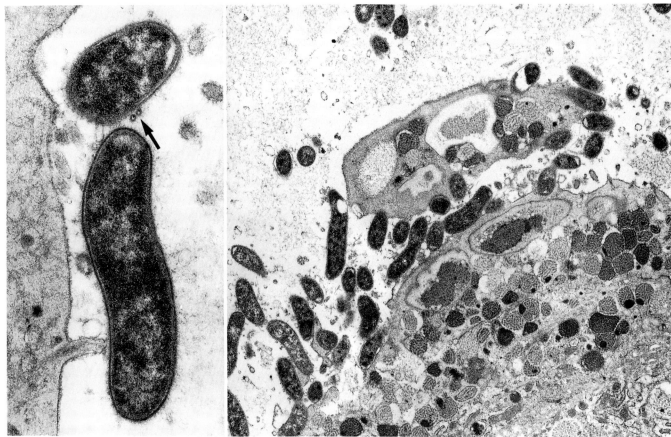

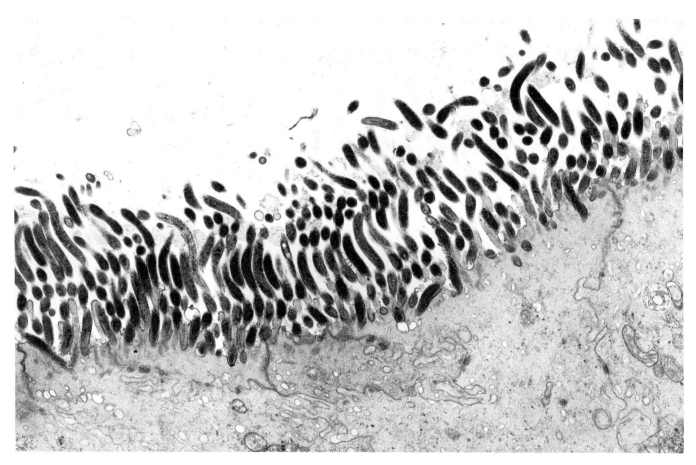

Fig. 9.23 Intestinal spirochaetosis: surface spirochaetes in rectal biopsy. There is a heavy infestation by spirochaetes aligned parallel to the long axis of surface epithelial cell microvilli and projecting into the lumen. The organisms are sigmoid with slightly tapering ends, and they measure 2–6 × 0.2 μm. (× 12 000) (See also Figs 14.13 and 14.14)

Fig 9.22 (Facing page) *Helicobacter pylori*: gastric antral colonization. Endoscopic biopsy from a patient with active chronic gastritis and duodenal ulceration. Multiple spiral bacteria make close contact with mucinous epithelial cell surface concavities (adherence pedestals). Microvilli have virtually disappeared, and in the subjacent cytoplasm, out of the illustrated field, mucin granules were considerably reduced. (× 8000) *Inset* Higher magnification demonstrates a smooth bacterial surface and the presence of sheathed flagella in transverse section (arrow). (× 30 000) (Case contributed by Dr J A Armstrong)

The close association between *Helicobacter pylori* (formerly *Campylobacter*) and active chronic gastritis has recently been established, but any causal role in peptic ulceration and non-ulcer dyspepsia remains controversial. The organism appears adapted to life on the surface of antral mucous cells, where it is protected by the overlying mucus, and is non-invasive. Its presence within canaliculi of resting-phase parietal cells has also been described. Appropriate therapy leads to reversal of the epithelial lesions and disappearance of the bacteria but recurrence is common. Its fatty acid composition and four to six sheathed flagella with terminal bulbs appear unique to *Helicobacter*. *Campylobacter fetus* subspp. *jejuni* and *intestinalis* (which can cause diarrhoea and rarely septicaemia), usually possess only a single terminal non-sheathed flagellum arising from a pit-like surface depression, have a rugose surface and are found within cells as well as being attached to surface glycocalyx.

Adherence pedestals also develop between enterocytes and enteropathogenic strains of *Escherichia coli*, which produce lesions similar to those produced by *H. pylori* without invasion. Connection by fimbriae, on the other hand, appears to be more important with enterotoxigenic *E. coli*. References: 122, 139, 140, 153, 161, 166, 174 and 177.

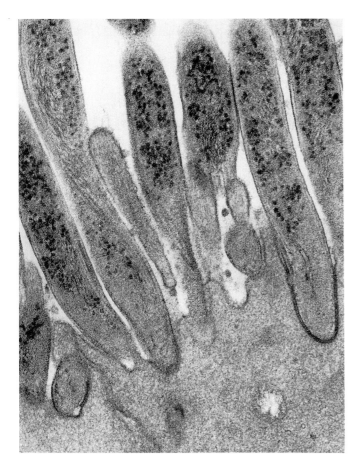

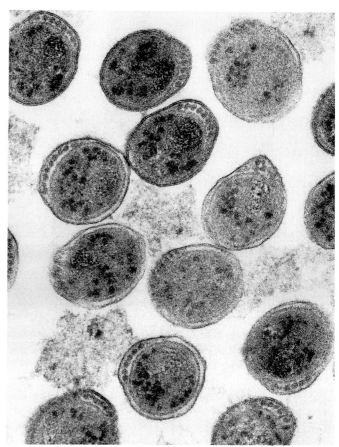

Fig. 9.24 Intestinal spirochaetes: epithelial attachment. Although epithelial penetration has been described, intestinal spirochaetes almost always remain extracellular with their tips lying within invaginations of the epithelial cells. A thin layer of electron-dense material may be identified beneath the epithelial plasma membrane at points of contact. The spiral course of the internal flagella is evident in some organisms. (× 62 000)

Fig. 9.25 Intestinal spirochaetes: transverse section. The characteristic internal sheathed flagella lying in the periplasmic space between the plasma membrane-cell wall complex and the asymmetric unit membrane of the outer sheath are evident. Four flagella originate from each pole of the cell and overlap at the centre. (× 93 000)

Spirochaetes, for which the name *Brachyspira aalborgi* has been proposed, have long been recognized as occasional inhabitants of the human intestinal tract but their clinical significance is unsettled and the involved epithelium rarely shows any ultrastructural abnormality. Although likewise generally extracellular, *Treponema pallidum* has been found within cells in penile and cervical chancres. Internal flagella (also termed periplasmic fibrils or axial filaments) are found only in members of the Order Spirochaetales. Spiral bacteria such as *Vibrio*, *Spirillum* and *Campylobacter*, which resemble spirochaetes at the light microscopic level, possess external flagella. References: 115, 132, 142–147, 170–171, 172 and 179.

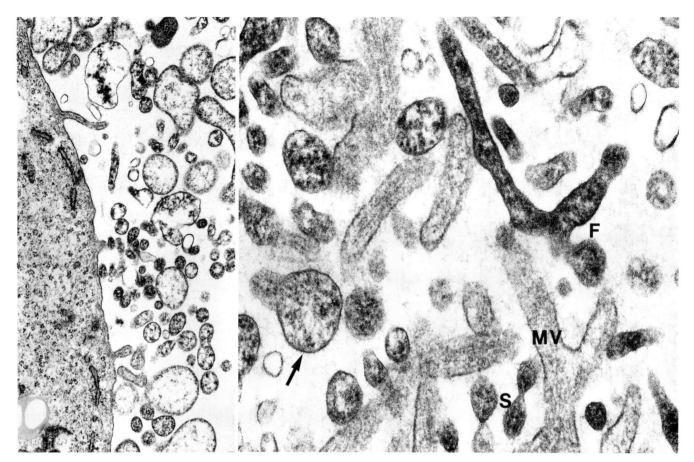

Fig. 9.26 Tissue culture cells from an undifferentiated carcinoma: *Mycoplasma* infection. Although cell-associated mycoplasmas tend to be less pleomorphic than those grown on artificial media, considerable morphologic variation is found nevertheless. Most are roughly spherical, up to 0.5 μm in diameter and bounded by a unit membrane with a coating of minute spikes (arrow). The cytoplasm contains numerous ribosomes, a fibrillar nuclear region and sometimes an occasional vacuole. Denser, smaller spherules (S), some of which appear to be dividing, and fibrillary forms (F) are also present. The latter differ from the culture cell microvilli (MV) in their greater density and ribosomal content, but it may be difficult to distinguish between larger mycoplasmas and shed fragments of degenerate cells. (× 56 000; Inset, × 20 000)

Mycoplasmas bind avidly to plasma membranes, and a specialized terminal organelle appears to be responsible for the attachment of *Mycoplasma pneumoniae* to ciliated epithelial cells of the human respiratory tract; however, it is questionable whether they can actually penetrate into cells. Contamination of cell cultures by mycoplasmas may affect experimental systems through interference with plasmalemmal or other biochemical activities, as well as by the presence of unwanted nucleic acids. No morphological alterations occur in the affected cells, so that EM has proved useful in detecting mycoplasmas; cultural identification is frequently unavailable in tissue culture laboratories, and is slow and sometimes difficult. However, immunodiagnostic methods are becoming more widely available. References: 108, 111, 112, 117, 123, 124, 128, 130, 135, 152, 162 and 165.

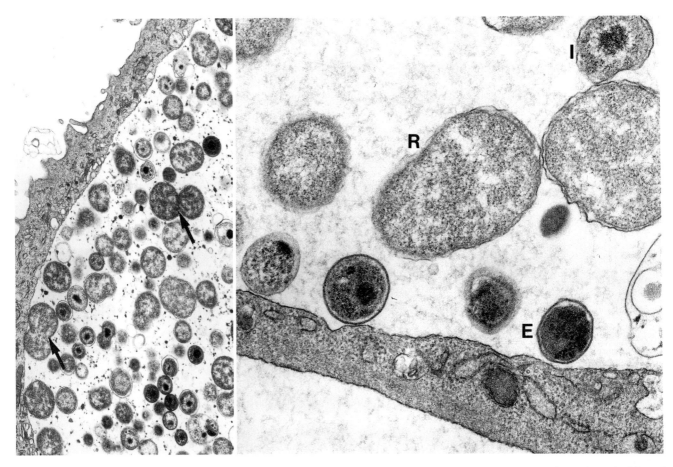

Fig. 9.27 *Chlamydia psittaci* in McCoy cells. The mature inclusion vacuole occupies most of the host cell cytoplasm and contains large numbers of chlamydiae at each stage of the growth cycle. Elementary bodies (E), the infectious form of the organism, are rigid spherical structures 200–300 nm in diameter with two closely apposed unit membranes and a dense DNA core. After entry by endocytosis they transform into metabolically active reticulate bodies (R) which divide by binary fission (indicated by arrows in inset) within the protected environment of the cytoplasmic vacuole. The structure of reticulate bodies is essentially that of Gram-negative bacteria 800–1000 nm in diameter. Approximately 20 hours after infection some reticulate bodies undergo reorganization into elementary bodies, passing through an intermediate body stage (I). Release is by cell lysis but particle budding through the plasma membrane has also been described. The membranous and granular background material (inset) contains antigens shed from the chlamydial surface. At bottom right, an intracisternal budding A-type particle is evident (see also Fig. 9.52). (× 47 000; inset, × 11 000)

Chlamydia psittaci is a common animal pathogen which occasionally causes pneumonia in humans. *Chlamydia trachomatis* is responsible for trachoma, inclusion conjunctivitis, lymphogranuloma venereum and many cases of sexually transmitted disease. Although most ultrastructural studies have involved in vitro systems, the same growth cycle can be recognized in infected columnar endocervical cells from cervical biopsies. From these and immunohistochemical studies it has become evident that the presence of cytoplasmic vacuoles and inclusions in histological sections and cytology smears is an unsatisfactory diagnostic criterion. The most reliable means of diagnosis remains isolation in tissue culture cells. References: 114, 125, 133, 169, 173 and 178.

Fig. 9.28 (Facing page) Molluscum contagiosum: molluscum body. Skin biopsy from a young boy with widespread molluscum contagiosum complicating the Wiskott–Aldrich syndrome. The altered nucleus and most of the remaining cytoplasmic components have been pushed to the periphery of this keratinocyte by a molluscum body, an example of a cytoplasmic inclusion consisting almost entirely of virus. Particles are formed in 'virus factories' within the narrow trabeculae between aggregates of mature virions. The inclusions increase in size as the cells migrate towards the skin surface and virus is released with exfoliation. (× 8 000) (Case contributed by Prof D W Henderson)

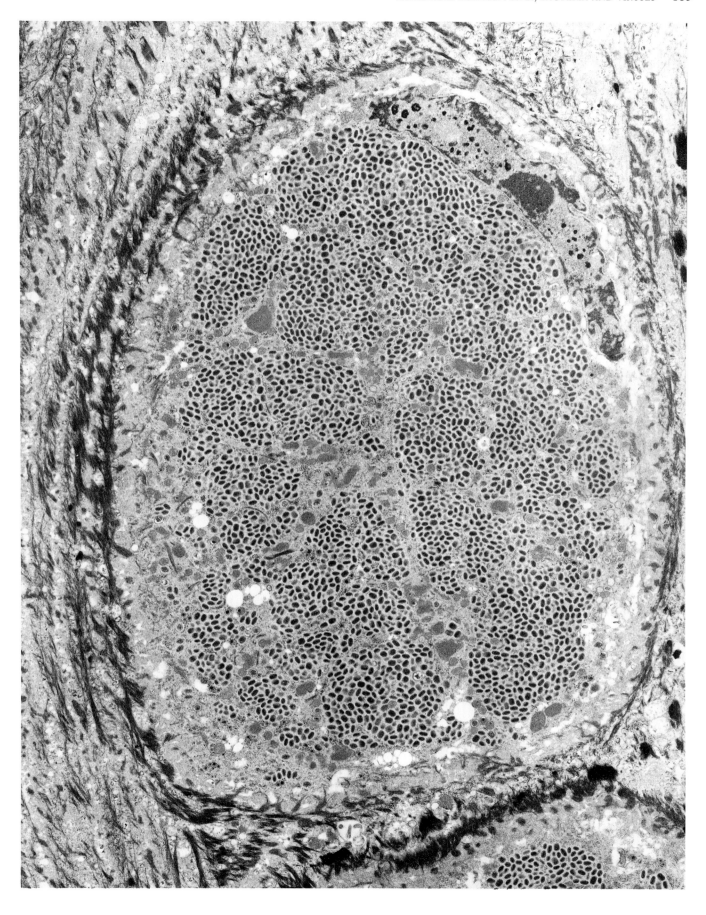

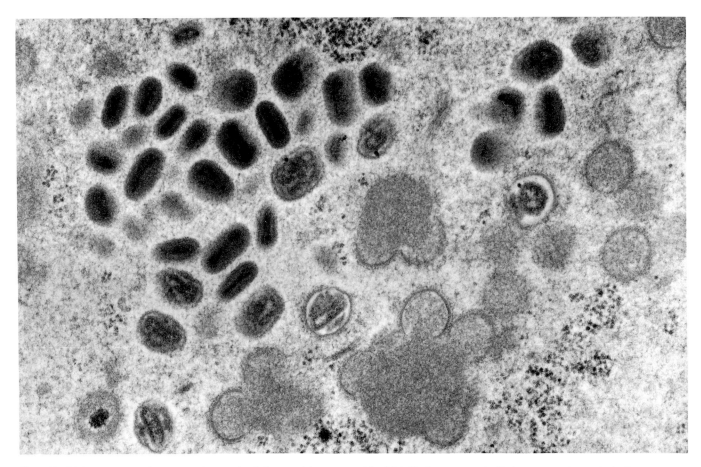

Fig. 9.29 Molluscum contagiosum: morphogenesis of virus particles. Virus particles assemble in the cytoplasmic matrix of the upper stratum spinosum and, to a lesser extent, the stratum granulosum, by the enclosure of finely granular viroplasm within double-layered arcuate membranes covered externally by spicules. In synthesizing their own lipoprotein envelope de novo (rather than acquiring it by budding through a host cell membrane), pox viruses are unique. The surrounding ribosomes may participate in viral protein synthesis. Completion of the membrane shell yields spherical immature particles with unstructured granular contents or electron-opaque nucleoids around the periphery of virus factories. Subsequent maturation produces the typical brick-shaped particle with rounded corners measuring approximately 300 × 200 × 100 nm. Although antigenically ungrouped, molluscum contagiosum virus demonstrates the typical morphology of other pox viruses, with a layered core containing viral DNA that appears dumbbell-shaped in transversely sectioned particles, together with an intermediate coat that expands into two lateral bodies and a laminated outer envelope. A small electron-opaque granule may be visible between the envelope and intermediate coat. Mature particles are separated by fine filamentous material. (× 52 000) (Case contributed by Prof D W Henderson) References: 1, 187, 188–189, 215 and 270.

Fig. 9.30 (Facing page, top) Ecthyma contagiosum (orf): degenerate keratinocytes. Ballooning degeneration apparent by light microscopy is the result of cytoplasmic swelling, vacuolation and lysis of keratin. Scattered immature and mature virus particles appear to be floating in the rather flocculent remains of the cytoplasm. At bottom right, widening of the intercellular space by oedema fluid has produced a small intra-epidermal vesicle. (× 14 000)

Fig. 9.31 (Facing page, bottom left) Orf: intracellular virions. Orf virus, a member of the paravaccinia group, is smaller (200–380 × 150–250 nm in ultrathin sections) and more ovoid than other pox viruses. The DNA-containing core is surrounded by a bilayered capsid with complex symmetry, external to which is the envelope. The spirally wound surface filament is visible in transverse section at centre field and is seen below in grazing surface section, where the criss-cross pattern that is so prominent in negatively stained particles is evident. (× 100 000)

Orf is an uncommon infection generally occurring on the hands of veterinarians (as in the illustrated case) or agricultural workers after contact transmission from infected sheep or goats. Virus isolation is extremely difficult, and biopsy specimens may be taken for the diagnosis of early lesions or the later proliferative stage that may simulate a neoplastic process. References: 182 and 284.

Fig. 9.32 (Facing page, bottom right) Adenovirus infected cells: survey. Adenovirus sialadenitis in a patient who developed painful submandibular swelling following conjunctivitis. Salivary gland tissue showed diffuse acute inflammation and virus-containing ductular and secretory epithelial cells in necrotic foci. In the two cells depicted, virus is organized into small crystalline arrays within nuclei which have undergone degenerative margination of chromatin, flocculation of nucleoplasm, focal nuclear envelope disruption and the accumulation of small, irregular electron-opaque inclusions. There is striking vesicular degeneration of the cytoplasm. (× 6000) (Case contributed by Dr J A Armstrong)

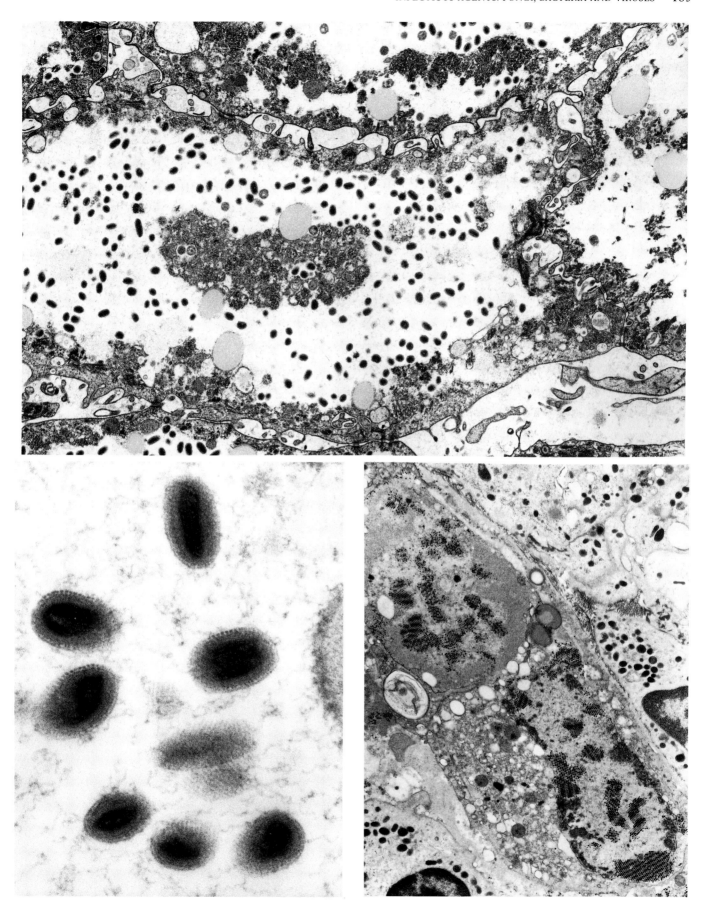

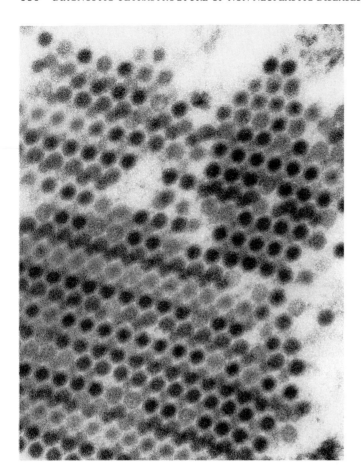

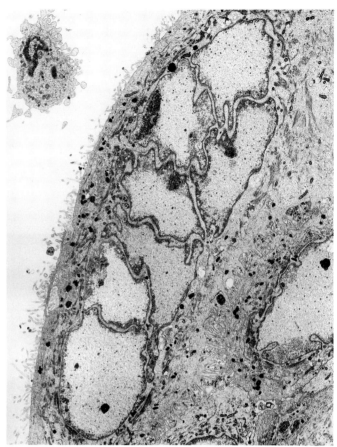

Fig. 9.33 Adenovirus sialadenitis: intranuclear virus crystal. Adenoviruses are non-enveloped DNA viruses that replicate in the nucleus with frequent formation of lattice arrays. The reported diameter of individual virions has ranged from 65 to 90 nm. The hexagonal contour in section reflects icosahedral symmetry whose distinctive substructure of non-vertex capsomers (hexons) and vertex capsomers (pentons) with attached fibres is revealed by negative staining. ($\times$ 75 000) (Case contributed by Dr J. A. Armstrong.)

Adenoviruses are a frequent cause of transient upper respiratory and eye infections but specimens from these sources are rare. However, case reports of some of the less common manifestations of adenovirus infection include fatal pneumonia, subacute encephalitis, intussusception and infantile gastroenteritis. The various intranuclear inclusions whose fine structure has been elaborated (particularly in tissue culture systems) can be correlated to some extent with those seen by light microscopy. Eosinophilic inclusions which are separated from a distinct nuclear membrane by a halo contain 'early' proteins and, with some virus types, crystals formed of excess capsid components not incorporated into virions. 'Smudge-cell' basophilic or amphophilic inclusions, in which there is no clear nuclear membrane and which are said to be characteristic of adenovirus infections, contain large numbers of mature virus particles. References: 4, 190, 207, 245, 248, 255, 279 and 285.

Fig. 9.34 Herpes simplex-induced cytopathic effect I: multinucleation. Cell fusion has produced a multinucleate giant cell at the base of a skin vesicle; such cells yield characteristic Tzanck smears. The relatively clear nuclei with marginated chromatin contain immature virus. ($\times$ 4000)

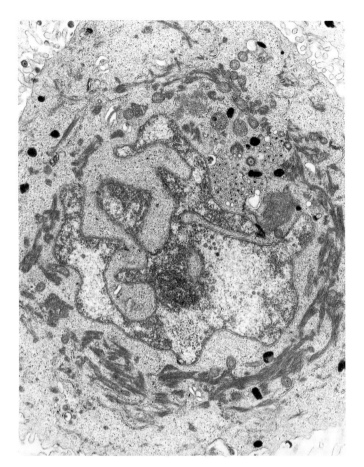

Fig. 9.35 Herpes simplex-induced cytopathic effect II: nuclear collapse. The nucleus of a detached keratinocyte is shrunken and convoluted, with chromatin clumped beneath the nuclear envelope. (× 11 000)

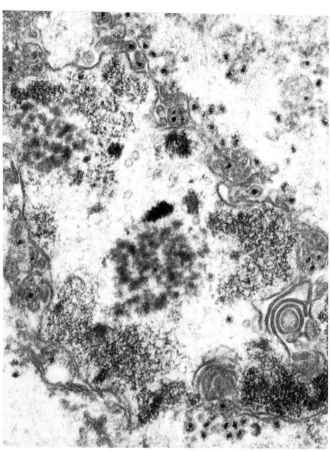

Fig. 9.36 Herpes simplex-induced cytopathic effects III: nuclear envelope changes in herpes oesophagitis. There is focal dissolution and extensive reduplication of the nuclear envelope with the formation of intranuclear whorls and complex folds extending into the cytoplasm. Granular inclusions and dense peripheral chromatin are also evident. (× 28 000) References: 182, 187, 189, 206, 237, 243, 253, 259 and 271.

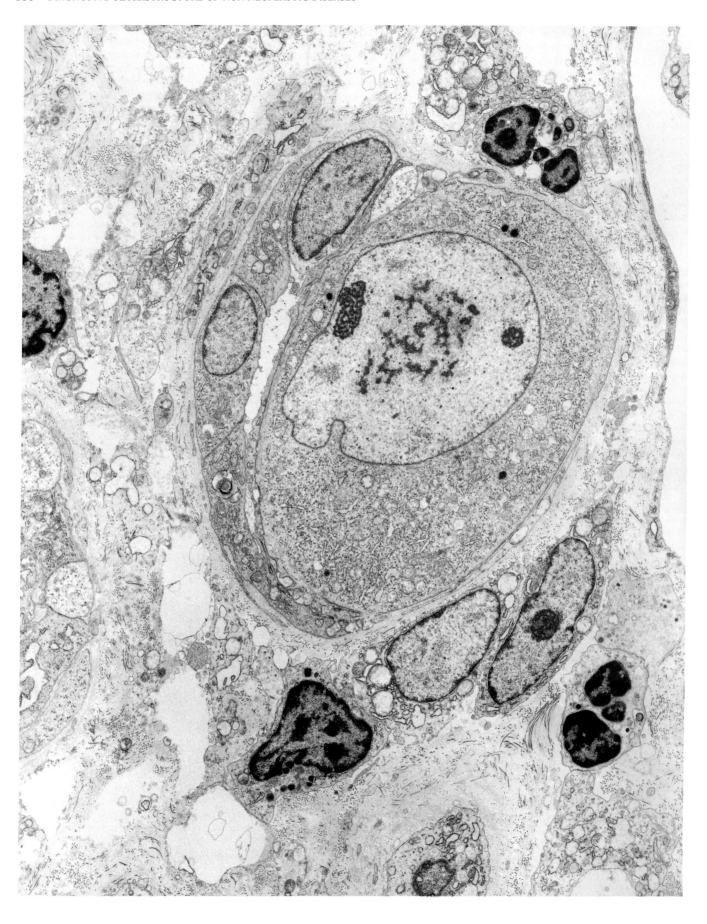

Fig. 9.37 (Facing page) Cytomegalovirus: cytomegalic inclusion cell. Both the nucleus and cytoplasm are enlarged. A reticulum of chromatin-like material in a fibrillar matrix forms the characteristic 'owl eye' intranuclear inclusion distinct from the nucleoli. The nuclear envelope is unaltered. Immature virus is dispersed through the nucleoplasm and the inclusion. Viral aggregates within vacuoles or in the ground substance may form cytoplasmic inclusions. (× 6000) Most cytomegalovirus infections occur in the fetal and neonatal periods but the virus is also an opportunistic pathogen of adults with AIDS or other immunosuppressed states. This infected capillary is from adult cytomegalovirus enterocolitis, an uncommon manifestation causing life-threatening haemorrhage and ulceration, with cytomegalic mesenchymal and ganglion cells. Epithelial cells of parenchymatous organs such as salivary glands, kidney, lungs or liver are commonly affected in generalized disease. References: 1, 194, 198, 199, 213, 221, 236, 244, 247, 256 and 301.

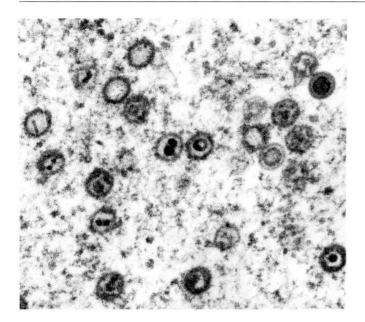

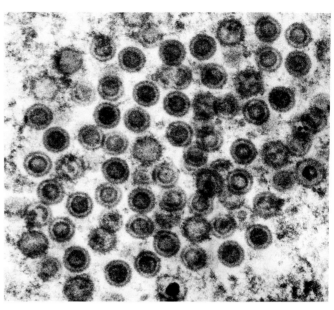

Fig. 9.38 Morphogenesis of Herpes simplex I: immature particles. Incomplete particles with or without cores lie amongst nuclear granular material. The capsid has icosahedral symmetry but may appear hexagonal, pentagonal or spherical in ultrathin sections. Depending on the plane of section and degree of maturation, the core of DNA wound around protein cylinders is round, polygonal, bar- or star-shaped. (× 75 000)

Fig. 9.39 Morphogenesis of Herpes simplex II: nucleocapsids. An aggregate of nucleocapsids is present in the nucleoplasm. (× 75 000)

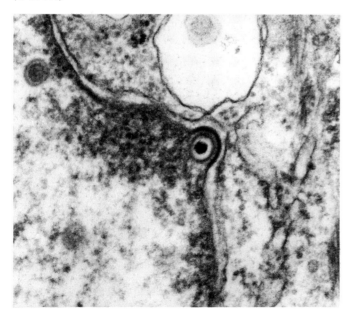

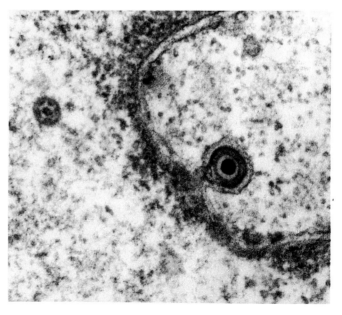

Fig. 9.40 Morphogenesis of Herpes simplex III: envelopment. The loose envelope is derived by budding at a virus modified patch of nuclear inner membrane. Envelopment by intranuclear membranous invaginations and budding at cytoplasmic membrane systems or the plasmalemma have also been described. (× 75 000)

Fig. 9.41 Morphogenesis of Herpes simplex IV: envelopment. Late stage of the budding process before the mature particle is pinched off and released into the perinuclear space. (× 75 000)

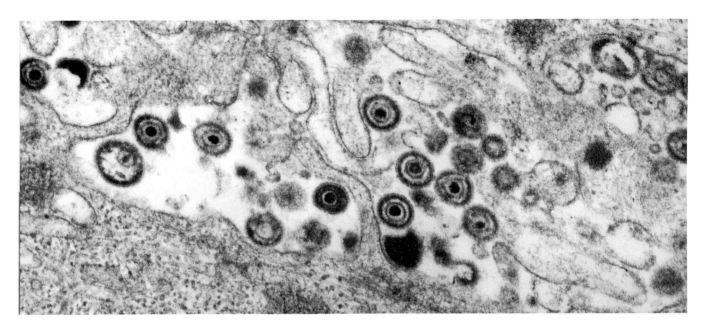

Fig. 9.42 Morphogenesis of Herpes simplex V: extracellular particles. Particles in the widened space between keratinocytes demonstrate the envelope, capsid and core components of mature herpes. The envelope is trilaminar with short surface spikes. The tegument layer outside the capsid contains large viral proteins while nucleocapsid protein may be included in the pericore zone between capsid and core. Published measurements of sectioned particles have varied from 35 to 50 nm for cores, 70 to 130 nm for capsids, and 120 to 160 nm for envelopes. (× 50 000) References: 4, 189, 190, 193, 250, 253, 259 and 271.

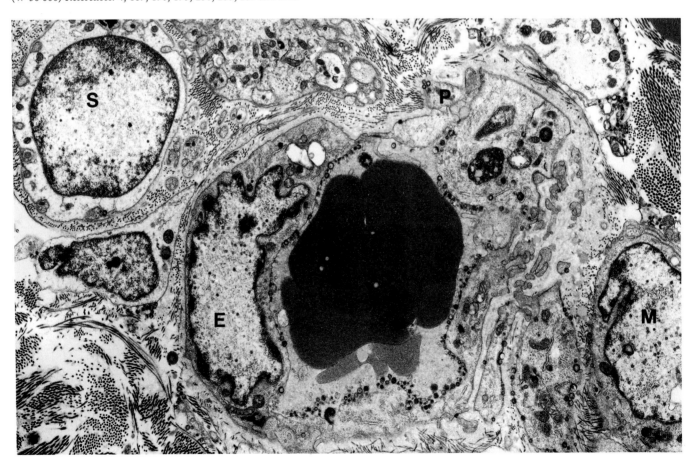

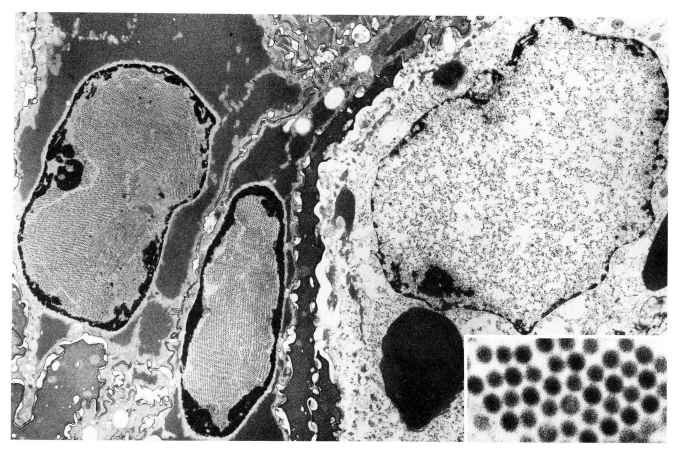

Fig. 9.44 Human papillomavirus (HPV) infection I: plantar wart. Crystalline arrays of virus occupy most of the two nuclei at left; particles are more dispersed on the right. In cutaneous warts, the virus replicates in keratinizing cells and is found in the outer stratum spinosum and more superficially (where it produces the basophilic intranuclear inclusions seen in histological sections). Disordered keratinization produces giant keratohyaline granules (right) that are eosinophilic by light microscopy. From a reprocessed paraffin block. (× 7000) *Inset* Small crystal of hexagonally packed HPV particles in a verruca vulgaris. Virions are non-enveloped, spherical and 40–50 nm in diameter. The electron-opaque DNA-containing core is surrounded by a capsid with cubic symmetry demonstrable by negative staining. (× 140 000)

Fig. 9.43 (Facing page)   Cutaneous herpes infection. In this area of the dermis underlying a skin vesicle, small rounded virus particles are evident in endothelial cells (E), pericytes (P), a Schwann cell (S) and a macrophage (M). (× 7500)

Herpesviruses are the most ubiquitous of viruses, infecting not only humans and other mammals but also reptiles, birds, amphibians and fish. Although most often involving the skin and mucosa, Herpes simplex and, to a lesser extent, varicella-zoster, may produce disseminated infection. Visceral disease may become evident for the first time in histological sections, and the use for electron microscopy of material stored in formalin or embedded in paraffin has proved valuable for retrospective diagnosis. EM is also helpful with brain biopsies in suspected herpes encephalitis. In all sites the diagnostic cells are best sought at the periphery of lesions, and familiarity with the morphology of immature viruses as well as the complete virus is essential. References: 2–4, 182, 187, 189, 193, 194, 206, 217, 231, 232, 237, 243, 253 and 271.

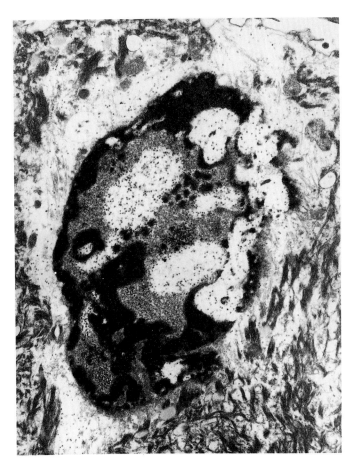

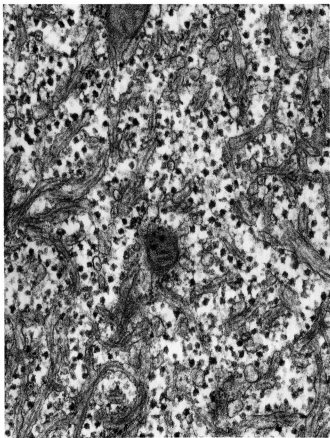

Fig. 9.45 HPV infection II: cervical condyloma. This superficial cell, histologically recognizable as a koilocyte, shows perinuclear clearing with compression of the remaining cytoplasmic organelles at the cell periphery. The nucleus is irregular in outline with marginated clumped chromatin. Virus is associated with both dense and clear nucleoplasm and has gained entry to the cytoplasm at sites of nuclear rupture. Koilocyte change is regarded as a cytopathic effect pathognomonic of HPV infection but only a small proportion of such cells contain virus. Clear cells with a similar fine structure also occur in skin warts. (× 12 000)

Early ultrastructural studies of papovavirus infections (the term is an acronym of papilloma, polyoma and vacuolating agent) were encouraged by inability to culture the virus. Particle frequency can be correlated to some extent with the lesion produced: virus is usually profuse in common or plantar warts and epidermodysplasia verruciformis but is sparse or absent in anogenital warts and laryngeal papillomas. Current nucleic acid hybridization studies are greatly expanding these observations and further uncovering the oncogenic potential of specific HPV types. Viruses of the polyoma subgroup (including the agent of progressive multifocal leucoencephalopathy) are smaller (33–38 nm in thin sections) and have both filamentous and spherical morphology. References: 2, 4, 187–190, 193, 194, 196, 203, 205, 208, 214, 216, 218, 222, 238, 240, 241, 251, 254, 258, 260, 266, 276, 280, 281 and 286.

Fig. 9.46 Hepatitis B: hepatitis B surface antigen (HBsAg) in hepatocyte endoplasmic reticulum. Proliferated SER in a chronic active hepatitis biopsy contains filaments of varying length, 20–30 nm in diameter and circular in cross section. Expanded SER of any origin produces ground glass hepatocytes in H & E stained sections but intracisternal filaments, demonstrable by Shikata's orcein or immunostaining, are diagnostic of hepatitis B. (× 32 000) (See also Figs 15.6–15.8)

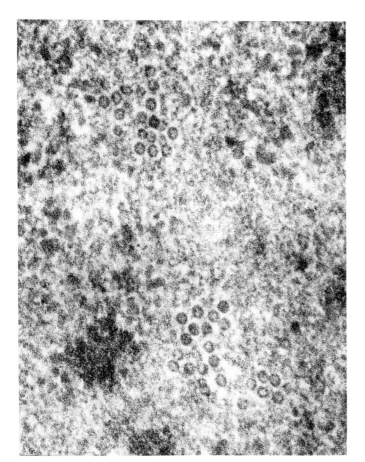

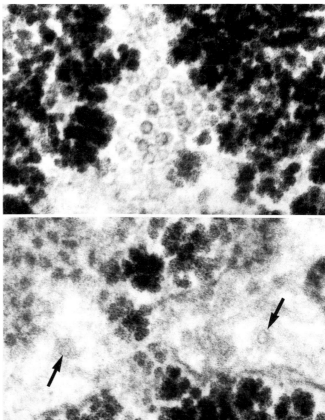

Fig. 9.47 Heptatitis B: intranuclear core antigen (HBcAg). HBcAg particles are 20–25 nm in diameter and most resemble empty shells; less than 10% have a DNA-containing core. They are usually sparse but aggregation may produce a 'sanded' pattern by light microscopy. Core particles are scarcer than HBsAg filaments and as a rule the two do not co-exist within the same cell. Liver biopsy from an infant carrier of maternally transmitted HB Ag. (× 140 000)

Fig. 9.48 Hepatitis B: core and surface antigens. **Upper** Core particles are occasionally found in cytoplasmic ground substance, Disse's space or bile canaliculi; the particles may appear naked — as depicted here — or they may have a fluffy coat of obscure nature. (× 140 000) **Lower** Coated, 35–40 nm bodies (arrows) resembling Dane particles in SER cisternae. Both from hepatitis B-related cirrhosis. (× 140 000)

Spherical particles of HBcAg are assembled in the nucleus then migrate to the cytosol, enter the SER and are coated with locally produced HBsAg to form complete virus (Dane particles). These are released by exocytosis into the blood along with excess surface antigen. Coating at the plasma membrane has also been proposed. For practical purposes, particulate antigens are never seen in acute hepatitis B but may be profuse in asymptomatic carriers, chronic active disease and cirrhosis. The virus is not directly cytopathic and damage may be due to cellular or humoral immune responses to hepatocyte surface neoantigens. Inadequate defence mechanisms may permit persistent infection. References: 193, 201, 211, 223, 227, 233, 234, 239, 249, 261–263, 267, 268, 282 and 283.

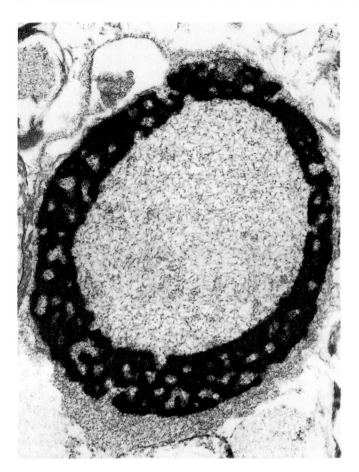

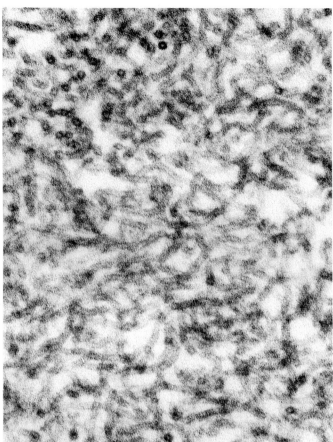

Fig. 9.49 Subacute sclerosing panencephalitis (SSPE): nuclear inclusion. Chromatin is aggregated at the periphery of a nucleus which is otherwise occupied by viral nucleocapsids. From a post-mortem brain specimen. (× 28 000)

Fig. 9.50 SSPE: nucleocapsids. The RNA-containing nucleocapsids are of variable length (up to 1 μm when isolated) and tubular in form, with a diameter of 17 nm and a central 7 nm hole. Transverse striations indicate the helical symmetry revealed by negative staining. (× 140 000)

The detection of intranuclear tubules resembling measles nucleocapsids by EM in 1965 paved the way for the isolation of the SSPE agent 4 years later. Nuclear inclusions in neurons and glial cells had been long recognized by light microscopy. Cytoplasmic nucleocapsids, usually with a fuzzy coating of viral internal proteins, are found less often. Inclusions of both types also occur in SSPE retinopathy and subacute measles encephalitis. Although morphologically and antigenically similar to measles, the defective SSPE virus does not acquire an envelope in vivo by the usual budding at the plasma membrane through inability of the host cell to synthesize viral matrix protein. Direct cell-to-cell transmission of virus seems likely. Other paramyxo- and myxo-viruses produce only cytoplasmic nucleocapsids, making their presence in the nucleus virtually pathognomonic of measles infection. As with certain other paramyxoviruses, cell fusion with polykaryon formation is a prominent cytopathic effect of productive measles virus infection both in culture and in vivo, with multinucleated epithelial cells containing intranuclear nucleocapsids occurring in the skin rash and Koplik's spots of acute measles, giant cell pneumonia and fatal generalized measles. References: 194, 202, 204, 220, 232, 235, 252, 265 and 269.

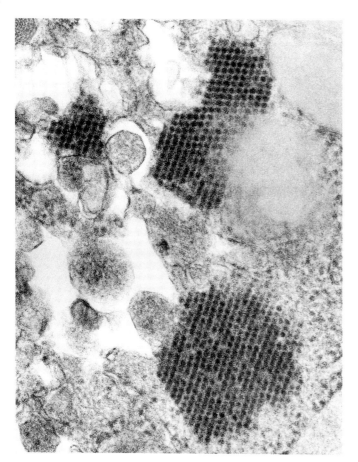

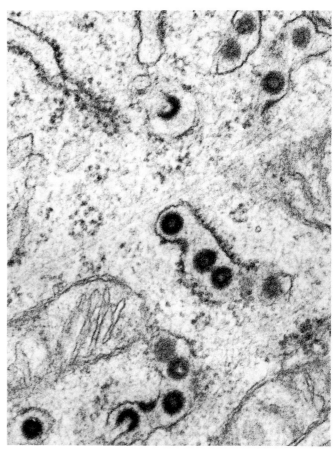

Fig. 9.51 Picornavirus: Rhinovirus in tissue culture cells. Rhinovirus particles form crystalline arrays in the cytoplasmic matrix of a human embryo lung cell inoculated with a throat swab. Individual spherical virions 27 nm in diameter are resolved best at the top of the field where there is no overlap. Although a few appear empty, the majority are uniformly opaque. (× 75 000) (Case contributed by Dr J. A. Armstrong.)

The picornaviruses, a family of small naked RNA viruses include enteroviruses (polio, echo, hepatitis A and coxsackie viruses) that are transient inhabitants of the alimentary tract before invading target organs. Rhinoviruses — causative agents of the common cold and other respiratory infections — are another member of this family. Although they have been much studied in tissue culture and experimental animals, there are few authentic illustrations of these viruses in human infections. Their small size and simple form have caused confusion with ribosomes or glycogen (Fig. 9.62), and their organization into crystals or linear arrays on fine filaments is much less common in vivo than in culture.
References: 182, 190, 193, 224, 228, 230 and 272.

Fig. 9.52 Oncoviruses I: intracisternal A-type particles in McCoy cell. A-type particles are doughnut shaped with an electron-lucent centre surrounded by two concentric shells, the inner staining more intensely than the outer. Intracisternal forms develop by budding into the endoplasmic reticulum and are of unknown significance. A-type particles also occur in the cytoplasmic matrix as precursors of B-type particles. (× 75 000)

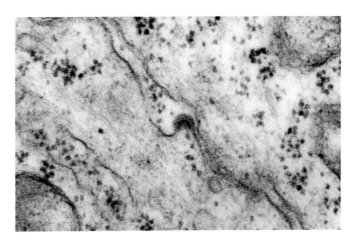

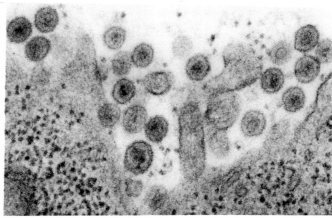

Fig. 9.53 Oncoviruses II: C-type particles in human ovarian carcinoma heterotransplant in nude mouse. ***Upper*** Budding commences with the formation beneath a virus-modified protrusion of the plasma membrane of a dense crescent destined to become the core of the particle. (× 75 000) ***Lower*** After separation, the immature particle has a central spherical core with an electron-lucent centre surrounded by an intermediate layer. The core becomes angulated with maturation and is darkly but irregularly stained. (× 75 000)

Oncoviruses (oncornaviruses) form a subfamily of retroviruses — RNA viruses possessing reverse transcriptase — and were originally classified by Bernhard as follows:

a. A-type particles, diameter 60–90 nm, occur within cells and may be intracisternal or intracytoplasmic.
b. B-type particles, diameter 125–130 nm, bud from the plasma membrane, and possess an eccentric core and surface glycoprotein spikes. The prototype is the mouse mammary tumour virus.
c. C-type particles, diameter 80–110 nm, have a central nucleoid and are associated with lymphomas, leukaemias and sarcomas in many species, to which the C-particles were subsequently added.
d. D-type particles, diameter 100–120 nm, which bud from the plasma membrane via ring-shaped precursors larger than A-type particles

and which have a bar-shaped core. The prototype is the Mason–Pfizer monkey virus.

Although many animal and avian oncoviruses are known, the search for human examples has been fraught with cautionary tales. Human tumour cells do not produce virus particles in vivo and it is only recently, following successful culture of leukaemic cells, that anybody has isolated a genuine human retrovirus. So far, the adult T cell leukaemia-lymphoma viruses HTLV-1 and HTLV-2, which show C-type morphology, are the only acceptable human viruses of this group.

Two practical situations where oncoviruses may present themselves are illustrated to underline the fact that animal and human viruses cannot be morphologically differentiated. Persistent infection has long been recognized in lines such as McCoy cells[1,28] and these organisms may turn up during the monitoring of laboratory cultures for contamination or identification of viruses that produce no cytopathic effect. More recently, oncoviruses have been found in human tumour heterotransplants in nude mice. They have been identified as endogenous xenotropic murine retroviruses carried by nude mice; following activation, they infect and replicate in the grafted tumour. References: 182, 186, 192, 200, 209, 210, 219, 257, 273, 275, 277 and 278.

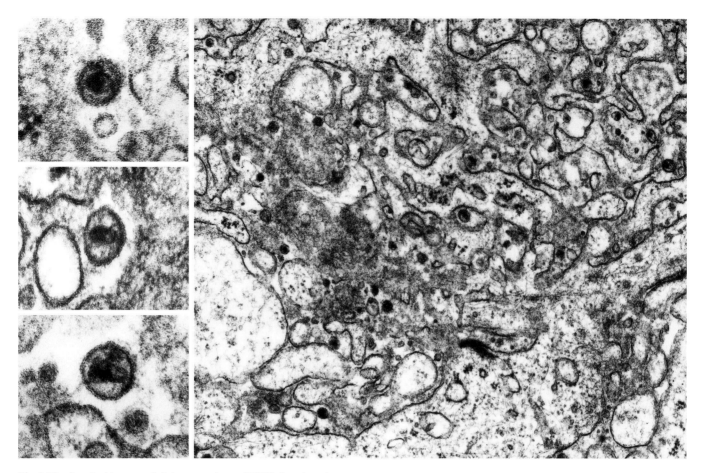

Fig. 9.54 Acquired immune deficiency syndrome (AIDS): lymph node. Follicular cell dendritic processes, many degenerate, form labyrinthine complexes in the enlarged germinal centre of a lymph node. Virus is sparsely scattered amongst other extracellular spherical microparticles. ($\times$ 28 000) *Insets* Mature human immunodeficiency virus HIV-1 particles are spherical, 90–120 nm in diameters, and have a distinctive core; depending on the plane of section, the core may be eccentric, ovoid or conical with a characteristic dense base and paler tapering tip. In morphology and nucleotide sequences HIV-1 most closely resembles the lentiviruses, a subfamily of retroviruses causing slow virus infections in ungulates. ($\times$ 100 000) (Case contributed by Dr J J Turner)

HIV-1 (formerly known as human thymus lymphotropic virus, HTLV-III, lymphadenopathy-associated virus, LAV, or AIDS-associated retrovirus, ARV) is found in lymph nodes both in AIDS and the AIDS-associated lymphadenopathy syndrome. Particles are most profuse in nodes with a histologically mixed pattern of follicular hyperplasia and involution, but with terminal lymphoid depletion they become scarce or absent, along with follicular dendritic cells. Prior to the availability of specific antibody testing, ultrastructural screening of lymph nodes was proposed for diagnosis; it has been stated that examination of two germinal centres is adequate to detect virus. Particles have also been reported in spleen, tonsil and brain. Although infected lymphocytes can be induced to produce virus in vitro, this is not apparent with clinical specimens. In lymph nodes, viral budding has been reported only from follicular dendritic cell surface membranes. In AIDS encephalopathy, virus is associated with multinucleated giant cells that are probably derived from macrophages (see also Ch. 29). References: 197, 212, 225, 226, 229, 242, 246, 264, 274 and 278.

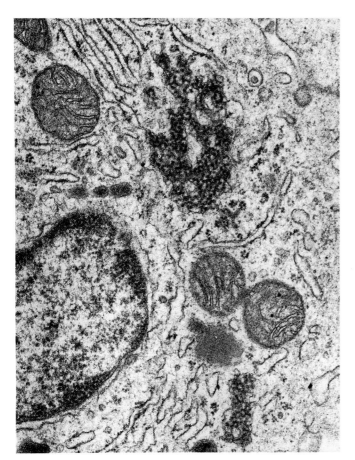

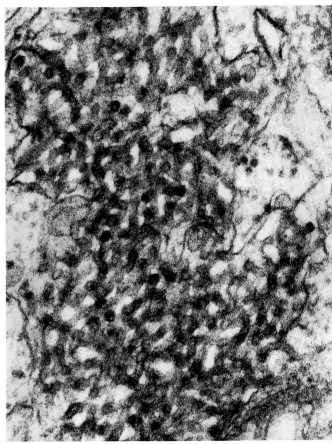

Fig. 9.55 'Virus-like' and 'virus-associated' structures IA: tubuloreticular inclusions (TRI). Also called undulating tubules, and various other names, TRI are reticular or undulating arrays of thick-walled tubules within dilated endoplasmic reticulum or cytoplasmic matrix. TRI occur in many infections, auto-immune disorders, lymphoid and other neoplasms, those illustrated being in an adenocarcinoma cell. More recently, TRI have been readily found in HIV-1 infected patients, and their formation linked with α and β type I interferons ($\times$ 35 000)

Fig. 9.56 'Virus-like' and 'virus-associated' sructures' IB: tubuloreticular inclusions (TRI). TRI have been frequently misidentified as 'myxovirus-like structures' (compare with Fig. 9.50), particularly in glomerular capillaries in systemic lupus erythematosus. Although also tubular with a lucent centre, TRI branch or anastomose, are wider (20–30 nm) with a denser, thicker (6 nm) wall than myxoviruses; in addition, they may be continuous with the endoplasmic reticulum in which they lie, they contain glycoprotein and lack nucleic acid. Lymphocyte of an HIV-1 seropositive subject. ($\times$ 100 000) References: 193, 195, 288, 289, 292, 301, 302, 306, 309, 315–318, 320 and 323.

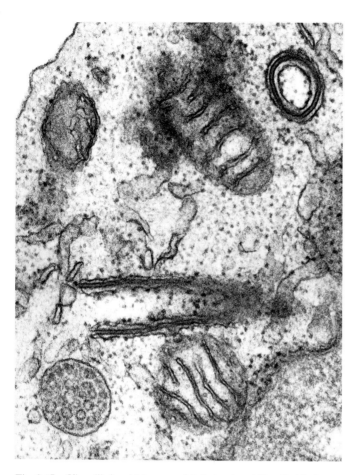

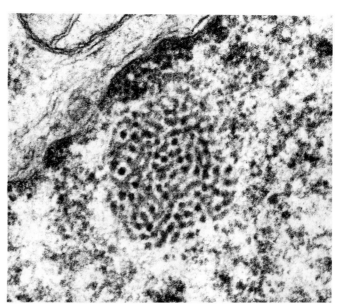

Fig. 9.58 'Virus-like' and 'virus-associated structures' III: vermicellar body. Nuclear bodies formed of granules, fibrils or combinations of both exist in many cells, and although there have been attempts at morphological classification and correlation with cell function, they are generally considered to be of no diagnostic significance. The vermicellar variety consists of intertwining beaded threads 20–30 nm in diameter and is most obvious in relatively thick sections; in thinner sections poorly defined granules are seen. This example from a small cell neuroendocrine carcinoma also contains granules resembling perichromatin granules. Vermicellar bodies were initially regarded as abnormal viral cores in herpes encephalitis and lately as markers of non-A, non-B hepatitis, but these claims have been disproved. They occur mostly in tumours. ($\times$ 75 000) References: 271, 295, 301, 314 and 322.

Fig. 9.57 'Virus-like' and 'virus-associated structures' II: cylindrical confronting cisternae (CCC) and multivesicular body (MVB). Initially considered unique to hepatocytes of chimpanzees infected with human non-A, non-B hepatitis, CCC occur in various disorders including AIDS. Derived from endoplasmic reticulum, they are parallel cisternae fused to an intervening 25 nm opaque layer. CCC are 150–300 nm in diameter, circular in cross section, and in apparent longitudinal section they assume the shape of an open cylinder or have one curved closed end ('test-tube and ring-shaped forms'). However, as illustrated in a lymphocyte from an HIV-1 antibody-positive patient, the test-tube form may be due to oblique sectioning. CCC may occur with TRI but their induction by interferon is less certain. The MVB (bottom left) is a form of lysosome. The regularity of the vesicles, sometimes darker than here, has led to erroneous assumptions of identity but nevertheless genuine virus particles may be present. 'Vesicular rosettes' of vesicles clustered around an ill-defined electron opaque centre in AIDS lymphocytes may be altered MVB. ($\times$ 57 000) References: CCC, 288, 301, 305, 309, 315, 316 and 320; MVB and vesicular rosettes, 294, 297, 300, 304, 315 and 325.

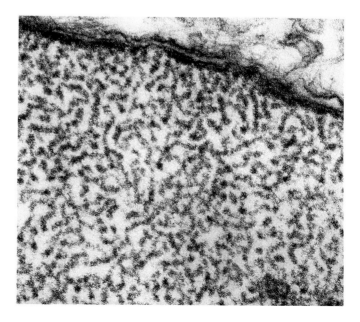

Fig. 9.59 (Right) 'Virus-like' and 'virus-associated' structures IV: altered chromatin filaments. Intranuclear filaments, subsequently shown to be derived from chromatin, were once proposed as the causative agent of acute multiple sclerosis. Some resemblance to paramyxovirus nucleocapsids notwithstanding (see Fig. 9.50), altered chromatin filaments usually fill the entire nucleus and are thicker (20–40 nm), denser, and more fuzzy in outline than paramyxovirus; in addition, they are only occasionally striated and are rarely tubular. The envelope may rupture with characteristic spillage of nuclear contents. The change appears to be related to cell injury and tissue processing methods, being commonest in formalin-fixed autopsy material. ($\times$ 75 000) References: 195, 311, 319 and 324.

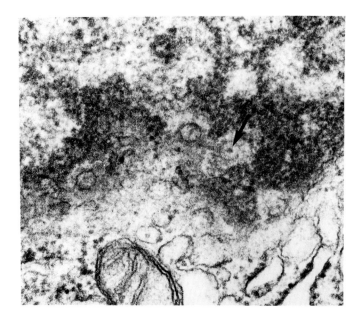

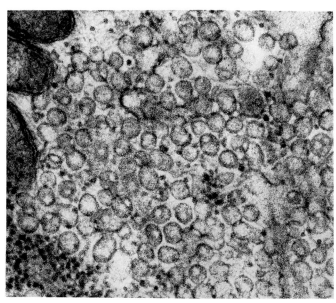

Fig. 9.60 'Virus-like' and 'virus-associated' structures V: nuclear pores. Pores formed by fusion of both layers of the nuclear envelope are normal structures whose number and distribution vary from one cell type to another. Viewed en face they appear as annuli 100–120 nm in diameter, sometimes with a central granule (arrow), which periodically leads to confusion with intranuclear herpes particles (Fig. 9.38). (× 75 000) References: 298, 301 and 304.

Fig. 9.61 'Virus-like' and 'virus-associated' structures VI: micropinocytosis vesicles. Tangential sectioning has obscured any relationship between these micropinocytosis vesicles and the plasma membrane. Electron opaque contents may simulate a viral core. (× 75 000) References: 298, 301 and 304.

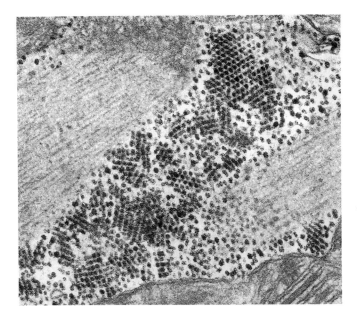

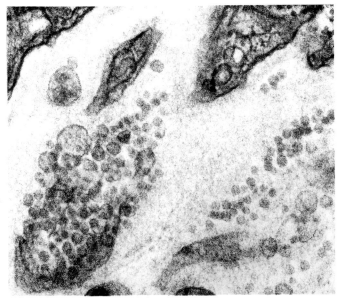

Fig. 9.62 'Virus-like' and 'virus-associated' structures VII: glycogen. Crystalline arrays of glycogen in muscle from a patient with idiopathic scoliosis. Often described in biopsy and postmortem specimens of pathological or even normal muscle as picornavirus-like, such particles have been identified as glycogen by amylase digestion and electron cytochemistry. Picornaviruses (see Fig. 9.51) are more uniform in size, outline and staining pattern than glycogen and rarely form crystals in vivo. (× 75 000) (Case contributed by Dr J M Papadimitriou) References: 184, 193, 293 and 307.

Fig. 9.63 'Virus-like' and 'virus-associated' structures VIII: spherical microparticles. Electron-opaque, membrane-bound spherical particles, occasionally found in connective tissue adjacent to normal cells, often form large aggregates in pathological glomerular basement membranes and mesangial matrix. The illustration is from a biopsy of the myocardium, another common site for these bodies, in congestive cardiomyopathy. Spherical microparticles are considered to be a form of cell debris associated with surface remodelling. Despite their wide size range (40–100 nm) and lack of internal structure resembling a nucleoprotein core, the unfortunate tendency of some nephrologists to call them C-type particles has not been laid to rest entirely. (× 75 000) References: 193, 195, 289, 299 and 301.

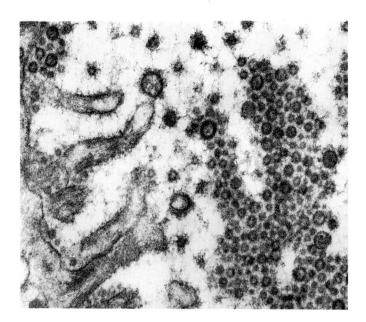

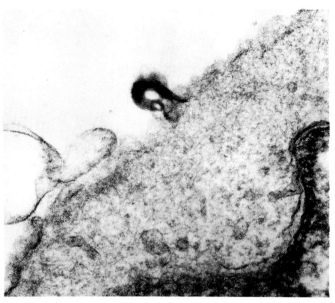

Fig. 9.64 'Virus-like' and 'virus-associated' structures IX: glycocalyceal bodies. Glycocalyceal bodies are spherical or ovoid membrane-bound vesicles with a diameter of 20–80 nm and a surface glycocalyx. Associated with the apical microvilli of normal or pathological colonic and respiratory epithelium or intestinal metaplasia, they are common in adenocarcinomas of the colon, as in this fine-needle aspirate from a bone metastasis. Although their nature and significance are unknown and their mode of formation arguable, glycocalyceal bodies appear to be a physiological rather than a degenerative phenomenon. (× 50 000) References: 287 and 312.

Fig. 9.65 'Virus-like' and 'virus-associated' structures X: myelin figures. Prolonged glutaraldehyde fixation may induce the formation of myelin figures, usually within mitochondria but sometimes in intracellular membrane systems or at the plasma membrane, as here, where they may superficially resemble budding virus particles (compare with Fig. 9.53). Their multilamellar structure is not always obvious. (× 75 000) References: 296 and 304.

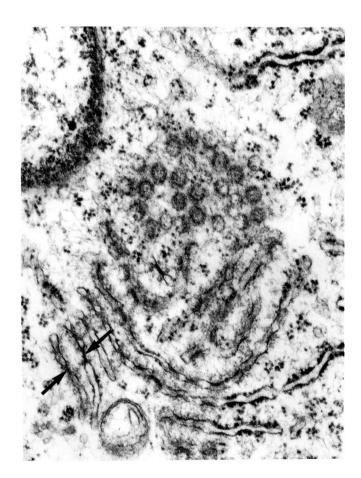

Fig. 9.66 (Right) 'Virus-like' and 'virus-associated' structures XI: annulate lamellae. First identified in oocytes but also found in other rapidly dividing cells, annulate lamellae play a conjectural role in growth and differentiation. These lamellae in a malignant lymphoma demonstrate annuli in profile within stacked cisternae (arrows) and en face; usually one aspect only is apparent. Continuity with the endoplasmic reticulum, seen here, and with the nuclear envelope has frequently been noted. Intranuclear examples occur occasionally. As with nuclear pores which they resemble (see Fig. 9.60), tangential sectioning may simulate clustered virus particles. (× 50 000) References: 184, 301, 306 and 308.

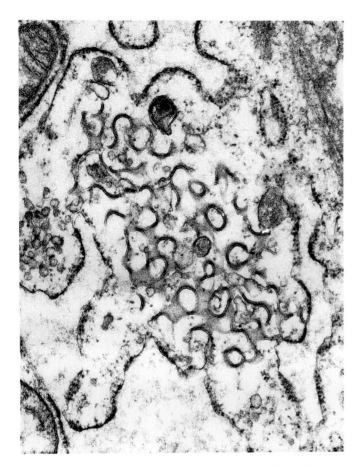

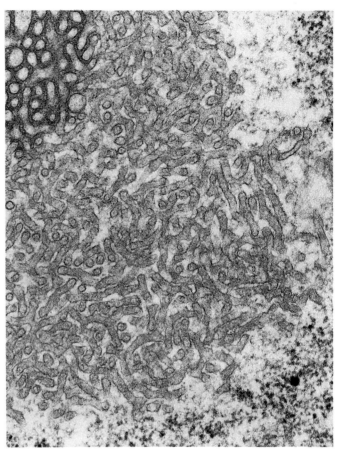

Fig. 9.67 'Virus-like' and 'virus-associated' structures XII: curvilinear membrane complexes. Probably related to tubuloreticular inclusions, these rarer complexes likewise develop from endoplasmic reticulum and consist of parallel closely paired unit membranes forming cytoplasmic lamellae with looped, wavy or circular profiles. Another proposed marker of non-A, non-B hepatitis in experimental chimpanzees, they also occur in tumours and histiocytes, particularly those of histiocytosis X. (× 35 000) References: 291, 301 and 313.

Fig. 9.68 'Virus-like' and 'virus-associated' structures XIII: intranuclear tubular inclusions. Unlike paramyxovirus nucleocapsids (see Fig. 9.50), these inclusions vary in diameter, branch or anastomose, lack transverse striations, are bound by a unit membrane and may be continuous with the nuclear envelope. Compound inclusions, with additional lamellar membranes, vesicles and condensed undulating tubules occur. Seen in bronchiolo-alveolar carcinomas (as in this instance) or reactive type II pneumocytes, these inclusions are regarded by some as restricted to type II cells and their corresponding tumours. Their relationship to the PAS-positive surfactant-specific apoprotein inclusions in bronchiolo-alveolar carcinomas is unsettled. (× 75 000) References: 301, 303, 306, 310 and 321.

10. Diagnostic ultrastructure of human parasites

A. Warton

INTRODUCTION

Despite the advances of modern medicine the prevalence of human parasitic diseases remains high and they are still the cause of much morbidity and mortality. In this context it is worth emphasizing that, according to some estimates,[103] parasitic diseases claim more lives than do all the malignant neoplasms combined.

Economic and social conditions affect the distribution of the parasites of man, and poverty and poor sanitation still play important roles in the transmission of several pathogenic species. However, some parasites, such as *Giardia*, *Toxoplasma* and *Trichomonas*, are seen in patients irrespective of their socio-economic status and are widely spread in both developing and developed countries. In addition, patients on immunosuppressive therapy are often targets of opportunistic parasitic infection which can, on occasion, prove fatal.

Differential diagnosis of parasitic diseases is of extreme importance. According to Sun,[103] 'with negligence or ignorance, ameboma can be misdiagnosed as carcinoma; toxocariasis as retinoblastoma; toxoplasmosis as lymphoma; giardiasis as non-tropical sprue; and paragonimiasis as tuberculosis. Rare though it may be, the loss caused by misdiagnosis to these patients and their families is, indeed, immeasurable, as patients can die, lose their eyes, or be subjected to many expensive yet unnecessary tests, as well as surgical procedures.'.

Since the clinical manifestations of parasitic diseases are often very general, diagnosis based upon symptomatology alone is inadequate. The final diagnosis and the adequate choice of treatment, however, require the precise identification of the parasite in the laboratory. Electron microscopy (EM) may be of great value in diagnosing or in confirming a light microscopic diagnosis of several parasitic diseases, especially those caused by Protozoa. In addition, the mechanism of pathogenicity of different human parasites and the changes in host tissues during the parasitic infection may be studied with electron microscopic methods.

Human parasites can be generally classified into four main phyla: Protozoa, Platyhelminthes, Nematohelminthes and Arthropoda. We will discuss the importance of electron microscopy in the diagnosis and the understanding of pathogenicity of some representatives of these groups.

PROTOZOA

Unicellular organisms can be divided into four classes on the basis of their locomotive patterns: Sarcodina (move by pseudopodia, e.g. *Entamoeba histolytica*), Mastigophora (move by flagella, e.g. *Trichomonas vaginalis*), Sporozoa (without any organ of locomotion, e.g. *Toxoplasma gondii*) and Ciliata (move by cilia, e.g. *Balantidium coli*). We shall discuss only those species of protozoa for which EM has been shown to be of help in diagnosis (or in understanding the pathogenicity) of the parasite.

Entamoeba

The diagnosis of amoebic infection rests on finding amoebae in stools or gastrointestinal tract biopsies or by detecting specific antibodies in serum.[46] Light microscopic observations of stools diluted with saline or examination of faecal smears are the most often used techniques in the recognition of amoebic infection. Amoebiasis is, however, often misdiagnosed. In fixed specimens leukocytes can be confused with parasites. Even experienced laboratory personnel have mistaken macrophages containing ingested red cells for protozoan parasites.[118] Although EM does not play a leading role in diagnosis of amoebiasis, nevertheless, ultrastructural techniques facilitate the recognition of amoebae in stools and biopsy specimens and, in addition, have elucidated the mechanisms of pathogenesis of this protozoan disease.

Electron microscopic studies[8,30,43,80,88,105,107] of *Entamoeba* of human origin revealed that this parasite is elongated or oval with an irregular surface (Fig. 10.1A). Many phagocytic and acid phosphatase-staining lysosomal vacuoles are found in the cytoplasm. The nucleus contains peripheral chromatin and a central, irregularly shaped karyosome. Mitochondria, rough endoplasmic reticulum or Golgi apparatus have not been identified in this protozoan, but aggregates of helically-arranged ribosomes are very characteristic. Dense, ovoid, membrane-limited bodies are present in the cytoplasm while glycogen particles are often clustered in bands or clumps (Fig. 10.1B).

Pathogenic and non-pathogenic strains of *Entamoeba* are morphologically indistinguishable. However, electron microscopic examination, combined with light microscopic studies, have revealed that pathogenic strains of *E. histolytica* display several cell surface properties that differ from those of non-pathogenic strains of the parasite. Strong agglutination induced by concanavalin A (con A), high con A surface binding, as seen by EM, and low surface charge are characteristic only for highly pathogenic strains of the parasite.[108] Host–parasite relationship in amoebiasis and its importance in the pathogenesis of the disease are, however, poorly understood. On the basis of electron microscopic studies, Eaton and coworkers[30] have suggested that the surface-active lysosomes of *Entamoeba* are involved in killing mammalian cells when the parasite contacts host tissues. Griffin & Juniper[43] hypothesized that the small, dense, ovoid bodies located in the cytoplasm of the parasite might contain concentrated toxic products which, when transported across the membrane, could cause the lysis of host cells. Pittman and coworkers[80] examined by EM sigmoid colonic mucosal biopsies from individuals with amoebic colitis and found that the surface epithelium contained swollen mitochondria and endoplasmic reticulum while microvilli were damaged, sparse, stunted and covered with little or no glycocalyx. Further, according to those authors, it is possible that 'once the surface epithelium is sloughed, amoebae gain access to blood vessels or lymphatic channels which carry them to deeper levels of the mucosa or to other organs of the body, especially the liver.' Damage to the surface epithelium may provide some explanation for the diarrhoea in patients with amoebic colitis.[80]

Tandon and coworkers[105] studied the ultrastructural appearance of human liver in hepatomegaly caused by amoebiasis. These authors found that, in contrast to normal liver, the specimens from all patients showed severe, widespread pathological changes in the organelles of hepatocytes. The endoplasmic reticulum and mitochondria were the principal targets of injury. The smooth endoplasmic reticulum appeared hypertrophic and dilated, while the rough endoplasmic reticulum (RER) was swollen and vacuolated with an apparent decrease in the number of bound ribosomes per unit area of membrane. The most striking changes were noticed in the mitochondria; paracrystalline, filamentous and tubular inclusions were observed in the matrix of large and bizarre-shaped mitochondria while the cristae were often destroyed.

Free-living pathogenic amoebae

During the last two decades human protozoal infections

to brain, skin, lung and eyes by the free-living amoebae *Acanthamoeba* and *Naegleria* have been reported.[15,16,20,35,41,42,66–70,116,117,131] *Naegleria* infection is characterized by a fulminant meningo-encephalitis producing death three to seven days after exposure. The portal of entry is the olfactory neuro-epithelium. The pathological changes consist of an acute haemorrhagic necrotizing meningo-encephalitis with scant purulent exudate, mainly on the base of the brain and cerebellum. Trophozoites can be seen within these lesions and are located mainly around blood vessels. *Acanthamoeba* produces a chronic or subacute granulomatous encephalitis, and trophozoites and cysts are present in the lesions. The portal of entry is probably the skin or respiratory tract, and the parasite reaches the central nervous system by haematogenous spread.

Electron microscopic studies of the trophozoite forms of *Naegleria*[16,68] have revealed a single, vesicular, relatively small nucleus with a centrally located nucleolus (Fig. 10.2). Endoplasmic reticulum in *Naegleria* trophozoites is poorly developed, but mitochondria are numerous and have a characteristic curved 'dumb-bell' shape — although 'cup-shaped' and 'oval' forms are also seen. Digestive vacuoles can be easily identified by their content of ingested material. Of the cytoplasmic inclusions, the most numerous and prominent are electron-dense fat globules, up to 1 μm in diameter. Virus-like particles have been seen in electron micrographs of some preparations of *Naegleria*;[96] their presence, however, was found to be unrelated to the presence of cytopathogens.[29]

In contrast to cases of *Naegleria* infections, which frequently occur in healthy young individuals with a history of recent water-related recreational activities, *Acanthamoeba* infection usually occurs in debilitated chronically ill, or immunosuppressed individuals. Martinez and coworkers[41,66,70,127] examined ultrathin sections of nasal mucosa and of central nervous tissue from patients infected with *Acanthamoeba*. Despite some postmortem autolysis of the tissue and preliminary fixation in formalin instead of glutaraldehyde, the amoebic trophozoites and cysts were well preserved (Figs 10.3 and 10.4). The cytoplasm of trophozoites contained numerous mitochondria with electron-dense cristae, vesicles of different sizes, vacuoles, lysosomes and glycogen granules (Fig. 10.3). Some trophozoites had a well developed Golgi system, and smooth and rough endoplasmic reticulum. The nucleus was eccentrically located and contained a dense nucleolus of irregular shape. Some trophozoites were found to be in a pre-encystment stage with the cytoplasm condensed all around the cytoplasmic membrane. The mean diameter of a mature *Acanthamoeba* cyst was about 10 μm. The cysts possessed a prominent, thick, wrinkled wall (Fig. 10.4)[70,127] which was occasionally composed of concentric parallel layers separated by irregular spaces. Sometimes, empty cysts were also observed.

Toxoplasma

Toxoplasma is a member of the subclass Coccidia which also includes the genera *Sarcocystis, Eimeria, Besnoitia, Frenkelia* and *Isospora*.[3,19,28,71] Although *Toxoplasma* was first discovered more than eighty years ago[75] and first reports of *Toxoplasma* infection in man were published half a century ago[130] the widespread interest in this protozoan parasite was evoked only recently in connection with the high incidence of serious *Toxoplasma* infection in patients with the acquired immunodeficiency syndrome (AIDS) and among those who were immunocompromised. *Toxoplasma* invades almost all cells regardless of their biological and physiological characteristics. Infection in man usually involves the brain, heart, lungs, lymphatic system and skin. Most infections in man are asymptomatic but at times the parasite causes devastating disease. Infection may be acquired congenitally or postnatally.[28]

According to recent data,[19,81,87,106] EM is valuable in confirming a histological diagnosis of *Toxoplasma* infection, and in some cases[106] it may be the diagnostic tool of choice. In cerebral toxoplasmosis the minute tachyzoite forms of the protozoan are scattered among the cellular debris but are easily detectable by EM (Fig. 10.5), although they are difficult to visualize by light microscopy — even with special stains. Cerezo and coworkers[19] report the case of a patient with AIDS in whom the specific diagnosis was established by EM which led to the timely initiation of effective treatment. Tang and collaborators[106] concluded on the basis of their experience that 'electron microscopy may be superior to other methods in the diagnosis of toxoplasmosis for many reasons: (1) EM demonstrates the organism directly, whereas immunologic methods only indirectly suggest the presence of the organism; (2) anti-sera for immunofluorescent assays are not widely available and their sensitivity in studying immunocompromised hosts with possible toxoplasmosis is unknown; (3) serologic studies are often negative in immunocompromised patients. Negative immunologic results should not detract from the value of positive EM findings; (4) with rapid EM processing techniques, the diagnosis of toxoplasmosis may be made by EM before immunologic tests or protozoan isolation can be accomplished; (5) *Toxoplasma gondii* is highly infective, and its isolation may be dangerous to laboratory workers.'.

Electron microscopic examination of brain biopsies reveals the cysts of *Toxoplasma* and numbers of tachyzoites both free and inside the host cells.[19,33,40,81,106,118] Variability of shape, size and stages of development seems to be characteristic of *Toxoplasma*. Usually the tachyzoites (rapidly dividing forms) of *Toxoplasma* are crescent-shaped, about 2 × 6 μm in size with a cone-shaped narrow anterior end (the conoid) and a rounded posterior (Figs 10.5–10.7). Intracellular tachyzoites are often ovoid. In addition to the usual cytoplasmic organelles such as mitochondria, endoplasmic

reticulum, vacuoles, Golgi apparatus and dense bodies, tachyzoites contain a polar ring, conoid, rhoptries and micronemes. The polar ring, which encircles a cylindrical, truncated cone (the conoid), is visible at the anterior end of the tachyzoite as an osmiophilic thickening of the inner membrane. The conoid consists of rods or tubules, and encloses 'gland-like' structures with an anterior narrow neck. These are called rhoptries, are 8–10 in number, and probably have a secretory function (hyaluronidase, lysosomal enzymes). Other characteristic organelles located at the anterior end of tachyzoites are toxonemes (micronemes) — numerous, convoluted, tube-like structures closely associated with the conoid. All these distinctive anterior-end organelles are thought to be associated with the process of host cell entry.[3,125,126] Tachyzoites, which divide by repeated endodyogeny (a specialized form of division in which two daughter cells are formed within the mother cell — the mother cell being destroyed during this process), fill the host cells, forming a membrane-bounded intracytoplasmic vacuole which is known as a parasitophorous vacuole.

Pseudocysts — host cells containing numerous tachyzoites — are often seen in necropsies and biopsies of brain infected with *Toxoplasma*. The tissue cysts — the resting stage of the parasite — contain bradyzoites (slowly multiplying forms of *Toxoplasma*) which differ structurally only slightly from tachyzoites (Figs 10.8 and 10.9). Cysts may remain in the host tissues throughout the lifespan of the host without causing any recognizable symptoms. Such cysts are sometimes found in brain and skeletal muscles at autopsy in patients dying of diseases other than toxoplasmosis. The presence in tissues, among the various developmental stages, of cysts with thick walls suggests that reactivation of a chronic infection may have occurred, probably as a result of alteration of immune function.

Although *Toxoplasma* affects particularly often the central nervous system, other tissues, especially cardiac muscle, lymph nodes and eye are also the target of this parasite. Myocarditis may occur in the acute, chronic or relapsing forms of toxoplasmosis. Rose and coworkers[87] described a patient with toxoplasmosis in whom infection had occurred from a donor heart during cardiac transplantation. Electron microscopy performed on endomyocardial biopsy showed the typical ultrastructural appearance of toxoplasmosis with the protozoan cells in different stages of development.

Electron microscopic studies of toxoplasmic retinochoroiditis have been performed on the eyes of patients without a history of immunosuppression,[84] on patients after high-dose corticosteroid administration[76] and in patients after radio- and chemo-therapy for systemic lymphoma.[132] Ultrastructural examination of the retina revealed numerous cysts of *Toxoplasma* in various stages of development and several tachyzoite forms. Numerous free *Toxoplasma* organisms were consistently present at the interface between necrotic and healthy retina. In these instances EM, according to

Nicholson & Wolchok[76] '... provided a useful technique for confirming the identity of the infecting organism in the absence of serologlc or culture data.'.

Nosema

Nosematosis — a disease caused by *Nosema* (Fig. 10.10), a common protozoan parasite of all major groups of animals — has been documented to occur also in man. Electron microscopy studies of this parasite in human tissue have been performed by Margileth et al,[64] and more recently by Pinnolis and coworkers.[79] *Nosema* organisms were seen singly or in small groups, both intracellularly and extracellularly. Sporont and sporoblast stages of the parasite were observed, but plasmodial stages were not identifiable. Tissue damage caused by the presence of the parasite and the ensuing inflammatory infiltrate were also observed. Since the biopsy material was inadequately prepared (electron microscopy was done on portions of the diaphragm previously embedded in paraffin for light microscopy), the parasite was identified only as *Nosema* without the species classification. Further studies of this parasite are needed, and, as Margileth and coworkers[64] indicate: 'biopsy specimens of diseased tissue and examination both by light and electron microscopy are indicated in suspected cases of nosematosis. Such studies may be worthwhile since sulfisonazole might be effective.'.

Babesia

The number of cases of human babesial infection has increased considerably during the last decade.[24,43,104] Diagnosis of babesiasis is usually made by the identification of intra-erythrocytic parasites in Giemsa-stained thick and thin smears of peripheral blood. While most cases of babesiasis were described in light microscopic studies, some authors have also used transmission and scanning electron microscopy to characterize the morphology of the infectious agent and the parasitized human erythrocytes.[86,104] *Babesia* infecting human erythrocytes display pronounced pleomorphism when studied by transmission electron microscopy (Figs 10.11–10.13), and all developmental stages are seen in both reticulocytes and mature erythrocytes.

The parasite can be of round, oval, elongated or amoeboid form. Soon after infecting a new erythrocyte, the parasite loses its thick inner membrane and is enclosed only by the thin outer membrane. Pinocytosis of the erythrocyte cytoplasm by the parasite is observed, and membrane-bound vacuoles with ingested haemoglobin are often seen within the parasites. Single, large, dense bodies called rhoptries, with a characteristic clear zone and numerous small organelles, called micronemes, are observed in the cytoplasm. The nucleus contains homogeneously dispersed chromatin but a nucleolus is absent. Scanning electron microscopy has demonstrated the presence in the peripheral blood of erythrocytes with characteristic protrusions and perforations.[104]

Plasmodium

Human malaria, a disease caused by the protozoan parasites *Plasmodium vivax*, *P. malariae*, *P. falciparum* or *P. ovale*, causes enormous morbidity and mortality in many areas of the world. The diagnosis of malaria is based upon the presence of detectable parasites in the peripheral blood. Usually, this is made by the examination of Giemsa- or Wright-stained blood smears. Light microscopy of plasmodia has enabled investigators to identify different species of malarial parasite and to describe several intracellular organelles. Although EM is practically not used for diagnostic purposes, numerous ultrastructural studies[1,2,4–6] have revealed many new intracellular features in *Plasmodium* (Figs 10.14 and 10.15) and permitted the characterization of the changes in host cells induced by malarial parasite infection. Here we present only a brief description of the exoerythrocytic and erythrocytic stages during the asexual part of the *Plasmodium* life cycle in man and briefly review the changes induced in host cells by malarial parasite infection.

The exoerythocytic stages of malarial parasites, although very similar morphologically to the erythrocytic stages, differs in some aspects from the latter.[5] The exoerythrocytic merozoite and its rhoptries appear to be somewhat elongated. The food vacuoles seen in the exoerythrocytic stages are small and electron-lucent. No typical mitochondria are found, although some species have doublemembrane-bound structures which are considered as the equivalent of mitochondria.[2] The processes of merozoite budding in exo-erythrocytic schizonts are similar to those of the erythrocytic stages, but merozoites are formed only in the former. Ribosomes are abundant in the merozoite cytoplasm, but endoplasmic reticulum is scanty and the Golgi apparatus inconspicuous.

The merozoite of the erythrocytic stage is oval and about 1.5 μm in length and 1 μm in diameter. Beneath the inner membrane of the merozoite a row of subpellicular microtubules originating from the polar ring of the apical complex can be observed. The cytostome — a circular structure through which food is ingested — is situated on the lateral side of the pellicle.[5] The large, round nucleus, with the chromatin clumped at the periphery is usually centrally located but a nucleolus is absent. The food vacuoles are bigger than those in the exoerythrocytic stage and are very electron-dense. Merozoites lack typical mitochondria; instead, doublemembrane-bound structures which are considered to be mitochondria equivalents are observed.[1,5]

Soon after entering into a new blood cell, the merozoite rounds-up; rapid degradation of the inner membrane and microtubules of the pellicular complex, rhoptries and micronemes occur and the trophozoite is formed. Trophozoites become irregular in shape showing often extensive protrusions and invaginations of the cytoplasm. The parasite, surrounded by only a single plasma membrane, is located within a parasitophorous vacuole which originates from the host cell. The chromatin of the trophozoite's single nucleus is more finely granular and filamentous than that in the nucleus of the merozoite. The cytoplasm of the trophozoite is coarsely granular and is filled with free ribosomes and polyribosomes. Host cell cytoplasm, ingested by the cytostome, is often seen in the food vacuoles. Nuclear divisions, which are the first evidence of schizogony, are sometimes observed. The schizont is larger than either the merozoite or trophozoite and possesses more than one nucleus. During schizogony, nuclear division and formation of the cytoplasmic organelles occur. The precursors of the cytoplasmic organelles, which had disappeared during trophozoite development (rhoptries, micronemes, subpellicular microtubules), appear again, and the process of merozoite budding progresses. After one or more schizogonies, some parasites develop into gametocytes (microgametocytes and macrogametocytes).

Gametocytes, when observed by EM,[5] differ from the asexual stages of malarial parasites since they are uninucleated, large parasites with the characteristic pellicle and osmiophilic bodies. The macrogametocytes, in turn, differ from microgametocytes: macrogametocytes possess more ribosomes, more developed endoplasmic reticulum and more osmiophilic bodies than the microgametes.[5]

Erythrocytes infected by malarial parasites show characteristic morphological alterations.[2,22,73] Such structures as caveolar–vesicle complexes, cytoplasmic clefts, nodules and excrescences are present in the erythrocytes infected with the asexual stages of plasmodia but are absent in uninfected red blood cells. The erythrocytes infected with gametocytes have caveola–vesicle complexes and cytoplasmic clefts but lack the excrescences and nodules. Some of these changes are species-specific, and others are not. The pits on the surface of erythrocytes infected with plasmodia can also be seen by scanning electron microscopy.[5] Exoerythrocytic malarial parasites also produce changes in the infected host cell, which increase in size and become distorted.[2]

Cryptosporidium

The interest in this coccidian protozoan parasite increased greatly during the last few years since the establishment of the role of *Cryptosporidium* in AIDS.[36] It is now recognized that this organism is an important cause of gastrointestinal infections in both normal and immunocompromised subjects throughout the world. *Cryptosporidium* can also infect other internal organs.[103] In normal subjects the symptoms may be both severe and persistent, while in immunocompromised patients the infection may be life threatening. Due to the increased number of patients with *Cryptosporidium* infection it is important to develop the appropriate diagnos-

tic techniques for organism recovery and identification. Tissue biopsy and the examination of stool specimens are recommended for diagnostic purposes. Several techniques for the identification of the parasite are recommended: acid-fast stain, the fluorescent auramine–rhodamine stain, PAS and the carbolfuchsin-negative stain.[37]

However, cryptosporidial organisms can easily be missed, and sometimes are difficult to recognize by light microscopy. Electron microscopy (Figs 10.16 and 10.17) can play an important role in detecting the parasite cells in biopsy material and faeces or simply in positively confirming the diagnosis.[10,17,39,45,60,61,98]

Cryptosporidia, like other coccidia, have a complicated life cycle that includes both asexual (schizonts) and sexual (micro- and macro-gamonts) forms.[28] Electron microscopic investigations showed that parasites are usually attached to the microvillar brush border of the epithelial cells, and it is usually possible to identify all cryptosporidial stages in biopsy material. The developing schizont has clearly identifiable nuclei with prominent nucleoli and well developed endoplasmic reticulum. The mature schizont contains fully formed merozoites attached to a residual body surrounded by a thin double-membraned wall. Mature merozoites are surrounded by a pellicle, have well developed RER, Golgi complex and clearly visible rhoptries and micronemes.[10,45,61] No mitochondria, microspores or subpellicular tubules are present. The cytoplasm of the macrogametocytes contains well developed RER and prominent polysaccharide and phospholipid granules. The microgametocyte can be clearly distinguished from the macrogametocyte by the regular, peripherally arranged budding microgametes.[10] The electron-dense nucleus of the mature microgamete is surrounded by a well defined endoplasmic reticulum. Tubular mitochondria can often be identified. Sometimes, zygotic formation can be observed in biopsy material.[10] Although it is usually difficult to find oocysts in biopsy material, oocysts containing developed sporozoites were identified ultrastructurally in human faecal specimens by Baxby and coworkers[9] and by Casemore and collaborators.[17]

Cryptosporidium infection causes several structural changes in the intestinal epithelial cells.[10,61] Many epithelial cells show degenerative changes: microvilli are damaged or absent, protozoan attachment sites show a characteristic dense plate-like thickening of the subplasmalemmal region, while epithelial membrane may enclose the parasite in a parasitophorous vacuole. Parasites on the other hand, develop membranous projections that penetrate into the host cell cytoplasm.

Pneumocystis

Pneumocystosis is the most important opportunistic infection in patients with AIDS,[11,74] occurring in more than 80% of patients with the disease. *Pneumocystis* is also the causative organism of a characteristic form of pneumonia seen in infants and children.[48,74] *Pneumocystis* is a unicellular organism without a definitely established taxonomic position. However, according to prevailing opinion it is a sporozoan of the toxoplasmid type.[31,91]

A variety of methods for diagnosing *Pneumocystis* infection have been described.[74,97] Most of them are based on light microscopic examination of transtracheal or transbronchial biopsies. The parasite cannot be identified in haematoxylin and eosin stains, but methanamine–silver nitrate stains cysts and trophozoites of *Pneumocystis*. It should be emphasized that pneumocystosis is a difficult infection to diagnose, and that histological diagnosis, even with methanamine–silver stains, is not straightforward. Because of this, some authors recommend electron microscopy for a definite diagnosis of *Pneumocystis* infection.[13,48] According to Hasleton and coworkers:[48] 'The rapid embedding technique, which can yield electronmicroscopic results in 3–4 hours, may be of use in the rapid diagnosis of pneumocystis pneumonia'. However, '...the resin used in the rapid embedding technique can sometimes fail to penetrate the specimen adequately and thus the relatively long conventional processing is a useful safeguard.'.[48]

The parasite is easily identified by electron microscopy (Figs 10.18 and 10.19) and several different stages of the protozoan can be recognized. The trophic forms are of two distinct types: the small (1–1.5 μm) round forms, and the large (2–5 μm and even up to 12 μm)[13,48,91] amoeboid forms. The small forms are surrounded by an electron-dense inner membrane and an external membrane which is less electron-dense. The surface of the small trophozoites is smooth, without invaginations. The nucleus is bounded by a double membrane and contains a nucleolus. The electron-dense cytoplasm contains a single mitochondrion with poorly developed cristae, well developed smooth and rough endoplasmic reticulum and a few osmiophilic bodies. A complex tubular structure which surrounds the pellicle of the small trophozoite becomes much more prominent in large trophozoites. The latter are very pleomorphic, have deep surface invaginations, a single nucleus with nucleolus, and poorly developed endoplasmic reticulum. The cytoplasm generally appears much less dense in large than in small trophozoites. The pellicle of large trophozoites lacks the outermost unit membrane which is present in small trophozoites. Very characteristic for the large trophozoites are prominent tubular surface structures which form a kind of pseudopodial surface extensions. These surface projections are probably parts of the parasite body,[48,91] and according to some investigators '...a definite continuity between the tubular surface projections and the trophozoites could be observed.'.[48] However, other authors[14,82] suggest that these structures are of host origin and are part of alveolar macrophage plasma membrane.

The precysts of *Pneumocystis* are oval or circular in shape, about 4 μm in diameter, with relatively smooth surfaces and devoid of surface projections.[102] Unlike the trophozoites, cysts do not contain a single nucleus but have a number of nuclear masses, usually bound by fragmented membranes derived from invaginated portions of plasmalemma. The wall surrounding the cyst is much thicker than that of the trophozoite and forms a multilaminated envelope. The precysts show no internal compartmentation but cysts contain (intracystic) bodies which structurally resemble the trophozoites. The mature cysts comprise a degenerating mother cell, composed of a thick-walled envelope with some cytoplasmic and mitochondrial remnants, and the newly formed intracystic bodies — the future trophozoites. Sometimes, up to eight intracystic bodies may be found lying within the mother cyst. Occasionally, cysts releasing the small trophozoites through a gap in the cyst wall can be observed.[48] Collapse of the empty cysts produce sickle- or crescent-shaped forms which are the most frequently observed and the most easily ultrastructurally identifiable forms in *Pneumocystis* infected tissues.

Giardia

This common parasite has been found in practically all areas of the world. *Giardia* infection of the small intestine is often responsible for outbreaks of diarrhoea and this protozoan is the most commonly identified human pathogenic intestinal parasite.[72,101] The parasite exists in either the cyst or the trophozoite form (Figs 10.20–10.22). A definitive diagnosis can be established only by the detection of the cyst or trophozoite of *Giardia*. The cysts are detected usually in formed stools, whereas the trophozoites can be seen in a loose or watery stool specimen, duodenal fluid and intestinal biopsy. Trichrome or iron–hematoxylin staining are normally used for diagnostic purposes.

Although EM is not used directly for the diagnosis of giardiasis, transmission and scanning electron microscopic studies of the parasite and of the infected small intestine have supplied new information of the morphology of this important pathogen and '...have allowed a deeper clinical evaluation of patients with *G. intestinalis* invasion and a choice of a most rational treatment.'.[56] Therefore, we will present here a brief description of the ultrastructural features of this ubiquitous parasite.

The ultrastructure of human *Giardia* cysts and trophozoites has been studied by several authors.[32,58,94,95,99] Cysts of *Giardia* (Fig. 10.22) are oval bodies with numerous lacunar spaces and vacuoles located at the periphery of the cytoplasm. Two or four nuclei are usually present. The cyst cytoplasm also contains axonemes of flagella, axostyles, median body, portions of the ventral disk and segments of RER.

Trophozoites of *Giardia* have a characteristic appearance (Fig. 10.21). In addition to two nuclei, eight kinetosomes, eight axonemes and eight flagella are arranged symmetrically in two groups. The ventral disc (striated disc), a kind of pressure-resistant microtubular skeleton supporting the domed chambers, is surrounded by the ventro-lateral flange which, in turn, is supported by two marginal plates. Each of the marginal plates is associated with one of the axonemes of the antero-lateral flagella. Microtubules of the striated disc are interconnected and attached to the cell membrane. The spiral formed by the ventral disc microtubules surrounds a central area which is devoid of microtubules and fibres but which encloses membrane-bound vacuoles. Located dorsally to the caudal axonemes is the median body — a microtubular structure typical of the genus. It consists of fascicles of microtubules, some of them equipped with a dense ribbon. In *Giardia intestinalis* the median body has a 'hammer-claw' shape and lies transversely in the middle portion of the cell body. The cytoplasm of *Giardia* trophozoites is filled with granules of glycogen, free ribosomes, polysomes and cisternae of the RER. Mitochondria and Golgi structures are absent.

Trichomonas

Three trichomonad species are human parasites: *Trichomonas vaginalis*, *T. tenax* and *Pentatrichomonas hominis*.[50] Only *T. vaginalis*, which inhabits the urogenital tract, is considered to be pathogenic for humans, and this species has attracted the greatest attention. *T. vaginalis* is detected by routine vaginal smear examination or by routine urinalysis. The parasite can be readily recognized by Giemsa and Leishman stains. Sometimes the cultivation of *T. vaginalis* *in vitro* is necessary for the identification of the parasite.

Electron microscopy is not used for diagnostic purposes in trichomoniasis; however, ultrastructural studies[12,52,55,77,78,121–124] have added considerably to our understanding of the parasite's structure, its interaction with human vaginal and cervical epithelial cells, and the action of antitrichomonadal drugs. At the electron microscopic level *T. vaginalis* has a very characteristic appearance (Figs 10.23–10.26). It is oval or pear-shaped, about 10–20 μm long and 5–10 μm in diameter. Four flagellae and an undulating membrane form the locomotion system. The cell nucleus, enclosed in a double envelope with a few pores, and usually surrounded by RER, is normally oval and located at the anterior part of the parasite. Pelta, costa and parabasal filaments as well as axostyl are the intracellular organelles found in all species of trichomonads. The most prominent among the cytoplasmic inclusions are the microbody-like granules (paraxostylar and paracostal granules) which play an important role in cell metabolism and which are called hydrogenosomes.[62] Mitochondria are absent in trichomonads. Data obtained in cytochemical investigations at the electron microscopic level show that there are some differences in the surface coat composition between pathogenic and mild strains of *T. vaginalis*.[122,123]

Leishmania

Leishmaniasis — a disease caused by a haemoflagellate of the genus *Leishmania* — is, in terms of morbidity and mortality, considered, among the human protozoan diseases, to be second in importance only to malaria.[59,65] *Leishmania* is a digenetic parasite — *i.e.* its life cycle can be completed only in two different hosts: a vertebrate and an insect. Three clinical types of diseases are distinguished: visceral (kala-azar); mucocutaneous (American leishmaniasis) and cutaneous leishmaniasis (oriental sore). Within human tissues, *Leishmania* exists in the amastigote (aflagellate) form (Figs 10.27–10.29). A specific diagnosis can be made by the identification of the leishmanias either in smears or biopsies. Parasites can be detected on Giemsa- or Wright-stained smears. Needle biopsies of the lymph nodes, spleen, liver or skin are used for diagnostic purposes. However, all *Leishmania* species are morphologically indistinguishable and they can be classifed only on the basis of clinical manifestations, epidemiological parameters, growth characteristic in culture media and serological tests.[59,129] Some workers[38,53,110] have suggested that species of the genus *Leishmania* can be distinguished on the basis of their ultrastructure. One of the morphological criteria proposed by Gardener and coworkers[38] was the number of subpellicular microtubules. However, the hope that electron microscopic data permit the clear separation of different species of *Leishmania* was not fulfilled. On the other hand, EM has revealed several details which were not obvious by light microscopy and has aided in the understanding of the host–parasite relationship in leishmaniasis.[21,85,133] In some cases electron microscopy can help in establishing the proper diagnosis; according to Daneshbod[26] 'Electron microscopy provides a simple, rapid method of differentiation of *Leishmania* from *Toxoplasma*, other protozoa, or fungi.'.

When examined with the electron microscope, the amastigote forms of the parasite are seen to be bounded by a two-layered membrane, beneath which a layer of peripheral fibrils is situated. The nucleus (about $1 \times 1.5 \mu$m in size) contains a well-defined nucleolus and peripherally located masses of chromatin. Well developed Golgi complex, RER and numerous ribosomes are present in the cytoplasm. The most interesting feature in representatives of the order Kinetoplastida in general (see: *Trypanosoma*) and *Leishmania* in particular is the kinetoplast — an organelle with a distinct fibrillar electron-dense band of DNA and highly branched 'mitochondrial sleeves' rich in cristae. Close to the kinetoplast there is the small reservoir ('flagellar pocket') with a short, rudimentary flagellum, which does not protrude through the surface of the protozoan.

Characteristic of cutaneous leishmaniasis is an initial heavy invasion of monocytes; later, the lesion is infiltrated by lymphocytes, plasma cells and macrophages. The parasite in its amastigotic form undergoes binary fission within the mononuclear phagocytes, and after rupture of the heavily parasitized cells, the liberated amastigotes spread and infect other macrophages. Ultrastructurally, up to 30 amastigotes may be seen within a single phagocyte.[85] Different types of parasitophorus vacuoles may be seen in the host macrophages.[21] Some vacuoles (type I — small; type II — large) contain a single amastigote. Very large parasitophorous vacuoles (type III) with multiple amastigotes adhering to the membrane have been also observed. When Chulay and coworkers[21] studied *Leishmania* parasites in splenic aspirates from patients with visceral leishmaniasis during treatment with stibogluconate, they noticed that amastigotes were reduced in size, had prominent irregularities of the cell outline, and characteristic changes occurred in their phagolysosomal system. Moreover, several amastigotes appeared to be undergoing autolysis.

Trypanosoma

Three species of the genus *Trypanosoma* are pathogenic to man: *T. cruzi* in America (Chagas' disease) and *T. gambiense* and *T. rhodesiense* in Africa (sleeping sickness). All members of the family Trypanosomidae have a complicated life cycle — they require an insect vector as an intermediate host and metamorphose during development. Both American and African trypanosomiasis are very important public health problems, and the vectors of these diseases have been studied intensively.[34,83,100,109,111–115] African trypanosomes multiply in the blood and other body fluids of man and of a variety of other mammals. *Trypanosoma cruzi* multiplies inside the host cells — mononuclear phagocytes, muscles and other tissues.

Since the clinical features of *Trypanosoma* infection are not typical, the diagnosis has to be made by demonstrating the parasite in blood, lymph fluid or cerebrospinal fluid or in biopsies of different body organs. Serological methods are also widely used for the diagnosis of both American and African trypanosomiasis. Xenodiagnosis is often used for the diagnosis of Chagas' disease. None of these methods, however, is fully successful for precise diagnosis. The best results are obtained by carrying out examinations by several methods in parallel.[109]

There are numerous publications available concerning the ultrastructure of *Trypanosoma*.[27,83,111–115] Although we could not find in the literature examples of EM being used for direct diagnostic purposes in trypanosomiasis, electron microscopic studies, in combination with techniques such as isoenzyme analysis, specific genetic probes, monoclonal antibodies application, have advanced our knowledge of the structure and pathogenicity of different species of *Trypanosoma* and of some aspects of the host–parasite relationships in trypanosomiasis.[27,114]

Electron microscopic studies of the successive stages in the life cycle of *Trypanosoma* revealed complex morphological changes in the parasite's architecture.[27,111] The basic cell structure of *Trypanosoma* (Figs 10.30–10.34) is essentially the same as that of *Leishmania*. The spindle-shaped cell is surrounded by a row of parallel microtubules located under the cell membrane. The flagellum is located in an invagination of the cell surface known as the flagellar pocket. The nucleus is in a central or slightly posterior position with the Golgi complex nearby. The kinetoplast has a very characteristic structure with extranuclear DNA occupying the centre of this organelle and a relatively poorly developed mitochondrial compartment. A variety of microbodies (lysosomes, glycosomes) are present in the cytoplasm. The surface coat (12–15 nm thick) forms a monolayer on the surface of the African trypanosomes and is clearly visible by EM. This surface coat is present during all mammalian stages of the parasite's life cycle but it disappears in the vector tissue. In the case of *Trypanosoma cruzi* the surface coat is less prominent. The changes in the glycoprotein composition (variant surface glycoproteins) of the surface coat of African trypanosomes play an important role in the survival strategy of these parasites.[100]

The mechanism of action of different antitrypanosomal drugs is still far from being resolved.[47,54] Macadam & Williamson[63] have investigated by EM the changes in the structure of *Trypanosoma* caused by different drugs. They found that the primary focus of trypanocides is the DNA core of the kinetoplast. After diamidine drug treatment, for example, the fibrillar lamellae disintegrate and highly opaque circular bodies appear.

OTHER PARASITES

Until now, we have concentrated on the ultrastructural analysis of the protozoan parasites. Numerous representatives of all other groups of human parasites have also been studied by EM. However, most of these investigations were performed on material from experimentally infected animals or *in vitro*. Very limited data are available on the ultrastructure of parasites from human tissues and on the ultrastructural changes in human organs infected by nematodes, trematodes or cestodes. Because of the relatively large size of the parasites belonging to these systematic groups, EM is rarely used in the diagnosis *sensu stricto*. However, information accumulated from ultrastructural investigations has thrown new light on many aspects of parasite structure, life cycle and host–parasite relationships during many parasitic infections of man.

Voge & Brown[119] studied by scanning and transmission EM the racemose cysts of cestodes from the human brain. They found that although the overall structure of the racemose cysticercus teguments and subtegumental areas were essentially the same as in other cestode teguments, some differences in the pattern of distribution of the internal structures were observed. The authors also discuss the possible function of the fine network of fibres connecting the microvilli. Damyanov and coworkers[25] employed electron microscopy for ultrastructural studies of hydatid disease of the liver in man. Electron microscopy was conducted in 15 cases of hydatid disease of the liver and various ultrastructural changes in diseased liver were described. An interesting case of the application of scanning electron microscopy for the identification of a cuterebra larva surgically removed from a human eye was described by Custis and coworkers[23] (Figs 10.35–10.37). According to the authors: 'The study demonstrates the usefulness of scanning electron microscopy for taxonomic identification of fly larvae. Since even small fragments of these organisms may contain characteristic features of external morphology, scanning electron microscopy may be useful in cases where the specimen is damaged or incomplete.'.

We do not expect that electron microscopy can be widely used in the diagnosis of parasitic infections other than those caused by protozoa. However, with the accumulation of ultrastructural data about different stages of parasites, both transmission and scanning electron microscopy may be sometimes of use for the definite diagnosis of these infectious agents.

REFERENCES

1. Aikawa M 1971 *Plasmodium*: the fine structure of malarial parasites. Experimental Parasitology 30: 284–320
2. Aikawa M 1977 Variations in structure and function during the life cycle of malarial parasites. Bulletin of the World Health Organisation 55: 139–156
3. Aikawa M, Komata Y, Asai T, Midorikawa D 1976 Transmission and scanning electron microscopy of host cell entry by *Toxoplasma gondii*. American Journal of Pathology 87: 285–296
4. Aikawa M, Miller L-M 1983 Structural alteration of the erythrocyte membrane during malarial parasite invasion and intraerythrocytic development. In: Evered D, Whelan J (eds) Malaria and red cell. CIBA Foundation Symposium 94. Pitman, London, pp 45–63
5. Aikawa M, Seed T M 1980 Morphology of plasmodia. In: Kreier J P (ed) Malaria, vol 1, Academic Press, New York, pp 285–344
6. Aikawa M, Sterling C R 1974 Intracellular parasitic protozoa. Academic Press, New York
7. Aikawa M, Suzuki M, Gutierrez Y 1980 Pathology of malaria. In: Kreier J P (ed) Malaria, vol 2. Academic Press, New York, pp 47–102
8. Aley S B, Scott W A, Cohan Z A 1980 Plasma membrane of *Entamoeba histolytica*. Journal of Experimental Medicine 152: 391–404
9. Baxby D, Getty B, Blundell N, Ratcliffe S 1984 Recognition of whole *Cryptosporidium* oocysts in feces by negative staining and electron microscopy. Journal of Clinical Microbiology 19: 566–567
10. Bird R G, Smith M D 1980 Cryptosporidiosis in man: parasite life cycle and fine structural pathology. Journal of Pathology 132: 217–233
11. Blaser M J, Cohn D L 1986 Opportunistic infections in patients with AIDS: clues to the epidemiology of AIDS and the relative virulence of pathogens. Reviews of Infectious Diseases 8: 21–30
12. Bonilla-Musoles F 1984 The destructive effect of Salco Trichovac-induced serum antibodies on *Trichomonas vaginalis*: an electron microscopic investigation. Gynakologische Rundschau, Basel 24: 38–43
13. Bouton C, Kernbaum S, Christol D, Trinh Dinh H, Vezinet F, Gutman L, Seman M, Bastin R 1977 Diagnostic morphologique du *Pneumocystis carinii*. Pathologie Biologie 25: 153–160
14. Brzosko W J, Madalinski K, Kawczynski K 1971 Immunochemistry in studies on the pathogenesis of *Pneumocystis* pneumonia in infants. Annals of the New York Academy of Sciences 177: 156–170
15. Carter R F 1969 Sensitivity to amphotericin B of *Naegleria* sp. isolated from a case of primary amoebic meningoencephalitis. Journal of Clinical Pathology 22: 470–474
16. Carter R F 1970 Description of a *Naegleria* sp. isolated from two cases of primary amoebic meningoencephalitis, and the experimental pathological changes induced by it. Journal of Pathology 100: 217–244
17. Casemore D P, Armstrong M, Sands R L 1985 The laboratory diagnosis of cryptosporidiosis. Journal of Clinical Pathology 38: 1337–1341
18. Cerezo L 1986 Cerebral toxoplasmosis. American Journal of Clinical Pathology 85: 757–758
19. Cerezo L, Alvarez M, Price G 1985 Electron microscopic diagnosis of cerebral toxoplasmosis. Journal of Neurosurgery 63: 470–472
20. Chang S L 1971 Small, free-living amebas: cultivation, quantitation, identification, classification, pathogenesis and resistance. Current Topics in Comparative Pathobiology 1: 201–254
21. Chulay J D, Fawcett D W, Chunge C N 1985 Electron microscopy of *Leishmania donovani* in splenic aspirates from patients with visceral leishmaniasis during treatment with sodium stibogluconate. Annals of Tropical Medicine and Parasitology 79: 417–429
22. Collins W E, Aikawa m 1977 Plasmodia of nonhuman primates. In: Kreier J P (ed) Parasitic Protozoa, vol 3. Academic Press, New York, pp 467–492
23. Custis P H, Pakalnis V A, Klintworth G K, Anderson W B, Machemer R 1983 Posterior internal ophthalmomyiasis. Identification of a surgically removed cuterebra larva by scanning electron microscopy. Ophthalmology 90: 1583–1590
24. Dammin G J, Spielman A, Benach J L, Piesman J 1981 The rising incidence of clinical *Babesia microti* infection. Human Pathology 12: 398–400
25. Damyanov B D, Stoyanov G I, Nikolova V A 1985 Hydatid disease of the liver: ultrastructural pathogenetic aspects and clinical and laboratory comparisons. Khirurgiya 25: 65–67 (in Russian)
26. Daneshbod K 1978 Localized lymphadenitis due to leishmania simulating toxoplasmosis, value of electron microscopy for differentiation. American Journal of Clinical Pathology 69: 462–467
27. De Souza W 1984 Cell biology of *Trypanosoma cruzi*. International Review of Cytology 86: 197–283
28. Dubey J P 1977 *Toxoplasma, Hammondia, Besnoitia, Sarcocystis* and other tissue cyst-forming Coccidia of man and animals. In: Kreier J P (ed) Parasitic protozoa, vol 3. Academic Press, New York, pp 101–237
29. Dunnebacke T H, Schuster F L 1977 The nature of a cytopathogenic material present in amebae of the genus *Naegleria*. American Journal of Tropical Medicine and Hygiene 26: 412–428
30. Eaton R D P, Meerovitch E, Costerton J W 1970 The functional morphology of pathogenicity in *Entamoeba histolytica*. Annals of Tropical Medicine and Parasitology 64: 299–304
31. Faust E C, Beaver P C, Jung R C 1975 Animals agents and vectors of human diseases, 4th edn. Lea and Febiger, Philadelphia, pp 118–121
32. Feely D E, Erlandsen S L, Chase D G 1984 Structure of the trophozoite and cyst. In: Erlandsen S L, Meyer E A (eds) *Giardia* and giardiasis. Biology, Pathogenesis and Epidemiology. Plenum, New York, pp 3–31
33. Fenzi F, Simonati A, Nardelli E, Novelli P, Galiazzo Rizzuto S, Rizzuto N 1982 Congenital toxoplasmosis: histological and ultrastructural study. Italian Journal of Neurological Sciences 1: 49–58
34. Fife H H 1976 Serodiagnosis of trypanosomiasis. In: Cohen S, Sailun E (eds) Immunology of parasitic infections. Blackwell Scientific, London, pp 49–58
35. Fowler M, Carter R E F 1965 Acute pyogenic meningitis probably due to *Acanthamoeba* sp.: a preliminary report. British Medical Journal 2:740–742
36. Gallo R C 1987 The AIDS virus. Scientific American 256: 46–56
37. Garcia L S, Bruckner D A, Brewer T C, Shimizu R Y 1983 Techniques for the recovery and identification of *Cryptosporidium* oocyst from stool specimens. Journal of Clinical Microbiology 18: 185–190

38. Gardener P J, Schory L, Chance M L 1977 Species differentiation in the genus *Leishmania* by morphometric studies with the electron microscope. Annals of Tropical Medicine and Parasitology 71: 147–155

39. Garone M A, Winston B J, Lewis J H 1986 Cryptosporidiosis of the stomach. American Journal of Gastroenterology 81: 465–470

40. Ghatak N R, Zimmerman H M 1973 Fine structure of *Toxoplasma* in the human brain. Archives of Pathology 95: 276–283

41. Gonzalez M M, Gould E, Dickinson G, Martinez A J, Visvesvara G, Cleary T J, Hensley G T 1986 Acquired immunodeficiency syndrome associated with *Acanthamoeba* infection and other opportunistic organisms. Archives of Pathology and Laboratory Medicine 110: 749–751

42. Griffin J L 1978 Pathogenic free-living amoebae. In: Kreier J P (ed) Parasitic Protozoa, vol 2. Academic Press, New York, pp 508–550

43. Griffin J L, Juniper K 1971 Ultrastructure of *Entamoeba histolytica* from human amebic dysentery. Archives of Pathology 21: 271–280

44. Gross T L, Wheat J, Bartlett M, O'Connor K W 1986 AIDS and multiple system involvement with *Cryptosporidium*. American Journal of Gastroenterology 81: 456–458

45. Guarda L A, Stein S A, Cleary K A, Ordonez N G 1983 Human cryptosporidiosis in the acquired immune deficiency syndrome. Archives of Pathology and Laboratory Medicine 107: 562–566

46. Guerrant R L 1986 The global problem of amebiasis: current status, research needs, and opportunities for progress. Review of Infectious Diseases 8: 218–227

47. Gutteridge W E 1985 Trypanosomiasis. Existing chemotherapy and its limitations. British Medical Journal 41: 162–168

48. Hasleton P S, Curry A, Rankin E M 1981 *Pneumocystis carinii* pneumonia: a light microscopical and ultrastructural study. Journal of Clinical Pathology 34: 1138–1146

49. Healy G R, Ruebush T K 1980 Morphology of *Babesia microti* in human blood smears. American Journal of Clinical Pathology 73: 107–109

50. Honigberg B M 1978 Trichomonads of importance in human medicine. In: Kreier J P (ed) Parasitic Protozoa, vol 2. Academic Press, New York, pp 275–454

51. Honigberg B M, 1978 Trichomonads of veterinary importance. In: Kreier J P (ed) Parasitic protozoa, vol 2. Academic Press, New York, pp 163–274

52. Honigberg B M Volkmann D, Entzeroth R, Scholtysek E 1984 A freeze-fracture electron microscope study of *Trichomonas vaginalis* Donné and *Trichomonas foetus* (Riedmüler). Journal of Protozoology 31: 116–131

53. Hoogstraal H, Heyneman D 1969 Leishmaniasis in the Sudan Republic. Final epidemiologic report. American Journal of Tropical Medicine and Hygiene 18: 1091–1210

54. Howells R E 1985 The modes of action of some anti-protozoal drugs. Parasitology 90: 687–703

55. Jodczyk K J, Kazanowska W, Zimnoch L, Karpowicz M J 1980 Diagnostic applications of electron microscopy in trichomoniasis. Patologia Polska 4: 524–531

56. Kociecka W, Gustowska L, Gawronski M, Blotna M, Knapowska M 1984 Evaluation of jejunal mucosa biopsy in patients with giardiasis. Wiadomosci Parazytologiczne 30: 311–319

57. Kocoshis S A, Cibull M L, Davis T E, Hinton J T, Seip M, Banwell J G 1984 Intestinal and pulmonary cryptosporidiosis in an infant with severe combined immune deficiency. Journal of Pediatric Gastroenterology and Nutrition 3: 149–157

58. Kulda J, Nohynkova E 1978 Flagellates of the human intestine and of intestines of other species. In: Kreier J P (ed) Parasitic protozoa, vol 2. Academic Press, New York, pp 2–138

59. Lainson R, Shaw J J 1978 Epidemiology and ecology of leishmaniasis in Latin America. Nature 273: 595–600

60. Le Charpentier Y, Galian A, Messing B, Andreani T, Modigliani R, Lavergne A, Hoang C, Puel F, Houin R 1982 Diagnostic ultrastructural d'une infection intestinale humaine à *Cryptosporidium* Sp. Annalles de Pathologie 2: 336–338

61. Lefkowitch J H, Krumholz S, Kuo-Ching Feng-Chen, Griffin P, Despommier D, Brasitus T A 1984 Cryptosporidiosis of the human small intestine: a light and electron microscopic study. Human Pathology 15: 746–752

62. Lindmark D A, Müller M 1973 Hydrogenosome, a cytoplasmic organelle of the anaerobic flagellate *Tritrichomonas foetus*, and its role in pyruvate metabolism. Journal of Biological Chemistry 235: 7724–7728

63. Macadam R F, Williamson J 1972 Drug effects on the fine structure of *Trypanosoma rhodesiense*: diamidines. Transactions of the Royal Society of Tropical Medicine and Hygiene 66: 897–904

64. Margileth A M, Strano A J, Chandra R, Neafie R, Blum M, McCully R M 1973 Disseminated nosematosis in an immunologically compromised infant. Archives of Pathology 95: 145–150

65. Marsden P D 1979 Current concepts in parasitology: Leishmaniasis. New England Journal of Medicine 300: 350–352

66. Martinez A J, Fultz D G, Amstrong C E 1976 The value of electron microscopy in the differential diagnosis of amebic meningoencephalitis. In: G W Bailey (ed) 34th Annual Conference of Electron Microscopy Society of America, Miami Beach 26: 226–227

67. Martinez A J, Kasprzak W 1980 Pathogenic free-living amoebae — a review. Wiadomosci Parazytologiczne 26: 495–522

68. Martinez A J, Nelson E C, Jones M M, Duma R J, Rosenblum W I 1971 Experimental *Naegleria* meningoencephalitis in mice. An electron microscope study. Laboratory Investigation 25: 465–475

69. Martinez-Palomo A, Gonzalez-Robles A, Chavez de Ramirez B 1976 Ultrastructural study of various *Entamoeba* strains. In: Sepulveda B, Diamond L S (eds) Proceedings of the International Conference on Amebiasis. IMSS, Mexico, pp 226–237

70. Martinez A J, Sotelo-Avila C, Garcia-Tamayo J, Moron J T, Willaert E, Stamm W P 1977 Meningoencephalitis due to *Acanthamoeba* sp. Pathogenesis and clinico-pathological study. Acta Neuropathologica 37: 183–191

71. Melhorn H, Frenkel J K 1980 Ultrastructural comparison of cysts and zoites of *Toxoplasma gondii*, *Sarcocystis muris* and *Hammondia hammondi* in skeletal muscle of mice. Journal of Parasitology 66: 59–67

72. Meyer E A, Radalescu S 1979 *Giardia* and giardiasis. Advances in Parasitology 17: 1–47

73. Miller L H 1972 The ultrastructure of red cells infected by *Plasmodium falciparum* in man. Transactions of the Royal Society of Tropical Medicine and Hygiene 66: 459–462

74. Mills J 1986 *Pneumocystis carinii* and *Toxoplasma gondii* infection in patients with AIDS. Reviews of Infectious Diseases 8: 1001–1011

75. Nicolle C, Manceaux L 1908 Sur un protozaire nouveau du gondi (*Toxoplasma* N. Gen). Archives Institute Pasteur Tunis 2: 97–103

76. Nicholson D H, Wolchok E B 1976 Ocular toxoplasmosis in an adult receiving long-term corticosteroid therapy. Archives of Ophthalmology 94: 248–254

77. Nielsen M H, Nielsen R 1975 Electron microscopy of *Trichomonas vaginalis* Donné: interaction with vaginal epithelium in human trichomoniasis. Acta Pathologica et Microbiologica Scandinavica Section B, Microbiology 83: 305–320

78. Ovcinnikov N M, Delektorskij V V, Turanova E N, Yashkova G N 1975 Further studies of *Trichomonas vaginalis* with transmission and scanning electron microscopy. British Journal of Veneral Diseases 51: 357–375

79. Pinnolis M, Egbert P R, Font R L, Winter F C 1981 Nosematosis of the cornea. Case report, including electron microscopic studies. Archives of Ophthalmology 99: 1044–1047

80. Pittman F E, El-Hashimi W K, Pittman J C 1973 Studies in human amebiasis. II. Light and electron-microscopic observations of colonic mucosa and exudate in acute amebic colitis. Gastroenterology 65: 588–603

81. Powel H C, Gibbs C J Jr, Lorenzo A M, Lampert P W, Gajdusek D C 1978 Toxoplasmosis of the central nervous system in the adult. Electron microscopic observations. Acta Neuropathologica 41: 211–216

82. Price R A, Hughes W T 1974 Histopathology of *Pneumocystis carinii* infestation and infection in malignant disease in childhood. Human Pathology 5: 737–752

83. Raadt P, Seed Y R 1977 Trypanosomes causing disease in man in Africa. In: Kreier J P (ed) Parasitic protozoa, vol 1. Academic Press, New York, pp 175–237

84. Rao N A, Font R L 1977 Toxoplasmic retinochoroiditis: electron-microscopic and immunofluorescence studies of formalin-fixed tissue. Archives of Ophthalmology 95: 273–277

85. Ridley M J, Wells C W 1986 Macrophage–parasite interaction in the lesions of cutaneous leishmaniasis. An ultrastructural study. American Journal of Pathology 123: 79–85
86. Ristic M, Conroy J D, Siwe S, Healy G R Smith A R, Huxsoll D L 1971 *Babesia* species isolated from a woman with clinical babesiosis. American Journal of Tropical Medicine 20: 14–22
87. Rose A G, Uys C J, Novitsky D, Cooper D K C, Barnard C N 1983 Toxoplasmosis of donor and recipient hearts after heterotropic cardiac transplantation. Archives of Pathology and Laboratory Medicine 107: 368–373
88. Rosenbaum R M, Wittner M 1970 Ultrastructure of bacterized and axenic trophozoites of *Entamoeba histolytica* with particular reference to helical bodies. Journal of Cell Biology 45: 367–382
89. Schuppli R 1982 Leishmaniasis: review. Dermatologica 165: 1–6
90. Schuster F L 1975 Ultrastructure of cysts of *Naegleria* sp. a comparative study. Journal of Protozoology 22: 352–359
91. Seed T M, Aikawa M 1977 *Pneumocystis*. In: Kreier J P (ed) Parasitic Protozoa, vol 4. Academic Press, New York, pp 329–357
92. Sheffield H G 1966 Electron microscope study of the proliferative form of *Besnoitia jellisoni*. Journal of Parasitology 52: 583–594
93. Sheffield H G 1970 Schizogony in *Toxoplasma gondii*: an electron microscope study. Proceedings of the Helmintological Society 37: 237–242
94. Sheffield H G 1979 The ultrastructural aspects of *Giardia*. In: Jakubowski W, Hoff J C (eds) Proceedings of the Symposium on Waterborne Transmission of Giardiasis. US Environmental Protection Agency, Cincinnati, pp 9–21
95. Sheffield H G, Bjorvatn B 1977 Ultrastructure of the cyst of *Giardia lamblia*. American Journal of Tropical Medicine and Hygiene 26: 23–30
96. Schuster F L 1969 Virus-like bodies in *Naegleria gruberi*. Journal of Protozoology 16: 724–727
97. Smith J W, Bartlett M S 1982 Laboratory diagnosis of *Pneumocystis carinii* infection. Clinics in Laboratory Medicine 2: 393–406
98. Soave R, Armstrong D 1986 *Cryptosporidium* and cryptosporidiosis. Reviews of Infectious Diseases 8: 1012–1023
99. Soloviev M M, Chentsov J S 1976 Ultrastructure of cysts of *Lamblia muris*. Parazitologiya 4: 510–514
100. Steinert M, Pays E 1985 Genetic control of antigenic variation in trypanosomes. British Medical Bulletin 41: 149–152
101. Stevens D P 1985 Selective primary health care: strategies for control of diseases in the developing world. XIX. Giardiasis. Reviews of Infectious Diseases 7: 530–535
102. Sueishi K, Hisano S, Sumiyoshi A, Tanaka K 1977 Scanning and transmission electron microscopic study of human pulmonary pneumocystosis. Chest 72: 213–216
103. Sun T 1982 Pathology and clinical features of parasitic diseases. Monographs in diagnostic pathology, vol 5. Masson, New York
104. Sun T, Tenenbaum M J, Greenspan J, Teichberg S, Wang R-T, Degnan T, Kaplan M H Morphologic and clinical observations in human infection with *Babesia microti*. Journal of Infectious Diseases 148: 239–248
105. Tandon B N, Tandon H D, Puri B K 1975 An electron microscopic study of liver in hepatomegaly presumably caused by amebiasis. Experimental and Molecular Pathology 22: 118–132
106. Tang T T, Harb J M, Dunne W M, Wells R G, Meyer G A, Chusid M J, Casper J T, Camitta B M 1986 Cerebral toxoplasmosis in an immunocompromised host. A precise and rapid diagnosis by electron microscopy. American Journal of Clinical Pathology 85: 104–110
107. Tchernov Y V 1984 Churayev M Y, Probeus T V, Gordeyeva L M 1984 Ultrastructural study of acid phosphatase activity in *Entamoeba histolytica* trophozoites. Meditzinskaya Parazitologiya i Parazytarnyje Bolezni 20: 3–6
108. Trissl D, Martinez-Palomo A, Arguello C, de la Torre M, de la Hoz R 1977 Surface properties related to Concanavalin A-induced agglutination. A comparative study of several *Entamoeba* strains. Journal of Experimental Medicine 145: 652–665
109. Van Meirvenne N, Le Ray D 1985 Diagnosis of American trypanosomiasis. British Medical Bulletin 41: 156–161
110. Veress B, Abdalla R E, El-Hassan A M 1981 Electron microscopic investigations on leishmaniasis in the Sudan: II. Ultrastructural morphology of macrophage–parasite interaction in human and

hamster infections in vivo. Annals of Tropical Medicine and Parasitology 75: 607–613
111. Vickerman K 1971 Morphological and physiological considerations of extracellular blood protozoa. In: Fallis A M (ed) Ecology and physiology of parasites. University of Toronto Press, Toronto, pp 58–91
112. Vickerman K 1972 Parasitic Protozoa: aspects of the host–parasite interface. In: Mettrich D F, Desser S S (eds) Parasites — their world and ours. Elsevier Biomedical Press, Amsterdam, pp 43–52
113. Vickerman K 1974 The ultrastructure of pathogenic flagellates. In: Trypanosomiasis and leishmaniasis with special reference to Chagas' disease. CIBA Foundation Symposium 20 (New Series). Associated Scientific Publishers, Amsterdam, pp 171–198
114. Vickerman K 1985 Developmental cycles and biology of pathogenic trypanosomes. British Medical Bulletin 41: 105–114
115. Vickerman K, Preston T M 1976 Comparative cell biology of the kinetoplastid flagellates. In: Lumsden W H R, Evans D A (eds) Biology of the Kinetoplastida. London, Academic Press, pp 35–130
116. Visvesvara G S, Callaway C S, Healy G R 1973 Light and electron microscopic studies on the mechanisms of pathogenesis of *Naegleria fowleri* in mouse brain and tissue culture. Journal of Protozoology 20: 438–499
117. Visvesvara G S, Jones D B, Robinson N M 1975 Isolation, identification and biological characterization of *Acanthamoeba polyphaga* from a human eye. American Journal of Tropical Medicine and Hygiene 24: 784–790
118. Vital A Dupont A, Guiot M C, L'homme D, Manier G, Castaing Y. 1983 Encéphalite toxoplasmique au cours d'un syndrome immunodeficitaire acquis (S.I.D.A.) Annales due Pathologie 3: 80–82
119. Voge M, Brown W J 1979 Fine structure of a racemose cysticercus from human brain. Journal of Parasitology 65: 262–266
120. Walsh J A 1986 Problems in recognition and diagnosis of amebiasis: estimation of the global magnitude of morbidity and mortality. Reviews of Infectious Diseases 8: 228–238
121. Warton A, Honigberg B M 1979 Structure of trichomonads as revealed by scanning electron microscopy. Journal of Protozoology 26:56–62
122. Warton A, Honigberg B M 1980 Lectin analysis of surface saccharides in two *Trichomonas vaginalis* strains differing in pathogenicity. Journal of Protozoology 27: 410–419
123. Warton A, Honigberg B M 1983 Analysis of surface saccharides in *Trichomonas vaginalis* strains with various pathogenicity levels by fluorescein-conjugated plant lectins. Zeitschrift für Parasitenkunde 69: 149–159
124. Warton A, Papadimitriou J M, Venaile T J, Mendis A H W, Robinson B W S 1988 Human amnion membrane as a model for studying the host-parasite relationship in trichomoniasis. International Journal for Parasitology 7: 1003–1005
125. Werk R 1985 How does *Toxoplasma gondii* enter host cells? Reviews of Infectious Diseases 7: 449–457
126. Werk R, Bommer W 1980 *Toxoplasma gondii*: membrane properties of active energy-dependent invasion of host cells. Tropenmedizine und Parasitologie 31: 417–420
127. Wiley C A, Safrin R E, Davis C E, Lampert P W, Braude A I, Martinez A J, Visvesvara G S 1987 *Acanthamoeba* meningoencephalitis in patients with AIDS. Journal of Infectious Diseases 155: 130–133
128. Willaert E 1974 Primary amoebic meningo-encephalitis. A selected bibliography and tabular survey of cases. Journal of Neurosurgery 54: 429–440
129. Williams P, Coelko M 1978 Taxomony and transmission of *Leishmania*. Advances in Parasitology 16: 1–42
130. Wolf A, Cowen D 1937 Granulomatous encephalomyelitis due to an encephalitozoon (encephalitozoic encephalomyelitis). A new protozoan disease of man. Bulletin of the Neurology Institute, New York 6: 306–335
131. Wong M M, Karr S L Jr, Balamuth W B 1975 Experimental infections with pathogenic free-living amebae in laboratory primate hosts: a study on susceptibility to *Naegleria fowleri*. Journal of Parasitology 61: 199–208

132. Yeo J H, Jakobiec F A, Iwamoto T, Richard G, Kreissig I 1983 Opportunistic toxoplasmic retinochoroiditis following chemotherapy for systemic lymphoma. A light and electron microscopic study. Ophthalmology 90: 885–898

133. Zuckerman A, Lainson R 1977 *Leishmania*. In: Kreier J P (ed) Parasitic protozoa, vol. 1. Academic Press, New York, pp 58–133

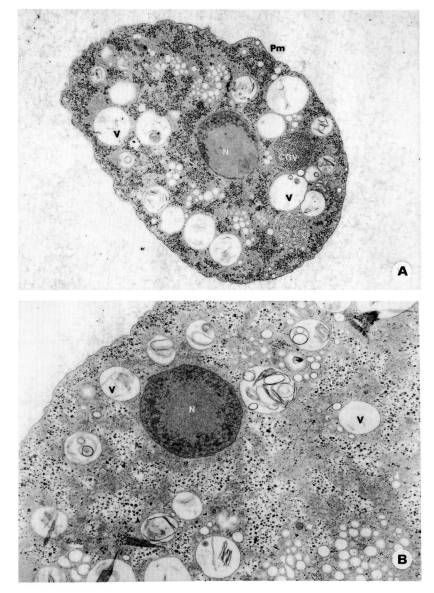

Fig. 10.1 **A** *Entamoeba histolytica*. Pm = plasma membrane; N = nucleus; V = vacuoles; CGV = chromatic granule-containing vacuoles. (× 3300) Unpublished micrograph, courtesy of Dr Chin Thack Soh, Wonkwang University Medical College, IRI, Korea. **B** *Entamoeba histolytica*. N = nucleus with peripheral chromatin; V = various types of vacuoles; glycogen masses (Gly) in cytoplasm are indicated by arrow heads. (× 5800) Unpublished micrograph, courtesy of Dr Chin Thack Soh, Wonkwang University Medical College, IRI, Korea.

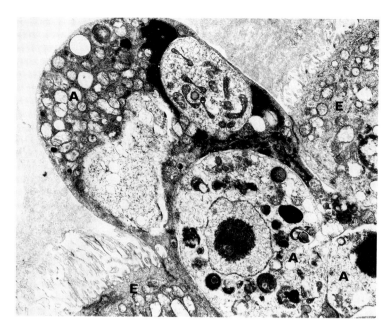

Fig. 10.2 *Naegleria fowleri.* A sustentacular cell of the olfactory epithelium engorged with amoebae. One amoeba contains typical dumb–bell-shaped mitochondria. Lack of microvilli may be related to increased volume of the cell during phagocytosis. A = amoebae; E = epithelial cells. (× 5500) Micrograph courtesy of Dr A Julio Martinez et al, reprinted with the permission of the publishers of Laboratory Investigation.

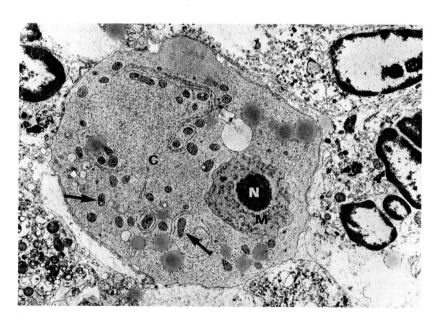

Fig. 10.3 *Acanthamoeba castellani:* trophozoite. A trophozoite encompassed by inflammatory cells and cellular debris in nasal mucosa. N = nucleolus; M = nucleus; C = cytoplasm; arrows point to mitochondria. (× 5600) Micrograph courtesy of Dr M M Gonzalez et al, reprinted with the permission of the publishers of Archives of Pathology and Laboratory Medicine.

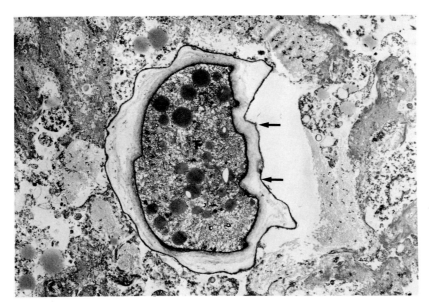

Fig. 10.4 *Acanthamoeba castellani*: cyst. A cyst in an intramuscular abscess is shown. T = condensed trophozoite inside the cyst; arrows point to double layer wall of cyst. (× 4000) Micrograph courtesy of Dr M M Gonzalez et al, reprinted with the permission of the publishers of Archives of Pathology and Laboratory Medicine.

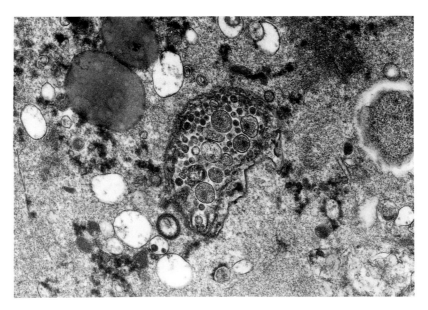

Fig. 10.5 *Toxoplasma gondii*: tachyzoite. A typical, crescent-shaped tachyzoite is clearly visible among the cellular debris of the necrotic area of the human brain. (× 19 800) Micrograph courtesy of Dr A Vital et al, reprinted with the permission of the publishers of Annales du Pathologie.

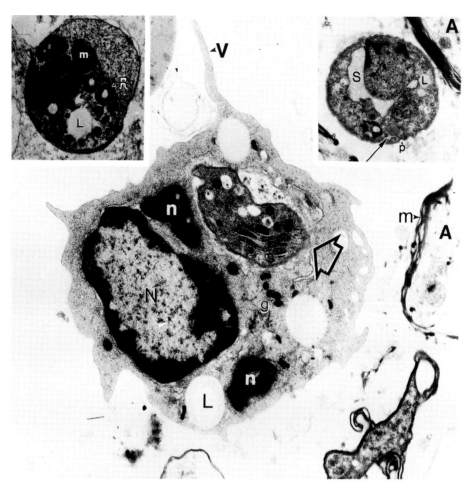

Fig. 10.6 *Toxoplasma condii*: tachyzoite. A tachyzoite (arrow) inside a neutrophil. The protozoan is ensconced within a parasitophorous vacuole. N = nucleus; n = segmented fragments of the nucleus; g = electron-dense storage granules; L = lipid droplets. A fragment of an axon (A) is also seen. (× 22 400) *Left inset* A cross section of a toxoplasmic tachyzoite with rhoptries (R), lipid droplets (L), and secretory granules (S). (× 15 800) *Right inset* A cross section of a tachyzoite with a multilayered pellicle (P), lipid droplets (L) and secretory granules (S). (× 11 500) Micrographs courtesy of Dr T T Tang et al, reprinted with the permission of the publishers of American Journal of Clinical Pathology.

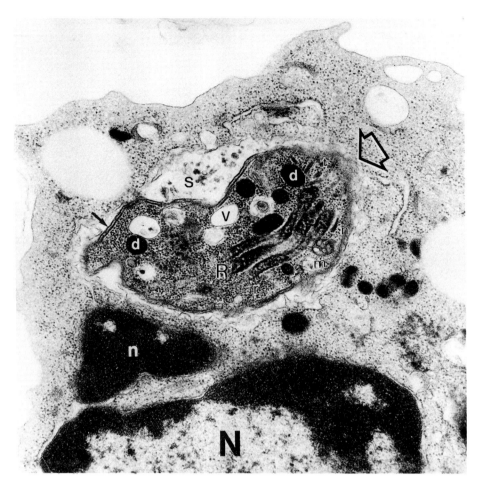

Fig. 10.7 *Toxoplasma gondii*: tachyzoite. An oblique section of a tachyzoite with an apical complex (open arrow). The cytoplasm is laden with abundant ribosomes (r), a few dense bodies (d), vesicles (v) and rare mitochondria (m). The sausage-like rhoptries (R) are clearly visible. The pellicle (solid thin arrow) is multilayered, with a distinct intervening space. Many secretory granules (S) are inside the membrane-lined parasitophorous vacuole. N and n = segmented nucleus of the neutrophil. (× 28 400) Micrographs courtesy of Dr T T Tang et al, reprinted with the permission of the publishers of American Journal of Clinical Pathology.

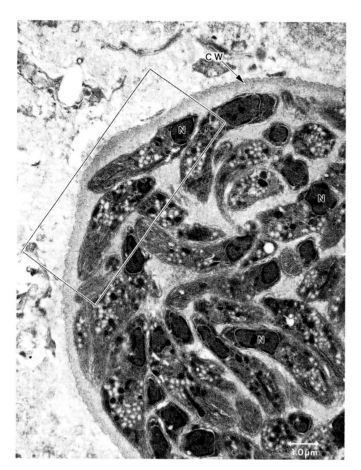

Fig. 10.8 *Toxoplasma gondii*: cyst. A cyst with numerous organisms.
N = nucleus; CW = cyst wall. (× 8000) Unpublished micrograph,
courtesy of Dr L Cerezo and Dr G Price, Orlando Regional Medical
Center, Florida, USA.

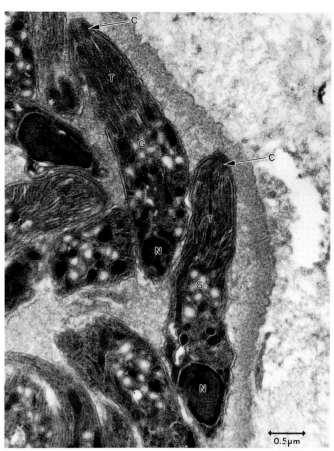

Fig. 10.9 *Toxoplasma gondii*: cyst wall. A higher magnification of the
previous micrograph. N = nucleus; G = storage granules; T =
toxonemes; C = conoid. (× 18 100) Unpublished micrograph courtesy of
Dr L Cerezo and Dr G Price, Orlando Regional Medical Center, Florida,
USA.

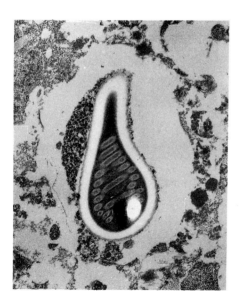

Fig. 10.10 *Nosema*. Pear-shaped organism within the cytoplasm of a
macrophage. Coiled polar filament showing 11 tubular coils is clearly
visible. Thick electron-lucent wall surrounds the parasite. (× 12 500)
Micrograph courtesy of Dr R L Font et al, reprinted with the permission
of the publishers of Archives of Ophthalmology.

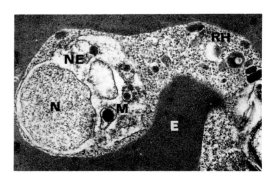

Fig. 10.11 *Babesia microti*: trophozoite. A maturing trophozoite in an
erythrocyte. Several micronemes (M), a single rhoptry (RH) with a
characteristic clear zone, and many free ribosomes are present. The
nuclear envelope (NE) of the nucleus (N) in this organism is enormously
expanded. Erythrocytic cytoplasm is indicated by E. (× 19 800)
Micrograph courtesy of Dr T Sun et al, reprinted with the permission of
the publishers of Journal of Infectious Diseases.

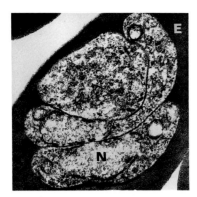

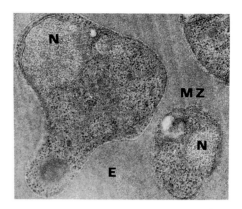

Fig. 10.12 *Babesia microti*: merozoites. Several merozoites (MZ) budding from a mature trophozoite. N = nucleus; E = erythrocytic cytoplasm. (× 21 800) Micrograph courtesy of Dr T Sun et al, reprinted with the permission of the publishers of Journal of Infectious Diseases.

Fig. 10.13 *Babesia microti*: gametocyte. An early gametocyte in an erythrocyte. This state is characterized by a convoluted cell with many free ribosomes. N = nucleus; E = erythrocytic cytoplasm. (× 18 800) Micrograph courtesy of Dr T Sun et al, reprinted with the permission of the publishers of Journal of Infectious Diseases.

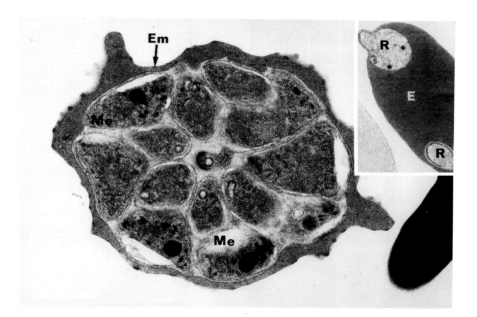

Fig. 10.14 *Plasmodium* sp. Advanced schizogony of the erythrocytic stages of the parasite. Em = erythrocytic membrane; Me = merozoites. (× 17 800) *Inset* Erythrocyte containing 'signet ring' stages of the parasite. E = erythrocyte; R = ring form of *P. falciparum*. (× 17 200) Unpublished micrograph courtesy of Dr D Stenzel, Queensland University of Technology, Brisbane, Australia.

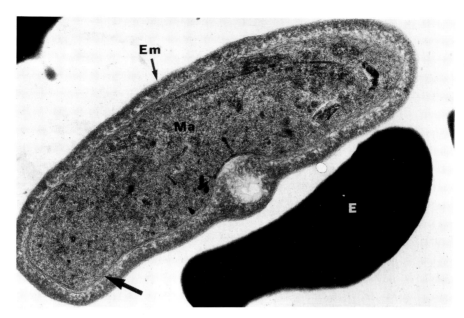

Fig. 10.15 *Plasmodium* sp. Macrogametocyte, the sexual form of the parasite, surrounded by three-layered membrane (arrow). Ma = macrogametocyte; Em = erythrocytic membrane; E = erythrocyte.

(× 15 800) Unpublished micrograph, courtesy of Dr D Stenzel, Queensland University of Technology, Brisbane, Australia.

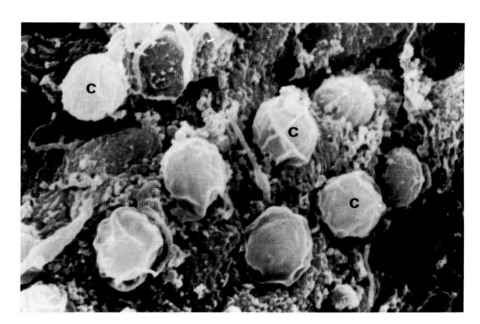

Fig. 10.16 *Cryptosporidium* sp. Scanning electron micrograph of numerous parasites on the surface of the small intestine of an AIDS patient. C = *Cryptosporidium*. (× 7100) Unpublished micrograph, courtesy of Drs M Vesk and A Romeo, University of Sydney, Australia.

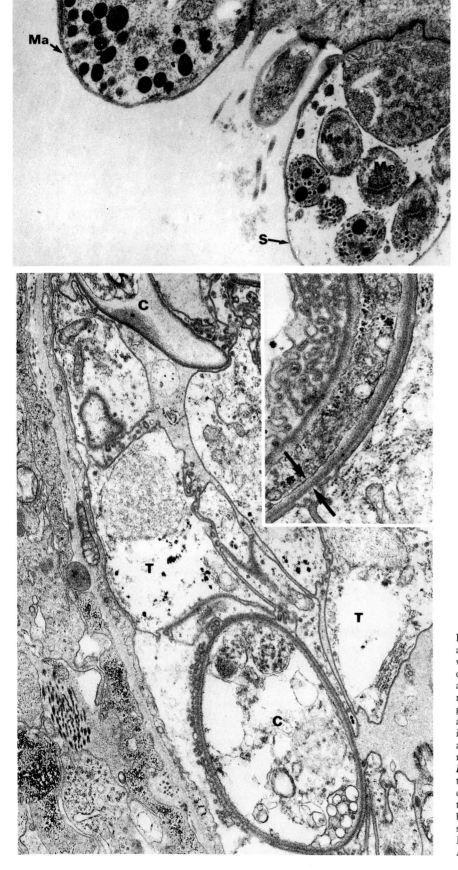

Fig. 10.17 *Cryptosporidium* sp. Transmission electron micrograph of a mature schizont (S) with fully developed merozoites (Me), and a macrogametocyte (Ma) with prominent electron-dense granules. (× 17 800) Unpublished micrograph, courtesy of Dr P O'Donoghue, Parasitology Section, Department of Agriculture, Adelaide, Australia.

Fig. 10.18 *Pneumocystis carinii*: trophozoites (T) and cysts (C) fill the alveolar lumen. Trophozoites vary from 1.5 to 5.0 μm in size. Nuclear organization varies, and the nuclear envelope is not always apparent. Cytoplasmic organelles include ribosomes, endoplasmic reticulum, mitochondria, glycogen granules and lipid droplets, but not Golgi apparatus and lysosomes. The cysts contain intracystic bodies resembling small trophozoites and membranous material that probably represents remnants of the mother cell. (× 15 800)
Inset Collapsed crescentic cyst between two trophozoites. The wall of the cyst has an outer dense and an inner paler layer (arrows). The trophozoites at the top and bottom of the field are bound by a plasma membrane and external layer similar to the outer cyst wall. (× 34 300) Micrograph courtesy of Dr E J Wills, Royal Prince Alfred Hospital, Sydney, Australia.

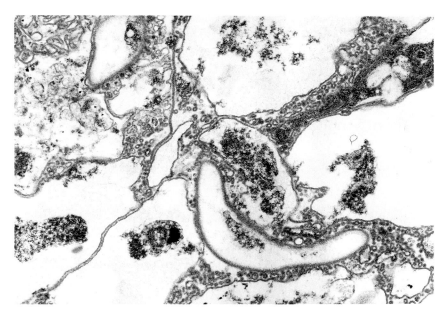

Fig. 10.19 *Pneumocystis carinii*: collapsed cysts are readily visible among tubulomembranous material. (× 13 200)

Micrograph courtesy of Dr E J Wills, Royal Prince Alfred Hospital, Sydney, Australia. (See also Figs 13.7–13.10)

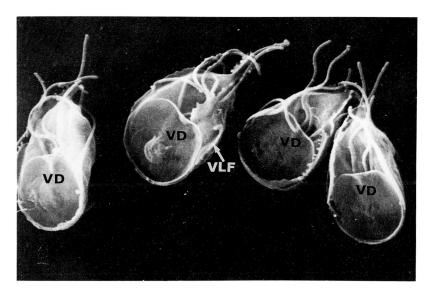

Fig. 10.20 *Giardia intestinalis*: trophozoites. Scanning electron micrograph of several trophozoites. The exposed ventral surface of the parasites reveals the adhesive ventral disc (VD) surrounded by the ventrolateral flange (VLF) and the paired ventral flagella (F). (× 5000)

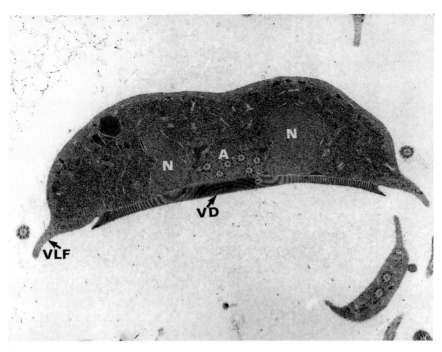

Fig. 10.21 *Giardia intestinalis*: trophozoite. A cross-section through the nuclear region of a trophozoite. The central disc appears flattened. Axonemes of posterior–lateral, ventral and caudal flagella can be seen between the nuclei. N = nucleus, A = axonemes; VD = ventral disc; VLF = ventrolateral flange. (× 12 300)

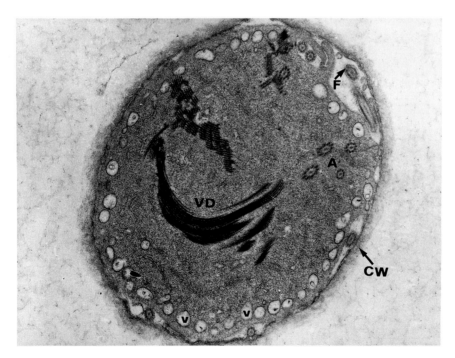

Fig. 10.22 *Giardia intestinalis*: cyst. Cross section of a cyst. The cyst wall and an extensive tubulo–vacular system beneath the cell membrane are clearly visible. Note the profiles of fragmented portions of the ventral disc, flagellar axonemes and free flagella. CW = cyst wall; V = vacuoles; VD = ventral disc; A = axonemes; F = flagella. (× 13 100)

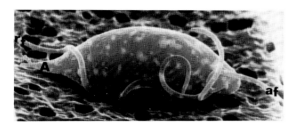

Fig. 10.23 *Trichomonas vaginalis*. Scanning electron micrograph of the parasite. A = axostyl; rf = recurrent flagellum; af = anterior flagella. (× 6500)

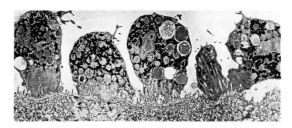

Fig. 10.24 *Trichomonas vaginalis*. Several trichomonads attached to human epithelial cells. The parasites form numerous cytoplasmic extensions which interdigitate with the microvilli of epithelial cells. Note that these extensions are formed by the protozoan cells only on the side adjacent to the surface of the epithelial cells. The opposite side of the parasite, where the recurrent flagellum is located, remains relatively smooth. (× 5400)

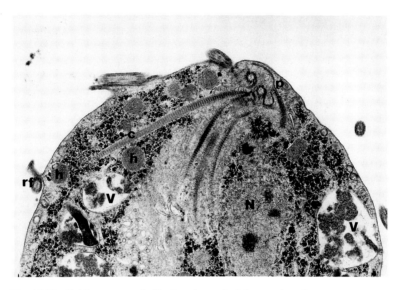

Fig. 10.25 *Trichomonas vaginalis*. Anterior end of the parasite. af = anterior flagellum; rf = recurrent flagellum; c = costa; p = pelta; k = kinetosome; v = vacuole. (× 13 700)

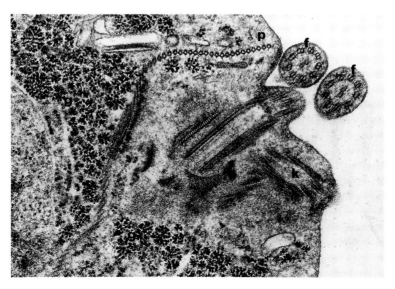

Fig. 10.26 *Trichomonas vaginalis*. Area of the flagellar pocket of the trichomonad. n = nucleus; f = flagellum; k = kinetosomes; p = pelta; h = hydrogenosome; g = glycogen granules. (× 31 700)

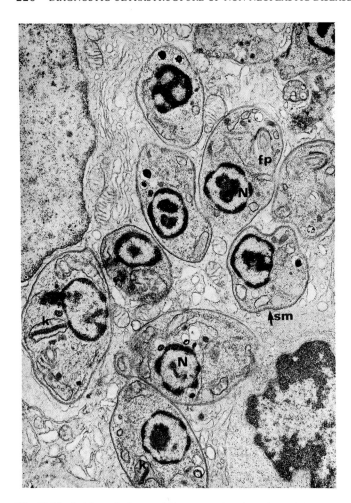

Fig. 10.27 *Leishmania donovani.* A cross section through several amastigotes within a parasitophorous vacuole of a macrophage. The kinetoplast–mitochondrion complex is clearly visible. A short rudimentary flagellum is present inside the flagellar pocket. A layer of subpellicular microtubules (arrow) is present under the plasma membrane. n = nucleus; k = kinetoplast; fp = flagellar pocket; sm = subpellicular microtubules. (× 10 600) Micrograph courtesy of Dr J D Chuleyer et al, reprinted with the permission of the publishers of Annals of Tropical Medicine and Parasitology.

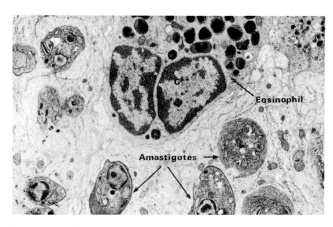

Fig. 10.28 *Leishmania donovani.* Several parasites inside a macrophage in the vicinity of an eosinophil. (× 5300) Micrograph courtesy of Dr J D Chulay et al, reprinted with the permission of the publishers of Annals of Tropical Medicine and Parasitology.

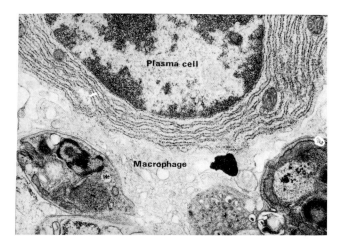

Fig. 10.29 *Leishmania donovani.* A macrophage containing a number of parasites is shown adjacent to a plasma cell. (× 10 400) Micrograph courtesy of Dr J D Culay et al, reprinted with the permission of the publishers of Annals of Tropical Medicine and Parasitology.

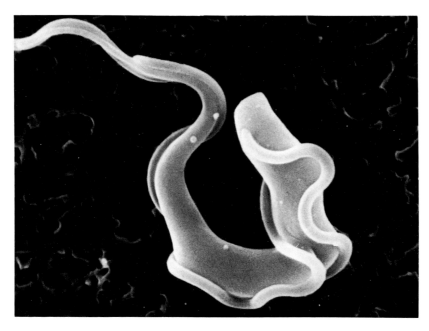

Fig. 10.30 *Trypanosoma rhodesiense*. Scanning electron micrograph of the bloodstream trypomastigote of the parasite. (× 9800)

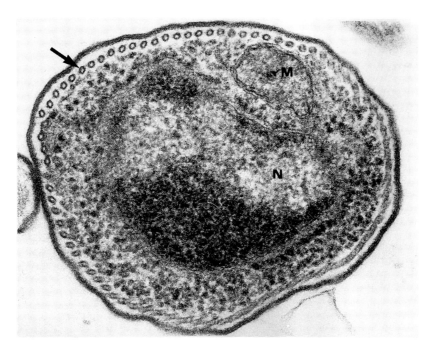

Fig. 10.31 *Trypanosoma* sp. Transverse section of a trypomastigote with a uniform, electron-dense surface coat covering the cell body. A prominent layer of subpellicular microtubes (arrow) is present under the plasma membrane. N = nucleus, M = mitochondrion. (× 75 200)

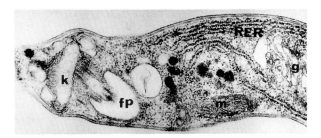

Fig. 10.32 *Trypanosoma* sp. A blood stream trypomastigote — longitudinal section through the parasite body. The kinetoplast (k) is seen within the mitochondrial matrix. Fragmented parts of mitochondrion (m) are observed. Well-developed rough endoplasmic reticulum (RER) with numerous ribosomes is visible. Plasma membrane is covered with an electron-dense surface coat. fp = flagellar pocket; G = Golgi apparatus. (× 21 100)

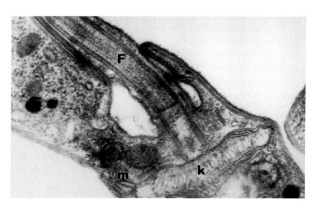

Fig. 10.33 *Trypanosoma* sp. Kinetoplast–mitochondrion complex and flagellar pocket of the trypomastigote. k = kinetoplast; m = mitochondrial part of the kinetoplast; f = flagella. (× 30 400)

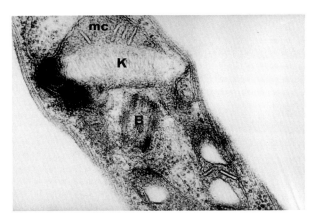

Fig. 10.34 *Trypanosoma* sp. Kinetoplast–mitochondrion complex with mitochondrial cristae clearly visible. Note the continuation of the kinetoplast body into mitochondrial sleeves. k = kinetoplast; mc = mitochondrial cristae; b = basal body of the flagellum. (× 31 700)

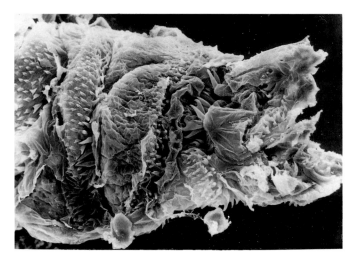

Fig. 10.35 *Cuterebra* sp. Scanning electron micrograph of a fly larva, surgically extracted from the human vitreous. The thoracoabdominal body segments covered by two types of spines arranged in rings perpendicular to the long axis of the organism are seen. (× 205) Micrograph courtesy of Dr R Machemer et al, reprinted with the permission of the publishers of Ophthalmology.

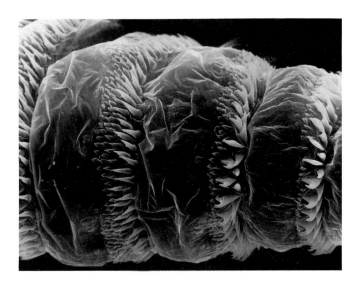

Fig. 10.36 *Cuterebra* sp. Scanning electron micrograph of the thoracoabdominal body segments of the fly larva. (× 330) Micrograph courtesy of Dr R Machemer et al, reprinted with the permission of the publishers of Ophthalmology.

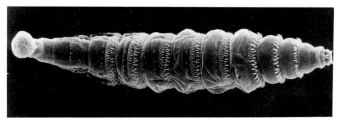

Fig. 10.37 *Cuterebra* sp. First instar larva of rodent botfly (*Cuterebra*) as seen by scanning electron microscopy. (× 330) Micrograph courtesy of Dr R Machemer et al, reprinted with the permission of the publishers of Ophthalmology.

11. Tumour-like disorders

D. W. Henderson   J. M. Papadimitriou   D. V. Spagnolo

INTRODUCTION

The potential ambit of this chapter is so broad that the selection of disorders for inclusion is necessarily arbitrary and arguable. The very expression 'tumour-like' poses problems, for it indicates that these disorders resemble neoplasms, but implies that they are not. However, the pathological status of a number of 'tumour-like' conditions is open to speculation: some are probably genuine neoplasms, while others fall into a twilight zone between inflammation and neoplasia.

Most tumour-like disorders are easily recognizable by light microscopy (LM), and electron microscopy (EM) can contribute little if anything to their diagnosis. Nevertheless, EM adds significantly to our understanding of the nature and pathogenesis of a number of these disorders, and it can clarify some of the features seen by LM. With this in mind we have concentrated on certain inflammatory and quasi-neoplastic disorders which have been elucidated by EM — including the myofibroproliferative disorders (myofibroblastoses), pigmented villonodular synovitis, hamartoma-like lesions and malakoplakia. Other tumour-like disorders are considered elsewhere in this book, in the tissue- and organ-based chapters.

MYOFIBROPROLIFERATIVE LESIONS: GENERAL REMARKS ON THE MYOFIBROBLAST

Myofibroblasts (MFB) were delineated as distinctive mesenchymal cells largely on the basis of EM and immunocytochemistry,[29,31] and they combine the characteristics of fibroblasts and smooth muscle cells, as indicated by their name.[55] Thus, their cytoplasm is characterized by both rough endoplasmic reticulum (RER) and actin-containing microfilaments.[29,31] Correlating with the cytomorphology, their functional properties include both collagen synthesis and cell contractility,[54,80,81] and they account at least in part for the phenomenon of wound contraction.[55]

The major ultrastructural features of MFB include the following:

1. Mesenchymal cell characteristics, with abundant RER typical of fibroblasts, and longitudinally orientated microfilaments with associated dense bodies — typical of the myofilamentous apparatus of smooth muscle (Figs 11.1 and 11.2). The lamellae of the RER are often thick, and the cisternae may be branched or dilated. The filaments typically measure 6–8 nm in diameter, but vimentin-containing intermediate (10 nm) filaments[79] may also be seen and they sometimes predominate.[54,80] The proportions of the RER and filaments appear to be related inversely to each other — RER predominating early in the evolution of MFB, and the microfilaments at a later stage.[18] In any single lesion containing MFB, a continuous spectrum may be evident — from predominantly fibroblastoid cells to filament-rich predominantly myoid MFB.[54] Myofibroblasts are usually spindle-shaped and they can be extremely slender and elongated (Figs 11.1 and 11.2),[61] but rounded cell profiles may be seen, depending on the plane of section. Both RER and microfilaments are essential for the identification of MFB, but the following characteristics are usually also present:

2. The nucleus is frequently folded or serrated as a result of a 'concertina' effect secondary to cell contraction, and nuclear bodies are often evident.[54] In addition, the nuclear fibrous lamina may be prominent (Figs 11.3 and 11.4).

3. Micropinocytotic vesicles, similar to those found in smooth muscle (Fig. 11.3).

4. Plasmalemma-related attachment plaques.

5. Intermediate and gap junctions between apposed plasma membranes of MFB (Fig. 11.3), like those occurring in smooth muscle.[32] Desmosomes do not occur on either smooth muscle cells[32] or MFB; the junctions and cytofilaments should not be misconstrued as desmosome-tonofilament complexes, and the MFB misidentified as epithelial cells as a result.[40] This distinction was not facilitated by the use of imprecise terminology for these junctions in some of the early literature on MFB — in which the junctions were designated as 'desmosomes'[29,30] or even

'junctional complexes of the macula adherens ("desmosome") and nexus (gap junction) types'.[77] (For a discussion on the correct nomenclature for intercellular junctions see Erlandson,[26] Ghadially,[33] Henderson et al[40] or Staehelin.[87])

6. Discontinuous external (basal) lamina (Fig. 11.3) which may be situated adjacent to the peripheral attachment plaques, producing so-called subplasmalemmal linear density complexes.[58]

7. Attachments of MFB to the surrounding stroma by microtendons (Fig. 11.2). 'Fibronexus' is another term introduced for the microtendon,[84] and these structures are thought to represent transmembrane associations of extracellular fibronectin-containing fibres with cytoplasmic microfilaments.[84]

8. Prominent Golgi complexes, occasional lysosomes and lipid droplets, mitochondria, polyribosomes and sporadic microtubules.[80]

Fibroblasts, smooth muscle and primitive mesenchymal cells have all been proposed as progenitors for MFB.[54] Experimental studies indicate that the macrophage–fibroblast–MFB progression constitutes the major pathway.[18,61,77] Observations on human granulation tissue,[76] fibro-contractive inflammatory disorders (Table 11.1) and maturing palmar fibromatosis[30,37] also suggest that MFB develop from fibroblasts. Therefore, it seems clear that smooth muscle cells are not necessary for the development of MFB. This view is supported by immunocytochemical analysis of MFB recovered from fibromatoses and the stroma of mammary carcinomas — which has demonstrated vimentin in the absence of desmin, suggesting that these cells are more akin to fibroblasts than smooth muscle.[79] Nevertheless, so-called synthetic-state vascular smooth muscle cells and MFB have morphological similarities,[18] and a number of observations suggest an alternative smooth muscle–MFB pathway.[54] These include the response of rat uterine smooth muscle to oestrogenic stimulation[74] and the development of MFB in regenerating ureteric smooth muscle following injury.[50] It seems likely that transformation of smooth muscle to MFB — if it occurs to a significant degree — is restricted to certain anatomical sites and follows injury to smooth muscle. Primitive mesenchymal cells represent a third potential source for MFB,[54] and RER is prominent in all developing smooth muscle cells,[32] producing a resemblance to MFB. In summary, it appears that macrophages-fibroblasts, smooth muscle and primitive mesenchymal cells can all act as progenitors for MFB, depending on the anatomical location and the nature of the factors inducing their development, but the macrophage-fibroblast-MFB pathway is almost certainly the most important.

The fate of MFB is not entirely clear. Some consider them to be transitional forms on the road from undifferentiated mesenchymal cells to smooth muscle,[85] and MFB can have predominantly myoid ultrastructural features. Although this line of development has been observed in certain normal

tissues,[54] it seems to be an unlikely progression in fibrocontractive inflammatory processes, since only fibroblasts are present in the sclerotic end-stage of these disorders.[54] In such circumstances it is likely that MFB are deleted from the tissue, either by reversion to fibroblasts or by cell death.[54]

MFB were originally identified in inflammatory processes, notably in granulation tissue.[29,55] Their presence has since been recognized in certain normal tissues,[80] and they are described in three main pathological settings:[80,81]

1. Inflammatory processes with contracting fibrous repair (Table 11.1)
2. Quasineoplastic fibroproliferative disorders (Table 11.1)
3. Neoplasms — either within the stroma of a variety of epithelial and other neoplasms,[82] or as an integral part of the neoplastic cell population in some mesenchymal tumours.[40]

In recent years the myofibroblast has generated a voluminous literature, yet in the light of current knowledge 'the notion of contractile fibroblasts seems almost anticlimactic', as Majno[55] has stated. Actin-containing microfilaments are well described in non-myoid cells (notably myoepithelium), and both actin and myosin are known to be present in almost every type of cell.[55] Actin in non-myoid cells is usually present in a disaggregated gel state rather than the polymerized filamentous form, and it may constitute up to 10–15% of the total protein content of the cells, having both cytoskeletal and contractile–locomotor functions.[40] As their occurrence in diverse pathological circumstances testifies, MFB have little or no diagnostic value by themselves. However, by enhancing our knowledge of a variety of inflammatory and low-grade fibroproliferative disorders, their importance cannot be overrated. The detailed reviews on MFB by Lipper et al[54] and Seemayer and associates[80] are recommended to the interested reader.

NODULAR FASCIITIS AND RELATED DISORDERS

Nodular fasciitis is a benign self-limiting circumscribed fibroproliferative disorder, usually affecting subcutaneous tissues, striated muscle or fascial planes; it is considered to be a reactive tumour-like lesion, although the exact cause is unknown.[4,25,92a] Because of its rapid growth, mitotic activity and cellularity, nodular fasciitis has been mistaken in the past for a sarcoma.[25] Misdiagnosis as sarcoma should never occur nowadays, and the lesion is recognizable by LM of either open tissue biopsies or fine-needle aspiration (FNA) specimens.[8,67] When the diagnosis is established by FNA cytology, surgical removal is unnecessary and spontaneous resolution can be expected.

Ultrastructural examination has virtually no place in the diagnosis of typical nodular fasciitis, although prominence of the nuclear fibrous lamina in the proliferative cells in some cases may correlate with the benign character of the lesion (Fig.11.3).[33,40] Instead, EM has been of value in elucidating

Table 11.1 Examples of inflammatory and tumour-like disorders containing myofibroblasts (MFB)*

Disorder	Remarks
Fibrogenic inflammatory disorders	
Miscellaneous inflammatory lesions	Include the following: granulation tissue; hypertrophic scars; scars around silicone implants in breasts; keloids; chronic otitis media;[13] post-tracheotomy tracheal stenosis; oesophageal stenosis; pseudo-intima developing in Dacron vascular grafts;[86] transected tendons; chronic Achilles paratenonitis in athletes;[52] carpal tunnel syndrome; stenosing tenosynovitis; ganglia of joints; ischaemic contracture of muscle; subendocardial fibrosis in the carcinoid syndrome; Winchester syndrome;[54] fibrosis in breast, oral mucosa and serosa of gall bladder;[62] transitional mucosa adjacent to colon carcinoma[9]
Scleroderma-like skin and subcutaneous lesions in the toxic oil syndrome in Spain[64]	MFB contained cytoplasmic microfilamentous inclusions identical to those characteristic of infantile digital fibromatosis (see below)
Fibrogenic lung diseases	Include sarcoidosis; fibrosing alveolitis; hypersensitivity pneumonitis;[47] and organizing pneumonia.[16] We have also observed MFB in asbestosis and pulmonary histiocytosis X. In the latter situation, some MFB extended extremely close to collections of folded basal lamina sequestered within the interstitium. It is conceivable that MFB exert traction on alveolar basal lamina and hence constitute one mechanism for alveolar obliteration
Fibrotic diseases of the liver	Including cirrhosis[15] and schistosomiasis (see Ch. 15)
Chronic renal diseases	We have observed MFB in the epithelioid crescents in crescentic glomerulonephritis (see Ch. 17)
Chronic ocular disorders	Including rubeosis iridis with closed-angle glaucoma; posterior capsule opacification in pseudophakic eyes;[56] and subcapsular region of anterior capsular cataracts.[66] In rubeosis iridis, the formation of a sheet of contractile MFB on the surface of the iris has been invoked as an explanation for the ectropion iridis in this disorder[46]
Reactive tumour-like lesions	
Intravenous pyogenic granuloma	—
Nodular fasciitis and its variants	See text, p 230, and Figs. 11.1–11.3
Myositis ossificans	MFB found in cental zone, together with macrophages and fibroblasts[68]
Elastofibroma	See text, p 232
Disseminated peritoneal leiomyomatosis	—
Inflammatory fibroid polyp of the gastrointestinal tract[133]	MFB may be rare[135]
Inflammatory pseudotumours of the urinary bladder	See text, p 232
Massive ovarian oedema	—
Plasma cell granuloma	See text, p 235
Giant cell reparative granuloma of jaw[132]	–
Pigmented villonodular synovitis	See text, p 233
So-called giant cell tumour of tendon sheath	See text, p 233
Fibroma of tendon sheath	—
Fibromatoses	
Fibrous hamartoma of infancy	See hamartomas below
Infantile myofibromatosis, solitary and multicentric types	See Fig. 11.4
Infantile digital fibromatosis	Characteristic cytoplasmic inclusions contain and are often continuous with microfilaments 5–7 nm in diameter. Presence of actin within the inclusions has been demonstrated by decorating the component filaments with heavy meromysin.[42] Growth of inclusions takes place by accretion of filaments
Juvenile hyaline fibromatosis	—
Juvenile aponeurotic fibroma	—
Nasopharyngeal angiofibroma	—
Dupuytren's contracture	See text, p 233
Desmoid fibromatosis	See text, p 232
Desmoplastic fibroma of bone	—
Cardiac fibroma (fibro-elastic hamartoma)	Ultrastructural studies have demonstrated a population of fibroblasts and MFB.[155,183] Because of an abundant extracellular matrix composed of numerous collagen and elastin fibres, Feldman & Meyer[155] designated these lesions as fibro-elastic hamartomas. However, Turi et al[183] emphasized their ultrastructural and behavioural similarities to soft tissue fibromatoses, and introduced the term 'cardiac fibromatosis'
Hamartomas and similar lesions	
Collagen naevus	—
Fibrous hamartoma of infancy	Alba Greco et al[3] observed fibroblasts and MFB in the fibrous and myxovascular areas, the fibroblasts being predominant. Adipose component contained lipocytes and fibroblastoid prelipocytes. Blood vessels of varying development and calibre were present, with possible rudimentary media formation around small channels. Ultrastructural appearances resembled developing fetal blood vessels and fat
Cardiac fibro-elastic hamartoma	See cardiac fibroma above
Congenital mesoblastic nephroma (fetal mesenchymal hamartoma of kidney)	Ultrastructural studies have revealed a population of undifferentiated mesenchymal cells, fibroblasts and MFB.[154,159,176,185] Shen & Yunis,[176] who evaluated seven cases by EM, found myofilaments in most cells. The cell population is less differentiated in cellular and recurrent lesions, and Fu & Kay[159] likened the cells in one recurrent case to fetal tendon fibroblasts
Lymphangiomyoma and lymphangiomyomatosis	—

*References: 1–3, 8–17, 19–25, 27–30, 34–44, 46–49, 52–57, 59, 60, 62–66a, 68, 70–73, 75, 77, 80, 81, 83, 85, 86, 88–96, 120–126, 132, 133, 135, 145, 154, 155, 159, 176 and 183–186.

the nature of the component cells, and has shown these to consist largely of MFB. The fine structure of nodular fasciitis is illustrated and discussed in Figs 11.1–11.3.

MFB have also been identified in proliferative fasciitis[22] and proliferative myositis,[63,80] and ultrastructural studies have established that the large ganglion-like cells characteristic of these lesions are modified myofibroblasts.[19,22,63] Ossifying fasciitis[23] and myositis ossificans[68] also contain MFB (see Table 11.l).

Recently, Nochomovitz & Orenstein[65] described two cases of inflammatory pseudotumours of the urinary bladder which resembled nodular fasciitis, but which were thought originally by some pathologists to be sarcomas. They contained eosinophilic strap-like cells resembling rhabdomyoblasts, but ultrastructural examination disclosed that these were MFB — which were the predominant cells in the lesions. The authors suggested that these pseudoneoplastic proliferations might represent the visceral counterpart of nodular fasciitis, and that they may be related to the postoperative spindle cell nodules of the genitourinary tract described earlier by Proppe et al;[69] however, only one of these postoperative nodules was studied by EM — which revealed fibroblastoid cells lacking the characteristics of MFB. Ro and associates[71a] have since reported similar observations on two lesions of the urinary bladder resembling nodular fasciitis, which they designated as 'pseudosarcomatous fibromyxoid tumours'. These lesions were initially misinterpreted as embryonal rhabdomyosarcomas by LM, but ultrastructural evaluation of tissue recovered from paraffin blocks revealed a population of fibroblasts with fewer MFB, and follow-up indicated that the lesions were benign.

In summary we consider EM to have almost no place in the recognition of nodular fasciitis and related lesions in soft tissues, where the criteria for diagnosis by LM are well established. However, EM may rarely be of value in the evaluation of similar pseudoneoplastic lesions in viscera, where the diagnosis may not readily be apparent by LM — or may be subject to dispute — because of the unusual anatomical location. In these circumstances EM may contribute to the correct diagnosis by:

1. Demonstrating a predominance of myofibroblasts in the lesion, or prominence of the nuclear fibrous lamina in the proliferating fibroblastoid–myofibroblastoid cells, thereby suggesting a reactive or low-grade neoplastic process and militating against a high-grade sarcoma.

2. Demonstrating that any eosinophilic strap-like or even ganglion-like cells in the lesion are devoid of the markers of rhabdomyoblastic differentiation[40] and that they represent MFB.

ELASTOFIBROMA

Elastofibroma is a distinctive degenerative pseudotumour occurring predominantly but not exclusively in the subscapular soft tissues, and probably resulting from repetitive subclinical tissue injury and repair.[44,48,70] By LM, elastofibromas are composed of intertwining collagen fibres and sclerotic masses, together with numerous elastin fibres and globules, and occasional fibroblastoid cells.[25,44,48] The swollen elastic fibres typically consist of a central dense linear core surrounded by elastic tissue showing periodic segmentation, resulting in a beaded or 'necklace'-like appearance.[25,48]

Ultrastructural studies have revealed a population of fibroblasts and myofibroblasts with long delicate cytoplasmic processes and a thick nuclear fibrous lamina.[2,24,48,70] Intermediate filaments may predominate in the cytoplasm,[70] and seemingly intracytoplasmic collagen fibres are recorded.[91] Dixon & Lee[24] also described dense granular cytoplasmic bodies and they suggested that these might represent elastin or an elastin precursor. The abnormal elastic fibres consist of a central core of one or more unaltered elastic fibres surrounded by an irregular mantle of fibrillary and granular elastic material[2,24,44,48,70] — although the elastin globules may lack a central core.[44] The masses of elastic tissue are often closely related to the fibroblastoid–myofibroblastoid cells,[11,91,93] and elastofibroma is thought to develop as a result of active and excessive synthesis of elastin,[2,24] with deposition around pre-existing elastic fibres followed by degeneration and fragmentation.[44,48] The diagnosis of elastofibroma is achieved by LM.

THE FIBROMATOSES

The concept of the fibromatoses encompasses a broad group of non-metastasizing fibro-proliferative disorders of similar microscopic appearance.[25,92a] Since by definition the fibromatoses do not metastasize, they should never be designated as low-grade fibrosarcomas,[5] and the concept excludes fibroma molle of the dermis, keloids and hypertrophic scars.[5] Allen[5] divides them into two major groups, namely, 'adult' and 'juvenile' fibromatoses, although Enzinger & Weiss[25] draw a subtle distinction and refer to the latter simply as 'fibrous proliferations of infancy and childhood' — while retaining the expression 'fibromatosis' for many of the individual entities in this group; the 'adult' group is further divided into Dupuytren and desmoid types.[5]

The fibromatoses display variable biological behaviour: some can be placed in an intermediate zone between reactive fibroproliferations and fibrosarcoma,[25,92a] and Allen[5] refers to them as tumours. For example, the desmoid fibromatoses appear to be tumour-like or neoplastic lesions as shown by their capacity for apparently semi-autonomous growth, destructive local infiltration of tissues and repeated local recurrences after attempted surgical removal.[5] However, they may stabilize after an initial period of rapid growth and even regress spontaneously, notably after the menopause.[92a] Other fibromatoses appear to enjoy a quasineoplastic status, while some may represent reactive lesions or hamartomas — and Navas-Palacios[63] considers the fibromatoses to be reactive tumour-like proliferations. Thus, Dupuytren's contracture has few of the attributes of neoplasia,[92a] and it is difficult to accept knuckle pads as 'tumours'. Similarly, fibromatosis colli (sternomastoid tumour) in infants never behaves aggressively, typically regresses spontaneously — albeit with residual fibro-contraction in some cases — and does not recur;[25] it has been suggested that this lesion may represent a reaction to perinatal tissue injury, and an association with breech or forceps delivery is recorded.[6,25] However, the LM features differ from those of fibrous repair or organizing haematomas, and Enzinger & Weiss[25] suggest that it may be a 'peculiar hamartomatous process'. For these reasons we consider the term 'fibromatosis' simply to be a convenient nosological umbrella for a variety of fibroproliferative disorders of diverse biological character, united mainly by an absence of metastatic potential.

Numerous ultrastructural studies of the fibromatoses have been reported (Table 11.1) and these have shown that all types are composed of varying proportions of fibroblasts and MFB, separated by varying amounts of collagenous stroma. In a fine-structural analysis of desmoid tumours, Goellner & Soule[36] found both fibroblasts and MFB in all eight cases; the relative proportions of these cell types varied and were apparently uninfluenced by clinical factors such as radiation therapy, or primary versus recurrent tumour status. MFB were rare in three tumours, but in the remainder they appeared to constitute the majority of the cell population. Gokel & Hubner[37] have reported an ultrastructural study of 21 cases of Dupuytren's contracture, in which they found that fibroblasts predominated during the proliferative phase, while MFB represented the majority of the cells in the involutional phase, but in a larger series of 43 cases MFB predominated in both of these phases.[43] Nevertheless, the myofibroblast content in Dupuytren's contracture is eventually depleted, and, in general, only fibroblasts can be found in the collagenous end-stage (residual phase),[37] which resembles mature scar tissue by LM. The MFB are thought to account for the fibro-contractive phenomena in some fibromatoses, notably Dupuytren's contracture,[30] and it has been suggested[37] that the stepwise shrinkage of the palmar fascia in this disorder is explicable by a cycle of:

1. Tissue contraction as a result of active contraction of MFB
2. Subsequent fixation of the tissue in a contracted state by deposition of collagen bundles.

MFB also predominate in congenital generalized and localized fibromatosis (Fig. 11.4)[53] and their predominance correlates with smooth muscle-like appearances by LM; accordingly, Chung & Enzinger[20] have re-designated this disorder as 'infantile myofibromatosis'. The fine structure of fibrous hamartoma of infancy is discussed briefly in Table 11.1.

It is our view that diagnosis of the fibromatoses is established by LM, and it is worth emphasizing that it is not possible to distinguish between desmoid tumours and highly differentiated fibrosarcomas by EM.[88] Electron microscopy has been of value mainly in elucidating the nature of the participating cells and some of the stromal components — but in so doing it has considerably influenced current concepts of the fibromatoses.

LOCALIZED NODULAR TENOSYNOVITIS AND PIGMENTED VILLONODULAR SYNOVITIS

Localized nodular tenosynovitis — more commonly known as giant cell tumour of tendon sheath (GCTTS) — and pigmented villonodular synovitis (PVNS) appear to be related disorders.[96] By LM both consist of a mixture of histiocytoid cells with spindle-shaped and foam cells, and with variable amounts of haemosiderin pigment.[96] They are distinguished mainly by their extent and their predilection for different anatomical sites. Thus, GCTTS typically forms a localized nodule in relation to a tendon sheath, especially in the fingers, whereas PVNS represents a diffuse villous and nodular arthropathy, usually affecting the knee joint.[117] Both are considered by most investigators to be reactive fibro-histiocytic lesions,[96,97,103,107,108] but some[110,119] regard them as true neoplasms, and PVNS does exhibit aggressive clinical behaviour in some cases, with local destruction of bone and extension into peri-articular soft tissues (Fig. 11.9).

Ultrastructurally, synovial membranes are normally lined by two cell types: type A cells resembling macrophages (with prominent Golgi complexes and pinocytotic vesicles, but little RER), and fibroblastoid type B cells (with abundant RER, but relatively few vesicles and Golgi complexes).[109] Intermediate forms combining these features also occur (type C cells), and several investigators believe that type A and B cells simply represent structural-functional modulations of a single cell line[106,116] — although there is evidence that type A cells originate from bone marrow whereas type B cells do not.[102] Accordingly, the proliferating cells in GCTTS and PVNS have been likened to synovial A and B cells.[96,97,103] This approach seems appropriate for the synovial intima in PVNS,[108] but one should not assume that the subsynovial cells in these disorders simply represent a local proliferation of synovial lining cells. Evidence indicates that after phagocytosis of material from the joint space, synovial lining cells migrate into the subsynovial connective tissue, where they would be regarded as macrophages.[108] Although these migratory cells constitute one potential source for the proliferating cells in GCTTS and PVNS, it is likely that many of the cells in these disorders represent macrophages and their derivatives originating from monocytes in the circulating blood[108] — and monocytoid and lymphocytic cells are described in GCTTS.[96] One can also speculate that even some of the synovial intimal cells in PVNS may originate from circulating monocytoid precursors. For these reasons we prefer to designate the cells resembling synovial A, B or C cells in GCTTS and PVNS simply as histiocytes (mononuclear phagocytes), fibroblasts or fibrohistiocytes respectively.

So-called giant cell tumour of tendon sheath. Ultrastructural studies of GCTTS have revealed varying proportions of histiocytoid and fibroblastoid cells (Fig. 11.5),[119a] with the former generally predominating.[96,103] Lysosomes and siderosomes (Fig. 11.6) are frequent in both cell types and intermediate junctions may be seen between apposed plasma membranes.[103] In addition, lipid-rich cells, polykaryons (Figs 11.7 and 11.8), myofibroblasts, and monocytoid and lymphocytic cells are described.[96,119a] Small blood vessels in the stroma of GCTTS are lined by swollen endothelium[96,103] and the lumen may be reduced to a slit-like space. Multilayering of the external lamina and extravasated erythrocytes are also recorded.[96,99]

Carstens[99] presented a dissenting viewpoint in an ultrastructural study of 11 cases of GCTTS, and reported osteoblast-like cells and giant cells resembling osteoclasts. He also recorded 'a few areas of osteoid and mineralized matrix' and suggested that GCTTS is 'derived from mesenchymal cells with partial osseous differentiation.' The evidence in support of this contention is not convincing and neither the osteoblast-like cells nor the 'mineralized matrix' are illustrated. Our own observations are similar to those of Alguacil-Garcia et al[96] and Eisenstein,[103] and we consider GCTTS to be a fibrohistiocytic lesion. Ushijima and associates[119a] reached the same conclusion in a large series comparing GCTTS localized to the digits with the form affecting large joints (localized nodular synovitis); although a greater abundance of cleft-like spaces was observed in the large-joint group by LM, the ultrastructural appearances in the two groups were essentially identical.

Pigmented villonodular synovitis. Ultrastructural studies of PVNS are confined to reports of single cases.[96,97,108,111] Alguacil-Garcia et al[96] described the cell population as more homogeneous and less differentiated than in GCTTS — with only occasional histiocytoid cells — and they also documented the presence of myofibroblasts. Ghadially and associates[108] found that the synovial intima in PVNS was composed of only rare type A cells but numerous foci of B cells, whereas the subintimal tissues were populated by innumerable macrophages containing frequent erythrophagosomes and siderosomes.

In their case of PVNS associated with psoriatic polyarthropathy, Archer-Harvey et al[97] observed erythrophagocytosis and fibrin extravasation by LM and EM. Both the intimal and subintimal tissues were composed predominantly of cells designated as 'mononuclear phagocytes with features intermediate between type A and type B cells' (fibrohistiocytic cells; Figs 11.9 and 11.10). Many contained erythrophagosomes in which erythrocytes could be seen in various stages of breakdown (Fig. 11.11), and there were numerous siderosomes (Fig. 11.12). In addition, a subpopulation of distinctive filament-containing mononuclear cells devoid of phagosomes was detected; representing about 5% of the total

cell population, they were characterized by predominantly perinuclear bundles of intermediate filaments (Fig. 11.14), which correlated with the presence of immunoreactive cytokeratins — whereas the predominant fibrohistiocytic cells contained lysozyme and α_1-antiprotease. The possible significance of these observations is discussed in the caption to Fig. 11.14.

Bhawan et al[98] have stressed the importance of microcirculatory changes in the pathogenesis of PVNS, and they suggested that the local microvascular endothelium may be the target of an immune response, possibly initiated by trauma — which appears to be a factor in about a quarter to a half of the cases.[105,114] The vascular abnormalities reported in PVNS include endothelial swelling, narrowing of capillary lumina, thickening and multilayering of the external lamina, the presence of fibrin within caveolar invaginations in endothelial cells, intraendothelial siderosomes[97,108] and widening of interendothelial spaces (Fig. 11.13). The microvascular pathology presumably accounts for extravasation of erythrocytes and fibrin into the interstitium, and hence provides a basis for siderosome formation. However, Ghadially[107] has suggested that the vascular changes may be the result and not the cause of PVNS — and vascular injury with multilayering of the external lamina is recorded in other disorders, for example rheumatoid synovitis.[107] Moreover, it seems unlikely that PVNS simply represents a florid fibro-histiocytic reaction to chronic or recurrent haemarthrosis, since unequivocal examples do not occur in haemophilic arthropathy or following experimentally induced haemarthrosis,[107] and Ghadially[107] has concluded that PVNS may be 'multifactorial in origin'.

From our own ultrastructural evaluation of GCTTS and PVNS, and a review of the literature, we have reached the following conclusions:

1. Ultrastructural studies are consistent with the notion that GCTTS and PVNS are related fibrohistiocytic disorders, and it is possible that they share similar pathogenetic factors. The differences between these conditions may reflect the intensity, duration, or localization of the initiating injury or the subsequent tissue reactions.

2. PVNS may result from synovial vascular injury modulated by other local or systemic factors, with extravasation of erythrocytes and plasma proteins, a secondary fibrohistiocytic inflammatory reaction, and subsequent erythrophagocytosis and siderosome formation. However, we incline to the alternative view that PVNS may represent a peculiar reactive or quasineoplastic arthropathy of unknown cause characterized by an accumulation of macrophages and fibrohistiocytic cells, which leads to the induction of secondary vascular injury and resultant haemosiderosis.

3. Although EM has been of value in elucidating the patterns of tissue reactions in GCTTS and PVNS and in giving some insight into their possible pathogenesis, the diagnosis of both is made by LM.

PLASMA CELL GRANULOMA

Plasma cell granuloma (PCG) is a polymorphous inflammatory lesion of unknown aetiology, composed of a variable admixture of 'inflammatory' cells, including mature plasma cells, and macrophages which are often laden with lipid (xanthoma cells).[120] Although PCG can develop in a variety of extrapulmonary sites,[121,122,124,126] it occurs predominantly in the periphery of the lung — where synonyms include the following: postinflammatory pseudotumour, xanthomatous pseudotumour, histiocytoma and fibroxanthoma. Predictably, the ultrastructural appearances are characterized by a variety of cell types — including plasma cells, lymphocytes, histiocytes, xanthoma cells, fibroblasts, myofibroblasts and undifferentiated mesenchymal cells.[120-123,125,126] Multilayering of the microvascular external lamina and capillaries with obliterated lumina lined by 'primitive' endothelial cells is also described.[120,121]

In the majority of cases the diagnosis of PCG by LM is reasonably straightforward and there is little point in recourse to EM. However, EM can occasionally contribute to the diagnosis by detecting the different cell types in the lesion, notably the histiocytes[122] — especially when the LM appearances are atypical or when the lesion is located in an unusual site. Thus, Chen et al[121] have reported a myxoid variant of PCG in which EM was useful in excluding nerve sheath cell differentiation and the myxoid variant of malignant fibrous histiocytoma. Similarly, West and associates[126] documented an intracranial PCG in which aggregates of epithelium-like cells surrounded by plasma cells were seen by LM, raising the possibility of the inflammatory variant of meningioma. Ultrastructural examination excluded meningioma by disclosing that the epithelioid cells were histiocytes devoid of intercellular junctions, and the authors suggested that 'cases considered to be meningiomas with conspicuous plasma cell-lymphocytic components must be studied by electron microscopy' to define their exact nature.

XANTHOMAS

Xanthomas of various types are reactive tumour-like lesions composed of lipid-laden histiocytes, and they may occur in any of the five subtypes of essential hyperlipidaemia or in other disorders accompanied by hyperlipidaemia — such as diabetes mellitus. The ultrastructure is characterized by histiocytes containing numerous lipid droplets and vacuoles.[138,140] EM plays no role in the diagnosis of xanthomas. For further information, the original articles detailing the fine structure of these lesions[137-143] should be consulted.

HAMARTOMAS AND HETEROTOPIAS

A hamartoma can be defined as a tumour-like developmental anomaly composed of multiple mature or partially differentiated tissues normally found at the site of occurrence. In contrast, tumour-like heterotopias (choristomas) are malformations consisting of differentiated tissue(s) foreign to the site of occurrence. Unlike neoplasms, the growth of true hamartomas does not exceed that of the normal tissues in which they are situated, unless they are complicated by some other factor such as haemorrhage or the accumulation of secretory products. Since heterotopias and many hamartomas are characterized by disorganization of normally differentiated tissues rather than disturbances of individual cell morphology or submicroscopic cell relationships, the vast majority are recognizable by LM alone. Perhaps because EM can contribute to their diagnosis only on exceptional occasions and because many are uncommon or rare lesions, the literature contains only sporadic ultrastructural studies of hamartomas, which include the following: hamartomatous intestinal polyps in the Peutz-Jeghers syndrome,[153] and the tuberous sclerosis complex (including the central nervous system lesions,[144,147,173] cardiac rhabdomyomas, renal angiomyolipomas and the pulmonary abnormalities[149]). Cardiac 'rhabdomyomas' and renal angiomyolipomas also occur as isolated lesions and are discussed below. Otherwise, if more detail on the hamartoma complexes is required, the original articles should be consulted. Instead, this account emphasizes the more common lesions, those in which EM may contribute to diagnostic evaluation, and those which have been elucidated recently by EM. The lymphangioleiomyomatosis syndrome[145,149,162,184,186] is illustrated and discussed in Chapter 13.

So-called chondromatous hamartoma of lung is the most common benign tumour encountered in the lung and is usually situated at the periphery, although up to 15% are endobronchial lesions within large bronchi.[150] The peripheral lesions appear to develop as interstitial growths, with secondary entrapment of airway epithelium at the circumference as the 'hamartoma' enlarges.[150] A loose myxoid fibrous component is consistently present[150] and may dominate the lesion. However, differentiation into cartilage, fibrous tissue and fat is usual within the myxofibrous tissue, and the appearances of such lesions are so characteristic that they can be recognized by LM at a glance. They are almost certainly not true hamartomas, for they do not occur in infancy or early childhood;[150] they are typically discovered during middle or even late adult life, and slow growth can sometimes be observed in serial chest X-rays. The weight of evidence indicates that they are benign fibromyxoid tumours, usually arising in peribronchial or peribronchiolar connective tissue,[146,171] with the capacity for multidirectional mesenchymal differentiation. The only virtue of the term 'hamartoma' is its brevity in comparison to the cumbersome alternatives proposed for this lesion.[150] The ultrastructural appearances are illustrated and discussed in Figs 11.15 and 11.16.

Pleomorphic pulmonary hamartoma. Gisser & Young[160] have reported an unusual pulmonary lesion associated with variant segmentation and anomalies of the vascular supply and bronchial passages, which they suggested may be a 'unique variant of pulmonary hamartoma'. By LM, the mass appeared undifferentiated, but EM was said to reveal immature mucin-secreting and ciliated epithelial cells in relation to mesenchyme, with a 'highly complex' organization. Unfortunately, the accompanying electron-micrographs are not very informative, but the authors suggested that EM may be of value in the diagnosis of similar lesions because of its capacity to identify epithelial elements undetectable by LM.

So-called multiple pulmonary leiomyomatous hamartomas. Ultrastructural studies have revealed the usual features of smooth muscle.[177] These lesions are now generally considered to represent 'benign metastasizing leiomyomas',[150] and accordingly they are not considered further.

So-called cardiac rhabdomyomas (glycogenic hamartomas) are ultrastructurally characterized by massive intracellular glycogen accumulation — accounting for the 'spider-web' appearance of the component myocytes by LM, and a myofilament content similar to that of extracardiac rhabdomyomas.[148,156,158,178,179,182] Apart from the obvious anatomical site differences, they are said to be distinguishable from adult rhabdomyomas of striated muscle by the presence of so-called zebra bodies, and the occurrence of desmosomes and gap junctions between cells. The 'zebra' bodies (leptomeres) consist of aggregates of parallel thin bands resembling Z-line material and spaced at intervals of 200 nm;[178] however, these structures are not specific for cardiac 'rhabdomyoma' and they have been described in various myopathies, and in both normal and strabismic extraocular muscles.[175]

Congenital endodermal heterotopia of the atrioventricular (AV) node is a rare polycystic epithelial lesion which can be responsible for cardiac conduction defects and sudden death. These lesions were originally designated as mesotheliomas of the AV node.[157] However, they have been shown to produce epithelial mucins and to contain carcinoembryonic antigen.[165,169] Ultrastructural investigations have revealed glandular epithelial cells with blunt microvilli and apical mucin granules, as well as cytoplasmic tonofibrils and a basal lamina.[165,169] Accordingly, these lesions are now thought to be epithelial heterotopias developing from foregut endoderm sequestered during cardiac organogenesis.[165,169]

Ectopic hamartomatous thymoma. Rosai and associates[174] have reported five examples of benign tumour-like lesions in the soft tissues of the lower neck in adults, which they suggested might represent a developmental anomaly, derived from the third branchial arch and composed of abnormal thymic tissue. Four components were identifiable in these masses by LM:

1. Cellular spindle-cell areas
2. Epithelial islands composed of solid nests, trabeculae, acini and cysts

3. Mature adipose tissue
4. Lymphocytes, which formed aggregates around epithelial nests in some areas, producing a resemblance to Hassall's corpuscles.

Ultrastructural examination of the epithelial islands and spindle-cell areas revealed cells with squamous characteristics in the form of cytoplasmic tonofibrils, desmosomes, and an adjacent basal lamina in those areas where the cells were bordered by stroma.

Mixed hamartoma of the liver. Rhodes et al[172] have described a hamartomatous hepatic mass in an infant which they suggested was distinguishable from focal nodular hyperplasia and liver cell adenoma by the following features:

1. Extremely broad fields of ductules on LM examination
2. The ultrastructural identification of hepatocytes with embryonic features — as expressed by wide intercellular spaces, more lateral microvilli and a greater abundance of RER than adult hepatocytes, and absence of dense bodies from peroxisomes.

Renal angiomyolipomas. Angiomyolipomas of the kidney are found in up to 80% of cases of tuberous sclerosis, but they also occur in association with the lymphangioleiomyomatosis syndrome or as an isolated phenomenon. There are few reports on the fine structure of angiomyolipoma, but these have revealed a mixture of glycogen-rich smooth muscle cells, lipocytes and fibroblasts.[151,166,170,181,187] Juxtaglomerular cells have also been observed.[170,187] The vascular component is abnormal:[187] the blood vessels lack a normal media and subendothelial collagen accumulation is described.[151]

Myoid hamartoma of the breast. EM has confirmed that the cells comprising these lesions have smooth muscle characteristics, although only rudimentary myoid features may be present.[152,163]

Miscellaneous mesenchymal hamartomas and hamartoma-like lesions. Ultrastructural studies of cardiac fibromatosis (fibroelastic hamartoma),[155,183] fibrous hamartoma of infancy,[3] omental–mesenteric myxoid hamartoma[161] and congenital mesoblastic nephroma[154,159,176,185] have revealed varying proportions of undifferentiated mesenchymal cells, fibroblasts and myofibroblasts; those containing MFB are discussed briefly in Table 11.1.

SO-CALLED TROPHOBLASTIC PSEUDOTUMOUR OF THE UTERUS

This entity is mentioned briefly here only because of its original nomenclature. 'Trophoblastic pseudotumour' was thought initially to be an exaggerated form of placental site reaction simulating neoplasia.[191] Subsequent reports have shown that some cases pursue a malignant course, with metastatic spread.[192] Accordingly, Scully & Young[192] proposed that the lesion be renamed 'placental site trophoblastic tumour'. The fine structure of the component cells resembles that of cytotrophoblast and syncytiotrophoblast;[188-190] for further detail the original articles should be consulted.

MALAKOPLAKIA AND SIMILAR LESIONS

Malakoplakia is an uncommon but distinctive inflammatory lesion composed of histiocytes known as von Hansemann histiocytes, which characteristically contain laminated calcospherites (Michaelis–Gutmann bodies) in their cytoplasm.[197] Malakoplakia typically forms plaque-like lesions replacing the urothelial lining of the bladder, but it also occurs elsewhere in the urinary tract, and cases have been recorded in a variety of anatomical sites.[196,197,203] The condition appears to represent an abnormal lysosomal response to bacterial infection — usually coliform organisms such as *E. coli* or *Klebsiella*.[202] Ultrastructural investigations have revealed Gram-negative bacilli in a proportion of cases, either intact or in various stages of disintegration, within phagolysosomes in the histiocytes.[194,200-202,205,213,214] Other bacteria — including Gram-positive cocci[208] and acid-fast bacilli[206] — have been observed or cultured on rare occasions. In other instances bacteria cannot be found by EM, but biochemical analysis of one such case affecting the prostate[211] revealed the presence of muramic acid — an amino sugar characteristic of bacterial cell walls — suggesting complete lysis of bacteria present at an earlier stage of the lesion. Apart from the detection of intracellular bacteria,

ultrastructural investigations have been directed largely towards elucidating the origin and evolution of the Michaelis–Gutmann (M–G) bodies characteristic of malakoplakia—which are illustrated and discussed in Figs 11.17–11.20.

Malakoplakia is generally recognizable by LM, but some cases pose diagnostic problems — especially if the lesion is situated in an unusual site, or the light microscopy appearances are atypical, or there are few if any M–G bodies.[196] In such circumstances ultrastructural examination can facilitate the diagnosis, and Lou & Teplitz[202] suggest that in the 'prediagnostic' LM phase[197] malakoplakia may be diagnosable by EM — by demonstrating Gram-negative bacilli or their remnants in phagolysosomes showing early evidence of calcium deposition.

The value of EM in detecting unusual infective disorders is further exemplified by the xanthogranulomatous vaginal pseudotumour reported by Strate et al[212] — which had ultrastructural similarities to malakoplakia and Whipple's disease (see Ch. 14), but lacked M–G bodies. This case presented with recurrent vaginal polyps resembling granular cell tumour by LM. EM revealed a population of histiocytes containing numerous phagolysosomes together with intracytoplasmic and extracellular Gram-negative bacteria. The bacterial cell bodies were surrounded by a lucent halo into which wispy strands of material projected, and culture revealed a mucoid strain of *E. coli*.

REFERENCES

Myofibroproliferative lesions, including nodular fasciitis and its variants, the fibromatoses and elastofibroma

1. Adler K B, Craighead J E, Vallyathan N V, Evans J N 1981 Actin-containing cells in human pulmonary fibrosis. American Journal of Pathology 102: 427–437
2. Akhtar M, Miller R M 1977 Ultrastructure of elastofibroma. Cancer 40: 728–735
3. Alba Greco M, Schinella R A, Vuletin J C 1984 Fibrous hamartoma of infancy: an ultrastructural study. Human Pathology 15: 717–723
4. Allen P W 1972 Nodular fasciitis. Pathology 4: 9–26
5. Allen P W 1977 The fibromatoses: a clinicopathologic classification based on 140 cases. Part 1. American Journal of Surgical Pathology 1: 255–270
6. Allen P W 1977 The fibromatoses: a clinicopathologic classification based on 140 cases. Part 2. American Journal of Surgical Pathology 1: 305–321
7. Austin P, Jakobiec F A, Iwamoto T, Hornblass A 1983 Elastofibroma oculi. Archives of Ophthalmology 101: 1575–1579
8. Azua J, Arraiza A, Delgado B, Romeo C 1985 Nodular fasciitis initially diagnosed by aspiration cytology. Acta Cytologica 29: 562–565
9. Balazs M, Kovacs A 1982 The 'transitional' mucosa adjacent to large bowel carcinoma — electron microscopic features and myfibroblast reaction. Histopathology 6: 617–629
10. Battifora H, Hines J R 1971 Recurrent digital fibromas of childhood. An electron microscopic study. Cancer 27: 1530–1536
11. Benish B, Peison B, Marquet E, Sobel H J 1983 Pre-elastofibroma and elastofibroma (the continuum of elastic-producing fibrous tumors). A light and ultrastructural study. American Journal of Clinical Pathology 80: 88–92
12. Benjamin S P, Mercer R D, Hawk W A 1977 Myofibroblastic contraction in spontaneous regression of multiple congenital

mesenchymal hamartomas. Cancer 40: 2342–2352
13. Berlinger N T, Schachern P 1983 Myofibroblasts in chronic otitis media. Laryngoscope 93: 1566–1568
14. Bhawan J, Bacchetta C, Joris I, Majno G 1979 A myofibroblastic tumor. Infantile digital fibroma (recurrent digital fibrous tumor of childhood). American Journal of Pathology 94: 19–36
15. Bhathal P S 1972 Presence of modified fibroblasts in cirrhotic livers in man. Pathology 4: 139–144
16. Bondi A, Mancini A M, Baldini N 1983 Occurrences of different types of contractile cells in some lung fibrosis. Applied Pathology 1: 66–75
17. Burry A F, Kerr J F R, Pope J H 1970 Recurring digital fibrous tumour of childhood: an electron microscopic and virologic study. Pathology 2: 287–291
18. Campbell G R, Ryan G B 1983 Origin of myofibroblasts in the avascular capsule around free-floating intraperitoneal blood clots. Pathology 15: 253–264
19. Chung E B, Enzinger F M 1975 Proliferative fasciitis. Cancer 36: 1450–1458
20. Chung E B, Enzinger F M 1981 Infantile myofibromatosis. Cancer 48: 1807–1818
21. Coalson J J 1982 The ultrastructure of human fibrosing alveolitis. Virchows Archiv A, Pathological Anatomy and Histology 395: 181–199
22. Craver J L, McDivitt R W 1981 Proliferative fasciitis. Ultrastructural study of two cases. Archives of Pathology and Laboratory Medicine 105: 542–545
23. Daroca P J Jr, Pulitzer D R, LoCicero J III 1982 Ossifying fasciitis. Archives of Pathology and Laboratory Medicine 106: 682–685
23a. Dini G, Grappone C, Del Rosso M, Lunghi F, Bartoletti R 1986 Intracellular collagen in fibroblasts of Peyronie's disease. Journal of Submicroscopic Cytology 18: 605–611

24. Dixon A Y, Lee S H 1980 An Ultrastructural study of elastofibromas. Human Pathology 11: 250–262
25. Enzinger F M, Weiss S W 1983 Soft tissue tumors. Mosby, St Louis
26. Erlandson R A 1981 Diagnostic transmission electron microscopy of human tumors. The interpretation of submicroscopic structures in human neoplastic cells. Masson, New York, pp 95–116
27. Farragiana T, Churg J, Strauss L, Voglino A 1981 Ultrastructural histochemistry of infantile digital fibromatosis. Ultrastructural Pathology 2: 241–247
28. Feiner H, Kaye G I 1976 Ultrastructural evidence of myofibroblasts in circumscribed fibromatosis. Archives of Pathology and Laboratory Medicine 100: 265–268
29. Gabbiani G, Hirschel B J, Ryan G B, Statkov P R, Majno G 1972 Granulation tissue as a contractile organ. A study of structure and function. Journal of Experimental Medicine 135: 719–734
30. Gabbiani G, Majno G 1972 Dupuytren's contracture: fibroblast contraction? An ultrastructural study. American Journal of Pathology 66: 131–146
31. Gabbiani G, Ryan G B, Lamelin J-P, Vassalli P, Majno G, Bouvier C A, Cruchard A, Luscher E F 1973 Human smooth muscle autoantibody. Its identification as antiactin antibody and a study of its binding to 'non-muscular' cells. American Journal of Pathology 72: 473–488
32. Gabella G 1981 Structure of smooth muscles. In: Bulbring E, Brading A F, Jones A W, Tomita T (eds) Smooth muscle: an assessment of current knowledge. Edward Arnold, London, pp 1–46
33. Ghadially F N 1980 Diagnostic electron microscopy of tumours. Butterworths, London
34. Ghadially F N 1983 Fine structure of synovial joints. A text and atlas of the ultrastructure of normal and pathological articular tissues. Butterworths, London
35. Ghadially F N, Mehta P N 1971 Multifunctional mesenchymal cells resembling smooth muscle cells in ganglia of the wrist. Annals of Rheumatic Diseases 30: 31–42
36. Goellner J R, Soule E H 1980 Desmoid tumors. An ultrastructural study of eight cases. Human Pathology 11: 43–50
37. Gokel J M, Hubner G 1977 Occurrence of myofibroblasts in the different phases of morbus Dupuytren (Dupuytren's contracture). Beiträge zur Pathologie 161: 166–175
38. Gokel J M, Hubner G 1977 Intracellular 'fibrous long spacing' collagen in morbus Dupuytren (Dupuytren's contracture). Beiträge zur Pathologie 161: 176–186
39. Henderson D W 1984 The morphogenesis and classification of diffuse interstitial lung diseases: a clinicopathological approach, based on tissue reaction patterns. Australian and New Zealand Journal of Medicine 14: 735–748
40. Henderson D W, Papadimitriou J M, Coleman M 1986 Ultrastructural appearances of tumours. Diagnosis and classification of human neoplasia by electron microscopy, 2nd edn. Churchill Livingstone, Edinburgh
41. Iwasaki H, Kikuchi M, Mori R, Miyazono J, Enjoji M, Shinohara N, Matsuzaki A 1980 Infantile digital fibromatosis. Ultrastructural, histochemical and tissue culture observations. Cancer 46: 2238–2247
42. Iwasaki H, Kikuchi M, Ohtsuki I, Enjoji M, Suenaga N, Mori R 1983 Infantile digital fibromatosis. Identification of actin filaments in cytoplasmic inclusions by heavy meromysin binding. Cancer 52: 1653–1661
43. Iwasaki H, Muller H, Stutte H J, Brennscheidt U 1984 Palmar fibromatosis (Dupuytren's contracture). Ultrastructural and enzyme histochemical studies of 43 cases. Virchows Archiv A, Pathological Anatomy and Histopathology 405: 41–53
44. Jarvi O H, Saxen A E, Hopsu-Havu V K, Wartiovaara J J, Vaissalo V T 1969 Elastofibroma — a degenerative pseudotumor. Cancer 23: 42–63
45. Johannessen J V 1982 Diagnostic electron microscopy. Hemisphere, Washington, pp 194–201
46. John T, Sassani J W, Eagle R C Jr 1983 The myofibroblastic component of rubeosis iridis. Ophthalmology 90: 721–728
47. Kawanami O, Basset F, Barries R, Lacronique J G, Ferrans V J, Crystal R G 1983 Hypersensitivity pneumonitis in man. Light- and electron-microscopic studies of 18 lung biopsies. American Journal of Pathology 110: 275–289
48. Kindblom L-G, Spicer S S 1982 Elastofibroma. A correlated light and electron microscopic study. Virchows Archiv A, Pathological Anatomy and Histology 396: 127–140
49. Kischer C W, Thies A C, Chvapil M 1982 Perivascular myofibroblasts and microvascular occlusion in hypertrophic scars and keloids. Human Pathology 13: 819–824
50. Kiviat M D, Ross R, Ansell J S 1973 Smooth muscle regeneration in the ureter. Electron microscopic and autoradiographic observations. American Journal of Pathology 72: 403–416
51. Kobayashi Y, Watanabe H, Suzuki H, Konno T, Yamamoto T Y 1981 Ultrastructural studies on congenital generalised fibromatosis regressed spontaneously. Tohoku Journal of Experimental Medicine 134: 431–445
52. Kvist M, Jozsa I, Jarvinen M, Kvist H 1985 Fine structural alterations in chronic Achilles paratenonitis in athletes. Pathology Research and Practice 180: 416–423
53. Liew S-H, Haynes M 1981 Localized form of congenital generalized fibromatosis. A report of 3 cases with myofibroblasts. Pathology 13: 257–266
54. Lipper S, Kahn L B, Reddick R L 1980 The myofibroblast. Pathology Annual 15, pt 1: 409–441
55. Majno G 1979 The story of the myofibroblasts. American Journal of Surgical Pathology 3: 535–542
56. McDonnell P J, Zarbin M A, Gree R 1983 Posterior capsule opacification in pseudophakic eyes. Ophthalmology 90: 1548–1553
57. Meister P, Gokel J M, Romberger K 1979 Palmar fibromatosis — 'Dupuytren's contracture'. A comparison of light, electron and immuno-fluorescence microscopic findings. Pathology Research and Practice 164: 402–412
58. Mirra S S, Miles M L 1982 Subplasmalemmal linear density: a mesodermal feature and a diagnostic aid. Human Pathology 13: 365–380
59. Mitchell M L, di Sant'Agnese P A, Gerber J E 1982 Fibrous hamartoma of infancy. Human Pathology 13: 586–588
60. Mortimer G, Gibson A A M 1982 Recurring digital fibroma. Journal of Clinical Pathology 35: 849–854
61. Mosse P R L, Campbell G R, Ryan G B 1985 A comparison of the avascular capsule surrounding free floating intraperitoneal blood clots in mice and rabbits. Pathology 17: 401–407
62. Nakanishi I, Kajikawa K, Okada Y, Eguchi K 1981 Myofibroblasts in fibrous tumours and fibrosis in various organs. Acta Pathologica Japonica 31: 423–437
63. Navas-Palacios J J 1983 The fibromatoses. An ultrastructural study of 31 cases. Pathology Research and Practice 176: 158–175
64. Navas-Palacios J J, Conde-Zurita J M 1984 Inclusion body myofibroblasts other than those seen in recurring digital fibroma of childhood. Ultrastructural Pathology 7: 109–121
65. Nochomovitz L E, Orenstein J M 1985 Inflammatory pseudotumor of the urinary bladder — possible relationship to nodular fasciitis. Two case reports, cytologic observations, and ultrastructural observations. American Journal of Surgical Pathology 9: 366–373
66. Novotny G E K, Pau H 1984 Myofibroblast-like cells in human anterior capsular cataract. Virchows Archiv A, Pathological Anatomy and Histopathology 404: 393–401
66a. Oertel Y C, Breckner M E, Engler W F 1986 Cytologic diagnosis and ultrastructure of fine-needle aspirates of ganglion cysts. Archives of Pathology and Laboratory Medicine 110: 938–942
67. Orell S R, Sterrett G F, Walters M N-I, Whitaker D 1985 Manual and atlas of fine needle aspiration cytology. Churchill Livingstone, Edinburgh, pp 205–232
68. Povysil C, Matejovsky Z 1979 Ultrastructural evidence of myofibroblasts in pseudomalignant myositis ossificans. Virchows Archiv A, Pathological Anatomy and Histology 381: 189–203
69. Proppe K H, Scully R E, Rosai J 1984 Postoperative spindle cell nodules of genitourinary tract resembling sarcomas. A report of eight cases. American Journal of Surgical Pathology 8: 101–108
70. Ramos C V, Gillespie W, Narconis R J 1978 Elastofibroma. A pseudotumor of myofibroblasts. Archives of Pathology and Laboratory Medicine 102: 538–540
71. Remberger K, Krieg T, Kunze D, Weinmann H-M, Hubner G 1985 Fibromatosis hyalinica multiplex (juvenile hyalin fibromatosis). Light microscopic, electron microscopic, immunohistochemical, and biochemical findings. Cancer 56: 614–624
71a. Ro J Y, Ayala A G, Ordóñez N G, Swanson D A, Babaian R J 1986

Pseudosarcomatous fibromyxoid tumor of the urinary bladder. American Journal of Clinical Pathology 86: 583–590

72. Rose A G 1974 An electron microscopic study of the giant cells in proliferative myositis. Cancer 33: 1543–1547
73. Rosenberg H S, Stenback W A, Spjut H J 1978 The fibromatoses of infancy and childhood. Perspectives in Pediatric Pathology 4: 269–348
74. Ross R, Klebanoff S J 1967 Fine structural changes in uterine smooth muscle and fibroblasts in response to estrogen. Journal of Cell Biology 32: 155–167
75. Roth L M, Deaton R L, Sternberg W H 1979 Massive ovarian edema. A clinicopathologic study of five cases including ultrastructural observations and review of the literature. American Journal of Surgical Pathology 3: 11–21
75a. Rudolph R, McClure W J, Woodward M 1979 Contractile fibroblasts in chronic alcoholic cirrhosis. Gastroenterology 76: 704–709
76. Ryan G B, Cliff W J, Gabbiani G, Irle C, Montandon D, Statkov P R, Majno G 1974 Myofibroblasts in human granulation tissue. Human Pathology 5: 55–67
77. Ryan G B, Cliff W J, Gabbiani G, Irle C, Statkov P R, Majno G 1973 Myofibroblasts in an avascular fibrous tissue. Laboratory Investigation 29: 197–206
78. Schürch W, Seemayer T A, Lagacé R 1981 Stromal myofibroblasts in primary invasive and metastatic carcinomas. A combined immunological, light and electron microscopic study. Virchows Archiv A, Pathological Anatomy and Histology 391: 125–139
79. Schürch W, Seemayer T A, Lagacé R, Gabbiani G 1984 The intermediate filament cytoskeleton of myofibroblasts: an immunofluorescence and ultrastructural study. Virchows Archiv A, Pathological Anatomy and Histopathology 403: 323–336
80. Seemayer T A, Lagacé R, Schürch W, Thelmo W L 1980 The myofibroblast: biologic, pathologic and theoretical considerations. Pathology Annual 15, pt 1: 443–470
81. Seemayer T A, Schürch W, Lagacé R 1981 Myofibroblasts in human pathology. Human Pathology 12: 491–492
82. Seemayer T A, Schürch W, Lagacé R, Tremblay G 1979 Myofibroblasts in the stroma of invasive and metastatic carcinoma. A possible host response to neoplasia. American Journal of Surgical Pathology 3: 525–533
83. Shelley W B, Shelley E D, Swaminathan R 1985 Myofibroblasts in a collagen nevus detected by electron microscopy. Journal of the American Academy of Dermatology 12: 917–921
84. Singer II 1979 The fibronexus: a transmembrane association of fibronectin-containing fibers and bundles of 5 nm microfilaments in hamster and human fibroblasts. Cell 16: 675–685
85. Sobel H J, Marquet E, Sobrinho-Simões M, Johannessen J V 1981 Tumors and tumor-like conditions of soft tissues. In: Johannessen J V (ed) Electron microscopy in human medicine, vol 4, Soft tissues, bones and joints. McGraw-Hill, New York, pp 143–256
86. Sottiurai V S, Batson B C 1983 Role of myofibroblasts in pseudointima formation. Surgery 94: 792–801
87. Staehelin L A 1974 Structure and function of intercellular junctions. International Review of Cytology 39: 191–283
88. Stiller D, Katenkamp D 1975 Cellular features in desmoid fibromatosis and well differentiated fibrosarcomas: an electron microscopic study. Virchows Archiv A, Pathological Anatomy and Histology 369: 155–164
89. Taxy J B, Battifora H 1980 The electron microscope in the study and diagnosis of soft tissue tumors. In: Trump B F, Jones R T (eds) Diagnostic electron microscopy, vol 3, Wiley, New York, pp 97–174
90. Ulbright T M, Santa Cruz D J 1980 Intravenous pyogenic granuloma. Case report with ultrastructural findings. Cancer 45: 1646–1652
91. Waisman J, Smith D W 1968 Fine structure of an elastofibroma. Cancer 22: 671–677
92. Wang N-S, Knaack J 1982 Fibromatosis hyalinica multiplex juvenilis. Ultrastructural Pathology 3: 153–160
92a. Weiss S W 1986 Proliferative fibroblastic lesions: from hyperplasia to neoplasia. American Journal of Surgical Pathology 10, suppl 1: 14–25
93. Winkelmann R K, Sams W M Jr 1969 Elastofibroma. Report of a case with special histochemical and electron-microscopic studies. Cancer 23: 406–415
94. Wirman J A 1976 Nodular fasciitis, a lesion of myofibroblasts. An ultrastructural study. Cancer 38: 2378–2389
95. Woyke S, Domagala W, Olszewski W 1970 Ultrastructure of a fibromatosis hyalinica multiplex juvenilis. Cancer 26: 1157–1168

Localized nodular tenosynovitis (giant cell tumour of tendon sheath) and pigmented villonodular synovitis

96. Alguacil-Garcia A, Unni K K, Goellner J R 1978 Giant cell tumor of tendon sheath and pigmented villonodular synovitis. An ultrastructural study. American Journal of Clinical Pathology 69: 6–17
97. Archer-Harvey J M, Henderson D W, Papadimitriou J M, Rozenbilds M A M 1984 Pigmented villonodular synovitis associated with psoriatic polyarthropathy: an electron microscopic and immunocytochemical study. Journal of Pathology 144: 57–68
98. Bhawan J, Joris I, Cohen N, Majno G 1980 Microcirculatory changes in post-traumatic pigmented villonodular synovitis. Archives of Pathology and Laboratory Medicine 104: 328–332
99. Carstens H B 1978 Giant cell tumors of tendon sheath. An electron microscopical study of 11 cases. Archives of Pathology and Laboratory Medicine 102: 99–103
100. Chase D R, Enzinger F M, Weiss S W, Langloss J M 1984 Keratin in epithelioid sarcoma. An immunohistochemical study. American Journal of Surgical Pathology 8: 435–441
101. Corson J M, Weiss L M, Banks-Schlegal S P, Pinkus G S 1983 Keratin proteins in synovial sarcoma. American Journal of Surgical Pathology 7: 107–109
102. Edwards J C W, Sedgwick A D, Willoughby D A 1981 The formation of a structure with the features of synovial lining by subcutaneous injection of air: an in vivo tissue culture system. Journal of Pathology 134: 147–156
103. Eisenstein R 1968 Giant-cell tumor of tendon sheath: its histogenesis as studied in the electron microscope. Journal of Bone and Joint Surgery 50A: 476–486
104. Erlandson R A 1984 Diagnostic immunohistochemistry of human tumors. An interim evaluation. American Journal of Surgical Pathology 8: 615–624
105. Fechner R E 1976 Neoplasms and neoplasm-like lesions of synovium. In: Ackerman L V, Spjut H J, Abell M R (eds) Bones and joints. International Academy of Pathology Monograph No 17. Williams & Wilkins, Baltimore, pp 157–186
106. Ghadially F N 1980 Overview article: the articular territory of the reticuloendothelial system. Ultrastructural Pathology 1: 249–264
107. Ghadially F N 1983 Fine structure of synovial joints. A text and atlas of the ultrastructure of normal and pathological articular tissues. Butterworths, London, pp 180–200
108. Ghadially F N, Ialonde J-M A, Dick C E 1979 Ultrastructure of pigmented villonodular synovitis. Journal of Pathology 127: 19–26
109. Graabaek P M 1982 Ultrastructural evidence for two distinct types of synoviocytes in rat synovial membrane. Journal of Ultrastructure Research 78: 321–339
110. Hajdu S I 1979 Pathology of soft tissue tumors. Lea and Febiger, Philadelphia, pp 165–226
111. Hirohata K 1968 Light microscopic and electron microscopic studies of individual cells in pigmented villonodular synovitis and bursitis (Jaffe). Kobe Journal of Medical Science 14: 251–279
112. Merkow L P, Frich J C Jr, Slifkin M, Kyreages C G, Pardo M 1971 Ultrastructure of a fibroxanthosarcoma (malignant fibroxanthoma). Cancer 28: 372–383
113. Miettinen M, Lehto V-P, Virtanen I 1982 Keratin in the epithelial-like cells of classical biphasic synovial sarcoma. Virchows Archiv B, Cell Pathology 40: 157–161
114. Myers B W, Masi A T 1980 Pigmented villonodular synovitis and tenosynovitis: a clinical epidemiologic study of 166 cases and literature review. Medicine (Baltimore) 59: 223–238
115. Osborn M, Weber K 1983 Tumor diagnosis by intermediate filament typing: a novel tool for surgical pathology. Laboratory Investigation 48: 372–394
116. Schmidt D, Mackay B 1982 Ultrastructure of human tendon sheath and synovium: implications for tumor histogenesis. Ultrastructural Pathology 3: 269–283

117. Spjut H J, Dorfman H D, Fechner R E, Ackerman L V 1971 Tumors of bone and cartilage. Atlas of tumor pathology, 2nd series, fascicle 5. Armed Forces Institute of Pathology, Washington, pp 400–410

118. Steiner G C 1981 Tumors and tumor-like conditions of bones and joints. In: Johannessen J V (ed) Electron microscopy in human medicine, vol 4, Soft tissues, bones and joints. McGraw-Hill, New York, pp 54–140

119. Stout A P, Lattes R 1967 Tumors of the soft tissues. Atlas of tumor pathology, 2nd series, fascicle 1. Armed Forces Institute of Pathology, Washington, p 47

119a. Ushijima M, Hashimoto H, Tsuneyoshi M, Enjoji M 1986 Giant cell tumor of the tendon sheath (nodular tenosynovitis). A study of 207 cases to compare the large joint group with the common digit group. Cancer 57: 875–884

Plasma cell granuloma

120. Buell R, Wang N-S, Seemayer T A, Ahmed M N 1976 Endobronchial plasma cell granuloma (xanthomatous pseudotumor). A light and electron microscopic study. Human Pathology 7: 411–426

121. Chen H P, Lee S S, Berardi R S 1984 Inflammatory pseudotumor of the lung. Ultrastructural and light microscopic study of a myxomatous variant. Cancer 54: 861–865

122. Eimoto T, Yanaka M, Kurosawa M, Ikeya F 1978 Plasma cell granuloma (inflammatory pseudotumor) of the spinal cord meninges. Report of a case. Cancer 41: 1929–1936

123. Kuzela D C 1975 Ultrastructural study of a postinflammatory 'tumor' of the lung. Cancer 36: 149–156

124. Maeda Y, Tani E, Nakano M, Matsumoto T 1984 Plasma-cell granuloma of the fourth ventricle. Case report. Journal of Neurosurgery 60: 1291–1296

125. Wentworth P, Lynch M J, Fallis J C, Turner J A P, Lowden J A, Conen P E 1968 Xanthomatous pseudotumor of lung. A case report with electron microscope and lipid studies. Cancer 22: 345–355

126. West S G, Pittman D L, Coggin J T 1980 Intracranial plasma cell granuloma. Cancer 46: 330–335

Other inflammatory pseudotumours: inflammatory polyps of the gastrointestinal tract and giant cell reparative granulomas

127. Adkins K F, Martinez M G, Hartley M W 1969 Ultrastructure of giant-cell lesions. A peripheral giant cell reparative granuloma. Oral Surgery, Oral Medicine and Oral Pathology 28: 713–723

128. Adkins K F, Martinez M G, Romaniuk K 1972 Ultrastructure of giant-cell lesions. Mononuclear cells in peripheral giant-cell granulomas. Oral Surgery, Oral Medicine and Oral Pathology 33: 775–786

129. Andersen L, Arwill T, Fejerskov O, Heyden G, Philipsen H P 1973 Oral giant cell granulomas. An enzyme histochemical and ultrastructural study. Acta Pathologica et Microbiologica Scandinavica Section A Pathology 81: 617–629

130. Anthony P P, Morris D S, Vowles K D J 1984 Multiple and recurrent inflammatory fibroid polyps in three generations of a Devon family: a new syndrome. Gut 25: 854–862

131. Bartel H, Piatowska D 1977 Electron microscopic study of peripheral giant-cell reparative granuloma. Oral Surgery, Oral Medicine and Oral Pathology 43: 82–96

132. El-Labban N G, Lee K W 1983 Myofibroblasts in central giant cell granuloma of the jaws: an ultrastructural study. Histopathology 7: 907–918

132a. Jessurun J, Paplanus S H, Nagle R B, Hamilton S R, Yardley J H, Tripp M 1986 Pseudosarcomatous changes in inflammatory pseudopolyps of the colon. Archives of Pathology and Laboratory Medicine 110: 833–836

133. Navas-Palacios J J, Colina-Ruizdelgado F, Sanchez-Larrea M D, Cortes-Cansino J 1983 Inflammatory fibroid polyps of the gastro-intestinal tract. An immunohistochemical and electron microscopic study. Cancer 51: 1682–1690

134. Sapp J P 1972 Ultrastructure and histogenesis of peripheral giant cell reparative granuloma of the jaws. Cancer 30: 1119–1129

135. Shimer G R, Helwig E B 1984 Inflammatory fibroid polyps of the intestine. American Journal of Clinical Pathology 81: 708–714

136. Williams R M 1981 An ultrastructural study of a jejunal inflammatory fibroid polyp. Histopathology 5: 193–203

Xanthomas

137. Depot M J, Jakobiec F A, Dodick J M, Iwamoto T 1984 Bilateral and extensive xanthelasma palpebrarum in a young man. Ophthalmology 91: 522–527

138. Dustin P, Tondeur M, Libert J 1978 Metabolic and storage diseases. In: Johannessen J V (ed) Electron microscopy in human medicine, vol 2, Cellular pathology, metabolic and storage diseases. McGraw-Hill, New York, pt 2, pp 151–245

139. Parker F, Odland G F 1968 Experimental xanthoma. A correlative biochemical, histologic, histochemical, and electron microscopic study. American Journal of Pathology 53: 537–565

140. Parker F, Odland G F 1973 Ultrastructural and lipid biochemical comparisons of human eruptive, tuberous and planar xanthomas. Israel Journal of Medical Sciences 9: 395–423

141. Ronan S G, Bolano J, Manaligod J R 1984 Verruciform xanthoma of penis. Light and electron-microscopic study. Urology 23: 600–603

142. Sanchez R L, Raimer S S, Peltier F, Swedo J 1985 Papular xanthoma. A clinical, histologic, and ultrastructural study. Archives of Dermatology 121: 626–631

142a. Seo I S, Min K W, Mirkin D 1986 Juvenile xanthogranuloma. Ultrastructural and immunocytochemical studies. Archives of Pathology and Laboratory Medicine 110: 911–915

143. Zemel H, Deeken J, Asel N, Packer J 1970 The ultrastructural features of normolipemic plane xanthoma. Archives of Pathology 89: 111–117

Hamartomas, heterotopias and related lesions

144. Arseni C, Alexianu M, Horvat L, Alexianu D, Petrovici A L 1972 Fine structure of atypical cells in tuberous sclerosis. Acta Neuropathologica (Berlin) 21: 185–193

145. Basset F, Soler P, Marsac J, Corrin B 1976 Pulmonary lymphangiomyomatosis. Three new cases studied with electron microscopy. Cancer 38: 2357–2366

146. Bateson E M 1973 So-called hamartoma of the lung — a true neoplasm of fibrous connective tissue of the bronchi. Cancer 31: 1458–1467

147. Bender B L, Yunis E J 1980 Central nervous system pathology of tuberous sclerosis in children. Ultrastructural Pathology 1: 287–299

148. Bruni C, Prioleau P G, Ivey H H, Nolan S P 1980 New fine structural features of cardiac rhabdomyoma: report of a case. Cancer 46: 2068–2073

149. Capron F, Ameille J, LeClerc P, Mornet P, Barbagellata M, Reynes M, Rochemaure J 1983 Pulmonary lymphangioleiomyomatosis and Bourneville's tuberous sclerosis with pulmonary involvement: the same disease? Cancer 52: 851–855

150. Carter D, Eggleston J C 1980 Tumors of the lower respiratory tract. Atlas of tumor pathology, 2nd series, fascicle 17. Armed Forces Institute of Pathology, Washington, pp 221–231

151. Chalvardjian A, Kovacs K, Horvath E 1978 Renal angiomyolipoma: ultrastructural study. Urology 12: 717–720

152. Daroca P J Jr, Reed R J, Love G I, Kraus S D 1985 Myoid hamartomas of the breast. Human Pathology 16: 212–219

153. Estrada R, Spjut H J 1983 Hamartomatous polyps in Peutz-Jeghers syndrome. A light-, histochemical, and electron-microscopic study. American Journal of Surgical Pathology 7: 747–754

154. Favara B E, Johnson W, Ito J 1968 Renal tumors in the neonatal period. Cancer 22: 845–855

155. Feldman P S, Meyer M W 1976 Fibroelastic hamartoma (fibroma) of the heart. Cancer 38: 314–323

156. Fenoglio J J Jr, Diana D J, Bowen T E, McAllister H A Jr, Ferrans V J 1977 Ultrastructure of a cardiac rhabdomyoma. Human Pathology 8: 700–706
157. Fenoglio J J Jr, Jacobs D W, McAllister H A 1977 Ultrastructure of the mesothelioma of the atrioventricular node. Cancer 40: 721–727
158. Fenoglio J J Jr, McAllister H A Jr, Ferrans V J 1976 Cardiac rhabdomyoma: a clinicopathologic and electron-microscopic study. American Journal of Cardiology 38: 241–251
159. Fu Y-S, Kay S 1973 Congenital mesoblastic nephroma and its recurrence. An ultrastructural observation. Archives of Pathology and Laboratory Medicine 96: 66–70
159a. Ghadially F N, Chisholm I A, Lalonde J-M A 1986 Ultrastructure of an intraocular lacrimal gland choristoma. Journal of Submicroscopic Cytology 18: 189–198
160. Gisser S D, Young I 1979 Pleomorphic pulmonary hamartoma. An apparently unique variant of pulmonary hamartoma. Human Pathology 10: 393–403
161. Gonzalez-Crussi F, de Mello D E, Sotelo-Avila C 1983 Omental-mesenteric myxoid hamartomas. Infantile lesions simulating malignant tumors. American Journal of Surgical Pathology 7: 567–581
162. Gray S R, Carrington C B, Cornog J L Jr 1975 Lymphangiomyomatosis: report of a case with ureteral involvement and chyluria. Cancer 35: 490–498
163. Huntrakoon M, Lin F 1984 Muscular hamartoma of the breast. An electron microscopic study. Virchows Archiv A, Pathological Anatomy and Histopathology 403: 307–312
164. Incze J S, Lui P S 1977 Morphology of the epithelial component of human lung hamartomas. Human Pathology 8: 411–419
165. Linder J, Shelburne J D, Sorge J P, Whalen R E, Hackel D B 1984 Congenital endodermal heterotopia of the atrioventricular node: evidence for the endodermal origin of so-called mesotheliomas of the atrioventricular node. Human Pathology 15: 1093–1098
166. Mori M, Ikeda T, Onoe T 1971 Blastic Schwann cells in renal tumor of tuberous sclerosis complex — an electron microscopic study. Acta Pathologica Japonica 21: 121–129
167. Pardo-Mindan F J, Vazquez J J, Joly M, Rocha E 1983 Splenic hamartoma, vascular type, with endothelial proliferation. Pathology Research and Practice 177: 32–40
168. Patrinely J R, Font R L, Campbell R J, Robertson D M 1983 Hamartomatous adenoma of the nonpigmented ciliary epithelium arising in an iris-ciliary body coloboma. Light and electron microscopic observations. Ophthalmology 90: 1540–1547
169. Paulsen S M, Kristensen I B 1981 So-called mesothelioma of the atrioventricular node. Journal of Submicroscopic Cytology 13: 667–674
170. Perez-Atayde A R, Iwaya S, Lack E 1981 Angiomyolipomas and polycystic renal disease in tuberous sclerosis. Ultrastructural observations. Urology 17: 607–610
171. Perez-Atayde A R, Seiler M W 1984 Pulmonary hamartoma. An ultrastructural study. Cancer 53: 485–492
172. Rhodes R H, Marchildon M B, Luebke D C, Edmondson H A, Mikity V G 1978 A mixed hamartoma of the liver: light and electron microscopy. Human Pathology 9: 211–213
173. Ribadeau Dumas J L, Poirier J, Escourolle R 1973 Ultrastructural study of cerebral lesions in tuberous sclerosis. Acta Neuropathologica (Berlin) 25: 259–270
174. Rosai J, Limas C, Husband E M 1984 Ectopic hamartomatous thymoma. A distinctive benign lesion of lower neck. American Journal of Surgical Pathology 8: 501–513
175. Schochet S S Jr 1981 Electron microscopy of skeletal muscle and peripheral nerve biopsy specimens. In: MacKay B (ed) Introduction to diagnostic electron microscopy. Appleton–Century–Crofts, New York, pp 131–169
176. Shen S C, Yunis E J 1980 A study on the cellularity and ultrastructure of congenital mesoblastic nephroma. Cancer 45: 306–314
177. Silverman J F, Kay S 1976 Multiple pulmonary leiomyomatous hamartomas. Report of a case with ultrastructure examination. Cancer 38: 1199–1204
178. Silverman J F, Kay S, Chang C H 1978 Ultrastructural comparison between skeletal muscle and cardiac rhabdomyomas. Cancer 42: 189–193
179. Silverman J F, Kay S, McCue C M, Lower R R, Brough A J, Chang C H 1976 Rhabdomyoma of the heart. Ultrastructural study of three cases. Laboratory Investigation 35: 596–606
180. Stone F J, Churg A M 1977 The ultrastructure of pulmonary hamartoma. Cancer 39: 1064–1070
181. Sun C N, White H J, Bissada N K 1975 Renal angiomyolipoma in a case of tuberous sclerosis, an electron microscopy study. Beiträge zur Pathologie 156: 401–410
182. Trillo A A, Holleman I L, White J T 1978 Presence of satellite cells in a cardiac rhabdomyoma. Histopathology 2: 215–223
183. Turi G K, Albala A, Fenoglio J J Jr 1980 Cardiac fibromatosis: an ultrastructural study. Human Pathology 11: 577–580
184. Vazquez J J, Fernandez-Cuervo L, Fidalgo B 1976 Lymphangiomyomatosis. Morphogenetic study and ultrastructural confirmation of the histogenesis of the lung lesion. Cancer 37: 2321–2328
185. Wigger H J 1975 Fetal mesenchymal hamartoma of the kidney. A tumor of secondary mesenchyme. Cancer 36: 1002–1008
186. Wolff M 1973 Lymphangiomyoma: clinicopathological study and ultrastructural confirmation of its histogenesis. Cancer 31: 988–1007
187. Yum M, Ganguly A, Donohue J P 1984 Juxtaglomerular cells in renal angiomyolipoma. Ultrastructural observation. Urology 24: 283–286

So-called trophoblastic pseudotumour

188. Berger G, Verbaere J, Feroldi J 1984 Placental site trophoblastic tumor of the uterus: an ultrastructural and immunohistochemical study. Ultrastructural Pathology 6: 319–329
189. Blackwell J B, Papadimitriou J M 1979 Trophoblastic pseudotumor of the uterus. Case report and ultrastructure. Cancer 43: 1734–1741
190. Gloor E, Hurlimann J 1981 Trophoblastic pseudotumor of the uterus. Clinicopathologic report with immunohistochemical and ultrastructural studies. American Journal of Surgical Pathology 5: 5–13
191. Kurman R J, Scully R E, Norris H J 1976 Trophoblastic pseudotumor of the uterus. An exaggerated form of 'syncytial endometritis' simulating a malignant tumor. Cancer 38: 1214–1226
192. Scully R E, Young R H 1981 Trophoblastic pseudotumor. A reappraisal. American Journal of Surgical Pathology 5: 75–76

Malakoplakia

193. Akhtar M, Ali M A, Robinson C, Harfi H 1985 Role of fine needle aspiration biopsy in the diagnosis and management of malacoplakia. Acta Cytologica 29: 457–460
194. An T, Ferenczy A, Wilens S L, Melicow M M 1974 Observations on the formation of Michaelis-Gutmann bodies. Human Pathology 5: 753–758
195. Charney E B, Witzleben C L, Douglas S D, Kamani M, Kalichman M A 1985 Medical management of bilateral renal malakoplakia. Archives of Disease in Childhood 60: 254–256
196. Colby T V 1978 Malakoplakia. Two unusual cases which presented diagnostic problems. American Journal of Surgical Pathology 2: 377–382
197. Damjanov I, Katz S M 1981 Malakoplakia. Pathology Annual 16, pt 2: 103–126
198. Finlay-Jones L R, Blackwell J B, Papadimitriou J M 1968 Malakoplakia of the colon. American Journal of Clinical Pathology 50: 320–329
199. Flint A, Murad T M 1984 Malakoplakia and malakoplakia-like lesions of the upper gastrointestinal tract. Ultrastructural Pathology 7: 167–176
200. Guccion J G, Thorgeirsson U P, Smith B H 1978 Malacoplakia of epididymis. Urology 12: 713–716
201. Hodder R V, St George-Hyslop P, Chalvardjian A, Bear R A, Thomas P 1984 Pulmonary malakoplakia. Thorax 39: 70–71
202. Lou T Y, Teplitz C 1974 Malakoplakia: pathogenesis and ultrastructural morphogenesis. A problem of altered macrophage (phagolysosomal) response. Human Pathology 5: 191–207
203. McClure J 1983 Malakoplakia. Journal of Pathology 140: 275–330

204. McClure J, Cameron C H S, Garrett R G 1981 The ultrastructural features of malakoplakia. Journal of Pathology 134: 13–25

205. McClurg F V, D'Agostino A N, Martin J H, Race G J 1973 Ultrastructural demonstration of intracellular bacteria in three cases of malakoplakia of the bladder. American Journal of Clinical Pathology 60: 780–788

206. Miranda D, Vuletin J C, Kaufman S L 1970 Disseminated histiocytosis and intestinal malakoplakia. Occurrence due to *Mycobacterium intracellulare* infection. Archives of Pathology and Laboratory Medicine 103: 302–305

207. Nistal M, Rodriguez Echandia E L, Paniagua R 1978 Septate junctions between digestive vacuoles in human malacoplakia. Tissue and Cell 10: 137–142

208. Price H M, Hanrahan J B, Florida R G 1973 Morphogenesis of calcium laden cytoplasmic bodies in malakoplakia of the skin. An electron microscopic study. Human Pathology 4: 381–394

209. Saraf P, di Sant'Agnese P, Valvo J, Caldamone A, Linke C 1983 An unusual case of malacoplakia involving the testis and prostate. Journal of Urology 129: 149–150

210. Sinclair-Smith C, Kahn L B, Cywes S 1975 Malakoplakia in childhood. Case report with ultrastructural observations and review of the literature. Archives of Pathology 99: 198–203

211. Sterrett G F, Heenan P J, Wyche P, Papadimitriou J M 1975 Malakoplakia of the prostate: a morphological and biochemical study. Pathology 7: 139–147

212. Strate S M, Taylor W E, Forney J P, Silva F G 1983 Xanthogranulomatous pseudotumor of the vagina: evidence of a local response to an unusual bacterium (mucoid *Escherichia coli*). American Journal of Clinical Pathology 79: 637–643

213. Tesluk H, Munn R J 1984 Malacoplakia of the uterus. Archives of Pathology and Laboratory Medicine 108: 692

214. Yang C C J, Huang T Y, Tsung S H, Han D C S 1983 Rectal malacoplakia in a patient with Hodgkin's disease. Report of a case and review of the literature. Diseases of the Colon and Rectum 26: 129–132

Fig. 11.1 (Facing page, top) Nodular fasciitis: survey of myofibroblasts. Subcutaneous nodule from the posterior neck region of an 8-month-old girl. Elongated bipolar cells traverse the field. One (F) is predominantly fibroblastic, with abundant RER and a paucity of microfilaments. Filaments in the other cells are not numerous, and are located mainly in the subplasmalemmal regions, but the cells in one area (arrows) contain a feltwork of filaments — which are not resolved at this magnification. (× 9200)

Although nodular fasciitis is one of the most common benign lesions of soft tissues, it has been the subject of remarkably few EM studies.[8,45,54,63,80,94] The most notable report is that of Wirman[94] who investigated eight cases by EM and found that the cells had the features of myofibroblasts. The nuclei were occasionally cleaved deeply, and intermediate filaments were observed in addition to the typical microfilaments — while the RER predominated over the filaments. Intermediate junctions (Fig. 11.3) were also present, and the interstitium contained extravasated erythrocytes without any evidence of surrounding endothelium. Nearby blood vessels were lined by prominent endothelium, and capillary buds with slit-like lumina were also present, but erythrocytes were not seen traversing the vessel walls. Giant cells with finger-like projections were evident in one case and were thought to resemble multinucleated histiocytes, their cytoplasm being characterized by elongated mitochondria, dense bodies (apparently lysosomes), residual bodies and numerous pinocytotic vesicles. References: 8, 45, 54, 63, 80 and 94.

Fig. 11.2 (Facing page, bottom) Nodular fasciitis: myofibroblasts. Microfilaments are not numerous in these MFB and are concentrated in the subplasmalemmal regions (arrows). Attachment zones and microtendons (arrowheads) are also evident. The extracellular matrix contains collagen fibres and proteoglycan granules (asterisk). (× 14 900)

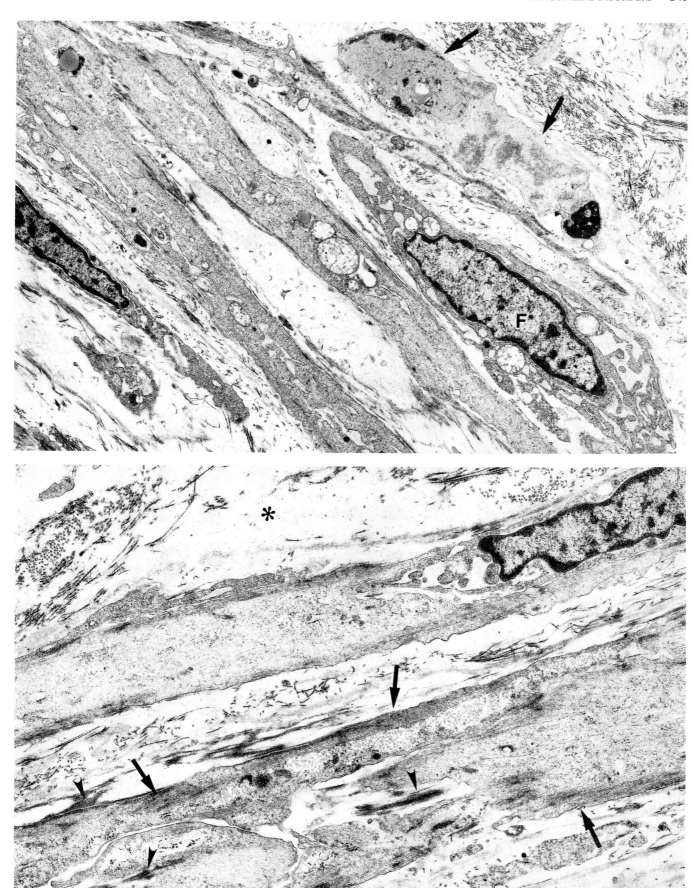

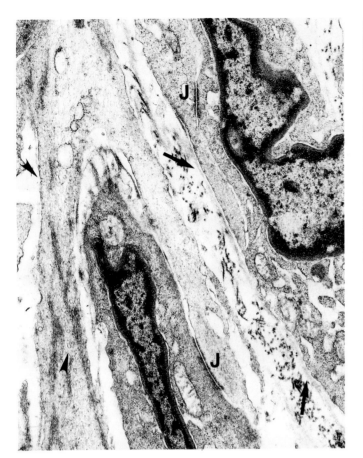

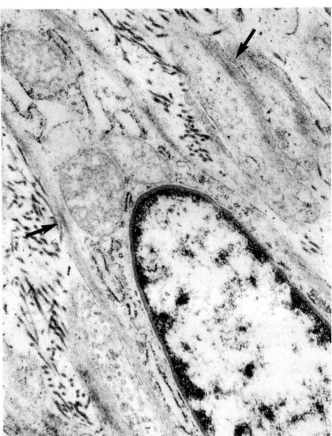

Fig. 11.3 Nodular fasciitis: myofibroblasts. Prominence of the nuclear fibrous lamina is a major feature of these MFB, while intermediate junctions (J) have formed between apposed plasma membranes. One cell contains a feltwork of microfilaments as well as micropinocytotic vesicles (arrowheads). External lamina (arrows) lies parallel to the plasma membrane of one cell. (× 15 600)

Fig. 11.4 Infantile myofibromatosis: myofibroblast. Solitary lesion from the scalp and calvarium of an infant aged 7 months. Microfilaments (arrows) are concentrated in the subplasmalemmal zones. Observe the prominent nuclear fibrous lamina. Myofibroblasts constituted the majority of cells in this case, but fibroblasts were also present. (Formalin fixation, × 23 000) (Case contributed by Dr P. W. Allen.) References: 5, 20, 25, 51, 53 and 73.

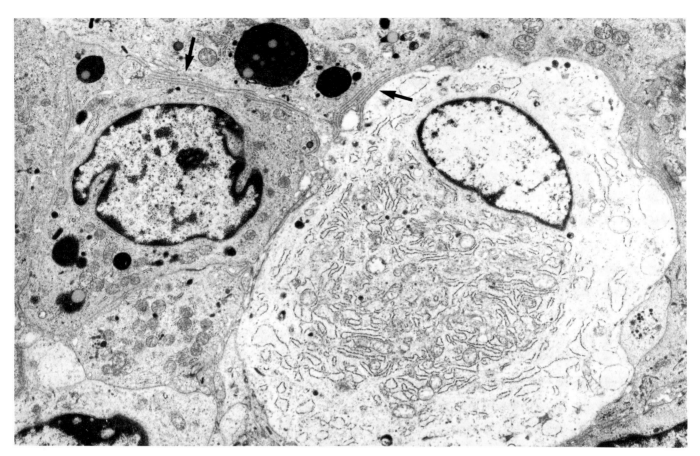

Fig. 11.5 So-called giant cell tumour of tendon sheath: histiocytic and fibroblastoid cells. Lesion from the index finger. The fibroblastoid cell depicted here has electron-lucent cytoplasm with abundant RER showing cisternal dilatation at the periphery of the cell. The histiocytic cells have denser cytoplasm with moderate numbers of siderosomes, and they also possess interdigitating cytoplasmic flaps (arrows). Whorled aggregates of intermediate filaments in histiocytoid cells and apparently intracytoplasmic collagen fibres in myofibroblasts were also seen in this case. The stromal blood vessels had narrow lumina and were lined by swollen endothelium. Erythrocyte extravasation was not seen. (× 8400)
References: 96, 99 and 103.

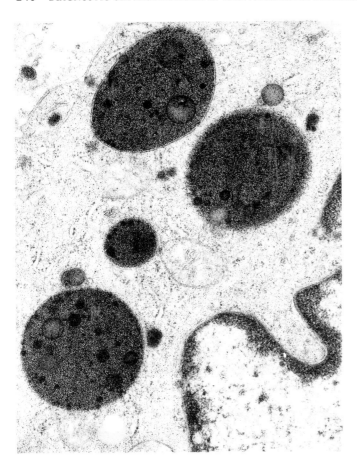

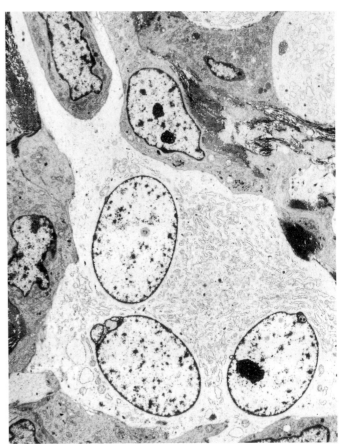

Fig. 11.6 Giant cell tumour of tendon sheath: siderosomes. The dense granular matrices of these lysosomal bodies are typical of siderosomes. The intervening cytoplasm is peppered with small iron-containing particles; note that these are not present in the vacuoles in the adjoining cell at the upper left corner. See also Fig. 11.12. (× 26 200)

Fig. 11.7 Giant cell tumour of tendon sheath: giant cell I. Two types of giant cells were found in this tumour. As depicted here, one had fibroblastoid characteristics, with pale cytoplasm containing abundant RER and inconspicuous lysosomes. Ramifying cytoplasmic projections were another feature of this type. (× 3100)

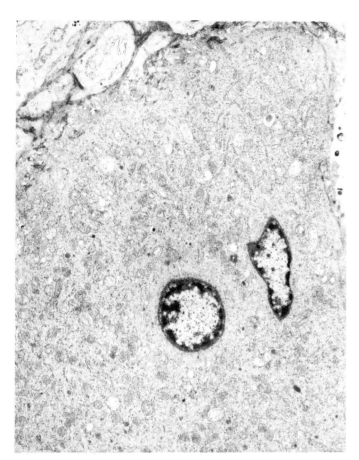

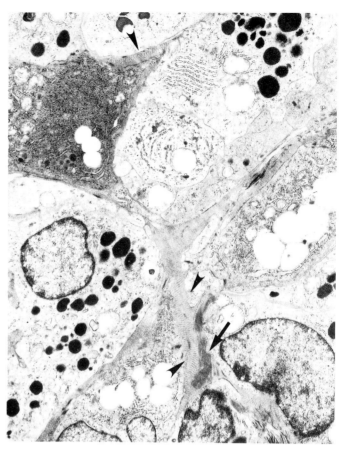

Fig. 11.8 Giant cell tumour of tendon sheath: giant cell II. The other type of giant cell was characterized by denser cytoplasm with a greater abundance of mitochondria. Once again, lysosomes are not conspicuous and there are no siderosomes. Instead of the elongated processes characterizing the fibroblastoid giant cells, the periphery of these cells formed shorter microvillous projections, which are not resolved at this magnification. (× 6000)

Fig. 11.9 Pigmented villonodular synovitis: subsynovial fibrohistiocytic cells. Case of PVNS associated with psoriatic polyarthropathy, from a 32-year-old woman. The lesion affected the right knee joint and, despite synovectomy on two occasions, it recurred stubbornly, with erosion of the lateral femoral condyle and extension into the musculature of the thigh. The patient was then treated by total excision of the knee joint with arthrodesis and postoperative radiotherapy, and there has been no subsequent recurrence. Electron-dense lysosomes and lucent lipid droplets are present in the subsynovial fibrohistiocytic cells occupying this field, and one cell possesses parallel lamellae of RER. The interstitium contains fibrous long-spacing collagen (arrowheads), native collagen fibres and fibrin (arrow). (× 6000) So-called desmosome-like junctions — which have only a tenuous resemblance to true desmosomes[107] — may be present between the subsynovial macrophages[108] but they were not evident in this case. Archer-Harvey and associates[97] also described two types of multinucleated giant cells, neither of which showed evidence of phagocytosis. The type I cells had crenated nuclei with prominent nucleoli, numerous mitochondria, plentiful RER and an irregular surface. The type II cells had smooth nuclear profiles, with few mitochondria and less RER than the type I cells. (Details of this case have been published elsewhere.[97]) References: 96, 97, 107, 108, 111 and 118.

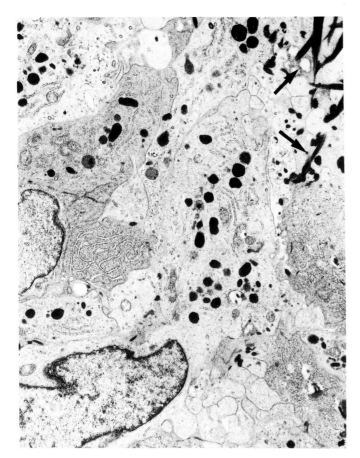

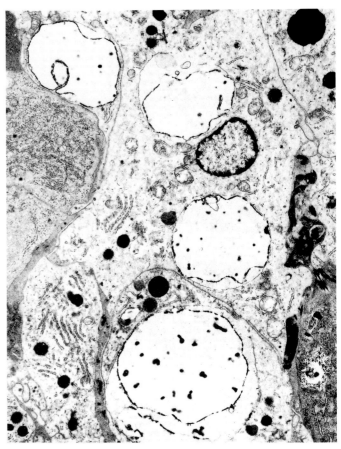

Fig. 11.10 Pigmented villonodular synovitis: subsynovial cells. In addition to numerous lysosomes, these fibrohistiocytic cells are characterized by complex interdigitation of cytoplasmic processes. Electron-dense fibrin tactoids are also evident (arrows). (× 6300)

Fig. 11.11 Pigmented villonodular synovitis: erythrophagocytosis. Four erythrophagosomes are depicted. Only ghosts of the ingested red cells remain, with partial collapse of their membranes. Most of the haemoglobin has been extracted; the residual haemoglobin is represented only by a thin submembranous dense layer, and small dense collections in the otherwise lucent interior of the erythrocytes. (× 6000)

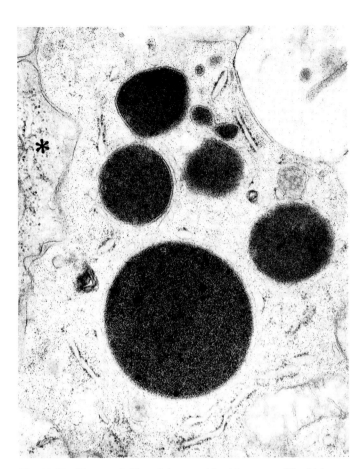

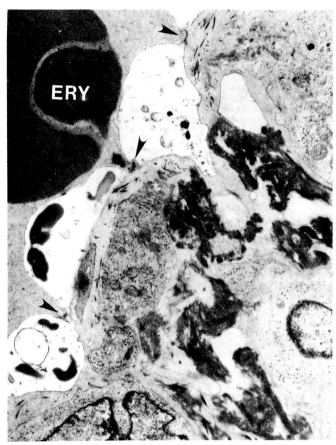

Fig. 11.12 Pigmented villonodular synovitis: siderosomes. The fairly uniform dense granularity of these bodies is typical of siderosomes. Note also the innumerable small iron-containing particles in the cytoplasm — but not in the mitochondria, the cisternae of the RER or an adjoining cell (asterisk). (× 27 700) Ghadially and associates[108] also observed an unusual conjunction of siderosomes and erythrophagosomes — in which small siderosomes were studded around the periphery of the erythrophagosomes, with continuity of their boundary membranes; these appearances were thought to reflect either fusion, or genesis of siderosomes from erythrophagosomes by budding.

Fig. 11.13 Pigmented villonodular synovitis: blood vessel. Erythrocytes (ERY) occupy the lumen. The swollen endothelium has lucent cytoplasm in which electron-dense material is evident; this material may be related to fibrin — which was seen in caveolar invaginations of the endothelium in other regions. The interendothelial spaces are widened (arrowheads) and numerous sheaves of fibrin are present in the perivascular area; at high magnification the characteristic transverse periodicity of 18–20 nm could be discerned in many of the fibrin tactoids. (× 7500)

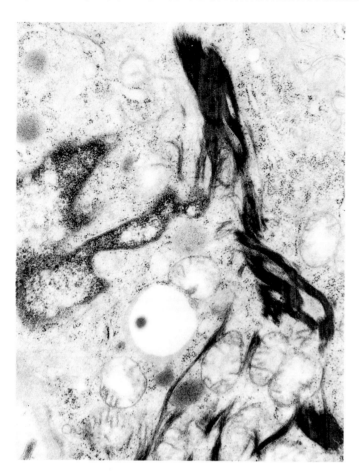

Fig. 11.14 Pigmented villonodular synovitis: tonofibrils. The cellular reaction in this case also included distinctive mononuclear cells containing bundles of intermediate filaments resembling tonofibrils; the filaments were often concentrated in the perinuclear territory and correlated with the immunocytochemical detection of cytokeratins. The irregular nucleus in this cell has been sectioned tangentially. A lucent lipid droplet is also present. Figs 11.9–11.14 are all from the same case. (× 22 000)

The identification of mononuclear cells expressing cytokeratin filaments (tonofilaments) in this case of PVNS[97] is of conceptual interest. Cytokeratins are considered to be a marker for epithelial cells[115] and they have not been reported in other cases of PVNS.[97] However, cytokeratins have been documented by immunocytochemical techniques in epithelioid sarcoma,[100] the tubular component of so-called synovial sarcoma[101,113] and monomorphic 'synovial' sarcoma.[104] In addition, intertwining filamentous bundles resembling tonofilaments have been illustrated in malignant fibrous histiocytoma,[112] and we have also observed perinuclear bundles of tonofilaments in a monomorphic fibrous 'synovial' sarcoma (Stirling & Henderson, unpublished observation). These findings do not by themselves indicate that any of these neoplasms are of synovial origin. Since they contain histiocytoid, fibroblastoid or fibrohistiocytic cells, such sarcomas may or may not be derived from synovium, but most probably are not because they occur in joint spaces, bursae and tendon sheaths only on extremely rare occasions. Moreover, as we have indicated above, the cells accumulating in PVNS may originate at least in part from extrasynovial sources, and cytokeratins are not a feature of normal synovial intimal cells. Instead, such an acquisition of cytokeratin filaments may be regarded as evidence of epithelial metaplasia in a mesenchymal lesion. There is evidence that all intermediate filament proteins share amino acid sequence homologies and they appear to be related members of a multigene family, usually expressed in a cell type-specific fashion.[115] Therefore, it is not entirely surprising that mesenchymal cells can express cytokeratin filaments under some circumstances, perhaps as a result of altered gene expression or gene re-arrangement accompanying neoplastic or quasineoplastic processes. We strongly believe that one cannot conclude that PVNS and the sarcomatoid tumours listed above are related disorders simply because they can express cytokeratins, when in contrast there are clear clinicopathological differences between these conditions — especially in regard to their morphology by LM and their predilection for different anatomical sites.

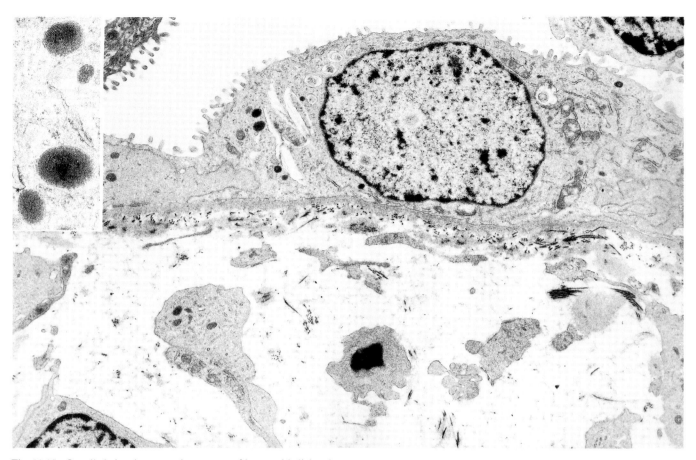

Fig. 11.15 So-called chondromatous hamartoma of lung: epithelial and subepithelial components. Peripheral 'coin' lesion from a 68-year-old man, which was seen to enlarge slowly in serial chest X-rays. This microvillous non-ciliated epithelial cell rests on a well-developed basal lamina and contains electron-dense granules. At higher magnification the granules display the characteristics of Clara cell granules (*inset*). Type II pneumocytes with lamelliform cytoplasmic granules were present in other areas. The subepithelial component consists of a flocculent proteoglycan-containing matrix traversed by mesenchymal cell processes. (× 8400, Inset, × 35 600)

Remarkably few ultrastructural studies of pulmonary chondromatous 'hamartoma' have been reported.[164,171,180] EM reveals that the epithelial element includes the cell types found normally in adult terminal bronchiolar and alveolar epithelium.[171,180] Interestingly, neuroendocrine cells have not been documented in the epithelial component,[171] but this may reflect the vagaries of tissue sampling and the paucity of cases evaluated by EM; we have since found them on one occasion (unpublished observation). In a report of three cases, Incze & Lui[164] observed intranuclear tubular inclusions in about 10% of the epithelial cells, and less frequent fibrillary inclusions within nuclei. In our experience these tubular inclusions are a useful marker for reactive and neoplastic bronchiolo-alveolar epithelium,[40] but we have not found them in any of our cases of 'hamartomas' and they were not reported by Stone & Churg;[180] however, Perez-Atayde & Seiler[171] observed frequent nuclear inclusions composed of amorphous debris and cholesterol clefts in their cases. Undifferentiated mesenchymal cells, fibroblasts and smooth muscle cells are described in the subepithelial myxofibrous tissue[171,180] and they may have strikingly stellate outlines.[171] The cells in the deeper chondroid tissue have the usual features of chondrocytes, with abundant surrounding cartilaginous matrix rich in proteoglycan granules (Fig. 11.16).[171,180]
References: 164, 171 and 180.

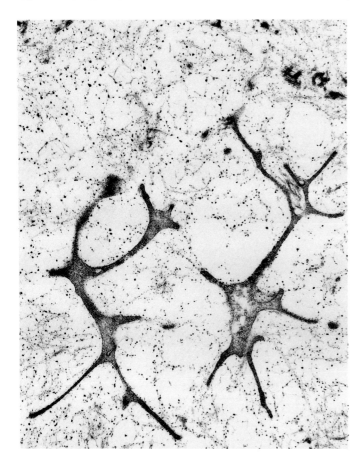

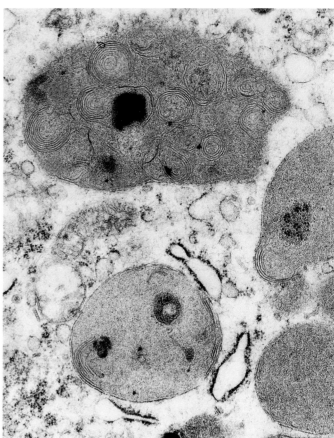

Fig. 11.16 Chondromatous 'hamartoma' of lung: chondroid tissue. Portions of two delicate branching chondrocyte processes are surrounded by cartilaginous matrix — in which innumerable proteoglycan granules and a network of filaments can be discerned. (× 14 800)

Fig. 11.17 Malakoplakia: Michaelis–Gutmann (M–G) body formation I. Case of malakoplakia of the prostate from a 58-year-old man; details of this case have been reported elsewhere.[211] This figure depicts an early stage of M–G body evolution. Portions of four phagolysosomes are evident, and these contain parallel curving membranes, forming myelinoid figures and imparting a finger print-like morphology. Small dense foci, consistent with early calcification, can be seen in relation to some of the myelinoid figures. On the basis of such appearances, Sterrett et al[211] suggested that calcification may be promoted by phospholipid hydrolysis, leading to high concentrations of phosphate ions in a lysosomal micro-environment of various enzymes and lipopolysaccharides. (Formalin fixation, × 25 100)

X-ray microanalysis in the electron microscope has demonstrated that M–G bodies contain hydroxyapatite,[197,208] and there is general agreement that they develop within phagolysosomes and cytosegrosomes. Before mineralization, these organelles typically possess a finely granular matrix and concentric membranous fragments.[208,211] In the initial stages of calcification, small dense particles appear both in the matrix and between the lamellae of the membranous fragments in the phagolysosomes.[208,211] The particles then aggregate to form a dense central body, and calcification proceeds by deposition of hydroxyapatite spicules at the periphery.[194] Individual spicules are often orientated radially, and the calcospherites characteristically possess multiple concentric layers — correlating with laminations evident by LM and suggesting that mineralization occurs in waves. Ultimately, the phagolysosomes are obliterated, and the M–G bodies may be released into the extracellular space. References: 193–195, 197–211, 213 and 214.

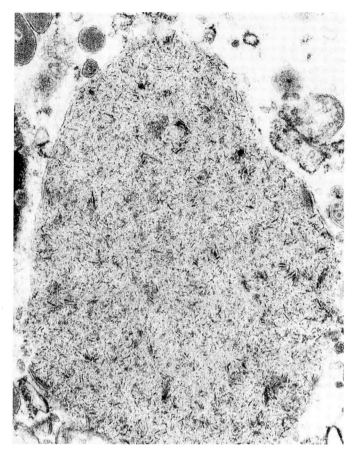

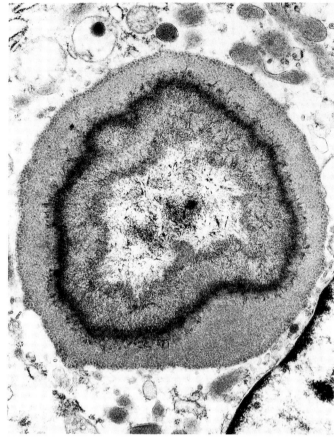

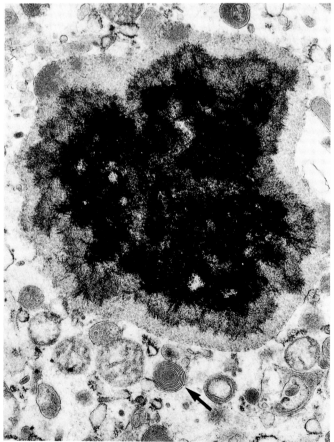

Fig. 11.18 Malakoplakia: Michaelis–Gutmann body formation II. The matrix of this lysosomal body is peppered with numerous haphazardly distributed electron-dense hydroxyapatite spicules. (Formalin fixation, × 27 100)

Fig. 11.19 (Top right) Malakoplakia: Michaelis–Gutmann body formation III. A laminated M–G body has developed within a membrane-bound lysosomal body. The central region of this M–G body is electron-lucent, while dense hydroxyapatite spicules are present at the periphery and show a radial orientation. (Formalin fixation, × 19 000)

Fig. 11.20 (Right) Malakoplakia: Michaelis–Gutmann body formation IV. In this M–G body there is a central extremely dense area of aggregated spicules. Individual spicules can be discerned at the periphery. A myelinoid whorl is present in an adjoining lysosome (arrow). (Formalin fixation, × 20 400)

12. Diagnostic electron microscopy of endomyocardial biopsies

Arline Albala   J. J. Fenoglio Jr

INTRODUCTION

The introduction of the endomyocardial biopsy has opened an entirely new area of surgical pathology of the heart. Virtually for the first time, portions of the myocardium that have not been subjected to prolonged periods of autolysis are available for study. The biopsy thus affords an unique opportunity to look at disease processes in their earliest stages and to characterize the ultrastructural changes associated with these diseases. This technique offers the promise of early diagnosis and perhaps new understanding of many cardiac diseases.[2,13,25,38]

Myocardial biopsies were first championed in the late 1950s and early 1960s using a variety of techniques; transthoracically using Menghini and Vim-Silverman needles, percutaneously with a catheter needle, or by open thoracotomy. The high morbidity and mortality associated with these procedures prevented their widespread use. Simultaneously in Japan, Konno & Sakakibara introduced a catheter bioptome utilizing a transvenous approach. Several modifications of this instrument were quickly developed, including the Caves-Shultz Stanford bioptome, the modified Olympus bioptome and the Kings endomyocardial bioptome. In the early 1970s, the technique was introduced at Stanford for monitoring rejection in cardiac allograft recipients.[2] During the ensuing fifteen years the technique has been widely applied and has proven both safe and effective.

Endomyocardial biopsy has been widely applied to all forms of cardiac disease and countless biopsies have been studied ultrastructurally.[25,38] The biopsy has remained the 'gold standard' in the diagnosis of cardiac rejection[2] and has proven extremely valuable in the diagnosis of myocarditis, anthracycline-induced cardiomyopathy, amyloid heart disease and selected types of cardiomyopathy.[38] Electron microscopy (EM) has proven of limited diagnostic value, although in a small percentage of biopsies (10–20%) it is the only means of establishing a diagnosis.[13] EM should be done on all cases in which a diagnosis cannot be established by light microscopy, in cases of suspected cardiotoxicity and in cases with possible small-vessel disease. EM has not proven helpful in evaluating cardiac rejection or suspected myocarditis. In spite of extensive screening by many investigators, viruses have not been identified ultrastructurally even in biopsy-proven cases of myocarditis.[22] This is not surprising since experimental evidence suggests that myocarditis is an immune-mediated, although virus-initiated, disease and that cardiac symptoms occur after virus has been cleared from the heart.

TECHNICAL CONSIDERATIONS

In order to obtain meaningful and reliable information, the biopsy must be properly handled and fixed.[2,13] Excessive handling of biopsies must be avoided and the samples should be fixed rapidly, preferably in the cardiac catheterization laboratory. Forceps should never be used to retrieve the biopsy from the bioptome; instead, the specimen should be removed from the bioptome with a sterile applicator or needle and placed immediately in fixative. Dividing the specimen, even with a single stroke of a sharp blade, will cause crush artefacts and is unnecessary prior to fixation. As the specimens are small (maximum size is usually 4 mm^3), fixation is rapid and complete without dividing the tissue.

We routinely fix *all* specimens in 2.5% phosphate-buffered glutaraldehyde (pH 7.35). The use of glutaraldehyde allows for the selection of any of multiple specimens or portion thereof for EM, assuring that fixation will be appropriate. Fixation is done only at room temperature, rather than in chilled fixative as is the general rule for EM, to minimize contraction artefacts. After fixation the tissue is divided into small blocks, rinsed in phosphate buffer and postfixed in 1.5% phosphate-buffered (pH 7.35) osmium tetroxide for one hour. The tissue is then dehydrated and embedded by any of a number of standard techniques.

BIOPSY INTERPRETATION

In order to interpret the electron-microscopic findings effectively, the investigator must be familiar both with the normal ultrastructure of the heart and the structural artefacts attendant on the procedure. The normal ultrastructure of ventricular myocardium is well documented in the literature.[11,35] Briefly, the myocytes are approximately 20 μm in width and 120 μm in length. The sarcoplasm is filled with contractile elements with the sarcomeres in register across the width of the myocyte. The sarcomeres are composed of thick (myosin) and thin (actin) filaments anchored by Z-bands which separate individual sarcomeres. The myofilaments are arranged to produce the characteristic banding pattern (A-band, M-band, H-band and I-band). Between arrays of sarcomeres, oval mitochondria are regularly dispersed, usually matched one to a sarcomeric unit. Interspersed through the sarcoplasm and between sarcomeres are abundant glycogen particles and sarcoplasmic reticulum tubules (SR). T-tubules associated with terminal cisternae of the SR are found adjacent to each Z-band. The nuclei are usually centrally placed and fusiform, with a distinct nucleolus. In the perinuclear region lysosomes, aggregates of lipofuscin pigment and a small Golgi apparatus are usually identified. The cells are separated by intercalated discs arrayed in step-like fashion across the myocyte. The myocyte is bound by a distinct sarcolemma which is often scalloped, and also by a thin but distinct basement membrane. The interstitial space between myocytes contains collagen, scattered fibroblasts and cardiac histiocytes, and small capillaries lined by a single endothelial cell. Larger vessels, small arteries and veins, are situated at the junctions of groups of myocytes. The endocardium, if present, consists of a single layer of endothelial cells beneath which is a distinct but narrow layer of dense collagen fibres and elastic fibres. The endocardium is separated from the myocardium by the subendocardium, a layer of loosely arranged collagen fibrils of varying thickness.

In evaluating the biopsy several artefacts must be carefully looked for and avoided.[9,13,26] The most important of these is the presence of contraction bands which are almost universally present in endomyocardial biopsies. These acidophilic bands in myocardial cells are an artefact of the procedure which can be minimized, but not eliminated, by fixation at room temperature and therefore they cannot be used as evidence of myocardial ischaemia. Ultrastructurally, the contraction of sarcomeres produces broad bands of clumped myofilaments across the width of the cell with sarcoplasmic clearing adjacent to areas of contraction. Areas of clearing of sarcoplasm must be distinguished from areas of myofibril loss in myocyte degeneration. More frequently the myocytes are uniformly contracted with loss of I-bands and marked scalloping of the sarcolemma. Sampling a previous biopsy site is a problem in patients undergoing multiple biopsies. Although in most instances EM is done only on first biopsies, this artefact must be considered when large areas of granulation tissue are identified ultrastructurally and emphasizes the importance of always examining the light microscopic sections before proceeding with EM. Finally, the extent of fibrosis must be evaluated with great care, since

tangential sections through the subendocardium can give the erroneous impression of extensive fibrosis.

CARDIOMYOPATHIES

The term cardiomyopathy refers to a group of diseases which affect heart muscle and are broadly grouped into three types; congestive, hypertrophic and restrictive cardiomyopathy. The diagnosis is one of exclusion and requires that other causes of cardiac dysfunction (namely hypertension, valvular heart disease and coronary artery disease) be ruled out before the diagnosis can be established.[10,12]

Congestive or dilated cardiomyopathy

This disease is characterized clinically by cardiomegaly and congestive heart failure for which no aetiology can be determined.[40] Unfortunately, endomyocardial biopsy has not been helpful in determining the aetiology of congestive cardiomyopathy in the majority of patients. The histological and ultrastructural changes are non-specific and consist primarily of interstitial fibrosis and myocardial cell hypertrophy and degeneration.[10,12,25] As in other forms of heart disease, the ultrastructural criteria of hypertrophy include: (1) increased cell size; (2) increased numbers of mitochondria and myofilaments; (3) abundant sarcoplasmic reticulum; (4) mitochondrial abnormalities; (5) accumulations of myelin figures and residual bodies; (6) invaginations of the sarcolemma, and (7) widened, convoluted intercalated discs. The ultrastructural criteria of degeneration include: (1) loss of myofilaments; (2) aggregation of glycogen, mitochondria and sarcoplasmic reticulum in areas of myofilament loss; (3) aggregation of abnormal Z-band material and cytoskeletal filaments; (4) mitochondrial abnormalities; (5) accumulations of myelin figures and residual bodies, and (6) cell atrophy. Furthermore, attempts to use these ultrastructural changes to predict prognosis have not proven reliable.[9,13,25]

In a small percentage of congestive cardiomyopathies, a definitive aetiology can be established structurally. In the majority of these cases, the cardiomyopathy is secondary to a metabolic or inherited disease[15] (see also Ch.6). The structural changes associated with these diseases are summarized in Table 12.1. In these patients, EM is always helpful and is frequently essential in establishing a diagnosis (Fig. 12.1). For cardiac lesions of a presumed metabolic nature, but for which the biochemical disorders have not been identified, the term basophilic degeneration is used. In basophilic degeneration there are deposits of PAS-positive material in the cytoplasm of the myocytes. Ultrastructurally, these deposits may be characterized by fibrils similar to those in Type IV glycogen storage disease or by large masses of finely granular material within which dense inclusions are seen.

Finally, congestive cardiomyopathy has been reported in neuromuscular diseases, endocrine abnormalities such as

Table 12.1 Distinctive structural features of cardiomyopathies associated with metabolic and inherited diseases*

Carnitine deficiency	Extensive lipid deposits free in the sarcoplasm of myocytes and in cytoplasm of fibroblasts and pericytes
Fabry's disease	PAS-positive, birefringent vacuoles in perinuclear zone on frozen section. Ultrastructurally, intralysosomal aggregates of concentric or parallel lamellae displace myofibrils to cell periphery
Generalized gangliosidosis (GM$_1$)	Membrane-limited vacuoles filled with granular or flocculent material in myocytes, endothelial cells and nerves
Glycogen storage disease	
type II (Pompe's disease)	Severe vacuolization of central portion of myocytes cells filled with glycogen by EM, displacing myofibrils to cell periphery; glycogen characteristically within lysosomes, and also free in cytoplasm
type III	Cardiac involvement rare; structurally, glycogen free in cytoplasm displacing myofibrils to cell periphery
type IV	Glycogen deposits strongly basophilic and resistant to digestion; glycogen in fibrillar form
Haemochromatosis	Iron deposits in membrane-bound granules (lysosomes) containing electron-dense particles embedded in electron-lucent matrix; particles also free in sarcoplasm; initially, deposits in perinuclear region
Mucolipidoses	
types II and III	Lipid-filled vacuoles in cells of interstitium; pleomorphic inclusions with concentric lamellae in clear areas of myocytes
Mucopolysaccharidoses	
type I (Hurler's syndrome, Scheie's syndrome)	Connective tissue cells contain clear vacuoles; by EM, perinuclear deposits of glycolipid with concentric or parallel lamellae in myocytes
Type III (Sanfilippo syndrome)	Vacuoles in myocytes; ultrastructurally, vacuoles either electron-lucent or filled with laminated osmiophilic material
Oxalosis	Yellow-brown birefringent crystals of calcium oxalate
Refsum's disease	Accumulation of fine lipid vacuoles around nuclei
Wilson's disease	Copper accumulation in myocytes

*See also Chapter 6.

thyrotoxicosis and myxoedema, and associated with ethanol abuse.[12] There are no structural findings to distinguish these cardiomyopathies from idiopathic congestive cardiomyopathy and the diagnosis can be established only on the basis of the clinical history. Similarly, hypertrophic cardiomyopathy is a clinical diagnosis, without specific morphological findings on endomyocardial biopsy.[10,12]

ANTHRACYCLINE-INDUCED CARDIOMYOPATHY

A valuable use of the endomyocardial biopsy is the monitoring of cardiotoxicity in patients treated with doxorubicin, daunorubicin hydrochloride, or related chemotherapeutic drugs.[3,37] The cardiotoxicity is clearly related to dosage in a linear fashion; however, some patients have rapidly progressive damage while others can tolerate large doses often up to 1000 mg/m^2 with minimal cardiac damage. Unfortunately, there is no way to predict how patients will respond to the drug without monitoring cardiac status.

The cardiotoxicity of anthracyclines can best be characterized as a cardiomyopathy.[8,14,20] The cellular lesions found on biopsy are not entirely unique to doxorubicin toxicity, and similar structural changes are occasionally seen in other cardiomyopathies. What is distinctive about the lesions is that, although focal, they are widespread throughout the myocardium and they are usually not associated with

hypertrophic changes. In the early stages of myocardial damage, the structural abnormalities can be adequately defined only by EM, and the grading of the extent of cardiotoxicity must be done ultrastructurally. Ideally, 5–10 plastic-embedded blocks should be evaluated.

The morphological changes induced by doxorubicin have been studied extensively in animal models.[8,20] In the acute phase, following a large dose, there is nucleolar fragmentation followed by nuclear chromatin clumping. This is followed by swelling of the sarcoplasmic reticulum and T-tubules which may coalesce to form large sarcoplasmic vacuoles. Mitochondrial swelling and myelin figures may also be seen. Following a larger cumulative dose myofibrillar loss (myocytolysis) is prominent.

In endomyocardial biopsy specimens from patients receiving doxorubicin (Fig. 12.2), two types of structural changes are prominent: swelling of the sarcoplasmic reticulum and T-tubular system, and myofibrillar loss.[4,5] The swelling of the sarcoplasmic reticulum and T-tubules creates membrane-bound vacuoles of varying size, often scattered through the myocyte. Occasionally, in severe cases, these vacuoles coalesce and can be seen on light microscopic sections of the biopsy. The myofibrillar loss involves both thick and thin filaments and may be present focally within individual myocytes or involve the entire myocyte. Characteristically, fragments of Z-band material remain, especially

Table 12.2 Morphological grading of anthracycline-induced cardiotoxicity*

Grade 0	=	Normal myocardial ultrastructural morphology
Grade 1	=	Isolated myocytes affected by distended sarcotubular system and/or early myofibrillar loss; damage to less than 5% of all cells
Grade 1.5	=	Similar changes to Grade 1, but with damage to 6–15% of all the cells
Grade 2.0	=	Clusters of myocytes affected by myofibrillar loss and/or vacuolization, with damage to 16–25% of all the cells
Grade 2.5	=	Many myocytes, up to 26–35% of all the cells affected by vacuolization and/or myofibrillar loss. (Only one more dose of anthracycline should be given without further evaluation.)
Grade 3.0	=	Severe and diffuse myocyte damage (more than 35% of all the cells affected by vacuolization and/or myofibrillar loss). (No more anthracycline should be given.)

*From Billingham et al.[5]

at the periphery of the myocyte. In areas of myofibrillar loss there is clumping of mitochondria, glycogen and sarcoplasmic reticulum. In endomyocardial biopsy specimens the nuclei are usually normal. Although there may be focal mitochondrial swelling and disruption of cristae, these changes are not a reliable indicator of cardiotoxicity. In advanced cases myelin figures are usually prominent and interstitial connective tissue is increased.

Assessment of both types of structural change is used to grade the severity of cardiotoxicity.[5] The extent of cellular damage is graded on a scale of 0 to 3 (Table 12.2) and this information is used to monitor treatment. Using this technique, heart failure due to doxorubicin therapy can virtually be eliminated.

AMYLOID HEART DISEASE

Cardiac amyloidosis describes a process characterized by the deposition of protein fibrils in a unique beta-pleated sheet.[18] The amyloid fibrils are usually derived from either immunoglobulin light chains (AL) or non-immunoglobulin protein (AA). Cardiac involvement may be present in systemic amyloidosis and organ-limited amyloidosis. Systemic amyloidosis is usually associated with immune disorders characterized by increased immunoprotein production, chronic diseases or heredo-familial syndromes (see also Ch. 5). In systemic amyloidosis, the deposits in the heart are usually of the AL type. Organ-limited amyloidosis is more common with ageing and is frequently termed senile amyloidosis. The deposits in the heart are usually of the ASc_1 and ASc_2 type (the former being closely related to human pre-albumin[33]) in organ-limited amyloidosis, and the heart may be the only organ involved.

Amyloid can be readily diagnosed by endocardial biopsy and this is the only reliable means of establishing the diagnosis in organ-limited amyloidosis.[10,12,32] Although less invasive techniques can usually be used to establish the diagnosis in patients with systemic amyloidosis, a significant number of patients present with congestive heart failure as the first symptom of systemic amyloidosis.[1] In these patients the diagnosis is usually established by endomyocardial

biopsy. The amyloid may be deposited in the interstitium, in the endocardium, or in the walls of myocardial blood vessels and is usually readily apparent by light microscopy. Characteristically the deposits ring individual myocytes and capillaries, and are glassy and amorphous in appearance. Usually the presence of amyloid can be confirmed with sulphated alcian blue, crystal violet or thioflavine T. Congo red is not reliably positive in cardiac biopsy tissue.

In early amyloid heart disease, and especially with systemic light chain disease,[29] EM is the most sensitive diagnostic method for demonstrating amyloid (Figs 12.3 and 12.4). By electron microscopy the fibrils are linear and non-branching, measuring 7.5 to 10 nm in diameter. The fibrils are aggregated in a random mesh. The amyloid fibrils are readily distinguished from connective tissue microfibrils — which are 13 nm or greater in diameter and usually associated with mature collagen. Deposition of amyloid in arterioles and around capillaries may be the first abnormality in amyloid heart disease[34] and should be looked for in all patients with unexplained congestive heart failure and normal-appearing myocardium on biopsy.

SMALL-VESSEL DISEASE

Whether small-vessel disease (i.e. disease of the coronary arterioles or capillaries) exists is controversial.[39] Several studies of autopsy material and myocardial biopsy specimens have unquestionably demonstrated the presence of abnormal intramyocardial coronary arteries both in the presence and absence of extramural coronary disease in patients with clinical symptoms of ischaemic heart disease.[23,31] The involvement may be selective, involving only arterioles or capillaries, or it may be generalized, involving vessels of all sizes. The degree of involvement may be evident only on electron-microscopic examination. Sampling error is a major problem in the diagnosis of small-vessel disease due to the small size of the sample obtained. In order to minimize this problem, a minimum of three samples is obtained from each patient. Multiple sections are carefully examined both by light and electron microscopy at all depths of the specimen. Despite this attention to detail, arterioles are not found in all biopsies.

The clinical presentation of patients with small-vessel coronary disease can be either chest pain, indistinguishable from coronary artery disease, unexplained congestive heart failure, or arrhythmias.[19] Heart failure may be severe and the clinical course is similar to that seen in patients with ischaemic cardiac disease secondary to epicardial coronary artery disease. In addition to congestive heart failure, ventricular arrhythmias and heart block may occur. Ventricular arrhythmias may be resistant to standard therapy. Sudden death occurs frequently.

Primary small-vessel disease

The aetiology and pathogenesis of primary small-vessel disease in the heart is unknown, in fact its very existence as a pathological entity has not been unequivocally proven.[7,23,31] The association between chest pain and small-vessel disease has been investigated by several groups,[7,27,30] and small-vessel disease has been reported in patients with aortic stenosis and chest pain in the absence of demonstrable coronary artery disease.[24]

By light microscopy, the biopsy findings are not specific.[19,21] Perivascular fibrosis, in the absence of interstitial or endocardial fibrosis, is usually the only finding. When identified, small arteries and arterioles appear to have markedly thickened walls. Increased fibrous tissue is often apparent within the walls of these vessels when they are stained with the Masson trichrome stain. Myocardial hypertrophy may or may not be present. The vessel changes must be confirmed by EM. Ultrastructurally, the subendothelial lamina of the arterioles and small arteries is markedly thickened. The normal thickness of the subendothelial lamina varies with age, comprising up to 37% of the vessel wall thickness in patients 57 to 64 years of age. By definition, in idiopathic small-vessel disease the subendothelial lamina comprises more than 50% of the thickness of the vessel wall. Since the normal range of subendothelial lamina of myocardial vessels has not been fully described, these findings must be considered as very preliminary. Ultrastructurally, the myocardial cells demonstrate accumulation of lipid droplets and glycogen and focal vacuolation of mitochondria. Degenerating myocardial cells are usually not found. These ultrastructural changes are suggestive of chronic ischaemia.

Diabetes mellitus

Cardiac disease is frequent in patients with diabetes mellitus. Many of these patients have typical ischaemic heart disease associated with coronary artery atherosclerosis. A number of patients with diabetes mellitus, however, have congestive heart failure in the absence of coronary artery disease or out of proportion to the degree of demonstrable coronary artery disease. The light microscopic changes on endomyocardial biopsy in these patients are usually non-specific and range from the typical findings of cardiomyopathy to findings suggestive of ischaemic heart disease. However, in a significant number of patients EM reveals thickening of capillary basement membranes.[6,28] The basement membranes range up to 150 nm in thickness; normal capillary basement membrane thickness is approximately 40 nm[6] (Fig. 12.5).

The specificity of basement membrane changes in diabetes is not known. Although capillary basement changes have been reported in patients with diabetes mellitus and cardiomyopathy, these changes are not universally present in patients with diabetes mellitus and unexplained heart disease.[39] Similar basement membrane changes may also be seen in patients without diabetes mellitus. Currently, however, capillary basement disease must be considered as a possible mechanism underlying congestive heart failure in patients with diabetes mellitus.

Radiation-induced cardiomyopathy

Endomyocardial biopsy has proven a valuable tool in diagnosing radiation-induced cardiomyopathy. Radiation-induced damage affects both the pericardium and myocardium and is a common sequel of mediastinal radiation for lymphoma.[36] Characteristically, radiation pericarditis will appear after a latent period of 3–7 years following exposure. The clinical presentation is often that of right heart failure characterized by systemic venous congestion and peripheral oedema and ascites. Clinically, it is impossible to differentiate between radiation-induced constrictive pericarditis and radiation-induced restrictive myocardial disease.

The sequel of radiation is fibrosis. In the myocardium the fibrosis is interstitial and perivascular and may be indistinguishable by light microscopy from the fibrosis in congestive cardiomyopathy. Extensive adventitial fibrosis of arterioles and small arteries is suggestive of radiation-induced damage, and when present in a patient known to have received mediastinal radiation, is diagnostic of radiation-induced cardiomyopathy.

The diagnosis of radiation-induced cardiomyopathy is readily established or confirmed by EM (Fig. 12.6). The hallmark of radiation change is thickening of capillary basement membranes.[39] In the early stages there is distinct duplication and triplication of the basement membrane. As the fibrosis becomes more extensive this replication of capillary basement membranes is often not apparent; rather the membranes are markedly thickened, measuring 100 nm or more in thickness. At this stage, basement membranes of the cardiac muscle cells are also markedly thickened. The thickening of the myocardial cell basement membrane distinguishes radiation injury from other diseases in which capillary basement membranes are thickened — notably diabetes mellitus.

REFERENCES

1. Bendixen B, Marboe C C, Ursell P C, Weiss M B, Fenoglio J J Jr 1984 Unsuspected amyloidosis first diagnosed by endomyocardial biopsy. Circulation 70 (suppl 2): 139
2. Billingham M E 1979 Some recent advances in cardiac pathology. Human Pathology 10: 367–386
3. Billingham M E, Bristow M R 1984 Evaluation of anthracycline cardiotoxicity. The predictive ability and functional correlation of the endomyocardial biopsy. Cancer Treatment Symposium 3: 71
4. Billingham M E, Bristow M, Glatstein E, Mason J W, Masek M A, Daniels J R 1977 Adriamycin cardiotoxicity: endomyocardial biopsy evidence of enhancement by radiation. American Journal of Surgical Pathology 1: 17–23.
5. Billingham M E, Mason J W, Bristow M R, Daniels J R 1978 Anthracycline cardiomyopathy monitored by morphologic changes. Cancer Treatment Reports 62: 865–872
6. Billingham M E, Schwartz B, Ruder A, Harrison D 1977 An ultrastructural study of age-related changes in intramyocardial arterioles. Laboratory Investigation 36: 331
7. Boucher C A, Fallon J T, Johnson R A, Yurchak P M 1979 Cardiomyopathic syndrome caused by coronary artery disease. III Prospective clinicopathological study of its prevalence among patients with clinically unexplained chronic heart failure. British Heart Journal 41: 613–620
8. Doroshow J H, Tallent C, Schecter J E 1985 Ultrastructural features of adriamycin-induced skeletal and cardiac muscle toxicity. American Journal of Pathology 118: 288–297
9. Edwards W D 1983 Endomyocardial biopsy and cardiomyopathy. Cardiovascular Reviews and Reports 7: 820–826
10. Edwards W D 1987 Cardiomyopathies. Human Pathology 18: 625–635
11. Fawcett D W, McNutt N S 1969 The ultrastructure of the cat myocardium. I. Ventricular papillary muscle. Journal of Cell Biology 42: 1–45
12. Fenoglio J J 1982 The cardiomyopathies: diagnosis by endomyocardial biopsy. In: Fenoglio J J (ed) Endomyocardial biopsy: techniques and applications. CRC Press, Boca Raton, Florida, pp 97–110
13. Fenoglio J J, Marboe C C 1987 Endomyocardial biopsy: an overview. Human Pathology 18: 609–612
14. Ferrans V J 1978 Overview of cardiac pathology in relation to anthracycline cardiotoxicity. Cancer Treatment Reports 62: 955–961
15. Ferrans V J, Boyce S W 1983 Metabolic and familial diseases. In: Silver M D (ed) Cardiovascular pathology. Churchill Livingstone, New York, pp 945–947
16. Fischer V W, Barner H B, Leskiw M L 1979 Capillary basal laminar thickness in diabetic human myocardium. Diabetes 28: 713–719
17. Geer J R, Bishop S P, James T N 1979 Pathology of small intramural coronary arteries. Pathology Annual 14: 125–154
18. Glenner G G 1980 Amyloid deposits and amyloidosis: the beta fibrilloses. New England Journal of Medicine 302: 1283–1292
19. Gorlin R 1983 Dynamic vascular basis in the genesis of myocardial ischemia. Journal of the American College of Cardiologists 1: 897–906
20. Jaenke R S 1974 An anthracycline antibiotic-induced cardiomyopathy in rabbits. Laboratory Investigation 30: 292–304
21. Koch F, Billingham M, Rider A, Mason J W, Cipriano P R, Hancock E W 1976 Pathophysiology of 'angina' with normal coronary angiograms. Circulation (suppl 2) 54: 173
22. Marboe C C, Fenoglio J J 1988 Biopsy diagnosis in myocarditis. In: Waller B F (ed) Contemporary issues in cardiovascular pathology. F A Davis Co, Philadelphia, pp 137–154
23. Mason J W, Strefling A 1979 Small vessel disease in the heart resulting in myocardial necrosis and death despite angiographically normal coronary arteries. American Journal of Cardiology 44: 171–176
24. Naeye R L, Liedtke A J 1977 Consequence of intramyocardial arterial lesions in aortic valvular stenosis. American Journal of Cardiology 85: 569–580
25. O'Connell J B, Subramanian R, Robinson J A, Henkin R E, Scanlon P J 1984 Endomyocardial biopsy. Techniques and applications in heart disease of unknown cause. Heart Transplantation 3: 132–143
26. Olmesdahl P J, Gregory M A, Cameron E W J 1979 Ultrastructural artifacts in biopsied normal myocardium and their relevance to myocardial biopsy in man. Thorax 34: 82–90
27. Parl R, Gutstein W H, Glasser M 1980 Relationship of small and large coronary artery disease to myocardial ischemia. Archives of Pathology and Laboratory Medicine 104: 70–74
28. Pearse M B, Bullock R T, Kizziar J C 1973 Myocardial small vessel disease in patients with diabetes mellitus. Circulation 8 (suppl 4): 6
29. Randall R E, Williamson W C, Mullinax F, Tung M Y, Still W J S 1976 Manifestations of systemic light chain deposition. American Journal of Medicine 60: 293–299
30. Richardson P J, Livesley B, Oram S, Olsen E G J, Armstrong P 1974 Angina pectoris with normal coronary arteries. Transvenous myocardial biopsy in diagnosis. Lancet ii: 677
31. Saphir O, Ohringer L 1956 Changes in intramural coronary branches in coronary atherosclerosis. Archives of Pathology 62: 159–170
32. Schroeder J S, Billingham M E, Rider A K 1975 Cardiac amyloidosis. Diagnosis by transvenous endomyocardial biopsy. American Journal of Medicine 59: 269–273
33. Sletten K, Westermark P, Natvig J B 1980 Senile cardiac amyloid is related to prealbumin. Scandinavian Journal of Immunology 12: 503–506
34. Smith R R L, Hutchins G M 1979 Ischemic heart disease secondary to amyloidosis of intramyocardial arteries. American Journal of Cardiology 44: 413–417
35. Sommer J R, Jenning R B 1986 Ultrastructure of cardiac muscle. In: Fozzard H A (ed) The heart and cardiovascular system. Scientific foundations. Raven Press, New York, pp 61
36. Stewart J R, Fajardo C F 1971 Radiation-induced heart disease. Clinical and experimental aspects. Radiological Clinics of North America 9: 511–531
37. Unverferth D V 1985 Anthracycline-induced heart disease. In: Unverferth D V (ed) Dilated cardiomyopathy. Futura, Mt Kisco, New York, pp 179–200
38. Ursell P C, Fenoglio J J 1984 Spectrum of cardiac disease diagnosed by endomyocardial biopsy. Pathology Annual 19: 197–219
39. Weiss M B, Fenoglio J J 1982 Small vessel disease: fact or fiction. In: Fenoglio J J (ed) Endomyocardial biopsy: techniques and applications. CRC Press, Boca Raton, Florida, pp 111–124
40. Wynne J, Braunwald E 1984 The cardiomyopathies and myocarditides. In: Braunwald E (ed) Heart disease: a textbook of cardiovascular medicine. Saunder, Philadelphia, pp 1399–1460

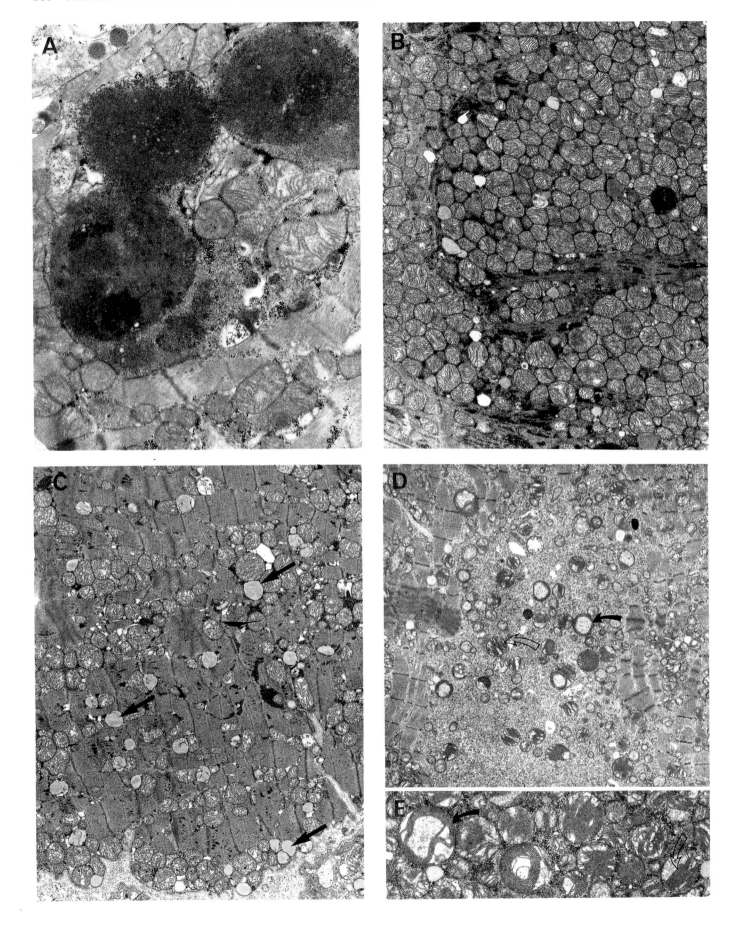

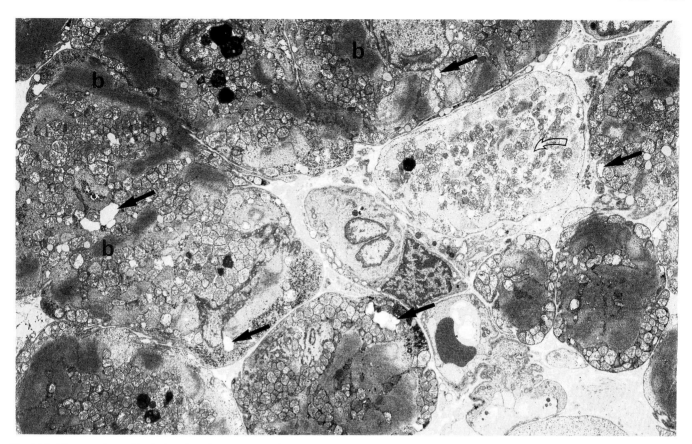

Fig. 12.2   Heart: anthracycline-induced cardiomyopathy. In
anthracycline-induced cardiomyopathy vacuoles are prominent (arrows).
The vacuoles consist of dilated segments of the sarcoplasmic reticulum
which may coalesce to form large vacuoles. Myofibrillar loss may also be
seen (open arrows). Frequently these changes are not present in the same
cell. The contraction bands (B) present through the photomicrograph are
an artefact of the procedure. (× 3400)

Fig. 12.1 (Facing page)   Heart: cardiomyopathy. Cardiomyopathies
occurring with metabolic diseases are associated with abnormal inclusions
and mitochondrial abnormalities. The large flocculent inclusions in panel
A are characteristic of gangliosidosis and basophilic degeneration.
Accumulations of mitochondria as in panel **B** are non-specific but are
associated especially with ethanol-related cardiomyopathy and so-called
'mitochondrial' cardiomyopathy. Lipid droplets (arrows) free in the
sarcoplasm (panel **C**) are characteristic of carnitine deficiency and
Refsum's disease but are also present in myocardial ischaemia. Inclusions
of concentric (closed arrows) and parallel (open arrows) lamellae (panels
D and **E**) in mitochondria and lysosomes are associated with a number of
metabolic cardiomyopathies (see Ch. 6). (A, × 13 320; B, × 8700;
C, × 4290; D, × 5120; E, × 7370)

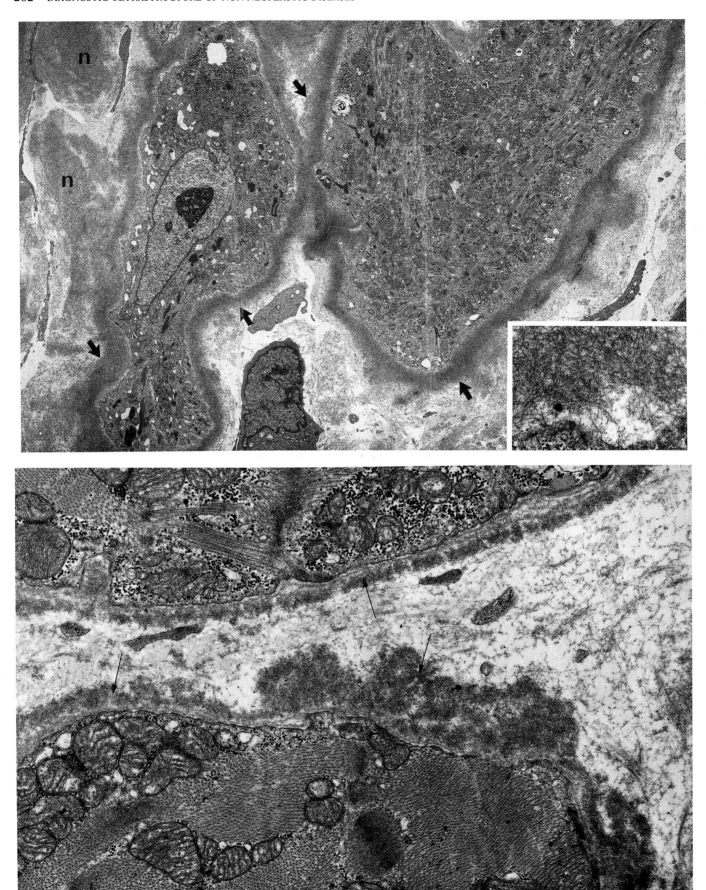

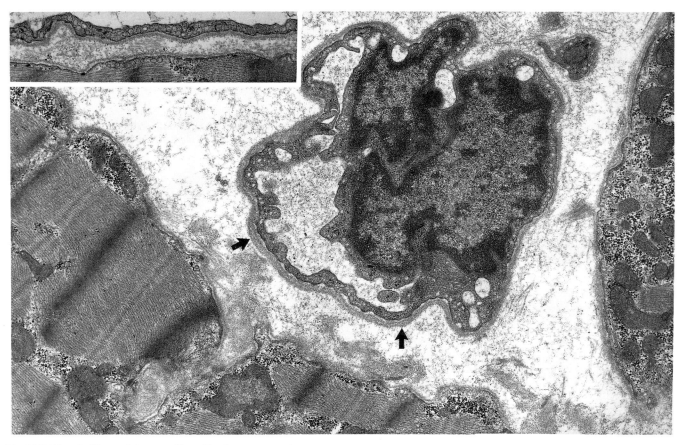

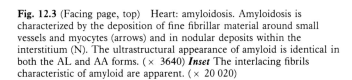

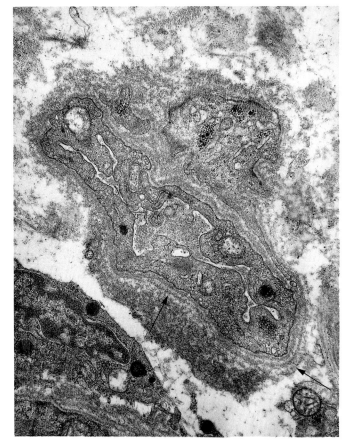

Fig. 12.5 (Above)   Heart: diabetes mellitus. The basement membrane thickening in diabetes mellitus, when present, involves the capillaries (arrows) and small arteries throughout the heart. The capillary basement membrane in the patient with diabetes mellitus measures 130 nm in thickness, roughly three times that of the normal. (× 13 440) *Inset* The normal capillary basement membrane measures approximately 40 nm in thickness. (× 15 670)

Fig. 12.6 (Right)   Heart: radiation-induced cardiomyopathy. In radiation-induced cardiomyopathy, in addition to fibrosis there is extensive basement membrane thickening involving capillaries and small vessels and myocytes. The thickening is characterized initially by duplication and triplication of the basement membrane (arrows) here seen ringing a capillary. This layering is lost with increasing thickening of the membrane. (× 14 830)

Fig. 12.3 (Facing page, top)   Heart: amyloidosis. Amyloidosis is characterized by the deposition of fine fibrillar material around small vessels and myocytes (arrows) and in nodular deposits within the interstitium (N). The ultrastructural appearance of amyloid is identical in both the AL and AA forms. (× 3640) *Inset* The interlacing fibrils characteristic of amyloid are apparent. (× 20 020)

Fig. 12.4 (Facing page, bottom)   Heart: light-chain disease. In light-chain disease the deposits are located around vessels and myocytes as in classic amyloidosis. The deposits contain fine fibrils embedded in flocculent material (arrows) and are frequently focal and irregular. (× 19 830)

13. Respiratory diseases

B. Corrin Ann Dewar

INTRODUCTION

The use of electron microscopy (EM) in the categorization of lung tumours is dealt with in the companion volume,[36] and its application to the identification of respiratory viruses in Chapters 8 and 9 — but this by no means exhausts its applications in the field of respiratory diseases.[71] EM is essential for identification of the various primary defects underlying the ciliary dyskinesia syndrome, is helpful in recognizing the Langerhans' cells characteristic of histiocytosis X, and is of inestimable value in the field of pneumoconioses — where electron microscopic analytical techniques are proving to be extremely valuable. In other areas of lung disease electron microscopy is not essential for diagnosis but nevertheless provides insight into basic disease processes, and these have therefore been included.

ABNORMALITIES OF CILIARY ULTRASTRUCTURE

Ciliary ultrastructure assumed clinical importance when it was realized that the respiratory infections in Kartagener's syndrome were the consequence of a developmental anomaly affecting certain components of cilia.[14] Kartagener's syndrome consists of situs inversus, bronchiectasis and sinusitis, but ultrastructural studies led to the realization that the ciliary defect was present in some patients with respiratory infections who did not have situs inversus; furthermore, affected male patients were infertile because sperm tails have a similar internal structure to cilia and the defect resulted in immotility of spermatozoa. The combination of respiratory infections due to defective cilia, and male infertility due to immotile spermatozoa — with or without situs inversus — was first named the immotile cilia syndrome.[28] However, the cilia are not always completely immotile, and the term primary ciliary dyskinesia was therefore substituted.[56] The diagnosis is largely dependent upon EM of either ciliated cells or spermatozoa. Cilia and sperm tails have an axial central pair of microtubules surrounded by an outer ring of nine equally spaced double microtubules (doublets) — the so-called '9 + 2' structure (Fig. 13.1).[60] Small dynein side

arms extend from the A microtubule of each doublet towards the next, and radial spokes connect each doublet with the central microtubules. The microtubules fuse near the tip, while near the base the central pair disappears. Just inside the cell body the doublets become triploid and fuse together as a cylinder which extends into the cytoplasm as the ciliary basal body. Cilia beat when the microtubular doublets, powered by adenosine triphosphate in the dynein arms, slide over each other. In respiratory epithelium there are between 200 and 300 cilia on the surface of each cell, each beating at about 1000 times per minute in a low viscosity aqueous hypophase beneath the surface mucus (Fig. 13.2). The cilia move the overlying mucus by their tips which are assisted in this in possessing minute terminal hooklets (Fig. 13.3).[41]

The first ciliary defect identified was an absence of dynein arms[28] (Fig. 13.4). Subsequently, it was recognized that the syndrome is caused occasionally by absence of ciliary spokes, or transposition of one of the outer microtubular doublets to replace the central pair (Figs 13.5 and 13.6).[64,65] These three developmental ciliary defects must not be confused with acquired ciliary abnormalities — such as compound cilia — which commonly result from infection or other injury. Recognition of the various primary abnormalities can require rather tedious electron microscopic quantification[30] or in vitro functional studies. Suitable cells for both functional and ultrastructural studies may be obtained by brushing the back of the nasal passages.[57] It is economical to limit EM to those specimens that show impaired ciliary motility in vitro.

PNEUMOCYSTIS CARINII PNEUMONIA

P. carinii was first described in the lungs of rodents in 1909 by Chagas, and soon after by Carini, after whom the organism is named. It was not identified as a cause of human disease until the middle of the century when outbreaks of what were described as interstitial plasma cell pneumonia were investigated. These occurred in east European orphanages housing malnourished children. Such epidemic *Pneu-*

mocystis pneumonia is no longer seen in Europe but is still encountered in parts of the world where poverty and malnutrition are rife.

Pneumocystis pneumonia was subsequently recognized as a complication of immunodeficiency states, both congenital and acquired. Until recently such immunodeficiency was generally due to lymphoproliferative disease or immunosuppressive therapy, but interest now centres on *Pneumocystis* pneumonia as being by far the commonest opportunistic infection in the acquired immunodeficiency syndrome (AIDS). *P. carinii* has now been found in a wide range of animals, inhabiting their lungs without giving rise to any apparent lesions. This probably also applies to man, the disease developing only when immunity is impaired.

Electron microscopy is not necessary for the diagnosis of this form of pneumonia but has provided informative data on the structure and life cycle of the causative organism (Fig. 13.7). EM has also contributed to our understanding of the nature of the parasite, now believed to be a protozoan rather than a fungus, and a sporozoan rather than a trypanosome. Finally, electron microscopy has been used to elucidate the pathogenesis of *Pneumocystis* pneumonia.[3,15,32,35,72]

P. carinii lives free and completes its life cycle within the lumen of its host's pulmonary alveoli, which may be filled with the parasite in various stages of development. This involves the development and proliferation of free-living trophozoites, followed by their encystment and subsequent release. EM shows that the cysts measure 3–6 μm in diameter and have a thick wall or pellicle (Fig. 13.8). The pellicle is triple-layered, consisting of an outer electron-dense zone about 75 nm in thickness, an electron-lucent 250 nm-thick intermediate zone and an inner 7 nm unit membrane. Numerous small tubular structures (filopodia) are associated with the inner layer. Also possibly derived from this membrane are up to eight nucleated intracystic bodies or sporozoa. Collapsed cysts are largely empty and the innermost membrane of the wall is either detached or absent (Fig. 13.9). The released intracystic bodies are known as trophozoites. These grow from about 1.5 to 6 μm, lack a pellicle, and are highly irregular in shape (Fig. 13.10). They possibly undergo binary fission before entering a pre-cyst stage in which they develop a pellicle. Cysts tend to be sparse near the alveolar walls which are bordered chiefly by trophozoites, suggesting that limitation of some nutritional factor promotes cyst formation. In successfully treated cases only empty cysts are found, indicating that all viable forms of the parasite, whether free-living or encysted, are vulnerable to chemotherapy. Although a heavy cellular reaction within the alveolus does not occur, degenerate cysts and trophozoites may be found within alveolar macrophages.

EM also shows that the trophozoites attach to type I alveolar epithelial cells, eventually causing these cells to slough away from the alveolar wall. Tracer studies show that there is increased permeability in the lung, even before epithelial cells are lost.[51,75]

IDIOPATHIC INTERSTITIAL PNEUMONIA AND FIBROSIS

This disease is of unknown cause but there are good reasons for suspecting an auto-immune basis. Thus, identical changes are found in the lung in diseases such as systemic sclerosis and rheumatoid disease, while serological markers of auto-immune disease such as rheumatoid and antinuclear factors are often present, even when disease is confined to the lung. Immune complexes are often present in the bloodstream[34] and may also be identified in bronchoalveolar lavage fluid.[29] Occasionally, immune complexes are identified in lung tissue by immunofluorescence microscopy, but this is generally limited to early cases.[58] An electron-microscopic study, limited to early cases in the hope of identifying electron-dense deposits, produced consistently negative results in this respect,[18] and this is the general experience. Abnormalities of possible pathogenetic significance have, however, been identified by EM in idiopathic interstitial fibrosis.[10,16,18,33,43,46]

In addition to providing merely higher magnifications of the interstitial inflammation and fibrosis recognizable by light microscopy, EM has identified interstitial oedema and abnormalities of both the alveolar capillary endothelium and the alveolar epithelium (Fig. 13.11). The alveolar capillary endothelium is frequently degenerate, as indicated by electron-lucent swelling of the cytoplasm (Fig. 13.11). Furthermore, the endothelial basal lamina is frequently thickened (Fig. 13.12) or multilayered, this being evidence of repeated endothelial regeneration.[70] Alveolar type I epithelial cells show degenerative changes similar to those in the endothelium (Fig. 13.11) and these sometimes proceed to frank necrosis, so that the underlying basement membrane is exposed to alveolar air (Fig. 13.13). Hyperplasia of type II cells is commonly observed (Figs 13.14 and 13.15); together with the finding of epithelial cells intermediate between types II and I (Fig. 13.16); this provides evidence of widespread alveolar epithelial cell injury. It is possible that the epithelium normally exerts an inhibitory influence on the underlying connective tissue cells, proliferation of which may proceed unchecked when there is long-standing injury to the epithelium. Furthermore, the endothelial damage might well augment the interstitial fibrosis as this is a recognized complication of prolonged interstitial oedema in diseases such as mitral stenosis. These observations provide no information on the cause of idiopathic interstitial fibrosis but provide insight into its pathogenesis; they are probably the consequence of cytotoxic mediators released by inflammatory and immune effector cells activated by auto-immune mechanisms.[8,18,24]

DIFFUSE ALVEOLAR DAMAGE

Diffuse alveolar damage is a pathological process seen in the lung as a result of a wide variety of noxious factors.[44] It represents acute cytotoxic injury and is essentially non-specific; recognized causes include shock,[2] viral pneumonia,[50] atmospheric pollutants,[11,50,63] oxygen at high concentration,[31] and chemical agents which may reach the lung via the blood stream after being ingested (for example, paraquat[67]).

The most delicate structures in the lung at the alveolar level are its epithelium and the capillary endothelium. In many respects the changes are similar to those just described under idiopathic interstitial fibrosis, to which it may progress, but the whole tempo of the disease is far faster. Epithelial necrosis and hyaline membranes consisting of necrotic debris and fibrin are its hallmarks (Fig. 13.17).

DESQUAMATIVE INTERSTITIAL PNEUMONIA

In many cases of idiopathic interstitial pneumonia, mononuclear cells accumulate in the alveolar lumen and sometimes this is the major abnormality; this appearance has been termed desquamative interstitial pneumonia, implying that the alveolar cells are derived from alveolar epithelium. EM shows that in nearly all cases the free alveolar cells are macrophages rather than desquamated epithelial cells (Fig. 13.18).[20,52] The changes would therefore be more correctly termed exudative rather than desquamative; luminal (as opposed to mural) is a further alternative.

Intranuclear virus-like inclusions are sometimes evident in alveolar lining cells in desquamative interstitial pneumonia. EM shows that the cells involved are type II alveolar epithelial cells and that the inclusions represent a nuclear degenerative process and are not of viral origin (see Ch. 9).[54]

GIANT CELL INTERSTITIAL PNEUMONIA

A rare variety of interstitial lung disease is that termed giant cell interstitial pneumonia. EM shows that in addition to multinucleated alveolar macrophages there are also giant multinucleated type II alveolar epithelial cells (Fig. 13.19). The giant cells of measles pneumonia are also multinucleated type II alveolar epithelial cells, but these are characterized by cytoplasmic and nuclear viral inclusions.[1] It has become apparent that many patients with giant cell interstitial pneumonia are hard metal workers and it is likely that some constituent of this alloy is responsible for the epithelial cell transformation.[26] On experimental grounds, cobalt has been identified as the constituent responsible for the interstitial fibrosis in hard metal workers' giant cell interstitial pneumonia.

MALLORY'S HYALIN IN ALVEOLAR EPITHELIUM

Hyaline inclusions, seemingly identical to those seen in the liver in alcoholic hepatitis, were first reported in the alveolar epithelium in asbestosis.[48] Electron microscopy shows that, as in the liver, they consist of a tangle of intermediate filaments (Fig. 13.20). They have since been identified in other interstitial lung diseases and must be regarded as evidence of non-specific alveolar injury.[74]

CIGARETTE SMOKE INCLUSIONS IN ALVEOLAR MACROPHAGES

Cigarette smoke is the most important cause of lung disease in developed countries but its principal consequences — cancer and obstructive airways disease — have either been dealt with elsewhere,[36] or have no diagnostic ultrastructural characteristics. Particulates of cigarette smoke itself can however be recognized in the lung by EM.[9,55] This depends upon the identification of certain inclusions within alveolar macrophages; not only are these cells increased in smokers, but their phagolysosomes are more numerous and contain tar bodies and characteristic small kaolinite crystals (Figs 13.21, 13.22).

SARCOIDOSIS

Sarcoidosis is a multisystem granulomatous disease of unknown cause, principally affecting the lungs and hilar lymph nodes. Electron microscopy plays no role in the diagnosis of sarcoidosis, but it provides interesting insights into the labile character of macrophages and the changes these cells undergo when they become epithelioid cells in the centre of a granuloma. Macrophages are phagocytic cells equipped with a rich complement of lysosomal dense bodies (Fig. 13.18), but when activated they may switch to become secretory. Two types of epithelioid cell can be recognized by electron microscopy: A and B.[40] The A type is also known as a plasmacytoid epithelioid cell, possessing an array of RER similar to that of a plasma cell, denoting the synthesis of protein destined for secretion. The B type of epithelioid cell is characterized by numerous granular vacuoles, presumably reflecting the storage of some as yet poorly characterized secretion. The type A is thought to mature into a B type, and Figure 13.23 shows an intermediate cell form. Mature granulomas consist mainly of vacuolated (B type) epithelioid cells. One secretory substance which has so far been localized to epithelioid cells by ultrastructural immunocytochemistry is dipeptidyl carboxypeptidase — the so-called angiotensin converting enzyme[59] which in this inflammatory process is probably inactivating kinins rather than activating angiotensinogen. Close apposition between lymphocytes and epithelioid cells (Fig. 13.24) supports the proposition that these cells have a functional relationship.

Broncho-alveolar lavage macrophages from patients with sarcoidosis have been examined by electron microscopy to see whether changes comparable to those described in tissue granulomas can be recognized.[25] Full-blown epithelioid conversion, as described above, is not identifiable, but certain ultrastructural changes indicate that the alveolar macrophages are activated in this disease. Thus, the macrophages are enlarged and possess more inclusions, which differ in their electron-density from the normal dense bodies. Ruffling of the cell membrane by prominent pseudopodia is also evident, and concentration of this change to one side of the cell indicates some sort of polarization process. Subplasmalemmal linear densities at contact points between macrophages are seen in both lavage fluid and tissue specimens from sarcoidosis patients (Fig. 13.25). Finally, contact points between activated macrophages and lymphocytes have been observed in lavage specimens from sarcoidosis patients (Fig. 13.26).

The inclusion bodies that characterize sarcoidosis and other granulomatous diseases have been studied by electron microscopy, but some of the results are conflicting. Asteroid bodies have been variously reported to represent inclusions of elastin or collagen, or to be derived from the interdigitating cell membranes of Langhans' giant cells; however, the most convincing reports favour exuberant synthesis of vimentin filaments and microtubules under the influence of hyperactive centrioles, the bodies consisting of densely packed intermediate filaments, microtubules, centrioles and paracentrioles, devoid of a unit membrane.[13] The laminated Schaumann (or conchoidal) bodies on the other hand appear to represent mineralized lysosomal residual bodies (Fig. 13.27).[42] In a few biopsies of patients with granulomatous lung disease that probably represents sarcoidosis, certain 'tadpole' structures have been identified (Fig. 13.28). The nature of these, and whether they represent an infective agent, is at present uncertain.[27,73]

HISTIOCYTOSIS X

This term is applied to a triad of diseases that may affect the lungs: Letterer–Siwe disease, Hand-Schüller–Christian disease and eosinophilic granuloma. The first two are generalized conditions whilst the last is usually limited to structures such as the lungs and skeleton. Whether the leukaemic-like Letterer–Siwe disease is the acute form of the indolent and frequently self-limiting eosinophilic granuloma is an open question, but EM has shown that all three diseases represent pathological proliferations of the Langerhans' histiocyte.[4,5] Recognition of the Langerhans' cell could initially be made with confidence only by electron microscopy, but immunocytochemistry for S-100 proteins — although less specific — now provides a simple alternative.

Recognition of the Langerhans' cell by EM depends on the presence of a marker organelle (the Birbeck granule), a pentalaminar rod-like cytoplasmic structure which sometimes communicates with the cell surface (Figs 13.29 to 13.32). The Langerhans' cell is a type of histiocyte which is thought to be concerned with the presentation of antigen to lymphocytes, and it seems to be implicated in cellular immunity and hypersensitivity. Whether or not the occasional continuity of the marker organelle with the cell surface is concerned with these immunological phenomena is unknown.

The Langerhans' cell is particularly well represented in the epidermis and is not found in the normal lung. It has been found in the lung only in histiocytosis X and occasional cases of interstitial fibrosis, neoplasia and hypersensitivity pneumonitis.[7,45] Its identification in broncho-alveolar lavage fluid in appreciable numbers is a pointer to histiocytosis X.

LYMPHANGIOLEIOMYOMATOSIS

This condition is generally widespread throughout the lungs and often also affects lymph nodes in the thorax and abdomen. As its name indicates, it represents a proliferation of smooth muscle derived from lymphatics, but the muscle cells are often immature so that at the light-microscopic level their nature may not be obvious and they may be mistaken for fibroblasts. Electron microscopy convincingly demonstrates their true nature (Fig. 13.33).[6]

PULMONARY ALVEOLAR LIPOPROTEINOSIS

A tissue diagnosis of lipoproteinosis can readily be made at the light-microscopy level but relatively non-invasive techniques such as lavage or sputum examination are being increasingly advocated and in these circumstances the extra detail afforded by EM is very helpful.[22] The fine structure of the alveolar material also correlates well with its chemical nature and contributes to our understanding of the pathogenesis of this disease.[19,37,49]

Alveolar lipoproteinosis is a metabolic disorder of unknown cause, in which the pulmonary alveoli become filled with a characteristic deposit. This is often described as being amorphous but is in fact finely granular, a point well demonstrated by electron microscopy. The granules are osmiophilic and lamellar (Figs 13.34 and 13.35), suggesting that the material is composed largely of complex polar lipids, the molecules of which take up such an arrangement *in vitro*. There is a distinct resemblance to the surfactant-containing secretory vacuoles of type II pneumocytes and to the surface layer of the biphasic alveolar lining film, which is believed to represent pulmonary surfactant. Alveolar macrophages are engorged with similar bodies (Fig. 13.36) and the disease is thought to represent a failure of alveolar clearance in the face of increased surfactant secretion. Occasionally the cause appears to be heavy dust exposure;[12,19,37] non-industrial cases have therefore been subjected to electron microprobe analysis and by this means a variety of dust particles has been identified.[53]

EFFECT OF AMPHIPHILIC DRUGS

Although drugs such as amiodarone, iprindole and chlorphentermine have widely differing pharmaceutical actions, they share common chemical groupings and all block the action of the lysosomal enzymes sphingomyelinase and phospholipase, leading to an accumulation of the lipidic substrates of these enzymes within lysosomes throughout the body. In the lung, virtually all cells are affected but the changes are particularly marked in the alveolar macrophages, the lysosomes of which contain numerous osmiophilic lamellar inclusions (Fig. 13.37).[21] In the experimental animal administered heavy doses of amphiphilic drugs, the changes progress: the alveolar macrophages break down and the alveoli become filled with their lamellar inclusions, mimicking the changes seen in alveolar lipoproteinosis.[68,69]

PULMONARY HAEMORRHAGE AND HAEMOSIDEROSIS

Pulmonary haemorrhage and haemosiderosis may be due to localized causes such as cancer, tuberculosis or Wegener's granulomatosis, to a generalized bleeding diathesis or to raised post-capillary resistance, as in mitral stenosis, pulmonary veno-occlusive disease or lymphangioleiomyomatosis. There remain three conditions that are best distinguished immunologically: immune-complex-mediated capillaritis (as in systemic lupus erythematosus; SLE), Goodpasture's syndrome and idiopathic pulmonary haemosiderosis (IPH). Immunofluorescence microscopy is helpful in distinguishing them and at the same time casting light on their pathogenesis; by this means immunoglobulin and complement have been identified in the alveolar capillary basement membrane in both SLE and Goodpasture's syndrome, the distribution of the immunoglobulin being focal in the former and diffuse in the latter. The aetiology of these two conditions is therefore believed to involve circulating immune complexes in the former and circulating antibasement membrane antibodies in the latter, while the aetiology of IPH remains uncertain. Electron microscopy has been applied to these conditions in the expectation that electron-dense deposits would be identified in the alveolar capillary basement membrane. This expectation has been realized in the case of SLE,[47] but not in either Goodpasture's syndrome or IPH. The immunofluorescence and ultrastructural findings are summarized in Table 13.1. Although no electron-dense deposits suggestive of immune complex disease are identifiable in IPH, non-specific degenerative changes in thecapillary endothelium, similar to those described above in idiopathic interstitial fibrosis, have been identified.[18a,39] Electron microscopy also shows extensive mineral deposition in the basement membranes, interstitial elastin bundles and alveolar macrophages (Fig. 13.38).

PULMONARY HYPERTENSION

Plexogenic arteriopathy — a feature of certain forms of pulmonary hypertension — has long puzzled histopathologists. Electron microscopy shows that the short spindle-shaped cells that separate the plexiform channels within certain dilatation lesions are of various types. As well as smooth muscle cells (Fig. 13.39) and fibroblasts, there are cells that possess numerous cytoplasmic filaments but lack the focal condensations and peripheral attachment points of smooth muscle, resembling certain cells that, in other situations, are described as vasoformative reserve cells (Fig. 13.40).[62] The plexiform lesions may therefore be considered to represent a reparative process following hypertensive damage to the vessel wall.[61]

TUBULORETICULAR STRUCTURES

Endothelial tubuloreticular structures are well-known in the kidney, particularly in systemic lupus erythematosus, but they may also be found in the lung (see Ch. 9, 17 and 29). Here they are a feature of several collagen vascular diseases and also of viral pneumonia,[33] but they are by no means specific for these conditions. The inclusions consist of membrane-bound interweaving tubules measuring approximately 20 nm in diameter. They have been shown to contain phospholipid and acidic glycoprotein. Their limiting membrane sometimes connects with that of the rough endoplasmic reticulum. Although their true nature remains obscure, it is now generally agreed that they do not represent viral inclusions. There is evidence that their formation can be induced by type I interferon.[33]

PNEUMOCONIOSES AND ANALYTICAL ELECTRON MICROSCOPY

Analytical electron microscopy is proving to be extremely valuable in relation to those diseases caused by inhaled

Table 13.1 Ultrastructural and immunofluorescent microscopic findings in immune complex-mediated lung haemorrhage (as in systemic lupus erythematosus), Goodpasture's syndrome and idiopathic pulmonary haemosiderosis.[18a,39,47]

	Electron microscopy	Immunofluorescence microscopy
Immune complex-mediated lung haemorrhage	Electron-dense deposits in kidney and lung.[47] Endothelial tubuloreticular arrays in SLE	Granular immunoglobulin deposits in kidney and lung
Goodpasture's syndrome	Normal basement membrane in kidney and lung	Linear immunoglobulin deposits in kidney and lung
Idiopathic pulmonary haemosiderosis	Thickened pulmonary capillary basement membrane[18a,39]	No immunoglobulin demonstrable in lung

inorganic dusts, whether it is applied to air samples, material obtained from the lung by lavage, or lung tissue.[23,66] The phagocytic capabilities of the various alveolar cells have been demonstrated by electron microscopy[17] (Fig. 13.41). Electron microscopy has also been used to study the fine structure of many dust particles,[38] including asbestos fibres and asbestos bodies (Figs 13.42 to 13.44).

By scanning electron microscopy, dust particles may be localized and analysed in relatively thick sections, so avoiding the difficulty of cutting ultrathin sections of tissue containing hard mineral particles. The back-scattered image may be used to detect dense materials beneath the surface of the tissue and energy dispersive X-ray spectroscopy may then be applied to individual particles to give an elemental analysis (Figs 13.45 and 13.46). The proportions in which various elements are associated can be identified and hence the nature of compound substances can be deduced. Finally, electron diffraction can be used to provide information on crystal structure (Fig. 13.47). Silica, for example, can be identified by X-ray spectroscopy and its quartz, cristobalite and tridymite forms distinguished by their electron diffraction patterns.

REFERENCES

1. Archibald R W R, Weller R O, Meadow S R 1971 Measles pneumonia and the nature of the inclusion-bearing giant cells: a light- and electron-microscope study. Journal of Pathology 103: 27–34
2. Bachofen M, Weibel E R 1977 Alterations of the gas exchange apparatus in adult respiratory insufficiency associated with septicemia. American Review of Respiratory Disease 116: 589–615
3. Barton E G, Campbell W 1967 Further observations on the ultrastructure of *Pneumocystis*. Archives of Pathology and Laboratory Medicine 83: 527–534
4. Basset F, Nezelof C, Ferrans V J 1983 The histiocytoses. Pathology annual 18, Part 2: 27–78
5. Basset F, Soler P, Jaurand M C, Bignon J 1977 Ultrastructural examination of broncho-alveolar lavage for diagnosis of pulmonary histiocytosis X. Thorax 32: 303–306
6. Basset F, Soler P, Marsac J, Corrin B 1976 Pulmonary lymphangiomyomatosis: three new cases studied with electron microscopy. Cancer 38: 2357–2366
7. Basset F, Soler P, Wyllie L, Abelauet R, Le Charpentier M, Kreis B, Breathnach A S 1974 Langerhans' cells in a bronchiolo-alveolar tumour of lung. Virchows Archiv A 362: 315–330
8. Bowden D H 1984 Unravelling pulmonary fibrosis: the bleomycin model. Laboratory Investigation 50: 487–488
9. Brody A R, Craighead J E 1975 Cytoplasmic inclusions in pulmonary macrophages of cigarette smokers. Laboratory Investigation 32: 125–132
10. Brody A R, Craighead J E 1976 Interstitial associations of cells lining air spaces in human pulmonary fibrosis. Virchows Archiv A, Pathological Anatomy and Histology 372: 39–49
11. Brown R F R, Clifford W E , Marrs T C, Cox R A 1983 The histopathology of rat lung following short term exposures to mixed oxides of nitrogen (NOx). British Journal of Experimental Pathology 64: 579–593
12. Buechner H A, Ansari A 1969 Acute silico-proteinosis. Diseases of the Chest 55: 274–284
13. Cain H, Kraus B 1977 Asteroid bodies: derivatives of the cytosphere. An electron microscopic contribution to the pathology of the cytocentre. Virchows Archiv, Cell Pathology 26: 119
14. Camner P, Mossberg B, Afzelius B A 1975 Evidence for congenitally non-functioning cilia in the tracheobronchial tract in two subjects. American Review of Respiratory Disease 112: 807–809
15. Campbell W G 1972 Ultrastructure of *Pneumocystis* in human lung. Archives of Pathology and Laboratory Medicine 93: 312–324
16. Coalson J J 1982 The ultrastructure of human fibrosing alveolitis. Virchows Archiv A, Pathological Anatomy 395: 181–199
17. Corrin B 1970 Phagocytic potential of pulmonary alveolar epithelium with particular reference to surfactant metabolism. Thorax 25: 110–114
18. Corrin B, Dewar A, Rodriguez-Roisin R, Turner-Warwick M 1985 Fine structural changes in cryptogenic fibrosing alveolitis and asbestosis. Journal of Pathology 147: 107–119
18a. Corrin B, Jagusch M, Dewar A, Tungekar M F, Davies D R, Kramer J O, Turner-Warwick M, Empey D 1987 Fine structural changes in idiopathic pulmonary haemosiderosis. Journal of Pathology 153: 249–256
19. Corrin B, King E 1970 Pathogenesis of experimental pulmonary alveolar proteinosis. Thorax 25: 230–236
20. Corrin B, Price A B 1972 Electron microscopic studies in desquamative interstitial pneumonia associated with asbestos. Thorax 27: 324–331
21. Costa-Jussa F R, Corrin B, Jacobs J M 1984 Amiodarone lung toxicity: a human and experimental study. Journal of Pathology 143: 73–79
22. Costello J F, Moriarty D C, Branthwaite M A, Turner-Warwick M, Corrin B 1975 Diagnosis and management of alveolar proteinosis: the role of electron microscopy. Thorax 30: 121–132
23. Crocker P R, Doyle D V, Levison D A 1980 A practical method for the identification of particulate and crystalline material in paraffin-embedded tissue specimens. Journal of Pathology 131: 165–173
24. Crystal R G, Gadek J E, Ferrans V J, Fulmer J D, Line B R, Hunninghake G W 1981 Interstitial lung disease: current concepts of pathogenesis, staging and therapy. American Journal of Medicine 70: 542–568
25. Danel C, Dewar A, Corrin B, Turner-Warwick M, Chretien J 1983 Ultrastructural changes in bronchoalveolar lavage cells in sarcoidosis and comparison with the tissue granuloma. American Journal of Pathology 112: 7–17
26. Davison A G, Haslam P L, Corrin B, Coutts I I, Dewar A, Riding W D, Studdy P R 1983 Interstitial lung disease and asthma in hard-metal workers; bronchoalveolar lavage, ultrastructural and analytical findings and results of bronchial provocation tests. Thorax 38: 119–128
27. Dewar A, Corrin B, Turner-Warwick M 1984 Tadpole shaped structures in a further patient with granulomatous lung disease. Thorax 39: 466–467
28. Eliasson R, Mossberg B, Camner P, Afzelius B A 1977 The immotile-cilia syndrome. A congenital ciliary abnormality as an etiologic factor in chronic airways infections and male sterility. New England Journal of Medicine 297: 1–6
29. Gelb A F, Dreisen R B, Epstein J D, Silverthorne J D, Bickel Y, Fields M, Border W A 1983 Immune complexes, gallium lung scans, and bronchoalveolar lavage in idiopathic interstitial pneumonia fibrosis. Chest 84: 148–153
30. Fox B, Bull T B 1981 Letter to editor, American Review of Respiratory Disease 123: 142–143
31. Gould V E, Tosco R, Wheelis R F, Gould N S, Kapanci Y 1972 Oxygen pneumonitis in man: ultrastructural observations on the development of alveolar lesions. Laboratory Investigation 26: 499–508
32. Ham E K, Greenberg S D, Reynolds R C, Singer D B 1971 Ultrastructure of *Pneumocystis carinii*. Experimental and Molecular Pathology 14: 362–372
33. Hammar S P, Winterbauer R H, Bockus D, Remington F, Sale G E, Meyers J D 1983 Endothelial cell damage and tubuloreticular structures in interstitial lung disease associated with collagen vascular disease and viral pneumonia. American Review of Respiratory Disease 127: 77–84

34. Haslam P L, Thompson B, Mohammed I, Townsend P J, Hodson M E, Holborow E J, Turner-Warwick M 1979 Circulating immune complexes in patients with cryptogenic fibrosing alveolitis. Clinical and Experimental Immunology 37: 381–390

35. Hasleton P S, Curry A, Rankin E M 1981 *Pneumocystis carinii* pneumonia: a light microscopical and ultrastructural study. Journal of Clinical Pathology 34: 1138–1146

36. Henderson D W, Papadimitriou J M, Coleman M 1986 Ultrastructural appearances of tumours: diagnosis and classification of human neoplasia by electron microscopy. 2nd edition. Churchill Livingstone, Edinburgh

37. Heppleston A G, Fletcher K, Wyatt I 1974 Changes in the composition of lung lipids and the 'turnover' of dipalmitoyl lecithin in experimental alveolar lipoproteinosis induced by inhaled quartz. British Journal of Experimental Pathology 55: 384–395

38. Herbert A, Sterling G, Abraham J, Corrin B 1982 Desquamative interstitial pneumonia in an aluminum welder. Human Pathology 13: 694–699

39. Jagusch M, Corrin B, Dewar A 1984 Personal observations

40. James V E M, Jones Williams W 1974 Fine structure and histochemistry of epithelioid cells in sarcoidosis. Thorax 29: 115–120

41. Jeffery P K, Reid L M 1975 New observations of rat airway epithelium: a quantitative electron microscopic study. Journal of Anatomy 120: 295–320

42. Jones Williams W, Williams D 1968 The properties and development of conchoidal bodies in sarcoid and sarcoid-like granulomas. Journal of Pathology and Bacteriology 96: 491–496

43. Katzenstein A-L A 1985 Pathogenesis of 'fibrosis' in interstitial pneumonia: an electron microscopic study. Human Pathology 16: 1015–1024

44. Katzenstein A-L A, Bloor C M, Leibow A A 1976 Diffuse alveolar damage — the role of oxygen, shock, and related factors. American Journal of Pathology 85: 210–224

45. Kawanami O, Basset F, Ferrans V J, Soler P, Crystal R G 1981 Pulmonary Langerhans' cells in patients with fibrotic lung disorders. Laboratory Investigation 44: 227–233

46. Kawanami O, Ferrans V J, Crystal R G 1982 Structure of alveolar epithelial cells in patients with fibrotic lung disorders. Laboratory Investigation 46: 39–53

47. Kuhn C 1972 Systemic lupus erythematosus in a patient with ultrastructural lesions of the pulmonary capillaries previously reported in the Review as due to idiopathic pulmonary hemosiderosis. American Review of Respiratory Disease 106: 931–932

48. Kuhn C, Kuo T-T 1973 Cytoplasmic hyalin in asbestosis. A reaction of injured alveolar epithelium. Archives of Pathology 95: 190–194

49. Kuhn C, Gyorkey F, Levine B E, Ramirez-Rivera J 1966 Pulmonary alveolar proteinosis. Laboratory Investigation 15: 492–509

50. Langloss J M, Hoover E A, Kahn D E 1977 Diffuse alveolar damage in cats induced by nitrogen dioxide or feline calicivirus. American Journal of Pathology 89: 637–648

51. Lanken P N, Minda M, Pietra G G, Fishman A P 1980 Alveolar response to experimental *Pneumocystis carinii* pneumonia in the rat. American Journal of Pathology 99: 561–588

52. Leroy E P 1969 The blood/air barrier in desquamative interstitial pneumonia. Virchows Archiv für pathologische Anatomie und Physiologie und für klinische Medizin 348: 117–130

53. McEuen D D, Abraham J L 1978 Pulmonary alveolar proteinosis: scanning electron microscopy and X-ray microanalysis results. Laboratory Investigation 38: 356

54. McNary W F, Gaensler E A 1971 Intranuclear inclusion bodies in desquamative interstitial pneumonia. Annals of Internal Medicine 74: 404–407

55. Pratt S A, Smith M H, Ladman A J, Finley T N 1971 The ultrastructure of alveolar macrophages from human cigarette smokers and non-smokers. Laboratory Investigation 24: 331–337

56. Rossman C M, Forrest J B, Lee R M K W, Newhouse M T 1980 The dyskinetic cilia syndrome. Ciliary motility in immotile cilia syndrome. Chest 78: 580–582

57. Rutland J, Cole P J 1982 Non-invasive sampling of nasal cilia for measurement of beat frequency and study of ultrastructure. Lancet ii: 564–565

58. Schwarz M I, Dreisen R B, Pratt D S, Stanford R E 1978 Immunofluorescent patterns in the idiopathic interstitial pneumonias. Journal of Laboratory and Clinical Medicine 91: 929–938

59. Silverstein E, Friedland J, Stanek A E, Smith P R, Deason D R, Lyons H A 1981 Angiotensin converting enzyme. Pathogenesis of sarcoidosis. Mechanism of angiotensin converting enzyme elevation: T-lymphocyte modulation of enzyme induction in mononuclear phagocytes; enzyme properties. In: Chretien J, Marsac J, Saltiel J C (eds) Sarcoidosis and other granulomatous disorders. Ninth International Conference Proceedings. Pergamon, Oxford, pp 319–325

60. Sleigh M A 1977 The nature and action of respiratory tract cilia. In: Brain J D, Proctor D F, Reid L (eds) Respiratory defence mechanisms, part 1, vol 5, Lung biology in health and disease. Dekker, New York

61. Smith P, Heath D 1979 Electron microscopy of the plexiform lesion. Thorax 34: 177–186

62. Stein A A, Mauro J, Thibodeau L, Alley R 1969 The histogenesis of cardiac myxomas: relation to other proliferative diseases of subendothelial reserve cells. Pathology annual, 4: 293–312

63. Strauss R H, Palmer K C, Hayes J A 1976 Acute lung injury induced by cadmium aerosol. American Journal of Pathology 84: 561–578

64. Sturgess J M, Chao J, Turner J A P 1980 Transposition of ciliary microtubules: another cause of impaired ciliary motility. New England Journal of Medicine 303: 318–322

65. Sturgess J M, Chao J, Wong J, Aspin N, Turner J A P 1979 Cilia with defective radial spokes. A cause of human respiratory disease. New England Journal of Medicine 300: 53–56

66. Terzakis J A 1985 X-ray microanalysis: problem solving in surgical pathology. Pathology Annual, 20 (Part 2): 59–81

67. Vijeyaratnam G S, Corrin B 1971 Experimental paraquat poisoning: a histological and electron-optical study of the changes in the lung. Journal of Pathology 103: 123–129

68. Vijeyaratnam G S, Corrin B 1973 Pulmonary alveolar proteinosis developing from desquamative interstitial pneumonia in long term toxicity studies of iprindole in the rat. Virchows Archiv A, Pathological Anatomy 358: 1–10

69. Vijeyaratnam G S, Corrin B 1974 Fine structural alterations in the lungs of iprindole treated rats. Journal of Pathology 114: 233–239

70. Vracko R, Benditt E P 1970 Capillary basal lamina thickening and duplication in relationship to endothelial cell death and replacement. Journal of Cell Biology 17: 281–285

71. Wang N-S 1983 Applications of electron microscopy to diagnostic pulmonary pathology. Human Pathology 14: 888–900

72. Wang N-S, Huang S-N, Thurlbeck W M 1970 Combined *Pneumocystis carinii* and cytomegalovirus infection. Archives of Pathology and Laboratory Medicine 90: 529–535

73. Wang N-S, Schraufnagel D E, Sampson M G 1981 The tadpole-shaped structures in human non-necrotising granulomas. American Review of Respiratory Disease 123: 560–564

74. Warnock M L, Press M, Churg A 1980 Further observations on cytoplasmic hyaline in the lung. Human Pathology 11: 59–65

75. Yoneda K, Walzer P D 1981 Mechanism of pulmonary alveolar injury in experimental *Pneumocystis carinii* pneumonia. British Journal of Experimental Pathology 62: 339–346

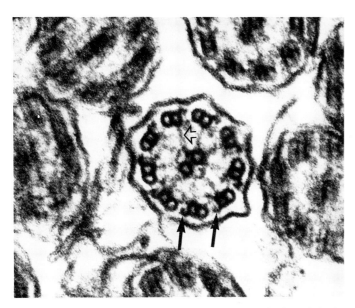

Fig. 13.1 Normal cilium: cross section. A central pair of microtubules is surrounded by a ring of nine outer doublets. The doublets are connected to the central pair by spokes (open arrow) while dynein arms (arrows) reach from one doublet to the next. (× 140 000)

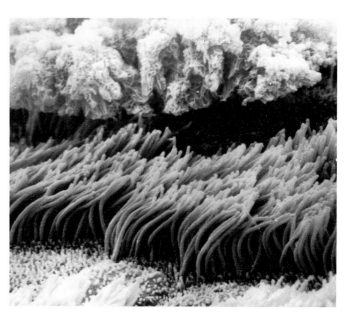

Fig. 13.2 Normal respiratory epithelium: cilia and hypophase. The cilia are covered by an overlying mucous blanket. The height of the aqueous hypophase in which the cilia beat is crucial to airway clearance: too high and the mucus is lifted off the cilia, too low and the mucus would impair ciliary movement. (Courtesy Dr P K Jeffery.) (× 5000)

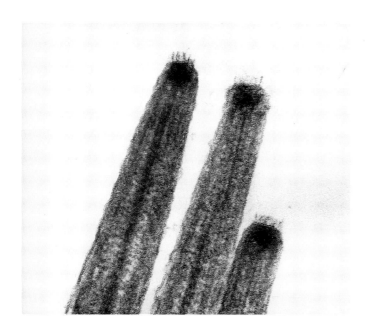

Fig. 13.3 Normal cilia in longitudinal section: terminal hooklets. A mucous blanket normally rests on the tips of the cilia and its propulsion is facilitated by small hooks on the ends of the cilia. (× 80 000)

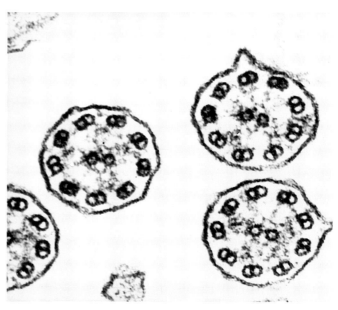

Fig. 13.4 Ciliary dyskinesia syndrome: absence of dynein arms. Dynein is associated with adenosine triphosphatase, which is believed to supply the energy required to power ciliary movement. The movement is effected by each microtubular doublet sliding on its neighbours. In this patient with ciliary dyskinesia dynein arms are absent. (Courtesy of Prof P Cole.) (× 140 000)

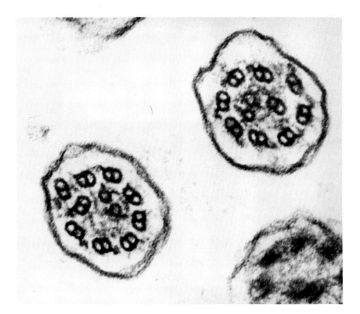

Fig. 13.5 Ciliary dyskinesia syndrome: absence of ciliary spokes. In this patient with ciliary dyskinesia, ciliary spokes are absent, allowing outer doublets to be displaced inwards. (Courtesy of Prof P Cole.) (× 140 000)

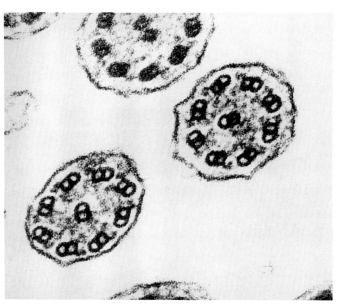

Fig. 13.6 Ciliary dyskinesia syndrome: transposition. In this patient with ciliary dyskinesia an outer microtubular doublet has taken up a central position to replace the normal central pair, which is absent. Note that there are only eight doublets in the outer ring and that the central microtubules are fused together, unlike a normal central pair. (Courtesy of Prof P Cole.) (× 140 000)

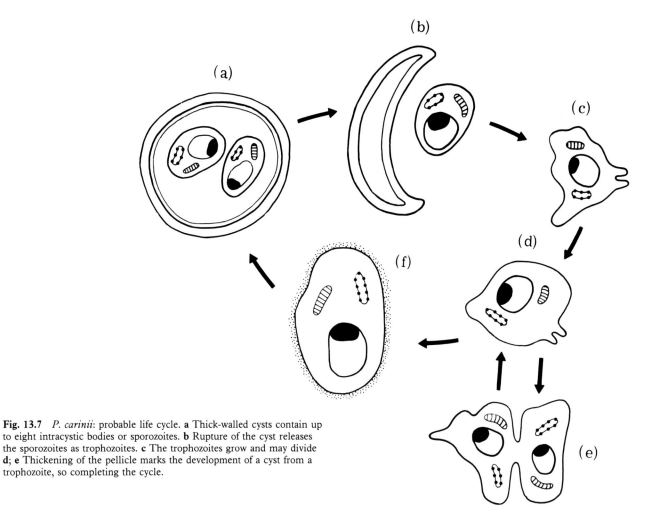

Fig. 13.7 *P. carinii*: probable life cycle. **a** Thick-walled cysts contain up to eight intracystic bodies or sporozoites. **b** Rupture of the cyst releases the sporozoites as trophozoites. **c** The trophozoites grow and may divide **d**; **e** Thickening of the pellicle marks the development of a cyst from a trophozoite, so completing the cycle.

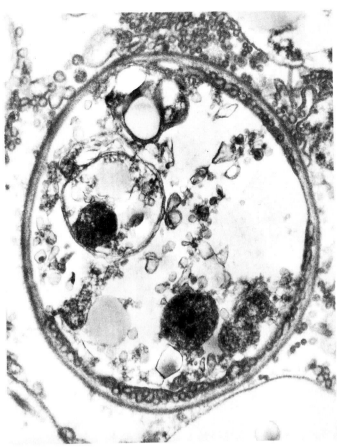

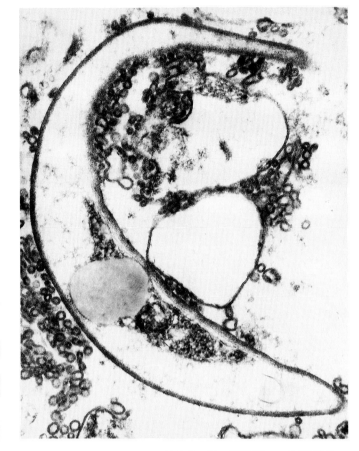

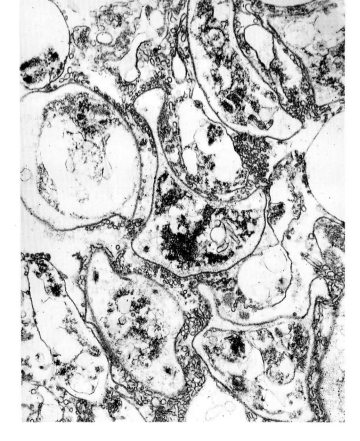

Fig. 13.8 (Above left) *Pneumocystis* pneumonia: cysts. The cyst form of
P. carinii. The cysts range from 3 to 6 μm across and are characterized by
a thick outer pellicle or cyst wall up to 350 nm in thickness. The cyst
wall is uniform and consists of three layers; an outer electron-dense zone
about 75 nm thick, an intermediate electron-lucent zone about 250 nm
thick, and an inner unit-type membrane about 7 nm in thickness.
Intracystic structures, possibly derived from the innermost layer of the
cyst wall, include up to eight intracystic bodies or sporozoites, one of
which is seen in this figure, and numerous small membranous tubular
structures. The intracystic body is nucleated and has a prominent
nucleolus. Both within the intracystic body and elsewhere in the cyst
there may be mitochondria, glycogen and fat. (× 21 000)

Fig. 13.9 (Above right) *Pneumocystis* pneumonia: membranous
complexes. Collapsed cyst form of *P. carinii* surrounded by numerous
membranous complexes derived from the cyst. The innermost membrane
of the cyst is detached from the rest of the cyst wall and contracted
around a little remaining glycogen and lipid. In successfully treated cases
only empty cysts are found, suggesting that all viable forms of the parasite
are susceptible to chemotherapy. (× 21 000)

Fig. 13.10 (Right) *Pneumocystis* pneumonia: membranous structures
and trophozoites. Densely packed membranous structures and
trophozoites of *P. carinii.* The latter are irregular in shape and measure
from 1.5 to 6 μm in length. They have a thin unit membrane wall until
they reach the pre-cyst stage which is marked by the fully mature
trophozoite acquiring on outer pellicle. Trophozoites tend to
preponderate near the alveolar walls and cysts in the centre of the
alveolar lumen, suggesting that limitation of some nutritional factor may
promote cyst formation. (× 12 000)

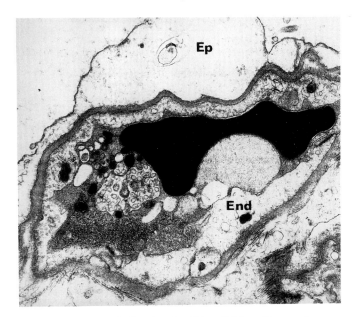

Fig. 13.11 Cryptogenic fibrosing alveolitis: cell injury. Electron-lucent cytoplasmic swelling indicative of non-specific cell injury is seen in both the endothelial (End) and type I epithelial (Ep) cells. Reproduced with permission from Corrin et al.[18] (× 10 000)

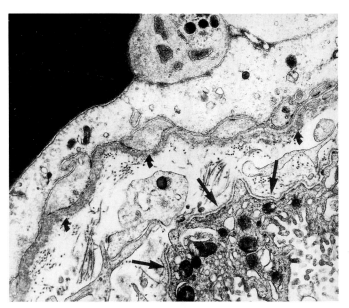

Fig. 13.12 Cryptogenic fibrosing alveolitis: endothelial basal lamina. The endothelial basal lamina (curved arrow), is greatly thickened, suggesting repeated endothelial injury and regeneration. Normally the endothelial basal lamina is the same thickness as the epithelial basal lamina (arrows). Reproduced with permission from Corrin et al.[18] (× 10 000)

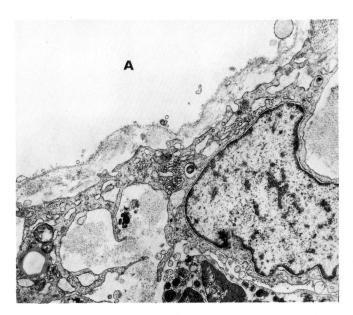

Fig. 13.13 Cryptogenic fibrosing alveolitis: interstitium. An interstitial fibroblast and adjacent collagen are separated from alveolar air only by basement membrane which is totally denuded of its epithelial membrane. (Reproduced with permission from Corrin et al.[18]) A = alveolus. (× 8000)

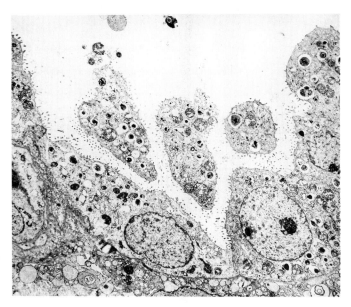

Fig. 13.14 Cryptogenic fibrosing alveolitis: type II pneumocyte hyperplasia. Type II epithelial cell hyperplasia is a common non-specific response to type II cell injury. (Reproduced with permission from Corrin et al.[18]) (× 2700)

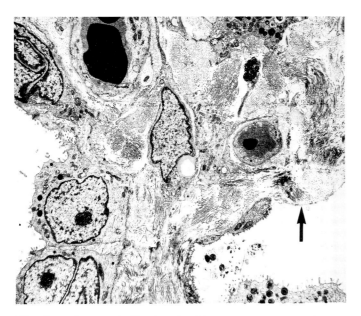

Fig. 13.15 Cryptogenic fibrosing alveolitis: pneumocyte hyperplasia and denudation. There is marked interstitial fibrosis with abundant collagen. On one side of the septum there is type II hyperplasia; on the opposite side the epithelial basement membrane is denuded of its cellular covering (arrow). (× 2700)

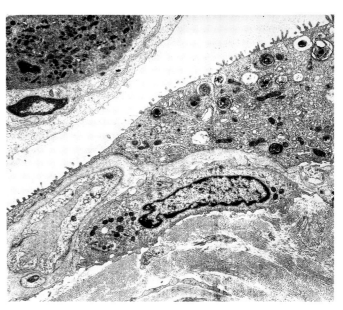

Fig. 13.16 Cryptogenic fibrosing alveolitis: intermediate pneumocyte. This shows an alveolar epithelial cell with the squamous form of a type I cell but the microvilli and lamellar vacuoles of a type II cell; such intermediate cells are indicative of epithelial regeneration. (Reproduced with permission from Corrin et al.[18]) (× 4700)

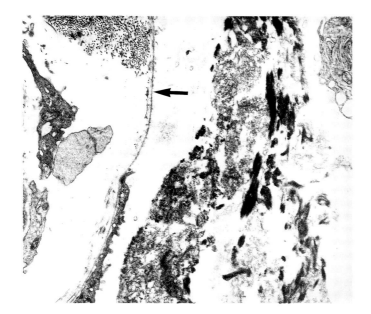

Fig. 13.17 Adult respiratory distress syndrome: diffuse alveolar damage. The alveolar epithelium is partly lost, so that its basement membrane (arrow) is bare except for a covering of necrotic debris and fibrin that corresponds to the hyaline membrane seen by light microscopy. This patient died of rapidly progressive respiratory failure (adult respiratory distress syndrome) complicating acute leukaemia treated by cytotoxic drugs, whole body irradiation and bone marrow transplantation. It is uncertain whether the cytotoxic factor responsible for the diffuse alveolar damage was the chemotherapy, irradiation, opportunistic infection or graft-versus-host disease, either alone or in combination. (× 7000)

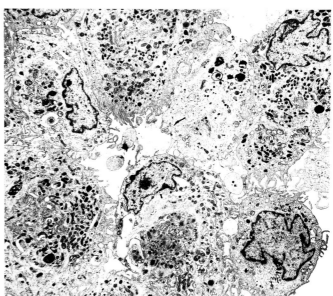

Fig. 13.18 Desquamative interstitial pneumonia: macrophage accumulation. The free alveolar cells are macrophages — recognizable by their wealth of lysosomal dense bodies and pseudopodia — rather than desquamated epithelial cells. (× 2700)

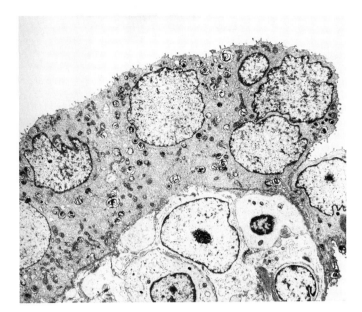

Fig. 13.19 Giant cell interstitial pneumonia in a hard metal worker: multinucleated type II pneumocytes. Electron microscopy demonstrates that many of the giant cells are multinucleated type II alveolar epithelial cells, recognizable by their microvilli and lamellar vacuoles. (× 3200)

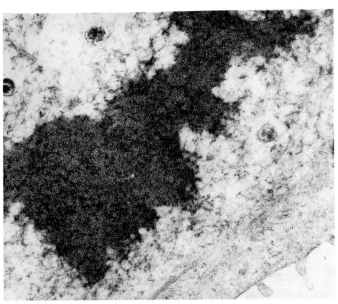

Fig. 13.20 Asbestosis: Mallory's hyalin in an alveolar epithelial cell. As in alcoholic hepatitis these bodies consist of tangled filamentous aggregates. (Courtesy of Prof D W Henderson) (× 28 800)

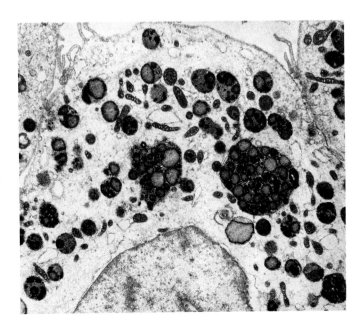

Fig. 13.21 Cigarette smoker: alveolar macrophages. Alveolar macrophages are increased in number in cigarette smokers, as are their lysosomal dense bodies which contain numerous 'tar bodies'. (× 6600)

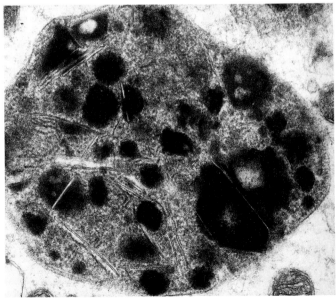

Fig. 13.22 Cigarette smoker: crystals of kaolinite. As well as the 'tar bodies', the macrophage lysosomes contain thin plate-like crystals of kaolinite. (× 53 000)

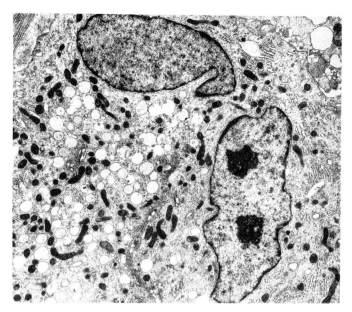

Fig. 13.23 Sarcoidosis: multinucleated epithelioid cell. Fusion of two epithelioid cells: to the right the cytoplasm contains abundant rough endoplasmic reticulum and the cell is evidently in a synthetic phase, while to the left the cytoplasm contains numerous vacuoles and the cell is in a storage phase. (× 4000)

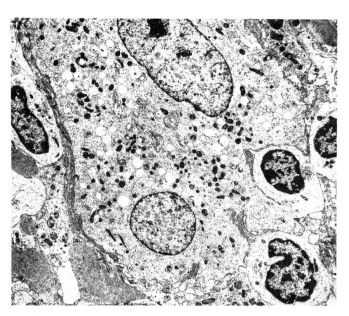

Fig. 13.24 Sarcoidosis: multinucleated epithelioid cell. A multinucleated (Langhans) epithelioid cell attended by several lymphocytes. Note the very close apposition between the lymphocytes and the giant cell. Reproduced from Danel et al.[25] (× 3000)

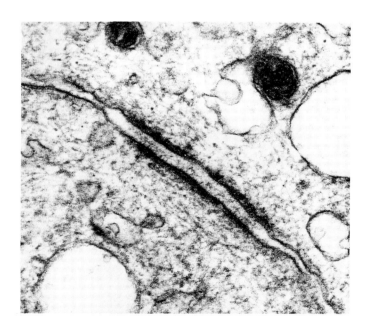

Fig. 13.25 Sarcoidosis: subplasmalemmal densities. Subplasmalemmal linear densities connect two macrophages. (× 80 000)

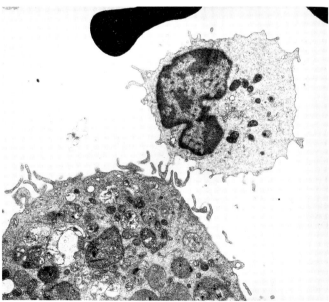

Fig. 13.26 Sarcoidosis: macrophage — lymphocyte apposition. Bronchoalveolar lavage from a patient with sarcoidosis, showing close apposition between the cell processes of a macrophage and those of a lymphocyte. Reproduced with permission from Danel et al.[25] (× 6000)

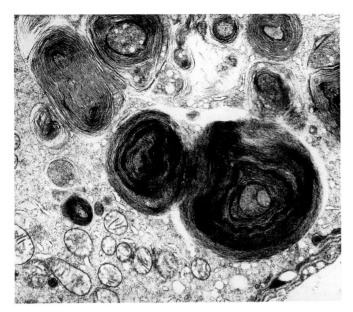

Fig. 13.27 Sarcoidosis: residual bodies in a Langhans cell. Part of a Langhans giant cell in which lysosomal residual bodies are particularly numerous. Schaumann bodies are thought to represent calcified residual bodies such as these.[42] (× 10 500)

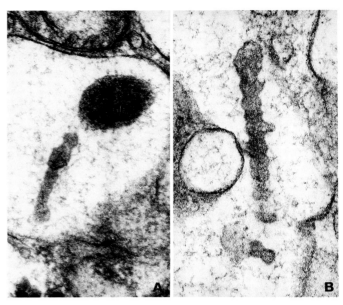

Fig. 13.28 Granulomatous lung disease: tadpole bodies. 'Tadpole'-shaped structures are seen within cell vesicles. They have electron-dense heads (**A**) and beaded tails (**A** and **B**). (Reproduced with permission from Dewar et al.[27]) (A, × 53 000; B, × 66 000)

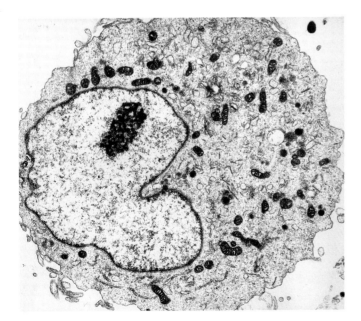

Fig. 13.29 Eosinophilic granuloma of lung: Langerhans' cell. A Langerhans' cell recovered by broncho-alveolar lavage from the lungs of a patient with pulmonary eosinophilic granuloma. There are few lysosomes but the cytoplasm contains many small rod-like structures, better seen in Figs 14.30–14.32. (Courtesy of Dr P H Haslam) (× 6000)

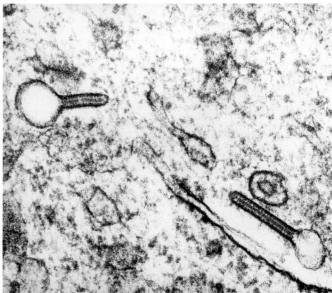

Fig. 13.30 Eosinophilic granuloma of lung: Birbeck granule. The characteristic rods of the Langerhans' cells often terminate in a vacuole. (× 93 000)

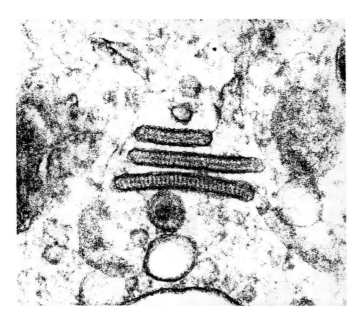

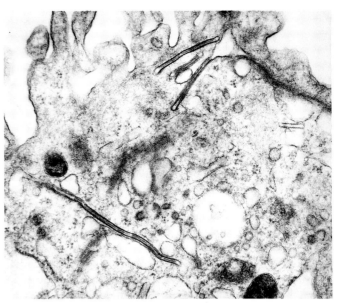

Fig. 13.31 Eosinophilic granuloma of lung: Birbeck granule. Further detail of the marker organelle of the Langerhans' cell (the Birbeck granule), which is a pentalaminar rod with cross striations. (× 100 000)

Fig. 13.32 Eosinophilic granuloma of lung: Birbeck granule. Langerhans' cell with particularly well developed Birbeck granules. (× 33 000)

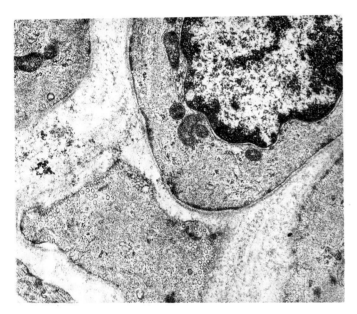

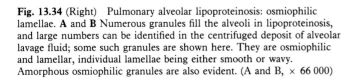

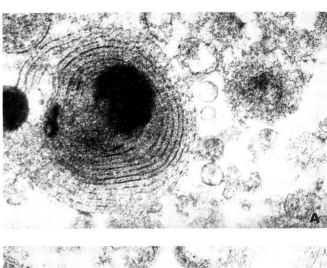

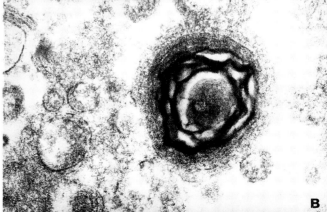

Fig. 13.33 Pulmonary lymphangioleiomyomatosis: leiomyocytes. Electron microscopy shows that the cellular infiltrate in the lung consists of smooth muscle cells, recognizable by their cytoplasmic filaments, attachment points and basement membrane. (Courtesy of Dr F Basset) (× 14 500)

Fig. 13.34 (Right) Pulmonary alveolar lipoproteinosis: osmiophilic lamellae. **A** and **B** Numerous granules fill the alveoli in lipoproteinosis, and large numbers can be identified in the centrifuged deposit of alveolar lavage fluid; some such granules are shown here. They are osmiophilic and lamellar, individual lamellae being either smooth or wavy. Amorphous osmiophilic granules are also evident. (A and B, × 66 000)

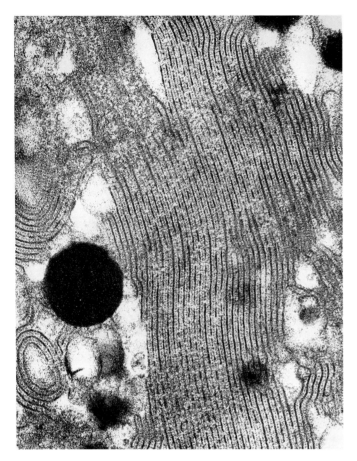

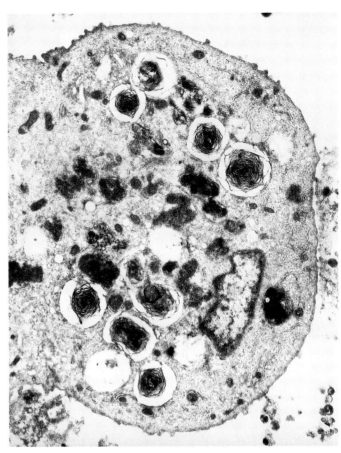

Fig. 13.35 Pulmonary alveolar lipoproteinosis: osmiophilic lamellae. Sheets of osmiophilic lamellar material are also found in the alveoli or, as depicted here, in alveolar lavage fluid. The intensely osmiophilic amorphous round body represents simple lipid while the lamellar material represents complex phospholipid or lipoproteins. Complex lipids take up such a lamellar configuration in vitro because hydrophilic and hydrophobic groupings repel each other and like seeks like. The lamellae represent sheets of lipidic molecules with all the molecules within one sheet aligned in a similar way. The molecular arrangement alternates in adjacent lamellae and this is probably responsible for the alternating pattern of electron-dense bands. (× 61 000)

Fig. 13.36 Pulmonary alveolar lipoproteinosis: alveolar macrophages. Alveolar macrophages with a foamy appearance at the light microscopic level are characteristically associated with the otherwise acellular deposit. Electron microscopy shows that their foamy appearance is due to numerous ingested lamellar bodies which are strongly osmiophilic and contained within cytoplasmic vacuoles. (× 9000)

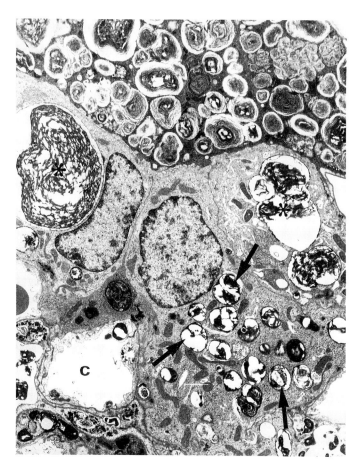

Fig. 13.37 Amiodarone lung: osmiophilic lamellae. This shows the lung of a rat treated with amiodarone; similar light-microscopic changes occur in man. An alveolar macrophage packed with lamellated bodies is seen. Several type II pneumocytes with a characteristic polygonal shape are also evident. These cells normally contain lamellated structures associated with surfactant (arrows), but also seen here are large lamellated drug-induced inclusions (asterisks). Such inclusions are also present in capillary endothelial cells. C: capillary. (Reproduced with permission from Costa-Jussa et al.[21]) (× 4200)

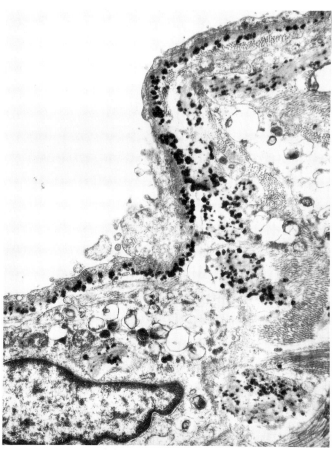

Fig. 13.38 Idiopathic pulmonary haemosiderosis: haemosiderin particles. Electron-dense haemosiderin particles are deposited in the lamina reticularis of the basement membrane and within interstitial elastin bundles. (× 8600)

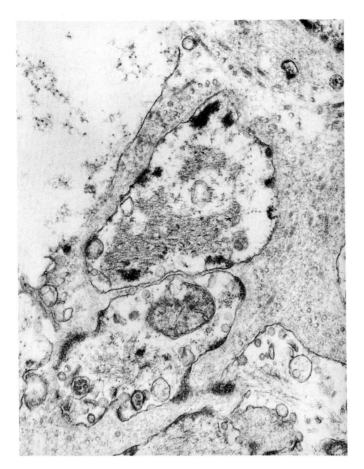

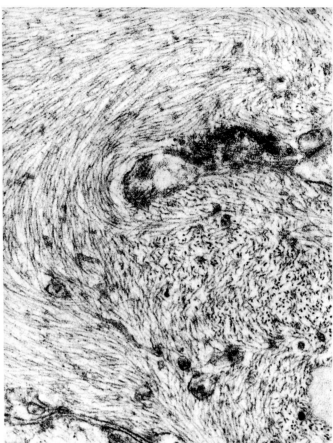

Fig. 13.39 Plexogenic pulmonary arteriopathy: leiomyocyte. Intimal proliferation in a muscular pulmonary artery includes cells which contain scanty bundles of short microfilaments, attachment points and focal condensations, features identifying them as smooth muscle. (Reproduced with permission from Smith & Heath.[61]) (× 25 000)

Fig. 13.40 Plexogenic pulmonary arteriopathy: vasoformative reserve cell. Some intimal cells contain numerous microfilaments but lack focal condensations and attachment points. (Reproduced with permission from Smith & Heath.[61]) (× 43 500)

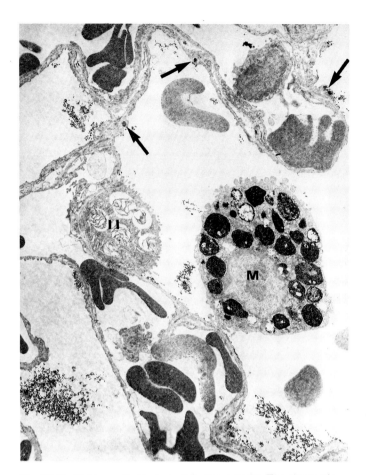

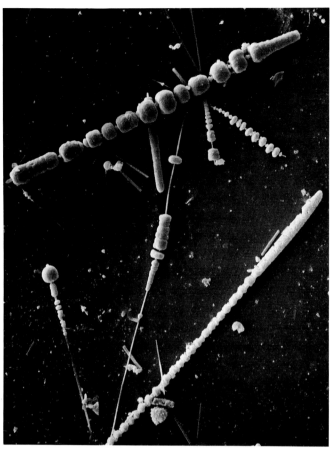

Fig. 13.41 Rat lung: phagocytosis of foreign material. The phagocytic potential of the various alveolar cells is illustrated in this portion of the lung of an experimental animal subjected to intratracheal injection of thorotrast. An alveolar macrophage (M) contains numerous thorotrast-laden phagosomes. A few small such phagosomes are seen in type I epithelial cells (arrows). A type II (II) cell is devoid of thorium. (Reproduced with permission from Corrin.[17]) (Unstained section, × 3000)

Fig. 13.42 Asbestosis: uncoated asbestos fibres and asbestos bodies. Scanning electron-micrograph of uncoated asbestos fibres and asbestos bodies obtained from the lung by tissue digestion. The long fibres probably represent an amphibole form of asbestos (e.g. crocidolite) as they are long and straight, in contrast to the serpentine form, chrysotile, which is curvilinear. Amphibole asbestos is also more likely to be coated and thereby form asbestos bodies. (Courtesy of Dr B Fox.) (× 1700)

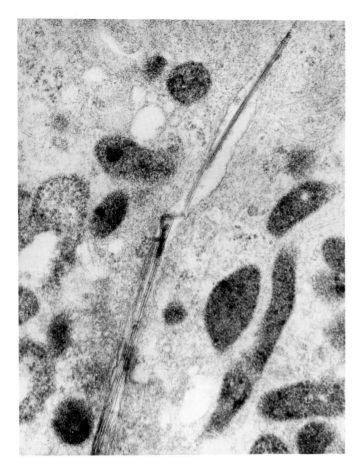

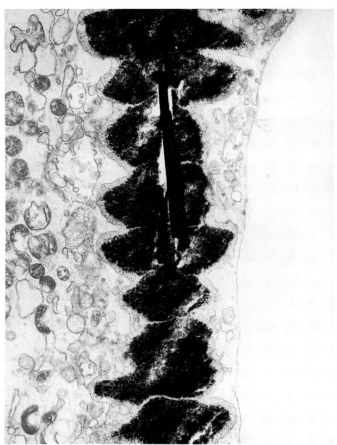

Fig. 13.43   Asbestosis: uncoated asbestos fibre. Transmission electron micrograph of an uncoated asbestos fibre within an alveolar macrophage. The fibre is contained within a membrane-bound phagosome and can be recognized as chrysotile from its characteristic clear central core. (× 38 000)

Fig. 13.44   Asbestosis: asbestos body. An asbestos body seen by transmission EM. The central rod-shaped asbestos fibre is surrounded by segmented granular electron-dense material rich in haemosiderin. (× 14 000)

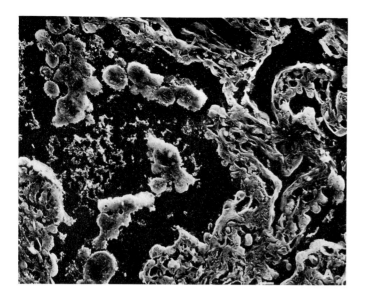

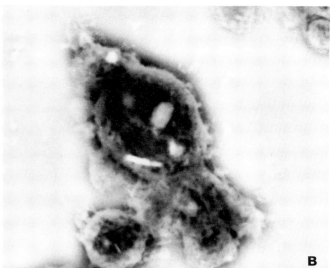

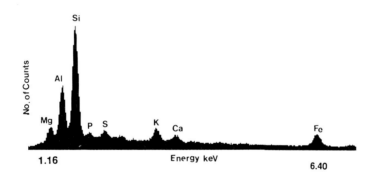

Fig. 13.45 Dust particles in lung: electron-microprobe analysis. Identification and analysis of dust particles in the lung. **A** The secondary (scanning) electron-microscopic image of a deparaffinized 5 μm thick section of lung showing clumps of macrophages in an alveolar lumen. (× 290) **B** Back-scattered scanning electron microscopic image showing several of the macrophages in the centre of **A** at higher power. Several bright particles are present in the cytoplasm. (× 1200) **C** X-ray energy spectrum of one of the brightest particles in **B** showing it to be a silicate. This analysis was done on a section mounted on a perspex slide which gives a negative background on X-ray energy spectroscopy. (Courtesy of Prof D A Levison and Mr P Crocker)

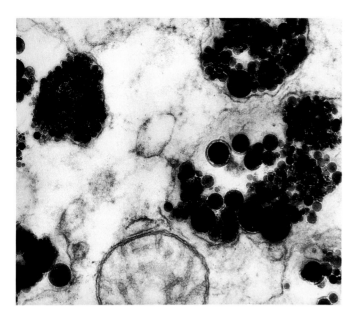

Fig. 13.46 Welder's lung: energy dispersive X-ray spectroscopy. Spherical electron-dense particles contained within membrane-bound vacuoles within pulmonary macrophages were identified as aluminium by energy dispersive X-ray spectroscopy. Reproduced with permission from Herbert et al.[38] (× 53 000)

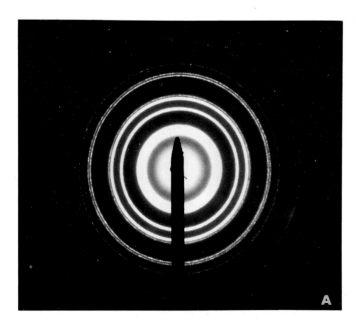
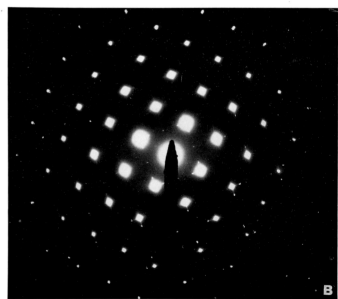

Fig. 13.47 **A** and **B** Electron-diffraction analysis: calibration. Electron-diffraction patterns of gold, used for calibration purposes and kindly provided by Dr M Wineberg. The ring pattern indicates that the material is polycrystalline, and the spot pattern indicates that it is a single crystal: amorphous materials give no regular pattern. The spacing of the rings gives information on crystalline structure and can be usefully applied to distinguish the various crystalline forms of silica (quartz, tridymite, cristobalite) for example.

14. The digestive system including biliary tract and pancreas

H. M. H. Kamel   S. M. Boyd   P. G. Toner   D. W. Henderson
J. A. Armstrong   T. M. Mukherjee

INTRODUCTION

The gastrointestinal tract is made up of a particularly complex assembly of tissue and cells. It has a wide variety of epithelial types, serving various specialized functions; it has an elaborately structured connective tissue framework for its support; it has a complex neuromuscular mechanism to supply motility; it has rich vascular and lymphatic networks to service its digestive and absorptive roles; and finally it is permeated by numerous lymphoid and other reactive cell types which provide defences against the ever-present risk of infection. This diversity is reflected in the many different pathologies that may be expressed within the framework of the gastrointestinal tract. Some of these may present in this site at a relatively early stage in their evolution, offering opportunities for clinically relevant diagnostic biopsies.

It is not surprising that many of the most significant gastrointestinal disorders are expressed in structural changes affecting the mucosa, the front line of defence in infective and allergic disease. The deeper connective tissues, muscle and nerve, may be involved in systemic disorders, such as amyloidosis, systemic sclerosis or storage diseases. These diseases may affect different parts of the gastrointestinal tract through essentially common pathogenetic mechanisms, and this is reflected in similar ultrastructural appearances at diverse sites. Interpretation, however, may be complicated by multiple interacting factors, such as primary and secondary infective agents, immunological mechanisms and vascular effects. Much of our standard classification of gastrointestinal disease relies on an admixture of aetiological factors, pathological pictures and clinical states. In such circumstances it is inevitable that disease concepts will overlap, a problem which is often reflected at the ultrastructural level.

In addressing the subject matter of this chapter we have adopted a predominantly tabular format with only a brief explanatory text, believing that this is the most practicable method for presenting a wide-ranging and heterogeneous body of reference material. With regard to electron micrographs, similar considerations have led us to illustrate in this chapter only those conditions in which electron microscopy has a significant diagnostic role. The reader will, however, be able to refer to the illustrations in the listed references for various other diseases.

THE ROLE OF ELECTRON MICROSCOPY

Most pathologists are familiar with the useful contribution which is made by electron microscopy to tumour diagnosis, notwithstanding the growing importance of immunostaining methods in routine practice. It is, however, fair to say that ultrastructural methods have made relatively little impact in routine diagnosis in non-neoplastic disease, an observation common to many other major body systems, apart from the kidney and skeletal muscle. Yet a cursory glance at the extensive literature referred to in this chapter shows no shortage of interest in ultrastructural findings. There are several possible reasons for the continuing low-profile role of routine diagnostic electron microscopy in gastrointestinal pathology.

Firstly, there is often a poor correlation between the clinical and the morphological manifestations of a particular disease. Although some conditions may present clinically at an early stage, clinical symptoms in others may demand investigation only after characteristic structural changes are so well developed that they are easily recognized by a combination of endoscopy and histology. In fact, the main interpretative problem may be the overshadowing of primary morphological changes by secondary alterations.

Secondly, there are the usual sampling problems which attend all pathological investigations, but which are particularly important in ultrastructural studies. Endoscopic biopsies are certainly readily available, and have transformed the practice of routine diagnostic gastrointestinal pathology, but the samples are at best superficial and biopsy size and orientation present problems. It is not customary to retain a portion of an endoscopic biopsy for possible subsequent electron microscopy: all tissue fragments are usually processed and examined at multiple levels, leaving little opportunity for retrospective ultrastructural examination, even in the occasional case of special interest. When a separate endoscopic biopsy is taken specifically for electron microscopy this may fail to show the feature of interest, owing to the chance of sampling. For these and other reasons, few routine diagnostic electron microscopy laboratories have the opportunity to develop any significant experience in the interpretation of such biopsies.

A third problem lies in tissue preservation and artefacts. In contrast to many of the other internal organs, the gut mucosa is constantly and intimately exposed to a hazardous environment, relying on its own structural and functional integrity to combat this threat. If this integrity is endangered, due to the primary disease, or even during the biopsy procedure, secondary changes in ultrastructural morphology may rapidly develop, particularly in sensitive tissues such as lining epithelial cells, lamina propria inflammatory components, or capillary vessels. Moreover, meaningful control material may be difficult to obtain. It is, therefore, often impossible to determine with certainty whether a particular ultrastructural finding represents an effect of the primary disorder, or a secondary phenomenon resulting from biopsy or fixation artefact.

Finally, it is in the nature of gastrointestinal disease that many disorders, such as volvulus or intussusception, are readily diagnosed by clinical presentation and gross morphology alone, and others, such as the common inflammatory disorders, by gross and light microscopic morphology. At our present level of knowledge the biopsy specimen that requires sophisticated further investigation is likely to represent a diagnostic rarity, submerged within a flood of commonplace pathology. This represents a fundamentally different situation from that seen in those low-volume specialities in which electron microscopy is routinely undertaken for diagnostic purposes, such as renal or muscle biopsy practice.

For these various reason, there are few centres or laboratories with an intensive experience of the application of electron microscopy in the diagnosis of a broad range of routine non-neoplastic gastrointestinal disorders. For the most part, the pathologist and the clinician are content to rely on routine histological techniques. Nevertheless, there are a few specific areas in which electron microscopy provides essential diagnostic assistance, whilst in many others characteristic ultrastructural features are present, although they may not be of critical diagnostic relevance. Electron microscopy may then be a useful confirmatory test, as well as offering possible insights into pathogenetic mechanisms. Finally, in a few areas of mucosal pathology, scanning electron microscopy has been used to explore cell surface morphology. Such applications are discussed in Chapter 3.

SAMPLING AND INTERPRETATION

In ultrastructural as in histopathological diagnosis, the preferred site of biopsy depends on the nature of the disease, its cause and its target. Ultrastructural interpretation may be constrained by sampling, especially in the case of the small endoscopic biopsy. It is also critically dependent on the distinction between primary and secondary subcellular alterations, which may be very difficult to make. Secondary changes, often referred to as 'non-specific degenerative alterations', include mitochondrial swelling, distension of the granular endoplasmic reticulum and the formation of cytoplasmic blebs. Evidence of increased cellular activity may also be a secondary effect of disease, resulting in an increase in the proportion of euchromatin, prominence of the Golgi apparatus or increased elaboration of the granular reticulum. Secondary changes such as these are more noticeable at the ultrastructural than the histological level and are encountered in various cell populations in many different pathological conditions. They should not be relied upon for diagnostic purposes.

The ultrastructural pathology of non-neoplastic gastrointestinal disease is far from being completely documented. In many diseases, the reported changes are limited to particular structures or cell types and may be derived from small series or individual case reports, an understandable problem in view of the ethical and practical limitations of tissue sampling and the rarity of various pathological conditions. This has resulted in a body of literature containing many fragmentary, incomplete or incidental observations, which may at times appear contradictory. In addition, ultrastructural studies often focus narrowly on specific cellular components or tissue compartments, to the detriment of the broader view of the disease in question. In this chapter the tabular presentation of reported findings highlights the gaps and limitations in our knowledge.

PATHOLOGICAL PROCESSES IN THE GASTROINTESTINAL TRACT

Familial disorders of enterocytes

Microvillous inclusion disease

In 1978, Davidson and associates[150] described an apparently familial enteropathy in infants, characterized by severe refractory diarrhoea in the neonatal period, which was shown by EM to be related to the presence of intracytoplasmic inclusions of brush-border microvilli within enterocytes, together with vesicular bodies.[145] The microvillous inclusions 'at times' took the form of complete brush borders surrounding a central lumen, with a microvillous membrane, surface glycocalyx, core microfilaments and a terminal web (Fig. 14.1; Table 14.4).[145,150] They were located either within the apical cytoplasm, or more deeply in the supranuclear territory. These abnormalities were first identified in jejunal biopsies, but similar microvillous inclusions may also be present in large-bowel enterocytes.[145]

Light microscopy of jejunal biopsies revealed villus atrophy with hypoplasia of crypts,[150] whereas the cell population within the lamina propria was normal or depleted.[145] Surface enterocytes 'lacked a well defined brush border', whereas fine apical vacuoles were evident, presumably corresponding to the inclusions observed by EM.[145]

The condition appears to represent an autosomal recessive disorder, and it carries a high mortality: eight of the nine patients reported by Cutz et al[145] died before the age of 18 months. The same authors[145] have proposed that microvillous inclusion disease may reflect an inborn abnormality of intracellular transport, causing aberrant assembly of enterocyte surface membrane components and defective brush-border formation. As they indicated, it is known that agents which disrupt microtubules, such as colchicine and cytochalasin, can produce abnormal assembly of microvillous borders.[109,145,511] Immunohistochemical studies in this condition have revealed normal immunostaining for low-molecular-weight cytokeratins, whereas staining for actin and villin appeared to be decreased, and myosin may also be depleted.[109] Accordingly, it has been suggested that the defect in this disorder may affect proteins that cross-link microtubules and membranes, such as kinesin.[145]

Infective and inflammatory conditions

General remarks

This is by far the largest category of gastrointestinal pathology. It includes gastrointestinal involvement in systemic disease, as well as specific primary gastrointestinal disorders. Many of these conditions are easily diagnosed by routine histological techniques, but electron microscopy may often be a useful confirmatory test and will occasionally prove essential for an accurate diagnosis. Since mucosal involvement is typical, an endoscopic biopsy is satisfactory for ultrastructural study. Many organisms, particularly viruses, can be recognized in this way (Ch. 9).

In some conditions where the identity of the histopathological picture is in doubt, electron microscopy may be essential to confirm the nature of the process. An example is the report by Shapen et al,[605] who demonstrated the presence of a Whipple's-like bacillus in a case presenting with sarcoid-like granulomata. On the other hand, cases caused by *Mycobacterium avium–intracellulare* can sometimes present with a Whipple's disease-like histopathological picture[645] and, again, electron microscopy can be a useful discriminator.[383] Rare, but potentially important examples of viral infection would include an unusual presentation of CMV infection, with or without a background history of HIV or graft-versus-host disease. On the other hand, for practical purposes, enteric viral infections are much more easily detected by routine virological screening of faecal suspensions using negative staining techniques, a procedure which has significant epidemiological applications.

Apart from the morphological recognition of an infective agent, whether as a primary or a secondary manifestation of

disease, electron microscopy has relatively little to contribute in strictly diagnostic terms. In most of the infective and inflammatory diseases of the gastrointestinal tract, the induced ultrastructural alterations, particularly in the epithelium, are best categorized as largely non-specific secondary changes which merely reflect the extent and severity of the underlying pathological process. The characteristic pathological picture in these conditions is often much better appreciated at the macroscopic and histological levels, as these offer a better representation of the structural interrelationships between the various cell and tissue components involved in the pathological process.

In this general area, electron microscopy has so far concentrated on the mucosal tissues, particularly the surface and crypt epithelium, the inflammatory infiltrate and the vascular endothelium. Increasingly, however, investigations are extending to include the structural appearances or alterations of neuro-endocrine cell populations in relation to conditions such as duodenal ulcer,[490] chronic atrophic gastritis,[79,80,553] and ulcerative colitis.[147] The morphology and distribution of various microbiological and parasitic agents[4,562,666] in various compartments of the gastrointestinal tract, as mentioned earlier, is another growing area of investigation.

The ultrastructural characteristics of various infective and inflammatory conditions are laid out in Table 14.1.

Helicobacter pylori and peptic ulceration

The microbial flora of the human gastric mucosa, for long considered of little pathogenetic significance, has aroused growing interest in recent years following isolation of a novel bacterial species from endoscopic biopsy specimens, originally named 'Campylobacter pyloridis' (later amended to *C. pylori*). This urease-producing spiral organism is now known to be of common occurrence in the human stomach worldwide. It is regularly associated with mucosal inflammatory changes and elicits a serological immune response. It has come to be accepted as a major cause of active chronic ('type B') gastritis, underlying many cases presenting as non-ulcer dyspepsia.[64,177,180,274,282,706] That it became known only recently can be attributed, partly at least, to fastidious cultural requirements and to the need for electron microscopy for precise morphological characterization of the organism and its relationship to the mucosal surface.[273,351,684] A combination of ultrastructural, biochemical and serological features showed it to be incompatible with the provisional classification, and it has now been assigned as type species of a new bacterial genus, Helicobacter.[276,278]

In thin sections, and by negative staining, *H. pylori* appears as a distinctive smooth-surfaced bacterium of Gram-negative type (Fig. 14.2; Table 14.1), about 0.5 μm wide and 3 to 4 μm long.[273,277,351] The cell shape is curved or gently spiral, the latter form rarely exceeding two to three wave-

Table 14.1 Ultrastructural features in inflammatory disorders of infective and non-infective origin

---

Disease or agent: Barrett's oesophagus in reflux disease.
Comments: The SEM shows a spectrum of characteristic appearances, of squamous or columnar mucosa and intestinal villi. Areas of micro-ulceration are sometimes present. TEM discriminates between different cell populations, such as squamous, columnar, parietal, Paneth, neuro-endocrine and intestinal goblet cells. The metaplastic columnar cells of Barrett's oesophagus may display ultrastructural features reminiscent of one or more of three main epithelial varieties, the gastric surface epithelium and mucous neck cells of normal gastric pits, the goblet cells of the small bowel and cells with features of both gastric mucus secreting cells and small bowel enterocytes.
References: 75, 418, 466 and 467.

Disease or agent: *Herpes simplex* virus infection.
Comments: Most parts of the gastrointestinal tract can be affected, but biopsies are commonly from mouth, oesophagus and large intestine, including anal mucosa. Characteristic 100 nm intranuclear herpesvirus particles are seen. Virus particles may also be present in the epithelial cell cytoplasm and intercellular spaces at the edges of ulcers.
References: 57, 82, 100, 272, 439 and 561.

Disease or agent: Cytomegalovirus infection.
Comments: Infection occurs mainly in mouth, salivary glands, oesophagus and large intestine. Characteristic nuclear and cytoplasmic viral inclusions are present in the capillary endothelial cells and also in pericytes, macrophages and fibroblasts in the granulation tissue at the ulcer base.
References: 12, 22, 51, 234, 241, 377, 461, 501, 644 and 703.

Disease or agent: HIV (Human immunodeficiency virus) infection.
Comments: All parts of the gastrointestinal tract can be affected, with alterations most noticeable in the mucosa of mouth, oesophagus, small and large intestines. Intra-epithelial lymphocytes appear activated with increased cell processes and organelles, including lysosomes. Tubuloreticular structures are described in endothelial cells, intra-epithelial lymphocytes, monocytes, lymphocytes and free in the capillary lumen. Degenerative changes and single cell necrosis may be present in the epithelium but these findings are not particularly prominent or diffuse. Other identifiable pathogens associated with AIDS include *Herpes simplex*, CMV, microsporidiosis and rectal spirochaetosis. Human T lymphotropic retrovirus-like particles are sometimes seen in homosexuals with or without AIDS. The similarities of the mucosal lesions in some AIDS cases to the changes seen in Whipple's disease have been highlighted in a few reports. EM can be useful in these cases.
References: 171, 193, 262, 363, 383, 385, 386, 416, 535, 618, 645, 714 and 721.

Disease or agent: Cryptosporidiosis.
Comments: The site of infection is mainly in the mucosa of the oesophagus, stomach, small and large bowel. On SEM, the ovoid 2–5 μm organisms are seen interspersed between the microvilli and attached to the epithelial surface. TEM identifies the various stages in the life cycle of the parasite, which is surrounded by crowded and fused microvilli. Mitochondrial swelling and clear cytoplasmic vacuoles occur in epithelial cells. Aggregation of lysosomes at apices of intestinal epithelial cells is sometimes seen. Occasional associated intranuclear and intracytoplasmic crystalline inclusions are identified, possibly viral in origin.
References: 60, 363, 412, 513, 535 and 689.

Disease or agent: *Campylobacter*-(*Helicobacter*)-associated inflammation.
Comments: The mucosa of stomach, jejunum or large bowel, including the anus, may be affected. In the epithelium there is loss of microvilli, depletion of intracellular mucin, and concavities on the epithelial surface where bacteria are adherent. Intracytoplasmic vacuoles, single cell necrosis and epithelial cell detachment from the basal lamina may be present. Regenerative undifferentiated cells may be observed in neck and low pit areas of gastric mucosa. Characteristic organism morphology is seen by SEM and TEM. S-shaped or elongated spiral forms lie in close contact with surface epithelial cells, either within or beneath the overlying mucus layer.
References: 4, 67, 68, 127, 274–278, 350, 351, 451–456, 512, 534, 557 and 684.

Disease or agent: Gastritis associated with other spiral organisms.
Comments: Helical (3.5–7.5 μm long and 0.9 μm in diameter) organisms with spiral form and truncated tips are present on the surface epithelium of the antral gastric mucosa. Gastrospirillum hominis has been proposed as a name for the organisms described by McNulty et al.[441]
References: 161, 441 and 557.

Disease or agent: Eosinophilic gastroenteritis.
Comments: There is a heavy eosinophil infiltration of the lamina propria, with associated mucosal ulceration. In areas of active inflammation, the eosinophils often have structurally altered granules, with loss of the electron density of the crystalline core. Dense reticular membranous structures may also be formed. Immunogold labelling has demonstrated the release of a major basic protein into the cell matrix, which may play some role in the observed damage.
Reference: 681.

Disease or agent: Acute diarrhoea due to *Vibrio cholerae*.
Comments: Changes in the small intestinal surface epithelium include widening of intercellular spaces, separation of junctional complexes, surface cytoplasmic projections and processes between microvilli and minor degenerative changes in organelles.
Reference: 28.

Disease or agent: Acute diarrhoea due to *Escherichia coli*.
Comments: The changes may be present in small and large intestine. Organisms adhere to the luminal border of the surface enterocytes and are partially surrounded by their plasma membranes. Microvilli may be distorted, with some loss of the glycocalyx. Other features sometimes observed are an increase in residual bodies in the apical cytoplasm, a widening of intercellular spaces and focal necrosis. Crypt epithelial cells tend to be less affected.
References: 104, 153, 214, 564, 565 and 666.

Disease or agent: Acute diarrhoea due to viruses: rotavirus, adenovirus, coronavirus, astrovirus, calicivirus etc.
Comments: Virus particles may be present in enterocytes or stool samples. Degenerative changes in enterocytes include widening of intercellular spaces, cell necrosis and desquamation.
References: 47, 61, 93, 94, 116, 128, 151–153, 179, 214, 231, 297, 315, 460, 507, 547, 610, 622 and 655.

Disease or agent: Giardiasis (*Giardia lamblia*).
Comments: The characteristic trophozoite morphology is identifiable by SEM and TEM in mucosa of small intestine, particularly the duodenum and jejunum. The trophozoites attach to the luminal border of epithelial cells by a concave striated adhesive disc. Cases with associated malabsorption sometimes show a mucoid pseudomembrane covering the epithelial cells.
References: 87, 303, 473, 478, 515, 523, 524, 526, 661 and 713.

Table 14.1 (continued)

Disease or agent: Tropical sprue.
Comments: Degenerative changes are seen in enterocytes of villi and crypts in the mucosa of the small intestine. Damaged enterocytes are subsequently replaced by less differentiated, or functionally immature cells.
References: 457 and 458.

Disease or infectious agent: Shigella dysentery (bacillary dysentery).
Comments: Effects are seen in the large intestinal mucosa. Non-membrane-bound bacterial bodies are present in surface enterocytes, in neutrophil polymorphs of the luminal exudate and in intercellular spaces. The extent of bacterial invasion does not necessarily correlate with the extent of cell damage. Surface and crypt cells have shortened or absent microvilli showing rarification or focal absence of glycocalyx. Nuclear and cytoplasmic degenerative changes are present, together with increased secondary lysosomes and fat droplets. In severe cases the cell membrane ruptures with resulting cell necrosis. The inflammatory infiltrate consists of activated lymphocytes, degranulated eosinophils, plasma cells and neutrophil polymorphs in various stages of disintegration. The macrophages display an increased number of lysosomes. In the lamina propria there is oedema, prominent dilated lymphatics, fibrin deposition and extravasated RBCs. The blood vessels have swollen endothelial cells, showing a paucity of pinocytotic vesicles. Sometimes the endothelial cells undergo necrosis and sloughing with aggregation of platelets and fibrin. Reduplication of capillary basal lamina may also be present.
References: 269, 367, 459 and 482.

Disease or agent: Intestinal spirochaetosis.
Comments: SEM and TEM show spiral organisms adherent to the luminal surface and neck of crypt epithelium and in the appendix and large bowel. The spirochaetes usually have one end embedded in an invagination of the cell membrane and the other end lying free at right angles to the surface epithelium. A cell-associated membrane density is often identifiable at the site of attachment of the spirochaetes. Spirochaetes may also be seen free within the cytoplasm, in lysosomes of macrophages and in Schwann cells.
References: 25, 140, 194, 255, 312, 313, 485 and 492.

Disease or agent: Histoplasma colitis (*Histoplasma capsulatum*).
Comments: The characteristic organisms are prsent in histiocytes in the lamina propria of both small and large bowel. They disappear following treatment, leaving some residual undigested fungal wall material within macrophages.
References: 182 and 370.

Disease or agent: Collagenous colitis.
Comments: A thick band of mature collagen fibres (20–30 nm diameter, axial periodicity of about 60 nm) is present beneath the surface epithelium, parallel to the basement membrane and concentrically encasing entrapped capillaries, which show reduplication of the basal lamina, hyperplasia of endothelial cells and loss of normal fenestration. The pericryptal sheath fibroblasts are increased in size although reduced in number. They appear separated from the crypt epithelium and may acquire myofibroblastic differentiation. Focal absence of the basal lamina beneath the surface epithelium has been described. Collagen deposition does not extend to surround crypts.
References: 41, 133, 217, 228, 248, 288, 289, 337, 668, 693, 725 and 741.

Disease or agent: Chemotherapy-induced colitis.
Comment: See Table 14.4

Disease or agent: Crohn's disease.
Comments: Affects any region, but EM studies have been carried out mainly in the small and large intestines. SEM observations in the small intestine include focal ulceration, formation of epithelial bridges between villi, change in villous size and shape, convolution and fusion of villi and goblet cell hypertrophy with increased secretion of mucus. There is irregular bulging of scattered enterocytes. On TEM the epithelial cells contain lysosomal inclusions of varying morphology. Epithelial tight junctions in cobblestone areas show severe disorganization. In areas of micro-ulceration there are less severe junctional alterations. It has been suggested that these alterations may contribute to the disturbed barrier function in Crohn's disease. Macrophages in the lamina propria and submucosa may contain large irregular secondary lysosomes with heterogenous inclusions, similar to those of the epithelial cells. These may represent digested organisms and luminal contents that have gained access to the tissues through a defective mucosal barrier. Autonomic nerves show widespread and extensive axonal degenerative changes, a feature claimed to be important in the differential diagnosis of Crohn's disease from other inflammatory disorders.
   Mucosal and submucosal lymphatics show thickening and reduplication of basal lamina with surrounding accumulation of collagen. Accumulation of protein-rich lymph at the abluminal surface of lymphatic capillaries may be seen. The lining endothelial cells can have increased cytoplasmic filaments. A combination of these changes may result in decreased permeability of the lymphatic wall and submucosal oedema.
References: 11, 15–17, 136, 184–192, 317, 387, 397, 421, 448, 449, 480, 499, 500, 503, 548, 639, 675 and 688.

Disease or agent: Malakoplakia.
Comments: Affected areas include the mucosa and submucosa in stomach, colon, and appendix. Characteristic cytoplasmic inclusions include dense laminated structures with a fingerprint appearance and Michaelis–Gutmann bodies of similar structure, but with deposition of electron-dense crystalline material.
References: 102, 165, 224, 420, 433, 435, 538, 555 and 641.

Disease or agent: Peptic ulcer.
Comments: EM has been applied to the study of gastric metaplasia in the duodenum in duodenal ulcers and of intestinal metaplasia in the stomach in gastric ulcers. Increased numbers of intra-epithelial lymphocytes are noted adjacent to the duodenal ulcers. Surface bacteria are noted in relation to the gastric type, but not the intestinal type of epithelium. Kidney- or S-shaped bacteria have been described by SEM on the surface of metaplastic gastric epithelium in the duodenal and prepyloric regions.
   Metaplastic gastric epithelial cells 3–8 mm from the edge of peptic ulcers range from fully differentiated, through various phases of metaplasia, to abnormal forms of the goblet cell pattern. Microvilli over gastric metaplastic cells often appear short and unevenly spaced, with discontinuity of the covering glycocalyx. Blebbing and branching of microvilli has been described. Increased and prominent basal granulated cells containing myelin figures are sometimes present in Brunner's glands. Fundic parietal cells in duodenal ulcer may be hypertrophied with dilated canaliculi.
References: 1–3, 157, 158, 286, 358, 490, 518, 636, 637, 740, 742 and 746.

Table 14.1 (continued)

Disease or agent: Healing duodenal ulcer.
Comments: The changes that occur during treatment and healing can be followed by SEM. Initial re-epithelialization of the ulcer base is associated with persistent microvillous changes. Stumpy villi may develop after a month, but persistently altered microvilli may still be seen. TEM of metaplastic epithelium reveals fundic parietal cells with a resting appearance and narrow canaliculi. This gradually transforms from gastric to duodenal pattern.
References: 1–3, 284, 285, 445, 476, 490, 491, 518, 560, 682, 683 and 746.

Disease or agent: Neonatal necrotizing enterocolitis.
Comments: The lesion involves the small intestine, colon and appendix, often to the full thickness of the bowel wall. In some cases, intracytoplasmic vesicles containing coronavirus-like particles have been described, along with microvillous alterations, in degenerating epithelial cells of the intestinal mucosa.
References: 566, 585 and 699.

Disease or agent: Solitary rectal ulcer.
Comments: Groups of fibroblasts entangled by prominent collagen fibres are present in the lamina propria.
Reference: 119.

Disease or agent: Chronic duodenitis.
Comments: There is evidence of enterocyte cell injury, with swollen endoplasmic reticulum, mitochondria and microvilli and focal severe loss of the ruthenium red stained filamentous component of the surface coat.
Reference: 146.

Disease or agent: Ulcerative colitis.
Comments: The epithelium in inflamed large bowel shows degenerative changes, including swollen mitochondria and endoplasmic reticulum, increased secondary lysosomes and dense bodies. Reticulum fibres show rarefaction or degeneration. Capillaries of the lamina propria are markedly dilated. With SEM there is irregular separation and decreased numbers of crypts, with variations in shape and size of cells. Microvilli are focally decreased in number. Studies of endocrine cells in biopsies of ulcerative colitis patients showed predominance of EC cells, PP, D1 and L cells in that order. Non-specific degenerative changes including degranulation of the dense core granules and vacuolization of the cytoplasm were observed in neuro-endocrine cells of some patients.
References: 147, 168, 176, 216, 269, 270, 332, 480 and 608.

Disease or agent: Whipple's disease.
Comments: The characteristic bacilli (2.5 × 0.25 μm) are seen in the lamina propria of the small and large bowel. They are present in macrophages and between and inside epithelial cells, lying free or within lysosomal inclusions. They may also be present in mast cell cytoplasm. The organisms are in various stages of degeneration and the epithelial cells show non-specific changes. Cell walls of degenerating bacteria form dense laminated inclusions. Other changes include occasional degranulating mast cells in close association with bacteria-containing macrophages. Lipid droplets may accumulate within the lamina propria.
References: 32, 123, 169, 170, 399, 444, 605, 632, 687 and 700.

Disease or agent: Gonococcal colitis.
Comments: EM is helpful in suspected cases showing negative light microscopic findings. Epithelial cells show severe and extensive degenerative changes. Ingested *Neisseria gonorrhoeae* organisms are identifiable within neutrophil leucocytes.
Reference: 504.

---

lengths. The ends are rounded, without polar pits. To one pole are attached four or five sheathed flagella, each with a prominent terminal bulb (Fig. 14.2, inset). Processing with tannic acid or ruthenium red (Fig. 14.3) reveals a polysaccharidic glycocalyx external to the cell wall unit membrane,[277,382] incorporating periodic peg-like projections and similar to the 'S-layers' of other unrelated bacteria.[277,278] Negative staining shows abundant annular surface subunits about 13 nm in diameter, which may be stacked in groups of four or five.[278,351]

In colonized endoscopic biopsy specimens[274,452,455,684] *H. pylori* organisms are scattered widely on the epithelial surface, mainly deep to the gastric mucus (Fig. 14.2). While usually most abundant on antral mucosa they may occur throughout the stomach and also in the duodenal cap, particularly in areas of gastric epithelial metaplasia. *H. pylori* exhibits a preferential affinity for the mucus-secretory cell type, coming into intimate contact with the epithelial microvilli and plasma membranes. The bacterial and epithelial glycocalyces appear to fuse, and distinctive pedestals (Fig. 14.4) are often discernible.[68,274,452,455,541] Microbial clustering is often prominent over the intercellular clefts and junctional complexes,[207] and in the gastric pits. Affected areas of mucosa exhibit characteristic ultrastructural changes in the epithelium, together with round cell and polymorph infiltrations of variable severity in the lamina propria.[510] The modified epithelium is intact but markedly uneven (Fig. 14.2), with depletion or complete loss of microvilli, irregular bulging of the apical plasma membranes, and disruption of the intracellular cytoskeletal web of microfilaments;[127,274,453,455,684] cellular mucin granules are depleted. Colonization is essentially extracellular. Apparently viable spiral organisms have been reported within canaliculi of glandular parietal cells,[127] but when observed in phagolysosomes of the epithelium or polymorphs they invariably show structural degradation. Therapeutic elimination of *H. pylori* from the stomach, employing antibacterial drugs, is followed by resolution of gastritis lesions, and reversion to normal epithelial ultrastructural patterns within a few weeks.[177,442,453,454]

The pathogenic mechanisms underlying *H. pylori* attachment and colonization are as yet poorly understood.

Haemagglutinating activity has been demonstrated in many clinical isolates,[207,209] and a fibrillar surface haemagglutinin has been proposed as a putative colonization factor antigen.[209]

Clinical studies and reviews from many centres have advanced the concept of *H. pylori*-related gastritis and duodenitis being important predisposing factors in the genesis and recurrence of peptic ulceration.[177,180,275,454,456,732] Should this prove to be so, then antibacterial measures aimed at lasting eradication of *H. pylori* from the stomach may assume an important place in the overall treatment of peptic ulcer disease.

Other gastric 'spirals'. Bacteria of spiral or bacillary form (Table 14.1), structurally resembling *H. pylori* and similarly associated with naturally occurring gastritis lesions, have now been recovered from the stomach of animals — including non-human primates, the ferret and pig.[92,236] The monkey isolates appear to be identical with human *H. pylori* isolates, whereas that from ferrets differs sufficiently to justify designation as a distinct but related species, *H. mustelae*.[276] It has regular rod-like rather than spiral form, and possesses sheathed flagella of both polar and lateral type. The *Helicobacter* organisms must be distinguished from a heterogeneous group of longer and more tightly coiled ('spirillum-like') bacteria which commonly inhabit the stomach and associated glands (Fig. 14.5) in dogs, cats and monkeys,[144,429,715] and which are now being recognized also as a sporadic finding among human patients undergoing gastric biopsy.[161,406,407] They are located generally within the gastric mucus rather than deep to it, do not adhere intimately to the epithelium, and are of doubtful pathogenic significance. A confusing situation arises in the presence of dual infestation by both *H. pylori* and the 'spirillum-like' forms, as described recently in a baboon.[144] Distinction between these two groups of micoorganisms should present little difficulty at the ultrastructural level.

Whipple's disease

This is a rare multisystem disease which typically extends throughout the small bowel — particularly affecting the jejunum[519] — and which is characterized by infiltrates of macrophages containing intensely PAS-positive cytoplasmic granules. By light microscopy, affected small intestinal villi are enlarged, distorted and club-shaped, due to an accumulation of the characteristic macrophages within the lamina propria.[519] In his original description of this disorder, Whipple[723] reported the presence of 'rod-shaped organisms' in Levaditi-stained specimens, and bacilliform bacteria are a consistent finding by EM (Figs 14.6 and 14.7).[160] As yet, these organisms have neither been classified nor isolated in culture; although a variety of bacteria have been recovered from affected tissue — including *Corynebacterium*, *Haemophilus*, *Klebsiella* and so forth — it seems that these represent contaminants.[519] However, cross-reactivity between anti-

bacterial sera and the granules within macrophages has recently been recorded, including antibodies to groups A, B and G streptococci and group B strains of *Shigella*.[56,181,210,519] EM has also shown that the PAS-positive diastase-resistant macrophage granules represent phagocytic vacuoles containing ingested bacilli in various stages of dissolution (Figs 14.8–14.12; Table 14.1), the PAS-positivity being attributable to residues of bacterial cell walls.[56,160]

Whipple's disease is perhaps the pre-eminent non-neoplastic disorder of the adult digestive system in which EM is of diagnostic importance, with three main applications in the assessment of this condition:

1. Confirmation of the clinicopathological diagnosis in typical cases, by demonstration of the characteristic bacilli (Figs 14.6 and 14.7)
2. Diagnosis of atypical cases, for example in extra-intestinal Whipple's disease,[7,444,447,632,730] which may seemingly be unassociated with gastrointestinal lesions on exceptional occasions[7,447] — or in cases where the histological appearances are atypical, including PAS-negative granulomatous inflammation[632,727]
3. Follow-up of known cases of Whipple's disease. Despite failure to isolate the infecting bacilli, antibiotic therapy — for example with tetracyclines — is known to be an effective treatment for Whipple's disease. Both extracellular and intracellular bacteria disappear rapidly from tissues with treatment, but the macrophages may persist for up to two years or longer, despite clinical resolution of the disorder.[160,444] Denholm and associates[160] studied a case of Whipple's disease with serial jejunal biopsies throughout a two-year period, and they divided the phagocytic vacuoles in macrophages into four stages, depending on the fine structure of their contents:

Stage I.   Vacuoles contained recognizable bacterial outlines (Figs 14.9 and 14.10)
Stage II.   Loose membranous aggregates in vacuoles (Figs 14.9 and 14.10)
Stage III. Fine, closely packed membranous aggregates in vacuoles (Figs 14.10 and 14.11)
Stage IV.   Homogeneous vacuole contents (Fig. 14.12).

In the biopsy taken at the time of diagnosis, Stage I–III vacuoles were found, but the early-stage vacuoles disappeared rapidly with treatment, and only Stage IV vacuoles were present six months after diagnosis.[160] The inference to be drawn from this study is that re-appearance of early-stage vacuoles or intact bacilli would constitute presumptive evidence of relapse.

Gastrointestinal mycobacteriosis in patients with the acquired immunodeficiency syndrome (AIDS) — especially *Mycobacterium avium-intracellulare* infection — can closely resemble Whipple's disease by light microscopy, including the presence of PAS-positive macrophages.[519] However, this infection is distinguishable from Whipple's disease by the clinical background, and the strongly acid-fast character of the mycobacteria in both Ziehl–Neelsen and Fite stains.[519] By EM, the mycobacteria have thicker walls than the bacilli of Whipple's disease, and they may 'crack out' of the section.

Intestinal spirochaetosis

This disease is characterized by spirochaetes arrayed perpendicularly along the surface of the colonic and rectal epithelium, where they are disposed between microvillous processes of the epithelial cells (Figs 14.13 and 14.14; Table 14.1). Penetration of the epithelium seems to be exceptional, and neither mucosal abnormalities nor clinical symptoms are attributable to their presence in most cases.[140,408] Nevertheless, Gebbers et al[253] have described the organisms within epithelial cells and subepithelial macrophages, and their patients had mild diarrhoea that was responsive to antibiotic therapy; the latter study also identified partly degranulated mast cells within the epithelium, and IgE-producing plasma cells in the lamina propria. Rodgers and associates[554] also found intracellular organisms, and diarrhoea in their patient was attributed to blunting and destruction of enterocyte microvilli.

The exact identity of the spirochaetes has not been established: some[159,312,554] have suggested that they may represent a *Brachyspira* or *Borrelia* species, whereas others consider them to be a *Treponema* species,[140] and Cooper et al[137] cultured a large anaerobic treponeme from their cases. Intestinal spirochaetosis has been recorded in about 5–16.5% of rectal biopsies[159,312] and in about 12% of otherwise normal-appearing vermiform appendices removed from patients with suspected appendicitis ('pseudo-appendicitis').[312] A higher incidence (36%) has been found in practising male homosexuals.[408,440] The diagnosis can be established on light microscopy examination of rectal biopsies using, for example, the Warthin–Starry stain for spirochaetes. Spiral organisms have also been recorded in the jejunum.[558]

Collagenous colitis

This uncommon form of colitis of obscure aetiology and pathogenesis, is characterized on light microscopy by a table of hyaline collagen about 7–100 μm in thickness (Widgren and associates[725] recorded a mean measurement of 19.5 ± 5.1 μm), situated immediately beneath the surface epithelium.[724,725] Types I and III collagen have been demonstrated in the hyaline zone by immunohistochemistry.[228]

Bamford et al[41] found that the epithelial basal lamina was thickened approximately two-fold and convoluted, but other ultrastructural studies have shown that the lamina is essentially normal in appearance,[39,228,725] while focal deficiencies have also been observed (Fig. 14.15; Table 14.1).[337] The collagen accumulates deep to the lamina, with encasement

of capillaries (Fig. 14.15).[39,41,668,724] Proliferation of pericryptal myofibroblasts with enhanced collagen fibre formation has also been described, as have mast cells (Figs 14.16 and 14.17).[39,228,337,725] However, Widgren et al[725] found that the mast cell counts did not differ significantly from their controls.

The reasons underlying the accumulation of the subepithelial collagen are obscure,[725] and it is notable that a similar collagen table does not occur in other chronic colitides such as ulcerative colitis and Crohn's colitis.[724] However, similar sublaminal collagen deposition occurs beneath bronchial mucosa in so-called chronic bronchitis and 'micropapillomatosis', and in asthma (where mast cells may also be seen).[436,479]

Crohn's disease

Dvorak and associates (for references, see Dvorak & Monahan-Earley[189]) have described a variety of ultrastructural abnormalities in Crohn's disease, (Table 14.1) especially widespread axonal necrosis affecting the myenteric plexuses and present at the ileal resection margins of every case studied, irrespective of disease activity at the site. In contrast, axonal necrosis was minimal or absent from ileal stomal biopsies in all other diseases investigated (previously resected ulcerative colitis; resected ulcerative colitis plus intercurrent viral gastroenteritis; ileocolectomy for multiple polyposis; small bowel biopsies from patients with a variety of inflammatory intestinal disorders; colonic stomas from patients with colectomies for colon cancer). From these studies they concluded that Crohn's disease may be an 'enteric autonomic neuropathy'. Although others[639] have supported this notion, we remain unconvinced. The inflammatory process in Crohn's enteritis is predominant and highly characteristic, and similar inflammatory changes do not occur in most gastrointestinal neuromuscular diseases such as Hirschsprung's disease, the familial visceral neuropathies, and the cathartic colon.[695] Moreover, the lymphoplasmacytic infiltrates seen in some neuromuscular disorders — notably inflammatory axonopathy and paraneoplastic visceral neuropathy[695] — differ both in composition and distribution from that of Crohn's disease. It is also worth emphasizing that apparent hypertrophy of enteric neural tissue occurs in a variety of chronic inflammatory bowel diseases, and that ultrastructural evidence of axonal injury — with ballooning of axons and an accumulation of dense bodies — has been recorded in melanosis coli.[39] Therefore, at our present state of knowledge, we consider that the neural abnormalities recorded in Crohn's disease are more likely to represent a secondary alteration. In future studies, it may be more meaningful to compare the neural tissue in Crohn's disease with other inflammatory disorders, in which the distribution of the inflammation is arguably more comparable than in the situations listed above — for example, chronic ischaemic enteritis. In the final analysis, the diagnosis of Crohn's disease is established by light microscopy and the clinicopathological background, and at present we consider that EM has little to offer in this exercise. A possible relationship to infection by mollicute-like organisms[348] awaits further investigation.

Mechanical and neuromuscular disorders

Strangulation, volvulus and intussusception are the three most common mechanical disorders and are essentially gross surgical and pathological diagnoses. In the case of the neuromuscular disorders, however, special investigations, including immunocytochemistry and electron microscopy, do have a contribution to make, since the gross and histological features of different entities may overlap.[533]

Electron microscopy may be a useful aid in differentiating between primary neural and muscular diseases, although with a few exceptions, individual conditions within these categories are not readily distinguished. Considerable over-lapping of histological features sometimes occurs in cases of neuromuscular disorder and intestinal pseudo-obstruction. Occasionally, however, characteristic ultrastructural features can be of diagnostic value. Venizelos et al,[701] reported two cases of chronic intestinal pseudo-obstruction with similar histological appearances, one due to systemic sclerosis and the other to visceral myopathy. The diagnosis of visceral myopathy was made by the demonstration of characteristic degenerative changes in smooth muscle cells. Disorders of the muscle also include hypertrophy, atrophy, non-specific degenerative changes and ultimately fibrous replacement.

Neural changes, affecting the nerve fibres and ganglionated plexuses, are often non-specific.

The main ultrastructural alterations in some of these diseases are summarized in Tables 14.2 and 14.3.

Malabsorption and malnutrition

General remarks

The end result of many disorders of the digestive system may be a malabsorption syndrome. This section, however, deals mainly with the primary malabsorptive diseases, in which the aetiological factors and the pathogenetic mechanisms often remain uncertain. This fact has prompted a variety of ultrastructural studies, which have undoubtedly contributed to our understanding. At the same time, it must be acknowledged that the additional resolution provided by electron microscopy may serve to magnify doubts as well as certainties. The close interrelationships between lympho-cytes and enterocytes in coeliac disease have been claimed as evidence of a cytotoxic process in action, but there remains a gulf between hypothesis and proof which cannot easily be bridged by morphological evidence alone, no matter what the level of magnification.

Certain fine-structural appearances are shared in conditions of malnutrition and malabsorption, regardless of the aetiological agent or pathognomonic features of the individual disease. These changes are present mainly in the villous epithelial cells and their underlying lamina propria and

Table 14.2 Diseases and agents causing mechanical and neuromuscular disorder mainly due to smooth muscle involvement

Disease or agent: Visceral myopathies, familial and sporadic.
Comments: Smooth muscle cells in any or all parts of the gastrointestinal tract may be affected. The changes affect the longitudinal muscle layer more than the circular layer. They may also be seen in the muscularis mucosae. Smooth muscle cells have increased electron-lucency due to cytoplasmic rarefaction related to the disorientation, disintegration and disarray of myofilaments. Degenerative changes include mitochondrial swelling, large perinuclear vacuoles, break-up of cell membranes resulting in cell disintegration and lysis, and excess collagen deposition. No neural changes are present and there is no significant increase in inflammatory cells.
References: 14, 227, 589–591, 593 and 701.

Disease or agent: Hypertensive oesophageal sphincter.
Comments: There are increased cytoplasmic organelles in interstitial cells of Cajal and in some smooth muscle cells. Nerve endings have a normal ultrastructure though they may be reduced in number.
Reference: 218.

Disease or agent: Amyloidosis (including familial variant with polyneuropathy).
Comments: It is mainly the small intestine and colon that are functionally affected, but deposits can be seen in all parts of the gastrointestinal tract. Rectal biopsy is used for diagnostic purposes. Deposits of amyloid are seen in the muscularis mucosae, submucosal blood vessels and layers of muscularis propria. A patchy decrease or absence of glycocalyx, with adherent bacteria, is described in familial amyloidosis with polyneuropathy. Submucosal and myenteric plexuses may also show deposits but usually to a lesser extent.
References: 131, 242, 252, 261, 265, 344, 371, 413, 521, 609, 635, 648 and 707.

Disease or agent: Progressive systemic sclerosis.
Comments: The entire gastrointestinal tract may be affected, but the functional effects are mainly due to involvement of the smooth muscle cells and capillaries of the oesophagus and intestine. There is replacement of smooth muscle cells by proliferating collagen and fibroblasts. In contrast with visceral myopathy, the changes are more prominent in circular than longitudinal muscles and there is no perinuclear vacuolation or cytoplasmic degeneration. Instead these cells may show thickening of dense bodies along myofilaments and of dense plaques along cell membranes. Characteristic capillary changes include lamination and thickening of basement membrane, endothelial swelling with cytoplasmic degeneration and adherent platelet aggregates. Nerve endings are not affected. The small intestinal mucosa may show dilated intercellular spaces and a paucity of nexus junctions between epithelial cells. Degenerative changes including fat droplets and cholesterol clefts are seen in epithelial cells and in the lamina propria. Collagenous encapsulation of Brunner's glands has also been described.
References: 148, 283, 311, 563, 570 and 701.

Table 14.3   Diseases and agents causing mechanical and neuromuscular disorder mainly due to neural involvement

Disease or agent: Achalasia.
Comments: Non-specific degenerative changes are seen mainly in neural elements, including nerve fibres of the vagal trunk, and in the myenteric plexus. Small nerve fibres are reduced in number and show fewer than normal neurosecretory granules. There is a reported decrease in interstitial cells of Cajal. Increased cytoplasmic organelles and myofilaments in smooth muscle cells have been described.
References: 7, 156, 218, 243 and 570.

Disease or agent: Diffuse oesophageal spasm.
Comments: Wallerian degeneration occurs in afferent vagal nerve fibres. There is also some reduction in small nerve fibres, which have a reduced content of neurosecretory granules. Smooth muscle cells may show increased cytoplasmic organelles in the perinuclear area.
References: 7, 101, 243 and 570.

Disease or agent: Chagas' disease.
Comments: Causes mega-oesophagus. Degenerative changes are seen in Auerbach's plexus, nerve fibres and the dorsal motor nucleus of the vagus. These are similar to achalasia and include degenerative changes in neurons and nerve fibres of Auerbach's and myenteric plexuses, axonal degenerative changes, infiltration of plexuses by lymphocytes and plasma cells and increased cytoplasmic organelles in smooth muscle cells, due to hypertrophy. The changes are present mainly in the lower two-thirds of the oesophagus and in the colon. Pseudocysts containing characteristic leishmanial forms of the parasite are seen in the muscle layer and degenerative changes are noted in the myenteric plexuses.
References: 31, 55, 195, 218, 235, 432, 650 and 676.

Disease or agent: Neuronal intranuclear disease (variant of familial visceral neuropathy).
Comments: The myenteric plexuses in the oesophagus, stomach and intestine contain neuronal intranuclear filamentous (straight or curved) inclusions. Some inclusions show a beaded periodicity at 15–20 nm. They are non-DNA non-RNA protein in nature. The inclusions can also be seen in submucosal neurones and this disease can therefore be diagnosed in rectal biopsies.
References: 227, 295, 506, 509, 589, 592–595 and 627.

Disease or agent: Sporadic visceral neuropathy.
Comments: The myenteric plexus in any part of the gastrointestinal tract may be affected, with variable degrees of neuronal degeneration. Early changes include electron-lucency of neurons due to fragmentation, loss of neurotubules and oedema, with aggregates of ribosomes and swollen mitochondria. Severe changes include cell membrane rupture and fragmentation and neuronal cytoplasmic vacuolation. Axons are swollen with or without fragmentation of the axolemma. There is a loss of neurotubules and a paucity or absence of organelles.
References: 589, 594 and 595.

Disease or agent: Inflammatory axonopathy.
Comments: Degenerative changes are seen in axons in myenteric plexuses of the gastrointestinal tract. Lymphocytes and plasma cells infiltrate the plexuses.
Reference: 388.

Disease or agent: Cytomegalovirus infection of myenteric plexus.
Comments: Neuronal intranuclear inclusions, degenerative changes in axons, inflammatory cells and Schwann cell hyperplasia are seen in the myenteric plexus.
References: 531 and 631.

Disease or agent: Cathartic colon.
Comments: The submucosal plexus of the large bowel shows axonal swelling and paucity of neurofilaments, neurotubules and nerve specific organelles. There may be a decrease in neurosecretory granules in nerve endings. For other changes of melanosis coli see Table 14.7.
Reference: 549.

include the occurrence of complex or branching forms of the surface microvilli, the accumulation of lipid droplets, autophagolysosomes and dense bodies in the cytoplasm, and the deposition of granular dense material or collagen bundles around the capillaries and the basement membrane. Most of these alterations are, however, reversible following treatment.

In some instances, electron microscopy is essential in the absence of a positive diagnosis by other methods, such as in congenital microvillous inclusion disease and Whipple's disease. Electron microscopy can contribute to a lesser extent in brown bowel syndrome, collagenous sprue, intestinal lymphangiectasia and paraprotein depositions, which may mimic amyloidosis. The ultrastructural features of some of these disorders are summarized in Table 14.4.

Coeliac disease

Despite numerous investigations over many years, the aetiopathogenesis of coeliac disease remains an enigma shrouded in mystery — although immune mechanisms have been implicated,[519,611,614] and its clinical responsiveness to a gluten-free diet is sufficiently consistent that it constitutes a therapeutic test of the diagnosis (gluten-sensitive enteropathy).[519] The flat small bowel mucosa which typifies the disorder (with a 'cerebral' appearance on dissecting microscopy)[169] is sometimes referred to as subtotal villus atrophy, yet evidence indicates that the flattening is the result of augmented crypt cell turnover, with elongation of crypts. The crypt cell population in the lower third of the crypts is similar to that found in normal small intestine, whereas the upper third corresponds to the normal villus base, and the middle third has intermediate or transitional features.[679]

Numerous intra-epithelial lymphocytes are usual in coeliac disease, on both light and electron microscopy. The surface microvilli of the enterocytes are flattened and often sparse (Figs 14.18 and 14.19; Table 14.4),[519] resulting in

Table 14.4 Ultrastructural features in disorders involving protein intolerance, malabsorption and malnutrition

Disorder or agent: Congenital microvillous atrophy or intractable diarrhoea syndrome (congenital microvillous inclusion disease).
Comments: The changes are present mainly in small intestinal enterocytes and to a lesser extent in the colon. Decreased cell height with increased cytolysosomes, secondary lysosomes and polyribosomes are seen, together with the formation of apical vesicular bodies. Paucity and shortening of microvilli are prominent. A characteristic feature is the occurrence of supranuclear inclusions composed of neatly organized, well formed microvilli, bounded by their terminal webs, but with no surrounding membrane. SEM reveals flattened mucosa interspersed by shallow mucosal ridges. It also shows the rounded apical surface of enterocytes and the formation of frequent cytoplasmic blebs. The paucity, shortening or absence of microvilli is easily spotted by SEM.
References: 145, 150, 281 and 516.

Disorder or agent: Coeliac disease (Gluten sensitive enteropathy).
Comments: The ultrastructural changes widely described involve the villous and crypt epithelium. Crypt cell hyperplasia is associated with a variable degree of morphological differentiation. Villous epithelial cells have irregular apical surfaces, short uneven microvilli and microvilli fused at their bases, with formation of small microvillous 'bunches'. Cytoplasmic vacuolation, swollen disrupted mitochondria and increased lysosomes are observed. There may be focal disruption of basal lamina, with increased collagen deposition. Re-duplication of the lamina densa may be present. Intra-epithelial lymphocytes are numerous and prominent plasma cells with dilated cisternae are present in the lamina propria, along with other inflammatory cells. Paneth cell deficiency has been observed in some cases.
    SEM shows various appearances reflecting the severity of the disease and the progress of recovery on withdrawal of gluten from the diet. These range from complete absence of villi and flattening of the mucosa in severe or untreated disease, to the formation of recognizable villi and ultimately the restoration of an essentially normal pattern in full remission on gluten-free diet. Distortion of enterocytes and marked irregularity of microvilli, with decrease, focal absence or rarefaction of glycocalyx and bifurcation of microvilli, may also be observed.
References: 19, 106, 130, 135, 143, 293, 294, 296, 301, 380, 428, 430, 443, 450, 508, 523, 524, 556, 568, 611, 612 and 640.

Disorder or agent: Soy protein intolerance.
Comments: SEM appearances are similar to those seen in coeliac disease.
References: 523 and 524.

Disorder or agent: Collagenous sprue.
Comments: Collagen bands and deposits are present beneath the epithelial basement membrane.
References: 717.

Disorder or agent: Intestinal lymphangiectasia.
Comments: Enterocytes contain lipoprotein droplets. Lymphatic endothelial cells of small intestinal mucosa contain increased filaments and are surrounded by a more prominent and thickened basal lamina than normal lacteals.
References: 29, 166, 169 and 387.

Disease or agent: Antibiotic- and chemotherapy-related malabsorption or colitis.
Comments: Disturbances in protein synthesis and direct toxic effects on cell membranes are thought to be responsible for prominent changes in the microvilli. Topographical alterations are visible by SEM in cases of antibiotic induced colitis. In cases of malabsorption there are increased numbers of macrophages in the small intestinal lamina propria. These macrophages contain large irregular dense inclusions the origin of which is not known, but fragments of degenerating crypt cells or neomycin particles are sometimes present.
References: 167, 520 and 619.

Disease or agent: Kwashiorkor.
Comments: There is a prominent accumulation of fat droplets in the cytoplasm of the enterocytes. No accumulation of fat droplets is, however, seen in the Golgi apparatus. There is evidence of non-specific cell damage. The findings are reversible on treatment and may be due to deficient lipoprotein synthesis.
References: 484, 670 and 678.

Disease or agent: Infantile marasmus.
Comments: Deposition of amorphous dense material and collagen beneath the epithelium and capillaries in the lamina propria of the small intestinal villi has been described in a number of cases. There may also be increased numbers of autophagolysosomes and dense bodies, together with branching microvilli in epithelial cells. These alterations regress following therapy.
References: 96, 484 and 678.

diminished absorptive surface area;[169] they may also be fused or broad, and the underlying terminal web is poorly developed.[179] These abnormalities of microvilli are also detectable by scanning EM.[301] Wheat-gluten challenge of patients maintained on a gluten-free diet has been shown to induce deterioration of microvillus architecture as soon as 2.5 hours after the challenge.[37] Lysosome-like granules and hypertrophic rough endoplasmic reticulum inhabit the apical cytoplasm (Figs 14.18 and 14.19),[39] where lipid droplets may also be found, suggesting 'exit-blockade' of lipids.[169]

The abnormalities afflicting the microvilli are thought to correlate with the clinical features of malabsorption and steatorrhoea. Even so, we emphasize that although these changes are characteristic, they are not specific for coeliac

disease:[679] they may also be encountered in other small intestinal disorders, and similar alterations of microvilli have been depicted in Whipple's disease, for example (see above).[169]

Abetalipoproteinaemia

Apart from the deficiency of β-lipoproteins in the blood, which gives this disorder its name, the other clinical manifestations include erythrocyte acanthosis, steatorrhoea, retinitis pigmentosa and neurological symptoms.[679] Although the surface brush border of small bowel enterocytes appears normal by EM,[679] lipid droplets accumulate in the apical cytoplasm, together with lysosomes,[169] whereas chylomicrons are absent from the intercellular spaces.[679] These appearances have been interpreted as indicative of defective lipid transport mechanisms, with impaired release of chylomicrons from enterocytes.[679]

Systemic disease

The gastrointestinal tract is involved in wide variety of systemic disorders, including infections, granulomatous and non-granulomatous inflammation, metabolic and storage diseases, immunologically-based and vascular disorders. Some of these have already been mentioned, whilst others are described more fully elsewhere (Ch 6, 8, 9 and 10). In some cases, the relative simplicity of an oral mucosal or endoscopic biopsy makes this a favoured initial screening test, being less invasive and potentially less hazardous than, for example, a brain biopsy.

Table 14.5 lists some of the systemic, predominantly non-gastrointestinal diseases, in which significant diagnostic or prognostic ultrastructural features can be detected in gastrointestinal biopsies.

Two specific areas can now be dealt with separately, the vascular and haemopoietic disorders and the diseases associated with immunological phenomena. The small blood vessels of the gastrointestinal tract are commonly involved in systemic vascular disorders, such as occur in hypertension, diabetes, collagen–vascular diseases, Henoch–Schonlein purpura and other vasculitic conditions, DIC, irradiation and certain drug effects and other vascular anomalies.[103,368,369,410,698] The ultrastructural alterations in some of these diseases are discussed in detail in other chapters. Certain other vascular disorders exert their effects particularly in the gastrointestinal tract, as in portal hypertension, gastric antral vascular ectasia, angiodysplasia and lymphangiectasia. Haematopoietic disturbances, however, are rarely addressed through a gastrointestinal biopsy.

Table 14.6 lists some of the diseases in these general categories in which gastrointestinal manifestations have

Table 14.5 Ultrastructural features of the gastrointestinal tract in systemic disorders

Disease or agent: Metabolic and storage diseases including; neuronal ceroid lipofuscinosis, gangliosidosis, Niemann–Pick disease, juvenile and infantile Batten's disease, mucopolysaccharidosis, fucosidosis, mannosidosis and aspartylglycosaminuria.
Comments: Rectal biopsies are ideal for diagnostic purposes and in screening non-symptomatic patients at risk. Characteristic inclusions of the individual diseases are predominantly present in macrophages in the lamina propria, but may also be seen in Schwann cells, capillary endothelial cells and smooth muscle cells (see Ch. 6).
References: 26, 62, 90, 105, 163, 205, 306, 338, 339, 540, 596, 695, 737 and 738.

Disease or agent: Tangier's disease (alpha-lipoproteinaemia).
Comments: Fat droplets are present in smooth muscle cells and Schwann cells in the lamina propria. These lipid vacuoles are more pronounced than in multiple lipid islands disease, and are intensely doubly refractile.
References: 543–545.

Disease or agent: Amyloidosis.
Comments and references: See Table 14.2.

Disease: Renal failure and dialysis patients.
Comments: Subcellular alterations in the duodenal mucosa may be a contributing factor in the development of impaired calcium absorption in renal failure patients. These changes include reduction in villous and crypt length and the presence of shortened and irregularly distributed microvilli. These changes are severe in renal dialysis patients and are reversible after treatment.
References: 267 and 338.

Disease or agent: Progressive systemic sclerosis.
Comments: See also Table 14.2. The observed changes in the jejunal mucosa may indicate an induced dysfunction of the jejunal absorptive epithelial cells. These cells show cytoplasmic condensation and contain fat droplets and cholesterol crystals. There is dilatation of the intercellular spaces, which contain deposits of fat droplets. Fat droplets are also present in the lamina propria, where there is a wide dilatation of the vascular spaces and a perivascular inflammatory infiltrate. In the muscularis propria there is smooth muscle atrophy with collagen deposition. These changes underlie the impaired peristalsis which enhances bacterial overgrowth and malabsorption.
Reference: 311.

Disease or agent: Systemic lupus erythematosus.
Comments: There may be a diffuse venulitis involving the vessels of the submucosa and the muscularis externa of the jejunum. The walls of veins and venules are disrupted by infiltrating inflammatory cells, including polymorphs and macrophages, which are seen between the endothelium and the basal lamina. The basement membrane of the villous epithelium is reported to be thickened by up to a factor of ten, due to C3 and fibrinogen deposition, with an associated significant increase in collagen.
References: 320 and 719.

Disease or agent: Cystic fibrosis.
Comments: SEM shows an unusual covering of the surface of the jejunal mucosa with sheets of mucus which obscure the underlying villi. These mucus sheets perhaps function as diffusion barriers to nutrients and result in malabsorption.
References: 523 and 524.

Disease or agent: Mast cell disease.
Comments: Changes in mast cells, which are present in the epithelial layer and lamina propria in the mucosa of the small intestine, include nuclear irregularity and binucleation with loss of the normal heterochromatin pattern and degranulation of the cytoplasm, which contains only a few residual granulated bodies and occasional whorled inclusions.
References: 88 and 598.

been recorded. In most of these instances, electron microscopy is not generally seen as having a significant diagnostic role, there being only a very few examples of rare haematopoietic and vascular diseases in which this can be claimed.

There is a growing interest in the possible pathogenetic significance of immunological phenomena in a wide range of gastrointestinal disease. The recognition of such factors in disorders traditionally classified according to presumed aetiology or predominant clinical features, highlights deficiencies in our present understanding of these diseases. It is, therefore, worthwhile for the ultrastructural pathologist to take account not only of alterations in obvious target cells, such as the enterocytes themselves, but also of the structural features and relationships of associated cells, such as the intra-epithelial lymphocytes, which may reflect unusual immunological reactivity. As mentioned above, morphological criteria are limited in this respect, but may at least serve

to focus attention on specific phenomena worthy of more detailed functional study. The growing sophistication of immunological labelling makes it increasingly possible to combine morphological and functional criteria at the ultrastructural level.

Graft-versus-host disease occurring in patients who have received allogenic bone marrow transplants is a major area of current interest. The organ systems mainly affected are the skin, the liver and the gastrointestinal tract. Studies of oral, gastric and intestinal mucosal biopsies from clinical cases and from experimental animals[208,245,250,400,477] have shown single cell coagulative necrosis, or apoptosis, amongst mucosal cells, particularly in the neck and basal regions of the gastric glands and intestinal crypts, the lumina of which were widened and contained necrotic debris. The severity and extent of these changes appeared to correlate with the severity of the disease.

A conspicuous reported feature is the presence of multiple

Table 14.6 Disorders related to the vascular system

Disease or agent: Gastric antral vascular ectasia.
Comments: Electron microscopy is helpful in demonstrating a proliferation of neuro-endocrine cells in the lamina propria and between epithelial cells in the antral gastric mucosa. The neurotransmitters produced by these cells are thought to be the underlying cause for the focal vascular dilatation and subsequent gastric bleeding that often occurs in these patients.
Reference: 434.

Disease or agent: Pseudoxanthoma elasticum.
Comments: The changes are seen in the small and medium sized arteries of the stomach and small intestine. There is fragmentation or absence of the internal elastic lamina with focal calcification in the subintimal tissue. This may also show alterations of collagen fibres including loss of normal periodicity, divergence of individual fibres and reduction of their usual electron-density.
Reference: 396.

Disease or agent: Lymphangiectasia.
Comments: There is a prominent basal lamina beneath endothelial cells of small bowel lacteals. An increased and prominent filamentous component may also be present in these endothelial cells. A prominent basal lamina also underlies absorptive epithelial cells. Lipid droplets are present between intestinal enterocytes near their bases and in the lamina propria.
References: 166, 169 and 387.

Disease or agent: Systemic lupus erythematosus.
Comments: See Table 14.5.

Disease or agent: Hypertensive varices.
Comments: Venules in the oesophagus and stomach show phlebosclerosis, characterized by a proliferation of medial smooth muscle cells and elastic fibres, together with fibrosis. The newly synthesized elastic fibres contain amyloid P component distributed with lysozyme. Intra-epithelial blood filled spaces have been associated with bleeding from these abnormal vessels.
References: 154 and 464.

Disease or agent: Gastric and colonic angiodysplasia.
Comments: The features are an abnormal proliferation, in mucosa and submucosa of stomach and colon, of small blood vessels lacking in elastic fibres.
References: 335, 395, 437, 539 and 542.

Disease or agent: Small-vessel disease.
Comments: The small blood vessels of the bowel wall are affected in several systemic disorders. Proliferative intimal hyperplasia is present in diabetes and essential hypertension. Obliterative microangiopathy is seen in several forms of collagen disease, in vasculitic disorders, in disseminated intravascular coagulation, in amyloidosis and as a result of irradiation and vaso-active drugs such as ergotamine.
References: 395, 437, 539 and 542.

Disease or agent: Malignant atrophic papulosis of Deyos.
Comments: There is fibrinoid necrosis in the walls of small vessels of the large bowel. Endothelial cells may show swelling and prominent cytoplasmic vacuolation.
Reference: 463.

Disease or agent: Diabetic micro-angiopathy as a risk factor in anastomotic leakage after gastrectomy.
Comments: The relationship between the severity of diabetic micro-angiopathy and the incidence of anastomotic leakage has been investigated by Kihara et al.[369] They found that the degree of severity of micro-angiopathy as evidenced by the increased thickness of the basement membrane of the gastric mucosal capillaries significantly correlated diabetic micro-angiopathy in the skin as well as the increased risk of anastomotic leakage after gastrectomy.
Reference: 369.

---

intimate point contacts between the epithelial cells and the intra-epithelial lymphocytic infiltrate, which is increased, particularly in the basal and lateral aspects of the crypts between the basal lamina and the basal face of the epithelium. Other features of lymphocyte–epithelial relationships include broad front contacts, interdigitation of membrane surfaces and occasional penetrating pseudopodia.[208,250,400] Non-specific changes including focal absence and reduplication of the basal lamina, the dropping of enterocytes into the lamina propria and alterations of crypt cells are also observed.[208,250]

These changes are not to be confused with other early post-transplantation mucosal alterations, which are due mainly to chemotherapy and radiotherapy and are most severe in the first three weeks. Intra-epithelial lymphocytes are usually sparse, randomly distributed, and show no point or close contacts or pseudopod formation in association with adjacent damaged epithelial cells, as is the case in graft-versus-host disease.

It has been proposed that point contacts between lymphocytes and epithelial cells in graft-versus-host disease are morphological evidence of a cytotoxic interaction. Similar changes have been reported in the skin. Fukii et al[245] using immuno-electron microscopic techniques, have shown evidence of damage in oral keratinocytes contacted by suppressor/cytotoxic T cells, whereas those contacted by helper T cells appeared normal. The lymphocytic infiltrate in these cases was found to consist mainly of the suppressor/cytotoxic subset. Close associations between lymphoid and epithelial cells have long been recognized in other bowel disorders, including coeliac disease, ulcerative colitis and shigellosis, perhaps suggesting the existence of some similar process.

Another immunologically-based disorder, selective IgA deficiency, has been studied by electron microscopy.[263] Focal flattening of the mucosa with surrounding villous ridges, increased mucus production, the presence of bacteria and surface debris and the loss of the glycocalyx in the mid-villus regions constituted the main topographical features. Enterocyte changes were largely non-specific, including shortening and branching of microvilli, increased apical lysosomes and alterations of mitochondria and endoplasmic reticulum. All of these changes, however, may be interpreted as secondary phenomena. The changes seen in HIV infection have been described earlier (see Table 14.1).

Abnormal pigmentation

This phenomenon may occur in association with a wide variety of conditions, including obstruction and ulceration of the gastrointestinal tract due to various causes, including carcinoma of the stomach, duodenal and jejunal diverticulosis and Crohn's disease. It has also been documented in chronic pancreatitis and fibrocystic disease, cholestasis and congenital biliary atresia and in various types of cirrhosis and hepato-biliary neoplasia.[78,355] The pigmentation in these disorders is, however, non-specific and the underlying conditions are usually obvious. The best known examples of abnormal pigmentation are smoker's melanosis of the oral mucosa, pseudomelanosis duodeni, melanosis coli and the 'brown bowel' syndrome. Electron microscopy, combined with energy-dispersive X-ray microanalysis, has assisted in the study of these conditions. Some of the findings are summarized in Table 14.7.

The 'brown bowel' syndrome has been encountered in several intestinal diseases characterized by malabsorption, particularly idiopathic steatorrhoea. It has been described in association with vitamin E deficiency, malnutrition, non-tropical sprue, Whipple's disease, lymphangiectasia, idiopathic hypoproteinaemia and abetalipoproteinaemia. It has been suggested that the underlying cause of the observed pigmentation in these conditions is the result of a deficiency of the fat-soluble vitamin E, with subsequent loss of its protective role against free radical-induced damage, together with other agents such as peroxidase, catalase and superoxide dismutase.[78,355] The ultrastructural observation of similar dense lipofuscin inclusions in the various diseases associated with brown bowel syndrome further supports a common, possibly mitochondrial origin (see Table 14.7), for this pigment, in keeping with this theory.

In contrast to the exceedingly common melanosis coli (Table 14.7), related to prolonged ingestion of anthraquinone laxatives,[38] pseudomelanosis duodeni is an extremely rare disorder, and most reports address single cases (see Pounder and associates[530] for review of the literature to 1982).[113,422,530] On gross or dissecting microscope examination, the affected mucosa displays punctate, linear or comma-shaped black foci. Conventional light microscopy reveals pigment-laden macrophages within the lamina propria. The mucosal epithelium appears normal by EM, with the possible exception of increased numbers of lysosomes in the apical cytoplasm (Fig. 14.20).[530] The pigment-containing mononuclear phagocytes contain pleomorphic lysosomes (Fig. 14.21), which vary from round, to elongated, to angular in shape. Angular and pleomorphic electron-dense particles are evident within the lysosomes (Fig. 14.21), and lipid droplets may also be present.[113,530] Although the nature of the particles cannot be ascertained by conventional transmission EM, electron-probe X-ray microanalysis has demonstrated the presence of iron and sulphur.[530] Pounder and associates[530] and Lee et al[409] have concluded that the pigment represents iron sulphide (FeS), and it has been suggested that the iron accumulates as a result of haemorrhage into the lamina propria.[530] The former workers[530] also identified small amounts of Ca, K, Al, Mg, Si and Ag, and they suggested that the Al, Mg and Si are derived from antacid medications.

Miscellaneous disorders

In the miscellaneous group (Table 14.8) are included various conditions which, in spite of ultrastructural and

Table 14.7 Abnormal pigmentation in the digestive system

Disease or agent: Smoker's melanosis.
Comments: Melanin-loaded keratinocytes are present in the gingival epithelium. The mucosa contains melanocytes with stage III and IV melanosomes in comparison with pigmented tissue of non-smokers where the melanocytes usually contain mainly stage II melanosomes.
Reference: 308.

Disease or agent: Gingival pigmentation beneath a metallic crown.
Comments: TEM and EDXA have confirmed that this pigmentation is due mainly to the deposition of melanin pigments in the epithelial and connective tissue cells and in the ground substance of the lamina propria of the gingiva. Only traces of metallic elements are found. It has been suggested that elements accidentally implanted during the therapeutic procedure may be responsible for the induced increased deposition of melanin pigments in these tissues. The differential diagnosis of conditions associated with increased melanin deposition in the oral mucosa includes melanoma, Albright's syndrome, Peutz–Jeghers' syndrome, Addison's disease and von Recklinghausen's disease.
Reference: 575.

Disease or agent: Brown bowel syndrome.
Comments: The smooth muscle cells in muscularis propria of oesophagus, stomach, small and large bowel are affected in cases of malabsorption. There is deposition of lipofuscin as osmiophilic granular inclusions or aggregates in the perinuclear area, or inside lacunae surrounded by filaments in muscle cells of the muscularis propria. The spectrum of morphology includes electron-dense myelinated figures, round to irregular homogeneous bodies of variable electron-density, and some forms showing possible mitochondrial derivation, perhaps due to free radical induced damage. Similar pigments have been described in the smooth muscle cells of the muscularis mucosae, and of the arterioles and venules of the gastrointestinal tract.
References: 233, 249, 319, 330, 331, 355, 398, 578 and 634.

Disease or agent: Pseudomelanosis duodeni.
Comments: Heterogeneous secondary lysosomes in macrophages of the duodenal lamina propria contain granular electron-dense material, which may also lie free in the cytoplasm. This pigmentation is thought to be due to ingestion of certain medications, such as some anti-hypertensive drugs. These have a benzene ring within their structure, which can produce a melanin-like compound under a tyrosinase-like action.[226,606] Alternatively, the pigment may be derived from iron compounds absorbed from the lumen.[360] Other associated diseases and agents include peptic ulceration, gastric haemorrhage, renal failure and antacid compounds.
References: 89, 113, 142, 226, 228, 291, 360, 530, 606 and 739.

Disease or agent: Melanosis coli.
Comments: Heterogeneous secondary lysosomes containing lipofuscin aggregates are presumed to be derived from organelles damaged by the anthracene group of purgatives. These inclusions are present in macrophages in the lamina propria of the large bowel.
References: 259, 260, 364 and 586.

---

other investigations, remain of uncertain origin or cannot easily be accommodated elsewhere. Radiation and drug-induced effects are also included under this heading, since the main bulk of information on these topics is derived from animal studies and is therefore not of direct diagnostic relevance.

Cell type and altered morphology

The main aim of electron microscopy in neoplasia is to identify and type tumour cells by means of ultrastructural markers of differentiation, in accordance with their presumed histogenetic origins. In non-neoplastic disorders, however, this is seldom required, since the cellular identity and anatomical relationships between different tissue compartments are generally well preserved. The ultrastructural identification of various cell types may, however, prove of value in the investigation of the neuroendocrine cell populations in conditions such as chronic atrophic gastritis, pernicious anaemia, gastric and duodenal ulcers and ulcerative colitis. Immuno-electron microscopy provides a powerful tool for the precise identification of endocrine cells, subclassified according to both morphological and functional criteria.[629,630] The study, for example, of gastric biopsies from patients with chronic atrophic gastritis and hypergastrinaemia has shown that enterochromaffin-like

cells are the most frequent cell type, followed by type D1 cells.[77,79,80] Another example of the value of electron microscopy is the identification of the mast cell, which can be reliably recognized by its ultrastructural features, regardless of fixative. The various stages of degranulation of mast cells, including the formation of dense lamellar residues, empty vesicles or crescent shaped forms, can be studied in conditions such as false and anaphylactic food allergy.[471] Table 14.9 enumerates some specific cell types and the relevant pathological conditions in which they are particularly prominent or deficient, or show significant structural alterations.

In general, however, the major role of electron microscopy in non-neoplastic diseases of the gut lies not in identifying specific patterns of differentiation, but in recognizing fine structural alterations which may be useful in diagnosis, prognostic evaluation and understanding of the mechanisms of disease. It is the study of cell alterations, therefore, rather than of cell types, which is the aim in most non-neoplastic disorders. The mucosal epithelial cells have undoubtedly dominated most of these studies to date, since they are the prime target in most of the inflammatory disorders and in many other diseases, whereas studies of mechanical and neuromuscular disorders have naturally concentrated on the muscle layers and the nerve plexuses.

Table 14.8   Miscellaneous disorders

Disease or agent: Multiple lipid islands disease.
Comments: The condition may affect the lamina propria of any part of the gastrointestinal tract including the oesophagus, stomach, duodenum, colon and rectum, but is most commonly seen in the rectum and colon as lipid proctitis or colitis. This condition is characterized by lipid vacuoles of various sizes and shapes present in histiocytes, fibroblasts, pericytes, smooth muscle cells and Schwann cells in the lamina propria.
References: 69, 544–546 and 643.

Disease or agent: Intestinal metaplasia.
Comments: Intestinal metaplasia occurs mainly in the stomach and oesophagus in association with some inflammatory conditions and regurgitation. The resulting topographical alterations can easily be traced and assessed by SEM examination. Whether in the stomach or in the oesophagus, there is a loss of ordinary topographic features in foci of metaplasia. At high power, intestinal features are revealed, such as the characteristic microvillous border with goblet cell mouths. Ciliated epithelial cells can also be demonstrated by SEM and TEM. The axonemal pattern of these cilia is often abnormal. SEM and TEM of foci of metaplasia may show a grading of the metaplastic process, with mixtures of mature, immature and occasional intermediate or combined forms of metaplasia.
References: 266, 394, 643, 664 and 731.

Disease or agent: Pneumatosis coli (pneumomatosis cystoides intestinalis).
Comments: There are different views in the literature regarding the nature of the lining of these cystic structures. Some emphasize the presence of a partial lymphatic endothelial cell lining, with no underlying basal lamina, in support of the notion that these cystic spaces originate in lymphatics. Other studies show the cysts lined by macrophages and giant cells, with no evidence of an endothelial lining. Fat globules lie free in the lamina propria and in the cells of the lining layer and in nearby histiocytes and giant cells.
References: 292, 517 and 626.

Disease or agent: Bezoars.
Comments: Examination in the SEM and elemental analysis by EDXA contribute to knowledge of their structural organization and elemental composition, from which the mechanism of formation may sometimes be inferred.
Reference: 419.

Disease or agent: Alcohol ingestion and cirrhosis.
Comments: The small intestinal enterocytes show surface blebbing, swelling and irregularity of the microvilli, cytoplasmic vacuolation and lipid droplet accumulation. Mitochondrial changes include swelling and formation of laminated structures. There is prominence of the smooth endoplasmic reticulum.
References: 164, 258, 528 and 567.

Disease or agent: Blind loops and jejunoileal bypass.
Comments: TEM studies show decreased numbers of epithelial cells involved in lipid absorption and decreased lipid droplets in their cytoplasm. The cells may also show some non-specific degenerative changes. Topographical variations, particularly in villous height have been reported by SEM in the small intestinal villi of the mucosa of the functioning and excluded segments of jejunoileal bypass.
References: 18 and 173.

Disease or agent: Effects of irradiation.
Comments: The described early effects of irradiation in man include widening of intercellular spaces and loosening of cell-to-cell contacts in the mucosal epithelial cells 1 to 3 days following radiotherapy. Cytoplasmic processes are seen to extend through gaps in the basal lamina and come in direct contact with the mesenchymal cells of the lamina propria. In general, very little work has been carried out regarding the detailed effects of irradiation in humans. Most ultrastructural studies have been carried out in experimental material.
References: 53, 54, 215, 498, 712 and 718.

Disease or agent: Acrodermatitis enteropathica.
Comments: A rate hereditary disease, of autosomal recessive inheritance, characterized by low plasma zinc, epidermal lesions and gastrointestinal symptoms including diarrhoea and failure to thrive. The Paneth cells of the small intestinal crypts contain pleomorphic secretory granules and fibrillar inclusion bodies. Although these Paneth cell abnormalities have been described as pathognomonic of this condition, similar appearances have been seen in other circumstances.
References: 72, 379, 431, 522, 647 and 710.

Table 14.9   Cell types with documented involvement in certain disorders

---

Cell type: Macrophages.
Diseases: Some inflammatory and infectious diseases, including Crohn's disease, Whipple's disease, malakoplakia, histoplasma colitis and some viral infections such as CMV; metabolic and storage diseases; pseudomelanosis duodeni; melanosis coli; multiple lipid islands disease; pneumatosis cystoides intestinalis.

Cell type: Mast cells.
Diseases: Mast cell disease of the small bowel; coeliac disease; cow's milk protein intolerance; Crohn's disease; false food allergy; anaphylactic food allergy.

Cell type: Intra-epithelial lymphocytes.
Diseases: Coeliac disease; graft-versus-host disease; HIV infection; duodenal ulcers.

Cell type: Neuro-endocrine cells.
Diseases: Chronic atrophic gastritis; pernicious anaemia; ulcerative colitis; duodenal and gastric ulcers.

Cell type: Paneth cells.
Diseases: Acrodermatitis enteropathica; coeliac disease.

Cell type: Eosinophils.
Diseases: Eosinophilic gastroenteritis.

ORAL AND DENTAL DISEASE

The oral cavity

In addition to diseases specific to the mouth, the oral mucosa shares several disorders with other body systems, in particular the gastrointestinal tract and the skin. Since it is easily accessible and safe to sample, it is an ideal site for diagnostic biopsies and a satisfactory source of tissue for ultrastructural diagnostic investigations. Some of these multi-system conditions have already been listed in Table 14.1, with particular reference to diseases of the gastrointestinal tract.

The ultrastructural features of many specific oral soft tissue lesions have been described in detail in the literature. The routine diagnosis of these conditions can generally be achieved without resorting to ultrastructural morphology. On the other hand, such studies have at times explained certain features of these diseases and have contributed to our knowledge of the aetiology of some and the pathogenesis of others.

Recurrent ulceration of the oral mucosa occurs in association with several pathological conditions (see Table 14.9). In patients with Behcet's syndrome and recurrent aphthous ulceration, the underlying mechanisms have been investigated by Honma[323] and by Honma et al.[327,328] Dark apoptotic prickle cells were described in the 'normal' oral epithelium of these patients. It has been noticed that in the pre-ulcerative stage of these conditions, there is an increased mononuclear inflammatory infiltrate as well as polymorphs in the oral epithelium[323,577] and that there is active engulfment of the apoptotic cells by these mononuclear cells.[328] Perhaps these events may mark the onset of ulceration through a sequence of events that includes the interaction of the intra-epithelial lymphocytes with the phagocytozing mononuclear inflammatory cells, the production of immunoglobulin, the formation of immune complexes and the subsequent activation of complement.[327,328]

Qualitative and quantitative variations have been described in the human gingival Langerhans' cells under normal and pathological conditions.[36,162,487,488,574] These include a relative increase or decrease in the two types of Langerhans' cells with variations in their cytoplasmic organelles and dendrites, as described, for example, in chronic periodontal inflammatory conditions and in relation to bacterial plaques. These observations reflect the immunological functions of Langerhans' cells. It has been reported that increases in the number of Langerhans' cells may be stimulated by the penetration of the oral and gingival epithelium by bacteria.[574] Such phenomena have been examined in detail in several periodontal and gingival diseases by both scanning and transmission electron microscopy.[107,271,488,571-574,726] The ultrastructural features of some of the pathological conditions of the oral cavity have been briefly reviewed in Table 14.10.

The dorsum of the tongue

The characteristic topographical morphology of the dorsum of the human tongue and the recognized changes which sometimes affect its structure have been studied particularly by scanning electron microscopy (SEM). In the SEM, the dorsal surface of the normal tongue has characteristic topographical features highlighted by hair-bearing filiform papillae and the round fungiform papillae. Several conditions can alter this normal morphology and produce specific topographical patterns.[359,390-393] Some of the patterns described are summarized in Table 14.11.

The dental hard tissues

There is an extensive literature, including numerous review articles,[83,107,108,222,571] on the use of various ultrastructural techniques in the study of pathological conditions of the dental hard tissues. Some of the main topics are summarized in Table 14.12. The reader is referred to the specialist literature for further information.

THE SALIVARY GLANDS

Common salivary gland disorders include various forms of obstructive or non-obstructive sialadenitis, calculi, infections and auto-immune disorders which may also involve the lacrimal glands. Salivary gland biopsy in these disorders is not a routine procedure and a diagnosis is often made by other investigations, most of the reported findings coming from case reports or experimental animal studies. The following is a brief review of observations reported in human material.

Sialadenitis

Ultrastructural studies in obstructive sialadenitis have noted an increased incidence of goblet cells and ciliated cells in the excretory ducts of the submandibular gland. In the ciliated cells there is an increased incidence of ciliary anomalies, particularly the formation of compound cilia.[155,552,704] The so-called epimyoepithelial islands described in conditions of auto-immune sialadenitis, such as Mikulicz's disease and Sjögren's syndrome have been investigated by both immuno histochemical and ultrastructural techniques, with results that favour an epithelial identity and cast doubt on the presence of a participating myoepithelial component.[76,121,175,372,576]

Cystic lesions

Lymphoepithelial cysts arising from the sublingual and minor salivary glands in the floor of the mouth and tongue display the characteristic ultrastructure of keratinized squamous epithelium in their lining and of orthokeratotic and parakeratotic cells in their lumina.[98,120]

Table 14.10 Ultrastructural features of lesions of the oral mucosa and soft tissues

Disease or agent: Gingivitis.
Comments: Features of a non-specific inflammatory reaction are present in the mucosal epithelium; they include widening of intercellular spaces between epithelial cells by oedema fluid, reduction in desmosomes and intercellular contact zones, and swelling or disintegration of cytoplasmic organelles. The underlying basal lamina may show focal or diffuse absence or focal re-duplication. An increased Langerhans' cell population correlated with the severity of the gingivitis in some reports.
References: 36 and 222.

Disease or agent: Periodontitis and juvenile periodontitis.
Comments: The fine structural alterations in the lower part of the gingival pocket are similar to those seen in gingivitis. Changes in the upper part include the presence of increased numbers of keratohyaline granules and prominence of the plasma membrane, with evidence of increased or incipient keratinization. Abnormalities in the plasma membranes of the blood polymorphonuclear leukocytes are described in freeze–fracture preparations from patients with a genetically determined variant of juvenile periodontitis.[579] Several SEM and TEM studies have investigated the roles of various inflammatory cells and their interaction with contaminant organisms and plaques.
References: 13, 198, 222, 300, 423, 502, 579, 599, 604, 607, 657 and 702.

Disease or agent: Chronic desquamative gingivitis.
Comments: The ultrastructural features are similar to those in the skin in cases of bullous pemphigoid and erythema multiforme. There is evidence of reduced keratinization in the epithelial cells, which are separated by intercellular oedema with disintegration of their lower cell layers. The basal lamina may show either focal absence or focal re-duplication and is intimately adherent either to the epithelial cells or the stromal elements, which contain electron-dense filamentous material.
References: 97, 222, 232, 483, 493 and 628.

Disease or agent: Necrotizing ulcerative gingivitis.
Comments: The frequent observation of spirochaetes on the surface of, and penetrating into the epithelial cells supports their possible aetiological role.
References: 141, 222 and 424.

Disease or agent: Herpetic gingivo-stomatitis.
Comments: Identification of characteristic *Herpesvirus hominis* particles in the oral lesions and in cultures is diagnostic. See also Table 14.3 for herpes infection elsewhere in the GIT.
References: 222 and 621.

Disease or agent: Oral candidiasis.
Comments: Fungi are present on the epithelial surface or penetrating and completely inside the epithelial cells, which show evidence of non-specific degenerative changes. Lack of tonofilaments in adjacent epithelial cells is attributed to keratolytic properties of *Candida albicans*.
References: 117, 222, 470, 472 and 726.

Disease or agent: Lichen planus.
Comments: Essentially similar to cutaneous lichen planus. Numerous nuclear bodies are often present in epithelial cells and there is focal absence, thickening or re-duplication of basal lamina. Degenerating epithelial cells with large numbers of tonofilaments are seen near or in the basal layer. Precipitation of dense granular material also occurs overlying or external to basement membrane.
References: 118, 199–202, 222, 305, 373 and 532.

Disease or agent: Lupus erythematosus, discoid and systemic.
Comments: There is fragmentation and lysis, or re-duplication and thickening of the basement membrane, with fine fibrillar and granular deposits. Paramyxovirus-like inclusion bodies are sometimes described in endothelial cells, lymphocytes, histiocytes and fibroblasts. See also Table 14.5.
Reference: 222.

Disease or agent: Leukoedema.
Comments: Abnormal keratohyaline granules occur within the cytoplasm of superficial epithelial cells, associated with numerous ribosomes and possibly representing aborted keratinization in damaged cells. Deeper cells have marked cytoplasmic vacuolation and abnormal mitochondria.
References: 696 and 697.

Disease or agent: Oral aphthous (Mikulicz) ulceration.
Comments: Extravasation of erythrocytes is present at the base and the margin of the ulcer. The inflammatory infiltrate at the base of the ulcer consists predominantly of polymorphs, together with some lymphocytes and macrophages containing lysosomal debris of polymorph origin. The infiltrate at the margin of the ulcer is located mainly beneath an intact basement membrane, as distinct from Behcet's syndrome. Immune complex vasculitis is suggested as a pathogenetic mechanism.
References: 323, 414, 415, 587 and 588.

Disease or agent: Oral aphthous (Behcet's) ulceration.
Comments: The extravasation of erythrocytes and the inflammation at the base of the ulcer are features similar to Mikulicz aphthous ulceration. There is, however, marked oedema in the epithelial and subepithelial connective tissue at the ulcer margin, which contains only sparse inflammatory cells. Intra-epithelial lymphocytes and focal defects in the epithelial basement membrane are other features. Immune complex vasculitis may be involved.
References: 323–327, 414, 577, 587 and 588.

Disease or agent: Oral aphthous (herpetic) ulceration.
Comments: The extravasation of erythrocytes and the inflammatory infiltrate in and around the ulcer is similar to that described in Mikulicz and Behcet's syndromes. Characteristic intranuclear inclusion bodies are usually present in epithelial cells.
References: 581, 587 and 588.

Disease or agent: Congenital epulis.
Comments: The cytoplasm of the granular cells of congenital epulis is packed with large numbers of membrane bound inclusions. These include laminated, particulate and vesicular structures, as seen in granular cell tumours elsewhere. The nuclei are irregularly indented. Intracytoplasmic collagen bundles have been described.[358]
References: 358 and 404.

Table 14.10 (continued)

Disease or agent: Atypical histiocytic granuloma.
Comments: The predominant cell type in this lesion shows ultrastructural features in keeping with a histiocytic origin. Eosinophils and lymphocytes may also be present. The differential diagnosis includes traumatic granuloma of tongue, which shows the same cell population but differs in the histological appearance, and malignant lymphoid neoplasms, in particular non-Hodgkin's lymphoma.
Reference: 211.

Disease or agent: Oral vegetable granuloma (pulse granuloma of the alveolar ridge, giant cell hyaline angiopathy).
Comments: Histologically, this oral lesion consists of collections of eosinophilic hyaline rings in association with foreign body giant cells, other inflammatory cells and granulation tissue. The ultrastructural appearance of the hyaline rings is similar to that of vegetable cells walls, with a surrounding superficial layer of collagen. These appearances suggest that vegetable remains induce an inflammatory foreign body type reaction, providing the pathogenetic mechanism for such lesions. SEM and TEM coupled with histochemical techniques and polarization microscopy are useful in the identification of vegetable foreign body reactions in the oral cavity.
References: 126, 183, 203, 302, 384 and 468.

Disease or agent: Ectopic calcifications in human gingiva and in regional odontodysplasia.
Comments: TEM and EDXA demonstrate calcospherites formed of needle-like units of apatite present within a non-collagenous matrix of tightly packed branching 12-nm diameter microfibrils. It has been suggested that this non-collagenous material may be implicated in the pathogenesis of ectopic calcification.
References: 34 and 582.

Disease or agent: Oral leukoplakia and oral submucous fibrosis.
Comments: Both conditions present with white patches in the oral mucosa, and both show essentially similar ultrastructural appearances. The basal epithelial cell layer sends multiple cytoplasmic projections containing tonofibrils into the subepithelial stroma. Basement membrane alterations include a multilamellar basal lamina and deposition of electron-dense atypical basement membrane material in variable degrees beneath the basal layer. Intercellular oedema and the deposition of fine granular electron dense material between epithelial cells are sometimes prominent. Intracytoplasmic desmosomes are also described. Crystalline or needle-like structures may be seen in intercellular spaces, particularly between upper epithelial layers. Aggregation of amorphous material may occur between bundles of fragmented collagen fibrils in the subepithelial stroma.
References: 43, 59, 132, 222, 543 and 623.

Disease or agent: Tylosis-related leukoplakia.
Comments: Intranuclear 90-nm diameter viral-like electron-dense particles are seen in all layers of the epithelium except the basal. Cells in upper layers show perinuclear degenerative changes. Keratohyaline granules have various shapes and sizes, as well as an abnormal or perforated texture.
References: 222 and 686.

Disease or agent: Possible viral-induced leukoplakia.
Comments: Some epithelial cells appear ballooned and contain aggregates of chromatin with diffusely distributed microtubules in their centres. These microtubules and chromatin aggregates are surrounded by prominent bundles of tonofibrils. Phagocytic bodies and intracellular desmosomes are present. Giant cells are also seen.
References: 221 and 222.

Disease or agent: Focal epithelial hyperplasia.
Comments: Intranuclear papova-like viral particles are present in epithelial cells. There is clumping and margination of the chromatin, with nuclear envelope defects, vacuolization of the cytoplasm and condensation of the tonofilaments in these cells. Other changes include intracellular desmosomes, prominent smooth endoplasmic reticulum and concentric forms of rough endoplasmic reticulum.
References: 99 and 222.

Disease or agent: Oral giant cell granuloma.
Comments: Giant cells show evidence of prominent cytoplasmic and nuclear activity, with increased mitochondria and endoplasmic reticulum, enlarged Golgi apparatus, numerous ribosomes and multiple nuclei. Defects observed in the vascular lining in this condition may be responsible for the noticeable extravasation of RBCs.
References: 8, 20, 21 and 222.

Disease or agent: Oral leprosy.
Comments: Intra-epithelial lymphocytes are present. Occasional epithelial cells have many intracytoplasmic keratohyaline granules and tonofilaments. Whole and degenerating bacteria are seen within subepithelial epithelioid cells, often associated with numerous secondary lysosomes. RER in epithelioid cells is prominent and dilated.
Reference: 543.

Table 14.11 SEM of the dorsal surface of the tongue in some tongue forms*

Tongue form	SEM appearances
Normal tongue	Characteristic distribution and shape of the filiform papillae with or without hairs, and interspersed round fungiform papillae
Filiform atrophy of tongue	Flattened or smooth surface, with low or absent papilliform elevations; short hair-like structures
Fissured tongue	Shallow grooves with flattened or smooth mucosa showing low elevations; loss of hairs from the papillae, which are enlarged and vary in size; knob-like structures seen between surface epithelial microplicae; wedge-shaped cracks between epithelial cells
Geographic tongue	Paucity and shortness or absence of hair in the filiform papilla

*References: 27, 81, 359 and 390–393.

Table 14.12 Some EM applications in dental disease

Disease or agent: Dental plaques and deposits, including the distribution of spirochaetes and other bacteria and microorganisms, have been investigated through ultrastructural techniques (TEM and SEM) in patients with various forms of periodontitis and denture stomatitis. Other workers have studied denture-related plaque formation.
References: 9, 13, 91, 108, 114, 115, 178, 196, 222, 237, 239, 271, 322, 489, 537, 571, 669 and 722.

Disease or agent: Enamel and dental caries.
References: 33, 178, 222, 247, 345, 347, 349, 475, 649 and 656.

Disease or agent: Dental fluorosis.
References: 222 and 620.

Disease or agent: Enamel hypoplasia and amelogenesis imperfecta.
References: 65, 264, 321, 365, 366, 424, 583 and 690–692.

Disease or agent: Periodontal diseases and the study of the cementum structure and distribution of the cementum associated with lipopolysaccharides as revealed by SEM immunohistochemistry.
References: 24, 45, 178, 223, 333, 423, 600–602 and 705.

Disease or agent: Problems related to instrumental therapy. Examples include the study of corrosion of silver cones and their contribution to black deposits observed in the cells of the peri-apical granuloma, and the identification of melanin pigment deposition in the gingival epithelial and connective tissues in cases of crown-related gingival pigmentation.
References: 30, 84, 87, 204, 238, 426, 575, 624, 638 and 743–745.

Disease or agent: Periodontal diseases characterized by inflammatory and reactive changes or involving defectively functioning inflammatory cells.
References: 13, 107, 122, 129, 178, 256, 271, 300, 334, 571–574, 674 and 694.

Disease or agent: Calcifying, keratinizing and non-keratinizing, odontogenic cysts.
References: 125, 197, 219, 222, 244, 246, 298 and 299.

In the benign lymphoepithelial cyst of the parotid gland, the cystic spaces[716] are lined by three distinct types of epithelial cells, polygonal squamoid cells containing tonofibrils and having luminal glycocalyx-covered microvilli, columnar cells containing mucous granules, and cells containing zymogen granules suggestive of acinar origin. Tight junctions and desmosomes are present between these cells.

Polycystic disease of the parotid gland[172] is a rare lesion in which the cystic structures are seen to contain eosinophilic bodies (spheroliths) with ultrastructural features consistent with amyloid. The cuboidal epithelial cells lining parts of some of these cysts show sparse microvilli and few cytoplasmic organelles, features reminiscent of the intercalated duct epithelium. The flattened cells which line other parts do not show specific features of differentiation, such as the presence of secretory granules. Hexagonal and rhombohedral crystalloids described in salivary duct cysts have been found by SEM and EDXA to contain high concentrations of sulphur.[654]

Calculi

The origin and pathogenesis of salivary calculi is still incompletely understood. In recent years there has been an increased interest in the application of scanning electron microscopy and EDXA techniques to calculi of both minor and major salivary glands in an attempt to elucidate the structure and interrelationships of their components.[22,23,206,318,340,356,469,660,692,734–736] These findings have contributed to a better understanding of the development of salivary concretions and of the possible mechanisms involved in their formation.

THE PANCREAS

Elective tissue biopsy in non-neoplastic pancreatic disease is rare, since pancreatic biopsy is not without risk, and an adequate assessment can usually be made without reference to a tissue diagnosis. Tissue for histopathological investigation may be obtained in conditions requiring surgical intervention, but here the pathological process is usually so well established that there is no diagnostic role for electron microscopy.

In the interpretation of more subtle ultrastructural alterations in the human pancreas, we are restricted by our limited knowledge of its normal ultrastructural morphology. In contrast with most other body organs, normal control pancreatic tissues are difficult to obtain free from artefact, and post mortem material is of limited use because of the rapid onset of autolytic changes. Much recorded information on the normal ultrastructural morphology of the pancreas is derived from animal studies and from nearby 'normal' pancreatic tissue in resected human pancreatic neoplasms. This problem is reflected in the literature, where certain structural features are recorded as normal by some authors and abnormal by others.[42,280]

The endocrine pancreas

In the case of the endocrine pancreas, combined ultrastructural and immunohistochemical techniques may be used to investigate non-neoplastic disorders characterized by an increase or decrease in a particular endocrine cell type and in the structural assessment of the affected cells. In nesidioblastosis or nesidiodysplasia, characterized by an increase in the beta cell mass, the distribution of beta cells can be ascertained by electron microscopic examination.[42,44,48,279,280,343,374,646] Beta cells have a characteristic ultrastructural morphology, due to the easily identifiable paracrystalline configuration of their granule cores. Endocrine cells with an admixture of conventional dense core and paracrystalline granules have also been described in this condition, suggesting the production of more than one type of hormone. Such cells, however, can also be found in the pancreas of the normal neonate. The presence, in this condition, of amphicrine cells, with both endocrine and exocrine features, can best be appreciated by ultrastructural examination.[44,48,279,280,343,374,646]

Diabetes

Diabetes mellitus does not require a tissue biopsy for diagnosis, but there are various reports available on the ultrastructure of the pancreas in this condition.[138,139,257,375] There is a paucity or complete absence of the B cells in the pancreatic islets, which instead may be populated by numerous A cells with occasional D cells. Type A cells are also described individually and in groups amongst the exocrine pancreatic tissue. Other reported features include the loss of insulin granules in surviving B cells, which may also contain prominent glycogen deposits. This latter change is reversible after treatment. Lymphocytes and eosinophils may be present. Deposits of amyloid have also been described between capillary basement membranes and islet cells.[134] A striking feature is the presence of intermediate or amphicrine cells in the exocrine pancreas, carrying the cytoplasmic components of both exocrine cells, such as zymogen granules and well developed RER and Golgi apparatus, and endocrine cells, such as the characteristic neurosecretory granules. These cells have also been described, though less frequently, in normal pancreas and other pancreatic conditions, most noticeably in the pancreas of infants with hyperinsulinaemic hypoglycaemia, as described earlier[48,279,343] and possibly in adults with pancreatitis.

The presence of such intermediate, amphiphilic, or exo-acinar mixed forms of pancreatic cells may be explained as an expression of disturbed differentiation of pluripotential pancreatic stem cells[48] which may be either inborn or acquired. Cell fusion has also been suggested as a mode of formation of intermediate forms.[316,378] The possibility that these mixed forms are the precursors of either the exocrine or the endocrine cells must also be considered.[343,462] Alternatively they may represent stages of transformation from the exocrine to the endocrine pattern.[279,343] Such uncertainty further highlights our relative unfamiliarity with the ultrastructure of normal control material.

The major role of electron microscopy in non-neoplastic pancreatic disease remains, however, in the investigation of pathogenetic mechanisms and the delineation of still unexplained subcellular phenomena. In diabetes mellitus, for example, characteristic tubular inclusions of uncertain significance have been demonstrated in the perinuclear cisterna of the duct cells of the human pancreas,[287] but such observations have no immediate diagnostic relevance. Similar inclusions have also been recently reported in cases of human acute pancreatitis.[728]

Biopsies from patients with dysfunctional pancreatic grafts and recurrence of diabetes have revealed several interesting ultrastructural phenomena. When residual beta cells were still present in the grafts, lymphocytes and macrophages were seen within and around the islets, in contact with both beta and alpha cells. These beta cells in contact with lymphocytes had only a few crystalline angulated secretory granules. Macrophages engulfing remnants of necrotic and degenerating beta cells or their characteristic granules were also described. In cases where no mononuclear inflammatory cell infiltrate was present, only alpha and delta cells were demonstrated. The ultrastructural features supported light microscopic and immunohistochemical observations and were in keeping with the hypothesis of a cytotoxic T cell directed immune response.[616] Such interactions between T lymphocytes and beta cells are reminiscent of similar phenomena described in other gastrointestinal diseases.

The exocrine pancreas

The human exocrine pancreas has been investigated in cases of chronic hypergastrinaemia and in cases of WDHA syndrome (watery diarrhoea, hypokalaemia, achlorhydria).[559] The reported ultrastructural alterations are essentially similar in both conditions. They comprise hyperplasia and enlargement of the ductular and centroacinar cells, with increased organelles, microfilaments and apical microvilli. There is also zymogen degranulation of the acinar cells, which contain a well developed Golgi apparatus and granular endoplasmic reticulum and occasionally display prominent lipofuscin deposits and filamentous cytoplasmic bodies. These changes have been attributed to increased functional demands on these cells due to hypersecretion of fluid and bicarbonates.[42,559]

The postulated role of the pancreas in the pathogenesis of the stages and sequelae of shock has prompted several studies to correlate morphological patterns with the type and stage of shock, including its duration and severity.[309,494] The observed changes, however, are largely of a non-specific, degenerative nature. The most prominent changes occur in the endoplasmic reticulum of the cells of the exocrine pancreas. It may become markedly swollen, with loss of its lamellar organization and surface ribosomes. Cytoplasmic vacuolation and surface protrusions are frequent. Mitochondrial changes include increased density or swelling, with fragmentation or dissolution of the inner cristae. Coalescence of the zymogen granules results in the formation of confluent forms, or in severe cases, their dissolution. Intracytoplasmic accumulations of fat are seen and interstitial oedema, cellular swelling, peripheral clumping of the nuclear chromatin and shortening or loss of the apical microvilli are also frequently observed. In more severe cases, evidence of frank cell necrosis is also present. While most of the developed acinar cell changes are reversible, mitochondrial rupture and fusion of the zymogen granules are thought to signal evidence of lethal damage.

In general, it appears that the intensity and extent of cell injury directly correlate with the severity and duration of shock rather than with its type.[174,229,309,352,353,494] The changes have been attributed to the hypoxaemia and local ischaemia that accompany shock. If these are allowed to continue for prolonged periods, the release of the pancreatic enzymes from their secretory granules may follow, with the development of autodigestive pancreatitis.[229,353,677,685]

Fine-structural changes seen in the pancreas in cases of acute or chronic pancreatitis sometimes also occur in association with other conditions, such as gallbladder and bile duct stones and during gallstone migration, in alcoholics with or without pancreatitis, and in ischaemia.[10,310,353,376,411,481,495–497,529,665,677,729] Ultrastructural examination reveals alterations of the exocrine pancreas, particularly the acinar cells, which are similar to those described above. This reflects the well known limitations in the available patterns of reaction in highly differentiated tissues.

Willemer et al[729] have studied the subcellular distribution of zymogen granules and of the secretory protein trypsinogen in the acinar cells of patients with acute pancreatitis, using combined immuno-electron microscopy and morphometric techniques. They showed a reduction in the number and size of the zymogen granules but there was no noticeable decrease in the intensity of their staining for trypsinogen. Intracellular release of zymogen was also noticed. There was, however, a significant reduction in trypsinogen labelling over the RER, the Golgi apparatus and the acinar lumina. The authors concluded that these observations may indicate a reduction in trypsinogen synthesis and secretion. They proposed that the disruption of zymogen granule membranes and their fusion with lysosomes may contribute to the pathogenesis of acute pancreatitis.

Duct-like tubular structures are described in various inflammatory pancreatic diseases, particularly chronic pancreatitis.[66,728] Their ultrastructure reveals acini lined by degenerating zymogenic cells, which have lost their secretory granules and elaborate cytoplasmic membrane systems. There is widening of their lumina, as the lining cells become low cuboidal or flattened. Immunohistochemical studies indicate that these cells have lost their pancreatic enzymes and have acquired increased amounts of cytoskeletal proteins, including keratin and actin.[66,728]

In kwashiorkor, the ultrastructure of the gland reflects the deprivation of protein nutrients, as evidenced by alterations in various cell organelles.[63,677] The acinar cells show fewer and smaller zymogen granules than normal, while the endoplasmic reticulum and the mitochondria are less abundant, though they may appear dilated or enlarged. Nuclear envelope alterations include dilatation of the perinuclear cisterna with evagination and blebbing of the outer and inner nuclear membrane.

THE GALLBLADDER AND EXTRAHEPATIC BILIARY SYSTEM

It is difficult to imagine a purely diagnostic role for electron microscopy in most of the non-neoplastic disorders of the gallbladder and extrahepatic biliary channels. Even in hepatic diseases which primarily affect the intrahepatic and extrahepatic biliary tract, the literature concentrates on intrahepatic changes. Furthermore, in these conditions, publications regarding even light-microscopic histopathology in the extrahepatic portion are sparse. Nevertheless, electron microscopy, along with immunohistochemistry and EDXA techniques, have played a significant role in the experimental investigation of various disorders of the gallbladder and extrahepatic biliary system.

Scanning electron microscopy and X-ray microanalysis have a special role in the study of biliary calculi. This includes the investigation of the external and cut surfaces of these stones and the identification of their elemental composition, in an attempt to elucidate the various stages and mechanisms of gallbladder and common bile duct stone formation.[49,58,361,536,569,625,662] The presence or absence of bacteria in various types of gallstones can easily be detected. These studies have also revealed that acute cholangitis occurs more often in association with stones which contain bacteria than those which do not. It has been reported that a considerable percentage of pigment stones contain bacteria, while cholesterol stones more often do not.[361,625] This may perhaps explain why gallbladder diseases may be more severe in association with pigments rather than non-pigment stones.

Investigation by SEM of blocked biliary stents has revealed large masses of various types of bacterial microcolonies on their luminal and external surfaces. The integrated elements in these bacterial biofilms have been identified by EDXA.[417,633]

The ultrastructure of the bile duct epithelial lining in cases of choledocholithiasis and bile duct obstruction has been investigated by Hopwood et al.[329] The reported changes included irregularity of the surface microvilli, accumulation of mucus droplets of variable number and density, vacuolation and increased numbers of small lysosomal structures in the apical cytoplasm and the presence of a prominent RER and Golgi apparatus. Aggregates of lipid droplets were noted adjacent to the basement membrane, which showed focal reduplication. Lipid-laden macrophages were present in the lamina propria and between epithelial cells.

In cases of chronic cholecystitis, Hussein et al[336] found an increase in the amount of glycosaminoglycans, stained with cuprolinic blue, in the basement membrane of the inflamed gallbladder. The authors concluded that the increase is proportionate to the severity of the inflammation. The fine structure of the gallbladder in cholesterolosis and the presence of cholesterol vacuoles of various sizes inside macrophages has been described by Nevalainen and Laitio.[486]

CONCLUSION

It is often argued that one of the main limitations of conventional electron microscopy is the small sample size of the tissue samples that can be examined. In considering the non-neoplastic disorders of the digestive system, however, even these limited samples may be difficult to obtain for various practical and ethical reasons. In addition, the routine diagnosis of most non-neoplastic diseases of the digestive system is largely dependent on conventional H & E sections, with little emphasis on immunohistochemistry or electron microscopy, which are perceived as being of little practical value. The net outcome, therefore, is that the ultrastructure of many of these diseases is far from being completely documented. Observations and incidental findings, from single case studies, coupled with lack of adequate samples and normal controls, have resulted in a fragmented literature, often with conflicting or non-specific conclusions.

It is thus fair to say that the impact of subcellular morphology on the routine diagnosis of the common non-neoplastic digestive system diseases has been insignificant. The diagnostic pathologist, however, should always be aware of those few diseases that can easily be missed and of certain conditions that can be mistaken or misdiagnosed, unless electron microscopic investigations are carried out. As a matter of general principle, electron microscopy is particularly recommended in those biopsies where apparently significant clinical disease is associated with negative findings or with a difficult differential diagnosis on routine histology.

Finally, irrespective of its diagnostic relevance, there is value in the ultrastructural investigation of any pathological process. Such investigation is essential to fill the gap between the clinical, the gross and the histological appearances on the one hand, and the molecular basis of disease on the other. A global understanding of the disease process should form the basis for any proper diagnostic or prognostic assessment, or for the undertaking of therapeutic trials. When the problem is stated in these terms, it is clear that our present ultrastructural knowledge of the digestive diseases is far from complete.

REFERENCES

1. Aase S, Roland M, Olsen B R 1976 Ultrastructure of parietal cells before and after proximal gastric vagotomy in duodenal ulcer patients. Scandinavian Journal of Gastroenterology 11: 55–64
2. Aase S, Roland M 1977 Light and electron microscopical studies of parietal cells before and one year after proximal gastric vagotomy in duodenal ulcer patients. Scandinavian Journal of Gastroenterology 12: 417–420
3. Aase S, Roland M, Liavag I, Dahl E 1985 Stereological analysis of human parietal cells before and 6 months after vagotomy. Scandinavian Journal of Gastroenterology 20: 257–267
4. Aase S, Elgjo K, Fausa O, Bjørneklett A, Nedenskov-Søvensen P, Bukholm G 1988 Bacteria of the gastric antrum and their relation to chronic gastritis. Acta Pathologica, Microbiologica, et Immunologica Scandinavica 96: 273–279
5. Abrams G D 1987 Surgical pathology of the infected gut. American Journal of Surgical Pathology 11 (suppl 1): 16–24
6. Adams C W M, Brain R H F, Trounce J R 1976 Ganglion cells in achalasia of the cardia. Virchows Archiv A, Pathological Anatomy and Histology 327: 75–79
7. Adams M, Rhyner P A, Day J, De Armond S, Smuckler E A 1987 Whipple's disease confined to the central nervous system. Annals of Neurology 21: 104–108
8. Adkins K F, Martinez M G, Robinson L H 1969 Cellular morphology and relationships in giant cell lesions of the jaws. Oral Surgery 28: 216–222
9. Adriaens P A, Edwards C A, De Boever J A, Loesche W J 1988 Ultrastructural observations on bacterial invasion in cementum and radicular dentin of periodontally diseased human teeth. Journal of Periodontology 59: 493–503
10. Aho H J, Nevalainen T J, Havia T V, Heinonen R J, Aho A J 1982 Human acute pancreatitis. A light and electron microscopy study. Acta Pathologica et Microbiologica Scandinavica A 90: 367–373

11. Albot G, Parturier-Albot M, Camilleri J P 1970 Crohn's disease of the colon IV. Cytological and ultrastructural study of the plasmocytic and epithelio-giant-cellular inflammatory infiltrates. Semaine des Hôpitaux de Paris 46: 1545–1566
12. Allen J I, Silvis S E, Sumner H W, McClain C J 1981 Cytomegalic inclusion disease diagnosed endoscopically. Digestive Diseases and Sciences 26: 133–135
13. Allenspach-Petrzilka G E, Guggenheim B 1983 Bacterial invasion of the periodontium: an important factor in the pathogenesis of periodontitis? Journal of Clinical Periodontology 10: 609–617
14. Alstead E M, Murphy M N, Flanagan A M, Bishop A E, Hodgson H J 1988 Familial autonomic visceral neuropathy with degeneration of muscularis mucosae. Journal of Clinical Pathology 41: 424–429
15. Aluwihare A P 1971 Electron microscopy in Crohn's disease. Gut 12: 509–518
16. Aluwihare A P 1971 The ultrastructure of the colon in Crohn's disease. Proceedings of the Royal Society of Medicine 84: 162–164
17. Aluwihare A P 1972 The electron microscope and Crohn's disease. Clinical Gastroenterology 1: 279–294
18. Ament M E, Shimoda S S, Saunders D R, Rubin C E 1972 Pathogenesis of steatorrhea in three cases of small intestinal stasis syndrome. Gastroenterology 63: 728–747
19. Anand B S, Piris J, Jerrome D W, Offord R E, Truelove S C 1981 The timing of histological damage following a single challenge with gluten in treated coeliac disease. Quarterly Journal of Medicine 50: 83–94
20. Andersen L, Arwill T, Fejerskov O, Heyden G, Phillipsen H P 1973 Oral giant cell granulomas. An enzyme histochemical and ultrastructural study. Acta Pathologica et Microbiologica Scandinavica A 81: 617–629
21. Andersen L, Fejerskov O, Theilade J 1975 Oral giant cell granulomas. An ultrastructural study of the vessels. Acta Pathologica et Microbiologica Scandinavica A 83: 69–76

22. Andrade J de S, Bambirra E A, Lima G F, Moreira E F, De Olivera C A 1983 Gastric cytomegalic inclusion bodies diagnosed by histologic examination of endoscopic biopsies in patients with gastric ulcer. American Journal of Clinical Pathology 79: 493–496

23. Anneroth G, Eneroth C M, Isaacsson G, Lundquist P G 1978 Ultrastructure of submandibular gland calculi. Scandinavian Journal of Dental Research 86: 182–192

24. Armitage G C, Christie T M 1973 Structural changes in exposed human cementum. II. Electron microscopic observations. Journal of Periodontal Research 8: 356–365

25. Antonakopoulos G, Newman J, Wilkinson M 1982 Intestinal spirochaetosis: an electron microscopic study of an unusual case. Histopathology 6: 477–488

26. Arsenio-Nunes M L, Goutieres F 1975 An ultramicroscopic study of the skin in the diagnosis of the infantile and late infantile types of ceroid–lipofuscinosis. Journal of Neurology, Neurosurgery and Psychiatry 38: 994–999

27. Arvidson K 1976 Scanning electron microscopy of fungiform papillae on the tongue of man and monkey. Acta Otolaryngologica 81: 496–502

28. Asakura H, Tsuchiya M, Watanabe Y, Enomoto Y, Morita A, Morishita T, Fukumi H, Ohashi M, Castro A, Uylanoge C 1974 Electron microscopic study on the jejunal mucosa in human cholera. Gut 15: 531–544

29. Asakura H, Miura S, Morishita T, Aiso S, Tanaka T, Kitahora T, Tsuchiya M, Enomoto Y, Watanabe Y 1981 Endoscopic and histopathological study of primary and secondary intestinal lymphangiectasia. Digestive Diseases and Sciences 26: 312–320

30. Asikainen S, Sandholm L, Sandman S, Ainamo J 1984 Gingival bleeding after chlorhexidine rinses with or without mechanical oral hygiene. Journal of Clinical Periodontology 11: 87–94

31. Atias A, Neghme A, Mackay L A, Jarpa S 1963 Megaesophagus, megacolon, and Chagas' disease in Chile. Gastroenterology 44: 433–437

32. Austin L L, Dobbins W O III 1982 Intraepithelial leukocytes of the intestinal mucosa in normal man and in Whipple's disease: a light and electron-microscopic study. Digestive Diseases and Sciences 27: 311–320

33. Awazava Y 1964 Electron microscopy of enamel caries. Journal of Nihon University School of Dentistry 6: 122

34. Bab I, Lustmann J, Azaz B, Gazit D, Garfunkel A 1985 Calcification of non-collagenous matrix in human gingiva: a light and electron microscopic study. Journal of Oral Pathology 14: 573–580

35. Baba S, Maruta M, Ando K, Teramoto T, Endo I 1976 Intestinal Behcet's disease: report of 5 cases. Diseases of the Colon and Rectum 19: 428–440

36. Baelum V, Fejerskov O, Dabelsteen E 1989 Langerhans' cells in oral epithelium of chronically inflamed human gingivae. Journal of Periodontal Research 24: 127–136

37. Bailey D S, Freedman A R, Price S C, Chescoe D, Ciclitira P J 1989 Early biochemical responses of the small intestine of coeliac patients to wheat gluten. Gut 30: 78–85

38. Balázs M 1986 Melanosis coli. Ultrastructural study of 45 patients. Diseases of the Colon and the Rectum 29: 839–844

39. Balázs M, Egerszegi P, Vadász G, Kovács A 1988 Collagenous colitis: an electron microscopic study including comparison with the chronic fibrotic stage of ulcerative colitis. Histopathology 13: 319–328

40. Balf C L 1951 The alimentary lesions in Henoch–Schonlein purpura. Archives of Diseases in Childhood 26: 20–27

41. Bamford M J, Matz L R, Armstrong J A, Harris A R C 1982 Collagenous colitis: a case report and review of the literature. Pathology 14: 481–484

42. Bani Sacchi T, Bani D, Biliotti G 1985 Nesidioblastosis and islet cell changes related to endogenous hypergastrinemia. Virchows Archiv B, Cell Pathology 48: 261–276

43. Banoczy J, Juhasz J, Albrecht M 1980 Ultrastructure of different clinical forms or oral leukoplakia. Journal of Oral Pathology 9: 41–53

44. Barrett-Dahm B, Landing B J, Blaskovics M, Roe T F 1980 Nesidioblastosis and other cell abnormalities in hyperinsulinemic hypoglycemia of childhood. Human Pathology 11: 641–649

45. Barton N S, Van Swol R L 1987 Periodontally diseased vs. normal roots as evaluated by scanning electron microscopy and electron probe analysis. Journal of Periodontology 58: 634–638

46. Baskerville A, Newell D G 1988 Naturally occurring chronic gastritis and C. pylori infection in the rhesus monkey: a potential model for gastritis in man. Gut 29: 465–472

47. Beards G M 1988 Laboratory diagnosis of viral gastroenteritis. European Journal of Clinical Microbiology and Infectious Diseases 7: 11–13

48. Becker K, Wendel U, Przyrenbel H, Tsotsalas M, Muentefering H, Bremer H J 1978 Beta cell nesidioblastosis. European Journal of Pediatrics 127: 75–89

49. Been J M, Bills P M, Lewis D 1977 Electron probe microanalysis in the study of gallstones. Gut 18: 836–842

50. Belcon M C, Collins S M, Castelli M F, Qizilbash A H 1980 Gastrointestinal hemorrhage in mastocytosis. Canadian Medical Association Journal 122: 311–314

51. Bennett M R, Fine A P, Hanlon J T 1985 Cytomegalovirus hemorrhagic colitis in a non-transplant patient. Postgraduate Medicine 77: 227–232

52. Berendd R C, Jewell L D, Shnitka T K, Manickavel V, Danyluk J 1989 Multicentric gastric carcinoids complicating pernicious anemia. Archives of Pathology and Laboratory Medicine 113: 399–403

53. Berthrong M, Fajardo L F 1981 Radiation injury in surgical pathology. Part II. Alimentary tract. American Journal of Surgical Pathology 5: 153–178

54. Berthrong M 1986 Pathologic changes secondary to radiation. World Journal of Surgery 10: 155–170

55. Bettarello A, Pinotti H W 1976 Oesophageal involvement in Chagas' disease. Clinical Gastroenterology 5: 103–117

56. Bhagavan B S, Hofkin G A, Cochran B A 1981 Whipple's disease: morphologic and immunofluorescence characterization of bacterial antigens. Human Pathology 12: 930–936

57. Biberfeld P, Petren A L, Eklund A, Lindemalm C, Barkhem T, Ekman M, Ablashi D, Salahuddin Z 1988 Human herpes virus-6 (HHV-6, HBLV) in sarcoidosis and lymphoproliferative disorders. Journal of Virological Methods 21: 49–59

58. Bills P M, Lewis D 1975 A structural study of gallstones. Gut 16: 630–637

59. Binnie W H, Cawson R A 1972 A new ultrastructural finding in oral submucosal fibrosis. British Journal of Dermatology 86: 286–290

60. Bird R G, Smith M D 1980 Cryptosporidiosis in man: parasite life cycle and fine structural pathology. Journal of Pathology 132: 217–233

61. Bishop R F, Davidson G P, Holmes I H, Ruck B J 1973 Virus particles in epithelial cells of duodenal mucosa from children with acute non-bacterial gastroenteritis. Lancet ii: 1281–1283

62. Black V H, Cornacchia L 1986 Stereological analysis of peroxisomes and mitochondria in intestinal epithelium of patients with peroxisomal deficiency disorders: Zellweger's syndrome and neonatal-onset adrenoleukodystrophy. American Journal of Anatomy 177: 107–118

63. Blackburn W R, Vinijchaikul K 1969 The pancreas in kwashiorkor. An electron microscopic study. Laboratory Investigation 20: 305–318

64. Blaser M J 1987 Gastric Campylobacter-like organisms, gastritis, and peptic ulcer disease. Gastroenterology 93: 371–383

65. Blomlof L, Hammarstrom L, Lindskog S 1986 Occurrence and appearance of cementum hypoplasias in localised and generalised juvenile periodontitis. Acta Odontologica Scandinavica 44: 313–320

66. Bockman D E, Boydston W R, Parsa I 1983 Architecture of human pancreas: implications for early changes in pancreatic disease. Gastroenterology 85: 55–61

67. Bode G, Malfertheiner P, Ditschuneit H 1987 Invasion of Campylobacter-like organisms in the duodenal mucosa in patients with active duodenal ulcer. Klinische Wochenschrift 65: 144–146

68. Bode G, Malfertheiner P, Ditschuneit H 1988 Pathogenetic implications of ultrastructural findings in Campylobacter pylori-related gastroduodenal disease. Scandinavian Journal of Gastroenterology 142 (suppl): 25–39

69. Boger A, Hort W 1977 The importance of smooth muscle cells in the development of foam cells in the gastric mucosa. An electron microscopic study. Virchows Archiv A, Pathological Anatomy and Histology 372: 287–297

70. Bogomoletz W V, Adnet J J, Birembaut P, Feydy P, Dupont P 1980 Collagenous colitis: an unrecognised entity. Gut 21: 164–168

71. Bogomoletz W V 1983 Collagenous colitis: a clinicopathological review. Survey of Digestive Disease 1: 19–25

72. Bohane T D, Cutz E, Hamilton J R, Gall D G 1977 Acrodermatitis enteropathica, zinc and the Paneth cell. A case report with family studies. Gastroenterology 73: 587–592

73. Bonvicini F, Maltarello M C, Versura P, Bianchi D, Gasbarrini G, Laschi R 1986 Correlative scanning electron microscopy in the study of human gastric mucosa. Scanning Electron Microscopy 2: 687–702

74. Bonvicini F, Zoli G, Maltarello M C, Bianchi D, Pasquinelli G, Versura P, Gasbarrini G, Laschi R 1985 Clinical applications of scanning electron microscopy in gastrointestinal diseases. Scanning Electron Microscopy 3: 1279–1294

75. Bonvicini F, Versura P, Pretolani S, Gasbarrini G, Laschi R 1989 Scanning electron microscopy in the study of Campylobacter pylori associated gastritis. Scanning Electron Microscopy 3: 355–365 (discussion 365–368)

76. Boquist L, Kumlien A, Ostberg Y 1970 Ultrastructural findings in a case of benign lymphoepithelial lesion (Sjögren's syndrome). Acta Otolaryngologica 70: 216–226

77. Borch K, Renvall H, Liedberg G 1985 Gastric endocrine cell hyperplasia and carcinoid tumours in pernicious anaemia. Gastroenterology 88: 638–648

78. Borchard D 1988 Letters to the case. Pathology Research and Practice 183: 75–79

79. Bordi C, Ferrari C, D'Adda T, Pilato F, Carfagna G, Bertelé A, Missale G 1986 Ultrastructural characterisations of fundic endocrine cell hyperplasia associated with atrophic gastritis and hypergastrinaemia. Virchows Archiv A, Pathological Anatomy and Histology 409: 335–347

80. Bordi C, Pilato F, Carfagna G, Ferrari C, D'Adda T, Sivelli R, Bertelé A, Missale G 1986 Argyrophil cell hyperplasia of fundic mucosa in patients with chronic atrophic gastritis. Digestion 35 (suppl 1): 130–143

81. Borovsky E V, Danilevsky N F 1984 Diseases of the tongue. In: Borovsky E V, Mashkilleison A L (eds) The diseases of mucosa of oral cavity and lips. Medicina, Moscow, pp 264–284

82. Boulton A J M, Slater D N, Hancock B W 1982 Herpesvirus colitis: a new cause of diarrhoea in a patient with Hodgkin's disease. Gut 23: 247–249

83. Boyde A 1970 The contribution of the scanning electron microscope to dental histology. Apex 4: 15–21

84. Brady J M, Del Rio C E 1975 Corrosion of silver cones in humans: a scanning electron microscope and X-ray microprobe study. Journal of Endodontics 1: 205–210

85. Brandberg L L, Tankersley C B, Gottlieb S, Barancik M, Sartor V E 1967 Histological demonstration of mucosal invasion by Giardia lamblia in man. Gastroenterology 52: 143–150

86. Brandborg L L, Goldberg S B, Breidenbach W C 1979 Human coccidiosis — a possible cause of malabsorption. The life cycle in small bowel mucosal biopsies as a diagnostic feature. New England Journal of Medicine 283: 1306–1313

87. Branemark P I, Adell R, Albrektsson T, Lekholm U, Lundkvist S, Rockler B 1983 Osseointegrated titanium fixtures in the treatment of edentulousness. Biomaterials 4: 25–28

88. Braverman D Z, Dollberg L, Shiner M 1985 Clinical, histological, and electron microscopic study of mast cell disease of the small bowel. American Journal of Gastroenterology 80: 30–37

89. Breslaw J 1980 Melanosis of the duodenal mucosa. Gastrointestinal Endoscopy 26: 45–46

90. Brett E M, Lake B D 1975 Reassessment of rectal approach to neuropathology in childhood. Review of 307 biopsies over 11 years. Archives of Diseases in Childhood 50: 753–762

91. Breininger D R, O'Leary T J, Blumenshine R V 1987 Comparative effectiveness of ultrasonic and hand scaling for the removal of subgingival plaque and calculus. Journal of Periodontology 58: 9–18

92. Bronsdon M A, Schoenknecht F D 1988 Campylobacter pylori isolated from the stomach of the monkey Macaca nernestreina. Journal of Clinical Microbiology 26: 1725–1728

93. Brooks R, Brown L, Franklin R 1988 Comparison of a protein-stabilized Rotazyme II test, with standard Rotazyme II, and electron microscopy for detection of rotavirus. Diagnostic Microbiology and Infectious Diseases 11: 205–208

94. Brooks R G, Brown L, Franklin R B 1989 Comparison of a new rapid test (TestPack Rotavirus) with standard enzyme immunoassay and electron microscopy for the detection of rotavirus in symptomatic hospitalized children. Journal of Clinical Microbiology 27: 775–777

95. Brooks S E H, Audretsch J, Miller C G, Sparke B 1970 Electron microscopy of Giardia lamblia in human jejunal biopsies. Journal of Medical Microbiology 3: 196–199

96. Brunser O, Castillo C, Araya M 1976 Fine structure of the small intestinal mucosa in infantile marasmic malnutrition. Gastroenterology 70: 495–507

97. Brusati R, Bracchetti A 1969 Electron microscopic study of chronic desquamative gingivitis. Journal of Periodontology 40: 388–397

98. Buchner A, Hansen L S 1980 Lymphoepithelial cysts of the oral cavity. A clinicopathologic study of thirty-eight cases. Oral Surgery 50: 441–449

99. Buchner A, Ramon Y 1975 Ultrastructural study of focal epithelial hyperplasia. Oral Surgery 39: 622

100. Burrig E-F, Borchard F, Feiden W, Pfitzer P 1984 Herpes oesophagitis II. Electron microscopical findings. Virchows Archiv A, Pathological Anatomy and Histology 404: 177–185

101. Byrnes C K 1963 Muscular hypertrophy of lower oesophagus. Read before the Societe International de Chirurgie, Rome

102. Callea F, Van Damme B, Desmet V J 1982 Alpha-1-antitrypsin in malakoplakia. Virchows Archiv A, Pathological Anatomy and Histology 395: 1–9

103. Camilleri M, Chadwick V S, Hodgson H J F 1984 Vascular anomalies of the gastrointestinal tract. Hepatogastroenterology 31: 149–153

104. Candy D C A, Leung T S M, Marshall W C, Harries J T 1983 Increased adhesion of Escherichia coli to mucosal cells from infants with protracted diarrhoea: a possible factor in the pathogenesis of bacterial overgrowth and diarrhoea. Gut 24: 538–541

105. Carpenter S, Karpati G, Andermann F 1972 Specific involvement of muscle, nerve and skin in late infantile and juvenile amaurotic idiocy. Neurology 22: 170–186

106. Carpino F, Ceccamea A, Magliocca F M, Familiari G, Lombardi M E, Bonamico M 1985 Scanning electron microscopy of jejunal biopsies in patients with untreated and treated coeliac disease. Acta Paediatrica Scandinavica 74: 775–781

107. Carranza F A Jr, Saglie R, Newman M G, Valentin P L 1983 Scanning and transmission electron microscopic study of tissue-invading microorganisms in localized juvenile periodontitis. Journal of Periodontology 54: 589–617

108. Carrassi A, Abati S, Santarelli G 1988 The role of scanning electron microscopy in periodontal research. Scanning Electron Microscopy 2: 1128–1138

109. Carruthers L, Dourmashkin R, Phillips A 1986 Disorders of the cytoskeleton of the enterocyte. Clinical Gastroenterology 15: 105–120

110. Caselli M, Bovolenta M R, Aleotti A, Trevisani L, Stabellini G, Ricci N 1988 Epithelial morphology of duodenal bulb and Campylobacter-like organisms. Journal of Submicroscopic Cytology and Pathology 20: 237–242

111. Caselli M, Trevisani L, Bighi S, AIeotti A, Balboni P G, Gaiani R, Bovolenta M R, Stabellini G 1988 Dead fecal yeasts and chronic diarrhea. Digestion 41: 142–148

112. Casemore D P, Sands R L, Curry A 1985 Cryptosporidium species, a 'new' human pathogen. Journal of Clinical Pathology 38: 1321–1336

113. Castellano G, Canga F, Lopez I, Colina F, Gutierrez J, Costa R, Solis-Herruzo J A 1988 Pseudomelanosis of the duodenum. Endoscopic, histologic, and ultrastructural study of a case. Journal of Clinical Gastroenterology 10: 150–154

114. Catalan A 1985 Superficie interna de protesis dentaria y placa bacteriana protesica: estudio al microscopio electronico de barrido (Denture plaque and denture surface: scanning electron microscope study.) Revista Anales de la Academia Alfonso Leng 3: 22–31

115. Catalan A, Herrera R, Martinex A 1987 Denture plaque and palatal mucosa in denture stomatitis: scanning electron microscopic and microbiologic study. Journal of Prosthetic Dentistry 57: 581–586

116. Caul E O, Paver W K, Clarke S K R 1975 Letter: Coronavirus particles in faeces in patients with gastroenteritis. Lancet ii: 1192

117. Cawson R A, Rajasingham K C 1972 Ultrastructural features of the invasive phase of *Candida albicans*. British Journal of Dermatology 87: 435–443

118. Cerimele D, de Rysky S, Ruggeri A 1973 Le lichen de la bouche. Observations au microscope electronique. Bulletin du Groupement International pour la Recherche Scientifique en Stomatologie et Odontologie 16: 269–277

119. Chanvitan A, Nopanitaya W 1986 Solitary rectal ulcer. Electron microscopy study of two cases. Diseases of the Colon and Rectum 29: 421–425

120. Chaudhry A P, Yamane G M, Scharlock S E, Sunderraj M, Jain R 1984 A clinico-pathological study of intraoral lymphoepithelial cysts. Journal of Oral Medicine 39: 79–84

121. Chaudhry A P, Cutler L S, Yamane G M, Satchidanand S, Labay G, Sunderraj M 1986 Light and ultrastructural features of lymphoepithelial lesions of the salivary glands in Mikulicz's disease. Journal of Pathology 148: 239–250

122. Chavrier C, Couble M L, Hartmann D, Grimaud J A, Magloire H 1987 Immunohistochemical study of types I, III and IV collagen in fibrosis of diseased gingiva during chronic periodontitis: a light and electron microscopic study. Journal of Periodontal Research 22: 29–36

123. Chears W C, Asworth C T 1961 Electron microscopic study of the intestinal mucosa in Whipple's disease. Gastroenterology 41: 129–137

124. Chen H C, Reyes V, Fresh J W 1971 An electron microscopic study of the small intestine in human cholera. Virchows Archiv B, Cell Pathology 7: 236–259

125. Chen S Y, Miller A S 1975 Ultrastructure of the keratinizing and calcifying odontogenic cyst. Oral Surgery 39: 769–780

126. Chen S Y, Fantasia J E, Miller A S 1981 Hyaline bodies in the connective tissue wall of odontogenic cysts. Journal of Oral Pathology 10: 147–157

127. Chen X G, Correa P, Offerhaus J, Rodriguez E, Janney F, Hoffmann E, Fox J, Hunter F, Diavolitsis S 1986 Ultrastructure of the gastric mucosa harboring *Campylobacter*-like organisms. American Journal of Clinical Pathology 86: 575–582

128. Choudari C P, Mathan M, Rajan D P, Raghavan R, Mathan V I 1985 A correlative study of etiology, clinical features and rectal mucosal pathology in adults with acute infectious diarrhea in southern India. Pathology 17: 443–450

129. Cianciola L J, Genco R J, Patters M R, McKenna J, Van Oss C J 1977 Defective polymorphonuclear leucocyte function in human periodontal disease. Nature 265: 445–447

130. Ciclitira P J, Evans D J, Fagg H L K, Lennox E S, Dowling R H 1984 Clinical testing of gliadin fractions in coeliac patients. Clinical Science 66: 357–364

131. Cohen A S, Connors L H 1987 The pathogenesis and biochemistry of amyloidosis. Journal of Pathology 151: 1–10

132. Cohen B, Poswillo D E, Woods D A 1971 The effects of exposure to chewing tobacco on the oral mucosa of monkey and man. Annal of the Royal College of Surgeons of England 48: 255–273

133. Colina F, Solis-Herruzo J A, Munoz-Yagne M T, Vazquez G, Perez-Barrios A 1982 Collagenous colitis: the clinical and morphological features. Postgraduate Medical Journal 58: 390–395

134. Constantinides P 1984 Ultrastructural pathobiology. Elsevier Press, London, Amsterdam

135. Contini D, Torti A, Monti M, Caputo R, Gasparini G, Vecchi M, de Franchis R 1986 A freeze-fracture study of the enteropathy associated with dermatitis herpetiformis: a comparative investigation with coeliac disease. Journal of Cutaneous Pathology 13: 293–300

136. Cook M G, Turnbull G J 1975 A hypothesis for the pathogenesis of Crohn's disease based on an ultrastructural study. Virchows Archiv A, Pathological Anatomy and Histology 365: 327–336

137. Cooper C, Cotton D W K, Hudson M J, Kirkham N, Wilmott F E W 1986 Rectal spirochaetosis in homosexual men: characterisation of the organism and pathophysiology. Genitourinary Medicine 62: 47–52

138. Cossel L, Schade J, Verlohren H J, Lohmann D, Mattig H 1983 Ultrastructural, immunohistological and clinical findings in the pancreas in insulin-dependent diabetes mellitus (IDDM) of long

duration. Zentralblatt für Allgemaine Pathologie und Pathologische Anatomie 128: 147–159

139. Cossel L, Binh T, Verlohren H J, Lohmann D, Mattig H 1984 Electron microscopic findings in A-cells of the islands of Langerhans in diabetes mellitus. Zentralblatt für Allgemaine Pathologie und Pathologische Anatomie 129: 323–341

140. Cotton D W K, Kirkham N, Hicks D A 1984 Rectal spirochaetosis. British Journal of Venereal Diseases 60: 106–109

141. Courtois G J, Cobb C M, Killoy W J 1983 Acute necrotizing ulcerative gingivitis. A transmission electron microscope study. Journal of Periodontology 54: 671–679

142. Cowen M L, Humphries T J 1980 Pseudomelanosis of the duodenum. Gastrointestinal Endoscopy 26: 107–108

143. Creamer B, Pink I J 1967 Paneth cell deficiency. Lancet i: 304–306

144. Curry A, Jones D M, Eldridge J 1987 Spiral organisms in the baboon stomach. Lancet ii: 634–635

145. Cutz E, Rhoads J M, Drumm B, Sherman P M, Durie P R, Forstner G G 1989 Microvillus inclusion disease: an inherited defect of brush-border assembly and differentiation. New England Journal of Medicine 320: 646–651

146. Czernial B, Marlicz K 1984 Surface coat of enterocytes in chronic duodenitis. Materia Medica Polona 16: 9–14

147. D'Abros W, Stachura J, Bogda J, Tarnawski A 1983 Ultrastructure of colonic endocrine cells in ulcerative colitis. Folia Histochemica et Cytochemica 21: 263–272

148. D'Angelo G, Stern H S, Myers E 1985 Rectal prolapse in scleroderma: case report and review of the colonic complications of scleroderma. Canadian Journal of Surgery 28: 62–63

149. D'Silva V, Nayak R P, Cherian K M, Mulky M J 1979 An evaluation of the root topography following periodontal instrumentation. A scanning electron microscopy study. Journal of Periodontology 50: 283–290

150. Davidson G P, Cutz E, Hamilton J R, Gall D G 1978 Familial enteropathy: a syndrome of protracted diarrhea from birth, failure to thrive, and hypoplastic villous atrophy. Gastroenterology 75: 783–790

151. Davidson G P, Goller I, Bishop R F, Townley R R W, Holmes I H, Ruck B J 1975 Immunofluorescence in duodenal mucosa of children with acute enteritis due to a new virus. Journal of Clinical Pathology 28: 263–266

152. Davidson G P, Barnes G L 1979 Structural and functional abnormalities of the small intestine in infants and young children with rotavirus enteritis. Acta Paediatrica Scandinavica 68: 181–186

153. Davidson G P, Barnes G L 1985 Ultrastructural study of alterations in the small intestinal epithelium of children with acute diarrhoea. Journal of Pediatric Gastroenterology and Nutrition 4: 682–689

154. Davies J D, Young E W, Mera S L, Barnard K 1983 Lysozyme is a component of human vascular elastic fibres. Experentia 39: 382–383

155. Davies K J, Garrett J R 1981 Ciliated ductal cells in obstructive sialadenitis. Journal of Microscopy 123: RP1–RP2

156. De la Fuente A, Garcia-Calvo M, Cajal R Y, Cuesta P G 1977 Alteraciones ultrastructurales de nervio vago en la acalasia del esofago. Revista Espaniola des las Enfirmedales del Aparato Digestivo 51: 659–660

157. Degtiareva I I, Matvienko A V, Rodonezhskaia E V 1984 Morphological changes in the gastric mucosa of peptic ulcer patients. Vrachebnoe Delo 11: 83–88

158. Degtiareva I I, Matvienko A V 1985 Histoenzymological and electron microscopy changes in the gastric mucosa of patients with peptic ulcer. Vrachebnoe Delo 2: 23–29

159. Delladetsima K, Markaki S, Papadimitriou K, Antonakopoulos G N 1987 Intestinal spirochaetosis. Light and electron microscopic study. Pathology Research and Practice 182: 780–782

160. Denholm R B, Mills P R, More I A R 1981 Electron microscopy in the long-term follow-up of Whipple's disease. Effect of antibiotics. American Journal of Surgical Pathology 5: 507–516

161. Dent J C, McNulty C A, Uff J C, Wilkinson S P, Gear M W 1987 Spiral organisms in the gastric antrum. Lancet ii: 96

162. DiFranco C F, Toto P D, Rowden G, Gargiulo A W, Keene J J, Connelly E 1985 Identification of Langerhans' cells in human gingival epithelium. Journal of Periodontology 56: 48–54

163. Dinari G, Rosenbach Y, Grunebaum M, Zahavi I, Alpert G, Nitzan

M 1980 Gastrointestinal manifestations of Niemann–Pick disease. Enzyme 25: 407–412

164. Dinoso V P, Ming Si-Chem, McNiff J 1976 Ultrastructural changes of the canine gastric mucosa after topical application of graded concentrations of ethanol. Digestive Diseases 21: 626–632

165. DiSilvo T, Bartlett E F 1977 Malakoplakia of the colon. Archives of Pathology 92: 167–171

166. Dobbins W O III 1966 Electron microscopic study of the intestinal mucosa in intestinal lymphangiectasia. Gastroenterology 51: 1004–1017

167. Dobbins W O III, Herrero B A, Mansbach C M 1968 Morphologic alterations associated with neomycin induced malabsorption. American Journal of Medical Science 255: 63–77

168. Dobbins W O III 1975 Colonic epithelial cells and polymorphonuclear leukocytes in ulcerative colitis: an electron microscopic study. American Journal of Digestive Diseases 20: 236–252

169. Dobbins W O III 1978 Diagnostic pathology of the intestine and colon. In: Trump B F, Jones R T (eds) Diagnostic electron microscopy, vol 1. John Wiley & Sons, New York, pp 253–339

170. Dobbins W O III, Kawanishy H 1981 Bacillary characteristic in Whipple's disease: an electron microscopic study. Gastroenterology 80: 1468–1475

171. Dobbins W O III, Weinstein W M 1985 Electron microscopy of the intestine and rectum in acquired immunodeficiency syndrome. Gastroenterology 88: 738–749

172. Dobson C M, Ellis H A 1987 Polycystic disease of the parotid glands: case report of a rare entity and review of the literature. Histopathology 11: 953–961

173. Doldi S B, Trabucchi E, Mukenge S, Baratti C, Colombo R, Zennaro F, Lattuada E, Basadonna G 1984 Morphologic study by scanning electron microscope of the mucosa of the functioning and excluded intestinal segments after jejunoileal bypass. Minerva Chirurgica 39: 1399–1404

174. Donath K, Mitsche H, Seifert G 1970 Ultrastrukturelle veranderugen am rattenpankreas beim. Beitrage zur Pathologische Anatomie 141: 33–51

175. Donath K, Seifert G 1972 Ultrastruktur und pathogenese der myoepithelialen siadenitis uber das vorkommen von myoepithelzellen bei der benignen lymphoepitheelialen lasion. Virchows Archiv A, Pathological Anatomy and Histology 356: 315–329

176. Donnellan W L 1966 Early histological changes in ulcerative colitis: a light and electron microscopic study. Gastroenterology 50: 519–540

177. Dooley C P, Cohen H 1988 The clinical significance of Campylobacter pylori. Annals of Internal Medicine 108: 70–79

178. Dourov N 1984 Scanning electron microscopy contribution in oral pathology. Scanning Electron Microscopy 1: 243–248

179. Dowe G, King S D, Maitland P B, Swaby-Ellis D E 1988 Laboratory investigations on rotavirus in infantile gastroenteritis in Jamaica. Transactions of the Royal Society of Tropical Medicine and Hygiene 82: 155–159

180. Drumm B, Sherman P, Cutz E, Karmali M 1987 Association of Campylobacter pylori on the gastric mucosa with antral gastritis in children. New England Journal of Medicine 316: 1557–1561

181. Du Boulay C E H 1982 An immunohistochemical study of Whipple's disease using the immunoperoxidase technique. Human Pathology 13: 925–929

182. Dumont A, Piche C 1969 Electron microscopic study of human histoplasmosis. Archives of Pathology 87: 168–178

183. Dunlap C L, Barker B F 1977 Giant-cell hyalin angiopathy. Oral Surgery 44: 587–591

184. Dvorak A M 1979 Letter: electron microscopy of plasma cells in Crohn's disease. Lancet i: 834

185. Dvorak A M 1979 Mast cell hyperplasia and degranulation in Crohn's disease. In: Pepys J, Edwards A M (eds) The mast cell. Pitman, London pp 657–662

186. Dvorak A M, Connell A B, Dickersin G R 1979 Crohn's disease. A scanning electron microscopic study. Human Pathology 10: 165–177

187. Dvorak A M, Dickersin G R 1979 Crohn's disease. Electron microscopic studies. Pathology Annual 14: 259–306

188. Dvorak A M, Monahan R A, Osage J E, Dickersin G R 1980 Crohn's disease. Transmission electron microscopic studies II. Immunologic inflammatory response. Alterations of mast cells, basophils, eosinophils, and the microvasculature. Human Pathology 11: 606–619

189. Dvorak A M, Monahan-Earley R A 1986 Diagnostic ultrastructural pathology. A wide ranging series of practical cases demonstrating the use of electron microscopy. EM Pathology Monograph No. 1. Philips Electronic Instruments, Mahwah, pp 28–54

190. Dvorak A M, Osage J E, Monahan R A, Dickersin G R 1980 Crohn's disease. Transmission electron microscopic studies III. Target tissues. Proliferation of and injury to smooth muscle and the autonomic nervous system. Human Pathology 11: 620–634

191. Dvorak A M 1980 Electron microscopy of Paneth cells in Crohn's disease. Archives of Pathology and Laboratory Medicine 104: 393–394

192. Dvorak A M, Silen W 1985 Differentiation between Crohn's disease and other inflammatory conditions by electron microscopy. Annals of Surgery 201: 53–63

193. Dworkin B, Wormser G P, Rosenthal W S, Heier S K, Braunstein M, Weiss L, Jankowski R, Levy D, Weiselberg S 1985 Gastrointestinal manifestations of the acquired immunodeficiency syndrome: a review of 22 cases. American Journal of Gastroenterology 80: 774–778

194. Dymock R B 1977 Pathological changes in the appendix: a review of 1000 cases. Pathology 9: 331–339

195. Earlam R J 1972 Gastrointestinal aspects of Chagas' disease. Digestive Diseases and Sciences 17: 559–571

196. Eastcott A D, Stallard R E 1973 Sequential changes in developing human dental plaque as visualized by scanning electron microscopy. Journal of Periodontology 44: 218–224

197. Eda S, Yanagisawa Y, Koike H, Yamamura T, Kato T, Noma H, Inagaki K, Kawashuma Y 1974 Two cases of calcifying odontogenic cysts associated with odontoma, with an electron-microscopic observation. Bulletin of the Tokyo Dental College 15: 77

198. Eide B, Lie T, Selvig K A 1984 Surface coatings on dental cementum incident to periodontal disease. II. Scanning electron microscopic confirmation of a mineralized cuticle. Journal of Clinical Periodontology 11: 565–575

199. el-Labban N G 1970 Light and electron microscopic studies of colloid bodies in lichen planus. Journal of Periodontal Research 5: 315–324

200. el-Labban N G, Kramer I R 1972 Nuclear bodies in oral lichen planus. Journal of Ultrastructure Research 40: 470–479

201. el-Labban N G, Kramer I R 1974 Civatte bodies and the actively dividing epithelial cells in oral lichen planus. British Journal of Dermatology 90: 13–23

202. el-Labban N G, Kramer I R 1975 Light and electron microscopic study of liquefaction degeneration in oral lichen planus. Archives of Oral Biology 20: 653–657

203. el-Labban N G, Kramer I R 1981 The nature of the hyaline rings in chronic periostitis and other conditions: an ultrastructural study. Oral Surgery 51: 509–515

204. Ellender G 1987 Abnormal reaction to subgingivally placed dental amalgam studied by transmission electron microscopy and microprobe analysis. Case report. Australian Dental Journal 32: 190–195

205. Elsner B, Pernsky A L 1969 Ultrastructure of rectal biopsies in juvenile amaurotic idiocy. Neurology 19: 834–840

206. Epivatianos A, Harrison J D, Dimitrious T 1987 Ultrastructural and histochemical observations on microcalculi in chronic submandibular sialadenitis. Journal of Oral Pathology 16: 514–517

207. Emödy L, Carlsson A, Ljunch A, Wadstriöi T 1988 Mannose-resistant haemagglutination by Campylobacter pylori. Scandinavian Journal of Infectious Diseases 20: 353–354

208. Epstein R J, McDonald G B, Sale G E, Shulman H M, Thomas E D 1980 The diagnostic accuracy of the rectal biopsy in acute graft-versus-host disease: a prospective study of thirteen patients. Gastroenterology 78: 764–771

209. Evans D G, Evans D J, Moulds J J, Graham D Y 1988 N-acetylneurominyllactose-binding fibrillar haemagglutinin of Campylobacter pylori: a putative colonization factor antigen. Infection and Immunity 56: 2896–2906

210. Evans D J, Ali M F 1985 Immunocytochemistry in the diagnosis of Whipple's disease. Journal of Clinical Pathology 38: 372–374

211. Eversole L R, Leider A S, Jacobsen P L, Kidd P M 1985 Atypical histiocytic granuloma. Light microscopic, ultrastructural and histochemical findings in an unusual pseudomalignant reactive lesion of the oral cavity. Cancer 55: 1722–1729

212. Ewen S J, Gwinnett A J 1977 A scanning electron microscopic study of teeth following periodontal instrumentation. Journal of Periodontology 48: 92–97

213. Faoagali J L, Troughton D, Aitken J, Gwynne J F 1986 *Campylobacter*-like organisms in gastric biopsies: a Christchurch study. New Zealand Medical Journal 99: 50–52

214. Fagundex-Neto U, Pacheco I P, Patricio F R, Wehba J 1984 Ultrastructural study of alterations in the small intestinal epithelium of children with acute diarrhoea. Journal of Pediatric Gastroenterology and Nutrition 3: 510–515

215. Fajardo L F 1982 Pathology of radiation injury. Masson, New York, pp 6–14, 47–76

216. Fanatsu T 1984 Evaluation of the healing of ulcerative colitis by colonic gland density. Nippon Shokakibyo Gakkai Zasshi 81: 1377–1387

217. Fausa O, Foerster A, Hovig T 1985 Collagenous colitis. A clinical, histological and ultrastructural study. Scandinavian Journal of Gastroenterology 107: 8–23

218. Faussone-Pellegrini M S, Cortesini C 1985 The muscle coat of the lower oesophageal sphincter in patients with achalasia and hypertensive sphincter. An electron microscopic study. Journal of Submicroscopic Cytology 17: 673–685

219. Fejerskov O, Krogh J 1972 The calcifying ghost cell odontogenic tumor — or the calcifying odontogenic cyst. Journal of Oral Pathology 1: 273–284

220. Fejerskov O 1973 Keratinized squamous epithelium of normal and wounded palatal mucosa in guinea pigs. A light and electronmicroscopical investigation. Journal of Periodontal Research 11 (suppl): 1–80

221. Fejerskov O, Roed-Petersen B, Pinkborg J J 1977 Clinical, histological and ultrastructural features of a possible virus induced oral leukoplakia. Acta Pathologica et Microbiologica Scandinavica A: 897–906

222. Fejerskov O, Anderson C, Philipson H P 1980 The oral cavity and salivary glands. In: Johannessen J V (ed) Electron microscopy in human medicine, vol 7. McGraw-Hill, New York, London, pp 1–84

223. Fine D H, Greene L S 1984 Microscopic evaluation of root surface associations *in vivo*. Journal of Periodontal Research 19: 152–167

224. Finlay-Jones L R, Blackwell J B, Papadimitriou J M 1968 Malakoplakia of the colon. American Journal of Clinical Pathology 50: 320–329

225. Fiocca R, Villani L, Turpini F, Turpini R, Solcia E 1987 High incidence of *Campylobacter*-like organisms in endoscopic biopsies from patients with gastritis, with or without peptic ulcer. Digestion 38: 234–244

226. Fisher S E, Kahn E, Ellis D 1983 Melanosis duodeni in a child with congenital hepatic fibrosis and renal failure. Journal of Pediatric Gastroenterology and Nutrition 2: 567–569

227. Fitzgibbons P L, Chandrasoma P T 1987 Familial visceral myopathy. Evidence of diffuse involvement of intestinal smooth muscle. American Journal of Surgical Pathology 11: 846–854

228. Flejou J F, Grimaud J A, Molas G, Baviera E, Potet F 1984 Collagenous colitis. Ultrastructural study and collagen immunotyping of four cases. Archives of Pathology and Laboratory Medicine 108: 977–982

229. Flenker H, Liehr H 1978 Schock manifestationen im magen, darm, pankreas und leber. Klinik und Pathologie. Verhandlugen der Deutschen Gessellschaft für Pathologie 62: 127–146

230. Flenker H, Otto H F 1978 Funktionelle und morphologische unterzuchungen am inselsystem der ratte im standarisierten homorrhagischen schock. Zentralblatt für Allgemeine Pathologie und Pathologische Anatomie 58: 492–502

231. Flewett T H, Bryden A S, Davies H 1973 Virus particles in gastroenteritis. Lancet ii: 1497

232. Flores de Jacoby L, Fromme H G, Diedrich P, Erpenstein H 1974 Ein Beitrag zur Gingivitis desquamativa. Deutsch Zahnaerztl Zeitschrift 29: 478–482

233. Foster C S 1979 The brown bowel syndrome: a possible smooth muscle mitochondrial myopathy? Histopathology 3: 1–17

234. Foucar E, Mukai K, Foucar K, Sutherland D E R, van Buren C T 1981 Colon ulceration in lethal cytomegalovirus infection. American Journal of Clinical Pathology 76: 788–801

235. Fox J E T, Daniel E E, De Faria C R, Rezendez J M, Rassi L, De Rezendez J Jr, Daniel V P 1983 Relationship of functional changes to structural changes in megaoesophagus of Chagas' disease. In: Roman C (ed) Gastrointestinal motility. MTP Press Ltd, Lancaster, pp 51–58

236. Fox J G, Edrise B M, Cabot E R, Beaucage C, Murphy J C, Prostak K S 1986 *Campylobacter*-like organisms isolated from gastric mucosa in ferrets. American Journal of Veterinary Research 47: 236–239

237. Frank R M, Wolff F, Gutmann B 1964 Microscopie eléctronique de la carie au niveau de la dentine humaine. Archives of Oral Biology 9: 163–179

238. Frank R M, Fiore-Donno G, Cimasoni G 1983 Cementogenesis and soft tissue attachment after citric acid treatment in a human. An electron microscopic study. Journal of Periodontology 54: 389–401

239. Frank R M, Steuer P 1985 Transmission electron microscopy of plaque accumulations in denture stomatitis. Journal of Prosthetic Dentistry 53: 115–124

240. Freedman H L, Listgarten M A, Taichman N S 1968 Electron microscopic features of chronically inflamed human gingiva. Journal of Periodontal Research 3: 313–320

241. Freedman P G, Weiner B C, Balthazar E J 1985 Cytomegalovirus esophagogastritis in a patient with acquired immunodeficiency syndrome. American Journal of Gastroenterology 80: 434–437

242. French J M, Hall G, Parish D J, Smith W T 1965 Peripheral and autonomic nerve involvement in primary amyloidosis associated with uncontrollable diarrhea and steatorrhea. American Journal of Medicine 39: 277–284

243. Friesen D L, Henderson R D, Hanna W 1983 Ultrastructure of the oesophageal muscle in achalasia and diffuse oesophageal spasm. American Journal of Clinical Pathology 79: 319–325

244. Frithiof L, Hägglund G 1966 Ultrastructure of the capsular epithelium of radicular cysts. Acta Odontologica Scandinavica 24: 23–34

245. Fukii H, Ohashi M, Nagure H 1988 Immunohistochemical analysis of oral lichen-planus-like eruption in graft-versus-host disease after allogeneic bone marrow transplantation. American Journal of Clinical Pathology 89: 177–186

246. Fukiwara K, Watanabe T 1988 Mucus-producing cells and ciliated epithelial cells in mandibular radicular cyst: an electron microscopic study. Journal of Oral and Maxillofacial Surgery 46: 149–151

247. Furseth R 1971 Further observations on the fine structure of orally exposed and carious and dental cementum. Archives of Oral Biology 16: 71–85

248. Galian A, Le Charpentier Y, Goldfain D, Chauveinc L 1982 La colite collagene. A propos d'un nouveau cas avec etude ultrastructurale. Gastroenterologie Clinique et Biologique 16: 365–370

249. Gallagher R L 1980 Intestinal ceroid deposition — 'brown bowel syndrome'. A light and electron microscopic study. Virchows Archiv A, Pathological Anatomy and Histology 389: 143–151

250. Gallucci B B, Epstein R, Sale G E 1982 The fine structure of human rectal epithelium in acute graft-versus-host disease. American Journal of Surgical Pathology 6: 293–305

251. Garone M A, Winston B J, Lewis J H 1986 Cryptosporidiosis of the stomach. American Journal of Gastroenterology 81: 465–470

252. Gear E V Jr, Dobbins W O III 1968 Rectal biopsy: a review of its diagnostic usefulness. Gastroenterology 55: 522–544

253. Gebbers J-O, Ferguson D J, Mason C, Crucioli V, Jewell D P 1987 Local immune reaction in intestinal spirochetosis. Schweizerische Medizinische Wochenschrift 117: 1087–1091

254. Gebbers J-O, Ferguson D J P, Mason C, Kelly P, Jewell D P 1987 Spirochaetosis of the human rectum associated with an intraepithelial mast cell and IgE plasma cell response. Gut 28: 588–593

255. Gebbers J-O, Marder H P 1989 Unusual *in vitro* formation of cyst-like structures associated with human intestinal spirochaetosis.

European Journal of Clinical and Microbiological Infectious Diseases 8: 302–306

256. Genco R J, Slots J 1984 Host responses in periodontal diseases. Journal of Dental Research 63: 441–451

257. Gepts W, LeCompte P M 1981 The pancreatic islets in diabetes. American Journal of Medicine 70: 105–115

258. Gerlovin E S H, Reiskanen A V, Iakhontova O I 1980 Ultrastructural changes in the epithelial cells of the small intestine mucosa in chronic liver diseases. Archives of Pathology 42: 27–31

259. Ghadially F N, Parry E W 1966 An electron-microscope and histochemical study of melanosis coli. Journal of Pathology and Bacteriology 92: 313–317

260. Ghadially F N, Parry E W 1967 Melanosis coli. Current Medicine and Drugs 8: 13–29

261. Gilat T, Revach M, Sohar E 1969 Deposition of amyloid in the gastrointestinal tract. Gut 10: 98–104

262. Gillin J S, Urmacher C, West R, Shike M 1983 Disseminated *Mycobacterium avium intracellulare* infection in acquired immunodeficiency syndrome mimicking Whipple's disease. Gastroenterology 85: 1187–1191

263. Giorgi P L, Catassi C, Sbarbati A, Bearzi I, Cinti S 1986 Ultrastructural findings in the jejunal mucosa of children with IgA deficiency. Journal of Pediatric Gastroenterology Nutrition 5: 892–898

264. Glas J E, Nylen M U 1965 A correlated electron microscopic and microradiographic study of human enamel. Archives of Oral Biology 10: 893–908

265. Glenner G G, Ein D, Eanes E D, Bladen H A, Terry W, Page D L 1971 Creation of 'amyloid' fibrils from Bence Jones proteins *in vitro*. Science 174: 712–714

266. Goldman H, Ming S C 1968 Fine structure of intestinal metaplasia and adenocarcinoma of the human stomach. Laboratory Investigation 18: 203–210

267. Goldstein D A, Horowitz R E, Petit S, Haldimann B, Massry S G 1981 The duodenal mucosa in patients with renal failure: response to 1,25(OH)2D3. Kidney International 19: 324–331

268. Gonzalez-Angulo A, Corral E, Garcia-Torres R, Quijano M 1965 Malakoplakia of the colon. Gastroenterology 48: 383–387

269. Gonzalez-Licea A, Yardley J H 1966 Comparative ultrastructural study of the mucosa in idiopathic ulcerative colitis, shigellosis and other human colonic diseases. Bulletin of the Johns Hopkins Hospital 118: 44–461

270. Gonzalez-Licea A, Yardley J H 1966 Nature of tissue reaction in ulcerative colitis: light and electron microscope findings. Gastroenterology 51: 825–840

271. Gonzalez S, Lobos I, Guajardo A, Celis A, Zemelman R, Smith C T, Saglie F R 1987 Yeasts in juvenile periodontitis. Preliminary observations by scanning electron microscopy. Journal of Periodontology 58: 119–124

272. Goodell S E, Quinn T C, Mkrtichian E, Schuffler M D, Holmes K K, Corey L 1983 Herpes simplex proctitis in homosexual men: clinical sigmoidoscopic and histopathological features. New England Journal of Medicine 308: 868–871

273. Goodwin C S, McCullock R K, Armstrong J A, Wee S H 1985 Unusual cellular fatty acids and distinctive ultrastructure in a new spiral bacterium (*Campylobacter pyloridis*) from the human gastric mucosa. Journal of Medical Microbiology 19: 257–267

274. Goodwin C S, Armstrong J A, Marshall B J 1986 *Campylobacter pyloridis*, gastritis, and peptic ulceration. Journal of Clinical Pathology 39: 353–365

275. Goodwin C S 1988 Duodenal ulcer, *Campylobacter pylori*, and the 'leaking roof' concept. Lancet ii: 1467–1469

276. Goodwin C S, Armstrong J A, Chilvers T, Peters M, Collins M D, Sly L, McConnell W, Harper W E S 1989 Transfer of *Campylobacter pylori* and *Campylobacter mustelae* to *Helicobacter gen. nov.* as *Helicobacter pylori* comb. nov. and *Helicobacter mustelae* comb. nov., respectively. International Journal of Systematic Bacteriology 39: 397–405

277. Goodwin C S, Armstrong J A, Peters M 1989 Microbiology of *C. pylori*. In: Blaser M J (ed) *Campylobacter pylori* in gastritis and peptic ulcer disease. Igaku-Shoin, New York, Tokyo, pp 25–49

278. Goodwin C S, Armstrong J A 1990 Microbiological aspects of *Helicobacter pylori* (*Campylobacter pylori*) — a review. European

Journal of Clinical Microbiology (in press)

279. Gould V E, Memoli V A, Dardi L E, Gould N S 1981 Nesidiodysplasia and nesidioblastosis of infancy: ultrastructural and immunocytochemical analysis of islet cell alterations with and without associated hyperinsulinemic hypoglycemia. Scandinavian Journal of Gastroenterology 16: 129–142

280. Gould V E, Memoli V A, Dardi L E, Gould N S 1983 Nesidiodysplasia and nesidioblastosis of infancy: structural and functional correlations with the syndrome of hyperinsulinemic hypoglycemia. Pediatric Pathology 1: 7–31

281. Goutet J M, Boccon-Gribod L, Chatelet F, Ploussard J P, Navarro J, Polonovski C I 1982 Familial protracted diarrhoea with hypoplastic villous atrophy: a report of two cases. Pediatric Research 16: 1045

282. Graham D Y, Klein P D 1987 *Campylobacter pyloridis* gastritis: the past, the present, and speculations about the future. American Journal of Gastroenterology 82: 283–286

283. Greenberger N J, Dobbins W O, Ruppert R D, Jesseph J E 1968 Intestinal atony in progressive systemic sclerosis (scleroderma). American Journal of Medicine 45: 301–308

284. Gregory M A, Moshal M G, Spitaels J M 1982 Changes in the morphology of villar epithelial cells adjacent to duodenal ulcers during the process of healing. Scandinavian Journal of Gastroenterology 17: 441–448

285. Gregory M A, Moshal M G, Spitaels J M 1982 The ultrastructural effect of tripotassium dicitrato bismuthate on the duodenal mucosa during ulceration. An ultrastructural study. South African Medical Journal 62: 52–55

286. Gregory M A, Spitaels J M 1987 Variations in the morphology of villous epithelial cells within 8 mm of untreated duodenal ulcers. Journal of Pathology 153: 109–119

287. Greider M H, Lacy P E, Kissane J M, Rieders E, Thomas G 1977 Pancreatic perinuclear inclusions in diabetes mellitus and other diseases. Diabetes 26: 793–797

288. Grouls V, Vogel J, Sorger M 1982 Collagenous colitis. Endoscopy 14: 31–33

289. Guarda L A, Nelson R S, Stroehlein J R, Korinek J H, Raymond A K 1983 Collagenous colitis. American Journal of Clinical Pathology 80: 503–507

290. Guarda L A, Stein S A, Cleary K A, Ordonez N G 1983 Human cryptosporidiosis in the acquired immune deficiency syndrome. Archives of Pathology and Laboratory Medicine 107: 562–566

291. Gupta T P, Weinstock J V 1986 Duodenal pseudomelanosis associated with chronic renal failure. Gastrointestinal Endoscopy 32: 358–360

292. Haboubi N Y, Honan R P, Hasleton P S, Ali H H, Anfield C, Hobbiss J, Schofield P F 1984 Pneumatosis coli: a case report with ultrastructural study. Histopathology 8: 145–155

293. Hager-Melecka B, Dyduch A, Karczewska K, Kasner J, Lukasik M, Wasowicz-Bober A, Pawelek-Krombholtz D 1982 Glycocalyx of the intestinal epithelial cells in children with celiac disease. Pediatria Polska 57: 465–470

294. Halter S A, Greene H L, Helinek G 1982 Gluten-sensitive enteropathy: sequence of villous regrowth as viewed by scanning electron microscopy. Human Pathology 13: 811–818

295. Haltia M, Somer H, Palo J, Johnson W G 1984 Neuronal intranuclear inclusion disease in identical twins. Annals of Neurology 15: 316–321

296. Halter S A, Greene H L, Helinek G 1980 Scanning electron microscopy of small intestinal repair following treatment for gluten sensitive enteropathy. Scanning Electron Microscopy 3: 155–161

297. Hamilton J R, Gall D G, Butler D G, Middlelan P J 1976 Viral gastroenteritis: recent progress, remaining problems. Ciba Foundation Symposium 42: 209–222

298. Hansen J, Kobayasi T 1970 Ultrastructural studies of odontogenic cysts. I Non-keratinizing cysts. Acta Morphologica Neerlando-Scandinavica 8: 29–51

299. Hansen J, Kobayasi T 1970 Ultrastructural studies of odontogenic cysts. II Keratinizing cysts. Acta Morphologica Neerlando-Scandinavica 8: 43–51

300. Happonen R P, Viander M, Pelliniemi L J 1984 Immunoelectron microscopic study of *Actinomyces* colony in odontogenic periapical infection. International Journal of Oral Surgery 13: 539–544

301. Hardoff D, Levanon D, Gitay H, Nir I 1986 Evaluation of microvilli in gluten-sensitive enteropathy by means of scanning and transmission electron microscopy. Journal of Pediatric Gastroenterology and Nutrition 5: 560–564

302. Harrison J D, Martin I C 1986 Oral vegetable granuloma: ultrastructural and histological study. Journal of Oral Pathology 15: 322–326

303. Hartong W A, Gourley W K, Arvanitakis C 1979 Giardiasis: a clinical spectrum and functional-structural abnormalities of the small intestinal mucosa. Gastroenterology 77: 61–69

304. Hashimoto K, Di Bella R J, Shklar G, Lever W F 1966 Electron microscopic studies of oral lichen planus. Giornale Italiano di Dermatologia 107: 765

305. Hashimoto K, Di Bella R J, Tarnowski W M, Shklar G 1968 Electron microscopic studies of oral benign leukoplakia. Oral Surgery, Oral Medicine, Oral Pathology 25: 901–913

306. Haynes M E, Manson J l, Carter R F, Robertson E 1979 Electron microscopy of skin and peripheral blood lymphocytes in infantile (Santavaori) neuronal ceroid lipofuscinosis. Neuropediatrics 10: 245–263

307. Hazell S L, Lee A, Brady L, Hennessy W 1986 *Campylobacter pyloridis* and gastritis: association with intercellular spaces and adaptation to an environment of mucus as important factors in colonization of the gastric epithelium. Journal of Infectious Diseases 153: 658–663

308. Hedin C A, Larsson A 1984 The ultrastructure of the gingival epithelium in smokers' melanosis. Journal of Periodontal Research 19: 177–190

309. Hegewald G, Nikulin A, Gmaz-Nikulin E, Plamenac P, Barenwald G 1985 Ultrastructural changes of the human pancreas in acute shock. Pathology, Research and Practice 179: 610–615

310. Helin H, Mero M, Markkula H, Helin M 1980 Pancreatic acinar ultrastructure in human acute pancreatitis. Virchows Archiv A, Pathological Anatomy and Histology 387: 259–270

311. Hendel L, Kobayasi T, Petri M 1987 Ultrastructure of the small intestinal mucosa in progressive systemic sclerosis (PSS). Acta Pathologica, Microbiologica et Immunologica Scandinavica A 95: 41–46

312. Henrik-Nielsen R, Orholm M, Pedersen J O, Hovind-Hougen K, Teglbjaerg P S, Thayssen E H 1983 Colorectal spirochetosis: clinical significance of the infestation. Gastroenterology 85: 62–67

313. Henrik-Nielsen R, Lundbeck F A, Teglbjaerg P S, Ginnerup P, Hovind-Hougen K 1985 Intestinal spirochetosis of the vermiform appendix. Gastroenterology 88: 971–977

314. Henry K, Bird R G, Doe W F 1974 Intestinal coccidiosis in a patient with alpha-chain disease. British Medical Journal 1: 542–543

315. Henson D 1972 Cytomegalovirus inclusion bodies in the gastrointestinal tract. Archives of Pathology 93: 477–482

316. Herman L, Sato T, Fitzgerald P J 1964 The pancreas. In: Kurtz S M (ed) Electron microscopy anatomy. Academic Press, New York, pp S59–S95

317. Heuman R, Boeryd B, Bolin T, Magnusson K E, Sjodahl R, Tagesson C 1980 Subcellular fractionation of human intestinal mucosa by large-scale zonal centrifugation. Separation of the organelles in disease ileum of a patient with Crohn's disease. Acta Chirurgica Scandinavica 146: 195–201

318. Hiraide F, Nomura K 1978 Morphological studies on salivary calculi. Jibiinkou 50: 241–248

319. Hitzman J L, Weiland L H, Ofredahl G L, Lie J T 1979 Ceroidosis in the 'brown bowel syndrome'. Mayo Clinic Proceedings 54: 251–257

320. Hoffman B I, Katz W A 1980 The gastrointestinal manifestations of systemic lupus erythematosus: a review of the literature. Seminars in Arthritis and Rheumatism 9: 237–247

321. Hohling H J, Erpenstein H 1967 Elektronenmikroskopische Untersuchungen erblicher Schmelzhypoplasien, beobachtet an zwei Sippen. Deutsch Zahnaerztl Zeifschrift 22: 501–513

322. Holt S C, Tanner A C R, Socransky S S 1980 Morphology and ultrastructure of oral strains of *Acinobacillus actinomycetemcomitans* and *Haemophilus aphrophilus*. Infection and Immunity 30: 588–600

323. Honma T 1976 Electron microscopic study on the pathogenesis of recurrent aphthous ulceration as compared to Behcet's syndrome. Oral Surgery 41: 366–377

324. Honma T 1980 Electron microscopic observations of infiltrating neutrophils in aphthous ulceration in Behcet's disease. Acta Dermatologica and Venerealogica 60: 521–524

325. Honma T, Bang D, Saito T, Nakagawa S, Ueki H, Lee S 1987 Ultrastructure of lymphocyte-mediated fat-cell lysis in erythema nodosum-like lesions of Behcets's syndrome. Archives of Dermatology 123: 1650–1654

326. Honma T, Bang D, Saito T, Nakagawa S, Ueki H, Lee S 1988 Appearance of membranocystic lesion (Nasu)-like changes in Behcet's syndrome. An electron microscopic study of erythema nodosum-like lesions. Acta Pathologica Japonica 38: 1001–1010

327. Honma T, Saito T, Fujuioka Y 1981 Intraepithelial atypical lymphocytes in oral lesions in Behcet's syndrome. Archives of Dermatology 117: 83–85

328. Honma T, Saito T, Fujuioka Y 1985 Possible role of apoptotic cells of the oral epithelium in the pathogenesis of aphthous ulceration. Oral Surgery, Oral Medicine, Oral Pathology 59: 379–387

329. Hopwood D, Wood R, Milen G 1988 The fine structure and histochemistry of human bile duct in obstruction and choledocholithiasis. Journal of Pathology 155: 49–59

330. Horn T 1985 Brown bowel syndrome. Ultrastructural Pathology 8: 357–361

331. Hosler J P, Kimmel K R, Moeller D D 1982 The 'brown bowel syndrome': a case report. American Journal of Gastroenterology 77: 854–855

332. Hughes B R, Horne J 1988 Epidermolysis bullosa acquisita and total ulcerative colitis. Journal of the Royal Society of Medicine 81: 473–475

333. Hughes F J, Auger D W, Smales F C 1988 Investigation of the distribution of cementum-associated lipopolysaccharides in periodontal disease by scanning electron microscope immunohistochemistry. Journal of Periodontal Research 23: 100–106

334. Hurlen B, Olsen I 1984 A scanning electron microscopic study on the microflora of chronic pericoronitis of lower third molars. Oral Surgery, Oral Medicine, Oral Pathology 58: 522–532

335. Hunt R H 1984 Angiodysplasia of the colon. In: Salmon P R (ed) Gastrointestinal endoscopy: advances in diagnosis and therapy. Chapman & Hall, London, pp 97–114

336. Hussein K A, Milne G, Hopwood D 1988 Glycosaminoglycans in human gallbladder basement membrane: nature and quantitative changes in chronic cholecystis. Histochemical Journal 20: 449–454

337. Hwang W S, Kelly J K, Shaffer E A, Hershfield N B 1986 Collagenous colitis: a disease of pericryptal fibroblast sheath? Journal of Pathology 149: 33–40

338. Iancu T C, Lerner A, Shiloh H 1987 Intestinal mucosa in nephropathic cystinosis. Journal of Pediatric Gastroenterology and Nutrition 6: 359–364

339. Ikeda S, Ushiyama M, Nakano T, Kikkawa T, Kondo K, Yanagisawa N 1986 Ultrastructural findings of rectal and skin biopsies in adult GM_1-gangliosidosis. Acta Pathologica Japonica 36: 1823–1831

340. Isacson G, Friskopp J 1984 The morphology of salivary calculi. A scanning electron microscopic study. Acta Odontologica Scandinavica 42: 65–72

341. Ito Y, Tatekawa I, Nishiyama F, Hirano H 1987 Ultrastructural localization of acetylcholinesterase activity in Hirschsprung's disease. Archives of Pathology and Laboratory Medicine 111: 161–165

342. Ito H, Yokozaki H, Tokumo K, Nakajo S, Tahara E 1986 Serotonin-containing EC cells in normal human gastric mucosa and in gastritis. Immunohistochemical, electron microscopic and autoradiographic studies. Virchows Archiv A, Pathological Anatomy and Histology 409: 313–323

343. Jaffe R, Hashida V, Yunis E J 1980 Pancreatic pathology in hyperinsulinemic hypoglycemia of infancy. Laboratory Investigation 42: 356–365

344. Janisch H D, Fischer C, Savaser N A, Kleist V D, Hampel K E 1984 Esophageal motility in amyloidosis: manometry — scintigraphy — histology. Gastroenterology 86: 1124

345. Jansma J, Vissink A, 's-Gravenmade E J, de Josselin de Jon E,

Jongebloed W L, Retief D H 1988 A model to investigate xerostomia-related dental caries. Caries Research 22: 357–361

346. Jensen J L, Erickson J O 1974 Hyaline bodies in odontogenic cysts: electron microscopic observations. Journal of Oral Pathology 3: 1–6

347. Johansen E 1963 Ultrastructural and chemical observations on dental caries. In: Sognnaes R F (ed) Mechanisms of hard tissue destruction. American Association for the Advancement of Science, Washington, pp 75–187

348. Johnson L A, Wirostko E, Wirostko W J 1989 Crohn's disease uveitis. Parasitization of vitreous leukocytes by mollicute-like organisms. American Journal of Clinical Pathology 91: 259–264

349. Johnson N W 1967 Transmission electron microscopy of early carious enamel. Caries Research 1: 356–369

350. Jones D M, Lessells A M, Eldridge J 1984 *Campylobacter*-like organisms on the gastric mucosa: culture, histological and serological studies. Journal of Clinical Pathology 37: 1002–1006

351. Jones D M, Curry A, Fox A J 1985 An ultrastructural study of the gastric *Campylobacter*-like organism '*Campylobacter pyloridis*'. Journal of General Microbiology 131: 2335–2341

352. Jones R T, Garcia J H, Mergner W J, Mergner W J, Prendergrass R E, Valigorsky J M, Trump B F 1975 Effects of shock on the pancreatic acinar cell. Cellular and subcellular effects. Archives of Pathology 99: 634–644

353. Jones R T, Trump B F 1975 Cellular and subcellular effects of ischaemia on the pancreatic acinar cell. *In vitro* studies of rat tissue. Virchows Archiv B, Cell Pathology 19: 325–336

354. Jones S J, Lozdan J, Boyde A 1972 Tooth surfaces treated *in situ* with periodontal instruments. British Dental Journal 132: 57–64

355. Kaiserling E, Schäffer R, Weckermann J 1988 Brown bowel syndrome with manifestation in the gastrointestinal tract and thyroid gland. Pathology, Research and Practice 183: 65–79

356. Kameyama T, Kita K, Sujaku C, Watanabe T, Tateyama H 1987 A comparison of crystallinity of calculi by X-ray diffraction line broadening analysis for bilateral and concurrent submandibular sialolithiasis. Kurume Medical Journal 34: 29–34

357. Kameyama Y, Mizohata M, Takehana S, Murata H, Manabe H, Mukai Y 1983 Ultrastructure of the congenital epulis. Virchows Archiv A, Pathological Anatomy and Histology 401: 251–260

358. Kamiya R, Ide C, Yokota R 1984 Myelin figures in the basal-granulated cells of human Brunner's glands. Archivum Histologicum Japonicum 47: 337–343

359. Kanerva L, Hietanen J 1984 Electron microscopy of composite and intranuclear keratohyalin granules in geographic tongue of psoriasis. Journal of Cutaneous Pathology 11: 149–153

360. Kang J Y, Wu A Y, Chia J L, Wee A, Sutherland I H, Hori R 1987 Clinical and ultrastructural studies in duodenal pseudomelanosis. Gut 28: 1673–1681

361. Kaufman H S, Magnuson T H, Lillemoe K D, Frasca P, Pitt H A 1989 The role of bacteria in gallbladder and common duct stone formation. Annals of Surgery 209: 584–591 (discussion 591–592)

362. Kawamata S, Kubota Y, Sawataishi M, Takaya K 1986 The fine structure of atypical ciliated cells in the human gastric epithelium. Virchows Archiv B, Cell Pathology 51: 363–374

363. Kazlow P G, Shah K, Benkov K J, Dische R, LeLeiko N S 1986 Esophageal cryptosporidiosis in a child with acquired immunodeficiency syndrome. Gastroenterology 91: 1301–1303

364. Kermarec J, Duplay H, Daniel R 1972 Etude histochimique et ultrastructurale comparative des pigments de la melanose colique et du syndrome de Dubin-Johnson. Annales de Biologie Clinique 30: 567–577

365. Kerébel B, Daculsi G 1976 Amelogenesis imperfecta. Etude structurale ultrastructurale et radiocristallographique. Journal de Biologie Buccale 4: 43–60

366. Kerébel B, Daculsi G 1976 Etude ultrastructurale et cristallographique de l'email humain dans la fluorose endemique. Journal de Biologie Buccale 4: 143–154

367. Keush G T, Donohue-Rolfe A, Jacewicz M 1982 Shigella toxin(s): description and role in diarrhoea and dysentery. Pharmacology and Therapeutics 15: 403–438

368. Khokholia V P, Medvetskii E B, Abrosimova L P, Bury A N 1985 Ultrastructural changes in the gastric mucosa in acute erosive-ulcerative lesions. Vrachebnoe Delo 4: 81–84

369. Kihara S, Mori K, Akagi M 1983 Electron microscopic observation

370. Kirk M E, Lough J, Warner H A 1971 Histoplasma colitis: an electron microscopic study. Gastroenterology 61: 46–54

371. Kisilevsky R 1983 Biology of disease. Amyloidosis: a familiar problem in the light of current pathogenetic developments. Laboratory Investigation 49: 381–390

372. Kjorell U, Ostberg Y 1984 Distribution of intermediate filaments and actin microfilaments in parotid autoimmune sialoadenitis of Sjogren syndrome. Histopathology 8: 991–1011

373. Klein-Szanto A J, Andersen L, Schroeder H E 1976 Epithelial differentiation patterns in buccal mucosa affected by lichen planus. Virchows Archiv B, Cell Pathology 22: 245–261

374. Kloppel G, Altenaehr E, Reichel W, Willig R, Freytagi G 1974 The ultrastructure of focal islet cell adenomatosis in the newborn with hypoglycemia and hyperinsulinemia. Diabetologia 127: 75–89

375. Kloppel G 1981 Endokrines pankreas und diabetes mellitus. In: Doerr W, Seifert G (eds) Pathologie der endokrinen organe, vol. 41/I. Springer, Berlin, Heidelberg, New York, pp 523–728

376. Kloppel G, Dreyer T, Willemer S, Kern H F, Adler G 1986 Human acute pancreatitis: its pathogenesis in the light of immunocytochemical and ultrastructural findings in acinar cells. Virchows Archiv A, Pathological Anatomy and Histology 409: 791–803

377. Knapp A B, Horst D A, Eliopoulos G, Gramm H F, Gaber L W, Falchuk K R, Falchuk Z M, Trey C 1983 Widespread cytomegalovirus gastroenterocolitis in a patient with acquired immunodeficiency syndrome. Gastroenterology 85: 1399–1402

378. Kobayashi K 1966 Electron microscope studies of the Langerhans islets in the toad pancreas. Archivum Histologicum Japonicum 26: 439–482

379. Kobayashi Y, Suzuki H, Konno T, Tada K, Yamamoto T Y 1983 Ultrastructural alterations of Paneth cells in infants associated with gastrointestinal symptoms. Tohoku Journal of Experimental Medicine 139: 225–230

380. Kohl D, Ashkenazi A, Ben-Shaul Y, Bacher A 1987 Tight junctions of jejunal surface and crypt cells in celiac disease: a freeze–fracture study. Journal of Pediatric Gastroenterology and Nutrition 6: 57–65

381. Kojimahara M, Kamita Y 1986 Endothelial cells in the rectal venous plexus. An electron microscopic study. Journal of Submicroscopic Cytology 18: 807–814

382. Konishi H, Hirose H, Nakazawa T, Kochiyama T, Shigeeda M, Takemoto T 1988 Electron microscopy of *Campylobacter pylori* on human gastric mucosa. In: Takemoto T (ed) Proceeding of the First Tokyo International Symposium on *Campylobacter pylori*. Taisho Pharmaceutical, Tokyo, pp 49–53

383. Kooijman C D, Poen H 1984 Whipple-like disease in AIDS. Histopathology 8: 705–708

384. Kopping H S, Koppang R, Solheim T, Aarnes H, Stolen·S O 1987 Identification of cellulose fibres in oral biopsies. Scandinavian Journal of Dental Research 95: 165–173

385. Kotler D P, Gaetz H P, Lange M, Klein E B, Holt P R 1984 Enteropathy associated with AIDS. American Journal of Internal Medicine 101: 421–428

386. Kotler D P, Weaver S C, Terzakis J A 1986 Ultrastructural features of epithelial cell degeneration in rectal crypts of patients with AIDS. American Journal of Surgical Pathology 10: 531–538

387. Kovi J, Duong H D, Hoang C T 1981 Ultrastructure of intestinal lymphatics in Crohn's disease. American Journal of Clinical Pathology 76: 385–394

388. Krishnamurthy S, Kelly M M, Rohrmann C A, Schuffler M D 1983 Jejunal diverticulosis: a heterogeneous disorder caused by a variety of abnormalities of smooth muscle or myenteric plexus. Gastroenterology 85: 538–547

389. Krishnamurthy S, Schuffler M D, Belic L, Schweid A 1986 An inflammatory axonopathy of the myenteric plexus causing rapidly progressive intestinal pseudo-obstruction. Gastroenterology 90: 754–758

390. Kullaa-Mikkonen A 1986 Geographic tongue: an SEM study. Journal of Cutaneous Pathology 13: 154–162

391. Kullaa-Mikkonen A 1986 Studies on lingua fissurata. Proceedings of the Finnish Dental Society 82 (suppl 4): 1–48

392. Kullaa-Mikkonen A, Sorvari T E 1986 A scanning electron microscopic study of fissured tongue. Journal of Oral Pathology 15: 93–97

393. Kullaa-Mikkonen A, Sorvari T, Kotilainen R 1985 Morphological variations on the dorsal surface of the human tongue. Proceedings of the Finnish Dental Society 81: 104–110

394. Kumagae Y, Sashojima K, Hashimoto M, Numajiri H, Tokunaga A, Tanaka N, Shirota A, Asano G 1981 Cytochemical localization of alkaline phosphatase in intestinal metaplasia of the human stomach. Histochemical Journal 13: 57–62

395. Kumar P J, Dawson A M 1972 Vasculitis of the alimentary tract. Clinical Gastroenterology 1: 719–743

396. Kundrotas L, Novak J, Kremzier J, Meenaghan M, Hassett J 1988 Gastric bleeding in pseudoxanthoma elasticum. American Journal of Gastroenterology 83: 868–872

397. Labeille B, Gineston J L, Denoeux J P, Capron J P 1988 Epidermolysis bullosa acquisita and Crohn's disease. A case report with immunological and electron microscopic studies. Archives of Internal Medicine 148: 1457–1459

398. Lambert J R, Luk S C, Pritzker K P 1980 Brown bowel syndrome in Crohn's disease. Archives of Pathology and Laboratory Medicine 104: 201–205

399. Lamberty J, Varela P Y, Font R G, Jarvis B W, Coover J 1974 Whipple's disease: light and electron microscopy study. Archives of Pathology 98: 325–330

400. Lampert I A, Thorpe P, Van Noorden S, Marsh J, Goldman J M, Gordon-Smith E C, Evans D J 1985 Selective sparing of enterochromaffin cells in graft-versus-host disease affecting the colonic mucosa. Histopathology 9: 875–886

401. Laschi R, Govoni E 1986 Cell ultrastructure in disease. Scanning Electron Microscopy 1: 193–198

402. Laschi R, Pasquinelli G, Versura P 1987 Scanning electron microscopy application in clinical research. Scanning Electron Microscopy 1: 1771–1795

403. Lasho D J, O'Leary T J, Kafrawy A H 1983 A scanning electron microscope study of the effects of various agents on instrumented periodontally involved root surfaces. Journal of Periodontology 54: 210–220

404. Lauriola L, Musiani P, Bracaglia R, Maggiano N, Dina M A 1984 Congenital epulis: an ultrastructural and immunohistochemical study. Applied Pathology 2: 153–159

405. Lee A, O'Rourke J L, Barrington P J, Trust T J 1986 Mucus colonization as a determinant of pathogenicity in intestinal infection by Campylobacter jejuni: a mouse cecal model. Infection and Immunity 51: 536–546

406. Lee A, Dent J, Hazell S, McNulty C 1988 Origin of spiral organisms in human gastric antrum. Lancet i: 300–301

407. Lee A 1989 Human gastric spirilla other than C. pylori. In: Blaser M J (ed) Campylobacter pylori in gastritis and peptic ulcer disease. Igaku-Shoin, New York and Tokyo, pp 225–240

408. Lee F D 1989 The anal region: specific and non-specific inflammatory lesions. In: Whitehead R (ed) Gastrointestinal and oesophageal pathology. Churchill Livingstone, Edinburgh, pp 541–549

409. Lee H H, O'Donnell D B, Keren D F 1987 Characteristics of melanosis duodeni: incorporation of endoscopy, pathology and etiology. Endoscopy 19: 107–109

410. Lee H C, Kay S 1958 Primary polyarteritis nodosa of the stomach and small intestine as a cause of gastrointestinal haemorrhage. Annals of Surgery 147: 714–725

411. Lee K T, Ching Sheen P 1988 Effect of gallstones on pancreatic acinar cells. An ultrastructural study. European Surgical Research 20: 341–351

412. Lefkowitch J H, Krumholz S, Feng-Chen K C, Griffin P, Despommier D, Brasitus T A 1984 Cryptosporidiosis of the human small intestine: a light and electron microscopic study. Human Pathology 15: 746–752

413. Legge D A, Wollaeger E E, Carlson H C 1970 Intestinal pseudo-obstruction in systemic amyloidosis. Gut 11: 764–767

414. Lehner T 1969 Pathology of recurrent oral ulcerations and oral ulceration in Behcet's syndrome: light, electron and fluorescence microscopy. Journal of Pathology 97: 481–494

415. Lehner T, Sagebiel R W 1966 Fine structural findings in recurrent oral ulceration. British Dental Journal 121: 454–456

416. Leport C, Bruneval P, Tricottet V, Leport J, Camilleri J P, Vilde J L 1984 Presence of ultrastructural markers of AIDS in rectal biopsies at the early stage of the disease. Gastroenterologie Clinique et Biologique 8: 983–984

417. Leung J W, Ling T K, Kung J L, Vallance-Owen J 1988 The role of bacteria in the blockage of biliary stents. Gastrointestinal Endoscopy 34: 19–22

418. Levine D S, Rubin C E, Reid B J, Haggitt R C 1989 Specialised metaplastic columnar epithelium in Barrett's oesophagus. A comparative transmission electron microscopic study. Laboratory Investigation 60: 418–432

419. Levison D A, Crocker P R, Boxall T A, Randall K J 1986 Coconut matting bezoar identified by a combined analytical approach. Journal of Clinical Pathology 39: 172–175

420. Lewin K J, Harrell G S, Lee A S, Crowley L G 1974 Malacoplakia. An electron microscopic study: demonstration of bacilliform organisms in malacoplakic macrophages. Gastroenterology 66: 28–45

421. Lewis D, Walker-Smith J A, Phillips A D 1984 Microvilli- and desmosome-associated bodies in Crohn's disease and other disorders in childhood: an ultrastructural abnormality of the small and large intestine. Journal of Pediatric Gastroenterology and Nutrition 3: 46–55

422. Lin H-J, Tsay S-H, Chiang H, Tsai Y-T, Lee S-D, Yeh Y-S, Lo G-H 1988 Pseudomelanosis duodeni. Case report and review of the literature. Journal of Clinical Gastroenterology 10: 155–159

423. Lindskog S, Blomlof L 1983 Cementum hypoplasia in teeth affected by juvenile periodontitis. Journal of Clinical Periodontology 10: 443–451

424. Listgarten M A 1965 Electron microscopic observations on the bacterial flora of acute necrotizing ulcerative gingivitis. Journal of Periodontology 36: 328–339

425. Listgarten M A 1967 A mineralized cuticular structure with connective tissue characteristics on the crown of human unerupted teeth in amelogenesis imperfecta. A light and electron microscopic study. Archives of Oral Biology 12: 877–889

426. Listgarten M A 1972 Electron microscopic study of the junction between surgically denuded root surfaces and regenerated periodontal tissues. Journal of Periodontal Research 7: 64–79

427. Listgarten M A 1976 Structure of the microbial flora associated with periodontal health and disease in man. A light and electron microscopic study. Journal of Periodontology 47: 1–18

428. Liu T H 1987 A scanning electron microscopic study of normal and diseased jejunal mucosa. Chung-hua Ping Li Hsueh Tsa Chi 16: 110–112

429. Lockard V G, Boler R K 1970 Ultrastructure of a spiralled microorganism in the gastric mucosa of dogs. American Journal of Veterinary Research 31: 1453–1462

430. Loft D E, Marsh M N, Sandle G I, Crowe P T, Garner V, Gordon D, Baker R 1989 Studies of intestinal lymphoid tissue. XII. Epithelial lymphocyte and mucosal responses to rectal gluten challenge in coeliac sprue. Gastroenterology 97: 27–37

431. Lombeck I, von Bassewitz D B, Becker K, Tinschmann P, Kastner H 1974 Ultrastructural findings in acrodermatitis enteropathica. Pediatric Research 8: 82–88

432. Lopes E R, Tafur W L, Chapadeiro E 1969 Estudo mortologico & quantitativo dos nucleos dorsal de vago & hipoglosso em Chagasicos eronicos com & sem megaesofago. Revista de Instituto de Medicina Tropical de Sao Paulo 11: 123–129

433. Lou T Y, Teplitz C 1974 Malakoplakia: pathogenesis and ultrastructural morphogenesis. Human Pathology 5: 191–207

434. Lowes J R, Rode J 1989 Neuroendrocrine cell proliferations in gastric antral vascular ectasia. Gastroenterology 97: 207–212

435. McClurg F V, D'Agostino N A, Martin J H, Race G J 1973 Ultrastructural demonstration of intracellular bacteria in three cases of malakoplakia of the bladder. American Journal of Clinical Pathology 60: 780–788

436. McDowell E M, Beals T F 1986 Biopsy pathology of the bronchi. Chapman & Hall, London, pp 140–191

437. McGregor D, Pierce G E, Thomas J H, Tilzer L L 1980 Obstructive lesions of the distal mesenteric arteries. Archives of Laboratory Medicine 104: 79–83

438. McGregor D H, MacArthur R I, Carter T 1986 Avitene granulomas of colonic serosa. Annals of Clinical and Laboratory Science 16: 296–302

439. McKay J S, Day D W 1983 Herpes simplex oesophagitis. Histopathology 7: 409–420

440. McMillan A, Lee F D 1981 Sigmoidoscopic and microscopic appearance of the rectal mucosa in homosexual men. Gut 22: 1035–1041

441. McNulty C A, Dent J C, Curry A, Uff J S, Ford G A, Gear M W, Wilkinson S P 1989 New spiral bacterium in gastric mucosa. Journal of Clinical Pathology 42: 585–591

442. McNulty C A M, Gearty J C, Crump B, Davis M, Donovan I A, Melikian V, Lister D M, Wise R 1986 Campylobacter pyloridis and associated gastritis: investigator blind, placebo controlled trial of bismuth salicylate and erythromycin ethylsuccinate. British Medical Journal 293: 645–649

443. Madara J L, Trier J S 1980 Structural abnormalities of jejunal epithelial cell membranes in celiac sprue. Laboratory Investigation 43: 254–261

444. Maizel H, Ruffin J M, Dobbins W O III 1970 Whipple's disease: a review of 19 patients from one hospital and a review of the literature since 1950. Medicine 49: 175–205

445. Malfertheine P, Bode G, Mader U, Baozako K, Stanescu A, Ditschuneit H 1985 Histological and ultrastructural findings in the healing phase of duodenal ulcer. Klinische Wochenschrift 63: 1061–1070

446. Mangla J C, Lee C S 1979 Scanning electron microscopy of Barrett's oesophageal mucosa. Gastrointestinal Endoscopy 25: 92–94

447. Mansbach C M II, Shelburne J D, Stevens R D, Dobbins W O III 1978 Lymph-node bacilliform bodies resembling those of Whipple's disease in a patient without intestinal involvement. Annals of Internal Medicine 89: 64–66

448. Marin M L, Greenstein A J, Geller S A, Gordon R E, Aufses A H Jr 1983 A freeze fracture study of Crohn's disease of the terminal ileum: changes in epithelial tight junction organisation. American Journal of Gastroenterology 78: 537–547

449. Marin M L, Greenstein A J, Geller S A, Gordon R E, Aufses A H Jr 1984 Freeze-fracture analysis of epithelial cell lysosomal inclusions in Crohn's disease. Ultrastructural Pathology 6: 39–44

450. Marsh M N 1981 Studies of intestinal lymphoid tissue: the cytology and electron microscopy of gluten-sensitive enteropathy, with particular reference to its immunopathology Scandinavian Journal of Gastroenterology (suppl) 70: 65–85

451. Marshall B 1983 Unidentified curved bacilli on gastric epithelium in active chronic gastritis. Lancet i: 1273–1274

452. Marshall B J, Royce H, Annear D I, Goodwin C S, Pearman J W, Warren J R, Armstrong J A 1984 Original isolation of Campylobacter pyloridis from human gastric mucosa. Microbios Letters 25: 83–88

453. Marshall B J, Warren J R 1984 Unidentified curved bacilli in the stomach of patients with gastritis and peptic ulceration. Lancet i: 1311–1314

454. Marshall B J, McGechie D B, Rogers P A, Clancy R J 1985 Pyloric campylobacter infection and gastroduodenal disease. Medical Journal of Australia 142: 439–444

455. Marshall B J, Armstrong J A, Francis G J, Nokes N T, Wee S H 1987 Antibacterial action of bismuth in relation to Campylobacter pyloridis colonization and gastritis. Digestion 37 (suppl 2): 16–30

456. Marshall B J, Goodwin C S, Warren J R, Murray R, Blincow E D, Blackbourn S J, Phillips M, Waters T E, Sanderson C R 1988 Prospective double-blind trial of duodenal ulcer relapse after eradication of Campylobacter pylori. Lancet ii: 1437–1442

457. Mathan M, Mathan V I, Baker S J 1975 An electron microscopic study of jejunal mucosal morphology in control subjects and in patients with tropical sprue in southern India. Gastroenterology 68: 17–32

458. Mathan M, Ponniah J, Mathan V I 1986 Epithelial cell renewal and turnover and its relationship to morphologic abnormalities in the jejunal mucosa in tropical sprue. Digestive Diseases and Sciences 31: 586–592

459. Mathan M M, Mathan V I 1986 Ultrastructural pathology of the rectal mucosa in Shigella dysentery. American Journal of Pathology 123: 25–38

460. Matson D O, Estes M K, Glass R I, Bartlett A V, Penaranda M, Calomeni E, Tanaka T, Nakata S, Chiba S 1989 Human calicivirus-associated diarrhoea in children attending day care centers. Journal of Infective Diseases 159: 71–78

461. Meiselman M S, Cello J P, Margaretten W 1985 Cytomegalovirus colitis: report of the clinical, endoscopic and pathologic findings in two patients with the acquired immune deficiency syndrome. Gastroenterology 88: 171–175

462. Melmed R N 1979 Intermediate cells of the pancreas, an appraisal. Gastroenterology 76: 196–201

463. Melski J W, Murphy G F 1980 Progressive neurologic disorder and abdominal pain in an 18 year old woman. New England Journal of Medicine 303: 1103–1111

464. Mera S L, Lovell C, Davies J D 1986 Light microscopy, immunohistochemistry and electron microscopy of actinic elastosis in the skin. Journal of Pathology 149: 253A

465. Meyer K, Lie T 1977 Root surface roughness in response to periodontal instrumentation studied by combined use of microroughness measurements and scanning electron microscopy. Journal of Clinical Periodontology 4: 77–91

466. Miller D R, Lamster I B, Chasens A J 1984 Role of polymorphonuclear leukocytes in periodontal health and disease. Journal of Clinical Periodontology 11: 1–15

467. Mills L R, Schuman B M, Assad R T, Spurlock B O, Drew P A 1989 Scanning electron microscopy of dysplastic Barrett's epithelium. Modern Pathology 2: 112–116

468. Mincer H H, McCoy J M, Turner J E 1979 Pulse granuloma of the alveolar ridge. Oral Surgery 48: 126–130

469. Miyake M, Ishii T, Andoh M, Takayama Y, Tohyama Y, Hori M, Fujuisaki Y, Asahina H, Tanaka H, Sato H 1987 Submandibular gland sialolithiasis-sialographic and pathologic findings with evaluation using SEM and EPMA analysis. Journal of Nihon University School of Dentistry 29: 112–123

470. Mohamed A H 1975 Ultrastructural aspects of chronic oral candidosis. Journal of Oral Pathology 4: 180–196

471. Moneret-Vautrin D A, De Korwin J D, Tisserant J, Grignon M, Claudot N 1984 Ultrastructural study of the mast cells of the human duodenal mucosa. Clinical Allergy 14: 471–481

472. Montes L F, Wilborn W H 1968 Ultrastructural features of host-parasite relationship in oral candidosis. Journal of Bacteriology 96: 1349–1356

473. Morecki R, Parker J G 1967 Ultrastructural studies of the human Giardia lamblia and subjacent jejunal mucosa in a subject with steatorrhoea. Gastroenterology 52: 151–164

474. Morgan P R, Johnson N W 1974 Histological, histochemical and ultrastructural studies on the nature of hyalin bodies in odontogenic cysts. Journal of Oral Pathology 3: 127

475. Mortimer K V, Tranter T C 1971 A scanning electron microscope study of carious enamel. Caries Research 5: 240–263

476. Moshal M G, Gregory M A, Pillay C, Spitaels J M 1979 Does the duodenal cell ever return to normal? A comparison between treatment with cimetidine and De Nol. Scandinavian Journal of Gastroenterology 14: 48–51

477. Mowat A M, Ferguson A 1982 Intraepithelial lymphocyte count and crypt hyperplasia measure the mucosal component of the graft-versus-host reaction in mouse small intestine. Gastroenterology 83: 417–423

478. Muller J C, Jones A L, Brandbogh L L 1973 Scanning electron microscope observations in human giardiasis. Scannning Electron Microscopy. 557–564

479. Müller K-M, Müller G 1983 The ultrastructure of preneoplastic changes in the bronchial mucosa. Current Topics in Pathology 73: 233–263

480. Myllarniemi H, Nickels J 1980 Scanning electron microscopy of Crohn's disease and ulcerative colitis of the colon. Virchows Archiv A, Pathological Anatomy and Histology 385: 343–350

481. Nagata A, Yoshizawa S, Homma T, Oda M 1977 Comparative studies of experimental pancreatic injuries with human chronic pancreatitis by electron microscopy. Japanese Journal of Gastroenterology 74: 1650–1659

482. Nagle G J, Kurtz S M 1967 Electron microscopy of the human rectal mucosa: a comparison of idiopathic ulcerative colitis with

inflammation of known aetiologies. American Journal of Digestive Diseases 12: 541–567

483. Nasemann T 1974 Viruskrankheiten der Haut, der Schleimhaute und des Genitales. Georg Thieme Verlag, Stuttgart

484. Nassar A M, El Tantawy S A, Khalifa S, Abdel Fattah S, Abdel Hamid J 1980 Ultrastructural changes in the mucosa of the small intestine due to protein–calorie malnutrition. Journal of Tropical Pediatrics 26: 62–72

485. Neutra M R 1980 Prokaryotic–eukaryotic cell junctions: attachment of spirochetes and flagellated bacteria to primate large intestinal cells. Journal of Ultrastructure Research 70: 186–203

486. Nevalainen T, Laitio M 1972 Ultrastructure of gall bladder with cholesterolosis. Virchows Archiv B, Cell Pathology 10: 237–242

487. Newcomb G M, Powell R N 1986 The ultrastructure of human gingival Langerhans cells in health and disease. Archives of Oral Biology 31: 727–734

488. Newcomb G M, Seymour G J, Powell R N 1982 Association between plaque accumulation and Langerhans' cell numbers in the oral epithelium of attached gingiva. Journal of Clinical Periodontology 9: 297–304

489. Newman M G, Saglie R, Carranza F A Jr, Kaufman A K 1984 Mycoplasma in periodontal disease. Isolation in juvenile periodontitis. Journal of Periodontology 55: 574–580

490. Nielsen H O, Hage E 1987 The antral gastrin-producing cells in duodenal ulcer patients. A light microscopic and ultrastructural study during long-term, low dose treatment with cimetidine. Virchows Archiv A, Pathological Anatomy and Histology 411: 99–101

491. Nielsen H, Madsen P E, Christiansen L A 1980 The parietal cells in duodenal ulcer patients. A quantitative ultrastructural study before and during treatment with cimetidine. Scandinavian Journal of Gastroenterology 15: 793–797

492. Nielsen R H, Orholm M, Pedersen J O, Hovind-Hougen K, Teglbjaerg P S, Thaysen E H 1983 Colorectal spirochetosis: clinical significance of the infestation. Gastroenterology 85: 62–67

493. Nikai H, Rose G G, Cattoni M 1971 Electron microscopic study of chronic desquamative gingivitis. Journal of Periodontic Research 6: 6–17

494. Nikulin A, Hegewald G, Gmaz-Nijulin E, Plamenac P 1981 Ultrastructural changes in human pancreas during the early shock phase. Berliner Akadamische Wissenschaften Slowenien pp 57–64

495. Noronha M, Almeida M J F D, Dreiling D A, Bordalo O 1981 Alcohol and the pancreas I. Clinical associations and histopathology of minimal pancreatic inflammation. American Journal of Gastroenterology 76: 114–119

496. Noronha M, Bordalo O, Dreiling D A 1981 Alcohol and the pancreas II. Pancreatic morphology of advanced alcoholic pancreatitis. American Journal of Gastroenterology 76: 12–14

497. Noronha M, Dreiling D A, Bordalo O 1983 Sequential changes from minimal pancreatic inflammation to advanced alcoholic pancreatitis. Zeitschrift für Gastroenterologie 21: 666–673

498. Novak J M, Collins J T, Donowitz M, Farman J, Sheahan D G, Spiro H M 1979 Effects of radiation on the human gastrointestinal tract. Journal of Clinical Gastroenterology 1: 9–39

499. Nyhlin H, Stenling R 1984 The small intestinal mucosa in patients with Crohn's disease assessed by scanning electron and light microscopy. Scandinavian Journal of Gastroenterology 19: 433–440

500. O'Connor J J 1972 An electron microscopic study of inflammatory colonic disease. Diseases of Colon and Rectum 15: 265–277

501. Onge G S, Bezahler G H 1982 Giant esophageal ulcer associated with cytomegalovirus. Gastroenterology 83: 127–130

502. Ongradi J, Sallay K, Kulcsar G, Dan P, Horvath J, Nasz I 1984 Absorption of viruses into oral lymphocytes and decreased antibacterial activity of oral polymorphonuclear leukocytes. Acta Microbiologica Hungarica 31: 179–185

503. Otto H F, Gebbers J O 1981 Electron microscopic, ultracytochemical and immunohistological observations in Crohn's disease of the ileum and colon. Virchows Archiv A, Pathological Anatomy and Histology 391: 189–205

504. Ovčinnikov N M, Delektorskij V V 1971 Electron microscope studies of gonococci in the urethral sections of patients with gonorrhoea. British Journal of Venereal Diseases 47: 419–479

505. Page R C, Sims T J, Greissler F, Atlman L C, Baab D A 1984 Abnormal leukocyte motility in patients with early onset periodontitis. Journal of Periodontal Research 19: 591–594

506. Palo J, Haltia M, Carpenter S, Karpati G, Mushynski W 1984 Neurofilament subunit-related proteins in neuronal intranuclear inclusions. Annals of Neurology 15: 322–328

507. Panikar C K J, Mathew S, Mathan M 1982 Rotavirus and acute diarrhoeal disease in children in a Southern Indian coastal town. Bulletin of the World Health Organisation 60: 123–127

508. Patane R, Bottaro G, Ricca O, Galasso S 1982 Scanning electron microscopy (SEM) aspects of intestinal mucosal surface in childhood coeliac disease. Pediatrica Medica Chirurgica 4: 257–262

509. Patel H, Norman M G, Perry T L, Berry K E 1985 Multiple system atrophy with neuronal intranuclear hyaline inclusions. Report of a case and review of the literature. Journal of Neurological Science 67: 57–65

510. Paull G, Yardley J H 1989 Pathology of *C. pylori*-associated gastric and esophageal lesions. In: Blaser M J (ed) *Campylobacter pylori* in gastritis and peptic ulcer disease. Igaku-Shoin, New York, Tokyo, pp 73–97

511. Pavelka M, Ellinger A, Gangl A 1983 Effects of colchicine on rat small intestinal absorptive cells. 1. Formation of basolateral microvillous borders. Journal of Ultrastructure Research 85: 249–259

512. Pead P J 1979 Electron microscopy of *Campylobacter jejuni*. Journal of Medical Microbiology 12: 383–385

513. Perrone T L, Dickersin G R 1983 The intracellular location of cryptosporidia. Human Pathology 14: 1092–1093

514. Philipsen H P, Fejerskov O, Donatsky O, Hjorting-Hansen E 1976 Ultrastructure of epithelial lining of kerato-cytes in nevoid basal cell carcinoma syndrome. International Journal of Oral Surgery 5: 71–81

515. Phillips A D 1981 Small intestinal mucosa in childhood in health and disease. Scandinavian Journal of Gastroenterology (suppl) 70: 65–85

516. Phillips A D, Jenkins P, Raafat F, Walker-Smith J A 1985 Congenital microvillous atrophy: specific diagnostic features. Archives of Diseases in Childhood 60(2): 135–140

517. Pietersen A S, Leong A S Y, Rowland R 1985 The mucosal changes and pathogenesis of pneumatosis cystoides intestinalis. Human Pathology 16: 683–688

518. Pillay C V, Moshal M G, Bryer J V, Booyens J 1977 Ultrastructure of duodenal epithelial cells in patients with active duodenal ulcers and after treatment with Cimetidine. South African Medical Journal 52: 1082–1085

519. Piris J 1989 The small intestine: Part III. Malabsorption and protein intolerance. In: Whitehead R (ed) Gastrointestinal and oesophageal pathology. Churchill Livingstone, Edinburgh, pp 468–496

520. Pittman F E, Humphrey C D, Charleston S C 1974 Colitis following oral lincomycin therapy. Archives of Internal Medicine 134: 368–372

521. Pittman F E, Pittman J C, Ferrans V J, Harkin J C, Weichert J C 1969 Secondary amyloidosis of human colonic mucosa: light and electron microscopic findings. American Journal of Digestive Diseases 14: 356–367

522. Polanco I, Nistal M, Guerrero J, Vazquez C 1976 Letter: acrodermatitis enteropathica, zinc and ultrastructural lesions in Paneth cells. Lancet i: 430

523. Poley J R 1983 Chronic non-specific diarrhoea in children. Investigations of the surface morphology of small bowel mucosa utilizing the scanning electron microscope. Journal of Paediatric Gastroentrology and Nutrition 2: 71–94

524. Poley J R 1983 The small bowel mucosa in disease states characterized by chronic diarrhoea: observations by scanning electron microscopy. Scanning Electron Microscopy 3: 1293–1306

525. Poley J R, Klein A W 1983 Scanning electron microscopy of soy protein-induced damage of small bowel mucosa in infants. Journal of Pediatric Gastroenterology and Nutrition 2: 271–287

526. Poley J R, Rosenfeld S 1982 Malabsorption in giardiasis: presence of a luminal barrier (mucoid peudomembrane). Journal of Pediatric Gastroenterology and Nutrition 1: 63–80

527. Poley J R 1988 Loss of the glycocalyx of enterocytes in small intestine: a feature detected by scanning electron microscopy in children with gastrointestinal intolerance to dietary protein. Journal

of Pediatric Gastroenterology and Nutrition 7: 386–394

528. Portela-Gomes G, Martins M M, Correia J P 1974 Ultrastructural changes in jejunal epithelial cells in liver cirrhosis. Scandinavian Journal of Gastroenterology 9: 657–663

529. Potashov L V, Sidorov A I, Nevorotin A I 1984 Degenerative changes in the cellular ultrastructure of the pancreas in patients with compression stenosis of the celiac trunk. Klinicheskaia Khirurgiia 11: 61–62

530. Pounder D J, Ghadially F N, Mukherjee T M, Hecker R, Rowland R, Dixon B, Lalonde J-M A 1982 Ultrastructure and electron-probe X-ray analysis of the pigment in melanosis duodeni. Journal of Submicroscopic Cytology 14: 389–400

531. Press M F, Riddel R H, Ringus J 1980 Cytomegalovirus inclusion disease: its occurrence in the myenteric plexus of a renal transplant patient. Archives of Pathology and Laboratory Medicine 104: 580–583

532. Pullon P A 1969 Ultrastructure of oral lichen planus. Oral Surgery 28: 365–371

533. Puri P, Fujimoto T 1988 Diagnosis of allied functional bowel disorders using monoclonal antibodies and electron microscopy. Journal of Pediatric Surgery 23: 546–554

534. Quinn T C, Corey L, Chaffee R G, Schuffler M D, Holmes K K 1980 Campylobacter proctitis in a homosexual man. Annals of Internal Medicine 93: 458–459

535. Rabaneck L, Boyko W J, McLean D M, McLeod W A, Wong K K 1986 Unusual esophageal ulcers containing enveloped virus-like particles in homosexual men. Gastroenterology 90: 1882–1889

536. Rajagopal U, Mathur S K, Kartha V B, Prasad G E 1988 Pigment calculi — structure and composition. Indian Journal of Gastroenterology 7: 9–11

537. Ramachandran Nair P N 1987 Light and electron microscopic studies of root canal flora and periapical lesions. Journal of Endodontics 13: 29–39

538. Ranchod M, Kahn L B 1972 Malacoplakia of the gastrointestinal tract. Archives of Pathology 94: 90–97

539. Rao R N, Hilliard K, Wray C H 1983 Widespread intimal hyperplasia of small arteries and arterioles. Archives of Pathology and Laboratory Medicine 107: 254–257

540. Rapola J, Haltia M 1973 Cytoplasmic inclusions in the vermiform appendix and skeletal muscle in two types of so-called neuronal ceroid–lipofuscinosis. Brain 96: 833–840

541. Rauws E A J, Langenberg W, Houthoff H J, Zanen H C, Tytgat G N J 1988 Campylobacter pyloridis-associated chronic active antral gastritis: prospective study of its prevalence and the effects of antibacterial and antiulcer treatment. Gastroenterology 94: 229–238

542. Reeders J W A J, Tytgat G N J, Rosenbusch G, Gratama S 1984 Ischaemic colitis. Martinus Nijhoff, Boston

543. Reichart P A, Metah D, Althoff J 1985 Ultrastructural aspects of oral and facial lepromatous lesions. International Journal of Oral Surgery 14: 55–60

544. Remmele W, Engelsing B 1984 Lipid islands of the esophagus. Case report. Endoscopy 16: 240–241

545. Remmele W, Beck K, Kaiserling E 1988 Multiple lipid islands of the colonic mucosa. A light and electron microscopic study. Pathology, Research and Practice 183: 336–346

546. Remmele W, Mayer R, Gnauck H, Bettendorf U, Kanzler G 1978 Lipidinseln der Magenschleimhaut. Leber, Magen, Darm 8: 191–197

547. Resta S, Luby J P, Rosenfeld C R, Siegel J D 1985 Isolation and propagation of a human enteric coronavirus. Science 229: 978–981

548. Riemann J F 1977 Further electron microscopic evidence of virus-like particles in Crohn's disease. Acta Hepatogastroenterologica 24: 116–118

549. Riemann J F, Schmidt H, Zimmermann W 1980 The fine structure of colonic submucosal nerves in patients with chronic laxative abuse. Scandinavian Journal of Gastroenterology 15: 761–768

550. Riemann J F, Schmidt H 1982 Ultrastructural changes in the gut autonomic nervous system following laxative abuse and in other conditions. Scandinavian Journal of Gastroenterology 71 (suppl): 111–124

551. Rijpstra A C, Canning E U, Van Ketel R J, Eeftinck Schattenkerk J K, Laarman J J 1988 Use of light microscopy to diagnose small-intestinal microsporidiosis in patients with AIDS. Journal of Infectious Diseases 157: 827–831

552. Riva F, Riva A, Puxeddu P 1987 Ciliated cells in the main excretory duct of the submandibular gland in obstructive sialadenitis: a SEM and TEM study. Ultrastructural Pathology 11: 1–10

553. Rode J, Dhillon A P, Papadaki L, Stockbrugger R, Thompson R J, Moss E, Cotton P B 1986 Pernicious anaemia and mucosal endocrine cell proliferation of the non-antral stomach. Gut 27: 789–798

554. Rodgers F G, Rodgers C, Shelton A P, Hawkey C J 1986 Proposed pathogenic mechanism for the diarrhea associated with human intestinal spirochetes. American Journal of Clinical Pathology 86: 679–682

555. Rodrigues M A, Mattar N J, De Campos J C, Mitidieri H A, De Camargo J L 1981 Malacoplakia of the ascending colon and appendix in children. Report of a case with ultrastructural observations. Archives of Gastroenterology 18: 25–29

556. Roggero P, Offredi M L, Mangiaterra V, Mosca F, Perazzani M, Borzani M, Vanlierde A, Careddu P 1983 Scannning electron microscopy of the small intestine in patients with gluten intolerance, coeliac disease, giardiasis, lymphangiectasis. Minerva Pediatrica 35: 571–578

557. Rollaston T P, Stone I, Rhodes J M 1984 Spiral organisms in endoscopic biopsies of the human stomach. Journal of Clinical Pathology 37: 23–26

558. Rolston D D K, Fairclough P D, Wilks M, Levison D A, Farthing M J G 1986 Spiral organisms in the human jejunum. Journal of Clinical Gastroenterology 8: 628–629

559. Romagnoli P, Bani D, Biliotti G C 1984 The exocrine pancreas of patients with WDHA syndrome. A light and electron microscopical study. Journal of Submicroscopic Cytology 16: 569–576

560. Romeo G, Sanfilippo G, Basile F, Catania G, Iannello A, Carnazza M L 1981 Ultrastructural study of parietal cells before and after vagotomy in patients with duodenal ulcer. Surgery, Gynecology and Obstetrics 153: 61–64

561. Rose A G, Becker W B 1972 Disseminated herpes simplex infection: retrospective study by light microscopy and electron microscopy of paraffin embedded tissues. Journal of Clinical Pathology 25: 79–87

562. Rosen P P 1976 Opportunistic fungal infection in patients with neoplastic diseases. Pathology Annual 11: 255–315

563. Rosson R S, Yesner R 1965 Perioral duodenal biopsy in progressive systemic sclerosis. New England Journal of Medicine 272: 391–394

564. Rothbaum R J, McAdams A J, Giannella R A, Partin J C 1982 A clinicopathologic study of enterocyte-adherent Escherichia coli: a cause of protracted diarrhea in infants. Gastroenterology 83: 441–454

565. Rothbaum R J, Partin J C, Saalfield K, McAdams A J 1983 An ultrastructural study of enteropathogenic Escherichia coli infection in human infants. Ultrastructural Pathology 4: 291–304

566. Rousset S, Moscovici O, Lebon P, Barbet J P, Helardot P, Mace B, Bargy F, Le Tan Vinh, Chany C 1984 Intestinal lesions containing coronavirus-like particles in neonatal necrotizing enterocolitis: an ultrastructural analysis. Pediatrics 73: 218–224

567. Rubin E, Rybak B J, Lindenbaum J, Gerson C D, Walker G, Lieber C S 1972 Ultrastructural changes in the small intestine induced by ethanol. Gastroenterology 63: 801–814

568. Rubin W L, Ross L, Sleisenger M H, Weser E 1966 An electron microscope study of adult coeliac disease. Laboratory Investigation 15: 1720–1747

569. Ruiz de Aguiar A, Medina Nunex J A, Lopez Domingo M I, Villacorta Patino J, Leguey Jimenez S 1988 Calcium carbonate in cholesterol gallstones. Journal of Hepatology 6: 71–79.

570. Russell M L, Friesen D, Henderson R D, Hanna W M 1982 Ultrastructure of the oesophagus in scleroderma. Arthritis and Rheumatism 25: 1117–1123

571. Saglie F R 1988 Scanning electron microscopy of intragingival microorganisms in periodontal diseases. Scanning Electron Microscopy 2: 1535–1540

572. Saglie F R, Carranza F A Jr, Newman M G 1985 The presence of bacteria within the oral epithelium in periodontal disease. I. A

scanning and transmission electron microscopic study. Journal of Periodontology 56: 618–624

573. Saglie F R, Newman M G, Carranza F A Jr, Pattison G L 1982 Bacterial invasion of gingiva in advanced periodontitis in humans. Journal of Periodontology 53: 217–222

574. Saglie F R, Pertuiset J H, Smith C T, Nestor M G, Carranza F A Jr, Newman M G, Rezende M T, Nisengard R 1987 The presence of bacteria in the oral epithelium in periodontal disease. III. Correlation with Langerhans cells. Journal of Periodontology 58: 417–422

575. Sakai T, Sakai H, Hashimoto N, Hirayasu R 1988 Gingival pigmentation beneath a metallic crown: light and electron microscopic observations and energy dispersive X-ray analysis. Journal of Oral Pathology 17: 409–415

576. Saku T, Okabe H 1984 Immunohistochemical and ultrastructural demonstration of keratin in epi-myoepithelial islands of autoimmune sialadenitis in man. Archives of Oral Biology 29: 687–689

577. Saito T, Hanoma T, Sato T, Fujioka Y 1971 Autoimmune mechanisms as a probable aetiology of Behcets syndrome; an electron microscopic study of the oral mucosa. Virchows Archiv A, Pathological Anatomy and Histology 353: 261–272

578. Saito K, Matsumoto S, Yokoyama T, Okaniwa M, Kamoshita S 1982 Pathology of chronic vitamin E deficiency in fatal familial intrahepatic cholestasis (Byler disease). Virchows Archiv A, Pathological Anatomy and Histology 396: 319–330

579. Sandholm L 1984 Cells and cellular interactions in gingival crevice washings from patients with juvenile periodontitis. Scandinavian Journal of Dental Research 92: 436–442

580. Sandholm L, Lounatmaa K, Saxen L 1984 Ultrastructure of freeze–fractured neutrophil leukocyte membranes in juvenile periodontitis. Journal of Periodontal Research 19: 269–278

581. Sapp J P, Brooke R I 1977 Intranuclear inclusion bodies in recurrent aphthous ulcers with a herpetiform pattern. Oral Surgery 43: 416–421

582. Sapp J P, Gardner D G 1973 Regional odontodysplasia: an ultrastructural and histochemical study of soft tissue calcification. Oral Surgery 36: 383–392

583. Sauk J J Jr, Cotton W R, Lyon H W, Witkop C J Jr 1972 Electron optic analysis of hypomineralized amelogenesis imperfecta in man. Archives of Oral Biology 17: 771–779

584. Schmitz J, Arnaud-Batrtandier F, Jos J, Triadou N, Ricour C 1983 L'atrophie microvillositaire congenitale, une cuse rare de diarrhee neonatale incoercible. Gastroenterologie Clinique et Biologique 7: 21A

585. Schnagal R D, Morey F, Holmes I H 1979 Rotavirus-and corona-virus-like particles in aboriginal and non-aboriginal neonates in Kalgoorlie and Alice Springs. Medical Journal of Australia 2: 178

586. Schrodt G R 1963 Melanosis coli: a study with the electron-microscope. Diseases of the Colon and Rectum 6: 277–283

587. Schroeder H E, Muller-Glauser W, Sallay K 1983 Stereologic analysis of leukocyte infiltration in oral ulcers of developing Mikulicz aphthae. Oral Surgery 56: 629–640

588. Schroeder H E, Muller-Glauser W, Sallay K 1984 Pathomorphologic features of the ulcerative stage of oral aphthous ulcerations. Oral Surgery, Oral Medicine, Oral Pathology 58: 293–305

589. Schuffler M D 1989 Neuromuscular abnormalities of small and large intestine. In: Whitehead R (ed) Gastrointestinal and oesophageal pathology. Churchill Livingstone, Edinburgh, pp 329–353

590. Schuffler M D, Lowe M C, Bill A H 1977 Studies of idiopathic intestinal pseudo-obstruction I. Hereditary hollow visceral myopathy: clinical and pathological studies. Gastroenterology 73: 327–338

591. Schuffler M D, Pope C E 1977 Studies of idiopathic intestinal pseudo-obstruction II. Hereditary hollow visceral myopathy family studies. Gastroenterology 73: 339–344

592. Schuffler M D, Bird T D, Sumi S M, Cook A 1978 A familial neuronal disease presenting as intestinal pseudo-obstruction. Gastroenterology 75: 889–898

593. Schuffler M D 1981 Chronic intestinal pseudo-obstruction syndromes. Medical Clinics of North America 65: 1331–1358

594. Schuffler M D, Jonak Z 1982 Chronic idiopathic intestinal pseudo-

obstruction caused by a degenerative disorder of the myenteric plexus: the use of Smith's method to define the neuropathology. Gastroenterology 82: 476–486

595. Schuffler M D, Leon S H, Krishnamurthy S 1985 Intestinal pseudo-obstruction caused by a new form of visceral neuropathy: palliation by radical small bowel resection. Gastroenterology 89: 1152–1156

596. Schwendemann G, Colmant H J, Elze K-L, Koepp P, Lagenstein I, Steinhausen H C 1978 Juvenile type of generalised ceroid-lipofuscinosis. (Speilmeyer-Sjogren syndrome). II Biopsy findings. Neuropaediatrie 9: 28–48

597. Schwendemann G, Arendt G, Noth J, Lange H W, Strauss W 1987 Diagnosis of juvenile–adult form of neuroaxonal dystrophy by electron microscopy of rectum and skin biopsy (letter). Journal of Neurology, Neurosurgery and Psychiatry 50: 818–821

598. Scott B B, Hardy G J, Losowsky M S 1975 Involvement of the small intestine in systemic mast cell disease. Gut 16: 918–924

599. Sela M N, Romano H 1983 Ultrastructural studies of the effect of human leukocyte extracts on periodontopathic bacteria. Inflammation 7: 213–226

600. Selvig K A 1966 Ultrastructural changes in cementum and adjacent connective tissue in periodontal disease. Acta Odontologica Scandinavica 24: 459–500

601. Selvig K A 1963 Ultrastructural changes in human dentin exposed to a weak acid. Archives of Oral Biology 13: 401

602. Selvig K A, Hals E 1977 Periodontally diseased cementum studied by correlated microradiography, electron probe analysis and electron microscopy. Journal of Periodontal Research 12: 419–429

603. Sethi P, Banerjee A K, Jones D M, Eldridge J, Hollanders D 1987 Gastritis and gastric Campylobacter-like organisms in patients without peptic ulcer. Postgraduate Medical Journal 63: 543–545

604. Shafik S S, Zaki A E, Ashrafi S H, Nour Z M, Elnesr N M 1988 Comparison of scanning and transmission electron microscopy of the epithelial pocket wall in juvenile and adult periodontitis. Journal of Periodontology 59: 493–503

605. Shapen H D, Segers O, De Wit N, Goossens A, Buydens P, Dierckx R, Somers G 1989 Electron microscopic detection of Whipple's bacillus in sarcoid-like periodic acid-Schiff-negative granulomas. Digestive Diseases and Sciences 34: 640–643

606. Sharp J R, Insalaco S J, Johnson I F 1980 'Melanosis' of the duodenum — associated with a gastric ulcer and folic acid deficiency. Gastrointestinal Endoscopy 78: 366–369

607. Shenker B J, Berthold P, Dougherty P, Porter K K 1987 Immunosuppressive effects of Centipeda periodontii: selective cytotoxicity for lymphocytes and monocytes. Infection and Immunity 55: 2332–2340

608. Shields N M, Bates M L, Goldman H, Zuckerman G R, Mills B A, Best C J, Bair F A, Goran D A, DeSchyver-Kecskemeti K 1985 Scanning electron microscopic appearance of chronic ulcerative colitis with and without dysplasia. Gastroenterology 89: 62–72

609. Shimizu S, Yoshinaka M, Tada M, Kawamoto K, Inokuchi H, Kawai K 1986 A case of primary amyloidosis confined to the small intestine. Gastroenterologica Japonica 21: 513–517

610. Shindarov L M, Dimitrov D H, Rangelova S, Popov G, Tcakov B, Tsilka E 1988 Five year study of rotavirus gastroenteritis in Bulgaria. Acta Virologica 32: 309–316

611. Shiner M 1973 Ultrastructural changes suggestive of immune reactions in the jejunal mucosa of coeliac children following gluten challenge. Gut 14: 1–12

612. Shiner M 1974 Electron microscopy of jejunal mucosa. Clinical Gastroenterology 3: 33–53

613. Shiner M 1983 Ultrastructure of the small intestinal mucosa. Normal and disease-related appearances. Springer-Verlag, Berlin

614. Shiner M, Shmerling D H 1970 The pathogenesis of coeliac disease. Gut 11: 1058–1059

615. Shroeder H E, Amstad-Jossi M 1986 Epithelial differentiation at the edentulous alveolar ridge in man. A stereological study. Cell and Tissue Research 243: 661–671

616. Sibley R K, Sutherland D E, Goetz F, Michael A F 1985 Recurrent diabetes mellitus in the pancreas iso and allograft. A light and electron microscopic and immunohistochemical analysis of four cases. Laboratory Investigation 53: 132–144

617. Siboni A, Horn T, Christensen N 1987 Lipofuscinosis of the

human uterus. Archives of Pathology and Laboratory Medicine 111: 771–772

618. Sidhur G S, Stahl R E, El- Sadr W, Zolla-Pazner S 1983 Ultrastructural markers of AIDS. Lancet i: 990–991

619. Siew S, Tedesco F J 1977 Scanning electron microscopy of human colonic biopsies as an aid in the diagnosis of clindamycin-associated colitis. Proceedings of the Annual Scanning Electron Microscopic Symposium II, IIT Research Institute, Chicago, pp 187–194

620. Silness I, Gustavsen F 1970 Some observations on the fine structure of fluorosed dental enamel. Acta Odontologica Scandinavica 28: 701–720

621. Silverman S, Bruemer J 1973 Primary herpetic gingivostomatitis of adult onset. Clinical laboratory and ultrastructure correlations identifying viral etiology. Oral Surgery 36: 496–503

622. Singh P B, Screenivasan M A, Pavri K M 1989 Viruses in acute gastroenteritis in children in Pune, India. Epidemiology and Infection 102: 345–353

623. Sirsat S M, Dafray N A 1974 Keratinization patterns in the human oral mucosa in relation to oral habits and malignancy II. Ultrastructure. Indian Journal of Cancer 11: 13–27

624. Skaug N, Johannessen A C, Nilsen R, Matre R 1984 *In situ* characterization of cell infiltrates in human dental periapical granulomas. 3. Demonstration of T lymphocytes. Journal of Oral Pathology 13: 120–127

625. Smith A L, Stewart L, Fine R, Pellegrini C A, Way L W 1989 Gallstone disease. The clinical manifestations of infectious stones. Archives of Surgery 124: 629–633

626. Snover D C, Filipovich A H, Ramsay N K C, Weisdorf S A, Kersey J H 1985 A histopathologic study of gastric and small intestinal graft-versus-host disease following allogenic bone marrow transplant. Human Pathology 16: 387–392

627. Soffer D 1985 Neuronal intranuclear hyaline inclusion disease presenting as Friedrich's ataxia. Acta Neuropathologica 65: 322–329

628. Sognnaes R F, Weisberger D, Albright J T 1956 Pathologic desquamation of oral epithelium examined by electron microscopy and histochemistry. Journal of the National Cancer Institute 17: 329–334

629. Solcia E, Polak J M, Pearse A G E, Forssmann W G, Larsson L-I, Sundler F, Lechago J, Grimelius L, Fujita T, Creutzfeldt W S, Gepts W, Falkmer S, Lefranc G, Heitz Ph, Hage E, Buchan A M J, Bloom S R, Grossman M I 1978 Lausanne 1977 classification of gastroenteropancreatic endocrine cells. In: Bloom S R (ed) Gut hormones. Churchill Livingstone, Edinburgh, pp 40–48

630. Solcia E, Polak J M, Larsson L-I, Buchan A M J, Capello C 1981 Update on Lausanne classification of endocrine cells. In: Bloom S R, Polak J M (eds) Gut hormones. Churchill Livingstone, Edinburgh, pp 96–106

631. Sonsino E, Mouy R, Foucaud P, Cesard J P, Algrain Y, Bocquat L, Navarro J 1984 Intestinal pseudo-obstruction related to cytomegalovirus infection of myenteric plexus. New England Journal of Medicine 311: 196–197

632. Spapen H D M, Segers O, De Wit N, Goossens A, Buydens P, Dierckx R, Somers G 1989 Electron microscopic detection of Whipple's bacillus in sarcoid-like periodic acid–Schiff-negative granulomas. Digestive Diseases and Sciences 34: 640–643

633. Speer A G, Cotton P B, Rode J, Seddon A M, Neal C R, Holton J, Costerton J W 1988 Biliary stent blockage with bacterial biofilm. A light and electron microscopy study. Annals of Internal Medicine 108: 546–553

634. Stamp G W H, Evans D J 1987 Accumulation of ceroid in smooth muscle indicates severe malabsorption and vitamin E deficiency. Journal of Clinical Pathology 40: 798–802

635. Steen L, Stenling R 1983 Relationship between morphological findings and function of the small intestine in familial amyloidosis with polyneuropathy. Scandinavian Journal of Gastroenterology 18: 961–968

636. Steer H W 1984 Surface morphology of the gastro-duodenal mucosa in duodenal ulceration. Gut 25: 1203–1210

637. Steer H W 1985 The gastro-duodenal epithelium in peptic ulceration. Journal of Pathology 146: 355–362

638. Steinberg A D, Willey R 1988 Scanning electron microscopy observations on initial clot formation on treated root surfaces. Journal of Periodontology 59: 403–411

639. Steinhoff M M, Kodner I J, DeSchryver-Kecskemeti K 1988 Axonal degeneration/necrosis: a possible ultrastructural marker for Crohn's disease. Modern Pathology 1: 182–187

640. Stenling R, Fredrikzon B, Engberg S, Falkmer S 1984 Surface ultrastructure of the small intestine mucosa in children with coeliac disease. I. Untreated disease and effects of long-term gluten elimination and challenge. Ultrastructural Pathology 6: 295–305

641. Stevens S, McClure J 1982 The histochemical features of the Michaelis-Gutmann body and a consideration of the pathophysiological mechanisms of its formation. Journal of Pathology 137: 119–127

642. Stockton M, McColl I 1983 Comparative electron microscopic features of normal intermediate and metaplastic pyloric epithelium. Histopathology 7: 859–871

643. Stolte M, Seifert E 1985 Lipidinseln im Osophagus. Leber, Magen, Darm 15: 137–139

644. Strayer D S, Phillips G B, Barker K H, Winokur T, DeSchryver-Kecskemeti K 1981 Gastric cytomegalovirus infection in bone marrow transplant patients. Cancer 48: 1478–1483

645. Strom R L, Gruninger R O, Roth R I, Owen R L, Keren D F 1983 AIDS with mycobacterium *avium-intracellulare* lesions resembling those of Whipple's disease. New England Journal of Medicine 309: 1323–1325

646. Sullivan M K, Taylor B J, Broadbent R S, Yun K, Lovell-Smith M, Donald R A 1988 Somatostatin analogue SMS 201-995 in the short-term management of neonatal hyperinsulinism due to nesidioblastosis. Australian Paediatric Journal 24: 375–378

647. Suzuki H, Igarashi Y, Konno T, Arai N 1979 Letter: inclusion bodies in Paneth cells in zinc deficiency. Lancet i: 734

648. Symmers W St C 1956 Primary amyloidosis. A review. Journal of Clinical Pathology 9: 187–211

649. Symons N B B 1970 Electron microscopic study of the tubules in human carious dentine. Archives of Oral Biology 15: 239

650. Tafur W L, Brenner Z 1966 Lesoes do sistema nervoso autonomo no camundonga albino na fase cronica da tropanossomiase cruzi experimental. Revista de Instituto de Medicina Tropical de Sao Paolo 8: 177–183

651. Takarada H, Cattoni M, Sugimoto A, Rose G G 1974 Ultrastructural studies of human gingiva. III. Changes of the basal lamina in chronic periodontitis. Journal of Periodontology 45: 288–302

652. Takarada H, Cattoni M, Sugimoto A, Rose G G 1974 Ultrastructural studies of human gingiva. II. The lower part of the pocket epithelium in chronic periodontitis. Journal of Periodontology 45: 155–169

653. Takarada H, Cattoni M, Sugimoto A, Rose G G 1974 Ultrastructural studies of human gingiva. I. The upper part of the pocket epithelium in chronic periodontitis. Journal of Periodontology 45: 30–42

654. Takeda Y, Ishikawa G 1983 Crystalloids in salivary duct cysts of the human parotid gland. Scanning electron microscopical study with electron probe X-ray microanalysis. Virchows Archiv A, Pathological Anatomy and Histology 399: 41–48

655. Takeuchi A, Hashimoto K 1976 Electron microscopic study of the experimental enteric adenovirus infection in mice. Infection and Immunity 15: 569–580

656. Takuma S, Ogiwara H, Suzuki H 1975 Electron-probe and electron microscope studies of carious dentinal lesions with a remineralized surface layer. Caries Research 9: 278–285

657. Tanaka A, Mayahara H, Wada S, Tomita J, Tsutsui M 1984 Ultrastructural localization of acid phosphatase activity in plasma cells containing Russell's bodies in periodontitis. Journal of Oral Pathology 13: 105–110

658. Tanaka M, Nagai T, Tasaki T, Miki M, Hirakawa K, Watanabe T, Kobayashi H, Kubota S, Abe T 1988 A study of the internal structure of gallstones based on the differences between the interactions to elements of thermal neutrons and X-rays. Radioisotopes 37: 685–686

659. Tanaka K, Yamano T, Shimada M, Ohno M, Onaga A, Saeki Y, Kodama S, Nishio H 1987 Electronmicroscopic study on biopsied rectal mucosa in adrenoleukodystrophy. Neurology 37: 1012–1015

660. Tandler B 1965 Electron microscopical observations on early

sialoliths in a human submaxillary gland. Archives of Oral Biology 10: 509–522

661. Tandon B N, Puri B K, Gandhi P C, Tewari S G 1974 Mucosal surface injury of jejunal mucosa in patients with giardiasis: an electron microscopic study. Indian Journal of Medical Research 62: 1838–1842

662. Tandon R K 1988 Pathogenesis of gallstones in India. Tropical Gastroenterology 9: 83–93

663. Tarnowski A, Stachura J, Hollander D, Sarfeh I J, Bogdal J 1988 Cellular aspects of alcohol-induced injury and prostaglandin protection of the human gastric mucosa. Focus on the mucosal microvessels. Journal of Clinical Gastroenterology 10 (suppl 1): S53–S45

664. Tarpila S, Tekkla S, Siurala M 1967 Ultrastructure of various metaplasias of the stomach. Acta Pathologica et Microbiologica Scandinavica 77: 187–195

665. Taura S, Tsunoda T, Yoshino R, Harada N, Akashi M, Ito T, Tsuchiya R 1975 Ultrastructural studies of human acute pancreatitis. Gastroenterologica Japonica 10: 132–140

666. Taylor C J, Hart A, Batt R M, McDougall C, McLean L 1986 Ultrastructural and biochemical changes in human jejunal mucosa associated with enterpathogenic Escherichia coli (0111). Journal of Pediatric Gastroenterology and Nutrition 5: 70–73

667. Taylor D E, Hargreaves J A, Ng L K, Sherbaniuk R W, Jewell L D 1987 Isolation and characterization of Campylobacter pyloridis from gastric biopsies. American Journal of Clinical Pathology 87: 49–54

668. Teglbjaerg P S, Thaysen E H 1982 Collagenous colitis: an ultra-structural study of a case. Gastroenterology 82: 561–563

669. Theilade J, Budtz-Jørgensen E 1980 Electron microscopic study of denture plaque. Journal de Biologie Buccale 287–297

670. Theron J J, Wittman W, Prinsloo J G 1971 The fine structure of the jejunum in Kwashiorkor. Experimental and Molecular Pathology 14: 184–199

671. Thilander H 1968 Epithelial changes in gingivitis. Journal of Periodontal Research 3: 303–312

672. Thilander H, Kempson A 1975 Ultastructure of the oral epithelium in leukoplakia associated with tylosis and esophageal carcinoma. Journal of Oral Pathology 4: 72–79

673. Thompson I W, Day D W, Wright N A 1987 Subnuclear vacuolated mucous cells: a novel abnormality of simple mucin-secreting cells of non-specialized gastric mucosa and Brunner's glands. Histopathology 11: 1067–1081

674. Thurre C, Robert M, Cimasoni G, Baehni P 1984 Gingival sulcular leukocytes in periodontitis and in experimental gingivitis in humans. Journal of Periodontal Research 19: 457–468

675. Thyberg J, Graf W, Klingenstrom P 1981 Intestinal fine structure in Crohn's disease. Lysosomal inclusions in epithelial cells and macrophages. Virchows Archiv A, Pathological Anatomy and Histology 391: 141–152

676. Todd I P, Porter N H, Morson B C, Smith B, Friedmann C A, Neal R A 1969 Chagas' disease of the colon and rectum. Gut 10: 1009–1014

677. Toner P G, Carr K E, McLay A L C 1980 The exocrine pancreas. In: Johannessen J V (ed) Electron microscopy in human medicine vol. 7, Digestive system. McGraw-Hill, London, pp 209–245

678. Toner P G, Carr K E, Al-Yassin J M 1980 The gastrointestinal tract. In: Johannessen J V (ed) Electron microscopy in human medicine, vol. 7. McGraw-Hill, New York, London, pp 85–207

679. Toner P G, Carr K E, Al Yassin T 1980 The gastrointestinal tract. In: Johannessen J V (ed) Electron microsocpy in human medicine, vol. 7. McGraw-Hill, New York, pp 87–207

680. Toner P G, Carr K E, Wyburn G M 1971 The digestive system — an ultrastructural atlas and review. Butterworths, London

681. Torpier G, Colombel J F, Mathieu-Chandelier C, Capron M, Dessaint J P, Cortot A, Paris J C, Capron A 1988 Eosinophilic gastroenteritis: ultrastructural evidence for a selective release of eosinophil major basic protein. Clinical and Experimental Immunology 74: 404–408

682. Tovey F I, Husband E M, Yiu Y C, Baker L, McPhail G, Lewin M R, Jayaraj A P, Clark C G 1989 Comparison of relapse rates and of mucosal abnormalities after healing of duodenal ulceration and after one year's maintenance with cimetidine or sucralfate: a light and electron microscopy study. Gut 30: 586–593

683. Trabucchi E, Foschi D, Belloli P, Montorsi F, Marchetti V, Mariscotti C, Diamantini S 1989 Medical therapy of peptic ulcer: problems and prospects. Minerva Dietologicae Gastroenterologica 35: 1–6

684. Tricottet V, Bruneval P, Vire O, Camilleri J P, Bloch F, Bonte N, Roge J 1986 Campylobacter-like organisms and surface epithelium abnormalities in active, chronic gastritis in humans: an ultrastructural study. Ultrastructural Pathology 10: 113–122

685. Trump B F, Verezesky I K, Collan Y, Kahng M W, Mergner W J 1976 Recent studies on the pathophysiology of ischemic cell injury. Beitrage zur Pathologie 158: 363–388

686. Tyldesley W R, Kempson A 1975 Ultrastructure of the oral epithelium in leukoplakia associated with tylosis and esophageal carcinoma. Journal of Oral Pathology 4: 49

687. Tytgat G N, Hoogendijk J L, Agenant D, Schellken's P 1977 Etiopathogenetic studies in a patient with Whipple's disease. Digestion 15: 309–321

688. Tytgat G N, Van Minnen A, Verhoeren A 1978 Electron microscopy study of granulomas in Crohn's disease. Tijdschrift voor Gastroenterologie 21: 465–480

689. Tzipori S 1983 Cryptosporidiosis in animals and humans. Microbiological Reviews 47: 84–96

690. Vahl J 1971 Gesunder und pathologisch veranderter Zahnschmelz. Barth, Leipsig

691. Vahl J, Hohlung H J, Plackova A, Bures H 1966 Elektronenmikroskopische Ultradunnschnittuntersuchungen an Zahnen mit Schmelzflecken herrührend von initialer Karies, artifizieller Karies und Mineralisationsstörungen. Deutsch Zalnaerzl Zeitschrift 21: 983–989

692. Vahl J, Pfefferkorn G, Hohling H J 1968 Sublichtmicroskopische untersuchungen am menschlichlichen spechelstein. Deutsch Zalnaerzl Zeitschrift 23: 39–44

693. Van den Oord J J, Geboes K, Desmet V J 1982 Collagenous colitis: an abnormal collagen table? Two new cases and review of the literature. American Journal of Gastroenterology 77: 377–381

694. Van Dyke T E, Levine M J, Genco R M 1985 Neutrophil function and oral disease. Journal of Oral Pathology 14: 95–120

695. Van Haelst U J G M, Gabreels F J M 1972 The electron microscopic study of the appendix as early diagnostic means in Batten-Speilmeyer-Vogt disease. Acta Neuropathologica 21: 169–175

696. Van Wyk C W, Ambrosio S C 1983 Leukoedema: ultrastructural and histochemical observations. Journal of Oral Pathology 12: 319–329

697. Van Wyk C W, Ambrosio S C, Van der Vyver P C 1984 Abnormal keratohyalin-like forms in leukoedema. Journal of Oral Pathology 13: 271–281

698. Varkonyi T, Wittman T, Varro V 1977 Effect of local circulatory arrest on the structure of the enterocytes of the isolated intestinal loop. Digestion 15: 295–302

699. Vaucher Y E, Ray C G, Minnich L L, Payne C M, Beck D, Lowe P 1982 Pleomorphic enveloped virus-like particles associated with gastrointestinal illness in neonates. Journal of Infectious Diseases 145: 27–36

700. Veloso F T, Vaz Saleiro J 1982 Mast cells in Whipple's disease. Journal of Submicroscopic Cytology 14: 515–520

701. Venizelos I D, Shousha S, Bull T B, Parkins R A 1988 Chronic intestinal pseudo-obstruction in two patients. Overlap of features of systemic sclerosis and visceral myopathy. Histopathology 12: 533–540

702. Verderame R A, Cobb C M, Killoy W J, Drisko C L 1989 Scanning electron microscopic examination of pocket wall epithelium and associated plaque in localized juvenile periodontitis. Journal of Clinical Periodontology 16: 234–241

703. Villar L A, Massanari R M, Mitros F A 1984 Cytomegalovirus infection with acute erosive esophagitis. American Journal of Medicine 76: 924–928

704. Vortel V, Sazama L 1977 Rasinkovy epitel ve vyvodech polcelistni slinne zlazy. Ceskoslovenska Patologie 13: 134–137

705. Vrahopoulos T P, Barber P, Liakoni H, Newman H N 1988 Ultrastructure of the periodontal lesion in a case of Papillo-Leefevre syndrome (PLS). Journal of Clinical Periodontology 15: 17–26

706. Waghorn D J 1987 Campylobacter pyloridis: a new organism to explain an old problem? Postgraduate Medical Journal 63: 533–537

707. Wald A, Kichler J, Mendelow H 1981 Amyloidosis and chronic intestinal pseudo-obstruction. Digestive Diseases and Sciences 26: 462–465
708. Walter B, Frank R M, Steuer P 1986 Ultrastructural development of dated plaque in case of denture stomatitis. Journal Biologie Buccale 14: 115–124
709. Walter B, Frank R M 1986 Ultrastructural relationship of denture surfaces, plaque and oral mucosa in denture stomatitis. Journal Biologie Buccale 13: 145–166
710. Walravens P A, Hambidge K M, Neldner K H, Silverman A, van Doorninck W J, Mierau G, Favara B 1978 Zinc metabolism in acrodermatitis enteropathica. Journal of Pediatrics 93: 71–73
711. Warren J R, Marshall B J 1983 Unidentified curved bacilli on gastric epithelium in active chronic gastritis. Lancet i: 1273–1275
712. Wattiovaara J, Tarpila S 1977 Cell contacts and polysomes in irradiated human jejunal mucosa at onset of epithelial repair. Laboratory Investigation 36: 660–665
713. Watson J H L, Goodwin J, Rajian K S 1979 Giardia-lamblia in human duodenum and bile. Micron 10: 61–64
714. Weber J R Jr, Dobbins W O III 1986 The intestinal and rectal epithelial lymphocyte in AIDS. An electron-microscopic study. American Journal of Surgical Pathology 10: 627–639
715. Weber A F, Schmithdiel E F 1986 Electron microscopic and bacteriologic studies of spirilla isolated from the fundii stomach of cats and dogs. American Journal of Veterinary Research 23: 422–426
716. Weidner N, Geisinger K R, Sterling R T, Miller T R, Yen T S 1986 Benign lymphoepithelial cysts of the parotid gland. A histologic, cytologic and ultrastructural study. American Journal of Clinical Pathology 85: 395–401
717. Weinstein W N, Saunders D R, Tygat G N, Rubin C E 1970 Collagenous sprue — an unrecognised type of malabsorption. New England Journal of Medicine 283: 1297–1301
718. Weisbrot I M, Liber A F, Gordon B S 1975 The effects of therapeutic radiation on colonic mucosa. Cancer 36: 931–940
719. Weiser M M, Andres G A, Brentjens J R, Evans J T, Reichlin M 1981 Systemic lupus erythematosus and intestinal venulitis. Gastroenterology 81: 570–579
720. Weiser M M, Andres G A, Brendtjens J R, Evans J T, Reichlin M 1981 Systemic lupus erythematosus and intestinal venulitis. Gastroenterology 81: 570–579
721. Weller I V D 1985 The gay bowel. Gut 26: 869–875
722. Westergaard J, Fiehn N E 1987 Morphological distribution of spirochetes in subgingival plaque from advanced marginal periodontitis in humans. Acta Pathologica Microbiologica et Immunologica Scandinavica B 95: 49–55
723. Whipple G H 1907 A hitherto undescribed disease characterised anatomically by deposits of fat and fatty acids in the intestinal and mesenteric lymphatic tissues (intestinal lipodystrophy). Bulletin of the Johns Hopkins Hospital 18: 382–391
724. Whitehead R 1985 Mucosal biopsy of the gastrointestinal tract, 3rd edn. Saunders, Philadelphia, pp 270–274
725. Widgren S, Jlidi R, Cox J N 1988 Collagenous colitis: histologic, morphometric, immunohistochemical and ultrastructural studies. Report of 21 cases. Virchows Archiv A, Pathological Anatomy and Histology 413: 287–296
726. Wilborn W H, Montes L F 1980 Scanning electron microscopy of oral lesions in chronic mucocutaneous candidiasis. Journal of the American Medical Association 244: 2294–2297
727. Wilcox G M, Tronic B S, Schecter D J, Arron M J, Righi D F, Weiner N J 1987 Periodic acid–Schiff-negative granulomatous lymphadenopathy in patients with Whipple's disease. Localization of the Whipple bacillus to non-caseating granulomas by electron microscopy. American Journal of Medicine 83: 165–170
728. Willemer S, Adler G 1989 Histochemical and ultrastructural characteristics of tubular complexes in human acute pancreatitis. Digestive Diseases and Sciences 34: 46–55
729. Willemer S, Kloppel G, Kern H R, Adler G 1989 Immunocytochemical and morphometric analysis of acinar zymogen granules in human acute pancreatitis. Virchows Archiv A, Pathological Anatomy and Histology 415: 115–123
730. Winberg C D, Rose M E, Rappaport H 1978 Whipple's disease of the lung. American Journal of Medicine 65: 873–880
731. Winborn W B, Weser E 1983 Scanning electron microscopy of intestinal metaplasia of the human stomach. Gastrointestinal Endoscopy 29: 201–207
732. Wyatt J I 1989 Relationship of C. pylori to duodenal ulcer disease. In: Blaser M J (ed) Campylobacter pylori in gastritis and peptic ulcer disease. Igaku-Shoin, New York & Tokyo, pp 99–114
733. Wysocki G P, Sapp J P 1975 Scanning and transmission electron microscopy of odontogenic keratocysts. Oral Surgery 40: 494–501
734. Yamamoto H, Sakae T, Takagi M, Otake S 1984 Scanning electron microscopic and X-ray microdiffractometeric studies on sialolith crystals in human submandibular glands. Acta Pathologica Japonica 34: 47–53
735. Yamamoto H, Sakae T, Takagi M, Otake S, Hirai G 1983 Weddelite in submandibular gland calculus. Journal of Dental Research 62: 16–19
736. Yamane G M, Scharlock S E, Jain R, Sunderraj M, Chaudhry A P 1984 Intraoral minor salivary gland sialolithiasis. Journal of Oral Medicine 39: 85–90
737. Yamano T, Shimada M, Okada S, Yutaka T, Kato T, Yabuchi H 1982 Ultrastructural study of biopsy specimens of rectal mucosa. Its use in neuronal storage diseases. Archives of Pathology and Laboratory Medicine 106: 673–677
738. Yamano T, Shimada M, Sugino H, Dezawa T, Loike M, Okada S, Yabucchi H 1985 Ultrastuctural study on a severe infantile sialidosis (beta-galactosidase-alpha-neuraminidase deficiency). Neuropediatrics 16: 109–112
739. Yamase H, Norris M, Gillies C 1985 Pseudomelanosis duodeni: a clinico-pathologic entity. Gastrointestinal Endoscopy 31: 83–86
740. Yanev P, Chifchiiski S 1986 Electron microscope studies of the ulcer-surrounding mucosa in stomach ulcers. Folia Medica 28: 5–15
741. Yeshaya C, Novis B, Bernheim J, Leichtmann G, Samara M, Griffel B 1984 Collagenous colitis. Report of a case. Diseases of the Colon and Rectum 27: 111–113
742. Zaitsev V T, Shapatova K V, Nevzorov V P 1985 Comparative characteristics of the gastric mucosa in duodenal peptic ulcer patients undergoing different types of surgical treatment. Khirurgiia 10: 49–51
743. Zielke D R, Brady J M, Del Rio C E 1975 Corrosion of silver cones in bone: a scanning electron microscope and microprobe analysis. Journal of Endodontics 1: 356–360
744. Zmener O 1984 Macrophages isolated from periapical granuloma: a scanning electron microscopic study. Oral Surgery, Oral Medicine, Oral Pathology 58: 330–335
745. Zmener O, Dominguez F V 1988 Silver accumulations in periapical granulomas. Report of five cases using the scanning electron microscope, the electron microprobe and other complementary methods. Oral Surgery, Oral Medicine, Oral Pathology 65: 94–100
746. Zoli G, Bonvicini F, Ercoli C, Gasbarrini G, Laschi R 1984 Ultrastructural aspects of duodenal mucosa repair during treatment of peptic disease. Acta Physiologica Hungarica 64: 385–392

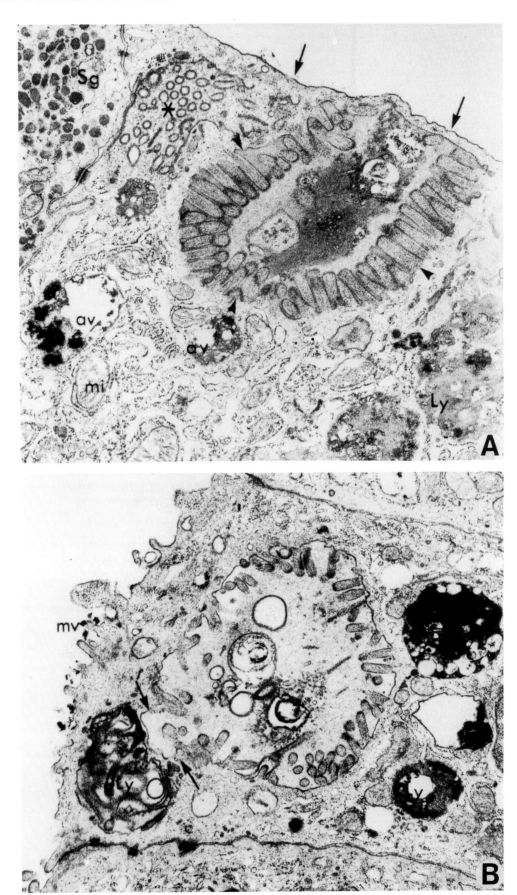

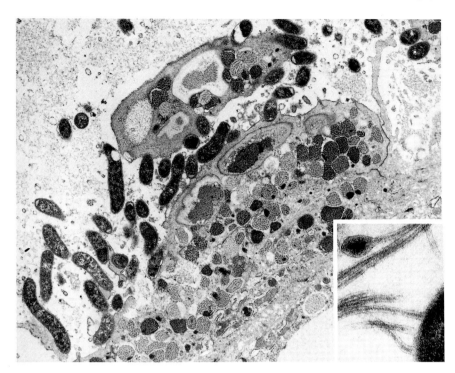

Fig. 14.2 *Helicobacter pylori* on the mucosa of the gastric antrum. Endoscopic biopsy specimen from a case of long-standing non-ulcer dyspepsia, showing *H. pylori* organisms scattered on the lumenal surface of antral mucosa. The mucous cells show typical bulging profiles and depletion of microvilli. (× 6300). *Inset* Close-up view of *H. pylori* sheathed flagella, and a terminal bulb, in the biopsy specimen. (× 64 000)

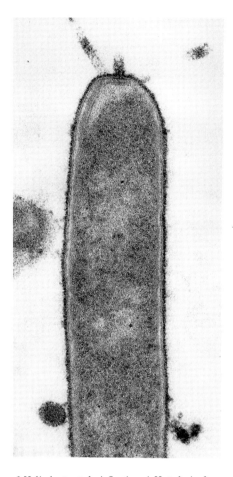

Fig. 14.3 Ultrastructure of *Helicobacter pylori*. Sectioned *H. pylori*, after processing with tannic acid — to show the presence of an external dense polysaccharidic layer, or glycocalyx. It extends over the flagella and their terminal bulbs. (× 64 600)

Fig. 14.1 (Facing page) Microvillus inclusion disease. **A** Per-oral duodenal biopsy. Apical cytoplasm of an enterocyte devoid of brush-border microvilli. An intracytoplasmic 'cyst' composed of invaginated brush border (arrowheads) is situated close to the surface plasmalemma (arrows). The microvilli comprising the inclusion possess a trilaminar plasma membrane, core microfilaments, and a thin surface layer of glycocalyx. Electron-dense material and debris inhabit the lumen of the inclusion. Intracellular microvilli in cross-section can be seen in the cytoplasm adjoining the 'cyst' (asterisk). Lysosomes (Ly) and autophagic vacuoles (av) are present in the same cell. Mitochondria (mi) are also depicted. Small pleomorphic secretory granules (Sg) occupy the apical cytoplasm of an adjacent cell. (× 21 000) **B** An intracytoplasmic micro-lumen in a different enterocyte is lined by microvilli that are less well developed. Lysosomes surround the 'cyst' and one is in close apposition, perhaps in the process of fusion with the membrane of the inclusion (arrows). The orientation of the cell and the presence of a few microvilli (mv) at its surface indicate that the lumen cannot be explained by an oblique plane of section. (× 17 000) (Reprinted with permission from the article 'Familial enteropathy: a syndrome of protracted diarrhea from birth, failure to thrive, and hypoplastic villus atrophy'.[150])

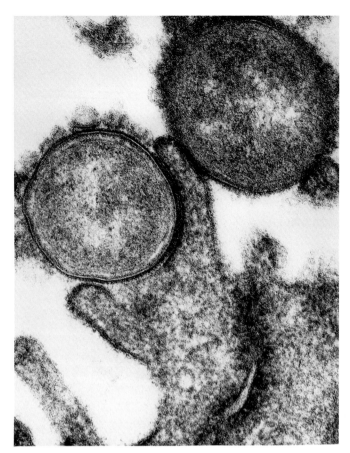

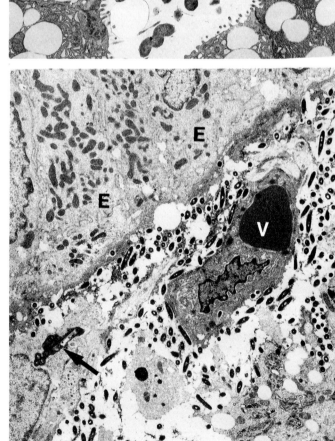

Fig. 14.4 (Above)   Ultrastructure of *Helicobacter pylori*. A raised adherence pedestal at the site of intimate attachment of *H. pylori* to an antral epithelial cell. Tannic acid processing. (× 106 600)

Fig. 14.5 (Above right)   Spiral organisms in the gastric mucosa. Endoscopic gastric biopsy specimen from a monkey (*Macaca mulatta*) showing typical 'spirillum-like' tightly spiral organisms lying free within the lumen of a gland in the gastric body mucosa. (× 6400)

Fig. 14.6 (Right)   Whipple's disease: survey. Fibre-optic duodenal biopsy from a 73-year-old man who presented with a 6-month history of weight loss, anorexia and intermittent diarrhoea. Myriad rod-like bacteria inhabit the extracellular space of the lamina propria deep to the enterocytes (E), where they surround a small blood vessel (V). Even at this magnification a few bacilli can be seen within a phagocytic vacuole in a macrophage (arrow). Enterocyte microvilli in this case were short and blunt, perhaps accounting for malabsorption. (× 7000)

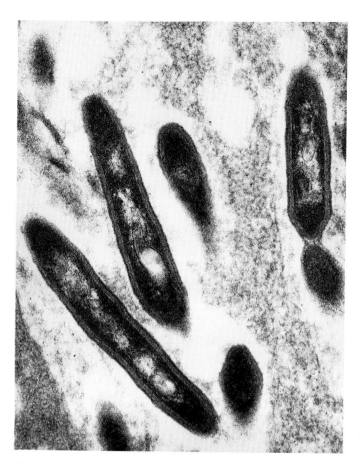

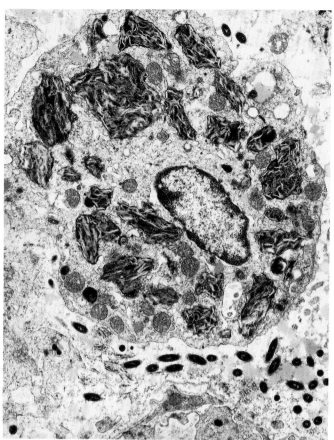

Fig. 14.7 (Above)   Whipple's disease: bacilli. The bacteria found in Whipple's disease typically measure 1–2 μm in length and 0.3 μm in diameter. ($\times$ 62 000)

Fig. 14.8 (Above right)   Whipple's disease: macrophage. A macrophage in the lamina propria. Numerous phagocytic vacuoles are evident, in which membranous contents are visible (stage II–III). Extracellular bacteria are also present. ($\times$ 10 000)

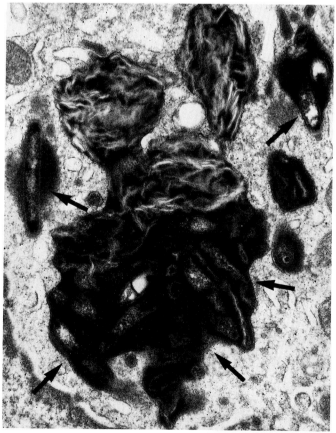

Fig. 14.9 (Right)   Whipple's disease: stage I–II phagocytic vacuoles. Bacteria are recognizable within the vacuoles (arrows), but elsewhere there is a transition to loose membranous material, conforming to stage II vacuolar contents. ($\times$ 23 000)

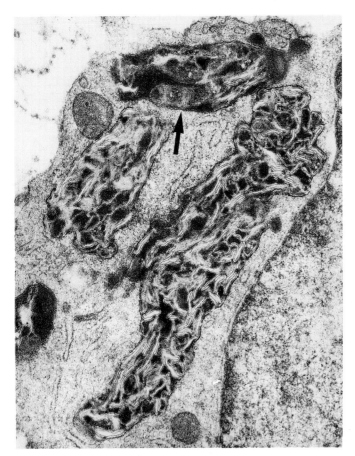

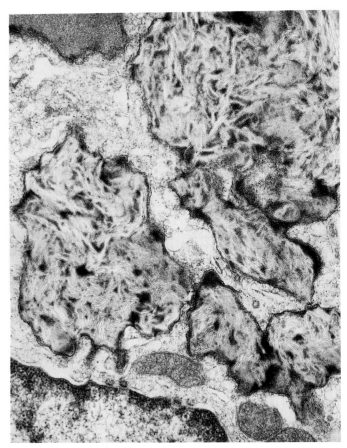

Fig. 14.10 (Above) Whipple's disease: stage I–III phagocytic vacuoles. Bacterial outlines are visible (stage I; arrow), but the contents in others consist of membranes which are not packed as tightly as in typical stage III vacuoles (stage II–III). (× 25 000)

Fig. 14.11 (Above right) Whipple's disease: stage III phagocytic vacuoles. The closely packed membranes depicted here are typical of stage III vacuoles. (× 24 000)

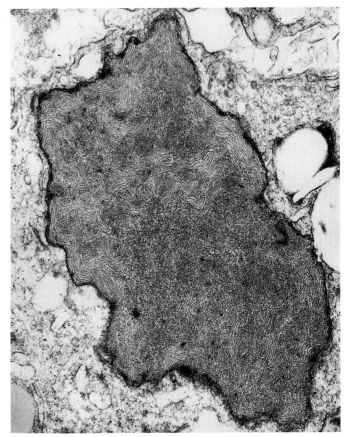

Fig. 14.12 (Right) Whipple's disease: stage IV phagocytic vacuole. The homogeneity of the contents is typical of an end-stage vacuole. (× 28 000)

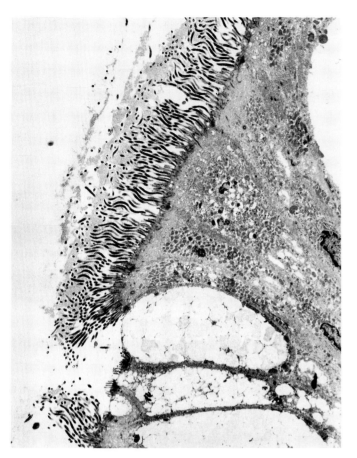

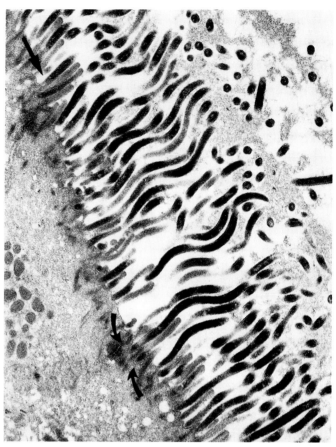

Fig. 14.13 Intestinal spirochaetosis: survey. Innumerable spirochaetes are arrayed along the apical surface of these rectal enterocytes, with sparing of the lucent goblet cells in the lower third of the micrograph. (× 4000)

Fig. 14.14 Intestinal spirochaetosis: spirochaetes. The undulant organisms are perpendicular to the free surface of the enterocytes, interleaving with the microvilli (arrow), and indenting the apical plasma membrane of the enterocytes (curved arrows). Characteristically, the organisms measure 2 to 4.8 μm in length and 0.2 μm in diameter, with a wavelength of 2 μm, and they display left-handed (anticlockwise) spirality. They have tapered ends, a triple-layered cytoplasmic membrane and a triple-layered outer membrane, and they also possess 4–5 flagella at each end (not shown here), best visualized in negatively-stained preparations. (× 12 000)

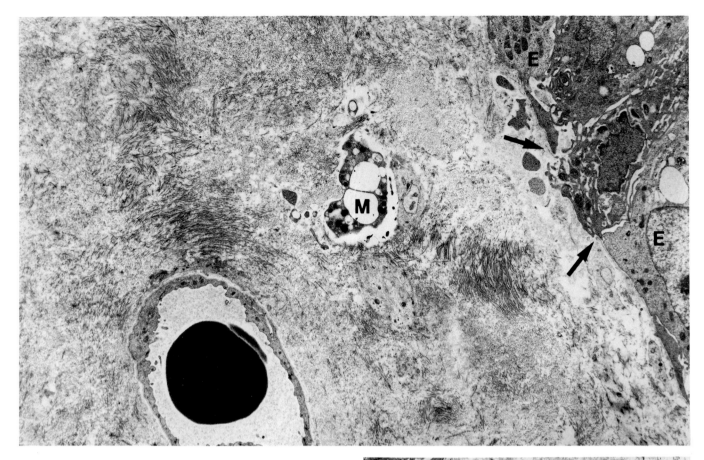

Fig. 14.15 Collagenous colitis: survey. A broad mantle of collagen lies adjacent to the crypt and its enterocytes (E), and extends around a small blood vessel at the lower left of centre. The external lamina surrounding the blood vessels appeared normal in this case, but multilayering of the lamina may be seen. The epithelial basal lamina appeared normal in most areas, but a breach is shown here, between the arrows. Portion of a mast cell (M) can also be seen. (× 5000)

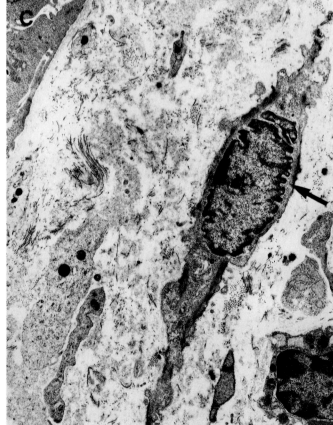

Fig. 14.16 Collagenous colitis: pericryptal myofibroblast. A relatively early stage of the disorder is depicted here, with less extensive accumulation of collagen alongside the crypt (C) than in the preceding figure. A myofibroblast is evident, showing focal serration of the periphery of the nucleus (arrow), and peripheral microfilaments in the cytoplasm, which are not resolved individually at this magnification. (× 7000)

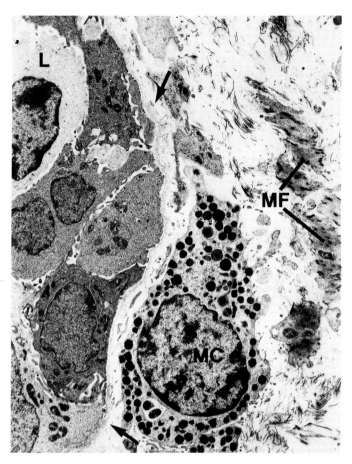

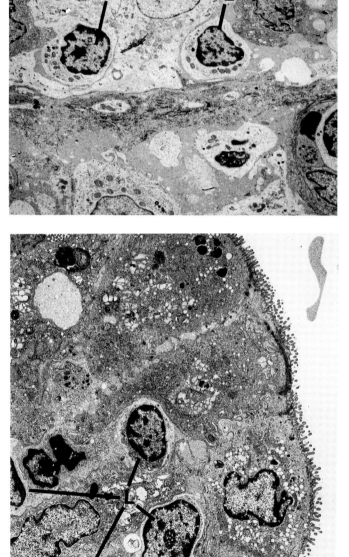

Fig. 14.17 (Above)   Collagenous colitis: pericryptal mast cell. The mast cell (MC) is in close proximity to the crypt epithelium, in which a lymphocyte (L) is evident. The basal lamina displays minor focal thickening (arrows), but in most areas it appeared normal (Figs 14.15 to 14.17 are all from the same case). Portion of a myofibroblast (MF) can also be seen. (× 5000)

Fig. 14.18 (Above right)   Coeliac disease: enterocytes and their microvilli — I. Small bowel biopsy from a 31-year-old woman with clinical evidence of malabsorption and IgA deficiency. The enterocytes are reduced in height and several intra-epithelial lymphocytes (L) are evident. The surface microvilli are short and in disarray. (× 3000)

Fig. 14.19 (Right)   Coeliac disease: enterocytes and their microvilli — II. The enterocytes and their surface microvilli are reduced in height, and the latter show loss of the normal polarity. Small lucent vesicles inhabit the enterocyte cytoplasm, and intra-epithelial lymphocytes are apparent (L). (× 4500)

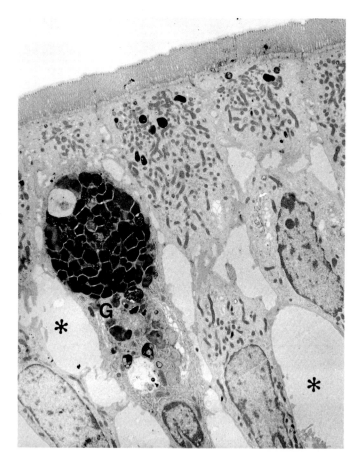

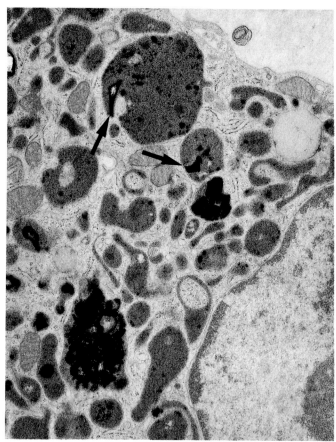

Fig. 14.20   Pseudomelanosis duodeni: mucosal epithelium. This case has been documented in detail by Pounder and associates.[530] The brush border appears normal. Electron-dense lysosomes are evident in the apical cytoplasm. A goblet cell (G) with moderately dense mucin granules is also present. The intercellular spaces (asterisks) are wide. (× 4000)

Fig. 14.21   Pseudomelanosis duodeni: lysosomes in macrophages. Pleomorphic lysosomes within a macrophage found in the lamina propria are depicted. In some regions the lysosomes have angular outlines, and angular electron-dense particles can be seen within them (arrows). (× 14 000)

15. The liver

K. Tanikawa

INTRODUCTION

The ultrastructural pathology of the liver is covered at length in at least two lavishly illustrated books[41,54] and several recent reviews.[40,55] For this reason only an overview is given here to highlight the contributions of electron microscopy to the investigation and diagnosis of hepatic disorders. For more detail these other accounts[40,41,54,55] should be consulted.

Needle biopsy of the liver is a relatively simple procedure, and recent ultrastructural studies on tissue secured by this technique have clarified the value of electron microscopy (EM) in the clinical diagnosis of hepatic disorders.[40,41,54,55,57] In addition, the basic fine-structural changes in the liver — such as reversible or irreversible hepatocyte injury, cholestasis, fibrosis, reactions of the sinusoidal cells (Kupffer cells, endothelial cells, fat-storing cells and pit cells) and cell infiltrates — are of considerable importance. Very often, a variety of tissue reactions are elicited by a single injurious agent, while on the other hand, a single histological picture can be produced by disparate causes. Thus, from the diagnostic point of view, accurate interpretation of fine-structural changes in the liver is often complex and may require considerable experience. For accurate interpretation of disordered hepatic fine structure, attention must be directed both to tissue–cellular variation within the lobule, and also to clinical data such as the patient's age, sex and social habits — including, for example, alcohol consumption and medications.

The fine structure of normal liver is well described and will not be dealt with here.[40,41,54,55] Of particular interest, however, are the recently described parasinusoidal fat-storing cells (Ito cell; Fig. 15.1)[24] and the pit cells (Fig. 15.2).[65] Located in the space of Disse, the Ito cells store vitamin A, and there has been much attention directed recently to their possible participation in hepatic fibrosis.[53] The pit cells, embedded in the endothelial lining, are considered to be liver-fixed natural killer cells.[27]

VIRAL HEPATITIS

Hepatitis A virus (HAV) and hepatitis B virus (HBV) have now been identified as causative agents of hepatitis. Much effort is now being directed to the identification of non-A, non-B hepatitis viruses — the presumed agents for hepatitis not caused by either HAV or HBV.

Acute hepatitis type A

The histological pattern in type A acute hepatitis is characterized by marked mononuclear cell infiltrates in portal tracts, together with prominent changes in hepatocytes and Kupffer cells located in the periportal zone. By electron microscopy, HAV particles can be found in liver biopsy specimens taken within 10 days after the clinical onset;[49,57] they take the form of rounded particles 27 nm in diameter and are found mostly within lysosomes in hepatocytes (Fig. 15.3) and Kupffer cells (Fig. 15.4). The hepatocytes appear to be markedly altered, with numerous electron-dense lysosomes containing HAV particles; such hepatocytes are often closely associated with swollen Kupffer cells, which are also replete with lysosomes containing HAV particles (Fig. 15.5). These morphological changes in Kupffer cells in the early stages of hepatitis suggest that they are dysfunctional, which is also supported by frequent clinical evidence of endotoxaemia and a high incidence of circulating immune complexes.[59] In addition, the development of hepatocyte necrosis appears to be closely related to the Kupffer cell changes.

Hepatitis type B

HBV particles are not easily found in human liver biopsy specimens taken from type B acute hepatitis. However, lymphocytes frequently appear to be in close contact with degenerating hepatocytes, implicating lymphocyte-mediated mechanisms in the development of hepatocyte necrosis (Fig. 15.6). In chronic hepatitis type B or the HBV carrier state, numerous HBc antigens are seen in the nucleus (Fig. 15.7); they are visualized as rounded particles 20 nm in diameter,[17,36] and some of them appear to pass through the nuclear pores.[11] In the cytoplasm, filamentous HBs antigens are abundant within distended cisternae of the smooth endoplasmic reticulum (SER; Fig. 15.8).[11,17,36] These HBV-associated antigens are diagnostic of the HBV carrier state. The complete Dane particles of HBV — double-shelled in appearance and 42 nm in diameter — are rarely found in the cytoplasm and seem to be completed by enwrapment of HBc by SER membranes, in which HVBs antigens are probably being synthesized.

Non-A, non-B hepatitis

No characteristic ultrastructural hallmarks have been found so far in human non-A, non-B hepatitis. In the nucleus of the hepatocyte, small rounded particles measuring about 20–27 nm in diameter are seen in clusters.[19] However, recent studies indicate that they are not specific.[12] In non-A, non-B hepatitis induced in chimpanzees, characteristic tubular structures have been noted in the cytoplasm,[48] but they are not found in human cases. These structures represent tubular confronting cisternae and are identical to those described in lymphocytes of patients with persistent generalized lymphadenopathy or AIDS (see Ch. 29). In infectious mononucleosis induced by Epstein–Barr virus, virus particles are reported to be found in both lymphocytes and hepatocytes.[46]

ALCOHOLIC LIVER INJURY

Alcohol is metabolized mainly in hepatocytes, and biochemical and fine-structural changes can be induced in these cells — even by an amount of alcohol which is 'non-toxic' in light microscopy terms. In alcoholics, proliferation of SER and enlarged mitochondria are characteristic features seen in hepatocytes. The increased SER correlates with induction of drug-metabolizing enzymes, while changes in the mitochondria may be related to inhibition of lipid metabolism in hepatocytes. The development of Mallory bodies in hepatocytes and characteristic patterns of fibrosis — such as pericellular fibrosis and perivenular fibrosis — may also be seen with alcoholic liver injury. Mallory bodies are often seen in alcoholic hepatitis and have a filamentous substructure (Fig. 15.9) which consists mainly of intermediate filament components representing cytokeratins, and they are classified into three types.[67] Typical and large Mallory bodies are easily found by light microscopy, but EM can reveal much smaller bodies which are found in hepatocellular damage produced by other causes. Accordingly, the finding of such small Mallory bodies by EM is of some value in suggesting an alcoholic basis for hepatitis, but it should be emphasized that Mallory bodies are also found infrequently in hepatocytes in non-alcoholic steatohepatitis,[23,31] primary biliary cirrhosis,[32] Wilson's disease,[50] Indian childhood cirrhosis,[35] prolonged cholestasis[16] and other disorders.

The hepatic fibrosis seen in alcoholic liver injury is characteristically pericellular and perivenular; pericellular fibrosis around hepatocytes can be demonstrated most clearly by electron microscopy (Fig. 15.10). Fine-structural observations suggest that hepatocytes and fat-storing cells play a joint role in the pathogenesis of this type of fibrosis.[58] In the sclerosis seen around central veins, increased numbers of myofibroblasts are characteristic (Fig. 15.11; see also Ch. 11)[5,34,44] and it has been postulated that the myofibroblast participates mainly in this type of fibrosis.[58]

DRUG-INDUCED LIVER INJURIES

Drug-induced liver injuries can be divided into two broad categories: one is predictable, and dose- and time-dependent, while in contrast the other is unpredictable, and independent of dosage or time. It is known that the predictable and dose-dependent drug-induced reactions result mainly from the generation of highly reactive metabolites, which bind to, and denature hepatocyte components; acetaminophen-induced liver damage is a typical example of this type of injury. The other is thought to be caused by a lymphocyte-mediated immune reaction to hepatocyte plasma membranes transformed by reactive metabolites, and is typified by halothane-induced hepatitis.

In predictable and dose-dependent drug-induced injury, the histological picture varies from fatty liver to fulminant forms of liver damage. In mild cases, in which fat droplets appear in combination with changes of RER — such as disarray or disruption — the formation of fat droplets is probably the result of disturbed lipoprotein synthesis in the RER. In acetaminophen- or carbon tetrachloride-induced liver injury, characteristic morphological changes include large membranous aggregates consisting of plump vesicles associated with an accumulation of dense material, which Trump and associates consider to be the result of membrane peroxidation.[1,60,61]

In cases with severe halothane-induced hepatitis, lymphocytes — probably cytotoxic in character — are in close contact with degenerating or necrotic hepatocytes, suggesting a lymphocyte-mediated reaction in the genesis of hepatocyte necrosis (Fig. 15.12).[62] In addition, hepatocyte mitochondria show characteristic alterations — such as large granules, diminished matrix density, or changes of the cristae.[62] Such mitochondrial alterations may explain the occurrence of anti-mitochondrial antibody in halothane-induced liver injury.

In phospholipidosis induced by the coronary dilator, 4,4'-diethylaminoethoxy hexestrol dihydrochloride, the hepatocyte is filled with numerous laminated electron-dense granules.[9,37] However, such laminated bodies are also described in a considerable number of drug-induced liver injuries,[43] and they seem to be non-specific.

In general, some pathogenetic processes in drug-related liver injury can be postulated from the fine-structural changes. However, it is frequently difficult or impossible to identify the causative agents in individual cases of drug-induced liver injury by EM.

CHOLESTASIS DUE TO VARIOUS CAUSES

Cholestasis represents one of the major pathological changes in the liver and two types — extrahepatic and intrahepatic — are well known. By electron microscopy the bile canaliculi are usually dilated, with loss or stunting of the lining microvilli, and the lumina often contain electron-dense bile thrombi which have finely granular, crystalline, lamellar or whorled configurations. The pericanalicular ectoplasm is usually widened due to an increased number of microfilaments. In the cytoplasm of the hepatocyte the mitochondria are often enlarged with occasional curling of cristae, and numerous electron-dense aggregates of finely granular and fibrillar material are found; these aggregates may represent either stagnated bile material or degenerated cytoplasmic components, the latter possibly resulting from the detergent action of bile acids accumulating in the cytoplasm. At the present time, however, it is usually impossible to distinguish extrahepatic from intrahepatic cholestasis by EM.

Byler's disease is a progressive familial intrahepatic cholestasis seen in young children, and by EM the bile canaliculi show remarkable changes, with thickening of pericanalicular ectoplasm.[10] However, the aberrations are basically similar to those seen in other types of cholestasis.

In primary biliary cirrhosis characteristic changes have been noted in bile ducts located in the portal tracts. Some of the ductal cells appear to be electron dense and shrunken, and they are often in close contact with lymphocytes (Fig. 15.13), suggesting lymphocyte-mediated mechanisms in the ductal damage. Usually the bile duct is surrounded by a thickened and irregular basal lamina which often contains electron-dense particles.

CIRRHOSIS

Provided that sufficient amounts of liver tissue are obtained by biopsy, the light microscopy diagnosis of cirrhosis is straightforward, but fragmented or insubstantial biopsies can make evaluation difficult. In such circumstances the fine-structural characteristics of hepatocytes or sinusoidal cells can facilitate the diagnosis. In general, hepatocytes in cirrhotic nodules are arranged in plates two to three cells wide, with expansion of the intercellular space surrounding the hepatocytes and development of microvilli on the entire plasma membrane (Fig. 15.14).[42] In addition, the sinusoids often appear to be capillarized, with the formation of a basal lamina beneath the endothelial cell (Fig. 15.15).[45]

In cirrhosis and chronic active hepatitis, mitochondria-rich hepatocytes (with deeply eosinophilic granular cytoplasm by light microscopy) have been noted,[15,29] but their significance is unclear.

FATTY LIVER

Two types of fatty liver are recognized: the common type is characterized by large fat droplets occupying most of the cytoplasm and displacing the hepatocyte nucleus to the periphery of the cell. In the development of the former, it appears that lipid synthesized and accumulating in the distended SER fuses to form large droplets,[52] but that other organelles in the cytoplasm are well preserved. In the second type of fatty liver, numerous small fat droplets are formed in association with distinct and characteristic alterations of the mitochondria (Fig. 15.16). This type of fatty liver is seen in Reye's syndrome[22,38,47] and acute fatty liver of pregnancy, and unless tissue has been taken for frozen section or osmication, electron-microscopic examination is the only means of making a definitive histological diagnosis. It has been reported that ultrastructural changes in the liver in salicylate intoxication are different from those of Reye's syndrome.[39]

CONSTITUTIONAL HYPERBILIRUBINAEMIA

At present, constitutional hyperbilirubinaemia (such as the Dubin–Johnson syndrome, the Rotor syndrome, or Gilbert's disease) can be diagnosed relatively easily by the history of chronic intermittent jaundice and conventional liver function tests. Rarely, however, there are difficulties in differentiating these disorders from acquired chronic liver disease or in distinguishing them from each other. Thus, knowledge of the characteristic ultrastructural features of these inherited disorders of bilirubin metabolism is of some importance,[56] but unfortunately most of the changes are non-specific.

On the basis of pathogenesis, Gilbert's disease can be divided into at least two types; one variety is due to a defect of bilirubin uptake at the sinusoidal plasma membrane of the hepatocytes and in its subsequent transport to the SER, in which bilirubin conjugation takes place, while the other type is due to a defect in the conjugation of bilirubin as a result of deficient glucuronyl transferase activity. The ultrastructural changes can also be divided into two varieties; one shows an increase in the volume of SER,[8] while in the other the SER appears normal.[25] However, confirmation of these observations by other studies is required.

In the Dubin–Johnson syndrome, electron-dense round or oval granules about 0.5 to 2.5 μm in diameter are characteristic (Fig. 15.17). They are frequently seen around the bile canaliculus, and they differ in their fine structure from other granules such as haemosiderin or lipofuscin; most Dubin–Johnson granules resemble lipofuscin bodies but are morphologically distinguishable from the latter, which often have lipid components. In addition, it should be emphasized that the bile canaliculi are slightly dilated with stunting or loss of microvilli, and about half the canaliculi contain intraluminal electron-dense granules which probably originate from the characteristic cytoplasmic granules.[55]

WILSON'S DISEASE AND HAEMOCHROMATOSIS

In Wilson's disease it is thought that the accumulation of copper in hepatocytes is caused by failure of excretion of this metal into the bile canaliculus, probably due to lysosomal abnormalities. During the asymptomatic phase, fatty change is frequently present. By EM, changes of hepatocyte mitochondria are prominent features and they include dense matrices, dilated cristae, prominent granules, irregularly shaped vacuoles, and separation of the outer and inner membranes.[50,51] Irregularly-shaped dense and large peroxisomes are also present. In this stage, copper is diffusely distributed in the cytoplasm of the hepatocytes, and the ultrastructural features seem to be similar to those seen in copper intoxication. Sometimes, it is difficult to distinguish Wilson's disease from chronic active hepatitis — not only by the clinical picture but also by light microscopy; therefore it is always important to consider Wilson's disease in children with chronic liver disease, and ultrastructural study may be helpful in making a diagnosis at this stage.

In the symptomatic stage, EM demonstrates numerous electron-dense lysosomes with several small vacuoles of similar size in hepatocytes (Fig. 15.18). Analytic studies indicate that these lysosomes contain a large amount of copper; concentration of copper within lysosomes seems to protect the hepatocyte from its toxic effects.

The hepatocytes in haemochromatosis are characterized by a considerable number of haemosiderin granules in the cytoplasm (Fig. 15.19). By electron microscopy, such granules are composed of fine iron-containing particles and they are surrounded by a single membrane;[4] close observation also discloses similar fine particles scattered throughout the cytoplasm.

In both Wilson's disease and haemochromatosis, elemental X-ray microanalysis can be used to demonstrate the presence of copper or iron in the respective characteristic granules.

STORAGE DISEASES AND OTHER CONGENITAL AND METABOLIC DISORDERS

Since the liver is a central organ in metabolism, it is affected in most of the storage diseases, and recent ultrastructural studies have demonstrated the characteristic findings in the liver of each (see also Ch. 6).

In glycogen storage disease the cytoplasm of the hepatocytes is occupied by excess glycogen granules, and in type II glycogenosis (Pompe's disease), abnormal lysosomes filled with glycogen particles are characteristic (see Ch. 6).[2,21] In alpha-1-antitrypsin deficiency a distinct and abnormal amorphous material is present in the greatly dilated endoplasmic reticulum of the hepatocytes.[13]

By EM, amyloid deposits are usually seen to be located in the space of Disse, and they are composed of fine fibrils measuring about 10 nm in diameter.

In the lipidoses, excess lipid accumulates in Kupffer cells, and sometimes also in hepatocytes and other cell components in the liver. Because the different types of lipidosis have distinct fine-structural features, EM is of diagnostic importance (see Ch. 6).[20,63] In Gaucher's disease, the so-called Gaucher cell contains many membrane-enclosed cytoplasmic bodies (lysosomes) filled with tubular structures (Fig. 15.20; see also Fig. 6.15).[14] In Niemann–Pick disease, numerous round or oval vacuoles filled with loosely arranged, sometimes concentric or parallel osmiophilic membranes are seen in hepatocytes and Kupffer cells.[64] In the mucopolysaccharidoses, numerous electron-lucid vacuoles bounded by a single membrane are observed in the hepatocytes (Fig. 15.21), Kupffer cells and bile duct epithelial cells.[7] Ultrastructural features of the liver in cholesterol ester storage disease take the form of numerous electron-lucent vacuoles or angularly shaped inclusions of cholesterol ester in Kupffer cells, hepatocytes and other cell components in the liver (Fig. 15.22).[28]

In the cerebrohepatorenal syndrome of Zellweger, peroxisomes in hepatocytes are greatly reduced in number or completely absent, while the mitochondria are abnormal, showing increased density of their matrices;[18,33] these changes are unique and are of diagnostic significance. Finally, in erythropoietic protoporphyria characteristic rosette-like aggregates of needle-like crystals can be observed in hepatocytes and Kupffer cells.[66]

MISCELLANEOUS DISORDERS

In reversible acute hypoxia the hepatocyte is characterized by depletion of glycogen particles, swelling of the mitochondria and dilatation of the endoplasmic reticulum, as well as by the appearance of large hypoxic vacuoles.[26] Electron microscopy can demonstrate talc particles as electron-dense, elongated particles with sharp edges, and sometimes with apparent lamination, in macrophages in the liver of narcotic addicts.[6] In a variant of multiple myeloma, kappa light-chain disease, granular and fibrillar electron-dense material is deposited in the space of Disse;[30] immunohistochemical study demonstrates the presence of kappa light chains.

REFERENCES

1. Arstila A U, Smith M, Trump B F 1972 Microsomal lipid peroxidation: morphological characterization. Science 175: 530–533
2. Baudhuin P, Hers H G, Loeb H 1964 An electron microscopic and biochemical study of type II glycogenosis. Laboratory Investigation 13: 1139–1152
3. Bernua D, Feldmann G, Degott C, Gisselbrecht C 1981 Ultrastructural lesions of bile ducts in primary biliary cirrhosis. Human Pathology 12: 782–793
4. Bessis M, Caroli J 1959 A comparative study of hemochromatosis by electron microscopy. Gastroenterology 37: 538–549
5. Bhathal P S 1972 Presence of modified fibroblasts in cirrhotic livers in man. Human Pathology 4: 139–144
6. Buschmann R J, Mir J 1979 Electron microscope identity of talc in the liver of a narcotic addict. Human Pathology 10: 736–739
7. Callahan W P, Lorincz A F 1966 Hepatic ultrastructure in the Hurler syndrome. American Journal of Pathology 48: 277–298
8. Dawson J, Carr-Locke D L, Talbot I C, Rosenthal F D 1979 Gilbert's syndrome: evidence of morphological heterogeneity. Gut 20: 848–853
9. De la Iglesia F A, Feuer G, Takada A, Matsuda Y 1974 Morphologic studies on secondary phospholipidosis in human liver. Laboratory Investigation 30: 539–549
10. De Vos R, De Wolf-Peeters C, Desmet V, Eggermont E, Van Acker K 1975 Progressive intrahepatic cholestasis (Byler's disease): case report. Gut 16: 643–650
11. De Vos R, Ray M B, Desmet V 1979 Electron microscopy of hepatitis B virus components in chronic active liver disease. Journal of Clinical Pathology 32: 590–600
12. De Vos R, Vanstapel M J, Desmyter J, De Wolf-Peeters C, De Groote G, Colaert J, Mortelmans J, De Groote J, Fevery J, Desmet V, 1983 Are nuclear particles specific for non-A, non-B hepatitis? Hepatology 3: 532–544
13. Feldman G, Bignon J, Chahinian P, Degott C, Benhamou J 1974 Hepatocyte ultrastructural changes in *alpha*-1-antitrypsin deficiency. Gastroenterology 67: 1214–1224
14. Fisher E R, Reidbord H 1962 Gaucher's diseases: pathogenetic consideration based on electron microscopic and histochemical observations. American Journal of Pathology 41: 679–692
15. Gerber M A, Thung S N 1981 Hepatic oncocyte. Incidence, staining characteristics and ultrastructural features. American Society of Clinical Pathologists 75: 498–503
16. Gerber M A, Orr W, Denk H, Schaffner F, Popper H 1973 Hepatocellular hyalin in cholestasis and cirrhosis: its diagnostic significance. Gastroenterology 64: 89–98
17. Gerber M A, Paronetto F 1974 Hepatitis B antigen in human tissues. In: Schaffner F, Sherlock S, Leevy C M (eds) The liver and its diseases. Intercontinental Medical Book Corporation, New York, pp 54–63
18. Goldfischer S, Moore C L, Johnson A B, Spiro A J, Valsamis M P, Wisniewski H K, Ritch R H, Norton W T, Rapid I, Gartner L M 1973 Peroxisomal and mitochondrial defects in the cerebro-hepato-renal syndrome. Science 182: 62–64
19. Grimaud J A, Peyrol S, Vitvitski L, Chevallier-Queyron P, Trepo C 1980 Hepatic intranuclear particles in patients with non-A, non-B hepatitis. New England Journal of Medicine 303: 818–819
20. Hers H G, Van Hoof F 1970 The genetic pathology of lysosomes. In: Popper H, Schaffner F (eds) Progress in liver diseases, vol III. Grune & Stratton, New York, pp 185–205
21. Hug G, Garancis J C, Schubert W K 1966 Glycogen storage disease, type II, III and IX. American Journal of Diseases of Children 111: 457–474
22. Iancu T C, Mason W H, Neustein H B 1977 Ultrastructural abnormalities of liver cells in Reye's syndrome. Human Patholology 8: 421–431
23. Itoh S, Matsuo S, Ichinoe A, Yamaba Y, Miyazawa M 1982 Nonalcoholic steatohepatitis and cirrhosis with Mallory's hyalin. Digestive Diseases and Sciences 27: 341–346
24. Ito T, Nemoto M 1952 Uber die Kupfferschen Sternzellen und 'die Fettspeicherungszellen' ('fat storing cells') in der Blutkapillarenwand der Menschilichen Leber. Folia Anatomica Japonica 24: 243–258
25. Jezequel A M, Mosca P G, Koch M M, Orlandi F 1980 The fine morphology of unconjugated hyperbilirubinemia revisited with stereometry. In: Okolicsanyi L (ed) Familial hyperbilirubinemia. John Wiley & Sons, Chichester, pp 69–79
26. Jozsa L, Reffy A, Demel S, Szilagyi I 1981 Ultrastructural changes in human liver cells due to reversible acute hypoxia. Hepato-Gastroenterology 28: 23–26
27. Kaneda K, Dan C, Wake K 1983 Pit cells as natural killer cells. Biomedical Research 4: 567–576
28. Kawaguchi M, Hidaka S, Ikejiri N, Maeyama T, Egucji N, Sato S, Abe H 1977 A case of cholesterol ester storage disease. Acta Hepatologica Japonica 18: 786–794
29. Lefkowitch J H, Arborgh B A M, Scheuer P J 1980 Oxyphilic granular hepatocytes: mitochondrion-rich liver cells in hepatic disease. American Society of Clinical Pathologists 74: 431–441
30. Linder J, Vollmer R T, Croker B P, Shelburne J 1983 Systemic kappa light-chain deposition: an ultrastructural and immunohistochemical study. American Journal of Pathology 7: 85–93
31. Ludwig J, Viggiano T R, McGill D B, Ott B J 1980 Nonalcoholic steatohepatitis. Mayo Clinic Proceedings 55: 434–438
32. MacSween R N M 1973 Mallory's (alcoholic) hyaline in primary biliary cirrhosis. Journal of Clinical Pathology 26: 340–342
33. Mooi W J, Dingemans K P, van Bergh Weerman M A, Jobsis A C, Heymans H S, Barth P G 1983 Ultrastructure of the liver in the cerebrohepatorenal syndrome of Zellweger. Ultrastructural Pathology 5: 135–144
34. Nakano M, Worner T M, Lieber C S 1982 Perivenular fibrosis in alcoholic liver injury; ultrastructure and histologic progression. Gastroenterology 83: 777–785
35. Nayak N C, Sagreiga K, Ramalingaswami M 1969 Indian childhood cirrhosis. The nature and significance of cytoplasmic hyaline of hepatocytes. Archives of Pathology 88: 631–637
36. Nazarewicz-de Mezer T, Krawczynski K, Michalak T, Nowoslawski A 1980 Intracellular localization of HB antigen in liver tissue. In: Bianchi L, Gerok W, Sickinger K, Stalder G A (eds) Virus and the liver. MTP Press, Lancaster, pp 85–95
37. Oda T, Shikata T, Naito C, Suzuki H, Kanetaka, T, Lino S, Miyake K, Sakai T, Onda H, Fujiwaka K, Yamanaka M, Shimuzu N, Yoshitoshi Y 1970 Phospholipid fatty liver; a report of three cases with a new type of fatty liver. Japanese Journal of Experimental Medicine 40: 127–140
38. Partin J C, Schubert W K, Partin J S 1971 Mitochondrial ultrastructure in Reye's syndrome (encephalopathy and fatty degeneration of the viscera). New England Journal of Medicine 285: 1339–1343
39. Partin J S, Daugherty C C, McAdams A J, Partin J C, Schubert W K 1984 A comparison of liver ultrastructure in salicylate intoxication and Reye's syndrome. Hepatology 4: 687–690
40. Pfeifer U 1983 Ultrastructural pathology of the human liver. In: Csomos G, Tahler H (eds) Clinical hepatology. Springer-Verlag, Berlin, pp 159–194
41. Phillips M J, Poucell S, Patterson J, Valencia P 1987 The liver. An atlas and text of ultrastructural pathology. Raven Press, New York
42. Phillips H, Steiner J W 1965 Electron microscopy of liver cells in cirrhotic nodules I. The lateral cell membrane. American Journal of Pathology 46: 985–1006
43. Poucell S, Ireton J, Valencia-Mayoral P, Downar E, Larratt L, Patterson J, Blendis L, Phillips M J 1984 Amiodarone-associated phospholipidosis and fibrosis of the liver. Gastroenterology 86: 926–936
44. Rudolph R, McClure W J, Woodward M 1979 Contractile fibroblasts in chronic alcoholic cirrhosis. Gastroenterology 76: 704–709
45. Schaffner F, Popper H 1963 Capillarization of hepatic sinusoids in man. Gastroenterology 44: 239–242
46. Schaffner F 1985 Epstein–Barr virus in chronic hepatitis. In: Bianchi L, Gerok W, Popper H (eds) Trends in hepatology. MTP Press, Lancaster, pp 209–216
47. Schubert W K, Partin J C, Partin J S 1973 Encephalopathy and fatty liver (Reye's syndrome). In: Popper H, Schaffner F (eds) Progress in liver diseases, vol IV. Grune & Stratton, New York, pp 489–510
48. Shimizu Y K, Feinstone S M, Purcell R H, Alter H J, London W T 1979 Non-A, non-B hepatitis: ultrastructural evidence of two agents in experimentally infected chimpanzees. Science 205: 197–200

49. Shimizu Y K, Shikata K, Beninger P R, Sata M, Setoyama M, Abe H, Tanikawa K 1982 Detection of hepatitis A antigen in human liver. Infection and Immunity 36: 320–324

50. Sternlieb I 1972 Evolution of hepatic lesion in Wilson's disease (hepatolenticular degeneration), In: Popper H, Schaffner F (eds) Progress in liver diseases, vol VI. Grune & Stratton, New York, pp 511–525

51. Sternlieb I 1983 Abnormalities of copper metabolism in disease states. In: Thomas H C, MacSween R N M (eds) Recent advances in hepatology I. Churchill Livingstone, Edinburgh, pp 115–129

52. Tanikawa K, Miyakoda U 1973 Etude au microscope electronique des mechanismes de depot et de disparition des lipides hepatiques dans la steatose ethylique. Annales de Gastroenterologie et Hepatologie 9: 411–422

53. Tanikawa K 1975 Ultrastructure of hepatic fibrosis and fat-storing cell. In: Popper H, Becker K (eds) Collagen metabolism in the liver. Stratton Intercontinental Medical Book, New York, pp 93–99

54. Tanikawa K 1979 Ultrastructural aspects of the liver and its disorders, 2nd edn. Igaku-Shoin, Tokyo

55. Tanikawa K 1979 Liver pathology. In: Trump B F, Jones R T (eds) Diagnostic electron microscopy, vol 2. John Wiley & Sons, New York, pp 15–46

56. Tanikawa K 1980 Pathology of jaundice and cholestasis at the ultrastructural level. In: Trump B F, Arstila A U (eds) Pathobiology of cell membranes II. Academic Press, New York, pp 381–420

57. Tanikawa K 1981 Application of electron microscopy to the clinical diagnosis of liver diseases. Journal of Clinical Electron Microscopy 14: 353–354

58. Tanikawa K, Ueno T 1975 Fine structural features and role of fat-storing cell and basement membrane in hepatic fibrosis. In: Hirayama C, Kivirikko K I (eds) Pathobiology of hepatic fibrosis. Excerpta Medica, Amsterdam, pp 3–11

59. Tanikawa K, Sata M, Setoyama H, Abe H 1986 Changes of the Kupffer cell and clinical manifestations in acute hepatitis type A. In: Kirn A, Knook D L, Wisse E (eds) Cell of the hepatic sinusoid, Vol 2. Kupffer Cell Foundation Rijewijk, The Netherlands. pp 371–376

60. Trump B F, Arstila A U 1971 Cellular and subcellular reactions of cells to injury. In: La Via N, Hill R (eds) Principles of pathobiology. Oxford University Press, New York, p 9

61. Trump B F, Dees J H, Sherburne J S 1973 The ultrastructure of the human liver cell and its common patterns of reaction to injury. In: Gall E A, Mostofi F K (eds) The liver. Williams & Wilkins, Baltimore, p 80

62. Uzunalimoglu B, Yardley J H, Boitnott J K 1970 The liver in mild halothane hepatitis. Light and electron microscopic findings with special reference to the mononuclear cell infiltrate. American Journal of Pathology 61: 457–478

63. Volk B H, Wellmann K F, Wallace B J 1970 Hepatic changes in various lipidoses: electron microscopic and histochemical studies. In: Popper H, Schaffner F (eds) Progress in liver diseases, vol III. Grune & Stratton, New York, pp 206–221

64. Volk W, Wallace B J 1966 The liver in lipidosis: an electron microscopic and histochemical study. American Journal of Pathology 49: 203–225

65. Wisse E, Van't Noordende J M, Van der Meulen J, Daems W T 1976 The pit cell: description of a new type of cell occurring in rat liver sinusoids and peripheral blood. Cell Tissue Research 173: 423–435

66. Wolff K, Wolff-Schreiner E, Gschnait F 1975 Liver inclusions in erythropoietic protoporphyria. European Journal of Clinical Investigation 5: 21–26

67. Yokoo H, Minick O, Batti F, Kent G 1972 Morphologic variants of alcoholic hyalin. American Journal of Pathology 69: 25–40

Fig. 15.1 (Top left) Normal liver: Ito cell. This fat-storing cell (Ito cell, lipocyte) is located in the space of Disse and has a fat droplet in the cytoplasm. The cell is surrounded by fibre bundles, and the prominence of RER and the Golgi apparatus in its cytoplasm confer a fine-structural resemblance to fibroblasts. ($\times$ 10 000) References: 24 and 53.

Fig. 15.2 (Top right) Normal liver: pit cell. The pit cell, embedded in the endothelial lining, contains characteristic granules and a few organelles which are all polarized to one side of the nucleus. ($\times$ 7300) References: 27 and 65.

Fig. 15.3 (Bottom left) Acute hepatitis type A: hepatitis A virus (HAV). Numerous HAV particles (arrow) are evident in the lysosome of the hepatocyte; they appear to be round, and measure 27 nm in diameter. ($\times$ 38 700) References: 49 and 57.

Fig. 15.4 (Bottom left) Kupffer cell: Hepatitis A virus (HAV) Liver biopsy specimen taken from a patient with acute hepatitis type A shows HAV particles (arrow) within a lysosome of the Kupffer cell. ($\times$ 26 700) References: 38 and 45.

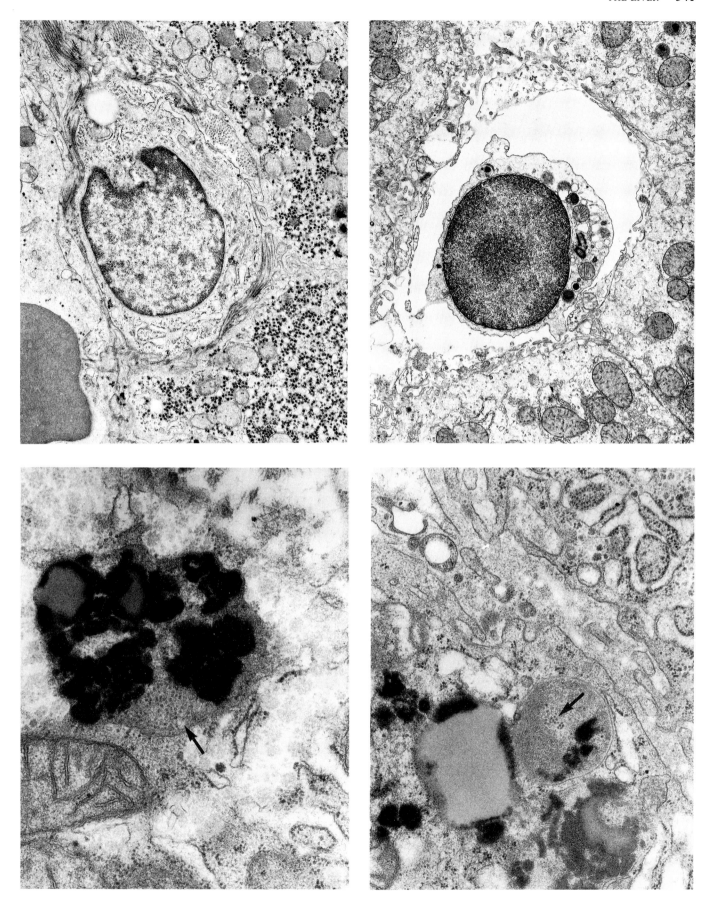

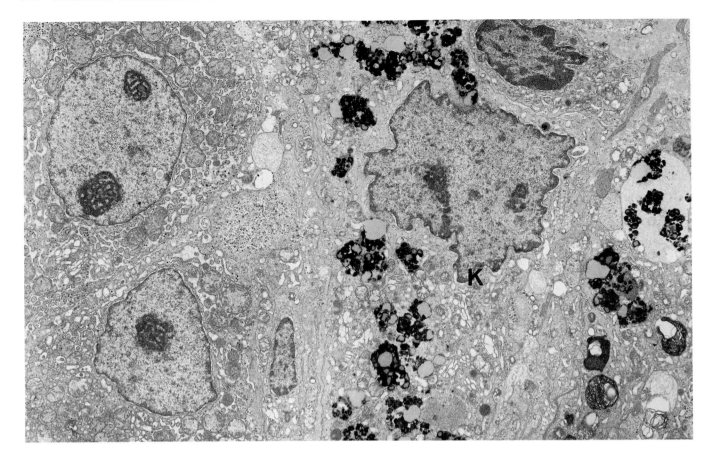

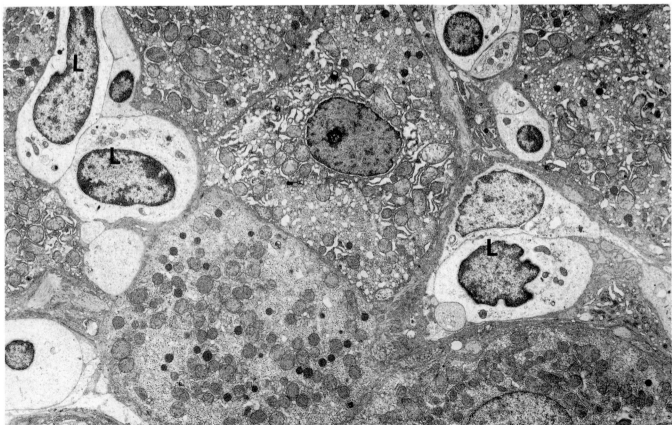

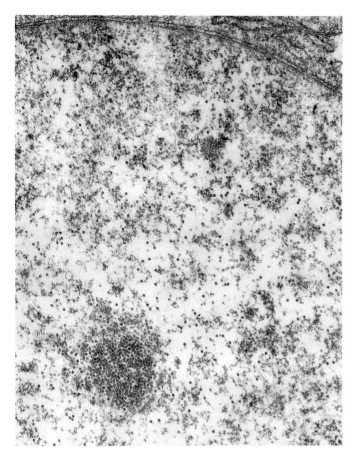

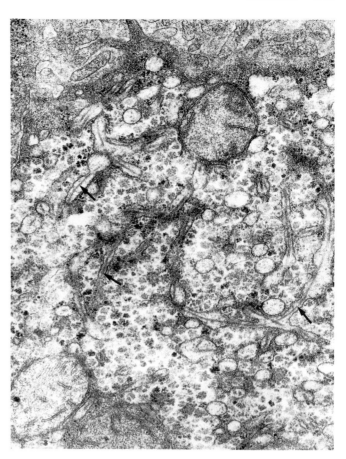

Fig. 15.7 Hepatocyte nucleus: HBc antigens. Numerous HBc antigen particles are scattered in the nucleus of this hepatocyte in a hepatitis B virus carrier; some of them form an aggregate (lower left). (× 30 000) References: 17 and 36.

Fig. 15.8 Hepatocyte cytoplasm: HBs antigens. A liver biopsy specimen taken from a hepatitis B virus carrier shows numerous filamentous HBs antigens (arrows) within the distended cisternae of the SER in the hepatocyte. (× 30 000) References: 11, 17 and 36.

Fig. 15.5 (Facing page, top) Kupffer cell: acute hepatitis type A. The Kupffer cell (K) is markedly enlarged and filled with numerous electron-dense lysosomes, some of which contain hepatitis A virus particles (not resolved at this magnification). Adjacent hepatocytes appear to be markedly altered. (× 5300) Reference: 59.

Fig. 15.6 (Facing page, bottom)   Acute hepatitis type B: lymphocytic infiltration. Lymphocytes (L) are in contact with hepatocytes which appear to be severely damaged, suggesting lymphocyte-mediated cell injury. (× 4000)

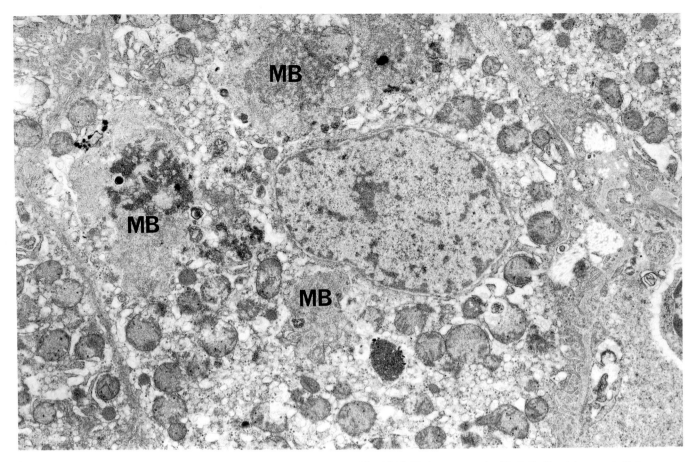

Fig. 15.9   Alcoholic hepatitis: Mallory body. Three Mallory bodies (MB) are seen in the hepatocyte. They are basically composed of filamentous materials (not resolved at this magnification), and some have dense central aggregates. Mitochondria appear to be enlarged or distorted (× 9300) Reference: 67.

Fig. 15.10 (Facing page, top)   Alcoholic liver injury: pericellular fibrosis. Pericellular fibrosis (F) is evident around a hepatocyte, while the hepatocyte plasmalemma adjacent to the fibre bundles appears to be flattened, with loss of its microvilli. (× 9300) Reference: 58.

Fig. 15.11 (Facing page, bottom)   Alcoholic liver injury: central sclerosis. In the central sclerosis around a central vein, myofibroblasts (MF; see also Figs 11.1 and 11.2) are increased in number and seem to participate in fibrosis at this site. They contain long microfilaments parallel to the plasma membrane. (× 1100) References: 5, 34 and 44.

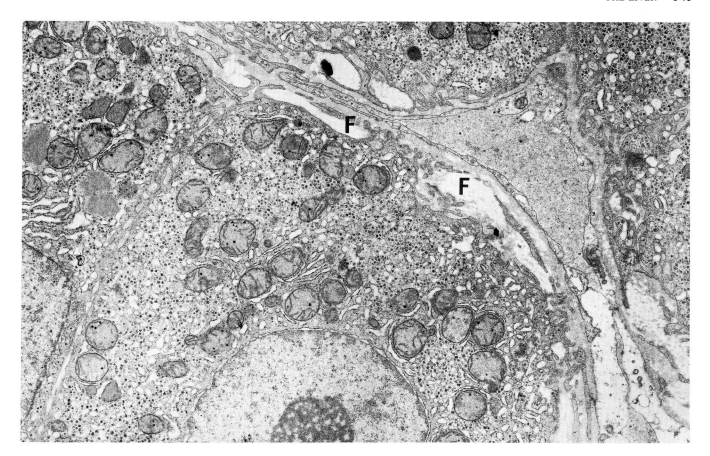

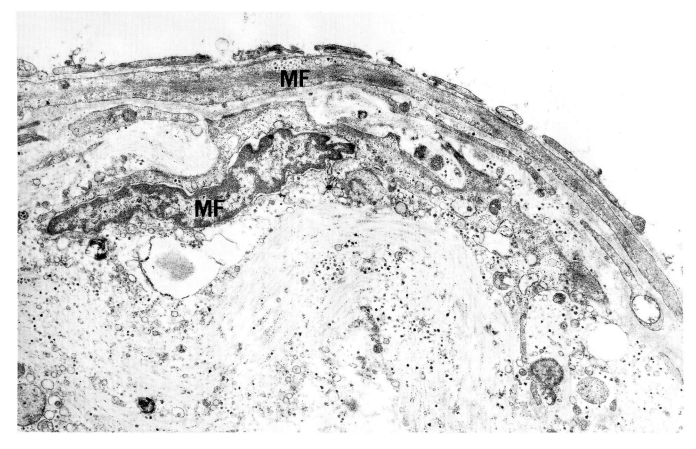

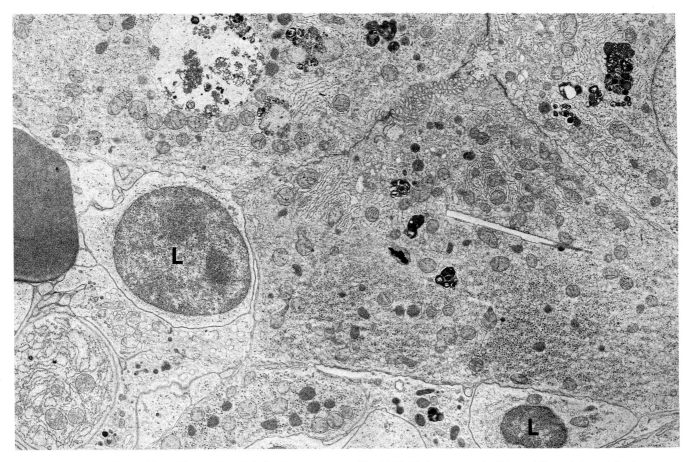

Fig. 15.12 Halothane-induced hepatitis: lymphocytic infiltration. Lymphocytes (L) are in close contact with hepatocytes, which appear to be markedly changed, with numerous electron-dense particles in the cytoplasm. (× 7300) Reference: 62.

Fig. 15.13 (Facing page, top)   Primary biliary cirrhosis: bile duct. The ductal cells appear to be markedly altered and are in close contact with lymphocytes (L), which migrate between the ductal cells. The bile duct is also surrounded by a thickened and irregular basal lamina. (× 5300)

Fig. 15.14 (Facing page, bottom)   Hepatocyte in cirrhotic nodule. Hepatocytes in cirrhotic nodule are arranged in plates two to three cells wide and the intercellular space is widened, with development of microvilli from the exposed plasma membrane of the hepatocyte. (× 6000) Reference: 42.

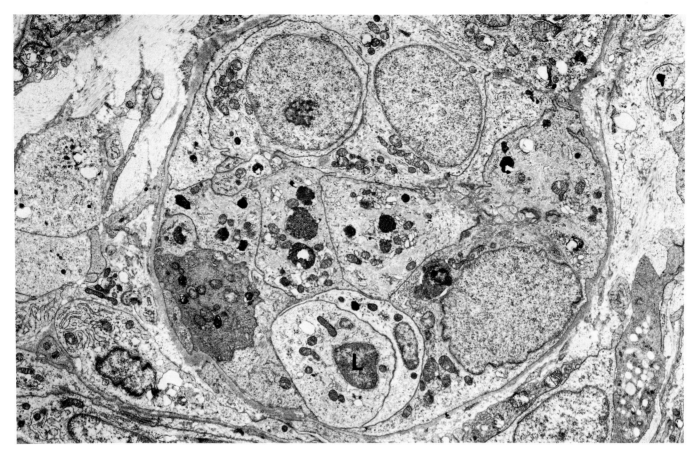

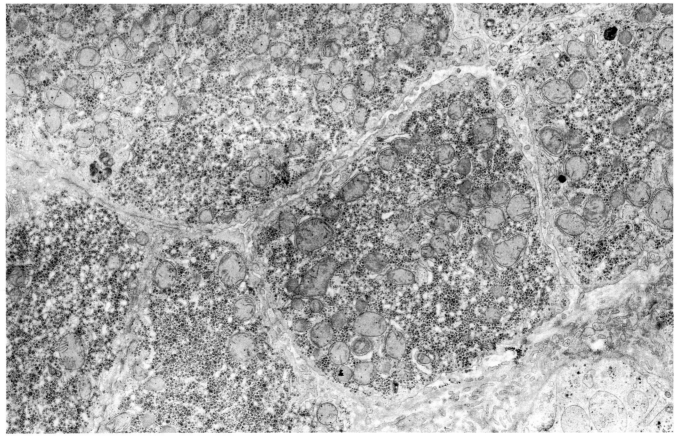

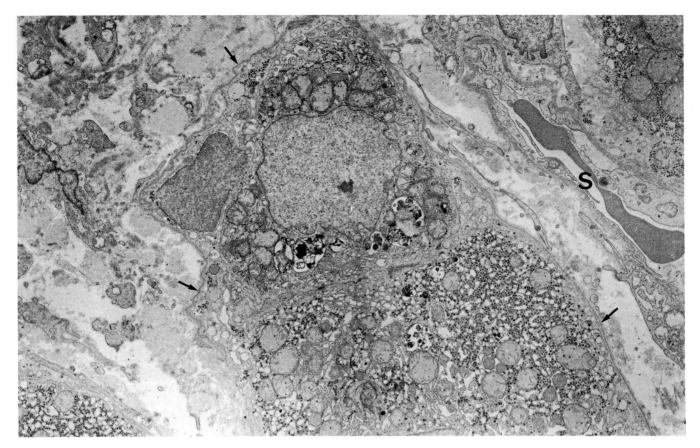

Fig. 15.15 (Above)   Liver cirrhosis: sinusoidal capillarization. The sinusoid (S) is capillarized, with the formation of a basal lamina beneath the endothelial cells. Basal lamina can also be seen very close to the hepatocytes (arrows). (× 5300) Reference: 45.

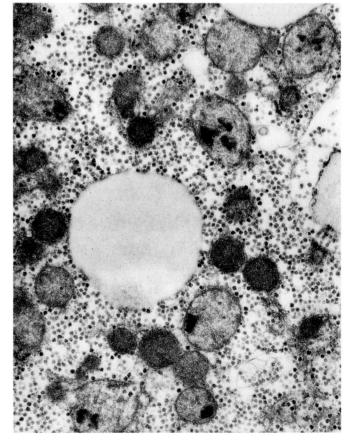

Fig. 15.16 (Right)   Reye's syndrome: hepatocytic lesions. Small fat droplets are evident in the cytoplasm of the hepatocyte, while the mitochondria are abnormal, showing prominent granules and a loss of cristae. (× 16 000) References: 38 and 47.

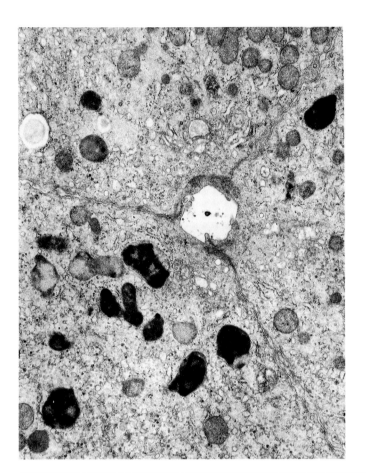

Fig. 15.17 (Left)   Dubin–Johnson syndrome: hepatocytic cytoplasm. Characteristic electron-dense granules are seen around the bile canaliculus, which is slightly dilated with stunting of microvilli, while its lumen contains small dense granules. (× 8000) Reference: 55.

Fig. 15.18 (Below)   Wilson's disease: hepatocytic cytoplasm. Numerous electron-dense granules with small vacuoles of similar size are present in the cytoplasm of the hepatocyte. Elemental X-ray microanalysis reveals the presence of copper in these granules. (× 13 000) References: 50 and 51.

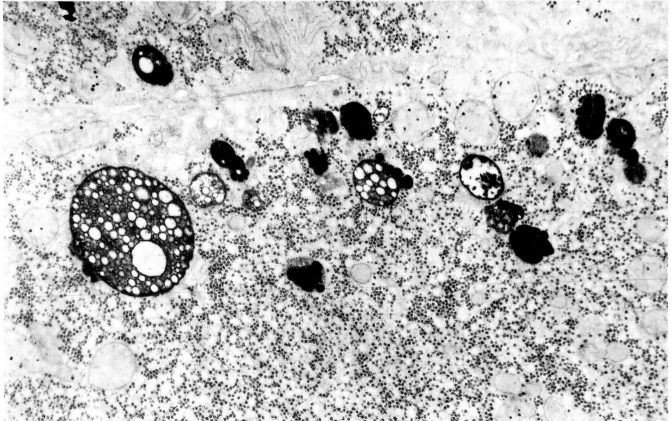

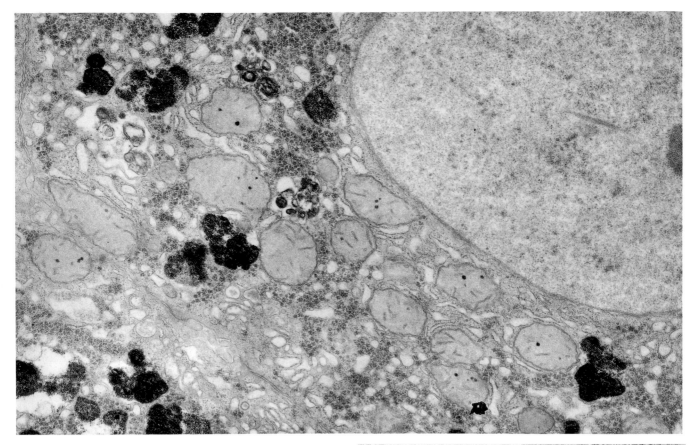

Fig. 15.19 Haemochromatosis: lysosomes. Hemosiderin granules, filled with fine iron-containing particles and surrounded by a single membrane, are numerous within the cytoplasm of this hepatocyte. (× 15 000)

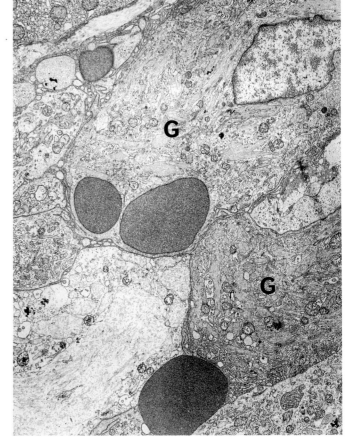

Fig. 15.20 Gaucher cell: lysosomes. Gaucher cells (G) in the liver are filled with characteristic intralysosomal tubular structures, enclosed by a single membrane. Erythrocytes are also shown to be taken up by the cell. (× 5300) Reference: 14.

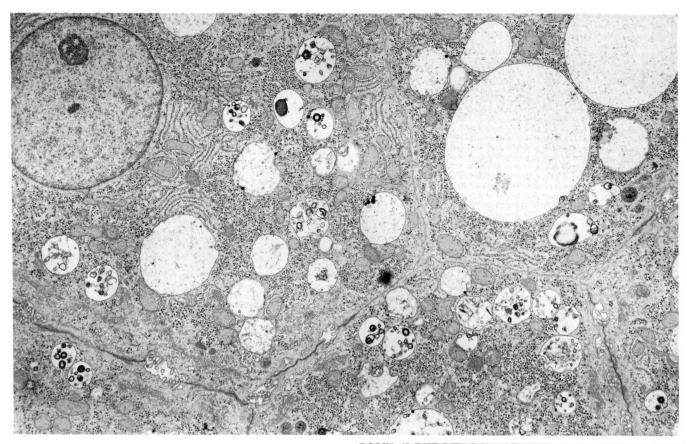

Fig. 15.21 Mucopolysaccharidosis: hepatocytic cytoplasm. Numerous electron-lucid vacuoles with small electron–dense granules are numerous within the cytoplasm of the hepatocyte; they represent accumulated acid mucopolysaccharide. (× 5300) Reference: 7.

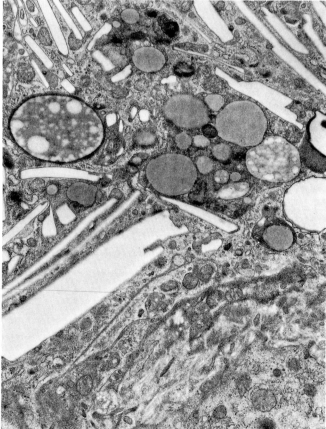

Fig. 15.22 Cholesterol ester storage disease: Kupffer cell. Numerous rounded and angulated inclusions of cholesterol ester are present in the Kupffer cell. (× 8000) Reference: 28.

16. The endocrine system

Sylvia L. Asa   Eva Horvath   K. Kovacs

INTRODUCTION

Electron microscopy (EM) is an important tool in the investigation of endocrine tissues in normal and abnormal conditions. Cells whose primary function is the secretion of hormones have characteristic subcellular features, with organelles specialized for hormone synthesis and release; the functional activity of endocrine cells is therefore reflected in their ultrastructural morphology. Most endocrine glands are composed of several cell types, and the identification of the constituent cells involved in disease processes is frequently based on specific structural characteristics. Recognition of changes in the ultrastructural appearances of various cell types is one means of studying the pathophysiology of non-neoplastic disorders and identifying the mechanisms of action of therapeutic agents.

This chapter is limited to a review of transmission EM. Other ultrastructural methods, including scanning EM, ultrastructural autoradiography, immuno-electron microscopy and freeze-fracture techniques are utilized in the morphologic study of endocrine tissues; however, they will not be dealt with here.

The scope of endocrinology has expanded to encompass parts of the hypothalamus, pineal gland and thymus in addition to the diffuse endocrine system, but these will not be discussed. The gonads, which are integral hormone-secreting glands, are described in other chapters.

ANTERIOR PITUITARY

Non-neoplastic diseases of the anterior pituitary are seen by the pathologist mainly at autopsy, and material obtained post mortem is not suitable for detailed electron-microscopic studies because pituitary tissue undergoes rapid autolysis after death. Surgical biopsies are rarely performed, as in the substantial majority of cases the correct diagnosis can be made on the basis of clinical and biochemical examinations. For these reasons, information on the ultrastructural features of non-neoplastic diseases of the anterior pituitary is limited (Fig. 16.1). Because of marked species differences in

the structural characteristics and functional responses of adenohypophyseal cells, no extrapolation from the animal pituitary to the human gland is justified. Thus, electron microscopic investigation of the pituitaries of various animal species provides little help in the better understanding of human disease.

Circulatory disturbances

Circulatory disturbances may lead to haemorrhage or infarction,[34] and in these cases ultrastructural findings are non-contributory. Hypoxia may cause changes in the endothelium (which is fenestrated under normal conditions in the anterior pituitary), with bleb formation, swelling, and evidence of injury to the nucleus and cytoplasmic organelles. If hypoxia is severe and prolonged the endothelial cells as well as pituitary cells undergo necrosis. Platelet aggregation and capillary thrombosis can easily be identified by electron microscopy.

Inflammatory conditions

Ultrastructural changes in infectious lesions and granulomatous inflammation are similar to those occurring in other organs and will not be described here. Lymphocytic hypophysitis[3] (Fig. 16.2) is thought to be an auto-immune phenomenon; lymphocytes, plasma cells and macrophages accumulate in the anterior pituitary, and adenohypophyseal cells close to the cellular infiltrate show varying degrees of damage. Pituitary cells interdigitate with activated lymphocytes; in severe cases, the plasmalemma becomes disrupted and the adenohypophyseal cells show evidence of necrosis. Some pituitary cells contain large lysosomal bodies fusing with secretory granules (crinophagy) and increased numbers of mitochondria, indicating oncocytic transformation.

Infiltrative disorders

Amyloid deposits,[6] iron accumulation[5] and calcification[26] may occur in the anterior pituitary. The electron-microscopic findings are no different from those found in other areas of the body.

Functional alterations

In contrast to abnormalities which involve the entire anterior lobe, or at least large areas of the organ, EM is more valuable in those conditions which are limited to single cells and are related to alterations in functional activity[25a].

It is claimed that, compared to normal adenohypophyseal cells, hyperactive cells are larger, and possess a more sizeable nucleus, with nucleolar prominence and abundant cytoplasm; the RER network and Golgi apparatus are conspicuous, while the secretory granules are sparse and small. In contrast, hypoactive cells are thought to be smaller, with a smaller nucleus, inconspicuous nucleolus and poorly developed cytoplasm; the RER and Golgi apparatus are not prominent. Secretory granules are either numerous and large or, alternatively, sparse and small. These assumptions, however, hinge on observations made in animal experiments, and how much can be extrapolated to the human pituitary is open to question. Very little is known about the morphological manifestations of increased or decreased functional activity in the human adenohypophysis.

The morphological responses of non-tumorous human somatotrophs and lactotrophs to stimulation or suppression have yet to be elucidated. In the rat,[20] lysosomes increase in number and size, and crinophagy becomes evident in lactotrophs after cessation of increased lysosomes are thought to participate in the disposal and degradation of unused secretory material. Hyperactive lactotrophs may exhibit enhanced exocytosis. It is not firmly established whether or not the release of secretory granules is increased simultaneously with increased secretory activity, and whether or not the intensity of hormone release is proportional to the number of exocytosis sites.

The ultrastructural changes in corticotrophs related to increased secretion are not clear. However, it is well established that corticotrophs show characteristic morphological alterations due to suppression of their functional activity. In cases of feedback inhibition, corticotrophs exhibit Crooke's hyaline change.[16,23,41,55] Deposition of Crooke's hyaline material (Fig. 16.3), which has been shown to contain immunoreactive cytokeratins by light microscopy,[49] is due to cortisol excess and it occurs in: non-tumorous corticotrophs of patients with Cushing's disease resulting from pituitary adrenocorticotrophin (ACTH)-producing adenoma; ectopic ACTH syndrome; and treatment with pharmacological doses of cortisol or its derivatives. By EM, Crooke's hyaline material corresponds to an accumulation of cytoplasmic type I filaments. These filaments are about 7-nm thick, form bundles, and possess no periodicity. In the early phases of Crooke's hyalinization, a few bundles of filaments are noticeable around the nucleus and Golgi complex. In more advanced Crooke's hyalinization, the filaments occupy a large part of the cytoplasm replacing other cytoplasmic constituents and secretory granules, except for a juxtanuclear spherical area containing the dilated Golgi complex as well as a group of secretory granules and a small rim beneath the plasmalemma; under the cell membrane, a few large secretory granules can still be recognized. Crooke's hyaline change is reversible; following the removal of cortisol excess, corticotrophs revert to their normal shape and all but a few filaments disappear.

Gonadotrophs show extensive changes following gonadectomy.[36] Castration eliminates the negative feedback inhibitory effect of gonadal steroids, leading to the overactivity of gonadotroph cells. EM reveals gonadectomy (castration) cells which represent stimulated gonadotrophs (Fig. 16.4). They are larger than normal, and show extensive dilatation of the RER; uneven dilatation of RER may result in the formation of a large vacuole displacing the nucleus and Golgi complex to one pole of the cell. These cells correspond to signet-ring cells seen by LM. The number and size of secretory granules are decreased. The formation of castration cells is reversible; they regress and revert to normal gonadotrophs when therapy replaces the missing gonadal steroids.

The ultrastructural changes in human gonadotrophs following inhibition by excess of gonadal steroids have yet to be explored. In Kallmann's syndrome, hypogonadism is due to a defect in the secretion of hypothalamic gonadoliberin. The functionally inactive gonadotrophs are small, and spherical or irregular. They have small central dense nuclei, and scanty cytoplasm which contains a few profiles of dilated RER. Golgi regions are poorly developed. Elongated or oval mitochondria may undergo degeneration of the internal compartment. Secretory granules are few and measure 50–150 nm. Large lysosomes and lipid droplets may be found.[42]

Thyrotrophs show characteristic ultrastructural changes in cases of protracted stimulation, seen in patients with long-standing primary hypothyroidism.[33] The removal of the negative feedback effect of thyroid hormones leads to stimulation of thyrotrophs with the formation of thyroidectomy or thyroid deficiency cells. In contrast to normal thyrotrophs, hyperactive thyroidectomy cells are larger and possess abundant cytoplasm characterized by dilated RER, together with conspicuous Golgi complexes and sparse small secretory granules. Such thyroidectomy cells transform into normal thyrotrophs if patients are treated with replacement doses of thyroid hormones.

The ultrastructural changes occurring in patients with thyroid hormone excess have not been investigated in detail; thus, no description of the ultrastructural appearance of suppressed human thyrotrophs can be given.

Hyperplasias

Hyperplasia is an increase in the number of constituent

cells; it can be monofocal, multifocal or diffuse, and it can involve one or more adenohypophyseal cell type[25a]. In order to assess objectively whether or not hyperplasia is present, large areas of the adenohypophysis have to be examined, and LM examination of the pituitary is necessary. It is important to emphasize that cell distribution in the adenohypophysis is not even; therefore, prominence of one or more cell types by EM can be misinterpreted as hyperplasia, whereas it may reflect only normal variation. Hyperplasia should also be differentiated from adenoma — a distinction which requires LM examination. The most important features of hyperplasia as opposed to adenoma are the maintenance of reticulin fibre network, preservation of architecture, intermingling of several different cell types, absence of demarcation, and lack of a pseudocapsule.[37]

Ultrastructural analysis can contribute to a better understanding of the disease process. Mammosomatotroph hyperplasia has been documented as a cause of gigantism of early onset,[48a] providing further evidence that this plurihormonal cell exists in the non-tumorous human gland. The presence of enlarged acini containing more cells than in the normal pituitary, the identification of several interspersed cell types, the preservation of the original architecture are consistent with and favour the diagnosis of hyperplasia. Hyperplastic cells may be larger than their normal counterparts and possess conspicuous Golgi complexes (Figs 16.5–16.9). Prominence of the Golgi apparatus in itself is, however, not pathognomonic and is not sufficient to establish a diagnosis of hyperplasia.[37]

NEUROHYPOPHYSIS

Clinically significant diseases of the neurohypophysis are uncommon; they include conditions caused by increased or decreased vasopressin secretion. While the ultrastructural morphology of the normal human neurohypophysis has been well documented,[35,66,67,69] the fine structural pathology of the human neurohypophysis has not been extensively studied.

Circulatory, inflammatory and traumatic lesions

Diabetes insipidus due to vasopressin deficiency is associated with many diverse disorders of the hypothalamus, pituitary stalk or posterior lobe, which cause tissue destruction or compression and interfere with vasopressin synthesis, transport or release. We shall not describe the ultrastructural features of traumatic injuries or inflammatory lesions (including granulomas) which can be implicated in this disorder. They all lead to atrophy of the constituents of the supraopticohypophyseal tract and the posterior lobe. In experimental animals, stalk transection leads to degeneration of axonal fibres; the more numerous type A fibres show an increase in the number of focal enlargements or swellings which contain abundant lysosomal bodies (type III

dilatations).[17] The human posterior lobe has not been studied by EM following stalk section, however, the LM changes are similar to those of the experimental lesions. Interference with blood flow may lead to infarction as well. Neurosecretory elements disappear and are replaced by dense collagenous sclerosis.

Functional alterations

Inappropriate excess secretion of vasopressin — the Schwartz–Bartter syndrome — may be due to ectopic hormone production by extrahypophyseal neoplasms or excessive hormone release from the posterior pituitary. The fine-structural alterations within the hypothalamus, stalk and posterior pituitary of this entity remain unidentified.

THYROID

Non-neoplastic diseases of the thyroid include several inflammatory conditions, functional alterations of colloid synthesis, storage or secretion, and hyperplasias.

Inflammatory conditions

Inflammatory lesions of the thyroid include a group of disorders thought to have an auto-immune aetiology.

Granulomatous (de Quervain's) thyroiditis is an infrequent lesion which is not often biopsied and relatively few EM descriptions of this entity have been recorded.[51,59,64,65,71] The predominant feature is the presence of mature activated lymphocytes and plasma cells in the interstitium, associated with accumulation of mature collagen fibres and microfibrils; occasionally, these cells are found within gaps in the follicular basal lamina and between epithelial cells. Multinucleated giant cells have irregular nuclei and abundant cytoplasm, with well developed RER and Golgi complexes, numerous mitochondria and lysosomes; these are assumed to be histiocytes.[65] The thyroid epithelium shows evidence of hyperactivity; the follicular epithelium contains dilated RER, numerous colloid droplets and lipid-containing phagolysosomes. The basal lamina is generally intact, but may be thickened; gaps and areas of reduplication have been described. Viruses have been thought to play a role in the aetiology of this disease. However, no viral inclusions have been demonstrated by EM, although controversial 'virus-like particles' have been reported.[64] The role of viruses in the pathogenesis of this disorder remains unproven.

Lymphocytic thyroiditis may be associated with chemical or mechanical trauma, radiation or other unknown factors; the most frequent type, Hashimoto's thyroiditis, is presumed to have an auto-immune pathogenesis. In this disorder, lymphoid follicles indistinguishable from those of lymphoid tissue are found within the thyroid parenchyma.[10] Plasma cells are present in variable numbers. The interstitium contains variable accumulations of mature collagen fibres and microfibrils. Follicular structures may be intact or may be partially destroyed and infiltrated by lymphocytes and plasma cells. Cytoplasmic projections of the inflammatory cells interdigitate with those of follicular cells, which undergo degenerative changes (Fig. 16.10). Some follicular epithelial cells have decreased numbers of microvilli, underdeveloped Golgi regions, loss of organelles, numerous lysosomes and an abundance of mitochondria; the latter gives rise to the characteristic oxyphilia of 'Hürthle' or 'Askanazy' cells by LM. The follicular basal lamina frequently has gaps or shows reduplication, and may contain electron-dense deposits which are thought to represent immune complexes.[27,30,31,50,59,71]

Ultrastructural examination does not contribute significantly to the diagnosis of Riedel's struma. In this lesion, accumulation of collagen in the interstitium is prominent. Follicular cells undergo degenerative changes of varying degrees.

Functional alterations

Goitre may result from various abnormalities of colloid synthesis, storage or secretion. The disorder may be congenital or acquired, and may be diffuse or may involve isolated foci, giving rise to a nodular goitre. EM reveals a spectrum of changes in the morphology of the thyroid follicular epithelium in involved areas.[46] Enlarged follicles are lined by flattened or cuboidal cells with reduced numbers of shortened and irregular microvilli. The dilated follicular lumen contains large amounts of electron-dense granular colloid. Follicular cell cytoplasm contains conspicuous dilated RER cisternae and large phagolysosomes; in contrast, Golgi complexes are poorly developed and mitochondria are few. The nuclei are bland, being round or oval with marginated chromatin and small nucleoli. Areas of hyperplasia are composed of follicular cells showing signs of increased stimulation (see below). Reduplication of the basal lamina is frequent.

Atrophy of the thyroid may be secondary to pituitary lesions which interfere with thyrotrophin secretion, or may be the result of iatrogenic administration of thyroid hormone. The morphological effects of hypophysectomy and chronic administration of thyroid hormone are similar in experimental animals.[46] Follicular epithelial cells have round or oval nuclei with dispersed chromatin and occasional nucleoli. Microvilli at the luminal surface are thin, short and reduced in number. Within the cytoplasm, few short profiles of poorly developed RER may contain a small amount of granular material. Golgi regions are small. Mitochondria are reduced in number and size, and may undergo vacuolar degeneration. Small dense granules may be observed, but colloid droplets are rare. Follicular basement membrane is intact and no changes are found in the interstitium.

Hyperplasias

Thyroid follicular hyperplasia may be diffuse or focal. The diffuse form of the disease is sometimes attributable to administration of iodine or various therapeutic agents; it may be secondary to excess thyrotropin secretion from pituitary adenomas. Congenital abnormalities of thyroid hormone synthesis result in compensatory hyperplasia. The most frequent diffuse hyperplasia is that of Graves' disease (exophthalmic goitre), which is thought to have an autoimmune basis and is related to Hashimoto's thyroiditis. Focal hyperplasia is seen in nodular goitres.[24,30,46,71]

By EM, hyperplastic thyroid tissue is composed of tall, columnar follicular cells arranged predominantly in a single layer, but there may be foci of multilayered epithelium. Follicular colloid is reduced, and some follicles may have an empty lumen. The nuclei are large and may show mild irregularity of contour; nucleoli are present and are often prominent. Microvilli are abundant, long and thin, and there may be large cytoplasmic projections into the follicular lumen. RER is dilated and contains fine granular material. Free ribosomes and polysomes are numerous, while Golgi complexes are prominent and mitochondria are abundant; the latter may exhibit swelling and may contain abnormal cristae. Complex phagolysosomes are usually present. Colloid droplets and dense bodies are found, most often in an apical position. Intracytoplasmic lumina are found within follicular cells, lined by membranes with well-developed microvilli. The basal cell contour is frequently convoluted; however, the follicles are encompassed by intact basal lamina that may be thickened and occasionally reduplicated; electron-dense deposits have been described within the thickened basal lamina in cases of Graves' disease.[30] The interstitium is usually vascular, and mature collagen fibres are rare. In Graves' disease lymphoid follicles and interstitial aggregates of lymphocytes and plasma cells may be found, reflecting the immunological nature of the disorder.

Treatment of hyperplastic conditions with therapeutic agents can alter the ultrastructural findings.[24,46] Iodine treatment has been reported to reduce the size and number of surface microvilli and cause dilatation of RER. Administration of thiouracil and its derivatives has been associated with irregularities of the basal aspect of follicular epithelium and reduplication of basal lamina. Carbimazole treatment apparently does not result in detectable structural changes.

Hyperplasia of parafollicular cells is associated with familial cases of medullary thyroid carcinoma; it may also occur with long-standing hypercalcaemia and in some cases of toxic goitre. The increased numbers of parafollicular cells are localized within the follicular basal lamina but are separated from the follicular lumen by the follicular epithelial cells. They may form nodules and may completely surround the follicles. Hyperplastic parafollicular cells have a round or oval nucleus with fine dispersed chromatin and a prominent nucleolus. The abundant cytoplasm contains well developed RER, large Golgi complexes, elongated mitochondria and spherical secretory granules 100–400 nm in diameter and of variable electron density; the granules are frequently aligned along the cell membrane. Some cells contain numerous large granules, apparently storing hormone; others contain few small granules and may represent actively secreting cells.[18]

PARATHYROID

Non-neoplastic parathyroid pathology is dominated by hyperplasias which are classified into several morphological subtypes and which may be primary or secondary to other underlying disorders. Hypoparathyroidism is usually associated with inadvertent surgical resection of the glands or compromised blood supply resulting in infarction. Idiopathic hypoparathyroidism maybe congenital or acquired.

Inflammatory disorders

Lymphocytic parathyroiditis has been observed in some patients with hypoparathyroidism and this has been interpreted as an auto-immune endocrinopathy. The ultrastructural features of experimental immune parathyroiditis in animals include lymphoplasmacytic infiltration and parenchymal destruction with cellular degeneration.[2,47] To our knowledge, the fine structure of lymphocytic parathyroiditis in humans has not as yet been reported.

Idiopathic hypoparathyroidism

The morphology of the parathyroid glands in idiopathic hypoparathyroidism is not well described. Some investigators have reported fatty replacement of parathyroid tissue, some have failed to identify parathyroid glands and others have identified histologically normal parathyroids.

Functional alterations

Non-tumourous parathyroid tissue resected from patients with a functionally active parathyroid adenoma is thought to be suppressed by hypercalcaemia, as is parathyroid tissue from patients with hypercalcaemia due to multiple myeloma or disseminated carcinoma.[11,19,53,63] The non-tumorous cells are small and have a smooth surface with reduced numbers of microvilli and interdigitations of plasma membranes. Nuclei are small and dense; the cytoplasm is depleted of organelles and accumulation of glycogen particles is noted. Lipid droplets may be numerous. In animals with experimentally suppressed glands, lysosome-like bodies are found, sometimes partly surrounding secretory granules; partially degraded granules may be seen within autophagic vacuoles.[11] These findings suggest a mechanism by which chief cells degrade secretory products in response to hypercalcaemia. In patients with medullary carcinoma of thyroid, the parathyroid glands may show a compensatory hyperactivity, possibly the reaction to hypocalcaemia.[53] Grossly and histologically normal glands are composed of cells with more extensive RER and fewer lipid inclusions than are seen in normal controls. There may also be an increase in transitional oxyphils (chief cells with slightly increased numbers of mitochondria).

Hyperplasias

Hyperplastic parathyroid glands may have a diffuse or a nodular growth pattern. Primary parathyroid hyperplasia is usually composed mainly of chief cells; the more rare water-clear cell hyperplasia is regarded as a distinct clinicopathological entity. Parathyroid chief cell hyperplasia may be secondary to chronic renal insufficiency, calcium malabsorption or vitamin D deficiency and is morphologically indistinguishable from primary chief cell hyperplasia.

In chief cell hyperplasia[1,7,8,9,11,19,21,53,61–63] chief cells are the main component, forming sheets and cords with complex cellular interdigitations and prominent microvilli (Fig. 16.11). The cells have regular nuclei with a loose chromatin network and conspicuous nucleoli; the cytoplasm shows evidence of active hormone synthesis and secretion (Fig. 16.11). Abundant lamellae of RER are stacked in parallel arrays; the Golgi region is large and well-developed, with numerous vesicles and occasional developing or immature secretory granules. Mature secretory granules may be numerous and are usually found at the cell pole closest to a capillary or the interstitium. Occasional cells harbour lipid vacuoles. Scattered among the dominant chief cells are cells which have clear cytoplasm by LM and contain abundant glycogen; some clear cells in cases of primary hyperplasia are thought to have large sacculi similar to those of water-clear cells (see below). Oxyphilic cells seen by light microscopy correspond to oncocytes with markedly increased numbers of mitochondria in addition to well developed endoplasmic reticulum, Golgi complexes and secretory granules (Fig. 16.12); transitional forms of chief cells with slightly increased numbers of mitochondria are seen.

There are few reports of the ultrastructure of the rare primary water-clear cell hyperplasia.[1,19,53,60] The water-clear cytoplasm of cells in this entity is due to the presence of numerous large cytoplasmic vacuoles which are lined by a triple membrane (Fig. 16.13). These vacuoles may appear empty, or may contain variable inclusions — such as amorphous or granular material, crystalline structures, myelin-like or thread-like figures. Some authors have suggested that these are derived from Golgi vesicles, dilated smooth endoplasmic reticulum, secretory granules or mitochondria. The remainder of the cytoplasm contains RER profiles, free ribosomes, mitochondria, and occasional secretory granules. In addition to the clear cells which constitute most of the hyperplastic glands, scattered chief cells and intermediate forms are seen; these findings support the theory that the two types of primary hyperplasia are related and are variants of the same disease.[60]

Pseudohypoparathyroidism — a disorder of renal response to parathyroid hormone — usually results in parathyroid chief cell hyperplasia.[61]

Persistence of hyperparathyroidism following longstanding secondary hyperfunction is known as tertiary parathyroid hyperplasia and is attributed to autonomy of hyperplastic parathyroid tissue. The morphological features are usually those of chief cell hyperplasia.[9,14,53,62] An unusual finding not reported in other disorders is the presence of regular, homogeneous dilatation of RER cisternae containing a linear sequence of globular particles attached to the inner surface of the limiting membrane.[14]

ADRENAL CORTEX

Non-tumorous lesions of the adrenal cortex include congenital dystrophies, circulatory and inflammatory conditions, infiltrative disorders, functional alterations and hyperplasias. In addition, specific drug effects have been described to have morphological correlates.

Congenital disorders

The rare adrenoleukodystrophy, a hereditary, sex-linked recessive disorder, represents a demyelinating disease. The specific aetiology has not been determined, but it is considered to be a form of lipid-storage disorder. The hypocorticism which accompanies it is associated with cytoplasmic ballooning of adrenocortical cells in the inner zona fasciculata and zona reticularis. By EM, the adrenal cells show cytoplasmic vacuolation with intracytoplasmic lamellae and lamellar-lipid profiles.[56,57]

Circulatory disturbances

The adrenocortical nodular change which is found incidentally, and is unassociated with hormone excess, is presumed to be a function of ageing and is correlated with arteriopathy of capsular vessels;[52] the ultrastructure of this entity has not been documented.

Infiltrative disorders

Amyloid, haemosiderin, and calcium salts are known to accumulate in the adrenal cortex in localized and systemic disease. The electron microscopic features are no different from those found in other areas of the body.

Functional alterations

Secondary involution of the adrenal cortex can result from hypopituitarism with primary ACTH deficiency, from feedback suppression by glucocorticoid hormone-secreting tumours, and from prolonged treatment with exogenous steroids. The ultrastructural morphology of the atrophic adrenal cortex is only scantily described.[47,48,52] The involuted non-tumorous cortex adjacent to adrenal glucocorticoid hormone-secreting tumours has been studied by EM. In this situation there is involution of the inner zones, while the zona glomerulosa is less affected. In the two inner zones, there is a conspicuous reduction in cell size and a marked decrease in the number and size of microvilli. The nucleus is dense with clumped chromatin. The cell cytoplasm is reduced and is almost completely filled by large lipid droplets (Fig. 16.14). There is little endoplasmic reticulum; Golgi regions are small and have collapsed membranes, while mitochondria are small and dark and reduced in numbers. Lysosomal accumulation is seen.

Lipid depletion of the adrenal cortex is the result of acute stress and ACTH stimulation. In the normal cortex, clear cells of the zona fasciculata predominate; their plentiful cytoplasm contains moderate amounts of smooth endoplasmic reticulum (SER), abundant osmiophilic lipid droplets and membrane-bound lipid vacuoles, variable numbers of lysosomes and spherical mitochondria with vesicular cristae. In response to stimulation, clear cells release stored hormone and increase steroid synthesis, thereby becoming morphologically compact cells with ultrastructural features of the zona reticularis.[13,47,48,52] The large cells have well-developed surface microvilli; the cytoplasm is filled with densely packed SER, few lipid vacuoles, numerous lysosomes and ovoid mitochondria with tubulovesicular cristae. The extent of this change is proportional to the degree of stimulation, and the features are reversible with reduction of ACTH levels.

Hyperplasias

Adrenocortical hyperplasia may occur in association with various forms of excess hormone secretion or it may be unassociated with endocrinopathy. The lesions may be primary in the adrenal or may be secondary to stimulation.

Diffuse hyperplasia of the cortex may be primary, but is usually secondary to prolonged severe stress, excessive pituitary secretion of ACTH, or ectopic ACTH secretion; it is frequently associated with Cushing's syndrome. The fine-structural changes in these conditions are similar and they cannot be reliably distinguished from each other by EM; however the extent and intensity of alteration may vary. The changes are most striking in cases of ectopic ACTH syndrome.[40,45,48,52,58,68] By EM, the fasciculata and reticularis cells are enlarged. The cell membranes are tortuous with multiple interdigitations between cells. Surface microvilli are increased in number and size. The cytoplasm is abundant and contains well developed organelles. The SER is conspicuous and the Golgi region is large (Fig. 16.15). In some cells RER may be present in significant quantities. There may be variable degrees of dilatation of endoplasmic reticular structures. Mitochondria are numerous and contain vesicular or tubulovesicular cristae; they may show rarefaction and cavitation of the internal compartment, associated with partial loss of cristae. Occasional pleomorphic mitochondria are found, some of which develop into giant forms. Lipid droplets are decreased in number and size (Fig. 16.16). The interstitium may contain an increased amount of collagen.

In cases of nodular hyperplasia, the cytological features are similar to those described in diffuse hyperplasia.[29,47,48,52,58,68] In addition, there is a marked prominence of collagen between the endothelium of capillaries and adrenocortical cells. Vascular and epithelial basal laminae are reported to be thickened. This lesion is usually unassociated with ACTH excess; however, it may also be secondary to stimulation and Cushing's syndrome is the most frequent clinical feature.

Hyperplasia of the zona glomerulosa is found in association with Conn's syndrome. The morphological findings are identical in those cases which are thought to be of primary adrenal aetiology and in various forms of secondary hyperaldosteronism, hyperreninism and adrenal hypertension.[52] By EM, zona glomerulosa cells seem to be enlarged. The cell membranes are tortuous and microvilli are prominent. There is accumulation of SER and the Golgi region is large (Fig. 16.17). Membrane-bound dense bodies are conspicuous. The mitochondria are frequently increased in number or size and may show cavitation of internal compartments. They contain lamellar cristae.

Drug effects

The effects of various drugs on the adrenal cortex have been described. The most important diagnostic change is induced by spironolactone (an anti-aldosterone agent), which has characteristic effects on cells of the zona glomerulosa and outer fasciculata.[15,39] Spironolactone administration results in the formation of round laminated bodies in these cells. By EM, spironolactone bodies are composed of concentric whorls of smooth membranes (Fig. 16.18). They frequently have an electron-dense central core (Fig. 16.19). Ribosomes may be found attached to the external profile of these membranous structures, suggesting derivation from the endoplasmic reticulum. The functional significance of these bodies is not known.

ADRENAL MEDULLA AND EXTRA-ADRENAL PARAGANGLIA

Hyperplasias

Hyperplasia of the adrenal medulla has been reported in association with multiple endocrine neoplasia (MEN) type II.[12] The medullary cells are arranged in cords or small nests; they are oval or polyhedral, and increased in size in comparison with normal cells. The nuclei are spherical or oval; the chromatin is usually finely granular and occasional chromatin clumps may be seen. Nucleoli are prominent. The cytoplasm contains well developed RER and Golgi regions (Figs. 16.20 and 16.21.) Immature secretory granules may be identified within Golgi sacculi and vacuoles. Mitochondria are usually elongated, with lamellar cristae. Lipid droplets and lysosomes may be found within the cytoplasm. Secretory granules are generally numerous; some cells are degranulated indicating active release of hormone. They may be spherical, oval or irregular in shape and usually measure between 100–400 nm in diameter. They have a dark core, a well-defined limiting membrane and frequently an electron-lucent halo. The two distinct granule populations which have been proposed to contain adrenaline and noradrenaline are both found within cells of the hyperplastic process. It has been proposed that the lighter, larger, inhomogeneous granules with symmetrical halos contain adrenalin, whereas the small, dense and homogeneous granules contain noradrenalin. Intermediate forms are found and it remains uncertain whether the morphological variations reflect differences in function.

Extra-adrenal paraganglia also undergo hyperplasia.[28] In this situation, the hyperplasia involves both elongated sustentacular and Schwann cells. These two cell types become more numerous than in normal paraganglia, forming concentric whorls around the chief cell nests. This change is associated with an increase in the number of axons.

GASTRO-ENTERO-PANCREATIC ENDOCRINE TISSUE

Non-tumorous disorders of the endocrine pancreas include degenerative lesions, usually associated with diabetes mellitus, and nesidioblastosis. Within the diffuse gastrointestinal endocrine tissues, hyperplastic processes predominate; due to the widespread distribution of this endocrine organ, there has been little investigation of the fine-structural pathology.

Circulatory disturbances

Peliosis of pancreatic islets has been reported in association with the MEN-I syndrome.[38] The lesion is focal, involving some islets with single or multiple peliotic sacs, which may replace most of the endocrine tissue. The blood-filled cavities of various sizes lack an endothelial lining and are not surrounded by basal lamina. They appear to be separate from capillaries, but may be continuous with a ruptured capillary lumen, indicating a site of extravasation of red blood cells.

Inflammatory disorders

Inflammatory lesions are recognized within the islets of Langerhans, with a spectrum from acute to chronic changes. Acute inflammation is similar to that seen in other organs; EM is not useful in the diagnosis of this entity. Chronic inflammation is felt to represent an auto-immune endocrine phenomenon; alternatively, a viral aetiology has been proposed. This lesion is associated with juvenile-onset diabetes mellitus. The predominant infiltrating cell is the lymphocyte. The inflammation is associated with variable degrees of fibrosis, suggesting that islet fibrosis is the end stage of insulitis. Complete or almost complete absence of B cells and reduction of islet volume associated with chronic insulin-dependent diabetes mellitus[44] may be attributable to a selective destructive process. The ultrastructural features of this lesion in humans are not well documented.

Infiltrative disorders

Fibrosis of islets may vary from a slight increase in interstitial fibrous tissue to a severe destructive lesion with diffuse collagen deposition and atrophy of cellular components.[44]

Amyloid deposition in the interstitial space of islets is associated with adult onset diabetes mellitus and has the typical fibrillary morphology seen in other sites[32,73] (see Chs. 5, 12 and 17). The non-branching, irregularly arranged fibrils measure 10 nm in thickness and are usually deposited between the basal lamina of endocrine cells and the islet capillary network. Similar fibres have also been identified within deep cytoplasmic invaginations of B cells and within B cells of insulinomas, suggesting that the source of this amyloid is the B cell.

Haemochromatosis results in deposition of haemosiderin within endocrine cells of the islets of Langerhans.[57a] Iron pigment is found preferentially in B cells. The other cell types are reported to be devoid of pigment but reduced in number (See also Fig. 15.19).

Hyperplasias

Nesidioblastosis is found in newborns with hyperinsulinaemic hypoglycaemia and is also associated with MEN-I. Endocrine cells are numerous and are found in disorganized clusters.[22,25,72] Islets are enlarged, and scattered cells are found singly and in small groups in relation to ducts and acinar tissue. The endocrine cells (Fig. 16.22) found within exocrine acini are predominantly in a basal position overlying a well-defined basal lamina. Endocrine cells and cytoplasmic processes of these cells can be interspersed among exocrine cells. The most frequently observed cell type is the insulin-producing B cell; usually it has a round to oval nucleus with peripheral chromatin and occasionally a prominent nucleolus. Profiles of RER are seen, and there is a well-developed Golgi region. The secretory granules have a characteristic appearance: they exhibit a dense centre with a para-crystalline appearance resulting in rhomboidal or cigar-shaped cores. Some granules within these cells have a variable morphology with a less well-defined core structure. The granules measure from 250 to 450 nm in diameter. In addition to the characteristic granules, B cells may harbour membrane-bound variegated structures which appear to contain some lipid and which may represent lysosomes; these have been called ceroid bodies. Typical glucagon-secreting A cells and somatostatin-producing D cells are also found as components of nesidioblastosis. The A cells have secretory granules measuring from 200 to 350 nm in diameter, which are characterized by electron-dense, often eccentric cores, a 'grey' halo, and a peripheral limiting membrane. D cells have granules of variable electron-density measuring upwards of 350 nm in diameter and usually lacking peripheral halos. A small percentage of the endocrine cell population is composed of pancreatic polypeptide hormone-secreting PP cells. These contain secretory granules with an average diameter of approximately 170 nm and uniform osmiophilic dense cores separated by a narrow clear halo from the limiting membrane.

Metaplastic and hyperplastic proliferations of endocrine cells have been observed in association with chronic pancreatitis and in pancreatic tissue surrounding tumours.[4,43] This proliferation may be florid, simulating neoplasia. Some investigators have described a disproportionate increase in the number of A cells as compared to B cells, while others have described a predominance of PP cells in this setting. The ultrastructural morphology of the endocrine cells in this entity is characteristic of the specific cell type. There is, in addition, a prominence of interstitial fibrosis with extensive collagen deposition underlying the basal lamina.

Selective hyperplasias of A and D cells have been described in the non-tumorous pancreas of patients with gastrin-secreting pancreatic tumours;[70] this may represent a gastrin-dependent secondary change. The cells involved have the typical features of A and D cells described above.

G cell hyperplasia in the gastric antrum has been reported as the cause of primary gastrin excess in the Zollinger–Ellison syndrome.[54] The endocrine cells are largely but not entirely confined to recognizable G cells whose ultrastructural morphology is not unlike that of normal G cells. Goblet-shaped cells contain secretory granules with a mean diameter of 350 nm; the granules are usually round, surrounded by a limiting membrane and contain variably electron-dense material. The mucosal surface of the cells possesses microvilli and the secretory granules are typically located between the nucleus and the basal lamina.

REFERENCES

1. Altenähr E 1972 Ultrastructural pathology of the parathyroid gland. Current Topics in Pathology 56: 1–54
2. Altenähr E, Jenke W, 1974 Experimental parathyroiditis in the rat by passive immunisation. Virchows Archiv A, Pathological Anatomy and Histopathology 363: 333–342
3. Asa S L, Bilbao J M, Kovacs K, Josse R G, Kreines K 1981 Lymphocytic hypophysitis of pregnancy resulting in hypopituitarism: a distinct clinicopathologic entity. Annals of Internal Medicine 95: 166–171
4. Bartow S A, Mukai K, Rosai J 1981 Pseudoneoplastic proliferation of endocrine cells in pancreatic fibrosis. Cancer 47: 2627–2633
5. Bergeron C, Kovacs K 1978 Pituitary siderosis. A histologic, immunocytologic and ultrastructural study. American Journal of Pathology 93: 295–306
6. Bilbao J M, Horvath E, Hudson A R, Kovacs K 1975 Pituitary adenoma producing amyloid-like substance. Archives of Pathology 100: 411–415
7. Black W C III 1969 Correlative light and electron microscopy in primary hyperparathyroidism. Archives of Pathology 88: 225–241
8. Black W C III, Haff R C 1970 The surgical pathology of parathyroid chief cell hyperplasia. American Journal of Clinical Pathology 53: 565–579
9. Black W C III, Slatopolsky E, Elkan J, Hoffstein P 1970 Parathyroid morphology in suppressible and non suppressible renal hyperparathyroidism. Laboratory Investigation 23: 497–509
10. Brandes D, Anton E, Orbegoso C M 1969 Hashimoto's thyroiditis. Johns Hopkins Medical Journal 124: 211–233
11. Capen C C, Roth S I 1975 Ultrastructural and functional relationships of normal and pathologic parathyroid cells. In: Sommers S C (ed) Endocrine Pathology dicennial 1966–1975. Appleton-Century-Crofts, New York, pp 267–319
12. Carney J A. Sizemore G W, Tyce G M 1975 Bilateral adrenal medullary hyperplasia in multiple endocrine neoplasia type 2. The precursor of bilateral pheochromocytoma. Mayo Clinic Proceedings 50: 3–10
13. Carr I 1961 The ultrastructure of the human adrenal cortex before and after stimulation with ACTH. Journal of Pathology and Bacteriology 81: 101–106
14. Cinti S, Osculati F, Parravicini C 1982 RER-associated structure in parathyroid glands removed because of tertiary hyperparathyroidism. Ultrastructural Pathology 3: 263–268
15. Davis D A, Medline N M 1970 Spironolactone (aldactone) bodies: concentric lamellar formations in the adrenal cortices of patients treated with spironolactone. American Journal of Clinical Pathology 54: 22–32
16. De Cicco F A, Dekker A, Yunis E J 1972 Fine structure of Crooke's hyaline change in the human pituitary gland. Archives of Pathology 94: 65–70
17. Dellmann H D, Stoeckel M E, Porter A, Stutinsky F 1974 Ultrastructure of the neurohypophysial glial cells following stalk transection in the rat. Experientia 30: 1220–1222
18. DeLellis R A, Nunnemacher G, Wolfe H J 1977 C-cell hyperplasia. An ultrastructural analysis. Laboratory Investigation 36: 237–248
19. Faccini J M 1978 The ultrastructure of parathyroid glands removed from patients with primary hyperparathyroidism: a report of 40 cases, including four carcinomata. Journal of Pathology 102: 189–199
20. Farquhar M G 1971 Processing of secretory products by cells of the anterior pituitary gland. In: Heller H, Lederis K (eds) Subcellular Organization and Function in Endocrine Tissues. Cambridge University Press, London, pp 79–122
21. Garcia-Bunuel R, Kutchemeshgi A, Brandes D 1974 Hereditary hyperparathyroidism. The fine structure of the parathyroid gland. Archives of Pathology 92: 399–403
22. Gould V E, Memoli V A, Dardi L E, Gould N S 1983 Nesiodiodysplasia and nesidioblastosis of infancy: structural and functional correlations with the syndrome of hyperinsulinemic hypoglycemia. Pediatric Pathology 1: 7–31
23. Halmi N S, McCormick W F, Dekker D A Jr 1971 The natural history of hyalinization of ACTH-MSH cells in man. Archives of Pathology 91: 318–326
24. Heimann P 1966 Ultrastructure of human thyroid. A study of normal thyroid, untreated and treated diffuse toxic goitre. Acta Endocrinologica 53 (suppl 110): 1–102
25. Heitz P U, Klöppel G, Häcki W H, Polak J M, Pearse A G E 1977 Nesidioblastosis: the pathologic basis of persistent hyperinsulinemic hypoglycemia in infants. Morphologic and quantitative analysis of seven cases based on specific immunostaining and electron microscopy. Diabetes 26: 632–642
25a. Horvath E, Kovacs K 1988 Fine structural cytology of the adenohypophysis in rat and man. Journal of Electron Microscopy Technique 8: 401–432
26. Ilse G, Ryan N, Kovacs K, Ilse D 1980 Calcium deposition in human pituitary adenomas studied by histology, electron microscopy, electron diffraction and X-ray spectrometry. Experimental Pathology 18: 377–386
27. Irvine W J, Muir A R 1962 An electron microscopic study of Hashimoto's thyroiditis. Quarterly Journal of Experimental Physiology 48: 13–26
28. Jago R, Smith P, Heath D 1984 Electron microscopy of carotid body hyperplasia. Archives of Pathology and Laboratory Medicine 108: 717–722
29. Josse R G, Bear R A, Kovacs K, Higgins H P 1980 Cushing's syndrome due to unilateral nodular adrenal hyperplasia: a new pathophysiological entity. Acta Endocrinologica 93: 495–504
30. Kalderon A E, Bogaars H A 1977 Immune complex deposition in Graves' disease and Hashimoto's thyroiditis. American Journal of Medicine 63: 729–734
31. Kalderon A E, Bogaars H A, Diamond I 1973 Ultrastructural alterations of the follicular basement membrane in Hashimoto's thyroiditis. American Journal of Medicine 55: 485–491
32. Kawanishi H, Akazawa Y, Machill B 1966 Islet of Langerhans in normal and diabetic humans. Ultrastructure and histochemistry with special reference to hyalinosis. Acta Pathologica Japonica 16: 177–197
33. Khalil A, Kovacs K, Sima A A F, Burrow G N, Horvath E 1984 Pituitary thyrotroph hyperplasia mimicking prolactin-secreting adenoma. Journal of Endocrinologic Investigation 7: 399–404
34. Kovacs K 1969 Necrosis of anterior pituitary in humans. Neuroendocrinology 4: 170–241
35. Kovacs K 1984 Pathology of the neurohypophysis. In: Reichlin S (ed) The neurohypophysis. Physiology and Clinical Aspects. Plenum, New York, pp 95–113
36. Kovacs K, Horvath E 1975 Gonadotrophs following removal of the ovaries. A fine structural study of human pituitary glands. Endokrinologie 66: 1–8
37. Kovacs K, Horvath E 1986 Tumors of the pituitary. In: Atlas of Tumor Pathology. Fascicle XXI, 2nd series. Armed Forces Institute of Pathology, Washington DC
38. Kovacs K, Horvath E, Asa S L, Murray D, Singer W, Reddy S S K 1986 Microscopic peliosis of pancreatic islets in a woman with MEN-I syndrome. Archives of Pathology and Laboratory Medicine 110: 607–610
39. Kovacs K, Horvath E, Singer W 1973 Fine structure and morphogenesis of spironolactone bodies in the zona glomerulosa of the human adrenal cortex. Journal of Clinical Pathology 26: 949–957
40. Kovacs K, Horvath E, Singer W, Lilienfield H 1977 Fine structure of adrenal cortex in ectopic ACTH syndrome. Endokrinologie 69: 94–102
41. Kovacs K, Horvath E, Stratmann I E, Ezrin C 1974 Cytoplasmic microfilaments in the anterior lobe of the human pituitary gland. Acta Anatomica 87: 414–426
42. Kovacs K, Sheehan H L 1982 Pituitary changes in Kallmann's syndrome: a histologic, immunocytologic, ultrastructural and immunoelectron microscopic study. Fertility and Sterility 37: 83–89
43. Klöppel G, Bommer G, Commandeur G, Heitz P U 1978 The endocrine pancreas in chronic pancreatitis. Immunocytochemical and ultrastructural studies. Virchows Archiv A, Pathological Anatomy and Histopathology 377: 157–174
44. Klöppel G, Drenck C R, Carstensen A, Morohoshi T, Oberholzer M, Heitz P U 1982 Ultrastructure and immunocytochemistry of the endocrine pancreas in diabetes. Medicina 2: 299–308
45. Li K H, Asa S L, Kovacs K, Murray D, Singer W 1990 The adrenal cortex in ectopic adrenocorticotropic hormone syndrome: a morphological study with histology, transmission and scanning

electron microscopy, flow cytometry and image analysis. Endocrine Pathology 1: 183–191

46. Lupulescu A, Petrovici A 1968 Ultrastructure of the thyroid gland. Heinemann, London

47. Lupulescu A, Petrovici A, Pop A, Heitmanek C 1968 Electron microscopic observations on the parathyroid gland in experimental hypoparathyroidism. Experientia 24: 62–63

48. Mackay A 1969 Atlas of human adrenal cortex ultrastructure. In: Symington T (ed) Functional Pathology of the Human Adrenal Gland. Churchill Livingstone, Edinburgh, pp 345–489

48a. Moran A, Asa S L, Kovacs K, Horvath E, Singer W, Sagman U, Reubi J-C, Wilson C B, Larson R, Pescovitz D H 1990 Pituitary mammosomatotroph hyperplasia associated with childhood gigantism. New England Journal of Medicine 323: 322–327

49. Neumann P E, Horoupian D S, Goldman J E, Hess M A 1984 Cytoplasmic microfilaments of Crooke's hyaline change belong to the cytokeratin class. American Journal of Pathology 116: 214–222

50. Nève P 1969 The ultrastructure of thyroid in chronic autoimmune thyroiditis. Virchows Archiv B, Cell Pathology 346: 302–317

51. Nève P 1970 Ultrastructure of the thyroid in DeQuervain's subacute granulomatous thyroiditis. Virchows Archiv B, Cell Pathology 351: 87–98

52. Neville A M, MacKay A M 1972 The structure of the human adrenal cortex in health and disease. Clinics in Endocrinology and Metabolism 1: 361–395

53. Nilsson O 1977 Studies on the ultrastructure of the human parathyroid glands in various pathological conditions. Acta Pathologica et Microbiologica Scandinavica A (suppl) 263: 1–88

54. Polak J M, Stagg B, Pearse A G E 1972 Two types of Zollinger–Ellison syndrome: immunofluorescent, cytochemical and ultrastructural studies of the antral and pancreatic gastrin cells in different clinical states. Gut 13: 501–512

55. Porcile E, Racadot J 1966 Ultrastructure des cellules de Crooke observées dans l'hypophyse humaine au cours de la maladie de Cushing. Comptes Rendus Hebdomadaires des Séances de l'Académie des Sciences 263: 948–951

56. Powers J M, Schaumburg H H 1974 Adreno-leukodystrophy (sex-linked Schilder's disease). A pathogenetic hypothesis based on ultrastructural lesions in adrenal cortex, peripheral nerve and testis. American Journal of Pathology 76: 481–500

57. Powers J M, Schaumburg H H 1974 Adreno-leukodystrophy: similar ultrastructural changes in adrenal cortical and Schwann cells. Archives of Neurology 30: 406–408

57a. Rahier J, Loozen S, Goebbels R M, Abrahem M 1987 The haemochromatotic human pancreas: A quantitative immunohistochemical and ultrastructural study. Diabetologia 30: 5–12

58. Reidbord H, Fisher E R 1968 Electron microscopic study of adrenal cortical hyperplasia in Cushing's syndrome. Archives of Pathology 86: 419–426

59. Reidbord H E, Fisher E R 1973 Ultrastructural features of granulomatous thyroiditis and Hashimoto's disease. American Journal of Clinical Pathology 59: 327–337

60. Roth S I 1970 The ultrastructure of water-clear cell hyperplasia of the parathyroid glands. American Journal of Pathology 61: 233–248

61. Roth S I, Capen C C 1974 Ultrastructural and functional correlations of the parathyroid gland. International Review of Experimental Pathology 13: 161–211

62. Roth S I, Marshall R B 1969 Pathology and ultrastructure of the human parathyroid glands in chronic renal failure. Archives of Internal Medicine 124: 397–407

63. Roth S I, Munger B L 1962 The cytology of the adenomatous, atrophic and hyperplastic parathyroid glands of man. A light-and electron-microscopic study. Virchows Archiv A, Pathological Anatomy and Histopathology 335: 389–410

64. Satoh M 1975 Virus-like particles in the follicular epithelium of the thyroid from a patient with subacute thyroiditis (De Quervain). Acta Pathologica Japonica 25: 499–501

65. Satoh M 1976 Ultrastructure of the giant cell in De Quervain's subacute thyroiditis. Acta Pathologica Japonica 26: 133–137

66. Seyama S, Pearl G S, Takei Y 1980 Ultrastructural study of the human neurohypophysis. I. Neurosecretory axons and their dilatations in the pars nervosa. Cell and Tissue Research 205: 253–271

67. Seyama S, Pearl G S, Takei Y 1980 Ultrastructural study of the human neurohypophysis. III. Vascular and perivascular structures. Cell and Tissue Research 206: 291–302

68. Tannenbaum M 1975 Ultrastructural pathology of the adrenal cortex. In: Sommers S C (ed) Endocrine Pathology Dicennial 1966–1975. Appleton–Century–Crofts, New York, pp 423–472

69. Takei Y, Seyama S, Pearl G S, Tindall G T 1980 Ultrastructural study of the human neurohypophysis. II. Cellular elements of neural parenchyma, the pituicytes. Cell and Tissue Research 205: 273–287

70. Vassallo G, Solcia E, Bussolati G, Polak J M, Pearse A G E 1972 Non-G cell gastrin-producing tumors of the pancreas. Virchows Archiv B, Cell Pathology 11: 66–79

71. Volpé R 1978 The pathology of thyroiditis. Human Pathology 9: 429–438

72. Weidenheim K M, Hinchey W W, Campbell W G 1983 Hyperinsulinemic hypoglycemia in adults with islet-cell hyperplasia and degranulation of exocrine cells in the pancreas. American Journal of Clinical Pathology 79: 14–24

73. Westermark P 1973 Fine structure of islets of Langerhans in insular amyloidosis. Virchows Archiv A, Pathological Anatomy and Histopathology 359: 1–18

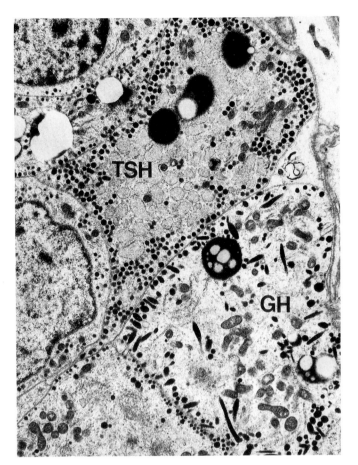

Fig. 16.1 (Left)   Adenohypophysis adjacent to adenoma: somatotrophs and thyrotrophs. Uninvolved part of a pituitary gland harbouring a prolactin cell adenoma in a middle-aged man. A portion of a somatotroph (growth hormone cell; GH) and thyrotrophs are depicted. Several secretory granules in the GH cell exhibit an abnormality which — via crystallization within the granular substance — results in the formation of elongated or geometrically shaped secretory granules. This anomaly is fairly common in adenomas but rarely occurs in normal somatotrophs. One of the thyrotrophs (TSH) shows marked dilatation of RER, which is a sign of hyperactivity. (× 9000)

Fig. 16.2 (Below)   Lymphocytic hypophysitis: survey view. The inflammatory process — resulting in marked enlargement of the gland and hyperprolactinaemia — mimicked a prolactin-secreting adenoma. Note the lymphocytes and plasma cells infiltrating and eventually destroying the parenchyma of the pituitary. (× 3200)

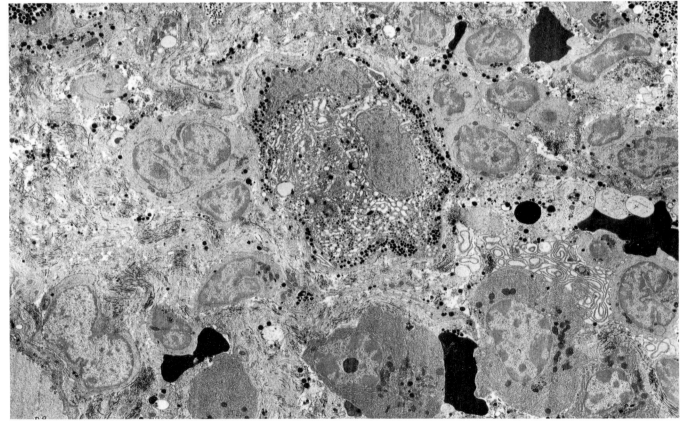

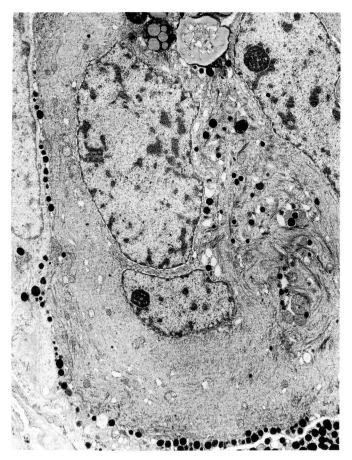

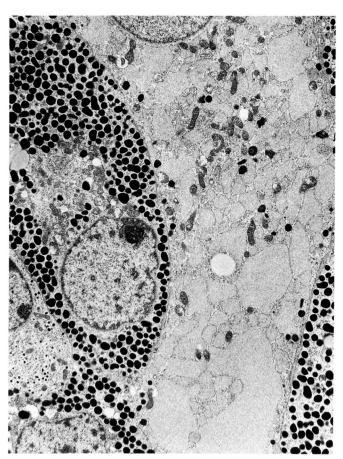

Fig. 16.3 Adenohypophysis: Crooke's hyaline. Crooke cell noted in the non-tumorous portion of a pituitary gland adjacent to a corticotroph adenoma causing Cushing's disease in a young woman. Most of the markedly enlarged cytoplasm is occupied by a massive deposition of filaments. The endoplasmic reticulum and Golgi complex are reduced to a few vesiculated membrane profiles; secretory granules are retained only in the Golgi area and at the extreme periphery of the cytoplasm. (× 5400)

Fig. 16.4 Adenohypophysis: gonadectomy cell in the pituitary gland of an ovariectomized woman who underwent therapeutic hypophysectomy. Note the markedly dilated RER containing an electron-lucent finely granular substance. At this stage of gonadectomy change, the secretory granules are scanty. (× 5600)

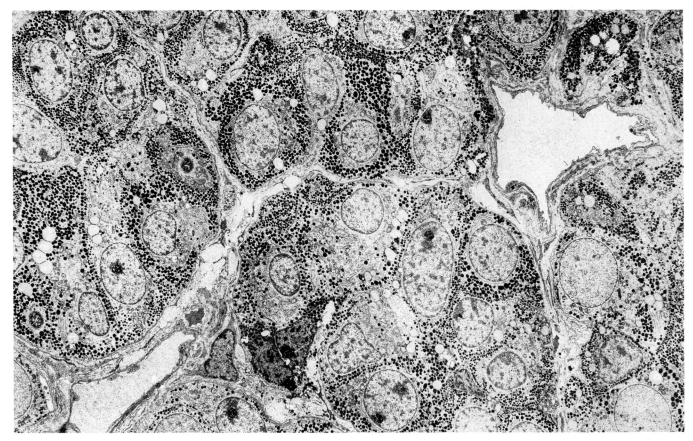

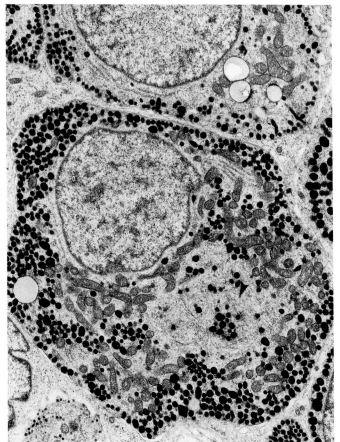

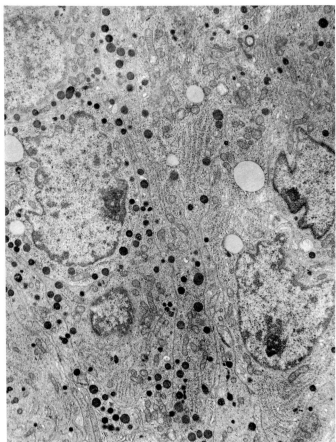

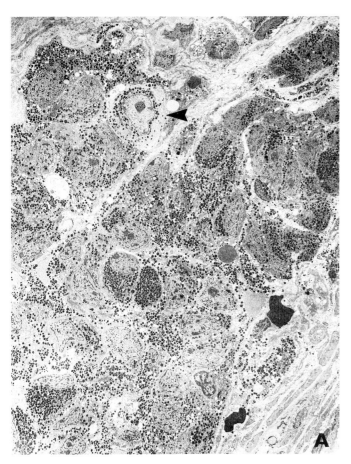

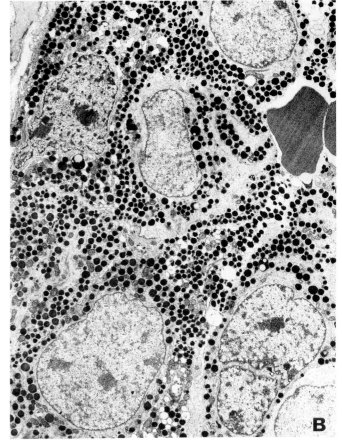

Fig. 16.8 (Above) **A** and **B** Adenohypophysis: corticotroph hyperplasia associated with Cushing's disease The reticulin network is preserved but the pattern is grossly distorted. The enlarged acini are populated by corticotrophs that are smaller than the normal densely granulated variety and contain variable numbers of filaments (arrowhead). In some cells, the accumulation of filaments reaches the extent seen in Crooke's cells (see Fig. 16.3). (A, × 1300; B, × 3500)

Fig. 16.5 (Facing page, top) Adenohypophysis: somatotroph hyperplasia. Focal nodular somatotroph hyperplasia with preserved reticulin pattern that appeared to be an adenoma at surgery in a young woman who also had a microprolactinoma. Immunohistochemistry detected scattered gonadotrophs and corticotrophs within the nodule as well. The majority of somatotrophs are heavily granulated with large, often slightly irregular granules. Note prominence of Golgi complexes. (× 2000)

Fig. 16.6 (Facing page, bottom left) Adenohypophysis: somatotroph hyperplasia. Same case as shown in Fig. 16.5. Mild accumulation of filaments (arrowheads) is seen in the Golgi region, but individual filaments are not resolved at this magnification; this is not known to occur in normal somatotrophs (× 6000)

Fig. 16.7 (Facing page, bottom right) Adenohypophysis: lactotroph hyperplasia. Focal lactotroph hyperplasia in the non-adenomatous area of a pituitary gland harboring a corticotroph cell adenoma. The membranous organelles are prominent in the overactive lactotrophs; the secretory granules are more numerous and larger (up to 450 nm) than in unstimulated prolactin cells. (× 6400)

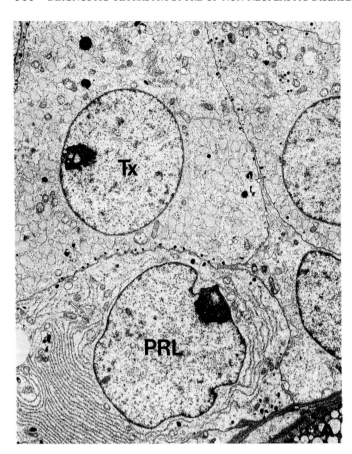

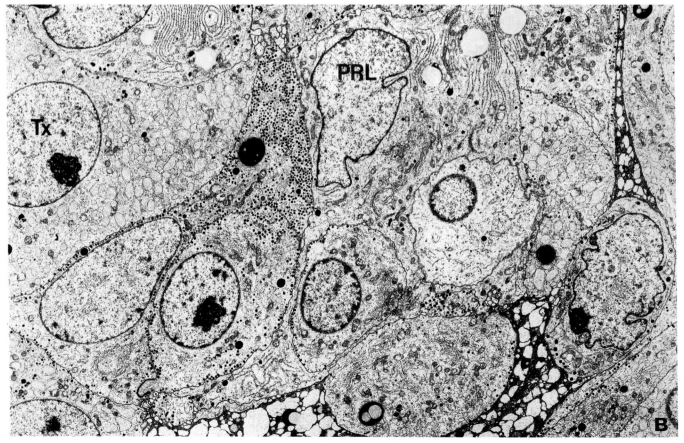

Fig. 16.9 A and **B** Adenohypophysis: thyrotroph hyperplasia in a case of untreated hypothyroidism. The hyperplasia resulted in a marked enlargement of the pituitary gland, mimicking adenoma. The enlarged acini are populated mostly by thyrotrophs showing the marked abundance and, often, dilatation of RER characteristic of 'thyroid deficiency cells' (Tx). Owing to sustained stimulation by thyrotropin-releasing hormone, overactive prolactin cells (PRL) are also noted. (A, × 3800; B, × 3400)

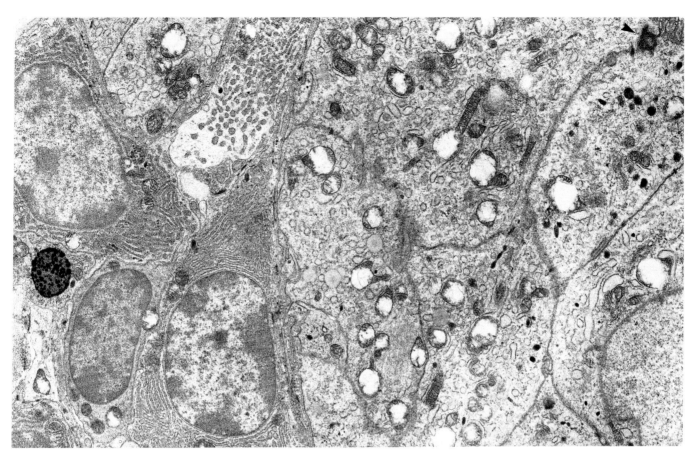

Fig. 16.10 Thyroid: Hashimoto's thyroiditis. The fine-structural
appearances of the follicular cells (right) are within normal limits. Note
obliquely cut junctional complex at the apical poles of cells (arrowhead at
top right). On the left of the picture, part of the lymphocytic-plasma cell
infiltrate is depicted. (× 6600)

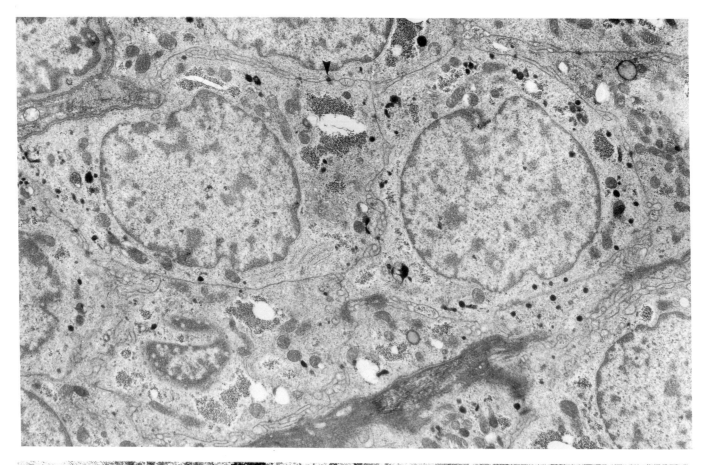

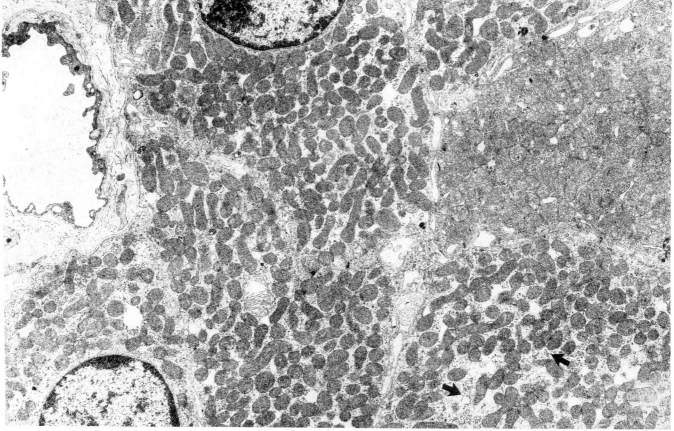

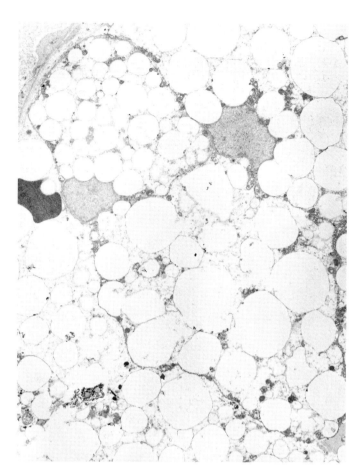

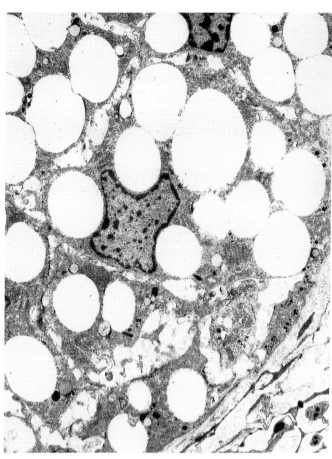

Fig. 16.13 Parathyroid: water-clear cell hyperplasia. The sole ultrastructural characteristic of this rare condition is the presence of membrane-bound vacuoles of varying size — probably representing endoplasmic reticulum —which occupy large areas of the cytoplasm. Except for the dark, deformed nuclei and a few scattered, small mitochondria, no other cell constituents are recognized. (× 2800) (Case contributed by Drs M. Coleman and D. W. Henderson.)

Fig. 16.14 Adrenal cortex: atrophy adjacent to a cortical adenoma causing Cushing's syndrome. Most of the small volume of cytoplasm is occupied by large lipid droplets, indenting the chromatin-rich nucleus. (× 5600)

Fig. 16.11 (Facing page, top) Parathyroid: chief cell hyperplasia of the parathyroid associated with primary hyperparathyroidism. The fine-structural features are similar to those of chief cell adenomas. The RER and Golgi complex are well developed; a modest number of secretory granules and several aggregates of glycogen-beta-particles are also present. Note the multiple foldings between cell membranes and prominent desmosomal attachments (arrowhead). (× 10 500)

Fig. 16.12 (Facing page, bottom) Parathyroid: oxyphil cell hyperplasia, associated with primary hyperparathyroidism. The obvious marker of this lesion is extensive oncocytic transformation. Clusters of glycogen beta-particles are visible (arrowheads), but other cytoplasmic constituents are obscured by the crowded mitochondria. Note fenestrated endothelium of the capillary. (× 7700)

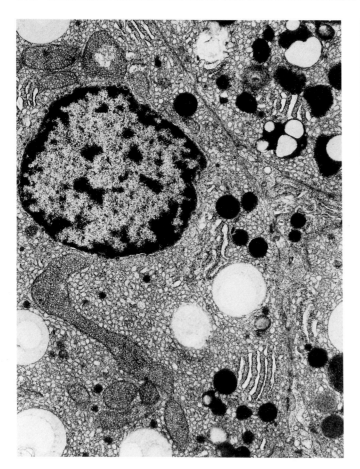

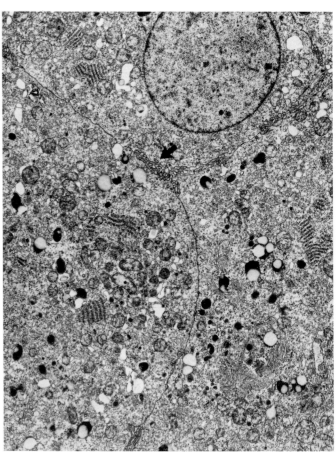

Fig. 16.15   Adrenal cortex: hyperplasia resulting in Cushing's syndrome. Note the hyperplastic smooth endoplasmic reticulum, prominent stacks of RER, vesicular mitochondria and numerous lysosomal dense bodies. (× 9000)

Fig. 16.16   Adrenal cortex: compact cell hyperplasia in ectopic ACTH syndrome. Note fine-structural signs of sustained stimulation: spherical nucleus with little heterochromatin, enlarged cytoplasm showing marked abundance of smooth endoplasmic reticulum, well- developed RER, prominent Golgi complex, as well as multiple interdigitations (arrowhead) between cell membranes. There are almost no lipid droplets. (× 4800)

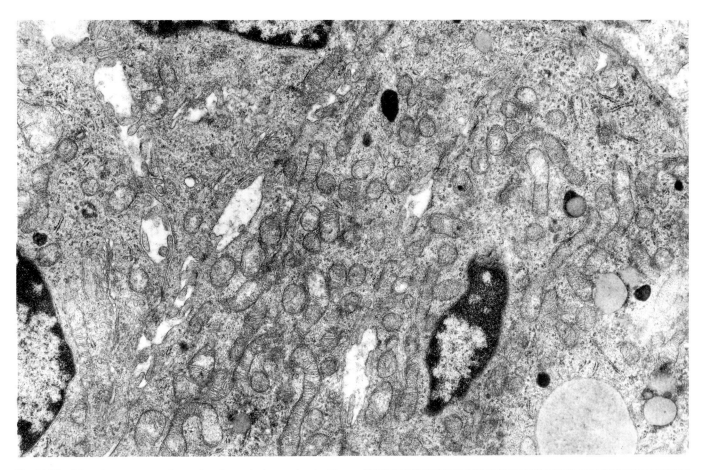

Fig. 16.17 Adrenal cortex: zona glomerulosa hyperplasia associated with Conn's syndrome. As opposed to the high lipid content of many tumours derived from the zona glomerulosa, this is a compact cell lesion. The RER, smooth endoplasmic reticulum and Golgi complex are prominent; polyribosomes are numerous. The elongated microvilli projecting into the intercellular space are numerous. The elongated mitochondria with lamellar cristae are typical of the zona glomerulosa. (× 9400)

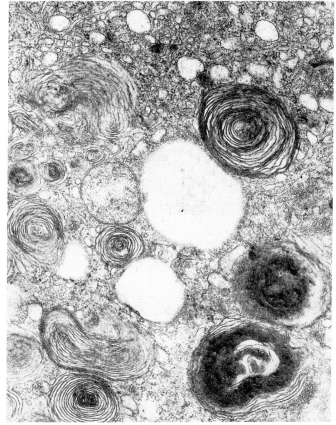

Fig. 16.18 Adrenal cortex: zona glomerulosa hyperplasia associated with Conn's syndrome, treated with spironolactone. A group of membranous whorls is shown, representing spironolactone bodies in early phases of their formation. (× 21 000)

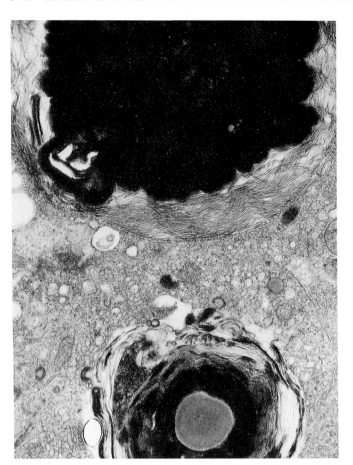

Fig. 16.19 (Left) Adrenal cortex: typical spironolactone bodies in a case of zona glomerulosa hyperplasia with Conn's syndrome. The central core consists of lipid-like, amorphous substance; the peripheral part is lamellar and the outermost membrane is continuous with the endoplasmic reticulum. (× 15 000)

Fig. 16.20 (Below) Adrenal medulla: hyperplasia in a case of MEN-2 syndrome. The well-differentiated phaeochromocytes possess light euchromatic nuclei, prominent RER and unusually numerous secretory granules. Note the uninvolved cortex at the bottom of the picture. (× 3500)

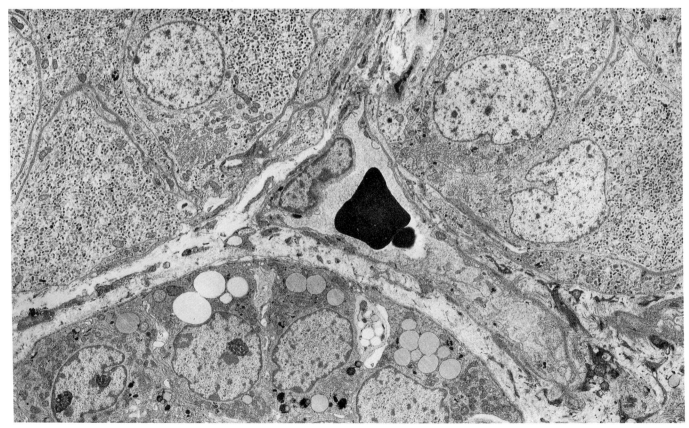

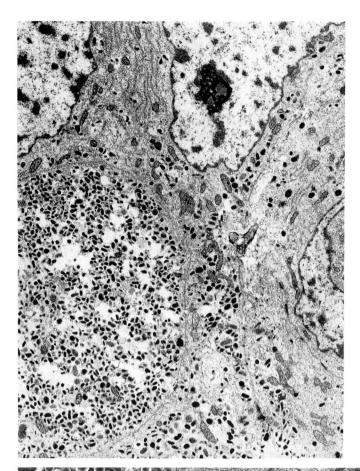

Fig. 16.21 (Left) Adrenal medullary hyperplasia: survey view. Same case as shown in Fig. 16.20. The well-differentiated cells contain abundant RER, well-developed Golgi apparatus (not shown) and a large population of secretory granules of variable morphology. (× 5200)

Fig. 16.22 (Below) Pancreas: nesidioblastosis associated with hyperinsulinism in an adult woman. The hyperplastic pancreatic islets contained all cell types indigenous to the organ (A = A cell; B = B cell; D = D cell). (× 11 400)

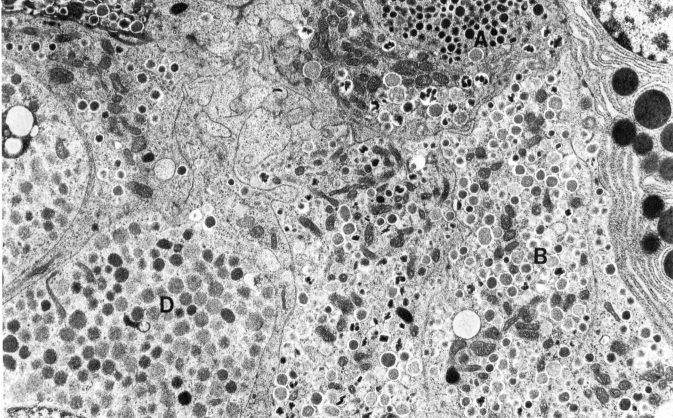

17. The kidney

M. Coleman   A. E. Seymour

INTRODUCTION

In the 25–30 years since the first ultrastructural studies of renal disease, electron microscopy (EM) has come to be recognized as an important component of renal diagnosis and, in particular, an integral part of the assessment of glomerular pathology.[39,187] The complexity of the technique has often sequestered EM interpretation from 'routine' histopathological diagnosis and this has, in many cases, complicated biopsy interpretation by preventing a unified approach. EM does not stand alone and frequently provides only non-specific information. To contribute most to renal diagnosis, therefore, ultrastructural data are best interpreted in conjunction with light microscopy (LM) and immunohistology (IH). Used in this way, EM provides a mechanism for more detailed assessment of the various morphological lesions of renal disease thus facilitating:

1. A better understanding of the changes seen by LM
2. More precise categorization of disease and, therefore, improved prognosis
3. Pathogenetic insight.

Early workers in renal pathology recommended that all renal biopsies be examined by EM. While this is desirable in investigative laboratories, accumulated experience now allows many commonly encountered renal diseases to be diagnosed by LM and IH. EM remains of major diagnostic value when LM is apparently normal, minimally perturbed, atypical or non-specific, and IH is non-specific, negative or unavailable. It is the sole method of specific diagnosis in hereditary glomerulopathies and so-called epithelial cell disease (minimal change disease), and often adds crucial diagnostic information in other disorders, such as lupus glomerulonephritis (GN), 'early' amyloidosis, membranous GN or diabetic nephropathy. EM examination is indicated in any biopsy in which LM changes are minimal or absent, or when the appearances are atypical and not easily categorized.

The aims of this chapter are to illustrate the ultrastructural morphology of renal disease, to summarize recent developments in some areas of renal diagnosis and to provide guides to the solution of specific problems. While a range of abnormalities may be seen in tubular and interstitial disorders, these are not of diagnostic value, and glomerular ultrastructure will constitute the major consideration of this chapter. EM does not contribute to routine assessment of non-neoplastic disease of the lower urinary tract except perhaps as an aid to the diagnosis of malakoplakia, which is considered in Chapter 11.

Familiarity with renal morphology and LM pathology will be presumed — details of references dealing with the general aspects of renal disease are included.[39,41,42,86,97,121,179,191,193,210–212,250] Only transmission EM will be discussed. Scanning EM has contributed considerable information to research studies but, so far, has little role to play in routine renal diagnosis.[25] Immuno-electron microscopy has great potential for the further study of renal disease but will not be considered here.[124,231]

TECHNIQUES

Standard processing schedules (see Ch. 2) are readily applicable to renal biopsy material.[6,212] Our personal preferences are for primary glutaraldehyde fixation, secondary osmication and Araldite or Epon embedding. Rapid processing schedules are available[156,212] but a standard 24-hour system provides excellent results and is satisfactory for routine diagnosis. Longer schedules are best avoided as they tend to isolate EM data from the early diagnostic process. We recommend, where possible, that tissue be retained for EM from all renal biopsies, and processed at least to block stage. LM remains the mainstay for renal diagnosis and provides the best prognostic information, but LM examination can be performed equally well with glutaraldehyde-fixed and plastic-embedded material[103] as with conventional paraffin sections. Indeed, some workers believe that careful scrutiny of toluidine blue sections can replace EM study in many biopsies.[96] Hence, when only limited material is obtained at biopsy, EM fixation and processing should be given preference to LM in some circumstances. If, however, there is strong clinical suspicion of glomerulonephritis, the tissue is best processed for LM as this will allow immunohistological examination. We believe that clinicopathological correlation is more effective, and interaction with our nephrological colleagues more fruitful, if the LM, EM and IH data are integrated into a single coherent report.

NORMAL ULTRASTRUCTURE

Normal renal ultrastructure is well described in standard texts and needs no reiteration.[95,97,119,167,200,212,227,246,250] However, there is considerable variation in renal ultrastructure, and deviation from the 'ideal' norm is commonly encountered. Processing methods may affect appearances; for example, the classical trilaminar structure of the glomerular basement membrane (GBM) is not apparent in glutaraldehyde-fixed, Araldite-embedded material. Commonly encountered but non-specific alterations include: striated membranous bodies (Fig. 17.4) and spherical microparticles (Figs 17.29 and 17.46)[15,16,30,72,102,191,212,250] (complement components have been demonstrated in these structures and in connective tissue matrices in normal kidneys[102]) as well as microfibrils (see below); microvillous transformation of endothelial and epithelial cells (Figs 17.24 and 17.25); short zones of foot process effacement; sporadic collagen fibril formation in mesangia or GBM; and fibrosis, calcification or dense deposit formation in Bowman's capsule.[95] Deposits and fibrillar collagen are often seen in the region of the glomerular base. Such findings are generally of no diagnostic significance when present as isolated phenomena. Obliquely sectioned normal structures may simulate pathological processes — for example, cross-cutting of mesangia mimics subendothelial mesangial interposition, and tangentially sectioned GBM simulates thickening of that structure. Oblique sectioning of the GBM is indicated by loss of definition of the membrane–plasmalemma interface and by the visualization of endothelial fenestrae. Careful morphometry is needed for the reliable assessment of GBM thickness.[4,49]

ARTEFACTS

Artefacts which may be observed include: intact or fragmented tubular epithelial cells forced into glomerular capillaries or the urinary space (Fig. 17.37) during the trauma of biopsy;[155,239] fibrin tactoids and platelet clumps (Fig. 17.10) resulting from coagulation initiated by the biopsy procedure; and changes reflecting delayed fixation (see Ch. 2) comprising mitochondrial vacuolation and ballooning, cellular swelling, loss of tubular cell brush border, cell rupture and interstitial oedema.[250]

GLOMERULAR DISEASE

The ultrastructural expressions of glomerular disease result from:

1. Alteration of intrinsic components
2. The infiltration of circulating inflammatory cells
3. The formation or deposition in the glomerulus of materials not normally present, such as immune complexes, amyloid or fibrin.

The repertoire of reaction patterns available to the glomerulus is limited and frequently non-specific, but distinctive patterns are often easily recognizable. EM study may provide diagnostic information distinguishing apparently identical LM patterns — for example, in the elucidation of the causes of capillary wall thickening — and sometimes discerns specific features before they can be seen by LM, as in amyloidosis or stage I membranous glomerulonephritis. Immune complex deposits are frequently seen in glomerulonephritis (GN) in distinctive arrangements — for example, the humps of acute post-infectious GN, or the mesangial deposits of IgA nephropathy. In addition, diverse reactive changes may accompany deposition such as 'spike' formation in membranous GN, mesangial interposition in mesangiocapillary GN, endothelial tubulo-reticular arrays in lupus nephritis, mesangial matrix lucencies in hepatic glomerulosclerosis and cellular proliferation or infiltration in a variety of nephritides. The hereditary nephropathies cannot be subclassified accurately without EM and are now being characterized more clearly through the use of ultrastructural morphometry (see below).

The various and often complicated reaction patterns of the glomerulus may be catalogued conveniently by anatomical site; that is, in terms of localization to the capillary lumen, capillary wall, mesangium and extracapillary space although many disease processes simultaneously involve more than one of these regions. Separate comments on some selected entities follow.

CAPILLARY LUMINAL REACTIONS

Inflammatory cells may occupy the lumina particularly in acute GN as exemplified by the neutrophil polymorph infiltration of post-infectious GN (Figs 17.36–17.38) in which endothelial ulceration and intimate apposition between neutrophils and GBM may be obvious. Luminal narrowing or occlusion by mononuclear cells (predominantly cytotoxic T-lymphocytes and monocytes) occurs in glomerular transplant rejection (Fig. 17.16).[13,99,228,229]

Thrombosis, with the formation of platelet/fibrin masses may accompany systemic intravascular coagulation, the haemolytic uraemic syndrome, accelerated hypertension,[116] hyperacute transplant rejection and any severe GN — particularly if necrotizing features are present.[212]

Massive or 'giant' immune deposits — corresponding to

the so-called 'hyaline thrombi' of LM which may fill capillary loops — are seen typically in systemic lupus erythematosus (SLE), macroglobulinaemia, and cryoglobulinaemia. Such deposits are actually probably subendothelial (Fig. 17.45) — their apparent intraluminal location being due to their large size and cross-cutting artefact.

Haematoxylin bodies, the pathognomonic structures of SLE, which consist of altered nuclear material, may occur anywhere within the glomerulus or in extraglomerular sites but may occupy the capillary lumen.

Fat vacuoles of fat embolism, bacteria, fungi, tumour cells and megakaryocytes may be apparent rarely in this site.[178,212,250]

CAPILLARY WALL

The glomerular capillaries are unique and specialized vascular channels the walls of which constitute the renal filter. While some conditions are characterized by capillary wall (CW) alterations which can be diagnosed only by EM, such as epithelial cell disease and so-called benign essential haematuria (see below), thickening is perhaps the most frequently observed alteration of the CW seen by LM. EM has made a major contribution to the elucidation of CW thickening by separating diagnostically distinct patterns which were confused by early workers — for example mesangiocapillary change and membranous GN. The differential diagnosis of CW thickening has been comprehensively reviewed by Seymour et al (1983).[191] Brief consideration is given below to some of the more important of these entities.

Membranous glomerulonephritis

The characteristic deposition patterns of this disease and its evolution are illustrated in Figs 17.1–17.6. Although the morphological expression of membranous GN is relatively constant,[33,64,80,129,132,136,170,191,212,222,251] the lesion may be the end point of diverse clinicopathological conditions including neoplasia,[7] drug toxicity, chronic infections and systemic diseases such as SLE.[7,33,131,170,188,212,222,245] The presence of atypical features may point to the secondary nature of the process (Fig. 17.19). For example, the presence of deposits in subendothelial or mesangial sites, fingerprint or tubular organization of deposits (Figs 17.46 and 17.47), and endothelial tubuloreticular arrays (Fig. 17.43) suggest SLE, and cytoplasmic aurisomes in proximal tubular epithelium indicate gold therapy (Fig. 17.22). Idiopathic membranous GN, however, remains the most common form of this condition and may result, in some patients, from glomerular interaction *in situ* between circulating antibodies and non-GBM glomerular antigens or 'planted' extraglomerular antigens.[52,53,136] There is increasing evidence suggesting that these mechanisms of immune complex formation may be more common than hitherto suspected in a variety of glomerulonephritides.[52,53,128,234]

Diabetic glomerulosclerosis

GBM thickening accompanied by mesangial matrix increase is the glomerular expression of diabetic microangiopathy (Fig. 17.7).[5,34,105,108,140,147,215,233,237] The increase in GBM width is typically uniform. Structural abnormalities of the GBM develop as early as two years after the onset of glucose intolerance[164–166] and in most cases the severity of glomerulosclerosis correlates approximately with duration and severity of disease.[98,105,140,238] However, the relationships between clinical expression of the disease and the various components of the glomerular lesion are variable. The morphometric studies of Mauer et al (1984)[140] demonstrated the following:

1. There was no strong relationship between either GBM thickness or mesangial expansion and duration of insulin-dependent diabetes mellitus.

2. There was only a weak relationship between GBM thickness and mesangial expansion.

3. The clinical manifestations of diabetic nephropathy related poorly, or not at all, to GBM thickness.

4. In contrast, all measures of mesangial expansion correlated strongly with the clinical state.

5. Mesangial expansion was strongly correlated inversely with capillary filtering surface area, suggesting that mesangial expansion could lead to functional deterioration by progessive narrowing and obliteration of glomerular capillaries.

Cases are encountered in which established GBM thickening is obvious in patients who have apparently normal glucose tolerance[154] but it is apparent from the above observations that GBM thickening alone is a poor indicator of disease. Further, this alteration is not specific for diabetes mellitus (DM). The pattern of diffuse glomerulosclerosis is reproduced in some situations leading to glomerular hypertrophy (glomerulomegaly) such as morbid obesity, chronic liver or pulmonary disease or, simply, loss of renal substance through nephrectomy or chronic nephropathy.[111,122] The nodular LM pattern of glomerulopathy, while being highly characteristic, may be closely mimicked by mesangial amyloid, light-chain nephropathy (see below), and mesangiocapillary GN.[161] Hence, although cases of diabetic glomerulosclerosis in the absence of clinically definable disease have been reported, such cases demand rigorous study, including EM, to exclude alternative diagnoses.[98,140]

Microproteinuria early in the course of DM depends more on functional than on structural changes[3,34,105,238] (although nephromegaly is common[105]), is related to an increase in glomerular filtration[105,233] and reduction of tubular reabsorption, and is exacerbated by exercise probably because of increased transcapillary pressure. This variable early microproteinuria predicts later nephropathy. That at least partial reversibility of some of these functional aberrations is associated with good control of hyperglycaemia has been documented by some workers[3,130,238] although not by others.[71] Late in the course of the disease, as glomerular structural abnormalities become overt, proteinuria becomes persistent, more severe, and clinically significant.[3] Ultimately, obliterative mesangial expansion terminates glomerular function.[3] That careful control of hyperglycaemia might alter the rate of progression of diabetic nephropathy is suggested by some authors[70,130] but this issue remains unresolved.[3] Because glomerular capillary hypertension or other haemodynamic aberrations might be implicated in the pathogenesis of this nephropathy, control of blood pressure may be at least as important as the maintenance of euglycaemia in the prevention of progressive disease.[140]

Rarely, proteinuria in a diabetic may be due to the presence of co-existent nephropathies.[27,35,141,174]

The characteristic mesangial nodules of DM develop on a background of diffuse GBM and mesangial disease.[5,28,108,161] Apparently, they represent nodular exaggeration of matrix accumulation, although other mechanisms for their formation have been suggested — such as mesangiolysis (see below) and organization of capillary aneurysms.[22,149] Microaneurysm formation has been ascribed variously to simple loop dilatation, mesangiolysis, and herniation of mesangial contents through ruptures of the paramesangial basement membrane.[22,149,233] Mesangial microfibrils have been recorded in some cases[28] (see below).

Mesangial/subendothelial interposition (mesangiocapillary change)

The CW thickening and GBM 'double contour' that characterize mesangiocapillary GN (MCGN) are consequences of the interposition of mesangial cells between the endothelium and GBM.[12,93,115,117,191,212,249] The outer argyrophilic contour seen by LM is shown by EM to be the original GBM. The inner contour comprises new matrix laid down by the mesangial cells invading the subendothelial potential space. Normally, this space is continuous with the mesangium and constitutes a functional pathway for the transport and disposal of macromolecules held up by the GBM.[145]

Mesangial interposition is most often secondary to mesangial proliferation, although by no means all mesangial proliferative GN is complicated by interposition. It may be partial or circumferential and is a non-specific reaction pattern common to many glomerular diseases. Sporadic short segments of interposition are frequently seen in many cases of GN but should not be confused with the appearances of cross-cut paramesangial or vascular pole regions which may mimic the lesion.

Widespread circumferential interposition typifies *MCGN type I* (subendothelial deposit variety, 'membranoprolifera-

tive GN') (Figs 17.8–17.10) which itself is the end point of numerous and disparate disease processes including chronic infections,[48] neoplasms, systemic connective tissue disorders (such as SLE — see Fig. 17.44), complement deficiencies and others.[93,117,191,212,249] Common to these conditions is immune complex deposition. The deposits in type I MCGN are conventionally referred to as subendothelial, but actually they are located in the mesangial structures of the interposition zone (Fig. 17.8). A variant pattern showing extensive centrimembranous deposition with dramatic GBM thickening and disruption is sometimes seen (*MCGN type III* — see Fig. 17.11).[9,217,218] Silver impregnation techniques may aid the ultrastructural elucidation of this variant.

Mesangiocapillary patterns may also occur in *dense-deposit disease* (DDD, so-called MCGN type II). Ultrastructurally, DDD is distinguished by a unique ribbon-like pattern of linear dense transformation of the GBM (Figs 17.12 and 17.13). The nature of DDD is obscure, but this condition is unrelated to the other varieties of MCGN.[37,59,60,63,75,92,157,198]

Circumferential mesangial interposition may be widespread in renal allografts as a manifestation of *transplant glomerulopathy* (Figs 17.15 and 17.21). The ultrastructural alteration in this situation is dramatic widening of the subendothelial space which appears to contain electron-lucent deposit of uncertain nature, sometimes with denser flocculent material and microfibrils (see below). Strands of new GBM-like material lie between this zone and the endothelium. The lucent substance also permeates and expands the mesangia which later become sclerotic.[107,138,139,191,228,229]

'Accelerated obsolescence'

Some cases of accelerated hypertension, the haemolytic uraemic syndrome (Fig. 17.14), thrombotic thrombocytopenic purpura, disseminated intravascular coagulation, progressive systemic sclerosis and radiation injury, develop a glomerulopathy characterized by the development of variably widespread subendothelial widening, producing luminal stenosis which may be dramatic. As in the transplant lesion described above, lucent deposit accumulates in the CW and, in the more florid cases, fibrin, erythrocytes, red cell fragments and other formed elements are seen in the subendothelial zone. Microfibrils (see below) may be found. An irregular layer of GBM-like material may form adjacent to the endothelium mimicking mesangial interposition.[113,116,191,195,196,202,212,226] Subsequent organization with new membrane replacing the deposit results in massive thickening of the CW and permanent luminal narrowing. Mesangial disruption by the lucent substance may be associated with mesangiolysis (see below).[149]

The pathogenesis of these changes is not established but it seems probable that the CW and mesangial changes are secondary to endothelial injury[113,226] with increased permeability allowing the egress of fluid, plasma proteins and, in severe cases, formed elements of the blood into the subendothelial tissues. Analogous lesions occur in extraglomerular blood vessels. The endothelial damage itself is probably multifactorial but may involve vasospastic phenomena and glomerular ischaemia[116] or direct toxic injury.[113] Transplant glomerulopathy (see above) may be closely related and secondary to endothelial injury mediated via humoral rejection. Similar mechanisms may also be implicated in the pathogenesis of vascular rejection which is usually found in concert with this glomerulopathy. Whether true mesangial interposition, or rather *in situ* formation of new GBM, occurs by some other mechanism as part of these phenomena is unclear.

The appellation 'accelerated obsolescence', a contraction of the term 'accelerated hypertensive obsolescence', has been applied to these glomerular lesions characterized by lucent subendothelial deposit.[116] This terminology is suboptimal since the lesion is without specificity and can develop in normotensive individuals; the alterations are dissimilar to the CW wrinkling and collapse of ischaemic obsolescence[143] — although glomerular sclerosis may be the end point — and the title lacks morphological precision.

Light-chain nephropathy

Several renal complications of multiple myeloma and related disorders are caused by the deposition or entrapment in the kidney of paraproteins or their derivatives emanating from the neoplastic lymphoplasmacytic clone.[7,19,77,148,172,212] These products may be entire immunoglobulin (Ig), Ig fragments, isolated heavy chains, light chains or immune complexes.[77] Modification of light chains may lead to amyloidosis (see below), long recognized as one of the major renal manifestations of myeloma. Recently, a nodular non-amyloid glomerulopathy has been recognized and related to the accumulation of light chains, nearly always of the kappa subtype and readily demonstrable by IH within basement membranes and mesangial matrix.[7,8,26,28,47,61,66,77–79,112,133,148,153,159,171–173,191,194,212,224,231] By LM the typical lesion mimics nodular diabetic glomerulosclerosis, and micro-aneurysm formation is described,[206] but affected glomeruli may appear normal,[191] show simple mesangial enlargement, GBM thickening,[79] endocapillary proliferation,[194] MCGN,[7] epithelial cell disease,[7] or, rarely, exhibit crescentic GN.[148]

Immunohistology dramatically demonstrates the presence of (monoclonal) light chains in mesangia and GBM as well as in Bowman's capsule, tubular basement membranes and blood vessels. Extraglomerular reactions sometimes predominate. The disease probably is systemic[133,173,212] in most cases, with involvement of liver, myocardium, spleen and other organs but this may be subclinical.

The ultrastructural hallmark of light chain deposition is the presence of finely granular, non-fibrillar deposits often as continuous bands or clusters[77] within basement membranes and glomerular mesangia (Figs 17.17 and 17.l8). Careful attention to the granular nature of the deposits should allow

distinction from dense-deposit disease with which they have been confused. Rare cases of kappa glomerulopathy with fibrillar deposits are recorded (see below), and an example with both kappa and lambda subtypes and both granular and fibrillar deposits is documented.[8a]

Although more than half of affected patients have myeloma at the time of diagnosis,[77,79,148] the condition has been described in association with other lymphoid malignancies or with monoclonal gammopathies but no other evidence of neoplasia. Light-chain nephropathy may precede other manifestations of plasma cell dyscrasia.

Kappa chains characterize most cases, but lambda light-chains and even heavy-chain deposition have been reported occasionally.[79]

Examples of immune complex GN have been described in which the deposited Ig has been shown to be monoclonal by possession of a single light-chain subclass.[8] Such cases are of interest because of the implication that they might be a consequence of clonal plasma cell activity and the production of monoclonal Ig with pathogenic antibody activity. These cases should not be confused with light-chain nephropathy.

The mechanism of deposition of light chains is not understood but may be related to the presence of molecular structural abnormalities or the promotion of polymerization by glycosylation,[79] or to intrinsic physicochemical differences in the subclasses — for example, lambda chains are more likely to be associated with amyloid deposition, possibly because they are more susceptible to proteolysis than are kappa chains.[7,48]

Fibrillar deposit formation

The characteristic extracellular feltwork of straight, non-branching fibrils (approximately 10-nm in diameter) of *amyloidosis* is well known and usually easily recognizable.[10,23,25,56,79,82,84,112,123,191,197,212] Amyloid typically involves the CW and permeates other glomerular and extraglomerular structures in an invasive, irregular and haphazard fashion (Figs 17.19 and 17.20). Rarely, confusion may be caused by the presence of other fibrillar materials including glomerular microfibrils, the fibrils of Congo red-negative amyloidosis-like glomerulopathy or so-called immunotactoid glomerulopathy, fibrillar deposits in light-chain disease, and organized deposits of cryoglobulinaemic GN (see below).

Microfibrils are ubiquitous components of the formed elements of connective tissue.[28,61,106,219,242] Three types have been described apart from unit collagen fibrils (30-nm diameter and greater): 'large' fibrils, 18–20-nm diameter, believed to be precursors of collagen fibres; 'small' fibrils, approximately 10-nm diameter, which may occur either alone or as components of elastic tissue; and 'thin filaments', 3–5-nm diameter, which may be related to basal lamina. Glomerular microfibrils have been found most commonly in conditions characterized by the formation of subendothelial lucent deposit (Fig. 17.21).

In a study of glomerular microfibrils, Hsu & Churg[106] demonstrated fibrils with an average diameter of 12-nm mainly under the endothelium of the CW, and in mesangia of renal biopsies from patients with transplant glomerulopathy, focal glomerulosclerosis, toxaemia of pregnancy, haemolytic–uraemic syndrome and accelerated hypertension. The microfibrils were most prevalent in zones of subendothelial lucency and widening which were common to these cases and, in general, the concentration of fibrils correlated with the degree of widening. Mesangial microfibrils were sometimes seen and were prominent in cases of mesangiocapillary GN and diabetic glomerulosclerosis. Sequential biopsies suggested that the fibrils gradually became incorporated into new GBM and mesangial matrix. Hsu & Churg speculated that the occurrence of microfibrils in these sites may be related to the presence of mechanical stress. A separate study of renal biopsies from children with a variety of diseases[242] showed that fibrils 17–35-nm in diameter may also be found.

Several authors[29,61,127,180,189,219] have described cases of renal fibrillosis, associated with glomerular immunoglobulin deposition (without evidence of paraproteinaemia or cryoglobulinaemia), which superficially resembled amyloidosis but in which, on close study, distinctive ultrastructural differences were discernible. The fibrils in most of these cases were curved, approximately 20-nm in diameter with a tubular, double contour cross-sectional structure, in loosely arranged aggregates. Tubule diameters were larger (up to 49 nm) in a few cases. Standard LM stains for amyloid were negative, there was no evidence of systemic amyloidosis, and many of the patients presented with nephritic clinical features and renal failure. A few were nephrotic.[61,180,189] Because of the highly organized crystalloidal structure of the immune deposits in these cases, the diagnostic term 'immunotactoid glomerulopathy' has been suggested.[127,189] A case of myeloma-associated paraproteinaemia with GN in which the deposits showed immunotactoid-type organization is illustrated in Fig. 17.48.

Congo red-negative deposits with fibrillar substructure, sometimes in orderly parallel arrays, have been documented in small numbers of cases of kappa light-chain disease. The fibril diameters reported have ranged between 10 and 14 nm.[28,78,133] Such material might represent polymerization of κ chains but the appearances suggest that at least some of these fibrillar deposits may be simply microfibril aggregates. Patients with co-existent typical amyloid and light-chain deposition are recorded also.[112]

Several patterns of organization of immune deposits may be seen in lupus GN,[38,191,199,212] and in cryoglobulinaemic GN.[68,77,160,191,212] In *lupus nephritis* (Figs 17.46 and 17.47), some or all of the deposits may exhibit a fingerprint pattern or contain small rod-like structures. The fingerprint pattern is almost specific for lupus with only rare exceptions (see below). The typical CW deposits of mixed *cryoglobulinaemia* may be organized into aggregates of cylindrical structures the individual tubules of which have diameters of 20–30 nm or more.[61] Fibrillar configurations may be seen in the rare monoclonal variant[68,77,191] and fingerprint patterns are recorded.[160] Not all cases of cryoglobulinaemic GN exhibit deposit organization and, conversely, this phenomenon may be seen in the absence of demonstrable cryoprecipitability. Granular and fibrillar–crystalline deposits have also been described in macroglobulinaemia.[77]

Epithelial cell disease (minimal change disease)

The diagnostic ultrastructural lesion of epithelial cell disease (ECD) is total or widespread foot process obliteration.[24,144,191,212,225,241,244] This phenomenon may be due to retraction of foot processes into the parent visceral cell bodies but individual cell integrity is maintained and cell fusion does not occur (Figs 17.23 and 17.24). The GBM is covered by cytoplasmic sheets and there is often a zone of increased cytoplasmic density immediately adjacent to the membrane. This pattern of increased density may mimic subepithelial deposits in some biopsies and, conversely, some examples of stage I membranous GN may be misinterpreted as epithelial cell disease unless the subepithelial region is carefully scanned for deposits. The epithelial cells typically exhibit microvillous surface transformation (Fig. 17.24), organellar prominence and may contain cysts. Focal epithelial disruption or ulceration is sometimes seen.[212,241]

The epithelial cell alterations are completely reversible and foot process integrity is restored during disease remission. It is important to appreciate that foot process effacement is without specificity and may be extensive in many forms of glomerulopathy. The diagnosis of ECD depends on the finding of complete or subtotal pedicel loss in the appropriate clinical and pathological context.

Nephrotic focal/segmental glomerulosclerosis

Idiopathic focal/segmental glomerulosclerosis (FGS) in nephrotic patients shares some pathological features with ECD and should not be diagnosed in the absence of diffuse foot process effacement.[55,85,122,125,162,190,191,212,225,230,236,241,244] The sclerotic lesions comprise capillary collapse and increase in mesangial matrix together with the accumulation of granular electron-dense material often containing lipid vacuoles (corresponding to LM hyaline deposits), foam cells and fibrillar collagen (Figs 17.25–17.27). Proliferation of epithelial cells related to these areas may be seen as part of the 'cellular lesion' of FGS (Fig. 17.28).[190]

Focal epithelial cell ulceration or detachment, sometimes accompanied by multilayered new membrane formation between the original GBM and detached epithelium, has been reported frequently in FGS (Fig. 17.26). This is not a specific phenomenon and is recorded in ECD as noted above, and in other glomerulopathies.[241] The presence of frequent podocyte vacuolation (Fig. 17.25) has been linked with progression to chronic renal failure.[244] Other non-specific findings which may be common in FGS include disturbances of GBM texture and contour, occasional electron-dense deposits, striated membranous structures, microvesicular bodies, 'lead shot' microparticles and microfibrils.[212,241] Segmental sclerosis caused by capillary collapse and consolidation is a common pathway of progressive glomerular damage and all of these changes may be seen complicating a range of primary and secondary glomerulopathies. Only in the nephrotic forms, however, is diffuse foot process obliteration a feature.

Hereditary glomerulopathies

Heterogeneous cystic, tubulo-interstitial and glomerular disorders are known to occur with increased frequencies in family groups.[21,40,87,90,110,191,212,235] Several inherited glomerular disorders, despite having normal or non-specific LM, show relatively specific ultrastructural features, the recognition of which is essential for diagnostic classification and prognosis.

Alport's syndrome (Figs 17.29 and 17.30) is characterized by GBM irregularity which is often, but not always, dramatic.[18,21,40,87,88,90,91,100,126,163,169,175,181-183,191,201,212-214,235,240,248] The membrane is irregular in contour, width and texture. Areas of marked thickening alternate with zones of attenuation. The textural aberrations comprise lucencies and longitudinal lamellation, sometimes producing 'basket weave' patterns. The inclusion of microparticles is typical. Foot process loss may be widespread. GBM changes are the only pathognomonic morphological features of Alport's syndrome. The fully developed lesion when widespread or diffuse is probably specific for this disease but similar changes may affect isolated loops in other glomerulopathies[49,100,126,150] and there is a considerable range of lesions in Alport's disease.[91] Early in the course of the syndrome, the GBM may be normal or show only attenuation; textural changes are often apparent by the age of 2 years but adult patients are described as showing only thinning (see below) or even normal GBM.[91] Tubular basement membranes also may be abnormal in Alport's syndrome but in adults these structures normally exhibit so much variability as to be unreliable indicators of disease.

The characteristic alteration of so-called *benign essential (familial) haematuria* (BEH)[21,49,57,100,163,169,177,183,220,235,243,248] is diffuse attenuation of the GBM without major textural disturbances (Figs 17.31 and 17.32). This condition is manifest clinically as recurrent haematuria and is almost always non-progressive. However, a few recent cases have been identified with renal functional impairment.[57] The status of these cases is uncertain and, indeed, the precise delineation of BEH is problematical because adult Alport kindred, fulfilling clinical criteria of the syndrome, have been described whose biopsies show only GBM thinning.[91] Although GBM attenuation in this context may indicate a relatively favourable prognosis,[91] this observation suggests that the diagnosis of BEH should not be made on morphological criteria alone but demands clinicopathological correlation. The number of reported cases of BEH is small but this nephropathy may be more prevalent than previously suspected.[49,57]

A recent morphometric study of cases with apparently idiopathic haematuria[49] has defined the morphological lesion of (putative) BEH in objective terms (Figs 17.33 and 17.34). This analysis showed that within a group of patients with idiopathic haematuria, the degree of GBM thinning was very variable from case to case and there was a continuum of results. Included were cases with severe attenuation which was easily identifiable subjectively, merging with cases with recognizable lesions but mean thicknesses approaching control values. In addition, this study identified cases showing small but significant measurable deviations from the control mean, the abnormality being recognizable only by objective assessment.

The characteristic GBM alterations of the *nail–patella syndrome* are illustrated in Fig. 17.35.

The kidney is involved in several lysosomal storage diseases.[250] These are detailed in Chapter 6 but some additional comments on *Fabry's disease* are worthy of note.[54,62,67,89,176,208] The kidney is invariably involved in Fabry's disease, the typical ultrastructural lesion being the presence of membrane-bound lamellated cytoplasmic inclusions exhibiting pleomorphic, concentric myelinoid profiles or stacked, zebra-like patterns in endothelium and, most characteristically in the kidney, in glomerular visceral epithelium. Other glomerular cells, tubular epithelium, and the interstitium may be involved. Although the inclusions have highly characteristic ultrastructural morphology, membranous cytoplasmic bodies which may mimic the inclusions of Fabry's disease can be seen in various nephropathies including other hereditary storage syndromes, and similar lysosomal alterations may be induced by drugs such as chloroquine,[62,208] and by other toxins as in silicon nephropathy.[14] Female carriers may be asymptomatic but can exhibit some features of the disease, usually in limited form. While inclusions are characteristically ubiquitous in hemizygotes, they are much less numerous and more irregular in distribution in carriers,[67,89,176] possibly on the basis of random X chromosome inactivation resulting in two cell populations.

Because the morphological features of Fabry's disease are not specific, the diagnosis must be confirmed by demonstration of the specific enzyme defect (e.g. in serum, urine or leukocytes). Levels of α-galactosidase are extremely low in affected males and are typically about 50% of normal (with wide variation) in heterozygous females.

MESANGIAL REACTIONS

Mesangial expansion is, perhaps, the commonest manifestation of glomerular disease.[120,145] It may be due to increases in cellular or matrix components, to inflammatory cell infiltration, or the deposition or formation of materials foreign to the normal glomerulus.

In acute GN (e.g. *post-infectious GN* — Figs 17.36–17.38)[76,101,179,212] mesangial alteration may be almost exclusively cellular. In this situation, the matrix bars are separated by proliferating, hypertrophic cells, typically accompanied by neutrophil polymorph infiltration. Recent immunohistological and histochemical investigations have shown that many or most of the proliferating cells in at least some forms of acute and chronic GN are macrophages.[104,134] Lymphocytes generally appear to be absent, at least in established disease, but transient infiltrates of T-lymphocytes have been shown to precede macrophage ingress and maximum glomerular injury in evolving experimental GN.[221]

The synthesis of new matrix is an almost inevitable accompaniment of mesangial disease and is a prominent feature of chronic glomerulopathies. Associated hypercellularity typifies GN but is usually (although not always) minimal or absent in non-nephritic glomerulosclerosis as, for example, in diabetic and cirrhotic glomerulosclerosis (see below). Fibrillar collagen formation is often seen in chronic mesangial sclerosis.

Mesangial deposition is characteristic of some forms of GN. The deposits of *IgA nephropathy* (Figs 17.39 and 17.40) may be relatively massive and typically form large paramesangial masses (which are often visible as hyaline nodules by LM).[43–45,65,83,158,179,204,205,212,247]

Mesangial expansion, whether acute or chronic, results in capillary luminal compromise which may be exacerbated by mesangial interposition. The increasing sclerosis of chronic disease may lead to permanent capillary obliteration.

Severe mesangial injury may lead to dissolution of matrix and degeneration of mesangial cells producing *mesangiolysis*.[113,149,195,196,202,203,205,206] This occurs in a variety of glomerular diseases and may be due to the effects of toxins (classically snake venom), chemical poisons, glomerular ischaemia, accelerated hypertension, thrombotic microangiopathies (Fig. 17.14), transplant rejection (Fig. 17.15), radiation and GN. Mesangiolysis has also been implicated in the pathogenesis of mesangial nodules and microaneurysms in diabetes mellitus. The swelling, lucency and dissolution of the matrix which precedes aneurysmal breakdown of capillary loops in this process is very similar to the alterations of 'accelerated obsolescence' described above.

Patients with chronic liver disease develop glomerulosclerosis in which mesangial matrix excess and GBM thickening develop together with a characteristic pattern of focal membrane and mesangial lucencies with variably dense centres (Fig. 17.41).[2,32,39,45,185,203,212] *Cirrhotic glomerulosclerosis* may be combined with glomerulonephritis, usually of IgA type.[2,32,39,45,203,212] Mesangiolysis with aneurysm formation is also recorded.[203]

EXTRACAPILLARY REACTIONS

Epithelial cell hypertrophy, microvillous surface transformation, protein droplet formation and foam cell transformation are common non-specific reactions which accompany diverse nephropathies.

Epithelial hyperplasia and crescent formation indicate more severe glomerular injury and are usually associated with capillary rupture and fibrin extravasation. The cellular composition of crescents is now a subject of controversy (see Figs 17.49–17.53).

TUBULO-INTERSTITIAL DISEASE

Ultrastructural assessment contributes little to the routine diagnosis of diseases of the tubules and interstitium of the kidney.[51] However, tubular basal laminal deposits are common in lupus nephritis,[168] cryoglobulinaemic GN and dense-deposit disease, and may be seen in other forms of GN.[142,212] Granular dense transformation of the GBM in light-chain nephropathy has been described above. Tubular epithelial cell alterations are sometimes discernible by EM. For example, gentamicin therapy results in the accumulation of myelinoid figures in epithelial cell cytoplasm,[250] abnormalities or loss of proximal tubule brush borders is described in the Fanconi syndrome,[137] crystals derived from immunoglobulin may be seen in tubular cells or in lumina in patients with myeloma,[212] and aurisomes develop secondary to chrysotherapy (see membranous GN). Vacuolar tubulopathy may follow the use of hypertonic agents and hypokalaemia, nuclear inclusions may be seen in cases of lead poisoning, and lysosomal inclusions accompany some lysosomal storage diseases.[250]

VASCULAR DISEASE

While EM is not the primary means of diagnosis of renal vascular disease, ultrastructural examination has contributed to the understanding of the pathogenesis of hyaline and hyperplastic arteriolosclerosis, the vascular lesions of progressive systemic sclerosis and the haemolytic uraemic syndrome.[212] EM has also elucidated the nature of the intimal cellular reaction following renal atheromatous embolism (Figs 17.54–17.56).[118,207] A peculiar 'capillarosclerosis' comprising multilamellar thickening of the medullary and lower urinary tract capillaries of analgesic abusers has been described as 'pathognomonic' of analgesic abuse.[146]

REFERENCES

1. Abraham P A, Keane W F 1984 Glomerular and interstitial disease induced by non-steroidal anti-inflammatory drugs. American Journal of Nephrology 4: 1–6
2. Abramowsky C, Dahms B, Swinehart G 1985 IgA-associated glomerular deposits in liver disease. Human Pathology 16: 1243–1246
3. Abrass C K 1984 Diabetic proteinuria. Glomerular or tubular in origin? American Journal of Nephrology 4: 337–346
4. Aherne W A, Dunnill M S 1982 Morphometry. Edward Arnold, London
5. Ainsworth S K, Hirsch H Z, Brackett N C Jr, Brissie R M, Williams A V Jr, Hennigar G R 1982 Diabetic glomerulonephropathy: histopathologic, immunofluorescent, and ultrastructural studies of 16 cases. Human Pathology 13: 470–478
6. Allen D E, Dowling J P 1981 Techniques for nephropathology. CRC Press, Florida
7. Alpers C E, Cotran R S 1986 Neoplasia and glomerular injury. Kidney International 30: 465–473
8. Alpers C E, Tu W-H, Hopper J, Biava C 1985 Single light chain subclass (kappa chain) immunoglobulin deposition in glomerulonephritis. Human Pathology 16: 294–304
8a. Alpers C E, Hopper J, Biava C G 1984 Light chain glomerulopathy with amyloid-like deposits. Human Pathology 15: 444–448
9. Anders D, Agricola B, Sippel M, Thoenes W 1977 Basement membrane changes in membranoproliferative glomerulonephritis: II. Characterization of a third type by silver impregnation of ultra thin sections. Virchows Archiv A, Pathological Anatomy and Histology 376: 1–19
10. Ansell I D, Joekes A M 1972 Spicular arrangement of amyloid in renal biopsy. Journal of Clinical Pathology 25: 1056–1062
11. Appel G B, Silva F G, Pirani C L, Meltzer J I, Estes D 1978 Renal involvement in systemic lupus erythematosus (SLE): a study of 56 patients emphasizing histologic classification. Medicine 57: 371–410
12. Arakawa M, Kimmelstiel P 1969 Circumferential mesangial interposition. Laboratory Investigation 21: 276–284
13. Axelsen R A, Seymour A E, Mathew T H, Canny A, Pascoe V 1985 Glomerular transplant rejection: a distinctive pattern of early graft damage. Clinical Nephrology 23: 1–11
14. Banks D E, Milutinovic J, Desnick R J, Grabowski G A, Lapp N L, Boehlecke B A 1983 Silicon nephropathy mimicking Fabry's disease. American Journal of Nephrology 3: 279–284
15. Bariéty J, Callard P 1972 Round virus-like extracellular particles in glomerular tufts. An electron microscopic study of 190 human renal biopsies. Virchows Archiv A, Pathological Anatomy and Histology 357: 125–135
16. Bariéty J, Callard P 1975 Striated membranous structures in renal glomerular tufts. An electron microscopic study of 340 human renal biopsies. Laboratory Investigation 32: 636–641
17. Bariéty J, Richer D, Appay M D, Grossette J, Callard P 1973 Frequency of intraendothelial 'virus-like' particles: an electron microscopy study of 376 human renal biopsies. Journal of Clinical Pathology 26: 21–24
18. Beathard G A, Granholm N A 1977 Development of the characteristic ultrastructural lesion of hereditary nephritis during the course of the disease. American Journal of Medicine 62: 751–756
19. Beaufils M, Morel-Maroger L 1978 Pathogenesis of renal disease in monoclonal gammopathies: current concepts. Nephron 20: 125–131
20. Bennett W M, Musgrave J E, Campbell R A, Elliot D, Cox R, Brooks R E, Lovrien E W, Beals R K, Porter G A 1973 The nephropathy of the nail–patella syndrome. American Journal of Medicine 54: 305–319
21. Bernstein J 1979 Hereditary renal disease. In: Churg J, Spargo B H, Mostofi F K (eds) Kidney disease: present status. Williams & Wilkins, Baltimore, pp 310–315
22. Bloodworth J M B Jr 1978 A re-evaluation of diabetic glomerulosclerosis 50 years after the discovery of insulin. Human Pathology 9: 439–453
23. Bohle A, Fischbach H, Gärtner H-V, Gise H V, Helmchen U, Potjan K, Wildhirt E 1978 Simultaneous occurrence of perimembranous glomerulonephritis and glomerular amyloidosis. Virchows Archiv A, Pathological Anatomy and Histology 378: 315–320
24. Bohman S-O, Jaremko G, Bohlin A-B, Berg U 1984 Foot process fusion and glomerular filtration rate in minimal change nephrotic syndrome. Kidney International 25: 696–700
25. Bonsib S M, Plattner B 1986 Acellular scanning electron microscopy of spicular renal amyloidosis. Ultrastructural Pathology 10: 497–504
26. Bradley J R, Thiru S, Evans D B 1987 Light chains and the kidney. Journal of Clinical Pathology 40: 53–60
27. Brulles A, Caralps A, Vilardell M 1977 Nephrotic syndrome with minimal glomerular lesions (lipoid nephrosis) in an adult diabetic patient. Archives of Pathology and Laboratory Medicine 101: 270
28. Bruneval P, Foidart J M, Nochy D, Camilleri J P, Bariéty J 1985 Glomerular matrix proteins in nodular glomerulosclerosis in association with light chain deposition disease and diabetes mellitus. Human Pathology 16: 477–484
29. Bürgin M, Hofmann E, Reutter F W, Gürtler B A, Matter L, Briner J, Gloor F 1980 Familial glomerulopathy with giant fibrillar deposits. Virchows Archiv A, Pathological Anatomy and Histology 388: 313–326
30. Burkholder P M, Hyman L P, Barber T A 1973 Extracellular clusters of spherical microparticles in glomeruli in human renal glomerular diseases. Laboratory Investigation 28: 415–425
31. Burkholder P M, Marchand A, Krueger R P 1970 Mixed membranous and proliferative glomerulonephritis. Laboratory Investigation 23: 459–479
32. Callard P, Feldmann G, Prandi D, Belair M F, Mandet C, Wiess Y, Druet P, Benhamou J P, Bariéty J 1975 Immune complex type glomerulonephritis in cirrhosis of the liver. American Journal of Pathology 80: 329–340
33. Cameron J S 1979 Pathogenesis and treatment of membranous nephropathy. Kidney International 15: 88–103
34. Carrie B J, Myers B D, Golbetz H 1980 Proteinuria and functional characteristics of the glomerular barrier in diabetic nephropathy. Kidney International 17: 669–676
35. Chihara J, Takebayashi S, Taguchi T, Yokoyama K, Harada T, Naito S 1986 Glomerulonephritis in diabetic patients and its effect on prognosis. Nephron 43: 45–49
36. Churg J, Dachs S 1966 Diabetic renal disease: arteriosclerosis and glomerulosclerosis. Pathology Annual 1: 148–171
37. Churg J, Duffy J L, Bernstein J 1979 Identification of dense deposit disease. A report for the International Study of Kidney Diseases in Children. Archives of Pathology and Laboratory Medicine 103: 67–72
38. Churg J, Grishman E 1972 Ultrastructure of immune deposits in renal glomeruli. Annals of Internal Medicine 76: 479–486
39. Churg J, Grishman E 1975 Ultrastructure of glomerular disease: a review. Kidney International 7: 254–270
40. Churg J, Sherman R L 1973 Pathologic characteristics of hereditary nephritis. Archives of Pathology 95: 374–379
41. Churg J, Sobin L H 1982 Renal diseases. Classification and atlas of glomerular diseases. Igaku-Shoin, New York, Tokyo
42. Churg J, Spargo B H, Mostofi F K, Abell M R 1979 Kidney disease: present status. In: Abell M R (ed) International academy of pathology monographs in pathology, vol 20. Williams & Wilkins, Baltimore
43. Clarkson A R, Seymour A E, Thompson A J, Haynes W D G, Chan Y-L, Jackson B 1977 IgA nephropathy: a syndrome of uniform morphology, diverse clinical features and uncertain prognosis. Clinical Nephrology 8: 459–471
44. Clarkson A R, Woodroffe A J, Bannister K M, Lomax-Smith J D, Aarons I 1984 The syndrome of IgA nephropathy. Clinical Nephrology 21: 7–14
45. Cohen A 1984 Renal pathology forum (case 3). Americal Journal of Nephrology 4: 388–390
46. Cohen A H, Zamboni L 1977 Ultrastructural appearance and morphogenesis of renal glomerular hematoxylin bodies. American Journal of Pathology 89: 105–118
47. Cohen J J, Colvin R B 1981 Case records of the Massachusetts General Hospital. A 53-year-old woman with nodular glomerular disease and renal failure. New England Journal of Medicine 304: 33–43
48. Coleman M, Burnett J, Barratt L J, Dupont P 1983 Glomerulonephritis associated with chronic bacterial infection of a

dacron arterial prosthesis. Clinical Nephrology 20: 315–320
49. Coleman M, Haynes W D G, Dimopoulos P, Barratt L J B, Jarvis L R 1986 Glomerular basement membrane abnormalities associated with apparently idiopathic hematuria: ultrastructural morphometric analysis. Human Pathology 17: 1022–1030
50. Comerford F R, Cohen A S 1967 The nephropathy of systemic lupus erythematosus. An assessment by clinical, light and electron microscopy criteria. Medicine 46: 425–473
51. Cotran R S 1983 Tubulo-interstitial nephropathies. In: Brenner B M, Stein J H (eds) Contemporary issues in pathology, vol 10. Churchill Livingstone, New York
52. Couser W G 1985 Mechanisms of glomerular injury in immune-complex disease. Kidney International 28: 569–583
53. Couser W G, Salant D J 1980 Editorial review: in situ immune complex formation and glomerular injury. Kidney International 17: 1–13
54. Dawson D M, Miller D C 1984 Case records of the Massachusetts General Hospital. Case 2-1984. New England Journal of Medicine 310: 106–114
55. Diamond J R, Karnovsky M J 1986 Focal and segmental glomerulosclerosis following a single intravenous dose of puromycin aminonucleoside. American Journal of Pathology 122: 481–487
56. Dikman S H, Churg J, Kahn T 1981 Morphologic and clinical correlates in renal amyloidosis. Human Pathology 12: 160–169
57. Dische F E, Weston M J, Parsons V 1985 Abnormally thin glomerular basement membranes associated with haematuria, proteinuria or renal failure in adults. American Journal of Nephrology 5: 103–109
58. Dombros N, Katz A 1982 Nail patella-like renal lesions in the absence of skeletal abnormalities. American Journal of Kidney Disease 1: 237–240
59. Droz D, Nabarra B, Noel L-H, Liebowitch J, Crosnier J 1979 Recurrence of dense deposits in transplanted kidneys: I. Sequential survey of the lesions. Kidney International 15: 386–395
60. Droz D, Zanetti M, Noel L-H, Liebowitch J 1977 Dense deposit disease. Nephron 19: 1–11
61. Duffy J L, Khurana E, Susin M, Gomez-Leon G, Churg J 1983 Fibrillary renal deposits and nephritis. American Journal of Pathology 113: 279–290
62. Dustin P, Tondeur M, Libert J 1978 Metabolic and storage diseases. In: Johannessen J V (ed) Electron microscopy in human medicine, vol 2. Cellular pathobiology. Metabolic and storage diseases. McGraw-Hill, New York, part 2
63. Eddy A, Sibley R, Mauer S M, Kim Y 1984 Renal allograft failure due to recurrent dense intramembranous deposit disease. Clinical Nephrology 21: 305–313
64. Ehrenreich T, Churg J 1968 Pathology of membranous nephropathy. Pathology Annual 3: 145–186
65. Emancipator S N, Gallo G R, Lamm M E 1985 IgA nephropathy: perspectives on pathogenesis and classification. Clinical Nephrology 24: 161–179
66. Fang L S T 1985 Light chain nephropathy. Kidney International 27: 582–592
67. Farge D, Nadler S, Wolfe L S, Barré P, Jothy S 1985 Diagnostic value of kidney biopsy in heterozygous Fabry's disease. Archives of Pathology and Laboratory Medicine 109: 85–88
68. Feiner H, Gallo G 1977 Ultrastructure in glomerulonephritis associated with cryoglobulinemia: a report of six cases and review of the literature. American Journal of Pathology 88: 145–162
69. Feinfeld D A, Olesnicky L, Pirani C L, Appel G B 1984 Nephrotic syndrome associated with the use of non-steroidal anti-inflammatory drugs. Case report and review of the literature. Nephron 37: 174–179
70. Feldt-Rasmussen B, Mathiesen E R, Deckert T 1986 Effect of two years of strict metabolic control on progression of incipient nephropathy in insulin-dependent diabetes. Lancet ii: 1300–1304
71. Feldt-Rasmussen B, Mathiesen E R, Hegedüs L, Deckert T 1986 Kidney function during 12 months of strict metabolic control in insulin-dependent diabetic patients with incipient nephropathy. New England Journal of Medicine 314: 665–670
72. Ferrans V J, Thiedemann K U, Maron B J, Jones M, Roberts W C 1976 Spherical microparticles in human myocardium: an ultrastructural study. Laboratory Investigation 35: 349–368
73. Fisher K A, Luger A, Spargo B H, Lindheimer M D 1981

Hypertension in pregnancy: clinicopathological correlations and remote prognosis. Medicine 60: 267–276
74. Gabbert H, Thoenes W 1977 Formation of basement membrane in extracapillary proliferates in rapidly progressive glomerulonephritis. Virchows Archiv B, Cell Pathology 25: 265–269
75. Galle P, Mahieu P 1975 Electron-dense alteration of kidney basement membranes. American Journal of Medicine 58: 749–764
76. Gallo G R, Emancipator S E 1983 Postinfectious glomerulonephritis. In: Rosen S (ed) Pathology of glomerular disease. Churchill Livingstone, New York, pp 66–77
77. Gallo G R, Feiner H D, Buxbaum J N 1982 The kidney in lymphoplasmacytic disorders. In: Sommers S C, Rosen P P (eds) Pathology annual pt 1, vol 17. Appleton–Century–Crofts, Connecticut, pp 291–317
78. Gallo G R, Feiner H D, Katz L A, Feldman G M, Correa E B, Chuba J V, Buxbaum J N 1980 Nodular glomerulopathy associated with non-amyloidotic kappa light chain deposits and excess immunoglobulin light chain synthesis. American Journal of Pathology 99: 621–644
79. Ganeval D, Noël L-H, Preud'Homme J-L, Droz D, Grünfeld J-P 1984 Light-chain deposition disease: its relation with AL-type amyloidosis. Kidney International 26: 1–9
80. Gartner H V, Watanabe T, Ott V, Adam A, Bohle A, Edel H H, Kluthe R, Renner E, Scheler F, Schmulling R M, Sieberth H G 1977 Correlations between morphologic and clinical features in idiopathic perimembranous glomerulonephritis: a study on 403 renal biopsies of 367 patients. Current Topics in Pathology 65: 1–29
81. Geary D, Thorner P, Arbus G S, Baumal R 1985 Minimal lesion disease followed by membranous glomerulopathy in two children with nephrotic syndrome. Clinical Nephrology 23: 258–264
82. Gise H V, Helmchen U, Mikeler E, Bruning L, Walther C, Christ H, Mackensen S, Bohl A 1978 Correlations between the morphological and clinical findings in a patient recovering from secondary generalised amyloidosis with renal involvement: light and electron microscopic investigations on serial biopsies. Virchows Archiv A, Pathological Anatomy and Histology 379: 119–129
83. Glassock R J, Kurokawa K, Yoshida M, Sakai O, Okada M, Shigematsu H, Ohno J, Sakai H 1985 IgA nephropathy in Japan. American Journal of Nephrology 5: 127–137
84. Glenner G G 1980 Amyloid deposits and amyloidosis: the β-fibrilloses. New England Journal of Medicine 302: 1283–1292, 1333–1343
85. Grishman E, Churg J 1975 Focal glomerular sclerosis in nephrotic patients: an electron microscopic study of glomerular podocytes. Kidney International 7: 111–122
86. Grundmann E 1976 Glomerulonephritis. Current Topics in Pathology, vol. 61
87. Grünfeld J-P 1985 The clinical spectrum of hereditary nephritis. Kidney International 27: 83–92
88. Grünfeld J-P, Noël L-H, Hafez S, Droz D 1985 Renal prognosis in women with hereditary nephritis. Clinical Nephrology 23: 267–271
89. Gubler M C, Lenoir G, Grünfeld J-P, Ulmann A, Droz D, Habib R 1978 Early renal changes in hemizygous and heterozygous patients with Fabry's disease. Kidney International 13: 223–235
90. Gubler M C, Levy M, Naizot C, Habib R 1980 Glomerular basement membrane changes in hereditary glomerular diseases. Renal Physiology 3: 405–413
91. Habib R, Gubler M-C, Hinglais N, Noël L-H, Droz D, Levy M, Mahieu P, Foidart J-M, Perrin D, Bois E, Grünfeld J-P 1982 Alport's syndrome: experience at Hôpital Necker. Kidney International 21 (suppl 11): S20–S28
92. Habib R, Gubler M C, Loirat C, Ben Maiz Z, Levy M 1975 Dense deposit disease: variant of membranoproliferative glomerulonephritis. Kidney International 7: 204–215
93. Habib R, Levy M 1983 Membranoproliferative glomerulonephritis. In: Rosen S (ed) Pathology of glomerular disease. Churchill Livingstone, New York, pp 151–160
94. Hancock W W, Atkins R C 1984 Cellular composition of crescents in human rapidly progressive glomerulonephritis identified using monoclonal antibodies. American Journal of Nephrology 4: 177–181
95. Haynes W D G 1981 The normal human renal glomerulus. Virchows Archiv B, Cell Pathology 35: 133–158
96. Heaton J M, Turner D R, Cameron J S 1977 Localization of

glomerular 'deposits' in Henoch–Schönlein nephritis. Histopathology 1: 93–104

97. Heptinstall R H 1983 Pathology of the kidney, 3rd edn. Little, Brown & Co., Boston

98. Herf S, Pohl S L, Sturgill B, Bolton W K 1979 An evaluation of diabetic and pseudodiabetic glomerulosclerosis. American Journal of Medicine 66: 1040–1045

99. Hiki Y, Leong A S-Y, Mathew T H, Seymour A E, Pascoe V, Woodroffe A J 1986 Typing of intraglomerular mononuclear cells associated with glomerular transplant rejection. Clinical Nephrology 26: 244–249

100. Hill G S, Jenis E H, Goodloe S Jr 1974 The non-specificity of the ultrastructural alterations in hereditary nephritis: with additional observations on benign familial hematuria. Laboratory Investigation 31: 516–532

101. Hinglais N, Garcia-Torres R, Kleinecht D 1974 Long-term prognosis in acute glomerulonephritis. American Journal of Medicine 56: 52–60

102. Hinglais N, Kazatchkine M D, Bhakdi S, Appay M-D, Mandet C, Grossetete J, Bariéty J 1986 Immunohistochemical study of the C5b–9 complex of complement in human kidneys. Kidney International 30: 399–410

103. Hoffmann E O, Flores T R 1981 High resolution light microscopy in renal pathology. American Journal of Clinical Pathology 76: 636–643

104. Hooke D H, Hancock W W, Gee D C, Kraft N, Atkins R C 1984 Monoclonal antibody analysis of glomerular hypercellularity in human glomerulonephritis. Clinical Nephrology 22: 163–168

105. Hostetter T H 1985 Diabetic nephropathy. New England Journal of Medicine 312: 642–643

106. Hsu H-C, Churg J 1979 Glomerular microfibrils in renal disease: a comparative electron microscopic study. Kidney International 16: 497–504

107. Hsu H-C, Suzuki Y, Churg J, Grishman E 1980 Ultrastructure of transplant glomerulopathy. Histopathology 4: 351–367

108. Huang T W 1980 The nature of basal lamina alterations in human diabetic glomerulosclerosis. American Journal of Pathology 100: 225–238

109. Ihle B U, Dowling J P, Kincaid-Smith P 1984 Hydralazine and lupus nephritis. Clinical Nephrology 22: 230–238

110. Imbasciati E, Paties C, Scarpioni L, Mihatsch M 1986 Renal lesions in familial lecithin-cholesterol acyltransferase deficiency. Ultrastructural heterogeneity of glomerular changes. American Journal of Nephrology 6: 66–70

111. Inglefinger J R, Cohrin R B 1985 A 13-year old boy with aniridia and proteinuria 11 years after nephrectomy for a Wilms' tumour. New England Journal of Medicine 312: 1111–1119

112. Jacquot C, Saint-Andre J-P, Touchard G, Nochy D, D'Auzac de Lamartinie C, Oriol R, Druet P, Bariéty J 1985 Association of systemic light-chain deposition disease with amyloidosis: a report of three patients with renal involvement. Clinical Nephrology 24: 93–98

113. Jain S, Seymour A E 1987 Mitomycin C associated hemolytic uremic syndrome. Pathology 19: 58–61

114. Jennette J C, Hipp C G 1986 The epithelial antigen phenotype of glomerular crescent cells. American Journal of Clinical Pathology 86: 274–280

115. Jones D B 1963 The nature of scar tissue in glomerulonephritis. American Journal of Pathology 42: 185–199

116. Jones D B 1974 Arterial and glomerular lesions associated with severe hypertension: light and electronmicroscopic studies. Laboratory Investigation 31: 303–313

117. Jones D B 1977 Membranoproliferative glomerulonephritis: one or many diseases. Archives of Pathology and Laboratory Medicine 101: 457–461

118. Jones D B, Iannaccone P M 1975 Atheromatous emboli in renal biopsies. An ultrastructural study. American Journal of Pathology 78: 261–276

119. Karnovsky M J 1979 The ultrastructure of glomerular filtration. Annual Review of Medicine 30: 213–224

120. Kashgarian M 1985 Mesangium and glomerular disease. Laboratory Investigation 52: 569–571

121. Kashgarian M, Hayslett J P, Spargo B H 1977 Renal disease.

(Teaching monograph.) American Journal of Pathology 89: 183–272

122. Kasiske B L, Napier J 1985 Glomerular sclerosis in patients with massive obesity. American Journal of Nephrology 5: 45–50

123. Katafuchi R, Taguchi T, Takebayashi S, Harada T 1984 Proteinuria in amyloidosis correlates with epithelial detachment and distortion of amyloid fibrils. Clinical Nephrology 22: 1–8

124. Kerjaschki D, Sawada H, Farquhar M G 1986 Immunoelectron microscopy in kidney research: some contributions and limitations. Kidney International 30: 229–245

125. Kida H, Takeda S, Yokoyama H, Tomosugi N, Abe T, Hattori N 1985 Focal glomerulosclerosis in pre-eclampsia. Clinical Nephrology 24: 221–227

126. Kohaut E C, Singer D B, Nevels B K, Hill L L 1976 The specificity of split renal membranes in hereditary nephritis. Archives of Pathology and Laboratory Medicine 100: 475–479

127. Korbet S M, Schwartz M M, Rosenberg B F, Sibley R K, Lewis E J 1985 Immunotactoid glomerulopathy. Medicine 64: 228–243

128. Lange K, Seligson G, Cronin W 1983 Evidence for the in situ origin of poststreptococcal glomerulonephritis: glomerular localization of endostreptosin and the clinical significance of the subsequent antibody response. Clinical Nephrology 19: 3–10

129. Latham P, Poucell S, Koresaar A, Arbus G, Baumal R 1982 Idiopathic membranous glomerulopathy in Canadian children: a clinicopathologic study. Journal of Pediatrics 101: 682–685

130. Leslie N D, Sperling M A 1986 Relation of metabolic control to complications in diabetes mellitus. Journal of Pediatrics 108: 491–497

131. Libit S A, Burke B, Michael A F, Vernier R L 1976 Extramembranous glomerulonephritis in childhood: relationship to systemic lupus erythematosus. Journal of Pediatrics 88: 394–402

132. Lin J T, Wada H, Maeda H, Hattori M, Tanaka H, Uenoyama F, Suehiro A, Noguchi K, Nagai K 1983 Mechanisms of hematuria in glomerular disease. An electron microscopic study in a case of diffuse membranous glomerulonephritis. Nephron 35: 68–72

133. Linder J, Vollmer R T, Croker B P, Shelburne J 1983 Systemic kappa light-chain deposition. An ultrastructural and immunohistochemical study. American Journal of Surgical Pathology 7: 85–93

134. Magil A B 1984 Monocytes and glomerulonephritis associated with remote visceral infection. Clinical Nephrology 22: 169–175

135. Magil A B 1985 Histogenesis of glomerular crescents. Immunohistochemical demonstration of cytokeratin in crescent cells. American Journal of Pathology 120: 222–229

136. Mallick N P, Short C D, Manos J 1983 Clinical membranous nephropathy. Nephron 34: 209–219

137. Manz F, Waldherr R, Fritz H P, Lutz P, Nützenadel W, Reitter B, Schärer I C, Schmidt H, Trefz F 1984 Idiopathic de Toni-Debré-Fanconi syndrome with absence of proximal tubular brush border. Clinical Nephrology 22: 149–157

138. Maryniak R K, First M R, Weiss M A 1985 Transplant glomerulopathy: evolution of morphologically distinct changes. Kidney International 27: 799–806

139. Mathew T H, Mathews D C, Hobbs J B, Kincaid-Smith P 1975 Glomerular lesions after renal transplantation. American Journal of Medicine 59: 177–190

140. Mauer S M, Steffes M W, Ellis E N, Sutherland D E R, Brown D M, Goetz F C 1984 Structural–functional relationships in diabetic nephropathy. Journal of Clinical Investigation 74: 1143–1155

141. Mazzuco G, Dogliani M, Castello R, Monga G 1983 Essential mixed cryoglobulinaemic glomerulonephritis associated with diabetic glomerulosclerosis. Light, immunofluorescence, and ultrastructural study of two cases. Archives of Pathology and Laboratory Medicine 109: 1036–1039

142. McCluskey R T 1983 Immunologically mediated tubulo-interstitial nephritis. In: Cotran R S, Brenner B M, Stein J H (eds) Contemporary issues in nephrology. Churchill Livingstone, New York, pp 121–149

143. McManus J F A, Lupton C H Jr 1960 Ischemic obsolescence of renal glomeruli: the natural history of the lesions and their relation to hypertension. Laboratory Investigation 9: 413–434

144. Meyrier A, Simon P, Perret G, Condamin-Meyrier M-C 1986 Remission of idiopathic nephrotic syndrome after treatment with cyclosporin A. British Medical Journal 292: 789–792

145. Michael A F, Keane W F, Raij L, Vernier R L, Mauer S M 1980 Editorial review: the glomerular mesangium. Kidney International 17: 141–154
146. Mihatsch M J, Torhorst J, Amsler B, Zollinger H U 1978 Capillarosclerosis of the lower urinary tract in analgesic (phenacetin) abuse. An electron-microscopic study. Virchows Archiv A, Pathological Anatomy and Histology 381: 41–79
147. Mogensen C E 1982 Diabetes mellitus and the kidney. Kidney International 21: 673–675
148. Morel-Maroger L, Verroust P, Preud'Homme J-L 1983 Glomerular lesions in plasma cell dyscrasias. In: Rosen S (ed) Pathology of glomerular disease. Churchill Livingstone, New York, pp 207–224
149. Morita I, Churg J 1983 Mesangiolysis. Kidney International 24: 1–9
150. Morita T, Kimura K, Ohnishi Y 1985 Polypoid change of the glomerular basement membrane in patients with congenital heart disease. Clinical Nephrology 24: 228–231
151. Morita T, Laughlin L O, Kawano K, Kimmelstiel P, Suzuki Y, Churg J 1973 Nail-patella syndrome: light and electron microscopic studies of the kidneys. Archives of Internal Medicine 131: 271–277
152. Morita T, Suzuki Y, Churg J 1973 Structure and development of the glomerular crescent. American Journal of Pathology 72: 349–368
153. Nakamato Y, lmai H, Hamanaka S, Yoshida K, Akihama T, Miura A B 1985 IgM monoclonal gammapathy accompanied by nodular glomerulosclerosis, urine concentrating defect and hyporeninemic hypoaldosteronism. American Journal of Nephrology 5: 53–58
154. Nash D A, Rogers P W, Langlinais P G, Bunn S M 1975 Diabetic glomerulosclerosis without glucose intolerance. American Journal of Medicine 59: 191–199
155. Ne'eman Z, Rosenmann E 1983 Tubular cell emboli in the glomerulus, a needle biopsy artifact. Ultrastructural Pathology 5: 109–112
156. Nesland J, Millonig G, Wilson A, Johannessen J V 1982 Technical review: rapid techniques in diagnostic electron microscopy. Ultrastructural Pathology 3: 295–300
157. Nevins T E 1985 Lectin binding in membranoproliferative glomerulonephritis. Evidence for N-acetylglucosamine in dense intramembranous deposits. American Journal of Pathology 118: 325–330
158. Ng W L, Chan K W, Yeung C K, Kwan S 1984 Peripheral glomerular capillary wall lesions in IgA nephropathy and their implications. Pathology 16: 324–330
159. Noel L H, Droz D, Ganeval D, Grunfeld J P 1984 Renal granular monoclonal light chain deposits: morphological aspects in 11 cases. Clinical Nephrology 21: 263–269
160. Ogihara T, Saruta T, Saito I, Abe S, Ozawa Y, Kato E, Sakaguchi H 1979 Fingerprint deposits of the kidney in pure monoclonal IgG kappa cryoglobulinaemia. Clinical Nephrology 12: 186–190
161. Olsen S 1972 Mesangial thickening and nodular glomerular sclerosis in diabetes mellitus and other diseases. Acta Pathologica et Microbiologica Scandinavica 80A(suppl 223): 203–216
162. Olson J L, De Urdaneta A G, Heptinstall R H 1985 Glomerular hyalinosis and its relation to hyperfiltration. Laboratory Investigation 52: 387–398
163. Osawa G, Kimmelstiel P, Seiling V 1966 Thickness of glomerular basement membranes. American Journal of Clinical Pathology 45: 7–20
164. Østerby R 1972 Morphometric studies of the peripheral basement membrane in early juvenile diabetes. I. Development of initial basement membrane thickening. Diabetologia 8: 84–92
165. Østerby R 1972 The number of glomerular cells and substructures in early juvenile diabetes: a quantitative electron microscopic study. Acta Pathologica et Microbiologica Scandinavica 80A: 785–800
166. Østerby R 1973 A quantitative electron microscopic study of mesangial regions in glomeruli from patients with short-term juvenile diabetes mellitus. Laboratory Investigation 29: 99–110
167. Ota Z, Makino H, Miyoshi A, Hiramatsu M, Takahashi K, Ofuji T 1979 Molecular sieve in glomerular basement membrane as revealed by electron microscopy. Journal of Electron Microscopy 28: 20–28
168. Park M H, D'Agati V, Appel G B, Pirani C L 1986 Tubulointerstitial disease in lupus nephritis: relationship to immune deposits, interstitial inflammation, glomerular changes, renal function and prognosis. Nephron 44: 309–319
169. Piel C F, Biava C G, Goodman J R 1982 Glomerular basement membrane attenuation in familial nephritis and benign hematuria. Journal of Pediatrics 101: 358–365
170. Ponticelli C, Garella S 1986 Prognosis and treatment of membranous nephropathy. Kidney International 29: 927–940
171. Preud'Homme J L, Morel-Maroger L, Brouet J C, Cerf M, Mignon F, Gugliermi P, Seligmann M 1980 Synthesis of abnormal immunoglobulins in lymphoplasmacytic disorders with visceral light chain deposition. American Journal of Medicine 69: 703–710
172. Preud'Homme J L, Morel-Maroger L, Brouet J C, Mihaesco E, Mery J P, Seligmann M 1980 Synthesis of abnormal heavy and light chains in multiple myeloma with visceral deposition of monoclonal immunoglobulin. Clinical and Experimental Immunology 42: 545–553
173. Randall R E, Williamson W C Jr, Mullinax F, Tung M Y, Still W J S 1976 Manifestations of systemic light chain deposition. American Journal of Medicine 60: 293–299
174. Rao K V, Crosson J T 1980 Idiopathic membranous glomerulonephritis in diabetic patients: report of three cases and review of the literature. Archives of Internal Medicine 140: 624–627
175. Reznik V M, Griswold W R, Vazquez M D, Mendoza S A, Borden M, Wilson C B 1985 Glomerulonephritis with absent glomerular basement membrane antigens. American Journal of Nephrology 5: 296–298
176. Rodriguez F H Jr, Hoffmann E O, Ordinario A T, Baliga M 1985 Fabry's disease in a heterozygous woman. Archives of Pathology and Laboratory Medicine 109: 89–91
177. Rogers P W, Kurtzman N A, Bunn S M Jr, White M G 1973 Familial benign essential hematuria. Archives of Internal Medicine 131: 257–262
178. Rosen S (ed) 1983 Pathology of glomerular disease. Contemporary issues in surgical pathology, vol I. Churchill Livingstone, New York
179. Rosenberg H G 1986 Primary glomerular diseases. (Primary glomerulopathies.) Pathology Research and Practice 181: 489–523
180. Rosenmann E, Eliakin M 1977 Nephrotic syndrome associated with amyloid-like glomerular deposits. Nephron 18: 301–308
181. Rumpelt H-J 1980 Hereditary nephropathy (Alport's syndrome): correlation of clinical data with glomerular basement membrane alterations. Clinical Nephrology 13: 203–207
182. Rumpelt H J 1983 Hereditary nephropathy (Alport's syndrome): spectrum and development of glomerular lesions. In: Rosen S (ed) Pathology of glomerular disease. Churchill Livingstone, New York, pp 225–238
183. Rumpelt H J, Langer K H, Schärer K, Straub E, Thoenes W 1974 Split and extremely thin glomerular basement membranes in hereditary nephropathy (Alport's syndrome). Virchows Archiv A, Pathological Anatomy and Histology 364: 225–233
184. Sabnis S G, Antonovych T T, Argy W P, Rakowski T A, Gandy D R, Salcedo J R 1980 Nail-patella syndrome. Clinical Nephrology 14: 148–153
185. Sakaguchi H, Dachs S, Grishman E, Paronetto F, Salomon M, Churg J 1965 Hepatic glomerulosclerosis: an electron microscopic study of renal biopsies in liver diseases. Laboratory Investigation 14: 533–545
186. Salinas-Madrigal L, Pirani C L, Pollack V E 1970 Glomerular and vascular insudative lesions of diabetic nephropathy: electron microscopic observations. American Journal of Pathology 59: 369–398
187. Schwartz M M 1983 Electron microscopy in renal pathology. Ultrastructural Pathology 4: iii–iv
188. Schwartz M M, Kawala K, Roberts J L, Humes C, Lewis E J 1984 Clinical and pathological features of membranous glomerulonephritis of systemic lupus erythematosus. American Journal of Nephrology 4: 301–311
189. Schwartz M M, Lewis E J 1980 The quarterly case: nephrotic syndrome in a middle-aged man. Ultrastructural Pathology 1: 575–582
190. Schwartz M M, Lewis E J 1985 Focal segmental glomerular sclerosis: the cellular lesion. Kidney International 28: 968–974
191. Seymour A E, Canny A, Spargo B H 1983 Thickening of glomerular capillary walls: a guide to differential diagnosis by

electron microscopy. Ultrastructural Pathology 4: 123–143

192. Seymour A E, Petrucco O M, Clarkson A R, Haynes W D G, Lawrence J R, Jackson B, Thompson A J, Thomson N M 1976 Morphological and immunological evidence of coagulopathy in renal complications of pregnancy. In: Lindheimer M D, Katz A I, Zuspan F P (eds) Hypertension in pregnancy. Wiley, New York, pp 139–153

193. Seymour A E, Spargo B H, Penska R 1971 Contributions of renal biopsy studies to the understanding of disease. American Journal of Pathology 65: 549–598

194. Seymour A E, Thompson A J, Smith P S, Woodroffe A J, Clarkson A R 1980 Kappa light chain glomerulosclerosis in multiple myeloma. American Journal of Pathology 101: 557–580

195. Shigematsu H, Dikman S H, Churg J, Grishman E 1978 Glomerular injury in malignant nephrosclerosis. Nephron 22: 399–408

196. Shigematsu H, Dikman S H, Churg J, Grishman E, Duffy J L 1976 Mesangial involvement in the hemolytic–uremic syndrome: a light and electron microscopic study. American Journal of Pathology 85: 349–362

197. Shirahama T, Cohen A S 1967 High-resolution electron microscopic analysis of the amyloid fibril. Journal of Cell Biology 33: 679–708

198. Sibley R K, Kim Y 1984 Dense intramembranous deposit disease: new pathologic features. Kidney International 25: 660–670

199. Silva F G 1983 The nephropathies of systemic lupus erythematosus. In: Rosen S (ed) Pathology of glomerular disease. Churchill Livingstone, New York, pp 79–124

200. Simpson L O 1980 Basement membranes and biological thixotropy: a new hypothesis. Pathology 12: 377–389

201. Simpson L O 1986 Is current research into basement membrane chemistry and ultrastructure providing any new insights into the way the glomerular basement membrane functions? Nephron 43: 1–4

202. Sinclair R A, Antonovych T T, Mostofi F K 1976 Renal proliferative arteriopathies and associated glomerular changes: a light and electron microscopic study. Human Pathology 7: 565–588

203. Sinniah R 1984 Heterogeneous IgA glomerulonephropathy in liver cirrhosis. Histopathology 8: 947–962

204. Sinniah R 1985 IgA mesangial nephropathy: Berger's disease. American Journal of Nephrology 5: 73–83

205. Sinniah R, Churg J 1983 Effect of IgA deposits on the glomerular mesangium in Berger's disease. Ultrastructural Pathology 4: 9–22

206. Sinniah R, Cohen A H 1985 Glomerular capillary aneurysms in light-chain nephropathy. An ultrastructural proposal of pathogenesis. Americal Journal of Pathology 118: 298–305

207. Smith M C, Ghose M K, Henry A R 1981 The clinical spectrum of renal cholesterol embolism. American Journal of Medicine 7l: 174–180

208. Sosa M A, Bertini F 1985 The effect of the lysosomotropic drug chloroquine on the binding of N-acyl-β-D-glucosaminidase to mannose 6-phosphate recognizing receptors of the liver. Biochemical and Biophysical Research Communications 131: 634–639

209. Spargo B, McCartney C P, Winemiller R 1959 Glomerular capillary endotheliosis in toxemia of pregnancy. Archives of Pathology 68: 593–599

210. Spargo B H 1975 Practical use of electron microscopy for the diagnosis of glomerular disease. Human Pathology 6: 495–520

211. Spargo B H, Seymour A E 1979 The value of electron microscopy in the study of glomerular disease. In: Black D, Jones N F (eds) Renal disease, 4th edn. Blackwell, Oxford, pp 185–218

212. Spargo B H, Seymour A E, Ordóñez N G 1980 Renal biopsy pathology with diagnostic and therapeutic implications. John Wiley, New York

213. Spear G S 1974 Pathology of the kidney in Alport's syndrome. Pathology Annual 9: 93–138

214. Spear G S 1984 Hereditary nephritis (Alport's syndrome) – 1983. Clinical Nephrology 21: 3–6

215. Steffes M W, Sutherland D E R, Goetz F C, Rich S S, Mauer M M 1985 Studies of kidney and muscle biopsy specimens from identical twins discordant for type I diabetes mellitus. New England Journal of Medicine 312: 1282–1287

216. Stejskal J, Pirani C L, Okada M, Mandelanakis M D, Pollak V E 1978 Discontinuities (gaps) of the glomerular capillary wall and basement membrane in renal diseases. Laboratory Investigation 28: 149–169

217. Strife C F, Jackson E C, McAdams A J 1984 Type III membranoproliferative glomerulonephritis: long-term clinical and morphological evaluation. Clinical Nephrology 21: 323–334

218. Strife C F, McEnery P T, McAdams A J, West C D 1977 Membranoproliferative glomerulonephritis with disruption of the glomerular basement membrane. Clinical Nephrology 7: 65–72

219. Sturgill B C, Bolton W K, Griffith K M 1985 Congo red-negative amyloidosis-like glomerulopathy. Human Pathology 16: 220–224

220. Tina L, Jenis E, Jose P, Medani C, Papadopoulou Z, Calgano P 1982 The glomerular basement membrane in benign familial hematuria. Clinical Nephrology 17: 1–4

221. Tipping P G, Neale T J, Holdsworth S R 1985 T lymphocyte participation in antibody induced experimental glomerulonephritis. Kidney International 27: 530–537

222. Törnroth T 1983 Membranous glomerulonephritis. In: Rosen S (ed) Pathology of glomerular disease. Churchill Livingstone, New York, pp 125–150

223. Törnroth T, Skrifvars B 1975 The development and resolution of glomerular basement membrane changes associated with subepithelial immune deposits. American Journal of Pathology 79: 219–236

224. Tubbs R R, Gephardt G N, McMahon J T, Hall P M, Valenzuela R, Vidt D G 1981 Light chain nephropathy. American Journal of Medicine 71: 263–269

225. Turner D R, Rosen S 1983 Lipoid nephrosis (minimal change nephropathy); focal and segmental glomerulosclerosis. In: Rosen S (ed) Pathology of glomerular disease. Churchill Livingstone, New York, pp 195–205

226. Tuttle S E, Sharma H M, Bay W H, Hebert L H 1985 Glomerular basement membrane splitting and microaneurysm formation associated with nitrosourea therapy. American Journal of Nephrology 5: 388–394

227. Urizar R E, Tinglof B O, Smith F G, McIntosh R M 1974 Persistent asymptomatic proteinuria in children. Functional and ultrastructural evaluation with special reference to glomerular basement membrane thickness. American Journal of Clinical Pathology 62: 461–471

228. Verani R 1983 Transplant glomerulopathy and glomerulonephritis in renal transplants. In: Rosen S (ed) Pathology of glomerular disease. Churchill Livingstone, New York, pp 249–268

229. Verani R R, Bergman D, Kerman R H 1983 Glomerulopathy in acute and chronic rejection: relationship of ultrastructure to graft survival. American Journal of Nephrology 3: 253–263

230. Verani R R, Hawkins E P 1986 Recurrent focal segmental glomerulosclerosis. A pathological study of the early lesion. American Journal of Nephrology 6: 263–270

231. Viale G, Dell'Orto P, Colombi R, Coggi G 1986 Ultrastructural localisation of extracellular immunoglobulins in immune-complex-mediated glomerulonephritis. Immunoelectron microscopy of Epon-embedded human renal biopsies using the immunogold staining procedure. Histochemistry 84: 1–4

232. Viol G W, Minielly J A, Bistricki T 1977 Gold nephropathy: tissue analysis by X-ray fluorescent spectroscopy. Archives of Pathology and Laboratory Medicine 101: 635–640

233. Vogler C, McAdams A J, McEnery P 1986 Glomerular membranopathy in adolescents with insulin-dependent diabetes. Human Pathology 17: 308–313

234. Vogt A 1984 New aspects of the pathogenesis of immune complex glomerulonephritis: formation of subepithelial deposits. Clinical Nephrology 21: 15–20

235. Waldherr R 1982 Familial glomerular disease. Contributions to Nephrology 33: 104–121

236. Weening J J, Beukers J J B, Grond J, Elema J D 1986 Genetic factors in focal segmental glomerulosclerosis. Kidney International 29: 789–798

237. Westberg N G 1980 Diabetic nephropathy: pathogenesis and prevention. Acta Endocrinologica 94 (suppl 238): 85–101

238. Wiseman M J, Saunders A J, Keen H, Viberti G 1985 Effect of blood glucose control on increased glomerular filtration rate and

kidney size in insulin-dependent diabetes. New England Journal of Medicine 312: 617–621

239. Yamase H T, Gillies C G 1985 Embolic tubular epithelial cells in percutaneous renal biopsies. American Journal of Clinical Pathology 83: 716–719

240. Yoshikawa N, Cameron A H, White R H R 1981 The glomerular basal lamina in hereditary nephritis. Journal of Pathology 135: 199–209

241. Yoshikawa N, Cameron A H, White R H R 1982 Ultrastructure of the non-sclerotic glomeruli in childhood nephrotic syndrome. Journal of Pathology 136: 133–147

242. Yoshikawa N, Cameron A H, White R H R, Standring D M 1982 Microfibrils in glomerulopathies of children: an ultrastructural study. Journal of Pathology 136: 123–131

243. Yoshikawa N, Hashimoto H, Katayama Y, Yamada Y, Matsuo T, Okada S 1984 The thin glomerular basement membrane in children with haematuria. Journal of Pathology 142: 253–257

244. Yoshikawa N, Ito H, Akamatsu R, Hazikano H, Okada S, Matsuo T 1986 Glomerular podocyte vacuolation in focal segmental glomerulosclerosis. Archives of Pathology and Laboratory Medicine 110: 394–398

245. Yoshikawa N, Ito H, Yamada Y, Hashimoto H, Katayama Y, Matsuyama S, Hasegawa O, Okada S, Hajikano H, Yoshizawa H, Mayumi M, Matsuo T 1985 Membranous glomerulonephropathy associated with hepatitis B antigen in children: a comparison with idiopathic membranous glomerulonephropathy. Clinical Nephrology 23: 28–34

246. Yoshikawa N, Uehara S, Yamana K, Ikeuchi H, Hiraumi M, Matsuo T, Okada S 1980 Clinicopathological correlations of persistent asymptomatic proteinuria in children. Nephron 25: 127–133

247. Yoshikawa N, Yoshiara S, Yoshiya K, Matsuo T, Okada S 1986 Lysis of the glomerular basement membrane in children with IgA nephropathy and Henoch–Schönlein nephritis. Journal of Pathology 150: 119–126

248. Yum M, Bergstein J M 1983 Basement membrane nephropathy: a new classification for Alport's syndrome and asymptomatic hematuria based on ultrastructural findings. Human Pathology 14: 996–1003

249. Zamurovic D, Churg J 1984 Idiopathic and secondary mesangiocapillary glomerulonephritis. Nephron 38: 145–153

250. Zollinger H U, Mihatsch M J 1978 Renal pathology in biopsy. Light, electron and immunofluorescent microscopy and clinical aspects. Springer-Verlag, Berlin

251. Zucchelli P, Cagnoli L, Pasquali S, Casanova S, Donini U 1986 Clinical and morphologic evolution of idiopathic membranous nephropathy. Clinical Nephrology 25: 282–288

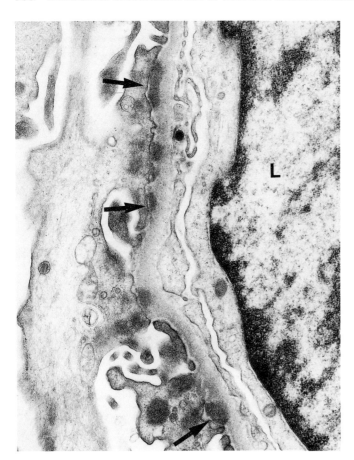

Fig. 17.1 (Left)   Membranous GN, stage I, associated with penicillamine therapy. Renal biopsy from a proteinuric 66-year-old man with rheumatoid arthritis, after 3 years of penicillamine therapy. Deposits (arrows) are small and sparse and are embedded in the GBM in subepithelial locations. Foot processes are partly effaced. There is minimal membrane reaction. Such lesions are undetectable by LM. A lymphocyte (L) occupies the capillary lumen. (× 18 300)

Fig. 17.2 (Below)   Idiopathic membranous GN, stage II. Biopsy from a nephrotic 18-year-old man. Epimembranous deposits (arrows) are very numerous and are covered by dense epithelial cytoplasm. The pattern of deposits with uniform density moulded by the overlying cytoplasm suggests recent and active deposit formation. Foot processes are lost. Irregular 'spike'-like protrusions of new basement membrane material (arrowheads) separate many of the deposits. L = capillary lumen. (× 12 300)

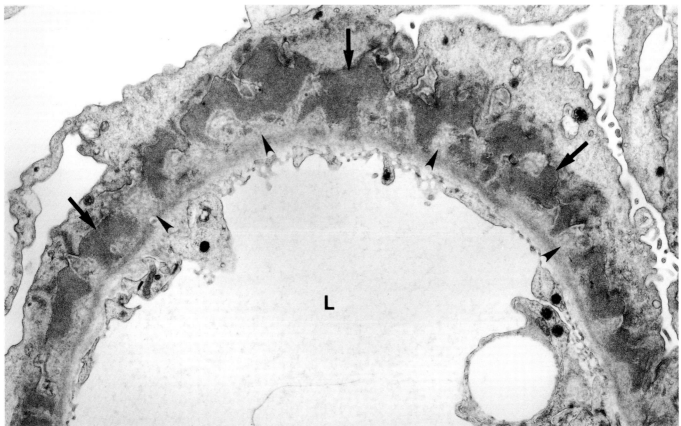

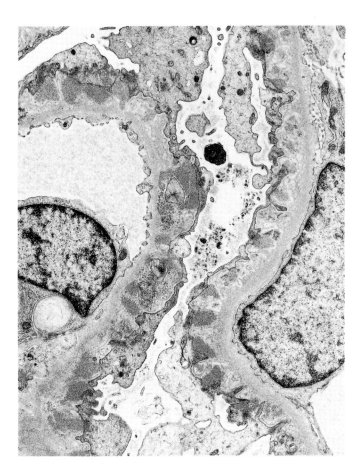

Fig. 17.3 (Left) Idiopathic membranous GN, stage II: partial deposit resolution. The complex pattern of dense and partially lucent or granular deposits, with associated membrane reaction, suggests persistent disease with concurrent deposit formation and dissolution. (× 7400)

Fig. 17.4 (Below) Idiopathic membranous GN, stage III. Deposits with variegated textures, some incorporating striated membranous structures (arrowheads), are enclosed within grossly thickened basement membrane. Intervening bars (arrows) reflect earlier spike formation. Thickening and calcification of Bowman's capsule (B) is a common non-specific finding and bears no direct relationship to glomerular disease. L = capillary lumen. (× 7500)

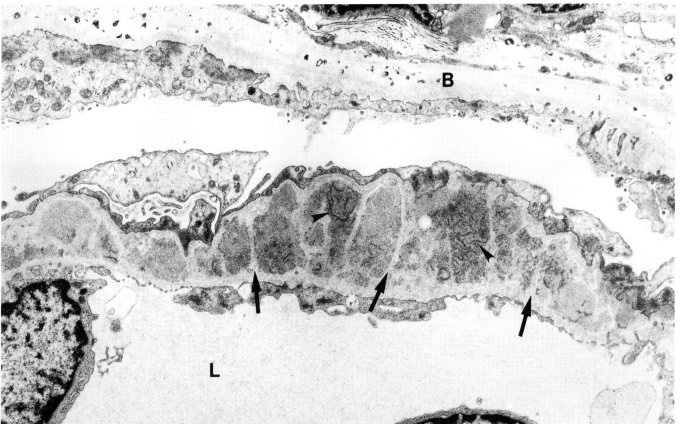

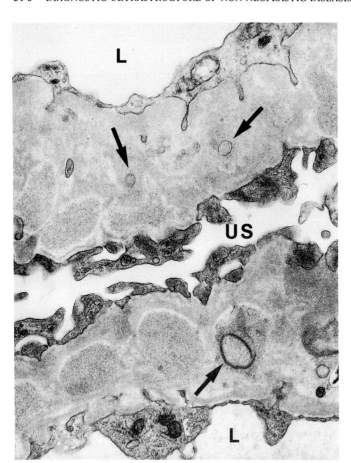

Fig. 17.5 (Left)   Idiopathic membranous GN, stage IV. Advanced disease with lucent, granular deposits in greatly disorganized and thickened membrane. Some deposits include membranous residues (arrows). L = capillary lumen; US = urinary space. (× 16 600)

Fig. 17.6 (Below)   Idiopathic membranous GN: further evolution. Sites of previous deposit formation are indicated by poorly circumscribed zones of lucency and rarefaction. Elsewhere in this biopsy some dense deposits were evident and immunohistology demonstrated capillary wall IgG and C3 in patterns typical of membranous GN indicating active disease. E = visceral epithelial cell cytoplasm; L = capillary lumen. (× 33 500)

Considerable variations in deposit density and membrane reaction are the rule in most biopsies of membranous GN. In general the appearances reflect disease duration and the intensity and fluctuations of deposition and disease activity. However, although the degree of proteinuria in a given case may correlate with deposit density, the ultrastructural appearances of membranous GN correlate poorly with renal function and prognosis.[222] Disease remission can result in loss of deposits and gradual reconstruction of the GBM (stage V).[191,251] Complete morphological normalization may be observed particularly in secondary forms of the disease after elimination of the causative factor.[179] References: 7, 23, 31, 33, 64, 80, 81, 129, 131, 132, 136, 170, 174, 188, 191, 212, 222, 223, 245 and 251.

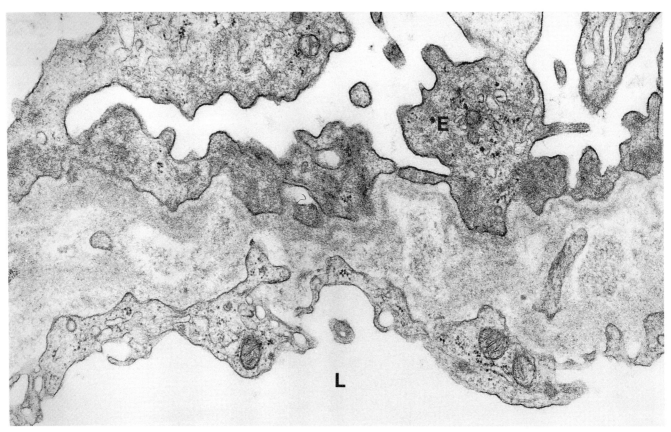

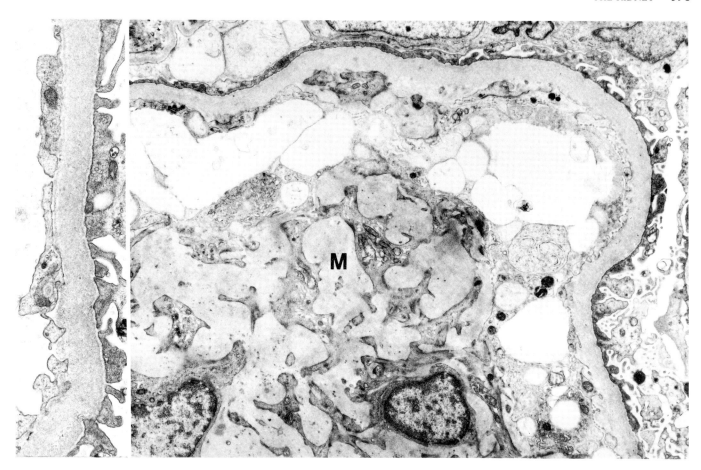

Fig. 17.7   Diabetic glomerulosclerosis: basement membrane and mesangial alterations. Portion of a greatly enlarged mesangium (M) and capillary loop in a biopsy from a nephrotic 20-year-old diabetic with severe retinopathy and impaired renal function. Mesangial expansion is due to excess of mottled matrix containing membrane debris and a few small deposits (corresponding to irregular reactions for IgM and C3). (× 6700) Basement membrane thickening is obvious and is shown in more detail in the **inset** which is from a 62-year-old proteinuric and hypertensive man with only mild glucose intolerance. (× 14 200)

Silver impregnation techniques have shown considerable textural disturbance of the GBM in diabetic patients. The abnormal laminae show disruption of the fibrillary meshwork and irregular, coarse laminations.[233] The morphological alterations may result from abnormal capillary haemodynamics associated with hyperfiltration, and derangements of membrane biochemistry[233] which might be related to abnormalities of collagen cross–linking secondary to non–enzymatic glycosylation.[130] References: 3, 5, 22, 27, 28, 34–36, 70, 71, 98, 105, 108, 130, 140, 141, 147, 154, 161, 164–166, 174, 186, 191, 212, 215, 233, 237 and 238.

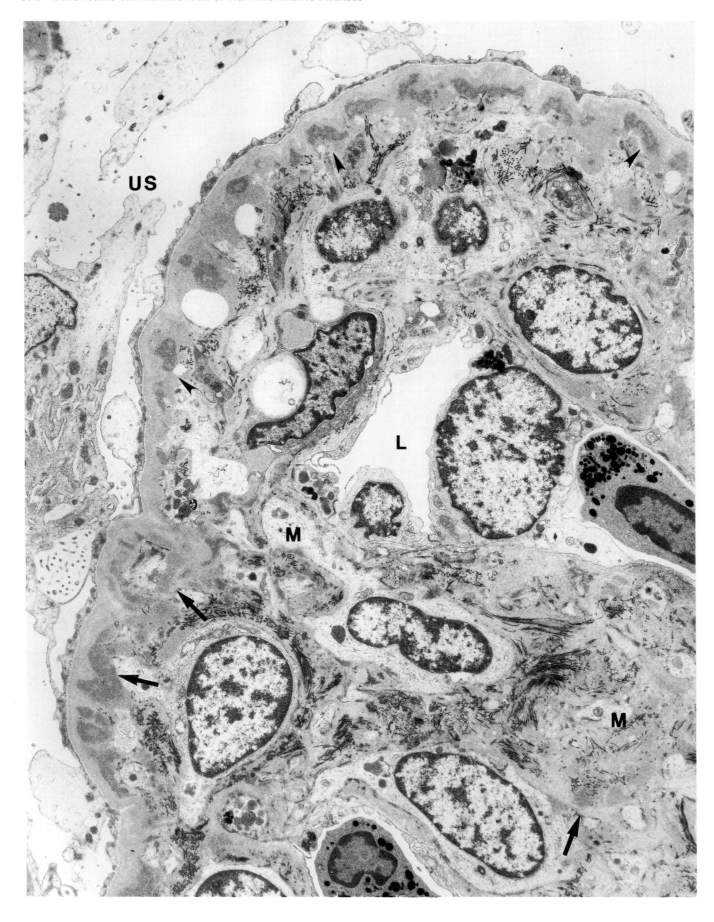

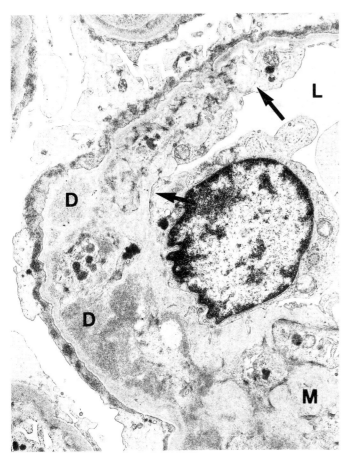

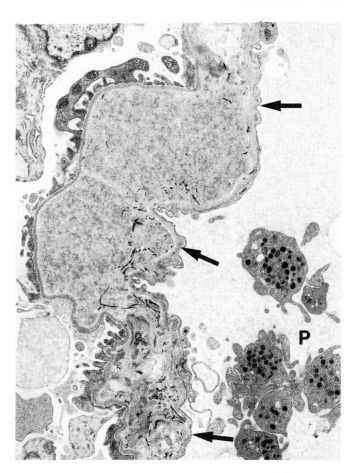

Fig. 17.9 Mesangiocapillary GN, type I: partial interposition. Incompletely developed interposition. Deposit is shown (D), and cytoplasmic extension is enclosed by new basement membrane-like material (arrows) which gradually merges with the true GBM. L = capillary lumen; M = mesangium. (× 8600)

Partial interposition — and even the completely developed lesion — is seen focally not uncommonly in a range of glomerulonephritides. Hence, the isolated presence of interposition does not, by itself, justify a diagnosis of MCGN which is a diagnosis dependent upon LM.

Fig. 17.10 Mesangiocapillary GN, type I: 'double contour'. The interposition zone in this micrograph is occupied mainly by flocculent deposit with fibrillar collagen. The subendothelial basement membrane-like layer is clearly visible (arrows). A cluster of luminal platelets (P) is also present. (× 6600) References: 12, 48, 93, 115, 117, 191, 212 and 249.

Fig. 17.8 (Facing page) Mesangiocapillary GN (type I; subendothelial deposit type). Circumferential mesangial interposition has resulted in dramatic capillary wall thickening and luminal (L) stenosis. Mesangial (M) cellular and matrix excess is also obvious, with the formation of abundant fibrillar collagen. Mesangial deposits (arrows) are located mainly in the paramesangial region. The capillary wall lesion is seen to be an extension of the mesangial abnormalities with cellular interposition and the complex laying down of matrix or basement membrane-like material, again with fibrillar collagen formation. It is apparent that the so-called 'subendothelial' deposit (arrowheads) is located mainly in the interposed submembranous mesangial structures. US = urinary space. (× 6900)

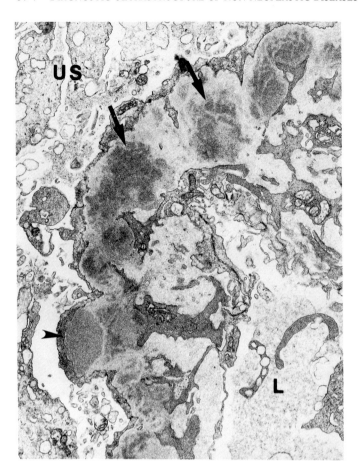

Fig. 17.11 (Left) Mesangiocapillary GN, type III. The deposit (arrows) is of variable density and tends to merge with the GBM which is irregularly thickened. Partial interposition is evident. The deposit lacks the smooth ribbon-like character which typifies dense deposit disease. Silver impregnation techniques in similar cases show basement membrane disruption. Epimembranous deposition may also be seen in this variant — a single subepithelial deposit (arrowhead) with poorly developed spike-like membrane reaction is present in this field. L = capillary lumen; US = urinary space. (× 8900) (Case contributed by Dr P W Allen and Mr D Gove.) References: 9, 217 and 218.

Fig. 17.12 (Below) Dense-deposit disease. The linear dense GBM transformation which typifies dense-deposit disease (DDD) is shown. Discontinuous, ribbon-like bands of electron-dense material can be seen in the GBM, and mesangial matrix involvement is conspicuous in contrast to pale, uninvolved segments of GBM and matrix (arrows). Mesangial interposition is present (arrowheads). (× 7300)

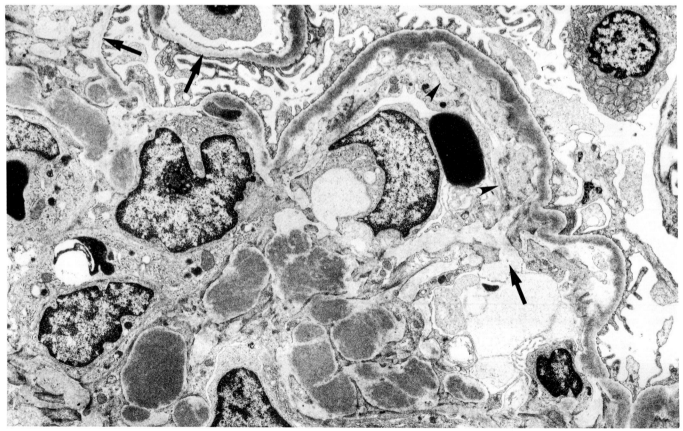

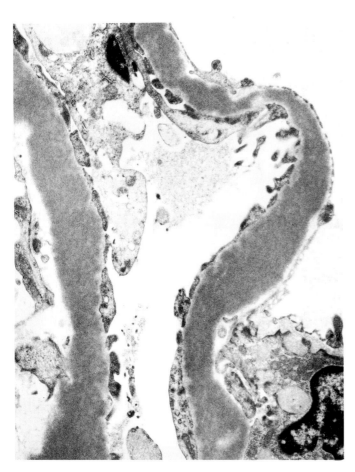

Fig. 17.13 (Left) Dense-deposit disease. Detail of thickened GBM containing linear, non-granular, dense deposits. Subendothelial lucency was focally prominent in this case. (× 10 400)

Similar laminar deposits may be seen in Bowman's capsule, and in tubular and vascular basal lamina in biopsies from patients with DDD. Granular glomerular subepithelial deposits may be superimposed on the main lesion. This disease occurs almost exclusively in children and young adults, some of whom have partial lipodystrophy. Profound hypocomplementaemia is usual. Patients may present with either nephritic or nephrotic syndromes and some develop rapidly progressive crescentic GN. Progression to renal failure is usual. MCGN patterns by LM are present in some but not all patients, and bright, refractile, eosinophilic, PAS-positive, ribbon-like thickening of basal laminae is characteristic. Immunofluorescence reactions are limited to C3 positivity apparently around, rather than within, the dense deposit. The deposits do not contain immunoglobulin. (Cases contributed by Dr I Aarons and Mr P Smith, and Dr G F Binns) References: 37, 59, 60, 63, 75, 92, 157, 191 and 198.

Fig. 17.14 (Below) Haemolytic uraemic-like syndrome associated with pregnancy — 'accelerated obsolescence'. Renal failure, with evidence of intravascular coagulation, developed in the 24th week of pregnancy in a previously healthy woman. Expansion and disruption of the mesangium (M) (mesangiolysis) is due to the accumulation of lucent and finely granular deposit. Similar material is present in subendothelial locations (arrows), and erythrocytic and other cytoplasmic fragments (arrowheads) are also present in a greatly expanded subendothelial zone. The changes result focally in considerable luminal stenosis. Fibrin strands or tactoids were present in other areas. (× 8000) References: 113, 116, 149, 191, 195, 196, 202, 212 and 226.

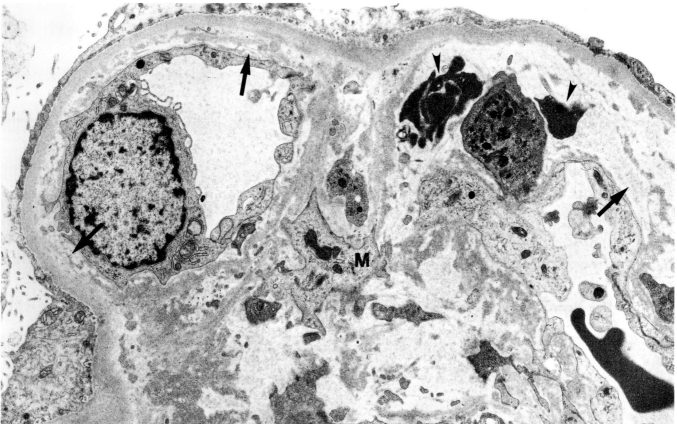

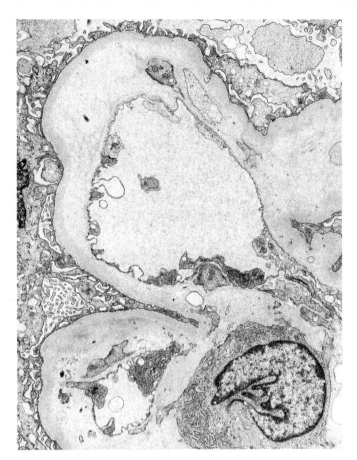

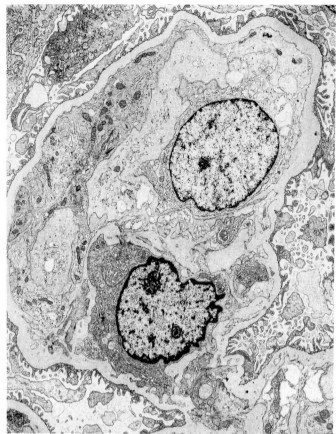

Fig. 17.15 (Above)   Transplant glomerulopathy. Widespread subendothelial lucency is the hallmark of transplant glomerulopathy. The subendothelial zone is occupied by finely granular material which typically extends into mesangia. The formation of new subendothelial basement membrane-like layers may be seen as double contours by LM. (× 5300) (Case contributed by Dr P W Allen and Mr D Gove) References: 107, 138, 139, 191, 228 and 229.

Fig. 17.16 (Above right)   Glomerular transplant rejection. Allograft biopsy following renal functional decline after transplantation. The lumen is occluded by portions of several mononuclear cells. (× 4100)

The segmental or global occlusion of allograft glomerular capillaries by swollen mononuclear cells appears to represent a distinctive form of glomerular rejection[13] mediated by cellular immunity. Immunohistological analysis has suggested that the lesion is mediated by T-lymphocytes, predominantly of the cytotoxic subset, and monocytes.[99] (Case contributed by Dr P W Allen and Mr D Gove) References: 13, 99, 228 and 229.

Fig. 17.17 (Right)   Kappa (K) light-chain nephropathy. Renal biopsy was performed on a 70-year-old woman to investigate unexplained loss of renal function. K light-chain excretion was found in the urine but the bone marrow was normal. Immunohistology demonstrated diffuse K chain deposition on tubular basement membranes, with minimal GBM involvement. This electron micrograph shows the granular dense transformation of basal laminae which is typical of light-chain disease. In addition to tubular laminal deposition (arrows), portion of an arteriolar wall (A) is included in which there is conspicuous alteration of arteriolar laminae (curved arrows). Most glomerular laminae were normal. (× 9500)

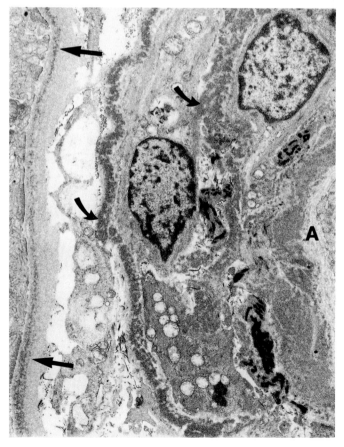

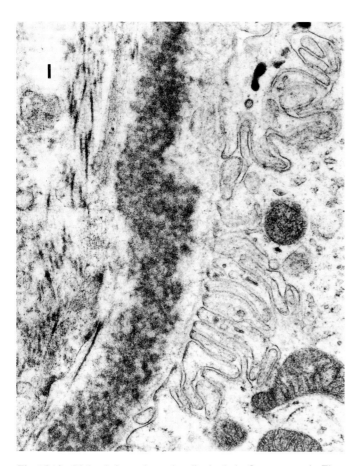

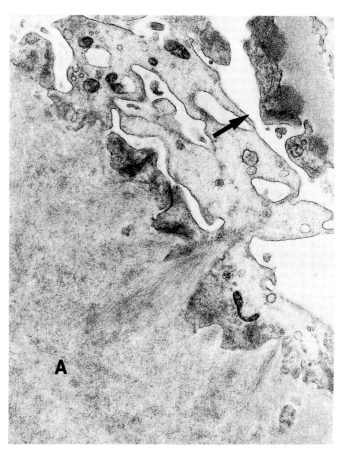

Fig. 17.18 Light-chain nephropathy: distal tubule. Same case as in Fig. 17.17. Detail of granular deposition in the basal lamina of a distal tubule. Portion of the adjacent interstitium (I) is included. (× 22 300)
References: 7, 8, 8a, 19, 26, 28, 47, 61, 66, 77–79, 112, 133, 148, 153, 159, 171–173, 191, 194, 206, 212, 224 and 231.

Fig. 17.19 Glomerular amyloidosis, complicated by stage I membranous GN, following penicillamine therapy. From a known case of renal amyloidosis complicating chronic rheumatoid arthritis. Proteinuria developed after a course of penicillamine. The edge of a grossly expanded mesangium is included. The matrix is replaced by a feltwork of amyloid fibrils (A) which are seen focally as approximately parallel arrays forming spicular deposits deforming the adjacent epithelial cytoplasm. In addition, three small epimembranous deposits are present in an adjacent capillary loop (arrow). The immunohistological features were typical of membranous GN. (× 16 300)

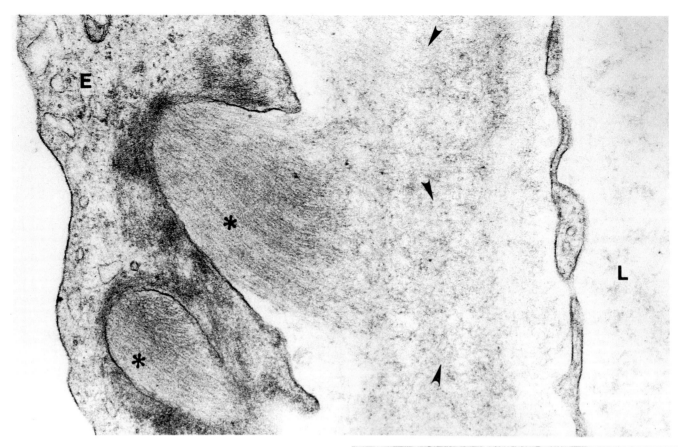

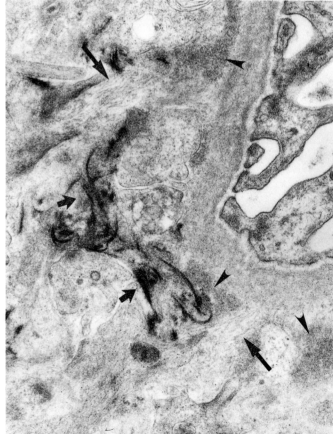

Fig. 17.20 (Above) Spicular glomerular amyloidosis complicating rheumatoid arthritis. Detail of two epimembranous amyloidotic basement membrane projections (asterisks) from a patient with chronic rheumatoid arthritis. The basement membrane is markedly thickened due to the accumulation of approximately 10-nm fibrils randomly orientated in the central membrane (arrowheads) but again showing parallelism in the spicular subepithelial projections. Note the condensation of epithelial cytoskeletal filaments over the amyloid masses. E = visceral epithelium; L = capillary lumen. (× 44 300)

The formation of reactive GBM between amyloid projections, or affinity for silver by the spicular deposits themselves,[25] may produce argyrophilic spikes by LM inviting confusion with membranous GN.[191] Proteinuria in patients with amyloidosis has been shown to correlate with detachment of the epithelium overlying GBM amyloid deposits.[123] There is no correlation between subtype of amyloidosis and variations in patterns of amyloid fibril deposition. References: 10, 23, 25, 56, 79, 82, 84, 112, 123, 191, 197 and 212.

Fig. 17.21 (Right) Glomerular microfibrils and collagen formation (transplant glomerulopathy). Allograft biopsy performed two years after renal transplantation. A complex glomerular lesion was present with evidence of *de novo* GN, and concomitant transplant glomerulopathy with frequent subendothelial widening and lucency. The figure displays part of a paramesangial region which was contiguous with lucent subendothelial deposit. Two types of fibril are depicted: (1) dark, curved, apparently aperiodic fibrils up to approximately 45-nm in diameter (short arrows) represent incompletely developed unit collagen; (2) two aggregates of approximately 18-nm microfibrils (long arrows) are seen in areas of lucency. Similar clusters were seen sporadically elsewhere in subendothelial locations. Finely granular deposits are shown also (arrowheads). (× 29 300) References: 28, 61, 106, 219 and 242.

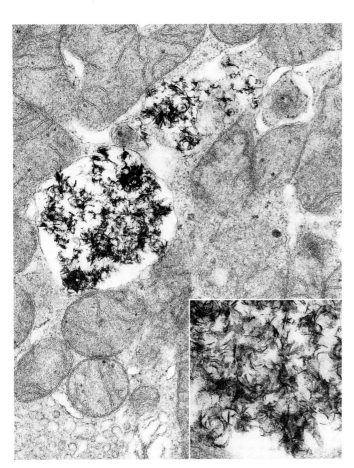

Fig. 17.22 (Left) Tubular epithelial aurisomes. Biopsy from a patient receiving gold therapy for rheumatoid arthritis. Multiple membrane-bound inclusions were present in tubular epithelium as depicted in this proximal tubular cell. ($\times$ 23 400) Typical electron-dense curvilinear lysosomal gold inclusions are illustrated in the *inset*. ($\times$ 54 200)

It is probable that all patients treated with gold compounds develop aurisomes. These inclusions are not inevitable indicators of toxicity or glomerular disease. Their presence in cases of gold-associated membranous GN does not necessarily indicate either that they are causative or that the glomerular lesion will be reversible. References: 212 and 232.

Fig. 17.23 (Below) Epithelial cell disease (ECD): foot process effacement. Steroid-responsive nephrotic syndrome in a 3-year-old boy. Epithelial foot processes are lost almost completely; the rare processes which persist are distorted and broadened. The GBM is covered by sheets of podocyte cytoplasm the density of which is increased adjacent to the membrane due to concentration of intermediate filaments. ($\times$ 13 500)

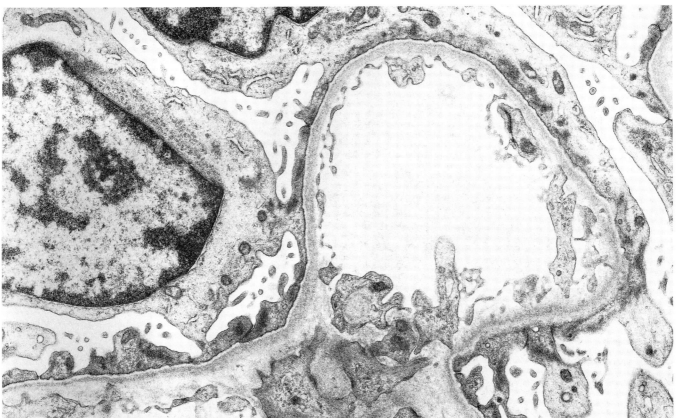

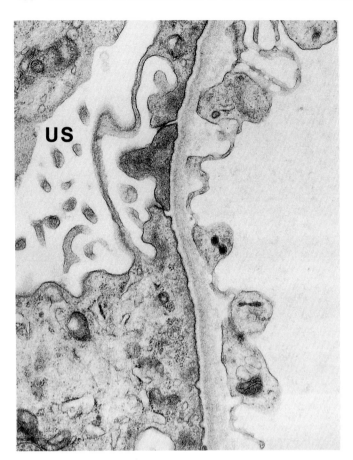

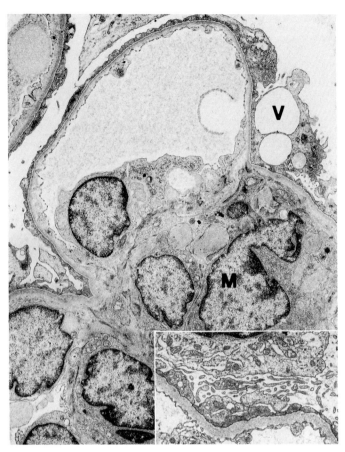

Fig. 17.24 Epithelial cell disease: preservation of cell junctions and slit pore regions, and microvillous transformation. Parts of three cell processes are included in the field. The plasmalemmal boundaries of each are clearly apparent and there is no 'fusion' of cytoplasm. The slit pores are visible but their overall length has been shown to be reduced in ECD.[24] Microvillus-like projections of the cell surfaces extend into the urinary space (US). (× 20 700)

Cases of epithelial cell disease have been described in association with lymphomas — usually Hodgkin's disease[7] — and following therapy with non-steroidal anti-inflammatory drugs, sometimes in combination with acute interstitial nephritis.[1,51,69] References: 1, 7, 24, 51, 69, 81, 144, 191, 212, 225, 241 and 244.

Fig. 17.25 Nephrotic focal/segmental glomerulosclerosis (FGS): mesangial expansion, foot process effacement, podocyte vacuolation and microvillous transformation. From a 67-year-old nephrotic woman. A small number of glomeruli contained segmental sclerosing lesions incorporating foam cells. This non-sclerotic area is affected by mesangial enlargement (M) due mainly to hypercellularity and foot process loss (which was near diffuse). One epithelial cell body contains vacuoles (V). (× 4900) *Inset* The non-specific phenomenon of podocyte microvillous surface transformation was a prominent feature in this example of FGS. (× 6100) See also Fig. 17.24.

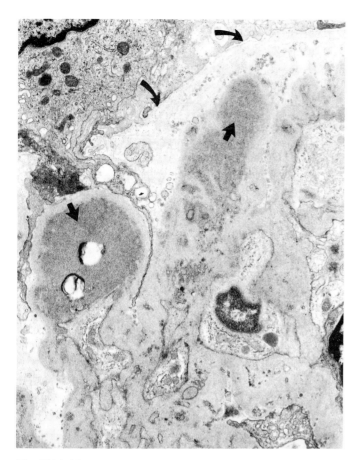

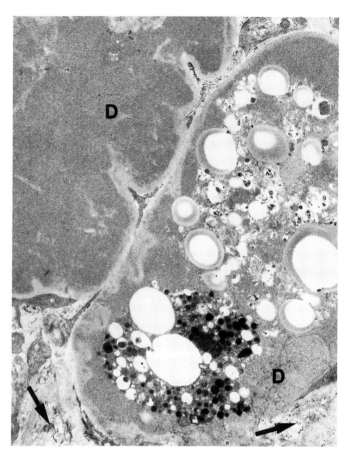

Fig. 17.26 Focal/segmental glomerulosclerosis: sclerotic region with hyalinosis and epithelial cell detachment. Increased amounts of mesangial matrix and basement membrane-like material typify sclerotic regions. Nodular masses of electron-dense deposit (bold arrows), in one instance containing lipid vacuoles, are the ultrastructural counterpart of hyalinosis. Such deposits are often mottled and variegated. A subepithelial zone of rarefaction and reticulation (curved arrows) represents a focus of presumed epithelial detachment and formation of new basement membrane. (× 8800) (Case contributed by Dr P W Allen and Mr D Gove.)

Fig. 17.27 (Non-nephrotic) focal/segmental glomerulosclerosis: hyalinosis in hereditary nephropathy — non-specificity of the segmental lesion. Part of a segmental sclerotic and hyalinotic glomerular lesion from a 48-year-old woman with a strong family history of chronic renal disease and an Alport-like glomerulopathy. Massive, nodular deposits are shown (D) and large amounts of lipid and membrane debris are incorporated in the material which appears to be surrounded by a GBM-like layer. Wisps of fibrillar collagen (arrows) are present in the intervening sclerotic regions. (× 7000) Segmental sclerosis and hyalinosis may be the end-points of diverse nephropathies (see text).

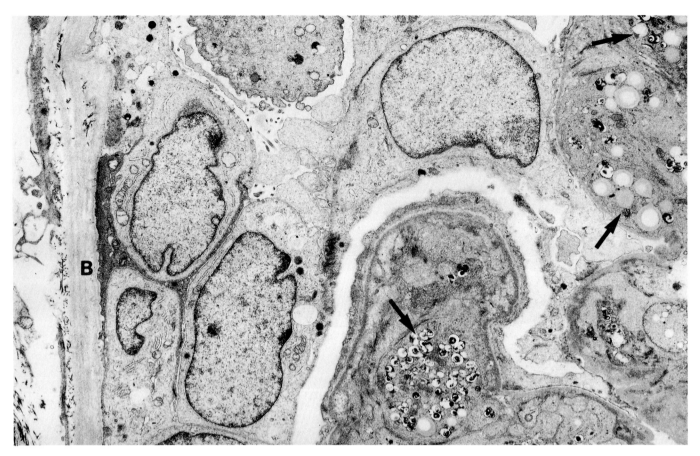

Fig. 17.28 (Above) Focal/segmental glomerulosclerosis: segmental sclerosis with associated epithelial proliferation — the 'cellular lesion' of FGS. Same case as in Fig. 17.25. This segmental lesion comprised loop collapse, sclerosis and endocapillary foam cell accumulation together with overlying epithelial proliferation resulting in the formation of a small cellular crescent. The micrograph depicts portions of the solidified capillary loops in which three foam cells are visible (arrows), with part of the adjacent epithelial lesion. B = Bowman's capsule. (× 6200)

The cellular lesion of FGS has been studied by Schwartz & Lewis[190] who described proliferative segmental lesions with both endo- and extra-capillary components in some patients with otherwise typical FGS. The endocapillary alterations included mesangial hypercellularity, foam cells, polymorphonuclear leukocytes and karyorrhectic debris. Overlying epithelial proliferation was characteristic. Such cellular lesions were often superimposed on, or associated with, more typical segmental scars. Temporal data demonstrated a relationship between cellular lesions and the onset of massive proteinuria, suggesting that such lesions may be antecedent to segmental scars. The authors postulated that the pathogenetic process leading to the fully developed lesion may begin with epithelial cell damage and that failure of epithelial cells to maintain normal capillary wall function might then lead to segmental collapse of the capillary tuft and glomerular scarring. Alternative pathogenetic mechanisms have been postulated. These implicate abnormal immune function, haemodynamic disturbances secondary to capillary hypertension or hyperperfusion, and mesangial overload.[179] Epithelial cell disease and nephrotic FGS may be related processes on the same continuum of disease — the outcome of which might depend on the degree of reversibility of the epithelial injury.[55,230] References: 55, 85, 122, 125, 162, 179, 190, 191, 212, 225, 230, 236, 241 and 244.

Fig. 17.29 (Facing page, top left) Alport's syndrome: glomerular basement membrane abnormalities. Renal biopsy from a 6-year-old boy with haematuria and severe nerve deafness. The micrograph is representative of the dramatic GBM disturbance which was seen diffusely in this case. The most obvious change is irregular increase in thickness, but areas of thinning are also present and there is profound alteration in membrane texture. The usual uniform density of the lamina is replaced by a pattern of rarefaction and reticulation, with occasional microparticles and included cytoplasm. L = capillary lumen; US = urinary space. (× 10 900)

Fig. 17.30 (Facing page, top right) Alport's syndrome: GBM textural disturbance; non-specificity of the isolated lesion. The main illustration is from the same case as in Fig. 17.29 and shows a region of lucency and lamellation with foot process effacement. (× 15 200) *Inset* GBM rarefaction and lamellation seen as an isolated phenomenon in a capillary loop from a case of otherwise typical IgA nephropathy. (× 17 100) See also Fig. 17.40.

Structural GBM abnormalities are present *sporadically* in many nephropathies. Typical Alport's syndrome is characterized by widespread or *diffuse* abnormalities of the type illustrated, but there is considerable variation in the degree of abnormality from case to case (see text). References: 18, 21, 40, 49, 87, 88, 90, 91, 100, 126, 163, 169, 175, 181–183, 191, 201, 212–214, 235, 240 and 248.

Fig. 17.31 (Facing page, bottom) So-called benign essential haematuria: basement membrane attenuation. Survey view representative of the ultrastructural appearances in a renal biopsy from a 42-year-old woman known to have had microscopic haematuria and minor proteinuria for at least 4 years before the investigation. Renal function was normal and remains normal 8 years later. There was no family history of renal disease. The singular abnormality is GBM thinning. Deposits are absent, the mesangium is normal and foot processes are preserved. (× 7300) The *inset* depicts a full thickness GBM defect found in this case (arrow) — but such lesions are exceptional and are found in non-haematuric patients. (× 17 100)

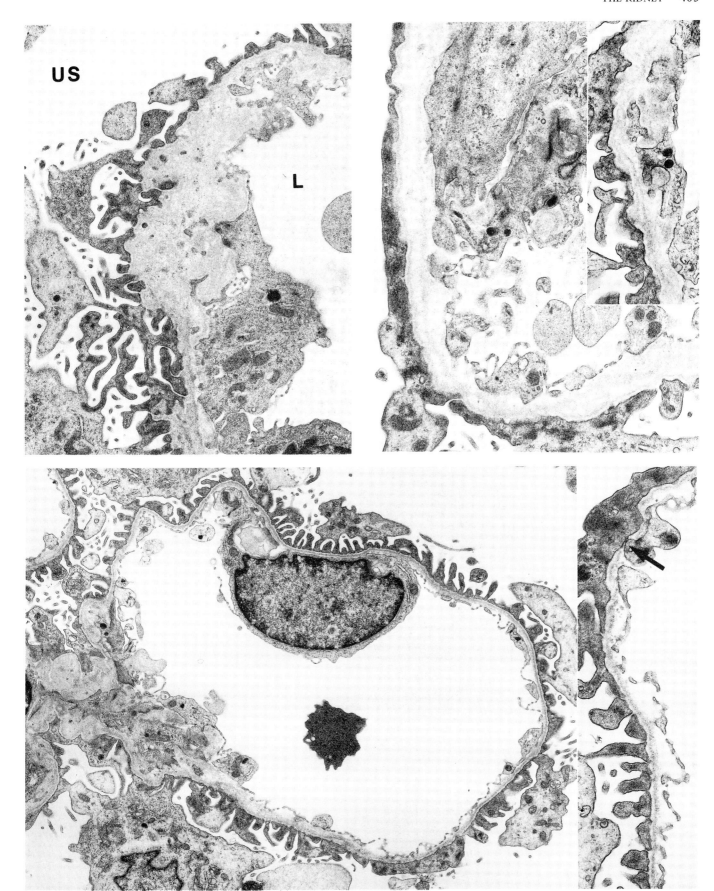

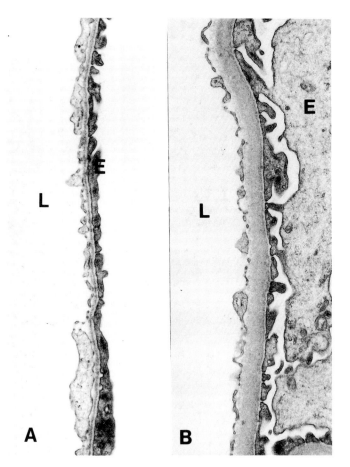

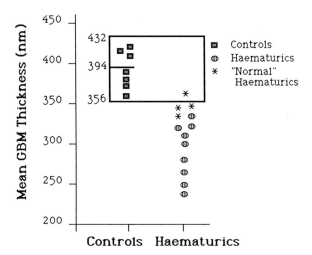

Fig. 17.33   So-called benign essential haematuria: glomerular basement membrane morphometry; mean GBM thickness. Coleman et al[49] have objectively characterized the GBM abnormality in renal biopsies from a group of patients presenting with apparently idiopathic haematuria. The mean results of measurement of GBM thickness are shown for 13 of the cases studied in contrast to 7 controls. The box delineates the normal range (overall control mean ± 2 SD). Included in the haematuric study group were cases in which GBM thinning was recognized subjectively during routine EM examination ('haematurics'). The case illustrated above corresponds to the haematuric case with the lowest mean value. The 4 "normal" haematuric cases were considered subjectively to have normal GBM ultrastructure. Measurement demonstrated pathological thinning in 3 of these cases. The fourth case had a low normal mean thickness; however, an excess of significantly thin GBM was shown by analysis of GBM thickness distribution (see below).

Fig. 17.32   So-called benign essential haematuria (BEH): extreme membrane thinning. Although there is a measurable continuum of thicknesses in cases of BEH, some examples are characterized by extreme attenuation as illustrated here (**A**; same case as in Fig. 17.31). Focal foot process loss is sometimes seen but textural disturbances are usually inconspicuous. Contrast these appearances with those of control material (**B**) shown at the same magnification (from a biopsy taken during nephrotomy for stone removal). L = capillary lumen; E = visceral epithelium. (× 11 500)

The nomenclature that has been applied to the syndrome(s) characterized by GBM attenuation is varied. Titles which include 'benign' and 'familial' are pathologically unsatisfactory (although clinically relevant). 'Thin membrane nephropathy', and 'basement membrane nephropathy (extensive attenuation type)' have been used in recent studies. The titles 'basal laminal nephropathy' or 'glomerular laminopathy (extensive attenuation type)' are suggested as alternatives but it is acknowledged that the more acceptable ultrastructural term 'basal lamina' is unlikely to replace the entrenched and traditional term 'basement membrane'.[49] References: 21, 49, 57, 100, 163, 169, 177, 183, 220, 235, 243 and 248.

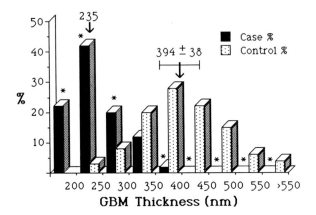

Fig. 17.34   So-called benign essential haematuria: glomerular basement membrane morphometry; GBM thickness distributions. In addition to measurement of mean GBM thickness, analysis of thickness distribution was undertaken also in the study described above. The figure depicts the distribution histogram for the haematuric case illustrated with the lowest mean thickness, in contrast to the histogram derived from pooled control data. It is apparent that thinning is the result of significant increases in the amounts of GBM in low-thickness categories at the expense of mid-range and high values. Results significantly different from the normal range (mean ± 2 SD) are indicated by asterisks ($P < 0.05$.) (Figures 17.33 and 17.34 are reprinted in modified form from Coleman et al[49]) Reference: 49.

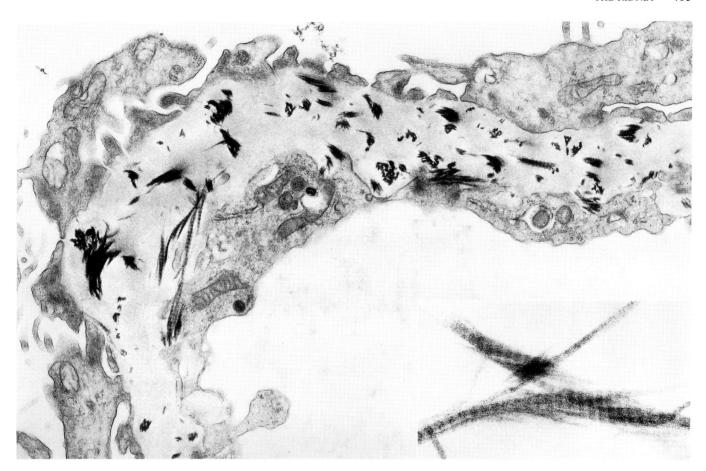

Fig. 17.35 Nail-patella syndrome: endomembranous fibrillar collagen formation. From a proteinuric 31-year-old man with skeletal abnormalities characteristic of the nail–patella syndrome. The GBM is irregularly thickened and contains numerous bundles of fibrillar collagen sometimes partly surrounded by faintly lucent regions. L = capillary lumen; US = urinary space. (× 19 200) Randomness of orientation within the membrane, and a transverse periodicity of approximately 60–65-nm are shown in the *inset*. (× 43 200) The deposition of such fibrils was seen in GBM and mesangia in a non-uniform manner; some parts of the glomeruli examined were unaffected.

The nail–patella syndrome (onycho-osteodysplasia) is a rare familial disorder transmitted as an autosomal dominant trait. Fingernail abnormalities are accompanied by bony lesions such as subluxation of the patellae and iliac spurs; some of the patients develop proteinuria and progressive renal dysfunction. The distinctive renal lesion can be visualized only by EM. As fibrillar collagen may form in glomeruli in a variety of chronic nephropathies, particularly in areas of glomerular sclerosis, the diagnosis of the nail–patella syndrome, in the absence of other evidence of the disease, should be considered only if the fibrils are found in clusters away from areas of scarring. References: 20, 21, 58, 151, 184 and 212.

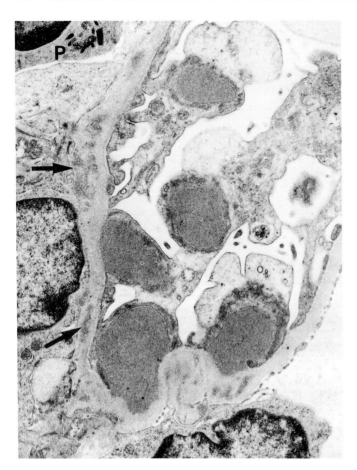

Fig. 17.37 (Facing page) Post-infectious glomerulonephritis: cellular mesangial reaction, mesangial and subendothelial deposit formation (with tubular epithelial cell artefact). The mesangial expansion typical of acute GN is mainly cellular. Part of a greatly enlarged mesangium is illustrated. The matrix bars (arrows) are sometimes indistinct and are spread apart by hypertrophic mononuclear cells, and neutrophils (N). Electron-dense deposit is obvious in the matrix, especially the paramesangial matrix, with smaller deposits in the subendothelial zone. The capillary lumen (L) is narrowed. In addition, the urinary space (US) is packed with fragments of epithelial cells extruded from the proximal tubule during the (needle) biopsy procedure.[155,239] Humps were moderately frequent elsewhere and are illustrated in Fig. 17.38. (× 6900)

Despite the dramatic alterations illustrated here, the patient (a 21-year-old man presenting with an acute nephritic syndrome) made a complete recovery — 5 years later the patient was normotensive; renal function, 24-hour urinary protein excretion and microurine examination were all normal. Reversibility presumably correlates with the cellular nature of the glomerular reaction in acute disease. There is some evidence that sporadic cases of acute post-infectious GN with atypical morphology may develop progressive disease but the long-term prognosis remains a matter of controversy.[76,179,212] In contrast to acute post-infectious disease, the GN associated with chronic visceral or systemic infection, or complicating infective endocarditis or the infection of indwelling intravascular cannulae ('shunt nephritis'), is characterized by heterogeneous morphology — although mesangial C3 deposition is seen in nearly all cases. It is noteworthy that recovery from chronic infection-associated GN is possible even when glomerular patterns develop which are usually associated with chronicity and progression (such as MCGN or crescentic GN), provided that the infection is completely eradicated.[48]

Fig. 17.36 Post-infectious glomerulonephritis: subepithelial 'humps'. The dome-shaped, protuberant deposits known as 'humps', projecting from the epithelial side of the GBM as illustrated in this case, are the hallmark of acute post-infectious GN. Additional deposits are always seen in other locations — small endomembranous deposits are also present in this field (arrows). Humps are often maximally concentrated in paramesangial locations and neutrophil polymorphs are sometimes seen in apposition with underlying GBM in areas of endothelial denudation (see Fig. 17.38). Part of an intraluminal polymorph (P) is included. (× 10 500)

Sporadic humps may be encountered in other forms of GN and are therefore not specific for post-infectious GN; however, the presence of frequent humps, in an appropriate clinico-pathological context, strongly suggests this diagnosis.

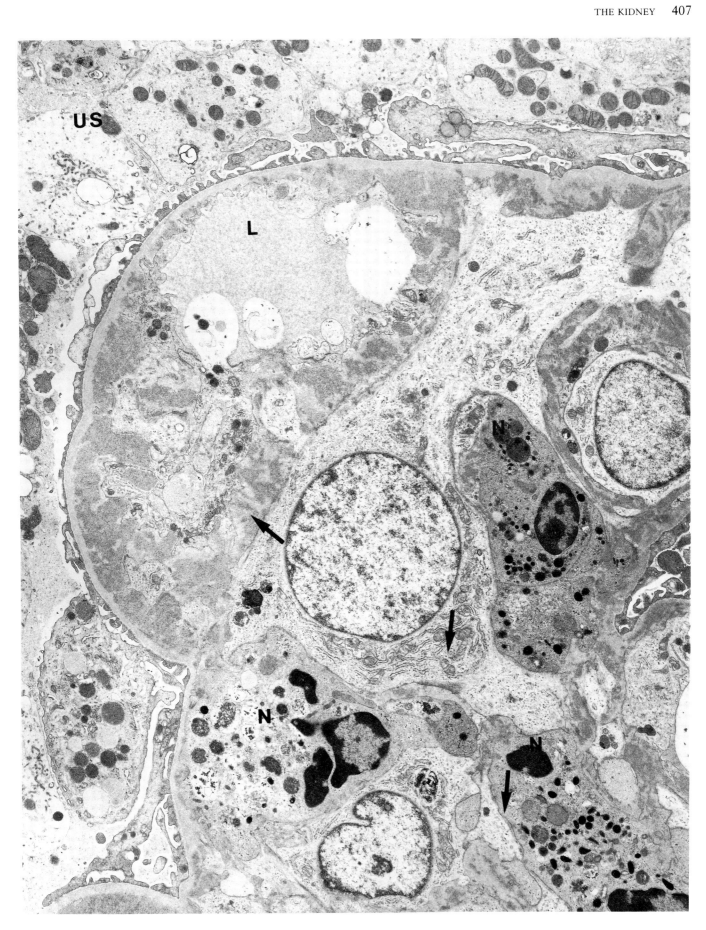

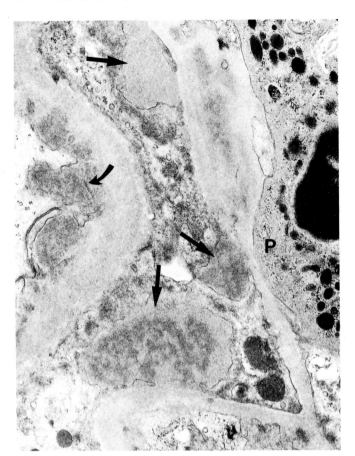

Fig. 17.38 (Left) Post-infectious glomerulonephritis: humps, subendothelial deposit and neutrophil polymorph. From the same case as in Fig. 17.37; portions of three humps (arrows), one with a variegated deposit texture, are present. Overlying foot processes are lost. Subendothelial deposit (curved arrow) is seen in an adjacent loop. An included polymorph (P) is closely applied to the GBM beneath one of the humps. (× 15 900) References: 48, 76, 101, 179 and 212.

Fig. 17.39 (Below) Mesangial proliferative GN with mesangial IgA deposits — IgA nephropathy. Profiles of three mesangial cell nuclei are seen in this markedly enlarged mesangium. Matrix bars are prominent and occupy much of the field at the expense of cytoplasm — excess of matrix accounts for most of the increase in mesangial volume in many examples of chronic GN; fibrillar collagen is commonly found also. Large amounts of electron-dense deposit are obvious. The pattern of deposition — in particular the formation of large paramesangial aggregates — is characteristic of IgA nephropathy. L = capillary lumen. (× 9500)

Inset A large, nodular, paramesangial deposit from another case of IgA disease. The presence of this pattern of deposition is most often seen in mesangia with less severe sclerosis, as in this case. (× 7200)

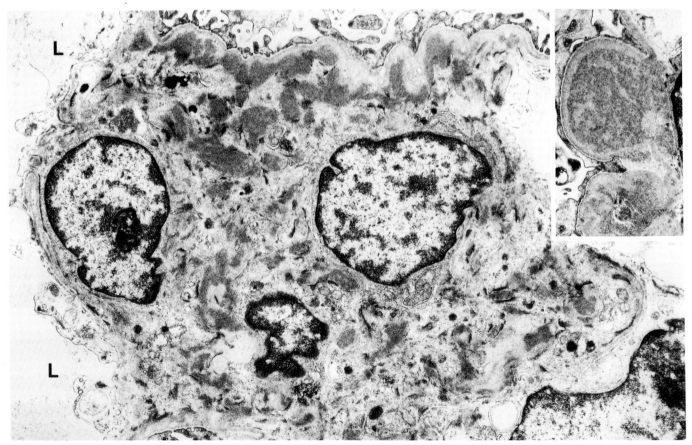

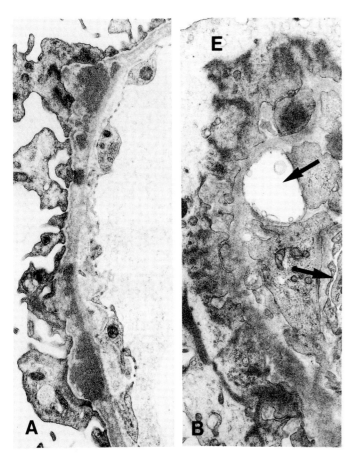

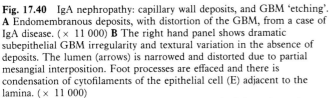

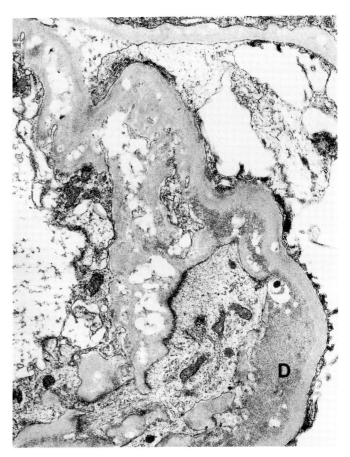

Fig. 17.40   IgA nephropathy: capillary wall deposits, and GBM 'etching'.
A Endomembranous deposits, with distortion of the GBM, from a case of
IgA disease. (× 11 000) **B** The right hand panel shows dramatic
subepithelial GBM irregularity and textural variation in the absence of
deposits. The lumen (arrows) is narrowed and distorted due to partial
mesangial interposition. Foot processes are effaced and there is
condensation of cytofilaments of the epithelial cell (E) adjacent to the
lamina. (× 11 000)

Whereas mesangial deposits are always present in IgA nephropathy,
capillary wall deposition is seen only in some loops of some cases.
Conversely, the presence of mesangial deposits containing IgA may be
seen in nephropathies other than primary IgA nephropathy. These
include Henoch–Schönlein purpura, systemic lupus erythematosus and
cirrhotic glomerulosclerosis. Mesangial IgA deposits have been described
also in association with mucin-secreting adenocarcinomas of the
respiratory and gastrointestinal tracts, and in patients with coeliac disease
and ankylosing spondylitis.[179,204] GBM lesions of the type illustrated (so-
called 'etching'), sometimes unassociated with deposit, are quite frequent
in IgA GN and Henoch–Schönlein purpura. Their pathogenesis is
obscure but they may result from polymorph mediated 'lysis' of the
membrane.[247] Correlations between 'lysis' or 'etching', or subepithelial
deposits, and progressive disease have been suggested.[83,179,247]
References: 43–45, 65, 83, 158, 179, 204, 205, 212 and 247.

Fig. 17.41   Cirrhotic glomerulosclerosis with mesangial IgA deposition
('cirrhotic glomerulonephritis'): mesangial deposit and lucencies. Renal
biopsy from an adult with hepatic cirrhosis. Diffuse mesangial IgA
reactions were demonstrated by immunofluorescence microscopy. The
edge of a mesangial region is shown including paramesangial deposit (D).
The scattered, irregular matrix lucencies — which rarely include dark
particles — are characteristic of cirrhotic glomerulosclerosis. Similar
lesions were present in the GBM. (× 10 400) (Case contributed by Dr I
Aarons and Mr P Smith) References: 2, 32, 39, 45, 185, 203 and 212.

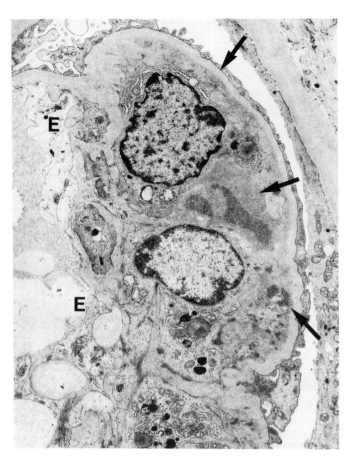

Fig. 17.42 (Left) Pre-eclamptic toxaemia: mesangial deposits. Biopsy from a 32-year-old pregnant woman who developed hypertension and proteinuria in the 32nd week of gestation. Part of a mesangial region is illustrated. There is mild increase in mesangial cell cytoplasm and irregular, mottled, light and dark deposits are present (arrows). The endothelium (E) is minimally swollen. (× 6800)

The pathogenesis of pre-eclamptic toxaemia (PET) of pregnancy is unknown. Disturbances of vascular responses, the coagulation system and the immunological relationships between mother and fetus have all been documented or proposed. The ultrastructural alterations accompanying PET include mesangial cellular hypertrophy often with the accumulation of lipid, mesangial interposition, and the formation of characteristic mottled deposits as shown in this case. Fibrin may be seen also. Endothelial swelling ('endotheliosis') has been recorded often but is rare in our material in which mesangial lesions are usually dominant. References: 73, 125, 191, 192, 209 and 212.

Fig. 17.43 (Below) Lupus nephritis: deposits and tubuloreticular arrays. From a patient with systemic lupus erythematosus (SLE) presenting with proteinuria and haematuria. Large, dense, mesangial (M) deposits are present and there are prominent subendothelial deposits (arrows). Endothelial tubuloreticular arrays were abundant in this case — two are included in the field (arrowheads); one of these is enlarged in the *inset*. (× 14 500; inset, × 50 600)

GN in SLE is mediated by the deposition of immune complexes. The location and amount of deposit usually correlate with the severity of the glomerular lesion. Patterns of deposition are highly variable but always involve the mesangium (except in the pure membranous variant), and often involve all parts of the glomerular tuft. Large subendothelial deposits correspond to the 'wire loop' lesions of LM. Tubuloreticular arrays are complex, branching, coiled, tubular structures found within dilated cisternae of the RER, most frequently in endothelial cells and rarely in other glomerular cells. While often present in large numbers in lupus nephritis, they are not specific for SLE and have been recorded in small numbers in many nephropathies, and in extra-renal situations, notably in tumours of diverse types.[17,131,212]

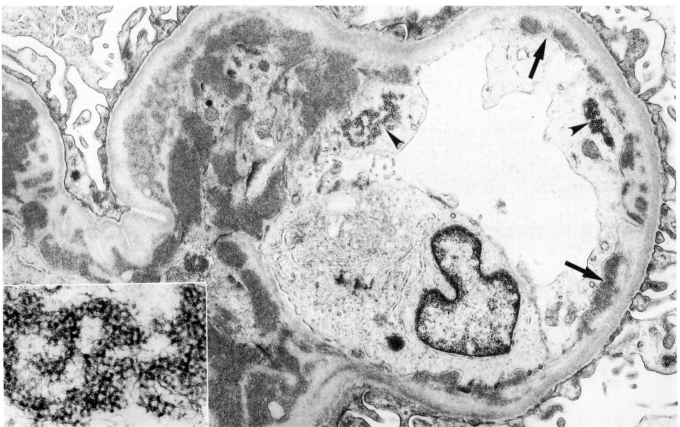

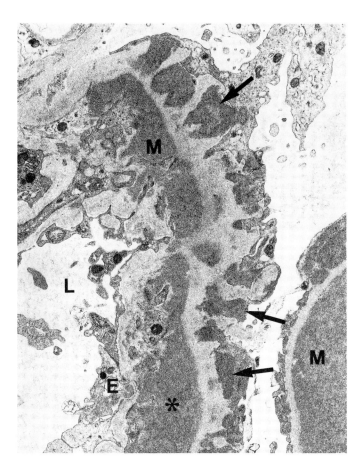

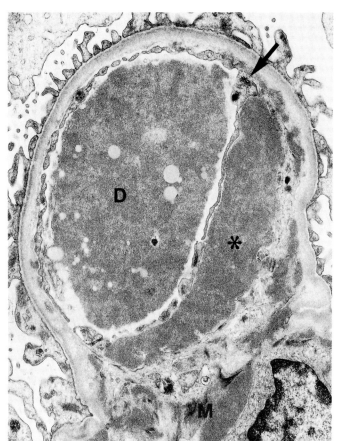

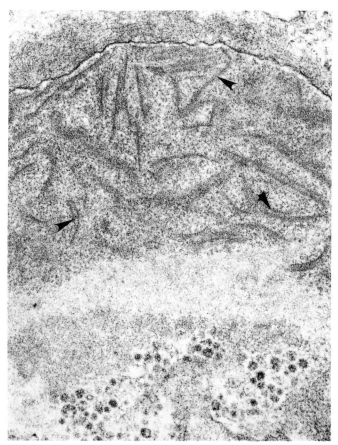

Fig. 17.44 (Above)   Lupus nephritis: deposits and interposition. The mesangial reactions accompanying mesangial (M) and subendothelial (asterisk) deposits of lupus nephritis may be associated with interposition as depicted in this micrograph. The capillary lumen (L) and endothelium (E) are indicated. In addition, subepithelial deposition is obvious (arrows) and is accompanied by the formation of epimembranous spikes similar to those seen in membranous GN. Epimembranous deposits predominate in some patients in patterns mimicking membranous GN ('pseudomembranous transformation'), and a pure membranous lesion may also be seen.[131,188,191,199] (× 7100)

Fig. 17.45 (Above right)   Lupus nephritis: massive apparently intraluminal deposit. Part of the deposit in this loop is clearly subendothelial (asterisk) and mesangial (M). The apparently intraluminal mass of variegated deposit (D) containing lipid-like vacuoles is probably further large subendothelial deposit in oblique section. This material corresponds to the so-called hyaline thrombi of LM. A tubuloreticular array is also present (arrow). (× 11 000)

Fig. 17.46 (Right)   Lupus nephritis: organized deposit, and spherical microparticles. Portion of a paramesangial deposit containing numerous straight and gently curved rod-like paracrystalline structures (arrowheads). Overlying foot processes are lost. Clusters of spherical microparticles are seen admixed with further deposit deeper in the mesangial matrix. (× 47 400) (Case contributed by Dr I Aarons and Mr P Smith)

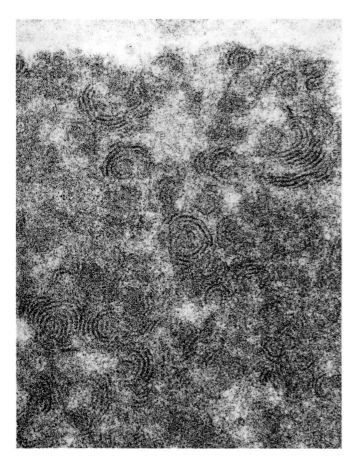

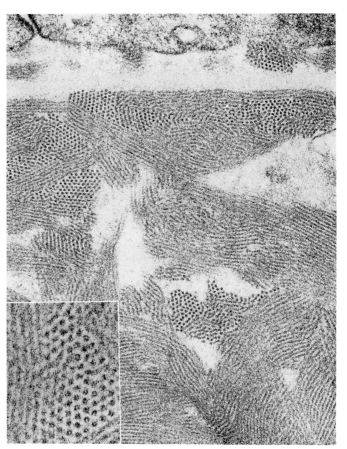

Fig. 17.47 Lupus nephritis: organized deposit. A whorling 'fingerprint'-like pattern of deposit organization was a prominent feature of this case of SLE. (× 46 800) References: 11, 17, 38, 46, 50, 109, 131, 188, 191, 199 and 212.

Fig. 17.48 Immunotactoid glomerulopathy: multiple myeloma with glomerulonephritis and organized deposit. Biopsy from a 69-year-old woman with multiple myeloma, IgA paraproteinaemia and an endocapillary proliferative GN with focal MCGN-like features. Circulating cryoglobulins could not be demonstrated. Immunofluorescence microscopy demonstrated strong, granular reactions, mainly for IgA, with mesangial and capillary wall involvement. Portion of a massive subendothelial deposit is illustrated (with smaller epimembranous deposits). The material has a highly organized substructure and consists of fibrillar–crystalline arrays in sheaves or lattice-like arrangements. Similar deposits frequently formed occlusive intraluminal 'thrombi' and smaller amounts were present in mesangia. (× 44 200) An apparently tubular configuration (approximate diameter 18-nm) is seen at higher magnification in the **inset**. (× 111 900)

Although the term 'immunotactoid glomerulopathy' was introduced in order to categorize glomerulopathies with organized immune deposits in patients without paraproteinaemia or systemic disease,[127,189] the case of IgA myeloma illustrated here is pathologically similar to the described cases so designated, and the term — as initially defined — is perhaps too restrictive. (Case contributed by Prof D W Henderson.) References: 29, 61, 77, 127, 180, 189 and 212.

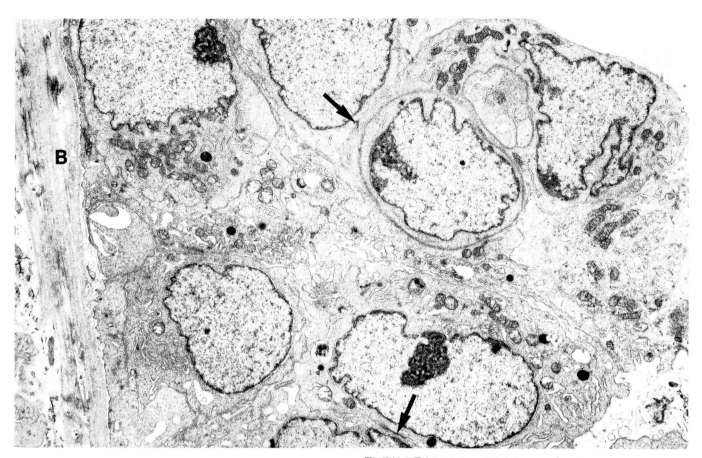

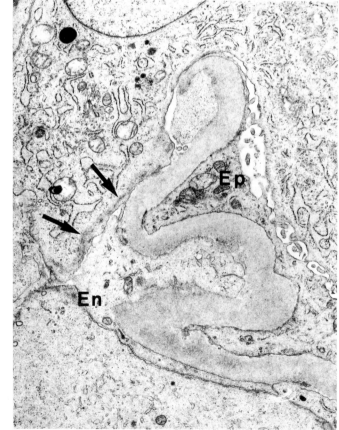

Fig. 17.49 (Above)   Crescentic glomerulonephritis: cellular crescent. From a case of anti-glomerular basement membrane antibody-mediated GN in a 23-year-old man. The illustration includes most of a small cellular crescent found in one of the glomeruli from this case. The cell mass is attached to Bowman's capsule (B) and rare, poorly formed, intercellular junctions (arrows) are present. (× 6900)

Traditionally, the crescent was regarded as composed of proliferating epithelial cells. Some recent studies, as detailed below, have suggested that macrophages participate in crescent formation but the extent to which this cell type contributes is not certain. Established crescents contain a variety of cells which can be difficult to type in routine preparations. The work of Hancock & Atkins[94] using monoclonal antibody cell markers indicated that, in cellular crescents, macrophages constituted the predominant cell, with lesser proportions of polymorphs and epithelial cells. Sclerosed crescents contained fewer macrophages but similar proportions of polymorphs and epithelial cells. The unlabelled cells in this study were considered to be probably fibroblasts (but see Figs 17.50, 17.52 and 17.53). The actual proportions remain uncertain[135] and there is now accumulating evidence that epithelial cells from Bowman's space are, in fact, in the majority.[114,135] It is apparent that the proportions in any given crescent will vary depending on the stage of formation and the degree of organization.

Fig. 17.50 (Right)   Crescentic glomerulonephritis: capillary loop rupture. Regardless of the nature of the underlying glomerular disease process, crescent formation is preceded by capillary loop rupture and the spillage of fibrinogen into the urinary space. The figure includes a segment of ruptured GBM enveloped by several cells. At least some of the cytoplasm most intimately applied to the lamina is probably epithelial (Ep) or endothelial (En), but the cell in the upper half of the field has fibroblastoid morphology with branching lamellae of RER and Golgi apparatus. In addition, there are faint peripheral cytoplasmic condensations (arrows) suggesting myofibroblastic properties. (See also Figs 17.52 and 17.53.) (× 10 100)

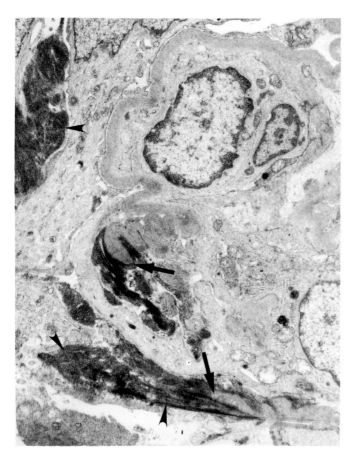

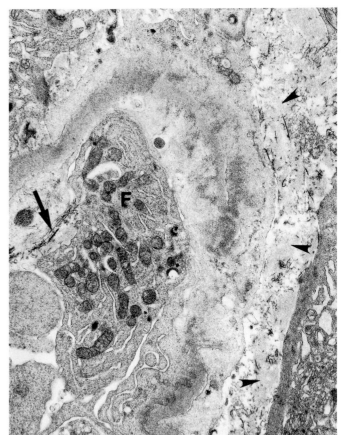

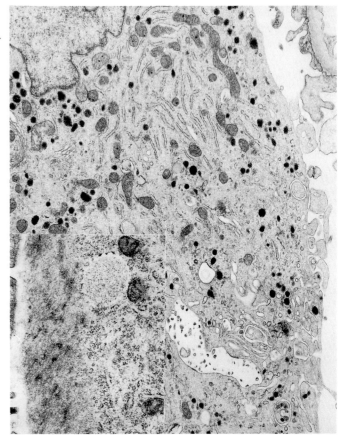

Fig. 17.51 (Above)   Crescentic glomerulonephritis: loop rupture and fibrin extravasation. The free ends of a ruptured capillary loop are shown (arrows), with fibrin (arrowheads) forming dense, irregular masses in the urinary space between cells of a crescent. (× 7000)

Fig. 17.52 (Above right)   Crescentic glomerulonephritis: crescent organization. Approximately seven or more days after the onset of crescent formation, organization of the crescentic cell mass may be seen. This field includes a disrupted capillary loop apparently undergoing dissolution. A fibroblast-like cell (F) has invaded the lumen, and fibrillar collagen (arrow) has formed in the adjacent space. The urinary space is now obliterated by accumulations of basal laminal material (arrowheads) with fibrillar collagen, together with fibroblastoid cells in apposition. The peripheral disposition of microfilaments with scattered condensations seen in the cell on the right suggests that this cell is a myofibroblast. (× 9800)

We have observed myofibroblasts in several cases of crescentic GN (and they occur in the renal interstitium in interstitial fibrosis). It is not surprising that organizing crescents might contain myofibroblasts as these cells with their contractile and synthetic properties are ubiquitous in reparative, fibrosing inflammatory lesions. Their presence would adequately explain the glomerular contracture and obliteration which follow crescent formation. (See also Fig. 17.53, and Ch. 11.)

Fig. 17.53 (Right)   Crescentic glomerulonephritis: macrophage and myofibroblast. Details of a macrophage, and a myofibroblast, found in two separate cases of crescentic GN. The macrophage is replete with pleomorphic lysosomes and exhibits the plasmalemmal ruffles which typify this cell. (× 10 200) The periphery of a myofibroblast is depicted in the **inset**. A few lamellae of the RER are included in the field. The subplasmalemmal zone is occupied by a mass of microfilaments within which focal condensations can be seen. These cells have properties intermediate between those of fibroblasts and smooth muscle. (× 16 500) References: 74, 94, 104, 114, 135, 152, 212 and 216.

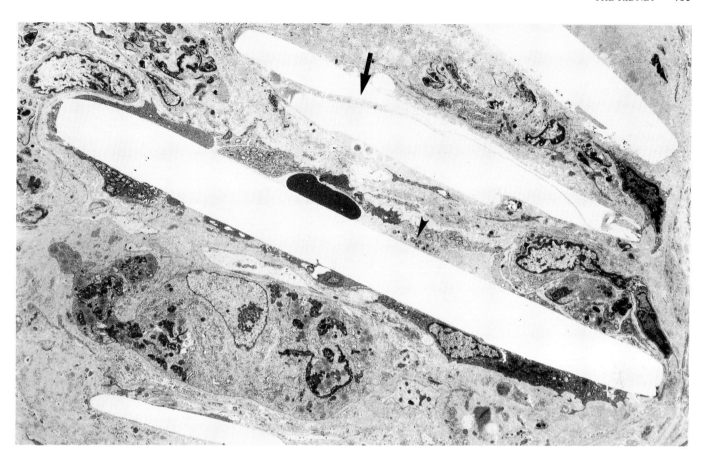

Fig. 17.54 Renal atheroembolism: arteriolar cholesterol emboli. From an elderly, hypertensive man who presented with declining renal function. This survey view includes portion of an arteriolar wall in transverse section and shows several elongated, clear clefts, the shape of which is characteristic of cholesterol crystals in section. One of the crystals is fractured (arrow). The largest crystal fills the lumen and is indenting the vessel wall. A platelet (arrowhead) can be seen adjacent to the cleft. The smaller crystals represent previous embolic episodes and have become incorporated into the thickened arteriolar wall. (× 3400)

Renal atheroembolism usually occurs in elderly patients with severe, complicated aortic arteriopathy and is a common complication of aortic surgery or arteriography. Affected patients may be asymptomatic or may develop clinically significant renal disease with infarction, acute and chronic renal failure, and hypertension as the most usual manifestations. The microemboli comprise flat, rhomboidal crystals (seen as clefts in routinely prepared sections processed through lipid solvents) often associated with thrombosis. With time, a cellular reaction ensues, sometimes with a phagocytic giant cell component, and the crystals become exteriorized and incorporated into neointimal tissues with or without luminal occlusion.

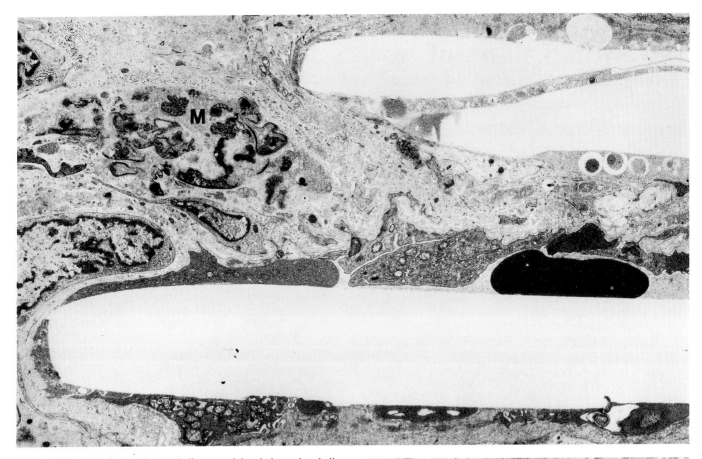

Fig. 17.55 (Above) Renal atheroembolism: arteriolar cholesterol emboli. Detail from Fig. 17.54. The luminal crystal abuts the endothelium in places and an erythrocyte is present in the narrowed lumen. The extraluminal crystal is surrounded by external lamina, including fibrillar collagen, and a macrophage (M) with pleomorphic lysosomes is nearby. The fracture is filled with cytoplasm. (× 6700)

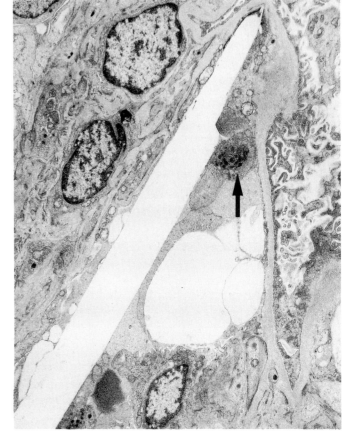

Fig. 17.56 (Right) Renal atheroembolism: glomerular embolus. Part of a capillary loop is shown with a cholesterol crystal impacted in the lumen. A platelet (arrow) is present in apposition with the cleft. (× 4800) References: 118 and 207.

18. Investigation of male infertility by electron microscopy: abnormal spermatozoa

Susan M. B. Stevens   R. A. Boadle

INTRODUCTION

Abnormal spermatozoa are present to a greater or lesser extent in all semen, including that of men of proven fertility, but are more frequent in the infertile[34] — where there may be gross changes in ultrastructure,[41] usually with considerable variation within the sperm population.[26,32,45,46] Careful examination of sperm morphology by light microscopy is essential in the evaluation of the semen of a patient presenting with infertility[27] and should be done together with other investigations as indicated by the initial clinical findings. Ultrastructural examination of spermatozoa becomes relevant when sperm show reduced, abnormal or complete immotility, but are demonstrated to be viable, if there is a high proportion of abnormal spermatozoa showing a similar defect throughout the population[33,46] or if 'normal' spermatozoa fail to fertilize *in vitro*.

PREPARATION OF SPERMATOZOA FOR ELECTRON MICROSCOPY

A low sperm count may accompany other abnormalities of spermatozoa, so a concentrated sample with minimum of artefact is the ideal of specimen preparation.[46] In our laboratory, fixation is by a modification of the method described by Pedersen[30] and encapsulation as described by Lazzaro[24] for fine needle aspirates.

Method for transmission electron microscopy

1. Mix two volumes of fixative (4% glutaraldehyde in 0.2 M cacodylate buffer, pH 7.4, containing 4% sucrose and 0.015% calcium chloride) with the fully liquefied semen at room temperature and fix at 4°C for 15 min without agitation.
2. Centrifuge at 500 *g* for 15 min at 4°C.
3. Remove supernatant and replace with an equal volume of 0.2 M cacodylate buffer, pH 7.4, containing 6.6% sucrose. Gently resuspend cells with a Pasteur pipette.
4. Centrifuge at 500 *g* for 15 min.
5. Repeat steps 3 and 4.
6. Remove buffer and add 2% cacodylate-buffered osmium tetroxide. Resuspend cells gently and fix for 1 h at room temperature with *gentle* agitation. Centrifuge at 500 *g* for 15 min.
7. Remove osmium tetroxide and wash with distilled water (resuspend the pellet gently with a Pasteur pipette) and centrifuge at 500 *g* for 15 min. Repeat washing.
8. Reduce volume of supernatant to about 0.3 ml and resuspend pellet gently. Transfer to a 400 μl polyethylene microcentrifuge tube and spin at 1500 r.p.m for 7 min in a microcentrifuge.
9. Remove supernatant and replace with approximately 0.2 ml 10% bovine serum albumin (fraction V Sigma A-4503) resuspending the cells gently with a Pasteur pipette.
10. Stand for 20 min at room temperature then centrifuge at 1500 r.p.m in a microcentrifuge for 7 min.
11. Remove supernatant and gently add 0.2 ml 2.5% buffered glutaraldehyde over the pellet without disturbing the cells. Fix at 4°C for 6 h (or overnight).
12. The pellet may be removed by cutting through the tube with a sharp blade and blocks selected and trimmed for further processing.
13. Blocks 1.0 mm thick are treated with 2% aqueous uranyl acetate for 1 h.
14. Dehydration is by a graded ethanol series, 50% for 10 min, 70% for 10 min, 90% for 10 min, 2 × absolute ethanol for 20 min, 2 × absolute acetone for 10 min.
15. Infiltration consists of 1:1 acetone:Spurr resin for 1 h at room temperature followed by 3 × 10 min changes of Spurr resin at 60°C.
16. Embedding is completed using suitable embedding moulds and polymerization at 60°C overnight.
17. Silver sections are collected on uncoated grids and stained with uranyl acetate and lead citrate.

Transmission electron microscopy (TEM) is essential to define abnormalities of the axoneme, and we have found the goniometer stage of great assistance to view cross-sections of the flagellum.

Method for scanning electron microscopy

Scanning electron microscopy (SEM) is particularly useful to visualize the whole length and configuration of the flagellum.[5,9,10,19]

A 1 ml aliquot of fixed washed semen is taken from the TEM protocol after the second buffer wash (step 5) and mixed with 1 ml of Ringer's solution or buffer and layered by centrifugation (500 *g* for 4–5 min) onto a suitable specimen support, such as a filter membrane or gold-coated coverslip.

The specimen is dehydrated using a graded ethanol series,

transferred to an intermediate fluid (Freon T.F.) prior to critical point drying from liquid CO_2. The dried specimen is attached to a suitable SEM stub using double-sided tape or silver paste and coated with a sputtered layer of gold or gold/palladium. Examination in a scanning electron microscope may then proceed.

IMMOTILE OR ABNORMALLY MOTILE SPERMATOZOA

Electron microscopy has contributed to the knowledge and understanding of normal sperm morphology,[21,46] in particular the axoneme; it has also defined abnormal sperm morphology and has linked this information to abnormalities of cilia and the associated clinical syndromes of immotile or dyskinetic cilia, typified by the earlier recognized Kartagener's syndrome[1,14] (see also Ch. 13).

A variety of changes have been described in the flagellum (Fig. 18.1) of immotile or poorly motile sperm.[2,16,46] A defect may be single but is frequently associated with other morphological changes.[16,25,45,46] Least motility is usually seen in sperm showing absence of both dynein arms from the microtubules[16] (Fig. 18.2), or absent radial spokes,[39] or with a defect of the inner dynein arm and peripheral junction complex.[16] Other defects described include absence of only the outer[2,16] or inner dynein arms,[2] transposition of the microtubules,[40] absence of the central pair of microtubules, the 9 + 0 defect[2,7] or of the whole axoneme.[9]

Other abnormalities of the flagellum include short tails[5,36] and absent tails.[39,46] Multi-tailed spermatozoa are frequently associated with large heads.[15,28,46] Abnormalities of the mid-piece have been described and are usually associated with defective or disorganized fibrous sheath and coarse accessory fibres[29,35,36,46] (see Ch. 20). In some cases where both cilia and spermatozoa have been examined, the same defect is not present in both[25] or one or the other may be normal by observation[7,23,44] or by implication.[37] Not all spermatozoa with abnormal motility show obvious ultrastructural changes[22,46] but increasingly refined morphometry is revealing subtle changes previously unrecognized.[17]

ROUND-HEADED SPERMATOZOA

The syndrome of round-headed spermatozoa (Figs 18.4 and 18.5) is the most frequently described of the conditions where a high percentage of abnormal sperm show a specific defect.[3,4,6,12,18,20,31,43] Most cases described lack an acrosome (compare Figs 18.3 and 18.5) necessary to penetrate the oolemma,[11,13,38,42] and also lack the post-acrosomal sheath, but occasional exceptions may be found.[3,4] Duplicate heads have also been described[43] (Fig. 18.4, inset). The nucleus may appear normal[20] or may show less condensation of chromatin than is usual[4,12] and be withdrawn from the nuclear membranes[12] (Fig. 18.5). The incompletely developed acrosome appears to have been either incorporated into the nucleus during spermatid differentiation[6] or left as residue in the Sertoli cells after release from the germinal epithelium.[12,20]

The flagellum of the round-headed sperm may be essentially normal.[6] However, it may be detached[4,43] or may be coiled in redundant cytoplasm[3,6,12,31,43] or the axoneme present may be abnormal.[6,31] Electron microscopy of testicular biopsy material contributes to the understanding of the development of abnormal spermatozoa, including the round-headed spermatozoa,[6,12,20] but diagnosis, including noting the presence or absence of the acrosome, can be done on ejaculated spermatozoa. Other abnormalities of the head noted in a high proportion of the sperm population have included double spermatozoa,[8] absent heads,[33] defective acrosomes[13,38,46] and large heads with multiple flagella.[15] Other non-specific abnormalities of the head of spermatozoa are considered in Chapter 20.

REFERENCES

1. Afzelius B A 1979 The immotile-cilia syndrome and other ciliary diseases. International Review of Experimental Pathology 18: 1–43
2. Afzelius B A, Eliasson R 1979 Flagella mutants in man: on the heterogeneity of the immotile-cilia syndrome. Journal of Ultrastructure Research 69: 43–52
3. Anton-Lamprecht I, Kotzur B, Schopf E 1976 Round-headed human spermatozoa. Fertility and Sterility 27: 685–693
4. Aughey E, Orr P S 1978 An unusual abnormality of human spermatozoa. Journal of Reproduction and Fertility 53: 341–342
5. Baccetti B, Burrini A, Pallini V, Renieri T, Rosati F, Menchini Fabris G F 1975 The short-tailed human spermatozoa. Ultrastructural alterations and dynein absence. Journal of Submicroscopic Cytology 7: 349–359
6. Baccetti B, Renieri T, Rosati F, Selmi M G, Casanova S 1977 Further observations on the morphogenesis of the round headed human spermatozoa. Andrologia 9: 255–264
7. Baccetti B, Burrini A G, Maver A, Pallini V, Renieri T 1979 '9 + 0' immotile spermatozoa in an infertile man. Andrologia 11: 437–443
8. Baccetti B, Fraioli F, Paolucci D, Selmi G, Spera G, Renieri T 1979 High prolactin level and double spermatozoa. Gamete Research 2: 193–199

9. Baccetti B, Burrini A G, Pallini V 1980 Spermatozoa and cilia lacking axoneme in an infertile man. Andrologia 12: 525–532
10. Baccetti B, Renieri T, Soldani P 1981 Scanning electron microscopy and human sperm pathology. Scanning Electron Microscopy 4: 151–156
11. Baccetti B, Burrini A G, Collodel G, Magnano A R, Piomboni P, Renieri T, Sensini C 1989 Crater defect in human spermatozoa. Gamete Research 22: 249–255
12. Castellani L, Chiara F, Cotelli F 1978 Fine structure and cytochemistry of the morphogenesis of round-headed human sperm. Archives of Andrology 1: 291–297
13. Courtot A M, Escalier D, Jouannet P, David G 1987 Impaired ability of human spermatozoa to penetrate zona-free hamster oocytes: is a postacrosomal sheath anomaly involved? Gamete Research 17: 145–156
14. Eliasson R, Mossberg B, Camner P, Afzelius B A 1977 The immotile cilia syndrome. A congenital ciliary abnormality as an etiologic factor in chronic airway infections and male sterility. New England Journal of Medicine 297: 1–6
15. Escalier D 1983 Human spermatozoa with large heads and multiple flagella: a quantitative ultrastructural study of 6 cases. Biology of the Cell 48: 65–74

16. Escalier D, David G 1984 Pathology of the cytoskeleton of the human sperm flagellum: axonemal and peri-axonemal anomalies. Biology of the Cell 50: 37–52
17. Escalier D, Serres C 1985 Aberrant distribution of the peri-axonemal structures in the human spermatozoon: possible role of the axoneme in the spatial organisation of the flagellar components. Biology of the Cell 53: 239–250
18. Flörke-Gerloff S, Töpfer-Petersen E, Müller-Esterl W, Mansouri A, Schatz R, Schirren C, Schill W, Engel W 1984 Biochemical and genetic investigation of round-headed spermatozoa in infertile men including two brothers and their father. Andrologia 16: 187–202
19. Fujita T, Miyoshi M, Tokunaga J 1970 Scanning and transmission electron microscopy of human ejaculate spermatozoa with special reference to their abnormal forms. Zeitschrift für Zellforschung und Mikroskopische Anatomie 105: 483–497
20. Holstein A F, Schirren C, Schirren C G 1973 Human spermatids and spermatozoa lacking acrosomes. Journal of Reproduction and Fertility 35: 489–491
21. Holstein A F, Roosen-Runge E C 1981 Atlas of human spermatogenesis. Grosse Verlag, Berlin, pp 194–219
22. Jaydot-Van de Casseye M, Schoysman R, Smets G, Gepts W 1980 Ultrastructural aspects of asthenospermia. International Journal of Andrology 3: 15–22
23. Jonsson M S, McCormick J R, Gillies C G, Gondos B 1982 Kartagener's syndrome with motile spermatozoa. New England Journal of Medicine 307: 1131–1133
24. Lazzaro A V 1983 Technical note: improved preparation of fine needle aspiration biopsies for transmission electron microscopy. Pathology 15: 399–402
25. Lungarella G, Fonzi L, Burrini A G 1982 Ultrastructural abnormalities in respiratory cilia and sperm tails in a patient with Kartagener's syndrome. Ultrastructural Pathology 3: 319–323
26. McClure R D, Brawer J, Robaire B 1983 Ultrastructure of immotile spermatozoa in an infertile male: a spectrum of structural defects. Fertility and Sterility 40: 395–399
27. Mortimer D 1985 The male factor in infertility. Part 1: semen analysis. Current Problems in Obstetrics, Gynaecology and Fertility 8: 1–87
28. Nistal M, Paniagua R, Herruzo A 1977 Multi-tailed spermatozoa in a case with asthenospermia and teratospermia. Virchow Archiv B, Cell Pathology 26: 111–118
29. Pedersen H, Rebbe H, Hammen R 1971 Human sperm fine structure in a case of severe asthenospermia — necrospermia. Fertility and Sterility 22: 156–164
30. Pedersen H 1974 The human spermatozoon. Danish Medical Bulletin 21 (suppl 1): 1–36
31. Pedersen H, Rebbe H 1974 Fine structure of round-headed human spermatozoa. Journal of Reproduction and Fertility 37: 51–54
32. Pedersen H, Hammen R 1982 Ultrastructure of human spermatozoa with complete subcellular derangement. Archives of Andrology 9: 251–259
33. Perotti M-E, Giarola A, Gioria M 1981 Ultrastructural study of the decapitated sperm defect in an infertile man. Journal of Reproduction and Fertility 63: 543–549
34. Pryor J P, Collins W P, Landon G, Tyler J P P 1981 The clinical application of electron microscopy and the heterologous ova penetration test to the assessment of spermatozoa from infertile men. British Journal of Urology 53: 660–663
35. Ross A, Christie S, Kerr M G 1971 An electron microscope study of a tail abnormality in spermatozoa from a subfertile man. Journal of Reproduction and Fertility 24: 99–103
36. Ross A, Christie S, Edmond P 1973 Ultrastructural tail defects in the spermatozoa from two men attending a subfertility clinic. Journal of Reproduction and Fertility 32: 243–251
37. Rott H-D 1979 Kartagener's syndrome and the syndrome of immotile cilia. Human Genetics 46: 249–261
38. Sauer M V, Bustillo M, Serafini P 1989 Transient acrosomal hypoplasia of spermatozoa and male infertility. Archives of Andrology 22: 95–98
39. Sturgess J M, Chao J, Wong J, Aspin N, Turner J A P 1979 Cilia with defective radial spokes. New England Journal of Medicine 300: 53–56
40. Sturgess J M, Chao J, Turner J A P 1980 Transposition of ciliary microtubules. New England Journal of Medicine 303: 318–322
41. Sun C N, White H J 1978 The variety of abnormal spermatozoa from patients with fertility problems, an ultrastructural study. I. Mature forms. Cytologia 43: 551–554
42. Syms A J, Johnson A R, Lipshultz L I, Smith R G 1984 Studies on human spermatozoa with round head syndrome. Fertility and Sterility 42: 431–435
43. Tyler J P P, Boadle R A, Stevens S M B 1985 Round-headed spermatozoa: a case report. Pathology 17: 67–70
44. Walt H, Campana A, Balerna M, Domenighetti G, Hedinger Chr, Jakob M, Pescia G, Sulmoni A 1983 Mosaicism of dynein in spermatozoa and cilia and fibrous sheath aberrations in an infertile man. Andrologia 15: 295–300
45. Williamson R A, Koehler J K, Smith W D, Stenchever M A 1984 Ultrastructural sperm tail defects associated with sperm immotility. Fertility and Sterility 41: 103–107
46. Zamboni L 1987 The ultrastructural pathology of the spermatozoon as a cause of infertility: the role of electron microscopy in the evaluation of semen quality. Fertility and Sterility 48: 711–734

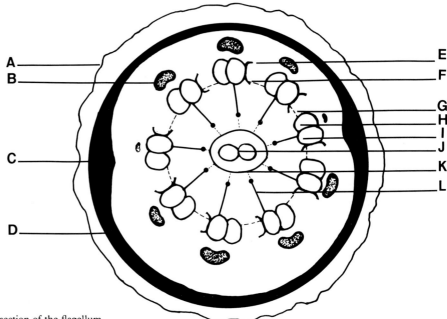

Fig. 18.1 Spermatozoon: diagram of a transverse section of the flagellum at the proximal end of the principal piece. A = cell membrane; B = accessory or dense fibre; C = longitudinal column; D = fibrous sheath; E = outer dynein arm; F = inner dynein arm; G = nexin link; H = microtubule B; I = microtubule A; J = central pair of microtubules; K = central sheath; L = radial spoke.

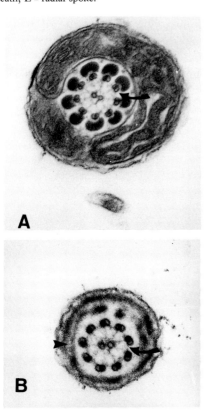

Fig. 18.2 Immotile spermatozoa: transverse sections of flagellum (**A**) at the level of the mid-piece, and (**B**) at the distal part of the principal piece. The specimen is from a 28-year-old male with 4 years primary infertility. Sperm count: 40–50 × 10^6 ml^{-1}; less than 1% motility with 65–70% viable sperm. Inner and outer dynein arms are absent from microtubule A (arrow) and there is some reduplication (arrowhead) of the fibrous sheath. (× 62 000)

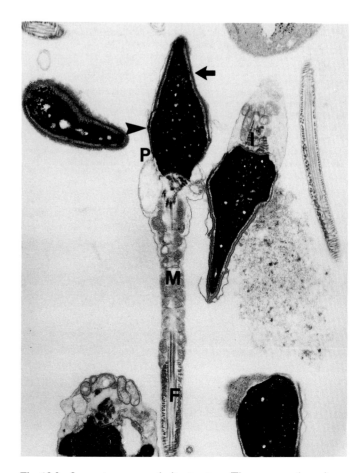

Fig. 18.3 Spermatozoa: normal ultrastructure. The acrosome (arrow), equatorial zone (arrowhead), post-acrosomal sheath (P), implantation site (I), mid-piece (M) and principal piece of flagellum (F) can be seen. (× 15 000)

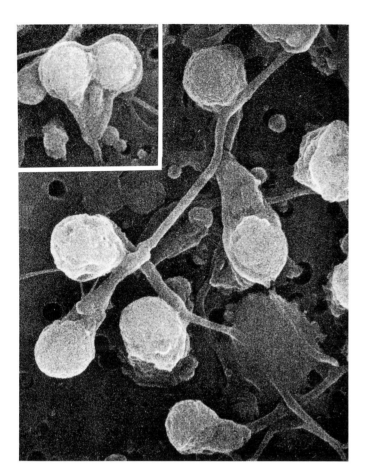

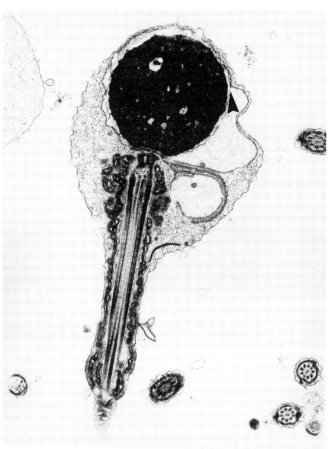

Fig. 18.4 Spermatozoa: round-headed abnormality. The specimen is from an otherwise healthy 28-year-old male with 18 months primary infertility. Semen volume 2.6–3.6 ml, spermatozoal density 25–44 M ml⁻¹, motility 21–39%. Light microscopy examination showed 90% with round heads. Scanning electron microscopy revealed spermatozoa which have round heads and lack the equatorial zone seen at the junction of the acrosome and post-acrosomal sheath. Many have redundant cytoplasm. *Inset* Double-headed variant. (× 6000)

Fig. 18.5 Spermatozoa: round headed abnormality. The circular nucleus lacks a covering acrosome and has separation of nuclear membranes (arrowhead) and redundant cytoplasm. (× 19 800)

19. Electron microscopy of the female genital tract

Suzanne Meleg Smith   Cecilia M. Fenoglio-Preiser

THE VULVA

The vulva is covered by keratinizing stratified squamous epithelium, the deepest layer of which contains elongated mitotically active basal cells forming the stratum germinativum. Ultrastructurally, basal cells have large nuclei and are attached to one another by desmosomes; hemidesmosomes attach the cells to the basal lamina. The cell membrane is convoluted and the cytoplasm contains dispersed tonofilaments, abundant free ribosomes, mitochondria, endoplasmic reticulum and Golgi apparatus. The overlying area, called the stratum spinosum, contains multiple layers of polyhedral cells attached to one another by intercellular bridges. The cells in the stratum spinosum are characterized by an increased cytoplasmic volume together with augmentation of the Golgi apparatus, rough endoplasmic reticulum and tonofilaments, in comparison to the basal layer. Lamellated keratinosomes, membrane-bound granules and keratohyaline granules appear and tonofilaments become more numerous. The next layer, the stratum granulosum, contains one or two layers of large granular cells with conspicuous keratohyaline granules.

Granular cells contain large bundles of tonofilaments associated with coalescent masses of keratohyaline granules. The cells are attached to one another by large desmosomal expanses. As the cells approach the horny layer they lose their desmosomal attachments, resulting in widening of the intercellular spaces and cellular desquamation. The most superficial and most differentiated layer is the stratum corneum which is composed of lamellated layers of horny cells devoid of nuclei. The surfaces of the squamous cells are covered by microvilli when the cells are immature; these convert to microridges with maturation. The epithelium also contains Langerhans' cells, recognizable by the presence of characteristic Langerhans' granules.[23]

NON-NEOPLASTIC VULVAR DISORDERS

Infections

Infections constitute one of the major disorders involving the vulva (Table 19.1),[6,7,9,11,14,18,22,26,33,37,49,50,53,54] and

Table 19.1 Selected infectious diseases of the lower female genital tract

Disorder	Causative agent	Histological features
Viruses		
Condyloma acuminatum Flat condyloma	Human papillomavirus	Koilocytosis, acanthosis hyperkeratosis, papillomatosis
Herpes genitalis	Herpes simplex II	Intranuclear inclusions, blisters, ulcers
Molluscum contagiosum	Poxvirus	Cytoplasmic inclusions
Cytomegalovirus infections	Cytomegalovirus	Nuclear inclusions
Bacteria		
Syphilis	*Treponema pallidum*	Chancre: ulcers, vasculitis, plasmacytis inflammation Condyloma lata: features of chancre and epithelial hyperplasia
Tuberculosis	*Mycobacterium tuberculosis*	Caseating granulomas containing acid-fast bacilli
Chancroid	*Hemophilus ducreyi*	Non-ceaseating granulomatous ulcers
Granuloma inguinale	*Calymmatobacterium*	Non-ceaseating granuloma, Donovan bodies, epithelial hyperplasia
Gonorrhoea	*Neisseria gonorrhoeae*	Acute and chronic inflammation
Chlamydial agents		
Lymphogranuloma venereum	*Chlamydia trachomatis* L$_1$, L$_2$, L$_3$	Thrombolymphangitis with focal necrosis
Non-gonococcal urethritis, cervicitis, salpingitis	*Chlamydia trachomatis* D–K	Acute and chronic inflammation

various diagnostic modalities can be used in their diagnosis. These include culture, serology, histopathology, immunohistochemistry, molecular hybridization reactions and electron microscopy. Herpetic vulvitis, HPV infections, vulvar warts, molluscum contagiosum and chlamydial infections are among the most commonly encountered infections. Histologically, productive herpes infections are characterized by suprabasal intra-epidermal vesicles filled with serum, degenerated epidermal cells and multinucleated giant cells, some of which contain intranuclear inclusions. Ultrastructurally, dissolution of cytoplasmic organelles with clumping of tonofilaments, loss of desmosomal attachments and widening of the intracellular spaces are seen, along with increased lysosomal activity. HSV virion[25,36] characteristics are listed in Table 19.2 (see also Ch. 9).

Vulvar warts are exophytic or flat lesions induced by members of the human papillomavirus (HPV) family. The typical histological features include the presence of koilocytotic atypia, acanthosis and hyperkeratosis. Cells containing viral particles show evidence of keratinization and large glycogen pools, with displacement of organelles to the periphery. Binucleated cells with hyperchromatic nuclei and cells with abnormal mitoses may all be encountered.[36,47] The viral characteristics are listed in Table 19.2.

Sato et al[53] compared the sensitivity of koilocytosis, immunocytochemistry and electron microscopy with DNA hybridization reactions in detecting HPV in condylomas and areas of intra-epithelial neoplasia. They found that HPV DNA was demonstrable in fresh tissues by Southern blot DNA hybridizations in all but one lesion of moderate dysplasia (98%). Koilocytosis was found in 80% of condylomas and in 20–89% of intra-epithelial neoplasias, depending on the grade. Immunocytochemistry was positive in 80% of condylomas and in 61% of intra-epithelial neoplasias, depending on the grade. Electron microscopy of preselected areas containing intranuclear inclusions demonstrated HPV particles in 90% of lesions.

Molluscum contagiosum is a virally induced lesion that may be venereally transmitted. It consists of hyperkeratotic and acanthotic lesions which histologically contain typical viral inclusions (molluscum bodies). These viral inclusions are most prominent in the upper horny layers. The characteristics of molluscum contagiosum virions are listed in Table 19.2 (see also Ch. 9).

Lymphogranuloma venereum is a contagious venereal disease prevalent in tropical countries and may involve the vulva. The lesion is caused by microorganisms in the Chlamydiacea group. These organisms undergo differentiation through three distinct phases. In the first phase, immature elementary particles consisting of DNA-containing nucleoids and surrounded by ribosomes and double limiting membranes are present. These transform into initial bodies with central fibrillar nucleoids that multiply by binary fission and multiple budding within the phagocytic vacuoles, forming polymorphic intracytoplasmic inclusions. Subsequent condensation of the initial bodies results in intermediary corpuscles which are transformed into elementary bodies initiating a new reproduction cycle.[17]

Other chlamydial infections are associated with severe inflammation, regenerative atypia and areas of cytoplasmic vacuolation. The organism can be stained with antibodies to *Chlamydia*.[11]

Bartholin's duct and Bartholin's duct cyst

The proximal two-thirds of the Bartholin's gland duct is lined by stratified transitional epithelium that is replaced by a stratified squamous epithelium as the duct approaches the vulvovestibular ostium. Transitional epithelium also lines the secretory ducts and ductules. The ultrastructure of the transitional ductal lining is identical to the transitional epithelium of the urinary tract. The cells nearer the basal lamina are low columnar and are relatively sparse in organelles. The middle layer contains enlarged cells, rich in cytoplasmic ribosomes, both free and bound. Perinuclear tonofilaments may be evident. The microvillous plasma membrane is connected by well-developed desmosomes resembling the spinous cells of the stratified squamous mucous membranes. Intracellular spaces are often dilated with numerous cytoplasmic projections. The desmosomes are small and randomly distributed. In the upper zone the

Table 19.2 Viral infections of the lower female genital tract

	Herpes*	CMV*	Human papillomavirus	Molluscum contagiosum
Viral type	DNA	DNA	DNA	DNA
Family	Herpesviruses	Herpesviruses	Papilloma	Poxviruses
Location of viral inclusions	Nuclei of superficial cells	Mononuclear cells, epithelium	Nuclei of: stratum spinosum stratum granulosum stratum corneum	Cytoplasmic inclusions predominantly in stratum corneum
Structure	Envelope 150–200 nm enclosing a 100 nm hexagonal capsid DNA core 50 nm	Identical to HSV	Groups round viruses	Compact brick-shaped, 230–300 nm envelope enclosing dumb-bell-shaped nucleocapsid

* Can be separated from one another only immunologically, by molecular probes, or by culture.

cells have abundant, smooth and rough endoplasmic reticulum, Golgi apparatus and prominent telolysosomes (autophagic lysosomes). The most superficial cells contain numerous lysosomes and are covered by stubby, irregular microvilli. Bartholin's glands are composed of cells that are histologically indistinguishable from those found in the endocervix. This mucinous epithelium contains numerous mucinous secretory granules and fibrillary bodies. Cells with a morphology intermediate between a transitional cell and a mucinous secretory cell are also present.[23]

Hyperkeratosis

Hyperkeratosis clinically appears as a whitish indurated plaque. Histologically and ultrastructurally a thickened keratinizing layer is present that is normal in its organization and there is no evidence of defective formation of the intracellular organelles or desmosomal attachments. Large masses of keratohyaline granules are evident.

THE VAGINA

Vaginal epithelium is exquisitely responsive to steroidal sex hormones (Table 19.3). Absence of oestrogens (as in the post-menopausal period) results in epithelial atrophy. A marked effect on the epithelium is also seen during pregnancy, when high levels of progesterone produce glycogen-rich intermediate cells as the predominant cell type.

Vaginal epithelium is non-keratinizing, but otherwise the cells ultrastructurally resemble those seen in the vulva. Epithelial renewal is the major function of the basal cells and is reflected in the prominence of cellular organelles. With maturation, the amount of cytoplasm increases and the nuclear size decreases. Bundles of tonofilaments as well as cytoplasmic organelles and large aggregates of glycogen are dispersed throughout the cytoplasm and are most prominent during the luteal phase of the menstrual cycle.[31] The nuclei become parallel to the surface; the surface microvilli transform into microridges. The most superficial cells have irregular, stubby surface projections and Döderlein bacilli may be attached to cell surfaces.[23]

Vaginal adenosis

Diethylstilboestrol and chemically related drugs were fre-quently administered to mothers of high-risk pregnancies during the 20-year period from 1940–1960,[43] and various structural non-neoplastic abnormalities are associated with their use (Table 19.4; Fig. 19.1). In addition, ultrastructural aberrations occur. Many of the cells in areas of adenosis resemble normal endocervical cells with the presence of fibrillogranular bodies. However, microvillous promontories (Fig. 19.1) on the surface of the cells, and cells with morphologies intermediate between endocervical cells and endometrial cells, are also present. The endometrial cells and the cells with a combined endometrial–endocervical morphology presumably are the precursors for the clear-cell carcinoma arising in the setting of vaginal adenosis.[21]

THE CERVIX

The native portio epithelium or ectocervix, like the vagina, is covered by non-keratinizing squamous epithelium responsive to steroid hormones in much the same way as the vaginal epithelium except that the former lacks the deep rete pegs seen in the latter. As in the vulva and vagina, the lowermost portion of cells adjacent to the basal lamina is referred to as the stratum germinativum.

At the time of menarche the transformation zone begins to form. This area represents centripetal replacement of the endocervical epithelium by squamous cells and generally occurs on the anterior and posterior cervical lips. As a result, the squamocolumnar junction moves inwardly with increasing age of the patient. Ultrastructurally, the transformation zone contains masses of stratified squamous epithelium that grow between the endocervical epithelium and its basal lamina.[23] These cells presumably arise from reserve cells within the transformation zone. The endocervical cells are replaced by the proliferating squamous cells and show evidence of degeneration. Eventually, desmosomal attachments occur between the squamous epithelium and the endocervical cells.

The endocervical canal contains mucin-secreting cells, scattered non-secretory cells and ciliated cells. The cyclic morphological changes that occur in the endocervical epithelium are not as conspicuous as those that occur in the endometrial canal or in tubal epithelium.[42] Endocervical secretory activity is both apocrine and merocrine. Mucinogenesis is initiated in the ribosome–endoplasmic reticulum–Golgi complex. Eventually, well-defined secretory granules

Table 19.3 Effect of hormones on vaginal epithelium

Oestrogens	Initiate proliferation
	Induce maturation
	Induce cornification
	Induce glycogen synthesis
Progestins	Induce partial proliferation
	Induce epithelial regression
	Induce glycogen synthesis

Table 19.4 Non-neoplastic conditions associated with diethylstilboestrol administration

| Adenosis |
| Cervical ectropion |
| Cervico-vaginal ridges |
| Structural abnormalities of the uterus |
| Structural abnormalities of the Fallopian tube |

are formed that are intermingled with granular fibrillar bodies. Glands are lined by single layers of mucus-secreting columnar epithelium with basally placed nuclei surrounded by a column of mucus. Typical mucus-secreting endocervical cells contain numerous tightly packed supranuclear secretory granules, fibrillar bodies and well developed Golgi apparatus. The luminal plasma membrane has numerous well developed branching microvilli. Ciliated cells lack evidence of mucin secretion but have well developed cilia and ciliary rootlets. Endocrine cells can be seen within this epithelium.

THE ENDOMETRIUM

Throughout reproductive life the endometrium undergoes cyclic alterations with concomitant characteristic histological and ultrastructural changes (Figs 19.2–19.5).[44,45] It is for this reason that histological features of endometrial biopsies are extensively used to classify and evaluate the physiological status of women with endocrinological abnormalities. Physiological doses of oestrogen stimulate the endometrium by increasing mitotic activity, cellular division and the rate of glandular, vascular and stromal growth.[34] This results from the binding of oestrogen to oestrogen receptors in the nucleus, and eventually DNA replication and synthesis of specific messenger RNAs and certain enzymes occurs.[20,27] As a result, the pre-ovulatory endometrium is characterized by active growth with the presence of mitoses in the glands, stroma and endothelial cells. As one might expect, during

the proliferative phase of the cycle one finds a proliferation of all cellular organelles associated with protein synthesis, which results in cellular hypertrophy (Figs 19.2 and 19.3; Table 19.5).

Endometrial cilia and microvilli are extraordinarily sensitive to physiological hormonal variations, and they reflect the presence of oestrogens within the cellular environment (Fig. 19.3).[3,4] Ciliated cells are thought to result from stem cell proliferation.[38] Ciliogenesis is associated with the presence of many dense proliferative elements called fibrous granules that are related to the Golgi apparatus. Later, both mono- and multi-ciliary vesicles are found.[34] The cells contain numerous mitochondria near the apical regions which are believed to provide the ATP necessary for ciliary movement. Glycogen aggregates appear also.

Other changes affecting endometrial cells include the transformation of the straight, lateral membranes to convoluted ones. At the time of ovulation invaginations are more frequent and extend more deeply into the cytoplasm than early in the proliferative phase. Junctional complexes occurring between the cells are similar to those seen in other epithelia. One may also find complex nuclear bodies, the formation of which is believed to result from high concentrations of oestrogen receptors.[34]

Once ovulation occurs progesterone levels begin to rise and the hormone binds to the progesterone receptor, inducing secretory differentiation of the glands and decidual transformation of the stroma, as well as cessation of DNA synthesis and mitotic activity. Within the endometrial epi-

Table 19.5 Ultrastructural features of the cycling endometrial epithelium

Organelle	Proliferative phase	Secretory phase
Microvilli	Numerous, straight, uniform	Degenerating
Cilia	Numerous	Degenerating
Nuclei	Oval, basal location, straight contours	Invaginated Nucleolar channel system
Mitochondria	Random distribution	Giant forms, pleomorphic Association with RER Cristae well developed
Giant lysosomes	Present	Present
Golgi	Poorly developed	Maximal development, then regression
RER	Scant	Well developed, contain fibrillar material
Microtubules and microfilaments	Scant; unorganized	Paranuclear bundles
Glycogen	Isolated small deposits	Abundant, apical
Free ribosomes	Abundant	Decreased
Lateral cell membrane	Straight	Convoluted
Annulate lamellae	Present	Absent
Lipid	Apical location	Increased
Autophagosomes	Rare	Numerous
Complex nuclear bodies	Present	Present, but few in number
Apoptotic vesicles	Absent	Present late
Mitoses	Present	Absent

thelial cells secretory differentiation is detected by a marked increase in the size of the Golgi apparatus, increased protein synthesis, and an increase in the number of free ribosomes and RER (Table 19.5). Secretory products begin to accumulate within the cells.

Histologically, the earliest recognizable post-ovulatory change is the appearance of subnuclear vacuoles on day 16 of the cycle. However, these structures are not indicative of ovulation as they may also be seen in hyperoestrogenic states.

At the ultrastructural level, ovulation is heralded by the appearance of the nucleolar channel system within the nucleolus (Fig. 19.4). It requires the presence of progestins for its development, and therefore is present only if ovulation has occurred or if progestational agents have been administered to the patient. The nucleolar channel system is a dynamic structure that is not seen before day 13 and disappears after day 26 of a standard 28-day menstrual cycle,[8,34,35] and is mobile within the nucleus.

Glycogen production is first found in a sub-nuclear location. However, as more glycogen is produced it accumulates on both sides of the nucleus (Fig. 19.5) and eventually is found only in a supranuclear location. It accumulates under the apical surface as small blebs in an area which is otherwise free of cellular organelles. These blebs become devoid of microvilli. Eventually the cell membrane ruptures, releasing the secretory product. Starting on day 25 of the cycle, the endometrium involutes, a process mediated by lysosomal enzymes. Autophagosomes form and there is breakdown of the glandular epithelium, stroma and vessels. Capillaries and arterioles rupture and apoptotic bodies increase. Apoptosis is believed to be a sensitive indicator of oestradiol withdrawal.[52] Ultrastructural changes in apoptotic cells include condensation and margination of the chromatin, cytoplasmic condensation, amoeboid changes in cell shape with the formation of pseudopods, and nuclear and cytoplasmic fragmentation. The cell fragments, also known as apoptotic bodies, accumulate near the basal lamina and are then phagocytosed by macrophages.[52]

Ultrastructure of stromal cells during the menstrual cycle

Even though the epithelial changes are the most dramatic, ultrastructural changes also occur within the stroma. The endometrial stroma contains numerous stromal cells, lymphocytes, macrophages, a mucoid matrix, collagen fibres, elastic fibres, plasma cells, and acute inflammatory cells. In addition, there are blood vessels, lymphatics and nerves. In the proliferative phase, the stroma undergoes changes that parallel those seen in the epithelium, with differentiation occurring toward a fibroblastoid morphology. The most oestrogen-sensitive change present in the stromal cells is proliferation of the rough endoplasmic reticulum, consistent with the induction of collagen synthesis by oestrogens.[34,58]

By the 20th day of the cycle the evidence of proliferation has disappeared and the cells assume a fully differentiated fibroblastoid morphology. On the 23rd day predecidual cells begin to form around the spiral arterioles. Pinocytotic vesicles are present along the cell membranes with abundant collagen synthesis being noted. Collagen bays are seen as early as day 10. Predecidual cells have luminous round nuclei and well developed Golgi, granular endoplasmic reticulum, mitochondria and free ribosomes. They are under the primary control of progesterone which is believed to stimulate stromal DNA-dependent RNA synthesis. Collagen synthesis is inconspicuous (Fig. 19.6) and numerous acid phosphatase-rich lysosomes contain fragments of partially digested collagen fibres.[16] Large bundles of undigested collagen fibres may be seen in the cytoplasmic matrix. Perivascular predecidual cells are separated from the endothelial cells by a narrow zone of collagenous stroma. Coincidentally with the formation of predecidua, the endothelium enlarges and perithelial cells with abundant microfilaments become conspicuous. The predecidual cells are bound together by gap (nexus) junctions.[23]

The endometrial granulocyte is thought to differentiate from native stromal cells during the luteal phase of the menstrual cycle and is also present during pregnancy. Liberation of relaxin from the granulocytes is believed to contribute to the dissolution of the stromal reticulin skeleton and aid in nidation.

Atrophy

Inactive or atrophic endometria obtained from postmenopausal women or from premenarchal girls consist of glands lined by uniform, low cuboidal cells with flattened surface plasma membranes covered by sparse, short microvilli (Fig. 19.7).[30,34] Secretions and cilia are absent. The cells contain numerous autophagic vacuoles, secondary lysosomes and residual bodies (Fig. 19.7). The overall thickness of the mucosa is reduced, as is the number of endometrial glands. The glands remaining are small and inactive. The type I cells have interdigitating lateral cell membranes and contain typical junctional complexes. The cells have rare cytoplasmic extensions, very rare cilia and transformation of the mitochondrial cristae into tubular forms. In addition, the RER is arranged in thread-like patterns. In type II cells one sees large numbers of organelles. The nuclei are elongated, often containing enlarged nucleoli, and the lateral borders show extensive interdigitations. Microvilli vary in shape and arrangement and are more numerous, longer and narrower on type II cells compared to type I cells. The ER is wider in these cells than in the type I cells.[30]

Endometrial metaplasias

Epithelial and mesenchymal metaplasias occur in the endometrium. Squamous, papillary, ciliated cell, mucinous, eosinophilic and hobnail patterns are seen with epithelial metaplasia.[28] Mesenchymal metaplasias include cartilaginous, osseous and smooth muscle cells. Squamous metaplasia resembles the squamous cells found in the area of the transformation zone of the cervix. Mucinous metaplasia consists of cells resembling those found in the endocervical canal, although they generally lack the typical fibrillogranular granules present in mucinous cells of the endocervical type. The ciliated epithelium resembles that seen in the fallopian tube.

Endometrium in patients with IUDs

Patients with IUDs may have focal erosion of the mucosa with the presence of large numbers of red blood cells, leukocytes and macrophages enmeshed in fibrin. The surfaces of the IUDs contain a crust composed of multiple layers of fibrinoid material and entrapped white and red blood cells.[3] Islands of atrophic endometrium may be interspersed with hypertrophic irregular cells.[34] Ciliated cells are reduced in number. Capillaries in the damaged surface of the endometrium contain fibrin thrombi. In addition there may be changes consistent with squamous metaplasia or chronic endometritis.

Endometritis

In patients with chronic endometritis, the endometrium may be out-of-phase and show both proliferative and secretory features. In addition, inflammatory cells, most notably plasma cells containing cytoplasmic immunoglobulin, are present.[10] The ultrastructure reflects the histological changes, with evidence of a proliferative, secretory or atrophic endometrium frequently co-existing. The epithelial cells may show evidence of degeneration and rupture with increased numbers of lysosomes. Intra-epithelial lymphocytes may be increased and the glandular basal lamina may be disrupted.

Changes with contraceptives

The histological and ultrastructural features associated with contraceptive steroids depend on the nature of the steroid used and whether the hormones are administered cyclically or continuously, whether they are given alone or in combination, the dose and duration of the hormone use, and the particular time of the cycle at which the tissue specimen is obtained for study.[34] Most oral contraceptives contain a mixture of oestrogens and progesterone. In patients who received the combined regime, subnuclear vacuoles appear earlier than in the normal cycle, usually by day 5. Secretory changes develop slowly and the glands may remain atrophic. Oestrogen-dependent functions are generally depressed, whereas the progresterone effects dominate the ultrastructural features. Large mitochondria, intranuclear canaliculi,

increased glycogen and RER characteristic of the secretory phase appear, although they are less prominent than in the normal endometrium. Patients on long-term contraceptive use have involutional changes. There is a marked decrease in the height of the endometrial cells as well as a reduction in the intracellular organelles.[24,59]

Hormone responses to oestrogen

The normal endometrium responds to oestrogens by proliferation, a response usually terminated by the antiproliferative effect of progesterone produced by the corpus luteum during the normal cycle. However, when ovulation does not occur, oestrogenic stimulation is unopposed and abnormal proliferations may result. Various terms have been used to describe these abnormal endometrial proliferations including anovulatory persistent proliferative endometrium (disordered proliferative endometrium), adenomatous hyperplasia, atypical adenomatous hyperplasia, dysplasia, atypia and carcinoma *in situ*. Since these changes represent a continuum of hyperproliferative abnormalities, the distinction between them may be difficult by light microscopy, immunocytochemistry and EM.[20] Furthermore, these abnormal proliferative responses occur most commonly in the same population of women likely to be taking exogenous oestrogens, making diagnosis even more difficult.

The treatment of the postmenopausal symptoms with exogenous oestrogens uninterrupted by progestins may promote growth of a proliferative endometrium which frequently deviates from the normal proliferative pattern. All of the endometrial components proliferate — including the glandular surface epithelium, the glandular luminal epithelium, stromal fibroblasts, and smooth muscle cells.[20,34] As a result, the total amount of endometrial tissue increases. The epithelial cells are columnar with nuclear pseudostratification and increased mitoses. Free ribosomes, RER, Golgi complexes, mitochondria, glycogen, lysosomes, cytoplasmic microfilaments, lipid bodies, surface microvilli and cilia are all increased and may become atypical (Table 19.6).[34] Endometrial glands bud and branch, resulting in the formation of a complex endometrial architecture. Active nucleic acid synthesis is associated with abundant euchromatin in the nucleus. The Golgi apparatus is often highly differentiated, often with little detectable glycogen in the cytoplasm. Large lipid accumulations may be encountered. Annulate lamellae may be present and found grouped within the cytoplasm.

If oestrogens are given during the postovulatory phase of the cycle the most prominent ultrastructural changes consist of disruption of the nucleolar channel system, with loss of the dense particles that are in immediate proximity to the channels and the particulate masses normally found in the nucleoplasm surrounding the channel systems. Giant mitochondria and glycogen are unaffected by the administration of oestrogens at this time, although less glycogen migrates to the apex of the cells than would otherwise normally occur.[1]

Table 19.6 Ultrastructural features of the continuum of endometrial proliferative states

Organelle	Proliferative	Disordered proliferation	Adenomatous hyperplasia	Carcinoma
Golgi apparatus*	+ +	+ + + +	+ + +	+ + +
RER*	+ +	+ + + +	+ + +	+ + +
Mitochondria*	+ +	+ + + +	+ + +	+ + +
Microfilaments*	+	+ +	+ +	+ + +
Cilia*	+ +	+ + + +	+ +	+
Microvilli*	+	+ + + +	+ + + +	+

*Show increasing pleomorphism and disorganization as lesion progresses towards carcinoma.

Stromal changes include prominence of the RER, Golgi apparatus and mitochondria, while stromal fibroblasts may contain lipids and lysosomal bodies. In fact, the presence of the lipid inclusions is characteristic of hyperoestrogenic states. Lipid-laden cells occur preferentially adjacent to small blood vessels.

Endometrial hyperplasia–carcinoma continuum

One can view endometrial hyperplasia and carcinoma as different points within the morphological continuum alluded to above, with progression through cystic glandular hyperplasia, adenomatous hyperplasia, atypical adenomatous hyperplasia, and carcinoma in situ and finally invasive carcinoma. At the extremes of the spectrum, the benign and malignant disorders are easy to diagnose. Diagnostic difficulties arise when one tries to distinguish adenomatous hyperplasia from well-differentiated carcinomas, or to attempt to define the specific point in this continuum where there is an abnormal morphology or ultrastructure that can be associated with aggressive pathological behaviour and evidence of clinical malignancy. Unfortunately, the changes seen within endometrial cells and their organelles by EM also represent a continuous spectrum, and therefore no objective standards exist for reproducibly defining this continuum into mutually exclusive subsets.

Endometrial hyperplasias can be divided into two biological phases: the proliferative and the remodelling phases.[20] The proliferative phase consists of increased numbers of cells and/or volume of the endometrium with only slight architectural distortion, and corresponds to the changes described above as disordered proliferative endometrium. Architectural distortions include focally dilated endometrial glands that can undergo concentric dilatation producing the characteristic changes of cystic glandular hyperplasia. It is presumed that some of the proliferating cells eventually escape oestrogenic control, accounting for their increased growth and the eventual development of adenomatous hyperplasia, resulting in more architectural and cytological abnormalities. The latter can be referred to as the remodelling phase which tends to progress and persist rather than regress, and may eventually develop into carcinoma.

By EM, the epithelium within the glands of disordered proliferative endometrium, cystic glandular hyperplasia and adenomatous hyperplasia shows progressive increases in oestrogen-related morphological and ultrastructural alterations, which basically represent an exaggerated normal proliferative response (Table 19.6; Fig. 19.8). Cilia, which represent one of the major oestrogen-dependent organelles, may show evidence of atypia. However, ciliar atypia is not helpful in recognizing abnormal proliferative states since it is also present in the normal endometrium.

Effect of progesterone

Endogenous or exogenous progesterone produces characteristic secretory changes within endometrial tissues. These include the appearance of giant mitochondria, the development of the nucleolar channel system, and the appearance of secretory activity as evidenced by the presence of multiple apical cytoplasmic protrusions and secretory droplets. Some authors have described the presence of progesterone-specific protein crystals that demonstrate a regular periodic pattern, which may be associated with the nuclear channel system or occasionally apposed to the mitochondria.[41] Progesterone induces the secretory conversion as well as the decrease in the length and number of microvilli, and ciliary loss.

The effect on the stromal cell results in the production of decidual cells resembling the decidua of normal pregnancy. Other stromal changes include nuclear enlargement with massive accumulations of the granular component, enlargement of the RER and increased free ribosomes.

If progesterones are administered during the early phases of the hyperproliferative continuum, the oestrogen-related morphological and ultrastructural alterations may be reversed. Progesterones inhibit ciliogenesis and microvillogenesis and transform the proliferative cells into cells with secretory activity.

Endometrial changes during pregnancy

Epithelial changes

Once fertilization occurs the usual endometrial cycling ceases and marked changes develop in the endometrial glands and stroma. At implantation the apical surface represents the association point with the primitive trophoblast of the blastocyst; it also serves as the interface between the maternal uterine lumen and the fetus. The apical ends of the epithelium undergo active endocytosis of fluid via the mechanism of pinocytosis with the formation of numerous pinopods.[19,39] This process plays a role in appositioning the blastocyst with the luminal epithelium and in interactions between the blastocyst and the endometrial stroma.

Early in pregnancy the Arias-Stella reaction occurs.[2] By EM the luminal surfaces are corrugated and the microvilli are less numerous and less regular than in normal secretory epithelium, with irregularities and thickenings. Cilia may be present but are abnormal. The cytoplasm membranes show great variability with complex interdigitations, or straight swollen membranes.[34] The intracellular organelles are well developed and mitochondria are small in contrast to those in other phases of the cycle. Glycogen is prominent and maintains an intimate association with the RER. The nucleus is generally irregular, with long finger-like projections of nucleoplasm and an increase in chromatin. Annulate lamellae may be present. As pregnancy progresses the epithelial cells become increasingly atrophic with low microvilli and prominent glycogen deposits. The nuclear changes result from nuclear polyploidy. These result from glandular hyperstimulation with oestrogens, progesterone and chorionic gonadotropin. The basal and lateral membranes show marked endocytic activity.[48]

Stromal changes

The most marked changes occur in the stroma-producing decidual cells, which have well developed RER. Gap junctions form between processes of the same cells to form structures known as reflexive gap junctions.[40] The cells have a large, pale nucleus with a homogeneous cytoplasm. The ER becomes maximally differentiated by six weeks. The plasma membrane develops projections containing electron-dense bodies resembling lysosomes that are associated with the formation of an extracellular coat material. Cells continue to differentiate until the 12th week. At the 22nd week of pregnancy stromal cells begin to degenerate with deposition of considerable basement membrane-like material, and at 28 weeks decidual cells contain short fragments of ER and Golgi complexes.[54] The mitochondria are small. At term, many of the stromal cells lie close to the epithelium and are surrounded by basal laminal material. Decidual cells may be binucleate and may contain multiple cilia with 2–4 ciliary processes. The cilia of endometrial stromal cells generally lack central filaments and they lack the dynein arms typically present in motile cilia.[56]

THE PLACENTA

Following implantation, the epithelium of the placenta organizes into cytotrophoblast and syncytiotrophoblast forming a complex system with multiple functions including synthesis, secretion and transport. Early in placental morphogenesis intervillous spaces form by the coalescence of lacunae in the primitive syncytium followed by the formation of primary, secondary and tertiary chorionic villi.[29] Primary villi are composed of cyto- and syncytiotrophoblasts (Fig. 19.9). Secondary villi result from the in-growth of fetal connective tissue, and tertiary villi are identifiable by the presence of their vascularized villous core. Once the syncytiotrophoblast of the primary villi invades the endometrial vascular structures, maternal placental–fetal circulation is established. Cytotrophoblastic cellular columns known as anchoring villi attach the terminal chorionic villi to the decidua and form the trophoblastic shell. Cytotrophoblast represents the generative compartment[51] for the mature syncytiotrophoblast whose function is the production of HCG and other hormones. Intermediate cell types are identifiable between the cytotrophoblast and the syncytiotrophoblast. At 8–12 weeks the immature chorionic villi are recognizable by the presence of an outer syncytial and an inner trophoblastic (Langerhans' cell) layer. They are supported by a loose myxoid villous core and larger trophoblastic villous sprouts are seen from the edges. Ultrastructurally the syncytiotrophoblast is non-dividing, and nuclei are dispersed at regular levels. The mid-portion of the cytoplasm, also known as the secretory zone, is filled with abundant dilated RER associated with free ribosomes, mitochondria, lipid droplets, glycogen and lysosomes. There are abundant organelles which are different from most steroidogenic cells.[4,12] The syncytiotrophoblast produces human chorionic gonadotropin, human placental lactogen and chorionic somatotropin. In addition to producing these hormones, numerous enzymes are present that contribute to the production and modification of the steroid hormones, principally progesterone, oestrogens, cortisone and aldosterone.[5,15,32,51] The syncytial cells form an uninterrupted cytoplasmic syncytium with the membranes attaching to the underlying cytotrophoblast by desmosomes. Cytotrophoblastic cells are lighter than the syncytial trophoblasts and represent the germinal layer. The free surface of the syncytium is covered by numerous microvilli of variable length, shape and number. These are well developed and microvillous promontories may be present.[23] The microvilli may also demonstrate branching and bulbous apices. In addition, active pinocytosis is present, providing a mechanism for the high levels of absorption related to the active fluid and ion transport occurring in the immature placenta (Fig. 19.9). Intermediate cells have more abundant organelles than those seen in cytotrophoblast, particularly with respect to rough endoplasmic reticulum. They are also intermediate in density between the dark cells and the lighter cells.

At term the cytotrophoblast is thin and almost inconspicuous. Similarly, the syncytial trophoblast is attenuated

(Fig. 19.10), but is still covered by numerous microvilli and microvillous promontories. The majority of the cells that are present represent syncytial cells with active pinocytosis, phagocytosis and prominent lysosomes.[23] Numerous capillaries are seen in association with the syncytial layer immediately subjacent to it, facilitating oxygen and fluid exchange (Fig. 19.11). The trophoblastic cells are separated from capillaries by a thick layer of basal laminal material. Large numbers of microfilaments are present within the syncytial trophoblastic cells, particularly located near the junction with the cytotro-

phoblast. The RER is quite prominent.

In the Nitabuch's striae, also known as the deciduotrophoblastic junctional zone, the adjacent decidual and syncytial cells degenerate and are separated by fibrin and amorphous fibrinoid material.[13,46,60] The fibrinoid is associated with numerous degenerating cells. Fibrinoid has a dense fibrillar structure composed of 30–45 nm fibrils with cross striations. The decidua contains large amounts of cytoplasmic microfibrils and dilated cisternae of the rough endoplasmic reticulum and Golgi (Fig. 19.12).

REFERENCES

1. Ancla M, de Brux J 1965 Occurrence of intranuclear tubular structures in human endometrium during the secretory phase and of annulate lamellae in hyperestrogenic states. Obstetrics and Gynecology 26: 23–33
2. Arias-Stella J 1954 Atypical endometrium associated with presence of chorionic tissue. Archives of Pathology 58: 112–128
3. Bank H L, Williamson H O, Manning K 1975 Scanning electron microscopy of copper containing intrauterine devices: long-term changes in utero. Fertility and Sterility 26: 503–512
4. Boyd J D, Hamilton W J 1967 Development and structure of the human placenta from the end of the 3rd month of gestation. British Journal of Obstetrics and Gynaecology 741: 161–226
5. Beck J S 1980 Time of appearance of human placental lactogen in the embryo. New England Journal of Medicine 283: 189–190
6. Blank H, Davis C, Collins C 1970 Electron microscopy for the diagnosis of cutaneous viral infections. British Journal of Dermatology 83: 69–80
7. Carinelli S G, Leopardi O, deVirgiliis G, Sideri M, Benzi G, Gilardi E M, Viali G, Dell Orto P 1984 Herpes viruses infections 1. The morphological spectrum of recent herpes virus type 2 infection of the cervix. Cytology, histology, immunochemistry, ultrastructure. Cervix 2: 127–134
8. Clyman M J 1963 A new structure observed in the nucleolus of the human endometrial epithelial cell. American Journal of Obstetrics and Gynecology 86: 430–432
9. Corey L, Spear P G 1986 Infections with herpes simplex viruses. New England Journal of Medicine 314: 686–691
10. Crum C P, Egawa K, Fenoglio C M, Richart R M 1984 Chronic endometritis: the role of immunohistochemistry in the detection of plasma cells. American Journal of Obstetrics and Gynecology 147: 821–851
11. Crum C P, Mitao M, Winkler B, Reumann W, Boon M E, Richart R M 1984 Localizing chlamydial infection in cervical biopsies with the immunoperoxidase technique. International Journal of Gynecological Pathology 3: 191–197
12. Dempsey E W, Luse S A 1971 Regional specialization in the syncytial trophoblast of early human placentas. Journal of Anatomy 108: 545–561
13. Dempsey E W, Lissey R A, Luse S A 1970 Electron microscopic observation on fibrinoid and histiotrophy in the junctional zone and villi of the human placenta. American Journal of Anatomy 128: 463–484
14. Douglas C P 1962 Lymphogranuloma venereum and granuloma inguinale of the vulva. British Journal of Obstetrics and Gynaecology 69: 871–880
15. Dreskin R B, Spiru S S, Griene W B 1970 Ultrastructural localization of chorionic gonadotropin in the human term placentas. Journal of Histochemistry and Cytochemistry 18: 862–874
16. Dyer R F, Sodek J, Heershe J N M 1980 The effect of 16B estradiol on collagen and noncollagenous protein synthesis in the uterus and some peridontal tissues. Endocrinology 107: 1014–1021
17. Eb F, Devauchelle G, Orfila J 1972 Etude ultrastructurele de l'agent de la lymphogranulomatose venerienne (Ricksiales, Chlamydiaceae). Journal de Microscopie 13: 47–55
18. Embil J A, Garner J B, Pereira L H, White F M M, Manuel F R 1985 Association of cytomegalovirus and herpes simplex virus infections of the cervix in four clinic populations. Sexually Transmitted Diseases 12: 224–228
19. Enders A C, Nelson D M 1973 Pinocytotic activity of the uterus of the rat. American Journal of Anatomy 138: 277–299
20. Fenoglio C M, Crum C P, Ferenczy A 1982 Endometrial hyperplasia and carcinoma. Are ultrastructural, biochemical and immunocytochemical studies useful in distinguishing between them? Pathology, Research and Practice 174: 257–284
21. Fenoglio C M, Ferenczy A, Richart R M, Townsend D 1976 Scanning and transmission electron microscopic studies of vaginal and cervical adenosis in DES progeny. American Journal of Obstetrics and Gynecology 126: 170–180
22. Ferenczy A, Miato M, Nagai N, Silverstein S S, Crum C P 1985 Latent papillomavirus and recurring genital warts. New England Journal of Medicine 313: 784–788
23. Ferenczy A, Richart R M 1974 Female reproduction system: dynamics of scan an transmission electron microscopy. John Wiley and Son, New York, pp 1–395
24. Flowers C E Jr, Wilborn W H, Enger J 1974 Effects of quingestanol acetate on the histology, histochemistry and ultrastructure of the human endometrium. American Journal of Obstetrics and Gynecology 120: 589–612
25. Friedrich E R, Cole W, Middelkamp J N 1969 Herpes simplex. Clinical aspects and electron microscopic findings. American Journal of Obstetrics and Gynecology 104: 758–779
26. Gissman L, Wolnik L, Ikenberg H, Koldovsky V, Schnurch H G, Zur Hausen H 1983 Human papillomavirus types 6 and 11 DNA sequences in genital and laryngeal papillomas and in some cervical cancers. Proceedings of the National Academy of Sciences 80: 560–563
27. Harkin J C 1956 Deoxyribonucleic acid (DNA) content of human endometrium. A microspectrophotometric study of the endometrial glandular nuclei in the physiologic cycle and in atrophy. Archives of Pathology 61: 24–30
28. Hendrickson M R, Kempson R C 1980 Surgical pathology of the uterine corpus. Major problems in pathology, vol 12. W B Saunders, Philadelphia, pp 1–580
29. Hertig A T 1968 Human trophoblast. In: Charles C. Thomas (ed) Springfield, Illinois, pp 1–363
30. Hopwood S, Levinson D A 1976 Atrophy and apoptosis in the cyclic human endometrium. Journal of Pathology 119: 159–166
31. Jaeger J 1969 New light and electron microscopic studies on cervical and vaginal epithelium. Archives of Gynecology 207: 55–58
32. Kaufmann P, Stark J 1972 Enzyme histochemical studies on mature placental villi. I. Differentiation and degeneration of the trophoblast. Histochemistry 29: 65–82
33. Kaufman R H, Faro S 1985 Herpes genitalis: clinical features and treatment. Clinical Obstetrics and Gynecology 28: 152–163
34. King G S, Yu X-R, Fenoglio-Preiser C M 1986 The normal and abnormal endometrium. In: Russor V I, Sommers S L (eds) Tumor diagnosis by electron microscopy. Field Rich and Associates, New York, pp 127–183
35. Kohorn E I, Rich S I, Hemperly S, Goreon M 1972 The relation of the structure of progestational steroids to nuclear differentiation in

human endometrium. Journal of Clinical Endocrinology and Metabolism 34: 257–264

36. Lutzner M A 1967 Virus diseases. In: Zelickson A C (ed) Ultrastructure of normal and abnormal skin. Lea and Febiger, Philadelphia, pp 365–387
37. Lynch P J, Minkin W 1968 Molluscum contagiosum of the adult. Archives of Dermatology 98: 141–143
38. More I A, Masterson R G 1975 The fine structures of the endometrial ciliated cell. Journal of Reproduction and Fertility 45: 343–348
39. Murphy C R, Swift J G, Mukherjee T M, Rogers A W 1982 Changes in the fine structure of the apical plasma membrane of endometrial epithelial cells during implantation in the rat. Journal of Cell Science 55: 1–12
40. Murphy C R, Swift J G, Mukherjee T M, Roger A W 1982 Reflexive gap junction on uterine epithelial cells. Acta Anatomica 112: 92–96
41. Nakao K, Meyer C J, Noda Y 1971 Progesterone specific protein crystals in the endometrium. An electron microscopic study. American Journal of Obstetrics and Gynecology 111: 1034–1038
42. Nilsson O, Westman A 1961 The ultrastructure of epithelial cells of the endocervix during the menstrual cycle. Acta Obstetrica et Gynecologica Scandinavica 40: 223–233
43. Noller K L, Fish C R 1974 Diethylstilbestrol usage: its interesting past, important present and questionable future. Medical Clinics of North America 58: 793–810
44. Noyes R W, Hertig A T, Rock J 1950 Dating the endometrial biopsy. Fertility and Sterility 1: 3–25
45. Noyes R W 1973 Normal phases of the endometrium. In: Norris H J, Hertig A T, Abell M R (eds) The uterus (IAP monograph 14). Williams & Wilkins, Baltimore, pp 110–125
46. Okudaira Y, Hashimoto T, Hamanaka N, Yoshinare S 1971 Electron microscopic study on the trophoblastic cell columns of human placenta. Journal of Electron Microscopy 20: 93–106
47. Oriel J D, Almeida J D 1970 Demonstration of virus particles in human genital warts. British Journal of Venereal Diseases 46: 37–42
48. Parr M B 1980 Endocytosis at the basal and lateral membrane of rat uterine epithelial cells during early pregnancy. Journal of Reproduction and Fertility 60: 95–99
49. Portnoy J, Ahronheim G A, Ghibu F, Clecner B, Joncas J H 1985 Recovery of Epstein–Barr virus from genital ulcers. New England Journal of Medicine 311: 966–968
50. Reid R J, Parkinson R P 1977 The histogenesis of molluscum contagiosum. American Journal of Surgical Pathology 1: 161–166
51. Richart R 1961 Studies of placental morphogenesis I. Radioautographic studies of human placenta utilizing tritiated thymidine. Proceedings of the Society for Experimental Biology and Medicine 106: 829–831
52. Sandow B A, West N B, Normal R L, Brenner R M 1979 Hormonal control of apoptosis in hamster uterine luminal epithelium. American Journal of Anatomy 156: 15–35
53. Sato S, Okagaki T, Clark B A, Twiggs L B, Fukushima M, Ostrow R S, Faras A J 1987 Sensitivity of koilocytosis, immunocytochemistry, and electron microscopy as compared to DNA hybridization in detecting human papillomavirus in cervical and vaginal condyloma and intraepithelial neoplasia. International Journal of Gynecological Pathology 5: 297–307
54. Sengel A, Stoebner P 1970 Ultrastructure of the normal human endometrium. II. The glandular cells. Zeitschrift für Zellforschung und Mikroskopische Anatomie 106: 245–259
55. Sehgal V N, Shyamprasad A L, Beohar P C F 1984 The histopathological diagnosis of donovanosis. British Journal of Venereal Diseases 60: 45–47
56. Tachi S, Tachi C, Lindner H R 1969 Cilia-bearing stromal cells in rat uterus. Journal of Anatomy 104: 295–308
57. Villee D B 1969 Development of endocrine function in the human placenta and fetus. New England Journal of Medicine 281: 493–533
58. Wienke E C Jr, Cavazos F, Hall D G, Lucas F V 1968 Ultrastructure of the human endometrial stromal cell during the menstrual cycle. American Journal of Obstetrics and Gynecology 102: 65–77
59. Wynn R M 1967 Intrauterine devices: effects on ultrastructure of human endometrium. Science 156: 1508–1510
60. Wynn R M 1969 Noncellular components of the placenta. American Journal of Obstetrics and Gynecology 103: 723–739

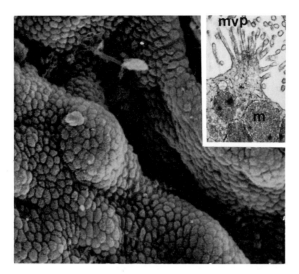

Fig. 19.1 (Left) Scanning electron micrograph of vaginal adenosis. The normal sheets of squamous epithelium are replaced by columnar cells which are largely endocervical and are covered by short microvilli. (× 265) *Inset* Part of the luminal aspect of a columnar cell displaying a well-formed microvillous promontory (mvp) and numerous mucin granules (m). (× 6600)

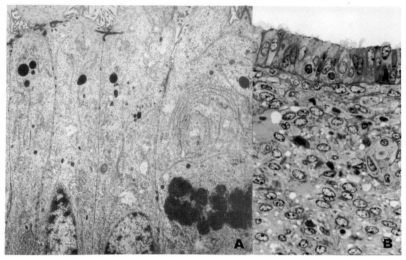

Fig. 19.2 Proliferative endometrium. **A** Ultrastructurally, mitotically active cells are present. The surfaces are covered with a sparse number of microvilli and cilia. The endoplasmic reticulum is proliferating and the cells which have straight, narrow borders are joined by numerous intercellular junctions. (× 3300) **B** The histological features of the proliferative endometrium are seen. (× 422)

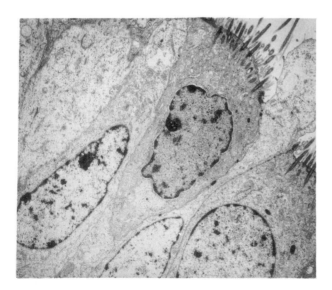

Fig. 19.3 Proliferative endometrium. Note the presence of numerous well-formed cilia and microvilli in between them. (× 4620)

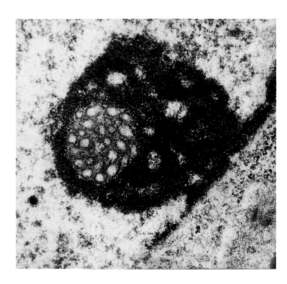

Fig. 19.4 Early secretory endometrium. A nucleolar channel system at high magnification. (× 39 600)

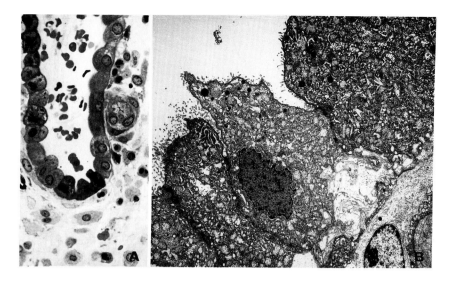

Fig. 19.5   Secretory endometrium. **A** The histological features as seen on thick section are demonstrated (× 422). **B** Ultrastructurally the presence of glycogen distributed throughout the cell, the appearance of numerous lysosomal bodies, irregular cell membranes, absence of cilia and decreased numbers of microvilli are seen. Secretory droplets are also evident. (× 2640)

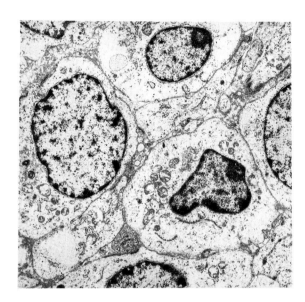

Fig. 19.6   Stroma during the secretory phase. Predecidual cells are evident. These cells have luminous nuclei and modest numbers of cellular organelles. (× 5280)

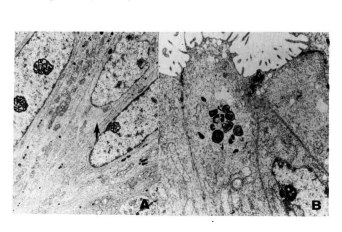

Fig. 19.7   Inactive endometrium. The cells are pseudostratified and contain numerous bundles of intermediate filaments distributed throughout the cell. The surface is covered by rudimentary microvilli and cilia are absent. Secretory activity is also absent. (× 3300)

Fig. 19.8 (Left)   Hyperplastic endometrium. **A** The nuclei are enlarged and contain active nucleoli. The intermediate filaments accumulate near the nucleus (arrow). (× 3300). **B** The presence of typical microvilli is shown. In addition, numerous lysosomal structures are present. The mitochondria are enlarged and pleomorphic in both pictures. (× 3000)

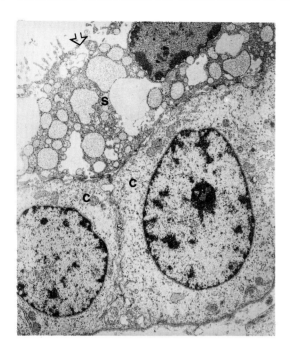

Fig. 19.9 Six-week pregnancy. Placenta demonstrating the presence of both cytotrophoblast (c) and syncytiotrophoblast (s). The syncytiotrophoblastic cells demonstrate the presence of active pinocytosis (arrow) with the formation of numerous pinocytotic vesicles. (× 5300)

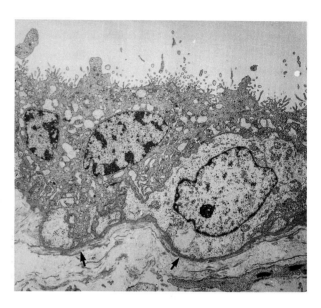

Fig. 19.10 Term placenta. The cytotrophoblastic cells are more compact than they are in the immature placenta and are covered by numerous irregular microvilli. The trophoblastic cells are separated from the underlying stroma by a thick basal lamina (arrows). (× 4000)

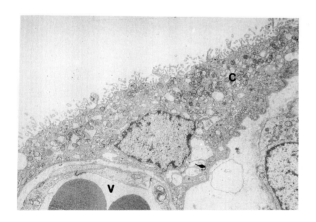

Fig. 19.11 Term placenta. The cytotrophoblastic cells (c) often overlie prominent vascular structures (v). (× 3300)

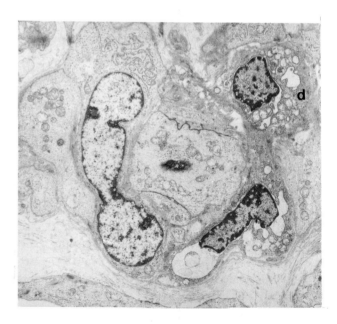

Fig. 19.12 Placenta. The decidual cells (d) in the stroma in the maternal portion of the placenta are markedly vacuolated. (× 4000)

20. Ultrastructural pathology of in vitro fertilization

A. H. Sathananthan

INTRODUCTION

Abnormalities of human in vitro fertilization (IVF) may occur at every stage of the procedure and lead to aberrant embryonic or fetal development, often culminating either in early abortion or the birth of an abnormal baby. Although the latter is very rare, the rate of clinical abortions is quite high, ranging from about 15 to 30% in major IVF centres.[27-29] However, many very early 'natural' spontaneous abortions go undetected, and 15% of all clinically recognized natural pregnancies are thought to terminate in spontaneous abortion. Furthermore, only 5–10% of embryos replaced in the uterus after IVF will actually result in a live birth.[28] Hence there is an inevitable embryonic mortality of 90–95% associated with IVF which can now be quantified and may be attributed to abnormal gametes, aberrant fertilization, abnormal development or to the IVF procedures in use — such as superovulation or culture conditions. Inherent genetic defects expressed by chromosomal aberrations such as triploidy, monosomy and trisomy, which can be diagnosed by amniocentesis or chorionic villus biopsies during early pregnancy, account for many.

Pike[13] has attempted to identify some of the biological risks associated with human IVF. The abnormalities in IVF may be expressed morphologically, biochemically or physiologically. Abnormal embryos may fail to develop in culture or they may slow down in development compared to normal viable embryos. Their gross morphological appearance observed by phase and interference microscopy and their rates of cleavage in culture are the main criteria used to assess their normality.[33] For a critical and objective assessment of the pathology of IVF one has to resort to transmission electron microscopy (TEM). Although invasive, TEM has been used extensively in our IVF programmes — initially to develop the technique, to diagnose gamete quality and function, and to provide clinical reports for patients having difficulties with IVF — and in ongoing research to improve and simplify existing techniques or to develop new techniques associated with IVF.

The normal morphology of ova, their penetration by spermatozoa and early embryo formation — including several abnormal features — have already been published,[17,22] and reference to these will be made. This chapter covers the ultrastructural aspects of abnormal oocyte maturation, gamete structure, fertilization and early embryonic development observed during human IVF since 1978, during which time over 600 ova and embryos, both normal and abnormal, have been examined by TEM. Some effects of the manipulation of ova will also be dealt with.

The human ovum is a fundamental, undifferentiated cell from which all other cells of the human body are derived after fertilization. Its abnormal structure and development might help towards a better understanding of the pathological process of various cells of the human body.

ABNORMALITIES OF OOCYTES AND MATURATION

Oocytes collected at laparoscopy or ultrasound-guided aspiration may already show degenerative changes (atresia), signs of ageing in culture or chromosomal aberrations associated with maturation.

Oocyte degeneration

Some oocytes have already degenerated in the follicle or may begin to degenerate during prolonged culture if they are not fertilized within 48–72 hours of collection. Those from follicles may be aspirated at the germinal-vesicle stage (prophase I) or at metaphase II — stages at which they are normally arrested during meiotic maturation. These ova show various degrees of vacuolar or lysosomal degeneration of the ooplasm.[22] The vacuoles, which are predominantly enlarged elements of smooth endoplasmic reticulum (SER) may be small and central in location (Fig. 20.1), or they may be very large, spreading throughout the ooplasm and eventually culminating in extensive or total disorganization of the ooplasm.[22] Germinal-vesicle oocytes often show secondary lysosomes, autophagic vacuoles and residual bodies. Nuclei and chromosomes of these oocytes may also degenerate presenting a pyknotic appearance (Fig. 20.2). About 99% of the two million or so oocytes formed in the fetal ovary and present at birth are destined to degenerate and are never ovulated during the lifetime of a fertile woman. Only about 400–500 oocytes mature and are expelled at ovulation.

Oocyte ageing and culture effects

Post-ovulatory oocytes may show subtle signs of ageing during prolonged periods of culture (24–72 hours after collection). Four different culture media have been used in this study,[22,33] which have similar effects. Hams F_{10}, Earle's, Whitten's and Whittingham's T_6 were the media used. Ageing unfertilized oocytes show progressive dilatation of vesicular SER, clumping of mitochondria, conglomeration of cortical granules at the surface and centripetal migration of these granules (Fig. 20.3). Oocytes more advanced in age have fewer surface microvilli — often stumpy and rounded in appearance — and show decreased pinocytotic activity as shown by the formation of caveolae at the oolemma (Fig. 20.4). Obviously these oocytes are physiologically inactive and may be on the verge of necrosis. Other ageing oocytes may occasionally reveal disorganization of the metaphase II spindle resulting in clumping or scattering of chromosomes in the ooplasm. The latter may eventually lead to formation of subnuclei or micronuclei (Fig. 20.5). These reflect chromosomal defects caused by ageing and may result in aneuploidy if the oocytes are fertilized. The incidence of chromosomal aberrations in the female is far in excess of that observed in the male because oocytes remain inactive within the ovary for as many as 12–45 years, arrested at prophase I of maturation, before they proceed to mature and ovulate. Furthermore, older women are more likely to produce abnormal oocytes and embryos resulting in trisomy or monosomy, causing major developmental defects such as Down's syndrome. More rarely, metaphase II chromosomes are deep-seated and may be associated with nucleolar inclusions and fewer microtubules (Fig. 20.6), which are normally organized into a superficial spindle in active pre-ovulatory oocytes.[18,22,40]

Oocyte maturation

Normally, germinal vesicle oocytes proceed to mature to metaphase II just prior to ovulation and fertilization.[18] Pre-ovulatory oocytes collected by aspiration are usually cultured for 3 to 7 hours or more before insemination to allow them to complete maturation. However, for unknown reasons, 10–20% of oocytes are arrested abnormally at metaphase I during culture; these do not extrude the first polar body, nor do they show a germinal vesicle, although they have resumed meiosis (Fig. 20.7). This may result in a considerable loss of maturing oocytes for IVF. Fertilization

of immature or postmature oocytes can result in polyspermy (vide infra).[14,17,22]

Another aberration of meiosis is nucleation of the first polar body (Fig. 20.8), which normally has naked chromosomes associated with residual microtubules, somewhat resembling the metaphase II spindle of the oocyte.[18,22,40] Such polar bodies may have one to five nuclear formations, and may occasionally also contain subnuclei. The second polar body which is formed at fertilization has a well-formed nucleus.[17,22,30]

Zona defects

These may be inherent or caused by physical stress during culture and handling of eggs. Normally the zona is composed of fibro-granular material embedded in a glycoprotein matrix and often shows a more compact and dense inner region.[22] Abnormal zonae show multiple fibrillar layers with intervening granular regions. Zona material may rarely be found trapped in polar bodies or within the cortical ooplasm.[22] Eggs sometimes show a compressed or distorted zona due to careless handling. The use of hyaluronidase indiscriminately to remove cumulus cells prior to insemination of oocytes in IVF[10] may erode the outer face of the zona, where the sperm initially bind before they penetrate the egg vestments.[4,17] The cumulus is removed to facilitate penetration of poor quality sperm or for micromanipulation of eggs. The zona protects the egg during the first week of development and prevents polyspermy at fertilization.[17,30]

Freezing damage

Excess oocytes recovered in IVF are now frozen by various methods for future use.[25,34] Initial ultrastructural studies reveal that some of the eggs have cracked zonae or may show extensive disorganization of the cell membrane and ooplasm.[25] These defects are caused by freeze–thawing and are mainly attributed to ice crystallization or osmotic effects of the cryoprotectants.[34] When the zona is damaged, follicle cells (Fig. 20.9) and supernumerary spermatozoa migrate into the perivitelline space of these oocytes, increasing the risk of polyspermy. Other subtle effects of freeze–thawing include possible loss of microtubules in metaphase II spindles and consequent scattering of chromosomes resulting in the formation of micronuclei as in pronuclear ova (see section on fertilization).

Microbial infections

A bacterial infection and virus-like particles have been detected in human oocytes recovered for IVF.[6,11] Three oocytes in culture were infected with a bacillus which was seen penetrating the zona pellucida and entering the perivitelline space. Particles similar to type C-virus have been observed in three other aspirated oocytes and were distributed along their cell membranes and surface microvilli.[6]

Spontaneous oocyte activation

Parthenogenetic activation is observed very rarely in human oocytes cultured in vitro.[14] These oocytes have a single pronucleus, may be haploid or diploid, and may proceed to cleave into two or four cell embryos. Normally fertilized oocytes have two distinct pronuclei (male and female) associated in the central or peripheral ooplasm.[17,21] Both nuclear activation and cortical granule release can be triggered by physical stimuli (heat, shock) and chemical stimuli (enzymes).[14]

Spontaneous cortical granule release has been occasionally observed in aspirated oocytes that were not inseminated for IVF.[15,20] The granules, which normally undergo exocytosis when the sperm fuses with the egg,[19] had spontaneously released their contents into the perivitelline space (Fig. 20.10). Oocytes accidentally punctured after collection discharge their cortical granules, showing that eggs have to be handled with caution. Cortical granules are involved in the cortical and zona reactions, which prevent polyspermy,[17,20,30] and their premature exocytosis might preclude fertilization. This, however, is not a problem in IVF.

ABNORMAL SPERMATOZOA AND PENETRATION

Various abnormalities can be observed in spermatozoa penetrating the vestments, cumulus and zona pellucida of the ovum. These include abnormal sperm-shapes and aberrations of the nucleus, acrosome, mid-piece and tail or various combinations of these features, often reported in semen[1] (see also Ch.18). Sperm may have double heads, pin heads, round heads or truncated heads and present a variety of abnormal forms.

Nuclear aberrations

These deformities include large bizarre vacuoles containing membranous profiles located centrally (Fig. 20.11) or peripherally (Fig. 20.12) pale chromatin or rarely partially decondensed chromatin. Sperm with abnormal nuclei may fuse with the ovum during polyspermic interaction[24] and these could cause genetic defects in the embryo.

Acrosomal abnormalities

Acrosomal defects include vacuoles within the acrosome, uneven thickenings (Fig. 20.13) or focal disruptions of this organelle, absence of the equatorial segment and rarely complete loss of the acrosome (Fig. 20.14). Sperm without acrosomes cannot penetrate the zona.[4,22] The acrosome produces hyaluronidase and acrosin, enzymes implicated in the penetration of the cumulus and the zona, respectively.[17]

Mid-piece and tail abnormalities

Defects of the mid-piece and tail are common and may severely impede sperm motility. Although sperm are used in large numbers and brought close to the ovum surface in IVF, hyperactivated motility acquired during the process of capacitation seems to be as important a factor as the acrosome reaction in penetrating the cumulus and zona.[17,22,39] The mid-piece may be totally absent, it may lack an axial axoneme or contain multiple axonemes. It may be devoid of a mitochondrial sheath or lack the full complement of mitochondria. Large vacuoles lined by membranes resembling annulate lamellae (Fig. 20.15) may be present. The tail may be absent or found in multiples fused to one another or to the head or mid-piece. Bizarre sperm forms may be seen penetrating the zona (Fig. 20.16). A variety of defects can be associated with the axoneme, including absence or disorganization of microtubules. Abnormal sperm penetration is more likely to occur in vitro than in vivo. Since many of our patients are subfertile, their semen contains more abnormal sperm than that of fertile men, which usually is in the range of 10 to 40%.

Sperm penetration

Both morphologically normal and abnormal sperm are phagocytosed by cumulus and corona cells during their penetration of the vestments. This may be an inbuilt mechanism to remove some of the weak or abnormal sperm before their interaction with the ovum. Abnormal sperm can bind to the zona and even penetrate it if the acrosome is functional. The acrosome reaction usually takes place by vesiculation of surface membranes (by intermittent fusion of plasma and outer acrosome membranes) as in normal sperm.[4,17,30] Sperm with intact acrosomes may find their way into the perivitelline space surrounding the ovum if the zona is punctured with a fine needle, but they are unable to fuse with the ovum (Fig. 20.17). Hence the acrosome reaction is an essential prerequisite to sperm–ovum membrane fusion, and sperm need to be washed and capacitated in vitro before they undergo this reaction.[19,24,39] Furthermore, a sperm injected into the perivitelline space by micromanipulation[7] is unable to fuse with the ovum unless its acrosome has reacted. There is also the chance of injecting an abnormal sperm during such micromanipulation because subtle sperm abnormalities cannot be detected by phase-contrast or interference microscopy.

ABNORMAL GAMETE FUSION

Various stages of polyspermic interaction with the human egg have been studied after mechanical removal or breaching of the zona.[24,30] This method has been useful in elucidating the events of gamete fusion, which appear to be more or less similar to those observed during monospermic interaction.[19] During polyspermic interaction, however, sperm approach the egg surface from all directions in the absence of the zona. Many penetrate the egg, usually head first (Fig. 20.18). When the zona is present, the sperm is held more or less tangentially close to the egg surface and is sometimes incorporated — posterior head region and tail first — which might suggest that sperm motility is not essential for sperm fusion and incorporation.[19] Totally immotile sperm from a patient with Kartagener's syndrome have been incorporated into zona-punctured human and hamster ova showing that sperm motility is not necessary for gamete fusion.[12] Sperm–oocyte membrane fusion usually occurs between the oocyte and mid-segment of the sperm, irrespective of the mode of sperm entry, followed by phagocytosis of the sperm by the ovum.[2,19,24] Thus the oocyte plays an active role in the incorporation of sperm during both monospermic or polyspermic interaction. The integrity of the plasma membrane over the mid-segment of the sperm head is essential for gamete fusion and any damage to it may be detrimental. Often the sperm plasma membrane appears to be damaged and this is frequently attributed to its sensitivity to fixatives used for TEM.

Gamete fusion has been observed with sperm showing nuclear defects and an abnormal sperm can be incorporated into an ovum (Fig. 20.19) during polyspermic interaction.[24] This proves beyond doubt that abnormal sperm can fertilize human oocytes and could give rise to abnormal embryos.

We have been able to fertilize human ova with epididymal sperm aspirated from the corpus epididymis[22] to produce a pregnancy in IVF.[32] Immature sperm have partially decondensed chromatin resembling that of spermatids[5] and are capable of zona penetration (Fig. 20.20). Both mature and immature sperm forms were observed in epididymal sperm aspirates and it is not certain which of these could have fertilized the egg. Immature sperm are also found occasionally in normal sperm ejaculates.

Sperm may penetrate degenerating oocytes but do not actually fuse with them.[17,22] These sperm have completed their acrosome reaction to penetrate the zona but do not form pronuclei, as their chromatin remains unexpanded in the disorganized ooplasm (Fig. 20.21). It is postulated that mature oocytes possess a sperm chromatin decondensing factor in their ooplasm.[30,39] This seems to be absent or inactive in immature oocytes and degenerating oocytes.

ABNORMAL FERTILIZATION

Polyspermy

The major problem associated with fertilization in vitro is the occurrence of polyspermy. About 2–10% of all oocytes inseminated and assessed for fertilization are multipronuclear[16,17,22,36–38] often caused by simultaneous penetration of two sperm (dispermy) or continued penetration by many supernumerary sperm. Polyspermy may be due to an inherent zona defect or an incomplete or delayed cortical reaction.[17,20,22] Dispermic ova have three pronuclei which may show incomplete incorporation of chromatin when arrested at this stage (Fig. 20.22). Other polyspermic ova (Fig. 20.23) may have up to 18 pronuclei crowded together, forming 'nests'. Polyspermy could be caused by insemination of immature or post-mature ageing oocytes.[16,36–38] These ova often show evidence of delayed cortical granule exocytosis, which consequently delays the zona reaction believed to prevent polyspermy.[17,22,30] Polyspermy may lead to abnormal or apparently normal cleavage[36] and is considered to be lethal in the human. Ova are usually assessed for fertilization 16–20 hours after insemination, and polyspermy can easily be detected with the laboratory microscope once the cumulus is removed. If this assessment is not done, one might inadvertently transfer two or four cell embryos derived from multipronuclear ova, which appear quite normal. Chromosomal studies confirm polyploidy and reveal that these ova have pronuclei with both X and Y chromosomes.[16] Suppression of second polar body formation or its incomplete abstriction can occur in multipronuclear ova.[22] When suppression occurs, the second meiotic spindle is deep-seated in the ooplasm and is not associated with chromosomes (Fig. 20.24). The second polar body is normally extruded at the moment the sperm fuses with the ovum.[17,19,22] Polyspermic eggs may begin to fragment early at the pronuclear stage (Fig. 20.25) or later during cleavage.

Micronuclear formation

Another nuclear aberration detected occasionally in IVF, particularly at the pronuclear stage, is the formation of micronuclei. These resemble pronuclei, and contain chromatin and even nucleoli.[22] Micronuclei could arise by incomplete incorporation of chromatin during pronuclear formation as observed in polyspermic ova (Fig. 20.22) or result from scattering of chromosomes in ageing oocytes, prior to fertilization (Fig. 20.5). Any change in chromosome number caused by non-disjunction during maturation or fertilization can lead to aneuploidy, and cause serious genetic defects.

Syngamy, regarded as the final stage of fertilization, may also show evidence of non-disjunction of chromosomes (Fig. 20.26). This stage, at which maternal and paternal chromosomes come together, is used for genetic studies if the embryo does not cleave after pronuclear formation.

Micromanipulation

Fertilization has been demonstrated by TEM for the first time with a single capacitated sperm introduced into the perivitelline space of a human ovum by micromanipulation.[7] Normal bi-pronuclear ova have been produced by this method. Such micromanipulation may become necessary for patients with the immotile cilia syndrome[12] (see Ch. 13 and 18), for those with very poor sperm motility, or for males having sperm without acrosomes, if they resort to IVF.

Fertilization of frozen oocytes

One of the most recent developments in IVF[25,34] is sperm–ovum fusion and sperm incorporation after insemination of frozen oocytes. The birth of a normal baby has been reported from an embryo developed from a frozen oocyte.[3] Gamete fusion occurs only when the oolemma is intact after freeze–thawing.[25] If damaged, spermatozoa penetrate the ooplasm but do not expand their chromatin as in the case of penetrated degenerating oocytes (Fig. 20.21). Hence both the oolemma and the sperm plasma membrane extending over its mid-segment must be present for successful gamete fusion.[19,24] Frozen oocytes show an increased incidence of polyspermy and micronuclei after fertilization.[25,34] Polyspermy seems to be due to zona damage (Fig. 20.9) while micronuclei (Figs 20.27 and 20.28) could be the result of disorganization of spindle microtubules of mature oocytes at metaphase II, which are sensitive to cooling.[9] Genetic aberrations may also be caused by 'solution effects' of toxic cryoprotectants used in cryopreservation.[34] Oocyte freezing is still in its infancy, and caution needs to be exercised before it is routinely integrated into an IVF programme. Critical methods of evaluation such as genetic analysis, electron microscopy, developmental studies using frozen mouse ova and appropriate clinical trials have to be conducted to validate the safety of the technique. Chorionic villus biopsies or amniocentesis should also be performed until a reliable method of oocyte freezing is developed.

ABNORMAL EMBRYOS

The main abnormalities of early development are associated with suboptimal or prolonged culture conditions, retarded or arrested cleavage and cleavage of polyspermic ova. Morphological changes observed in early embryonic cells are similar to those described for oocytes and may affect one or more blastomeres. Cleaving embryos from two to eight cell stages are usually replaced in the uterus after IVF. Gross morphological changes detectable by light microscopy include unequal, partially fragmented or multinucleated blastomeres. Asynchronous division of blastomeres may some-times result in abnormal embryos and occasionally cytokinesis may not occur after nuclear division.[17,22]

Culture effects

Effects of prolonged culture observed in early blastomeres are progressive swelling of vesicular SER and Golgi elements, and the formation of large vesicles associated with mitochondria[26,31,35] (Figs 20.29 and 20.30). Lipofuscin-like bodies, residual bodies and autophagic vacuoles may accumulate in ageing or degenerating blastomeres, similar to those seen in germinal vesicle oocytes.

Most abnormal embryos have anucleate cytoplasmic fragments or multinucleated blastomeres (Figs 20.30 and 20.31).[8,26,31,35] The nuclei resemble those of normal blastomeres and may occur in about 25% of the cells of a single embryo.[17,22] They can originate from polyspermic ova and possibly segregate passively into certain blastomeres during cleavage.[35,36] These embryos may continue to fragment, a process which begins in polyspermic ova (Fig. 20.25). In rare cases blastomeres may have micronuclei similar to those seen in pronuclear ova (Fig. 21.22). Partially fragmented embryos are not normally replaced in utero but some with small fragments, which are invariably found in most embryos, have given rise to successful pregnancies. It is conceivable that if there are one or two normal blastomeres in two to four cell embryos they may be viable, and a pregnancy might occur on transfer. One of the most difficult areas in IVF is the production of viable embryos with full developmental potential. The receptivity of the uterus to embryo implantation after hyperstimulation also plays an important role in determining a pregnancy.

Frozen embryos

Embryo cryopreservation also causes significant damage to cells of early embryos and affects their viability.[23] Embryos having more than half of their cells intact transferred to IVF patients have produced successful pregnancies.[34] Damage to embryos includes total destruction or disorganization of some cells while others survive freeze–thawing and show fairly good preservation of structure.[23] Subtle changes have also been noted in intact cells where varying degrees of disorganization or depletion of the cytosol is evident. These changes are possibly caused by ice crystallization and osmotic effects. The cytosol predominantly consists of water, and its disruption may also affect microtubules and microfilaments found in oocytes and embryonic cells. Micronuclei have also been detected in frozen embryos returned to culture after freeze–thawing.[23]

REFERENCES

1. Bartoov B, Eltes F, Weissenberg R, Lunenfeld B 1980 Morphological characterisation of abnormal spermatozoa using transmission electron microscopy. Archives of Andrology 5: 305–322
2. Bedford J M 1983 Form and function of eutherian spermatozoa in relation to the nature of egg vestments. In: Beier H M, Lindner H R (eds) Fertilization of the human egg in vitro: biological basis and clinical applications. Springer-Verlag, Berlin, pp 133–146
3. Chen C 1986 Pregnancy after human oocyte cryopreservation. Lancet i: 884–886
4. Chen C, Sathananthan A H 1986 Early penetration of human sperm through the vestments of human eggs in vitro. Archives of Andrology 16: 183–197
5. Holstein A F, Roosen-Runge E C 1981 Atlas of human spermatogenesis. Gross Verlag, Berlin
6. Larsson E, Nilsson B O, Sundstrom P, Widehn N 1981 Morphological and microbial signs of endogenous C-virus in human oocytes. International Journal of Cancer 28: 551–557
7. Laws-King A, Trounson A, Sathananthan A H, Kola I 1987 Fertilization of human oocytes by micromanipulation of a single sperm under the zona pellucida. Fertility Sterility 48: 637–642
8. Lopata A, Kohlman D, Johnston I 1983 Fine structure of normal and abnormal human embryos developed in culture. In: Beier H M, Lindner H R (eds) Fertilization of the human egg in vitro: biological basis and clinical applications. Springer-Verlag, Berlin, pp 189–210
9. Magistrini M, Szollosi D 1980 Effects of cold and of isopropyl-*N*-phenyl carbamate on the second meiotic spindle of mouse oocytes. European Journal of Cell Biology 22: 699–707
10. Mahadevan M, Trounson A 1985 Removal of cumulus cells around the human oocyte using bovine hyaluronidase. Fertility Sterility 43: 263–267
11. Ng S C, Edirisinghe W R, Sathananthan A H, Anandakumar C, Ratnam S S 1987 Bacterial infection of human oocytes during in vitro fertilization. International Journal of Fertility 32: 298–301
12. Ng S C, Sathananthan A H, Edirisinghe W R, Ho K C J, Wong P C, Ratnam S S, Ganatra S Fertilization of a human egg with sperm from a patient with immotile cilia syndrome: case report In: Ratnam S S, Teoh E S, Anandakumar C (eds) advances in Fertility and Sterility. Parthenon, Lancaster 4: 71–76
13. Pike I L 1984 Biological risks of in vitro fertilization and embryo transfer. In: Wood C, Trounson A (eds) Clinical in vitro fertilization. Springer-Verlag, Berlin, pp 137–146
14. Plachot M, Mandelbaum J, Junca A M, Salat-Boroux J, Cohen J 1985 Impairment of human embryo development after abnormal in vitro fertilizatlon. Annals of the New York Academy of Sciences 442: 336–341
15. Rousseau P, Meda P, Lecart C, Haumont S, Ferin J 1977 Cortical granule release in human follicular oocytes. Biology of Reproduction 16: 104–111
16. Rudak E, Dor J, Mashiach S, Nebel L, Goldman B 1984 Chromosome analysis of multipronuclear human oocytes fertilized in vitro. Fertility Sterility 41: 538–545
17. Sathananthan A H 1984 Ultrastructural morphology of fertilization and early cleavage in the human. In: Trounson A, Wood C (eds) In vitro fertilization and embryo transfer. Churchill Livingstone, London, pp 131–158
18. Sathananthan A H 1985 Maturation of the human oocyte: nuclear I. events during meiosis (an ultrastructural study). Gamete Research 12: 237–254
19. Sathananthan A H, Chen C 1986 Sperm oocyte membrane fusion in the human during monospermic fertilization. Gamete Research 15: 177–186
20. Sathananthan A H, Trounson A O 1982 Ultrastructure of cortical granule release and zona interaction in monospermic and polyspermic human ova fertilized in vitro. Gamete Research 6: 225–234

21. Sathananthan A H, Trounson A O 1985 The human pronuclear ovum: fine structure of monospermic and polyspermic fertilization in vitro. Gamete Research 12: 385–398
22. Sathananthan A H, Trounson A O, Wood C 1986 Atlas of fine structure of human sperm penetration, eggs and embryos cultured in vitro. Praeger Scientific, Philadelphia
23. Sathananthan A H, Trounson A 1986 Effects of culture and cryopreservation on human oocyte and embryo ultrastructure and function. In: Van Blerkom J, Motta P M (eds) Ultrastructure of Human gametogenesis and embryogenesis. Kluwer, Massachusetts, pp 181–199
24. Sathananthan A H, Ng S C, Edirisinghe R, Ratnam S S, Wong P C 1986 Human sperm–egg interaction in vitro. Gamete Research 15: 317–326
25. Sathananthan A H, Trounson A O, Freeman L 1987 Morphology and fertilizability of frozen human oocytes 16: 343–354
26. Sathananthan A H, Wood C, Leeton J 1982 Ultrastructural evaluation of 8–16 cell human embryos developed in vitro. Micron 13: 193–203
27. Schulman J D, Dorfmann A, Evans M I 1985 Genetic aspects of in vitro fertilization. Annals of the New York Academy of Sciences 442: 446–475
28. Seppala M 1985 The world collaborative report on in vitro fertilization and embryo replacement: current state of the art in January 1984. Annals of the New York Academy of Sciences 442: 558–563
29. Soules M R 1985 The in vitro fertilization pregnancy rate: let's be honest with one another. Fertility Sterility 43: 511–513
30. Soupart P 1980 Fertilization. In: Hafez E S E (ed) Human reproduction: conception and contraception. Harper and Row, New York, pp 453–470
31. Sundstrom P, Nilsson O, Liedholm P 1981 Cleavage rate and morphology of early human embryos obtained after artificial fertilization and culture. Acta Obstetrica Gynecologica, Scandinavica 60: 109–120
32. Temple-Smith P D, Southwick G J, Yates C A, Trounson A O, de Kretser D M 1986 Human pregnancy by in vitro fertilization (IVF) using sperm aspirated from the epididymis. Journal of In Vitro Fertilization and Embryo Transfer 2: 119–122
33. Trounson A 1984 In vitro fertilization and embryo development. In: Trounson A, Wood C (eds) In vitro fertilization and embryo transfer. Churchill Livingstone, London, pp 111–130
34. Trounson A 1986 Preservation of human eggs and embryos. Fertility Sterility 46: 1–12
35. Trounson A O, Sathananthan A H 1984 The application of electron microscopy in the evaluation of 2–4 cell human embryos cultured in vitro for embryo transfer. Journal of In Vitro Fertilization and Embyro Transfer 1: 153–165
36. Van Blerkom J, Henry G P, Porreco R P 1984 Pre-implantation human embryonic development from polynuclear eggs after in vitro fertilization. Fertility Sterility 41: 686–696
37. Van Der Ven H H, Al-Hasani S, Diedrich K, Hamerich U, Lehmann F, Krebs D 1985 Polyspermy in in vitro fertilization of human oocytes: frequency and possible causes. Annals of the New York Academy of Sciences 442: 88–95
38. Veeck L L 1985 Extracorporeal maturation: Norfolk, 1984. Annals of the New York Academy of Sciences 442: 357–367
39. Yanagimachi R 1981 Mechanisms of fertilization in mammals. In: Mastroianni L Jr, Biggers J D (eds) Fertilization and embryonic development in vitro. Plenum Press, New York, pp 82–182
40. Zamboni L, Thompson R S, Moore Smith D 1972 Fine morphology of human oocyte maturation in vitro. Biology of Reproduction 7: 425–457

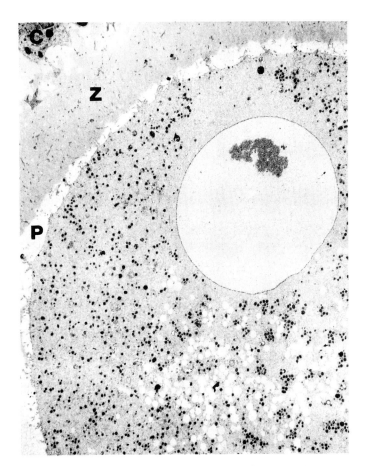

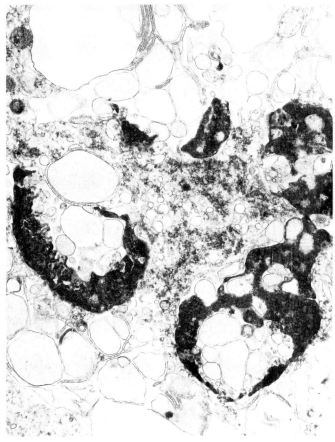

Fig. 20.1 (Above)   Immature oocyte: early atresia. Germinal-vesicle oocyte resuming meiosis after arrest at prophase I of maturation. The ooplasm shows centralized vacuolation indicating early atresia. The nucleus has condensed chromatin and has moved toward the periphery (3 h in culture). C = corona cell; P = perivitelline space; Z = zona pellucida. (× 2000) From Sathananthan et al.[22]

Fig. 20.2 (Above right)   Oocyte: degenerative changes. Oocyte at a more advanced stage of degeneration (66 h in culture). The chromatin is clumped and presents a pyknotic appearance, while the cytoplasm is extensively vacuolated. (× 13 100) From Sathananthan et al[22]

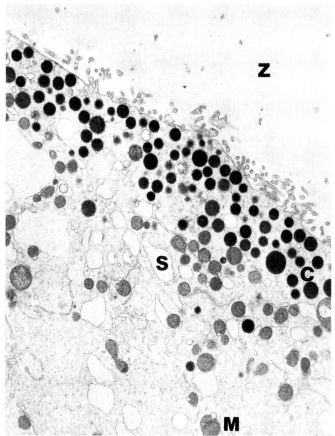

Fig. 20.3 (Right)   Maturing oocyte: aged in culture for 76 hours. Numerous cortical granules (C) are located close to the surface, and vesicular elements of SER (S) show progressive swelling to form larger vacuoles. M = mitochondria, Z = zona pellucida. (× 10 300) From Sathananthan et al.[22]

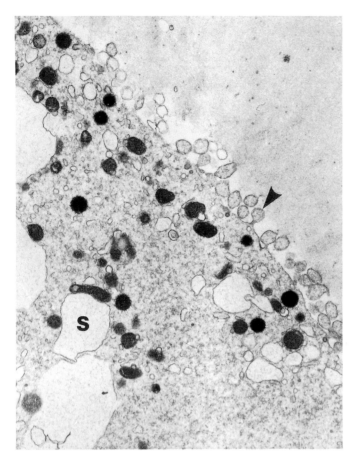

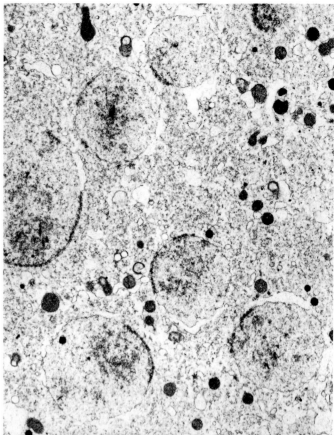

Fig. 20.4 (Above) Ageing oocyte: surface of ageing oocyte (66 h in culture). The microvilli are rounded and stumpy (arrow), while the vesicular SER (S) is dilated. (× 10 300) From Sathananthan et al.[22]

Fig. 20.5 (Above right) Ageing oocyte: in culture for 72 hours exhibiting many micronuclei. Each micronucleus has an envelope and specks of chromatin. (× 10 300) From Sathananthan et al.[22]

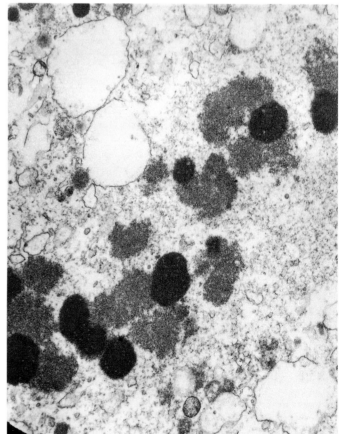

Fig. 20.6 (Right) Ageing oocyte: showing chromosomes associated with dense nucleolar bodies. The cytoplasm is vacuolated (66 h in culture). (× 13 100)

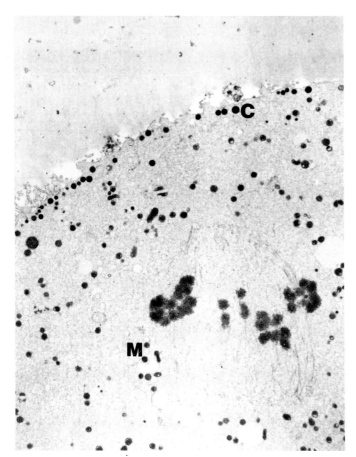

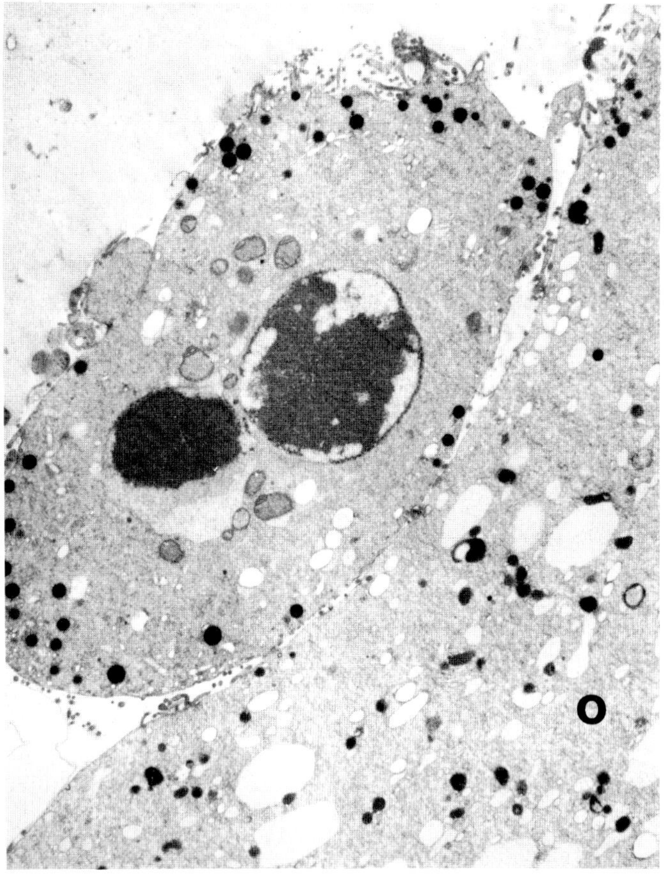

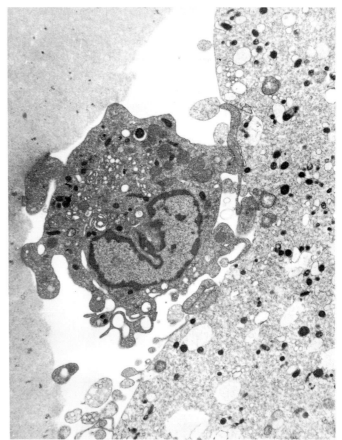

Fig. 20.7 (Above) Mature oocyte: arrested at metaphase I of meiosis (24 h in culture). The chromosomes seen in pairs are associated with spindle microtubules. There are no centrioles or asters in oocytes. C = cortical granules; M = mitochondria. (× 4700) From Sathananthan.[18]

Fig. 20.8 (Above right) Mature oocyte: nucleated polar body. Abnormal nucleated polar body of a mature oocyte (66 h in culture). The two nuclei have condensed chromatin. Note cortical granules at the periphery of the oocyte, which is normal. O = ooplasm. (× 4700)

Fig. 20.9 (Right) Frozen fast-thawed oocyte: cumulus cell. Cumulus cell that has migrated into the perivitelline space of an ovum; note the breach in the zona. The cell has pseudopod-like processes. Many sperm are also seen in this space. (× 7900) From Sathananthan et al.[25]

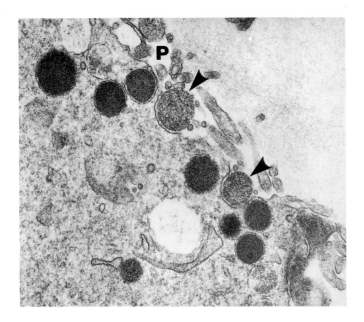

Fig. 20.10 Immature oocyte: cortical granule discharge. Spontaneous exocytosis (arrows) of cortical granules of an immature oocyte into its perivitelline space (P). Intact cortical granules are also seen close to the oolemma (not inseminated). (× 25 700) From Sathananthan et al.[22]

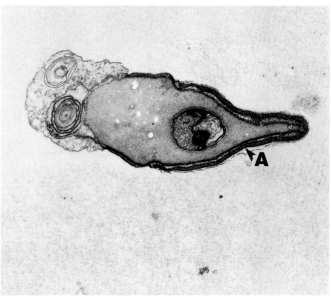

Fig. 20.11 Fertilized oocyte: abnormal sperm. Abnormal sperm bound to the zona of a fertilized ovum (3 h after insemination). Its nucleus has a central vacuole containing membranous and granular inclusions. The acrosome (A) is intact. (× 18 200)

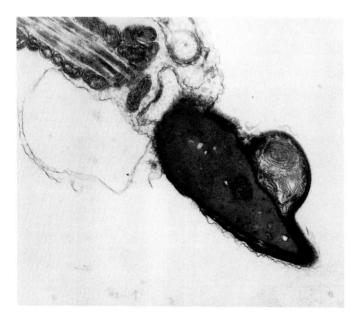

Fig. 20.12 Fertilized oocyte: abnormal sperm. Abnormal sperm entering the zona of a fertilized ovum (3 h after insemination). A peripheral vacuole with concentric lamellae, probably arising from the nuclear envelope, is seen beneath its acrosome. (× 18 200)

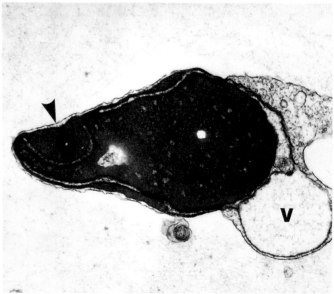

Fig. 20.13 Polyspermic oocyte: abnormal sperm. Abnormal sperm with an unevenly thickened acrosome in the outer zona of a polyspermic ovum (44 h post-insemination). Its plasma membrane is intact (arrow) and a distended vacuole (V) arising from the nuclear envelope is seen in the mid-piece. (× 23 800)

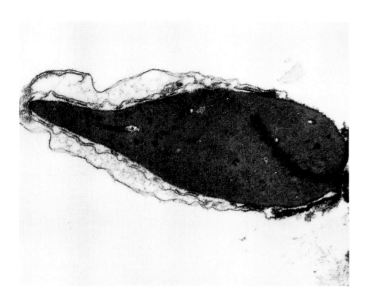

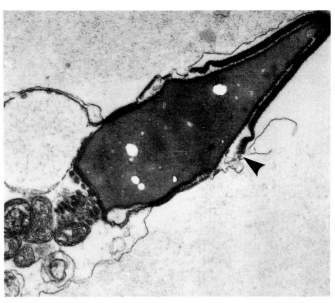

Fig. 20.14 Polyspermic ovum: abnormal sperm. Abnormal sperm at the surface of the zona of a polyspermic ovum (60 h post-insemination). It has no acrosome but the plasma membrane is intact. (× 23 800)

Fig. 20.15 Fertilized ovum: abnormal sperm. Sperm with an abnormal mid-piece in the outer zona of a fertilized ovum (3 h post-insemination). The mitochondrial sheath and the equatorial segment of the acrosome (arrow) are disorganized. (× 23 800)

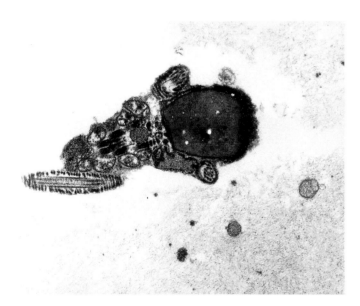

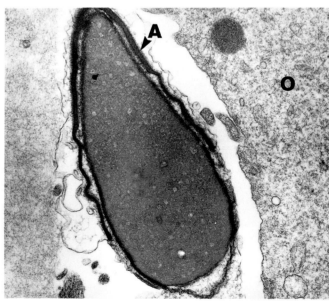

Fig. 20.16 Polyspermic ovum: abnormal sperm. Bizarre sperm attempting to penetrate the zona of a polyspermic ovum (60 h post-insemination). Its tail has fused with both sides of its head, which is truncated. (× 18 200) From Sathananthan et al.[22]

Fig. 20.17 Non-fertilized ovum: failure of sperm acrosome reaction. Sperm with an intact acrosome (A) within the perivitelline space of a zona-punctured oocyte (3 h after insemination). The sperm is unable to fuse with the ovum (O) because the acrosome has not reacted. (× 25 700)

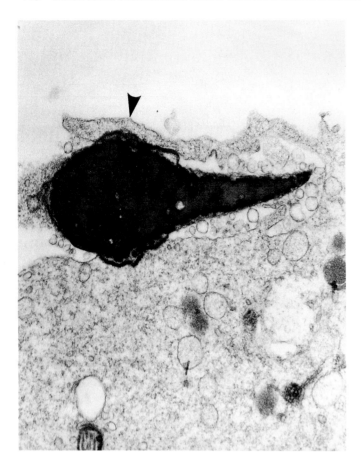

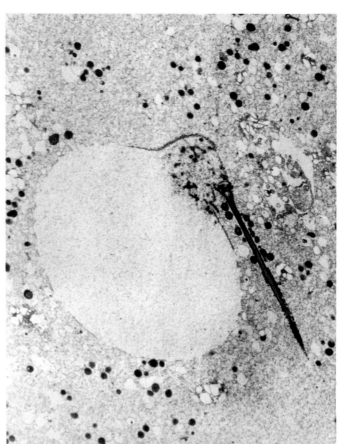

Fig. 20.18 Polyspermic ovum: gamete membrane fusion. Sperm–egg membrane fusion in a polyspermic ovum denuded of its zona (3 h after insemination). Gamete fusion has already taken place between the plasma membrane over the mid-segment of the sperm head (arrows) and the oolemma. The acrosome has just reacted by vesiculation, and the sperm is being engulfed by a process (arrow) extended by the ovum. (× 23 800) From Sathananthan et al.[24]

Fig. 20.19 Polyspermic ovum: abnormal sperm. Abnormal sperm incorporated into the ooplasm of the polyspermic ovum depicted in Fig. 20.18. The sperm is shaped like a shrimp and its nucleus has decondensed its chromatin to form a pronucleus. (× 4700)

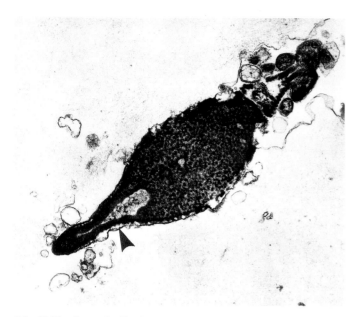

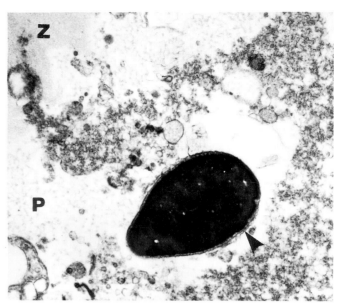

Fig. 20.20 Ovum: fertilization by immature sperm. An immature sperm aspirated from the corpus epididymis penetrating the outer zona of a fertilized pronuclear ovum (70 h post-insemination). Its acrosome has reacted by vesiculation exposing the inner acrosome membrane (arrow). Note that its chromatin has not fully condensed. (× 18 200) From Sathananthan et al.[22]

Fig. 20.21 Degenerated ovum: penetration by spermatozoon. Penetrated sperm within the ooplasm of a degenerated oocyte (60 h post-insemination). The post-acrosomal region of the sperm head is still intact (arrow) indicating that gamete fusion has not occurred. P = perivitelline space; Z = zona. (× 18 200) From Sathananthan et al.[22]

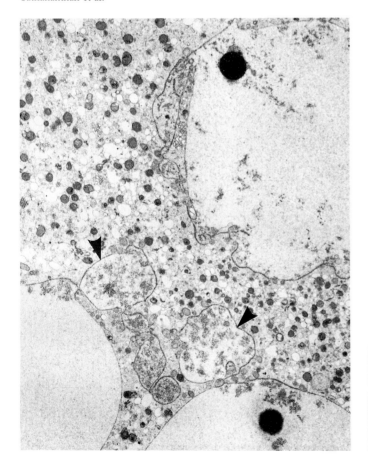

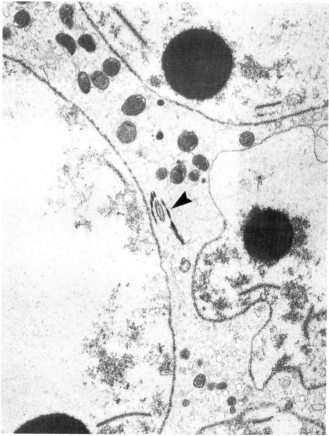

Fig. 20.22 Ovum: dispermy. Dispermic ovum showing three pronuclei and incomplete incorporation of chromatin (arrows) 60 hours after insemination. (× 4700) From Sathananthan.[17]

Fig. 20.23 Ovum: polyspermy. Four pronuclei of a polyspermic ovum associated with a sperm tail (arrow). Pronuclei have dense nucleoli associated with chromatin (60 h post-insemination). (× 10 300) From Sathananthan.[17]

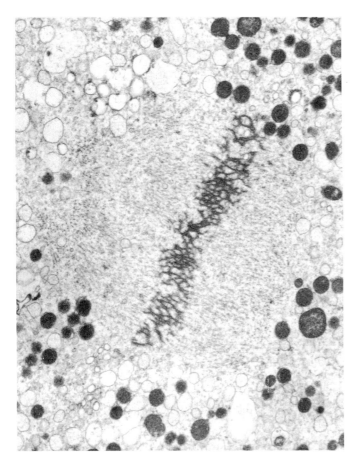

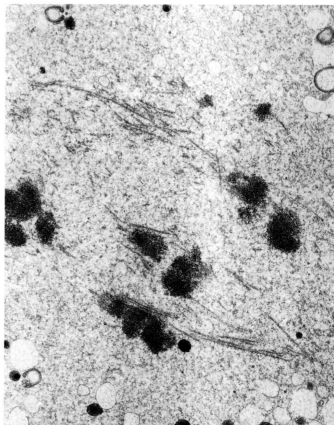

Fig. 20.24 (Above)   Ovum: polyspermy. Second meiotic spindle deep into the ooplasm of a polyspermic ovum denuded of its zona (3 h post-insemination). There were no chromosomes associated with spindle microtubules. The dense reticulum represents the interbody in oblique section. (× 13 100)

Fig. 20.25 (Above right)   Ovum: polyspermy. Cytoplasmic fragments of a polyspermic ovum (72 h post-insemination). These fragments have no nuclei, and were found adjacent to polar bodies. (× 4700)

Fig. 20.26 (Right)   Fertilized ovum: spindle. First cleavage spindle of a fertilized ovum arrested at syngamy (40 h post-insemination). Three pairs of chromatids are separating at the equator while the pair toward one pole has not separated (possible non-disjunction). The spindle microtubules are somewhat disorganized. (× 10 300) From Sathananthan & Trounson.[21]

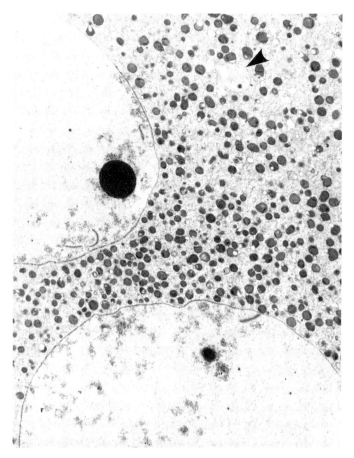

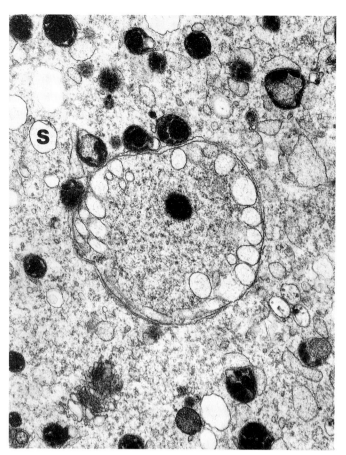

Fig. 20.27 (Above)   Fertilized ovum: two pronuclei. Abnormal bi-pronuclear ovum derived from a vitrified oocyte (18 h post-thaw insemination). A micronucleus (arrow) is seen in the ooplasm. (× 4700). From Sathananthan et al.[25]

Fig. 20.28 (Above right)   Vitrified oocytes: polyspermy, with micronucleus. A micronucleus in the ooplasm of a polyspermic ovum developed from a vitrified oocyte (18 h post-thaw insemination). It has an envelope, nucleolus and vesicular profiles similar to vesicular SER (S). (× 18 200) From Sathananthan et al.[25]

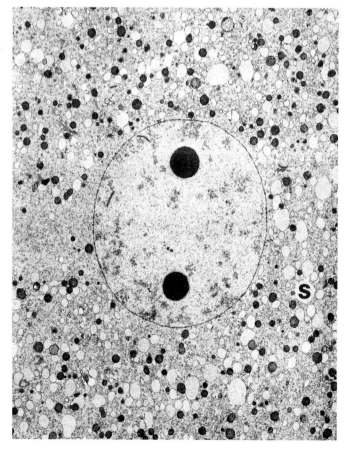

Fig. 20.29 (Right)   Two-cell embryo. Blastomere of a two-cell embryo showing progressive swelling of vesicular SER (S) in its cytoplasm (44 h post-insemination). (× 4700)

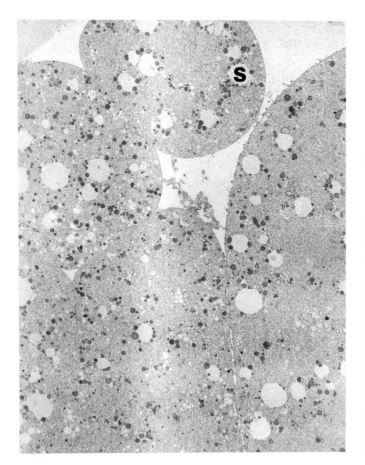

Fig. 20.30 Two-cell embryo: fragmented blastomere. Sixty hours post-insemination. The fragments are enucleated and are adjacent to the intact blastomere. The vesicles are dilated SER (s) associated with mitochondria. (× 2000) From Sathananthan et al.[22]

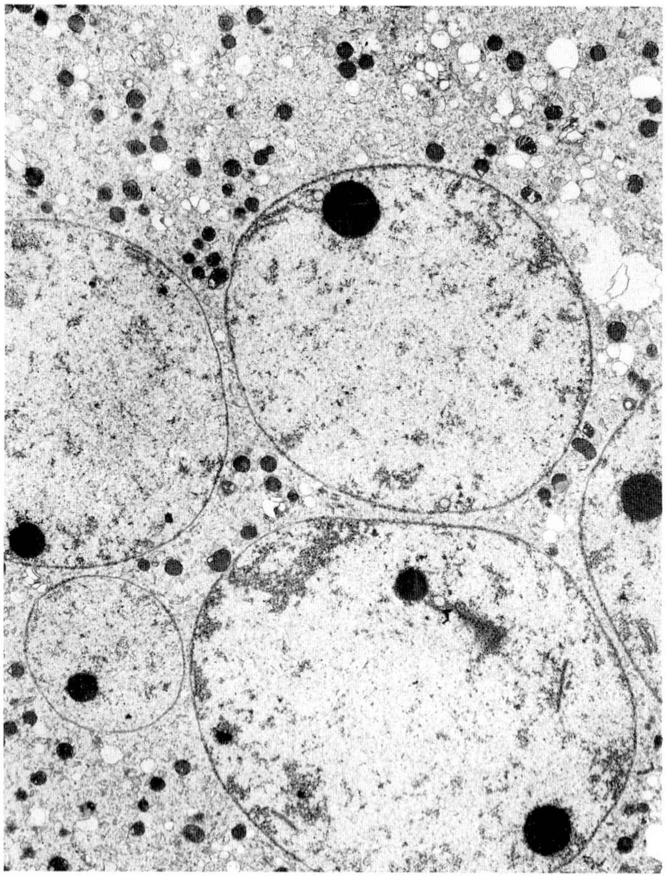

Fig. 20.31 Fragmented four-cell embryo: multinucleated blastomere. Sixty-five hours post-insemination. Each nucleus has dense compact nucleoli. (× 4700) From Sathananthan.[17]

21. The breast

A. Ahmed

INTRODUCTION

Ultrastructural appearances of human breast disease are now well-documented.[3,4,6,9,12,18,20] Although electron microscopy is not likely to be used as a routine technique in the diagnosis of breast lesions, the study of ultrastructural features of such lesions does invariably facilitate both the understanding and the accurate interpretation of the light microscopic features which form the basis of diagnostic histopathology.

In the present chapter, in addition to the normal ultrastructure of ducts and ductules in the resting breast, non-neoplastic changes of diagnostic importance are considered under the headings of epitheliosis (epithelial cell hyperplasia), sclerosing adenosis and apocrine metaplasia, as well as fat necrosis and radial scar and the rare microglandular adenosis.

NORMAL RESTING BREAST

Ducts and ductules of adult mammary gland are lined by luminal epithelial cells and peripheral myoepithelial cells. Intra-epithelial lymphocytes and macrophages can also be observed.[10]

In the resting epithelium, the cytoplasm is relatively sparse in organelles which include free ribosomes, occasional profiles of rough-surfaced endoplasmic reticulum (RER), a few mitochondria and poorly-developed Golgi complexes (Fig. 21.1).[25,26] Microvilli cover the luminal surface.

The myoepithelium, situated between the epithelial cells and the basal lamina, is characterized by the presence of thin cytoplasmic filaments arranged parallel to the basal lamina. These filaments exhibit dense bodies similar to those found in smooth muscle cells. The cytoplasm also contains occasional small mitochondria, free ribosomes a few profiles of RER and lipid bodies (Figs 21.2 and 21.3). The basal plasma membrane exhibits pinocytotic vesicles and presents distinctive club-like processes covered with hemidesmosomes (Figs 21.3 and 21.4). These two features are absent along the epithelial cell plasma membrane in contact with the basal lamina. Thus, the ultrastructural identification of myoepithelial cells requires the presence of cytoplasmic filaments with dense bodies, hemidesmosomes and pinocytotic vesicles.

Mammary ducts and ductules are surrounded by a continuous and uniform basal lamina beyond which there is a layer of loose collagen and elastic fibres. Surrounding this connective tissue there is a line of extremely attenuated fibroblasts termed 'delimiting fibroblasts', which, together with the epithelial and myoepithelial cell plasma membranes and the basal lamina, form 'the epithelial-stromal junction' (Fig. 21.2).[17]

The disruption of the epithelial–stromal junction has been suggested to be responsible for the histological manifestations of fibrocystic disease of the breast.[17,18,19]

EPITHELIOSIS

Epitheliosis is a term used to describe benign, non-papillary proliferation involving terminal ducts and sometimes ductules. In epitheliosis, there is proliferation of both epithelial and myoepithelial cells,[1] an important feature not easily appreciated by light microscopy. The proliferating myoepithelial cells intermingle with the epithelial cells and can be seen at the periphery of ducts and almost up to the luminal surface (Figs 21.5–21.7).

In the differentiation of epitheliosis from in situ carcinoma, it is important to recognize that, unlike epitheliosis, *no* myoepithelial cells are present among the carcinoma cells in ductal carcinoma in situ[1], apart from the obligatory peripheral layer of pre-existing myoepithelial cells.

SCLEROSING ADENOSIS

Sclerosing adenosis is a proliferative process involving myoepithelial, epithelial and stromal elements with associated fibrosis within the lobules.[1,3,11–15] In the early stages of sclerosing adenosis there is focal myoepithelial cell proliferation with resultant glandular distortion and loss of glandular lumina.[3] With progressive proliferation of myoepithelial cells, much of the glandular element becomes attenuated and is composed mainly of myoepithelial cells

452   DIAGNOSTIC ULTRASTRUCTURE OF NON-NEOPLASTIC DISEASES

(Fig. 21.8). The extremely elongated processes of proliferating cells can be readily identified as of myoepithelial origin (Fig. 21.9). Electron microscopy, therefore, facilitates the accurate diagnosis of sclerosing adenosis which, at light microscopic level, can be mis-diagnosed as infiltrating carcinoma.[16]

APOCRINE METAPLASIA

Apocrine metaplasia is characterized by epithelial cells with a granular, eosinophilic cytoplasm which, at the ultrastructural level, is rich in organelles — including increased numbers of mitochondria and round secretory granules (Fig. 21.10). Many of the secretory granules which are located in the apical cytoplasm are uniformly and intensely osmiophilic. Golgi complexes are often prominent[2,14,20,22] and small vesicles of dense osmiophilic material seen in relation with Golgi complexes suggest a possible site of granule formation.[20] The mitochondria exhibit dense matrices and a few — often incomplete — cristae (Fig. 21.11).[2,12] Another characteristic feature of apocrine cells is complex infolding of the basal plasma membrane (Fig. 21.11).[2,20]

The presence of focal apocrine metaplasia in borderline proliferative breast lesions denotes a non-neoplastic process. Thus the ultrastructural characterization of early apocrine metaplasia, not recognizable at light microscopy, could be of diagnostic value in such lesions.

FAT NECROSIS

Traumatic fat necrosis presents as a firm and indurated lesion. The damaged adipocytes release fat which activates a spindle-cell fibrous reaction. Electron microscopy of fat necrosis reveals a mixture of cells including active fibroblasts, early myofibroblasts and mature myofibroblasts as described in the stroma of infiltrating breast carcinomas.[5,27] The presence of a myofibroblastic reaction[5] in fat necrosis is clearly responsible for the focal sclerosis and retraction, and it accounts for the ability of fat necrosis clinically to mimic a carcinoma.

RADIAL SCAR

Radial scar (RS) is a proliferative lesion characterized by a central area of sclerosis with entrapped ducts surrounded by variable degrees of papillary or diffuse epithelial hyperplasia.[21] The clinical and histopathological importance of RS lies in its ability to mimic cancer. Grossly, the stellate and retracted appearance together with yellow streaks and flecks of elastosis can easily simulate a cancerous lesion. Histological appearance of RS can also resemble an infiltrating cancer, particularly tubular carcinoma.

Radial scar is considered to be the result of progressive myofibroblastic proliferation.[7] At the ultrastructural level numerous myofibroblasts, at various stages of maturation, are seen apposed to the compressed ductules (Fig. 21.12). The basal lamina is generally intact, but occasional defects can occur[5,7] (Fig. 21.12). Such basal lamina defects have been suggested to be related to the myofibroblastic proliferation.[5,7] In more advanced sclerotic lesions, the myofibroblasts are characterized by numerous cytoplasmic filaments and marked nuclear indentations indicative of a contractile state (Fig. 21.12).

In the differentiation of radial scar and tubular carcinoma it is important to note that both lesions are characterized by the presence of numerous myofibroblasts.[5] However, in contrast to the one-cell lined structures in tubular carcinoma,[3] ductules in radial scar are covered by two-cell type layers (Fig. 21.12). Also in tubular carcinoma, the basal lamina is completely absent.[3]

The morphological differences between radial scar and tubular carcinoma and the true nature of the spindle cells in these lesions can be accurately established only by electron microscopy.

MICROGLANDULAR ADENOSIS

Microglandular adenosis (MGA) is a rare lesion,[8,23] which can produce a palpable, well-demarcated mass. The distinctive histological pattern shows an increased number of ductular or acinar-like structures which widely infiltrate the connective and adipose tissues. Morphologically, MGA can resemble tubular carcinoma[8,23] and, at light microscopy, the differentiation of these lesions may prove to be difficult. Electron microscopy of MGA, however, reveals distinctive appearances (Fig. 21.13).

The associated stroma in MGA is almost devoid of stromal cells and in particular, unlike tubular carcinoma,[5] no myofibroblasts are found.

REFERENCES

1. Ahmed A 1974 The myoepithelium in cystic hyperplastic mastopathy. Journal of Pathology 113: 209–215
2. Ahmed A 1975 Apocrine metaplasia in cystic hyperplastic mastopathy; histochemical and ultrastructural observations. Journal of Pathology 115: 211–214
3. Ahmed A 1978 Atlas of the ultrastructure of human breast diseases. Churchill Livingstone, Edinburgh
4. Ahmed A 1980 Ultrastructural aspects of human breast lesions.

Pathology Annual 15 (pt 2): 411–443
5. Ahmed H 1990 The myofibroblast in breast disease. Pathology Annual 25 (pt 2): 237–286
6. Archer F, Omar M 1969 Pink cell (oncocytic) metaplasia in a fibroadenoma of the human breast: electron microscopic observations. Journal of Pathology 99: 113–117
7. Battersby S, Anderson T J 1985 Myofibroblastic activity of radial scars. Journal of Pathology 147: 33–40

8. Clement P B, Azzopardi J G 1983 Microglandular adenosis of the breast — a lesion simulating tubular carcinoma. Histopathology 7: 169–180
9. Fisher E R 1976 Ultrastructure of human breast and its disorders. American Journal of Clinical Pathology 66: 291–375
10. Ferguson D J P 1985 Intraepithelial lymphocytes and macrophages in the normal breast. Virchows Archiv A, Pathological Anatomy and Histology 407: 369–378
11. Joa W, Recant W, Swerdlow M A 1976 Comparative ultrastructure of tubular carcinoma and sclerosing adenosis of the breast. Cancer 38: 180–186
12. McCarty K S Jr, Douglas E P 1983 Ultrastructure of the human breast and its disorders. In: Trump B F, Jones R T (eds) Diagnostic electron microscopy, vol 4. John Wiley & Sons, New York, pp 249–318.
13. Murad T M, von Haam E 1968 Ultrastructure of the myoepithelial cells in human mammary gland tumours. Cancer 21: 1137–1149
14. Murad T M, von Haam E 1968 The ultrastructure of fibrocystic disease of the breast. Cancer 22: 587–600
15. Murad T M 1975 Evaluation of the different techniques utilized in diagnosing breast lesions. Acta Cytologica 19: 499–508
16. Nesland J M, Hoie J, Johannessen J V 1983 The fine structure of the human breast and its benign disorders. Diagnostic Histopathology 6: 51–67
17. Ozzello L 1970 Epithelial–stromal junction of normal and dysplastic mammary gland. Cancer 25: 586–600
18. Ozzello L 1971 Ultrastructure of the human mammary gland. Pathology Annual 6: 1–59
19. Ozzello L 1974 Electron microscopic study of functional and dysfunctional human mammary glands. Journal of Investigative Dermatology 63: 19–26
20. Ozzello L 1979 Breast. In: Johannessen J V (ed) Electron microscopy in human medicine, vol. 9. Urogenital system and breast. McGraw-Hill, New York, pp 409–452
21. Page D L, Anderson T J 1987 Diagnostic histopathology of the breast. Churchill Livingstone, Edinburgh, pp 89–103
22. Pier W J, Garancis J C, Kuzma J F 1970 The ultrastructure of apocrine cells in intracystic papilloma and fibrocystic disease of the breast. Archives of Pathology 89: 446–452
23. Rosen P P 1983 Microglandular adenosis: a benign lesion simulating invasive mammary carcinoma. American Journal of Surgical Pathology 7: 137–144
24. Saul K 1985 Microglandular adenosis of the female mammary gland: a study of a case with ultrastructural observations. Human Pathology 16: 637–640
25. Stirling J W, Chandler J A 1976 The fine structure of the normal resting terminal ductal-lobular unit in the female breast. Virchows Archiv A, Pathological Anatomy and Histology 372: 205–226
26. Stirling J W, Chandler J A 1977 The fine structure of ducts and subareolar ducts in the resting gland of the female breast. Virchows Archiv A, Pathological Anatomy and Histology 373: 119–132
27. Tamimi S, Ahmed A 1987 Stromal changes in invasive breast carcinoma: an ultrastructural study. Journal of Pathology 153: 163–170
28. Tavassolli F A, Norris H J 1983 Microglandular adenosis of the breast: a clinicopathological study of 11 cases with ultrastructural observations. American Journal of Surgical Pathology 7: 731–737

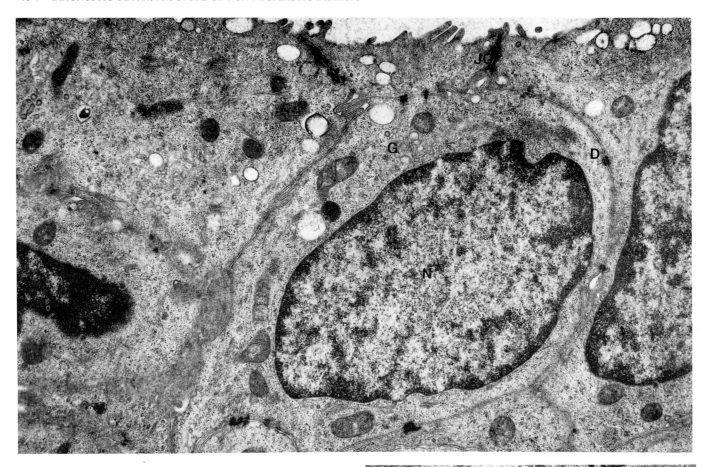

Fig. 21.1 (Above)   Normal resting breast: epithelium. The nucleus (N) shows an almost smooth nuclear membrane. The cytoplasm contains occasional profiles of endoplasmic reticulum, a few mitochondria and a Golgi complex (G). Note the junctional complexes (JC) towards the lumen and the desmosomal connections (D). (× 10 000)

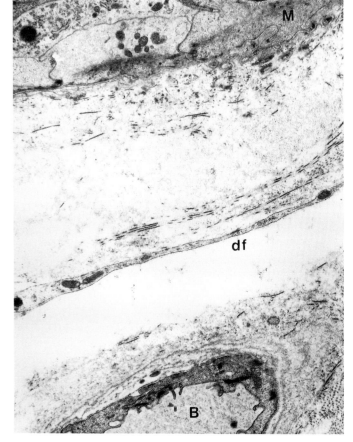

Fig. 21.2 (Right)   Normal resting breast: epithelial–stromal junction. The myoepithelial cell (M) characteristically exhibits hemidesmosomes. The attenuated processes of the delimiting fibroblasts (df) and a blood vessel (B) are present in the periductular connective tissue. (× 4000) Reference: 17.

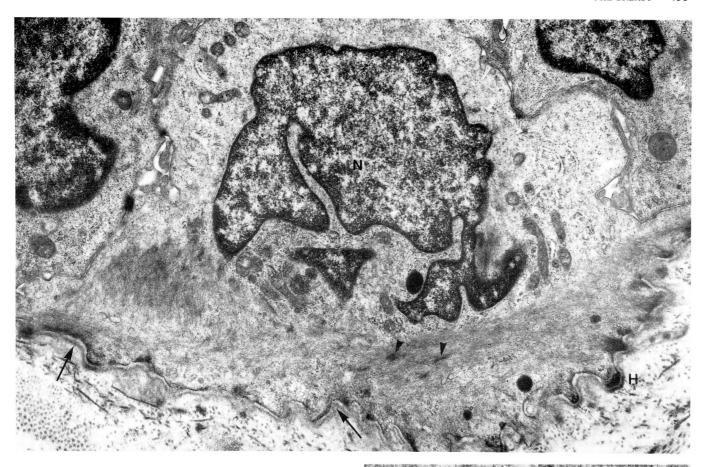

Fig. 21.3 (Above)   Normal resting breast: myoepithelium. The nucleus (N) is irregular and shows deep indentations. The cytoplasmic organelles are located in the paranuclear and apical zones. The cytoplasm contains the characteristic filaments with dense bodies (arrowheads). The basal plasma membrane forms club-like processes capped by hemidesmosomes (H). Note the basal lamina (arrows) along the plasma membrane. (× 10 000)

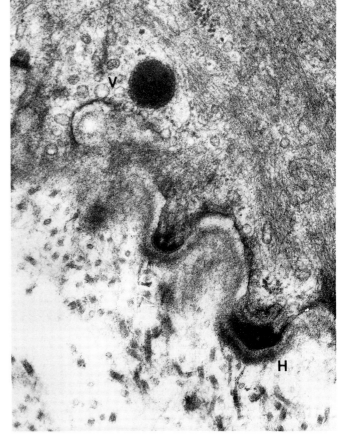

Fig. 21.4 (Right)   Myoepithelium: intracellular detail. The basal plasma membrane is characterized by numerous pinocytotic vesicles (V) as well as hemidesmosomes (H). (× 26 000)

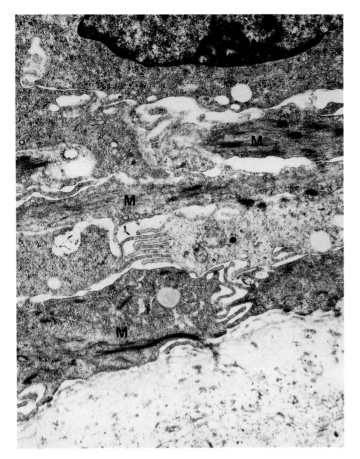

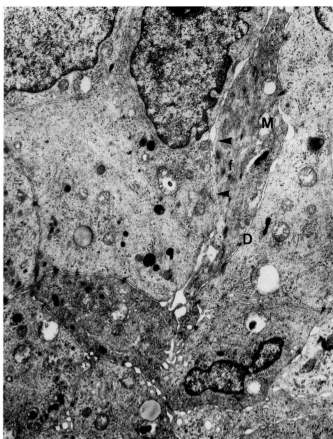

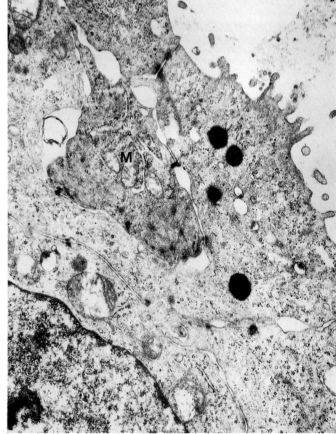

Fig. 21.5 (Above)   Epitheliosis: myoepithelial cell layering.
Myoepithelial cells (M) which normally occur singly along the periphery
of the ducts are seen forming multiple layers intermingling with the
epithelial cells. (× 7000)

Fig. 21.6 (Above right)   Epitheliosis: epithelial and myoepithelial cells.
A myoepithelial cell process (M) is present among proliferating epithelial
cells. Note the presence of characteristic cytoplasmic filaments (f) with
dense bodies and numerous pinocytotic vesicles (arrowheads) along the
plasma membrane of the myoepithelial cell. Desmosomes (D) connect the
myoepithelium with the adjacent epithelial cells. By light microscopy,
such myoepithelial cells in epitheliosis cannot be recognized with
certainty. (× 4200) Reference: 1.

Fig. 21.7 (Right)   Epitheliosis: myoepithelial cell. A myoepithelial cell
(M) is located almost at the luminal surface, well away from its normal
basal site. Note the desmosomal attachment to the adjacent epithelial
cells. Ultrastructural appearances confirm the proliferation of both
epithelial and myoepithelial cells in epitheliosis (× 7300). References: 1,
3 and 4.

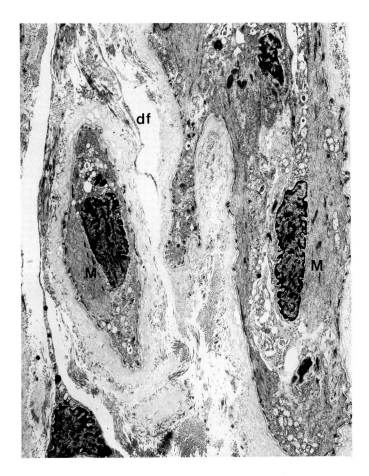

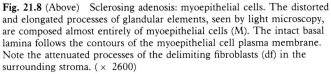

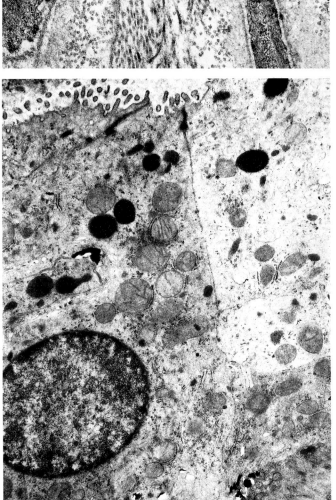

Fig. 21.8 (Above)   Sclerosing adenosis: myoepithelial cells. The distorted and elongated processes of glandular elements, seen by light microscopy, are composed almost entirely of myoepithelial cells (M). The intact basal lamina follows the contours of the myoepithelial cell plasma membrane. Note the attenuated processes of the delimiting fibroblasts (df) in the surrounding stroma. (× 2600)

Fig. 21.9 (Above right)   Sclerosing adenosis: myoepithelial cell processes. The progressive distortion and elongation produce extremely attenuated myoepithelial cell processes. Note that these processes still retain the basal lamina (arrowheads) and hemidesmosomes. Ultrastructural examination is essential for the accurate characterization of such processes which, by light microscopy, can easily be misinterpreted as fibroblasts. (× 10 000) Reference: 3.

Fig. 21.10 (Right)   Apocrine metaplasia: metaplastic apocrine cells. Apocrine metaplastic cells are characterized by increased numbers of mitochondria and numerous apically located osmiophilic bodies. Note the round, basally located, nucleus. (× 4800)

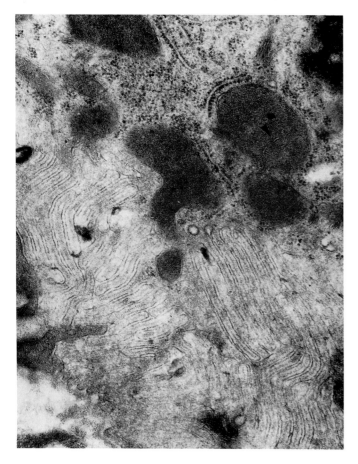

Fig. 21.11 (Above)   Apocrine metaplasia: cellular details. Apocrine cells show elaborate infoldings of the basal plasma membrane. The mitochondria exhibit an electron-dense matrix and incomplete cristae (arrowhead). Another frequently observed feature is the close association of profiles of RER and mitochondria. (× 14 400) The increased numbers of mitochondria in metaplastic apocrine cells has led to the suggestion that these cells are oncocytes,[5] similar to cells observed in salivary, parathyroid and thyroid glands. However, unlike oncocytes, the apocrine cells exhibit electron-dense mitochondria with incomplete cristae and possess elaborate basal plasma membrane infoldings similar to those seen in apocrine sweat gland cells. References: 2, 6, 9 and 18.

Fig. 21.12 (Above right)   Radial scar: ductule. The ductule is lined by epithelial (E) and myoepithelial cell (M). Note the adjacent intact basal lamina. The myofibroblasts contain a markedly indented nucleus (n) and numerous cytoplasmic filaments with dense bodies. (× 21 000)

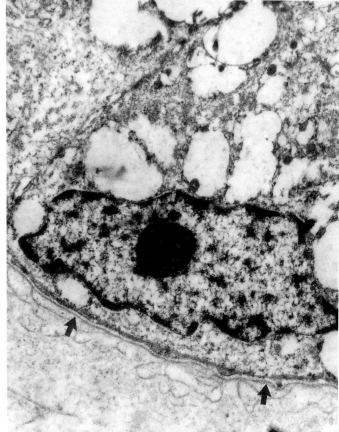

Fig. 21.13 (Right)   Microglandular adenosis: epithelial cell. The glandular structures are lined by a single layer of epithelial cells. The basally located nuclei often contain prominent nucleoli. Myoepithelial cells are absent[24,28] but unlike tubular carcinoma,[3] a distinct basal lamina (arrows) is a characteristic feature in MGA. The vacuolated cytoplasm contains scanty organelles. The lumina contain amorphous material and the luminal plasma membrane is irregular and lacks microvilli. (× 22 500)

22. The skin

Ingrun Anton-Lamprecht

INTRODUCTION

Dermatology has been a morphologically orientated speciality from the very beginning. In contrast to many other disciplines, where more indirect methods have to be applied, direct morphological observation, investigation and nosologic distinction have been important tools in dermatology since the time of its separation from general and internal medicine. With skin changes directly visible, the systematic clinical observation of skin lesions and their description disclosed a multitude of skin disorders and — from the viewpoint of the non-specialist — resulted in a confusing terminology. (See Appendix I, p. 494 for list of abbreviations used in this chapter.)

Though invasive, skin biopsies are easily performed without much harm, and therefore skin samples are readily accessible. Thus, the application of histopathology for diagnostic purposes in dermatology is still increasing. Technical improvements and supplementation with new methods, such as the use of monoclonal antibodies or of resin embedding for semithin sectioning, have contributed to this development. A large series of excellent textbooks and journals dedicated to dermatohistopathology reflects this situation.

Light microscopy (LM) has shown that, in spite of the large variation of the clinical appearance of skin disorders, the underlying tissue changes in many cases seem to be very similar and to reflect only a small repertoire of possible reaction patterns of the skin to a multitude of disturbances. 'Lumpers' and 'splitters', therefore represent the two poles in the spectrum of opinions among specialists on the possible uniformity or diversity of skin diseases. With apparent lack of histopathological distinction, lumpers tend to regard the clinical diversity among patients as a consequence of individual variation of a distinctive nosologic entity, whereas splitters consider such variations to indicate heterogeneity within a syndrome.

With the introduction of electron microscopy (EM) to the biomedical sciences in the late 1950s, ultrastructural investigations of normal and diseased skin were enthusiastically taken up in dermatology. Comparable to the early phase of light microscopy, this phase of descriptive EM of normal and abnormal skin characterized the two decades until the end of the 1970s, during which most of the common dermatological conditions were characterized by their EM features. In contrast to histopathology, however, the application of ultrastructural criteria to the diagnosis of skin diseases and in the classification of individual patients developed only slowly. [4,70,129,146]

Histiocytosis X was the first example — and for years the only one — thought to require ultrastructural demonstration of Langerhans' cell granules in the specific histiocytic cells of the infiltrate for definitive diagnosis. With diameters of about 30 nm and lengths of 0.1 to 0.5 μm, Langerhans' cell granules lie below the resolution of LM; therefore, EM proved to be indispensable in their identification. [42,97]

Genetic skin disorders became, and still are, the main field of diagnostic EM. [4] Systematic ultrastructural investigations of large series of patients suffering from keratinization disorders, such as the ichthyoses, or from mechanobullous disorders (epidermolysis bullosa) have revealed a much larger heterogeneity within these groups of genodermatoses than known or even expected from clinical impressions and histopathology. For most of these disorders the underlying biochemical defects are still unknown. Therefore, final diagnostic classification of most genodermatoses is possible only with the aid of EM based on specific ultrastructural criteria. In this context, *descriptive* and *diagnostic* EM have to be distinguished principally. During the investigation of tissue samples of a disease entity, many of the morphological features observed — though interesting from the viewpoint of morphology or in the course of the disease — may be of little or no diagnostic significance. In skin disorders, features of such low specificity may include inflammatory cell exudation, the enlargement of the intercellular spaces in the basal cell layer, multiplication of the epidermal basal lamina, deposition of fibrin, activation of complement, occurrence of fibrillar bodies (Civatte, colloid or hyaline bodies, composed of keratin filaments; see apoptosis), and pigmentary incontinence. It is therefore the aim of this chapter to set forth and to illustrate those features that may serve as distinctive and reliable diagnostic ultrastructural markers of skin disorders. It will be impossible to give a full description of the ultrastructural appearance in each of the disorders treated in this chapter. For a more complex description of the ultrastructural features of the various skin disorders the reader is referred to the original literature and to the respective textbooks. Moreover, only those dermatological disorders for which EM is an essential or an indispensable tool for diagnostic purposes are discussed. Many skin diseases can be identified and clearly diagnosed by means of classical histopathology alone. In other cases, such as bullous diseases of immunological origin, the principal diagnostic decision must be achieved by immunopathology; in special circumstances the final decision may remain questionable unless EM and/or immuno-EM are applied.

In those genodermatoses in which the underlying biochemical defect has been identified, the biochemical parameters are of greater diagnostic significance than ultrastructural features. As an example, X-linked recessive ichthyosis (XRI) with steroid sulphatase deficiency needs the biochemical or molecular genetic demonstration of the enzyme deficiency for its final proof, while EM (as well as transport velocity of the LDL fraction in lipid electrophoresis) only suggests the diagnosis of XRI, and it may be necessary to exclude other types of inherited ichthyoses.

Finally, there exist many skin disorders that reveal only non-specific morphological changes; as a consequence, LM and EM do not contribute significantly to their diagnosis.

GENODERMATOSES

1. Inborn errors of keratinization, keratinization disorders

The inherited ichthyoses, and later the palmoplantar keratoses, were investigated in the laboratories of the author in Heidelberg from 1968. These studies — initially aimed mainly at the clarification of the pathomorphogenesis of the common and well-known types of ichthyoses and at the classification of some unusual and poorly understood cases — were the first to reveal the considerable heterogeneity in the group of the ichthyoses that is still enlarging.[1-4,7,10,12,20,23,27,31,33,34]

Table 22.1 summarizes the most important features for the discrimination of this group of keratinization disorders. Additional remarks will highlight the significance and the diagnostic value of the various features.

Autosomal dominant ichthyosis vulgaris (ADI)

This is the only known keratinization disorder with a proven basic abnormality of keratohyalin (KH). The minute amounts of KH formed in the uppermost living epidermal keratinocytes (Figs 22.1 and 22.2) are not easily visible when glutaraldehyde–epoxy resin embedding techniques are used

because of the high contrast of the tonofilaments. This is especially true when phosphate-buffered glutaraldehyde, Karnovsky solution, and Araldite embedding are employed. It was by the application of an osmic acid fixation medium in combination with epon that the abnormal nature of this type of KH became demonstrable.[2] Similarly, combinations of glutaraldehyde-osmic acid double fixation with low-viscosity epoxy resin may be useful for visualizing minute KH amounts and for demonstrating the defective nature of KH (Figs 22.1 B and C, and 22.2).

Absence of one of the major polypeptides of KH or abnormalities preventing their polymerization or accumulation to normal-sized KH granules had been discussed as a basic defect.[2,27] This hypothesis was later proven by the absence of filaggrin and profilaggrin in ADI patients.[220]

Demonstration of the absence of this protein alone is, however, not sufficient to prove ADI in diagnostic cases because keratohyalin synthesis, and thus formation of filaggrin, can be suppressed almost completely under various conditions, while the typical crumbly appearance of keratohyalin (as compared to normal KH in control specimens and other ichthyoses such as X-linked ichthyosis (XRI) and congenital ichthyosis; Fig. 22.2D) is pathognomonic of ADI and may even be used as a genetic marker.[7] This defect is demonstrable in all parts of the skin where keratohyalin is found, including follicular epithelium, sebaceous gland ducts, and eccrine sweat ducts.

X-linked recessive ichthyosis (Wells–Kerr) with steroid sulphatase (STS) deficiency (XRI)

The gene has recently been mapped to the distal region of the short arm of the X-chromosome (STS locus, Xp 22.3) close to the Xg blood group and to the so-called pseudo-autosomal region (Xp-ter). Recent molecular genetic studies using specific clonal cDNA have demonstrated deletions in the region of the STS locus (Xp 22.3) in a high proportion of patients with XRI; these deletions are as yet below the resolution of HR banding techniques.[40,41]

Biochemical demonstration of the enzyme deficiency of STS[213] and molecular genetic proof of deletions (or abnormality) in the Xp-ter region (Xp 22.3, non-expression of STS locus) have the highest significance in the diagnosis, while increased velocity of the LDL fraction in serum lipid electrophoresis may be used as a simple screen for XRI. Ultrastructural features are of relative value: they may indicate XRI but are often rather non-specific. Increased numbers of transit cells, high numbers of desmosomes in the horny layer as well as increased amounts of keratohyalin per cell[3] may be explained in terms of a moderate or slight increase of the transit time available for differentiation. The accumulation of the horny layer is thought to be related directly to the increased amount of uncleaved cholesterol sulphate in the intercellular barrier lipids.[233] Patients with XRI often develop increased melanin synthesis ('ichthyosis nigricans'). The relationship to the STS deficiency is poorly understood. Most female carriers are normal with respect to skin scaling as the STS gene locus escapes Lyonization.

Prolonged or insufficient labour in the end-phase of the pregnancy during delivery is associated with STS deficiency in male pregnancies and has been ascribed to placental oestradiol insufficiency. Hypophyseal hypogonadism and cryptorchidism (with risk of seminoma)[217] are frequently associated with XRI. Combinations of XRI with other X-linked disorders have been reported as a result of larger deletions in the Xp-terminal region.[45,198] In the cases reported by Steuhl et al[217] co-segregation of XRI and epidermolysis bullosa simplex Köbner were observed.

Refsum's syndrome, heredopathia atactica polyneuritiformis (Refsum)

Defective phytanic acid alpha hydroxylation has been shown to be the basic defect in this severe genetic systemic lipid storage disease. The diagnosis demands the biochemical demonstration of phytanic acid accumulation and of the enzyme deficiency.[23,233] The ultrastructural features[23] are those of an ichthyosis secondary to a disturbance of lipid metabolism and are not specific. Keratohyalin is often significantly reduced or even absent, but that which is present is ultrastructurally normal, in contrast to that of ADI. Dietary treatment allows for clinical and morphological normalization and recovery (Table 22.1).

The ichthyosis congenita group (autosomal recessive congenital ichthyosis; non-bullous congenital ichthyosiform erythroderma; lamellar ichthyosis; ichthyosis congenita Riecke II)

Clinical variability with presence or lack of erythroderma, different degrees of severity, scale pattern and horny layer lipid composition pointed to two distinctive genetic types of what had been regarded as being one entity until recently.[233,234,235] In the European literature, erythrodermic and non-erythrodermic variants have always been distinguished, while in the Anglo–American literature all cases of congenital ichthyoses were termed lamellar ichthyosis collectively. Many, but not all of the subtypes of this group present as collodion babies at birth.[91,160]

EM analyses, systematically carried out in the author's laboratories on more than 130 cases of recessively transmitted congenital ichthyoses (recently also by Kanerva, Niemi and co-workers in Helsinki), have demonstrated a considerable degree of heterogeneity. Diagnostic distinction at present demands ultrastructural control, while the biochemical characterization of the different subtypes is underway[171,234,235] and the underlying basic defects are still unknown. It seems that most of the ichthyoses with recessive inheritance — if not all — are related to disturbances of the epidermal lipid metabolism.[16,23,33,34,76,77,171,197,213,233] In

the following, the Heidelberg classification will be used (Table 22.1).

Ichthyosis congenita type I. Corresponding to the erythrodermic cases of lamellar ichthyosis or non-bullous congenital ichthyosiform erythroderma, this is the classical type of hyperproliferative hyperkeratosis with considerable amounts of compact horny layer and acanthosis, increased mitotic activity, broad granular layer but suppression of specific keratinization proteins (low amounts of tonofilaments and keratohyalin per cell). Diagnostically significant is the demonstration of large amounts of lipid droplets[1] (neutral lipids, triglycerides, alkanes[234]) in the horny layer (Fig. 22.3). Parakeratosis is only occasionally found. Hyperproliferation-specific keratins (CK numbers 16 and 6; 48 and 56 kD) may be expressed in this subtype. Problems in the prenatal diagnosis of this type of congenital ichthyosis have recently been reported.[31,141]

Ichthyosis congenita type II, cholesterol type. Due to the variable degree of scaling and erythroderma, these cases correspond to either erythrodermic or non-erythrodermic lamellar ichthyosis. Patients are often born as classical collodion babies with pronounced ectropion and eclabium. The later course may lead to generalized polygonal — often dark-coloured — scales, or to rather mild and fine scaling. The skin mostly responds excellently to external ointments and oral retinoid treatment.

Hyperkeratosis, acanthosis and mitotic activity are less pronounced than in type I, with an often almost normal-appearing granular layer. Islands of cholesterol clefts in the horny layer are diagnostically distinctive ultrastructural markers (Fig. 22.4, A and B).[149]

Prenatal diagnosis of the cholesterol type is based upon abnormalities of horn cell contents in the follicular orifices of the fetal epithelium (Fig. 22.4D) at about week 20-21, while cholesterol clefts are not yet demonstrable at that age,[13,14,31,32] and fetal skin does not yet reveal continuous keratinization or even hyperkeratinization of the interfollicular epidermis, and no follicular plugging. Therefore, the prenatal diagnosis of this type of congenital ichthyosis demands extensive experience with normal and abnormal fetal skin. The same abnormality of the horn lamellae is later demonstrable in the follicular plugs in infants with the cholesterol type (Fig. 22.4C).

Ichthyosis congenita type III. Clinically non-erythrodermic, and characterized by a reticulate scale pattern, this type is distinctly different from the aforementioned ones. Acanthosis and hyperproliferation are insignificant with almost no increase in the mitotic rate. The amount of lipid droplets in the compact horny layer is low or minimal. Ultrastructural markers in the granular layer are (1) elongated perinuclear membranes (Fig. 22.5, A, B and D), often in association with adjacent empty spaces due to shrinkage phenomena during tissue dehydration; (2) empty membrane-bound vacuoles that reach sizes of LM resolution and sometimes contain one or a few abnormal keratinosomes

Table 22.1 Differential diagnosis of inherited ichthyoses (AD = autosomal dominant, XR = X-linked recessive; AR = autosomal recessive)

Term	Inheritance	Clinical features	Histopathology	EM features	Biochemistry/basic defect	Diagnostically significant parameters
Ichthyosis vulgaris group Autosomal dominant ichthyosis vulgaris	AD	Fine white scaling, flexures + face spared; ichthyotic hands (hyperlinearity of palms and soles); follicular keratosis; no palmo-plantar hyperkeratosis; frequently combined with atopic diathesis, atopic dermatitis, bronchial asthma or rhinitis	Orthohyperkeratosis, granular layer missing, no acanthosis, no hyperproliferation, no inflammatory infiltration; signs of eczema if combined with atopy	Orthohyperkeratosis: 40–60 layers; follicular plugging; isolated granular cells or one layer maximum; minute amounts of defective crumbly keratohyalin granules; no abnormalities of tonofilaments, keratinosomes or desmosomes	Disturbance of keratohyalin synthesis and/or polymerization; lack of filaggrin and profilaggrin	EM: abnormal ultrastructure of keratohyalin; biochemistry and/or immunoreaction for filaggrin–profilaggrin missing
X-linked ichthyosis	XR	Larger polygonal scaling, most pronounced on lower legs and abdomen; brown scaling due to hyperpigmentation: ichthyosis nigricans, great flexures and face spared, flexures of knees often only minimally spared; scaling of scalp skin; no palmo-plantar keratoses; often combined with cryptorchidism or hypogonadism	Orthohyperkeratosis, granular layer normal or decreased, keratohyalin amount normal or increased; Malpighian layer normal or moderate acanthosis; no hyperproliferation; no inflammatory infiltrate	Orthohyperkeratosis: 70–90 layers, horn cells densely packed, flat, with high numbers of desmosomes and with pigment granules; transit cells increased; keratohyalin of normal ultrastructure, amounts often increased; stimulation of melanin synthesis and transfer	Steroid sulphatase deficiency; arylsulphatase C deficiency; high amounts of cholesterol sulphate in horn cells; velocity of LDL-fraction mobility increased; intermediate values in female carriers (Lyonization)	Normal keratohyalin by EM; demonstration of increased LDL-velocity; demonstration of enzyme deficiency of steroid sulphatase
Refsum's syndrome	AR	Xerosis, mild to severe ichthyosis, generalized white scaling; progressive neurodegenerative disorder: polyneuropathia with inner ear hearing loss, atypical retinitis pigmentosa with night blindness, restriction of visual field, and progressive loss of vision; distal pareses, loss of deep tendon reflexes, high liquor proteins, cerebellar symptoms (ataxia)	Mild to pronounced orthohyperkeratosis; reduced granular layer (1–2 layers); low amount of keratohyalin, no acanthosis; no hyperproliferation; no inflammation in papillary dermis	Orthohyperkeratosis: 30–40 layers; delayed dissolution of desmosomal discs; normal keratohyalin, reduced amounts; lipid vacuoles (phytanic acid) in melanocytes, keratinocytes and dermal cell elements	Defective mitochondrial alpha-oxidation of lipids: storage of phytanic acid in serum, urine, and organ tissues including skin and horny layer due to absence of phytanic acid alpha-hydroxylation	Demonstration of phytanic acid in serum by gas chromatography; dietary management: chlorophyll-free diet

Ichthyosis congenita group

Ichthyosis congenita type I	AR	Pronounced severe generalized scaling, scales large or fine, varying degrees of erythroderma and inflammatory response; neonatal: collodion skin, ectropion, eclabium, pronounced scaling of scalp skin; face, palms and soles, large flexures involved; no additional neural involvement or internal abnormalities	Pronounced ortho- and parahyperkeratosis, horn masses dense and compact; hyperproliferative epidermis, acanthosis, hypergranulosis (up to six layers) or granular layer suppressed; mitotic rate increased; inflammatory infiltrate in dermis	Massive hyperkeratotic horny layer, only partly with nuclear remnants, high amounts of lipid droplets in horn cells; up to six layers granular cells; KH normal, low amounts, also of tonofilaments; mitoses frequent, few binuclear cells	Unknown; storage of alkanes and/or triglycerides in horny layer; defective epidermal lipid metabolism?
					Demonstration of lipid vacuoles in horn cells; biochemically: alkane accumulation?
Ichthyosis congenita type II (cholesterol type)	AR	Pronounced collodion skin at birth, parchment-like, severe ectropion and eclabium (often mistaken for harlequin ichthyosis); partial shedding leaves cap-like thick hyperkeratoses on scalp skin; involvement of large flexures, palms and soles (often severe hyperkeratoses); large polygonal scales on trunk, white or dark-brown; erythroderma mild, lacking or severe, some cases fitting CIE, some cases fitting LI; considerable variation in degree of severity and response to treatment	Mild to pronounced orthohyperkeratosis; compact, lamellar horny layer; granular layer normal or only slightly enlarged, normal amounts of keratohyalin; moderate hyperproliferation; mild or pronounced inflammatory infiltrate	Compact orthohyperkeratosis; low amounts of lipid droplets in horn cells, but groups of cholesterol clefts in the horny layer; no ultrastructural abnormalities of the Malpighian layer; variable degrees of mitoses and of inflammatory infiltrate; in the acro-infundibulum: ultrastructural abnormalities of horn cell contents, irregular membrane accumulations	Unknown; defective epidermal lipid metabolism, storage of cholesterol in the horny layer
					Demonstration of cholesterol clefts in stratum corneum by EM; prenatal diagnosis: demonstration of abnormal ultrastructure of horn cells lining the openings of the follicular acro-infundibulum
Ichthyosis congenita type III	AR	Mild to severe collodion skin, parchment-like; moderate ectropion and eclabium at birth; pronounced non-erythrodermic scaling in large polygonal patterns; ('lamellar ichthyosis') palms and soles hard and dry, slightly hyperkeratotic; no internal or neurological abnormalities; good response to topical and oral treatment	Mild to pronounced compact orthohyperkeratosis, 2–3 granular layers, normal amounts of keratohyalin, presence of ovoid vacuoles (semithin); moderate acanthosis; otherwise normal; no inflammatory infiltrate	Compact hyperkeratosis, variable amounts of lipid droplets; membranes and vesicular complexes in horn cells; elongated perinuclear membranes, vesicular complexes and membrane-bound vacuoles in granular cells, normal keratohyalin, some normal keratinosomes	Unknown; defective epidermal lipid metabolism – defective synthesis of polar lipids in keratinosomes? Abnormality of sphingolipids?
					Demonstration of (perinuclear) membranes and vesicular complexes in granular and horn cells

(Continued over)

Term	Inheritance	Clinical features	Histopathology	EM features	Biochemistry/basic defect	Diagnostically significant parameters
Ichthyosis congenita type IV	AR	Premature birth (ca. weeks 31–34); pronounced vernix caseosa; amnion fluid filled with horn cells (gruel-like); obstruction of trachea, nose and throat; perinatal death possible due to respiratory distress (asphyxia); ears deepsitting, malformed; pawlike hands; skin parchment-like, palms and soles hyperkeratotic, skin hystrix-like on front of legs and trunk; surviving cases with mild ichthyosis, skin hard, rough, no scaling; palms and soles free; no erythroderma	Compact or hystrix-like hyperkeratosis, moderate acanthosis; granular layer normal or thinned; no inflammatory reaction; histopathology of low specificity; semithin sections may be conspicuous	Moderate to pronounced orthohyperkeratosis; granular and horn cells with lentiform areas filled with membrane inclusions (polar lipids?), keratohyalin attached to them; highly specific ultrastructure, probably expressed in every granular and horn cell; lower epidermis inconspicuous; defective ultrastructure expressed in fetal skin (weeks 20–22) with onset of keratinization in follicular orifices	Unknown; disturbances of epidermal lipid metabolism?	Demonstration of masses of lipid membranes in lentiform paranuclear swellings of granular and horn cells by EM; prenatal diagnosis by ultrastructural demonstration of lentiform swellings with membrane accumulations in granular and horn cells lining follicular orifices (weeks 20–22)
Ichthyosis congenita type V	?	Perinatal condition unknown; no collodion skin; severe generalized scaling involving face and large flexures, fine on trunk, polygonal on lower legs; marked palmo-plantar hyperkeratosis; nails long and dyskeratotic; pronounced erythroderma; growth retardation	Massive parahyperkeratosis, acanthosis and hyperproliferation with increased mitotic rate; lack of granular layer; marked inflammatory infiltrate	Parahyperkeratosis, lipid vacuoles and nuclear remnants in horny layer; lack of granular layer, only few keratohyalin granules; severely suppressed keratinization, few thin tonofilaments; some scattered dyskeratotic cells; prickle cells large, pale, oedematous; many binuclear cells, tumour-like nuclei with indentations and granular inclusions; bowlform aggregations of finely filamentous material; basal cells small, hyperproliferative	Unknown	Demonstration of bowlform aggregations of filamentous material in hyperproliferative, often binuclear cells; tumourlike nuclei and suppressed keratinization

Disease	Inheritance	Clinical features	Histopathology	Ultrastructure	Biochemistry/pathogenesis	Diagnosis
Autosomal-dominant lamellar ichthyosis	AD	Birth at term, ichthyosis at birth; generalized hyperkeratoses with large brown scales including large flexures; pronounced plantar hyperkeratosis, palms less severely affected; lichenification on backs of hands and feet, wrists, knees, ankles; face relatively spared; no erythroderma; no blisters or erosions[224]	Marked hyperkeratosis, focal parakeratosis, increase of granular layer in ortho- and parakeratotic areas; acanthosis and slight papillomatosis, few mitotic cells; moderate perivascular mononuclear inflammatory infiltration	Mild hyperkeratosis, in part parakeratotic; only few lipid vacuoles; gradual transformation of granular cells (2–6 layers) retaining nuclei and organelles, lower-most granular cells normal; keratohyalin in the transforming cells with conspicuous spongy appearance between the compact tonofilament bundles[156]	Unknown; biochemical lipid composition of plantar scales: free fatty acids and triglycerides increased, n-alkanes elevated, free sterols and total ceramides decreased;[171] abnormality of one or more keratohyalin proteins?	Demonstration of abnormality (spongy appearance) of keratohyalin in increased transforming layer
Sjögren–Larsson syndrome (SLS)	AR	Generalized erythrodermic ichthyosiform scaling involving face, palms and soles, and great flexures; accentuation of lines of cleavage and of wrinkle lines, marked linear furrows and lichenification; oligophrenia; speech defects; seizures; spastic di- or tetraplegia; eyes: fundus abnormalities, macular degeneration, retinitis pigmentosa, 'glistening spots'; kyphosis; small stature; normal genital development[145,163,221]	Orthohyperkeratosis, acanthosis, inflammatory infiltrate; non-specific changes	Ultrastructurally non-specific: moderate to pronounced hyperkeratosis, few lipid droplets; no parakeratosis: no abnormalities of tonofilaments, keratohyalin, or keratinosomes	Abnormality of fatty alcohol cycle and metabolism: deficiency of fatty alcohol:NAD$^+$ oxidoreductase activity; impairment of fatty alcohol oxidation to fatty acids, accumulation of fatty alcohols,[197] intermediate levels of enzyme activity in heterozygotes; normal values for delta-6-fatty acid CoA-dehydrogenase (fatty acid desaturase) activity (fibroblast cultures)	Light and electron microscopy non-specific; diagnosis by clinical features, biochemically by fatty alcohol accumulation and deficiency of fatty alcohol:NAD$^+$ oxidoreductase activity[197]
Neutral lipid storage disease (Dorfman–Chanarin syndrome)	AR	Mild generalized erythroderma, fine white scaling, lichenification flexures and face involved; tautness of skin, ectropion; palmoplantar keratoderma; cataracts; neurosensory deafness; mild primary myopathy; abnormal serum muscle enzymes; aortic insufficiency; CNS abnormalities; diabetes mellitus; gluten enteropathy; fatty liver	Hyperparakeratosis hypergranulosis, and acanthosis; neutral lipid droplets in granular and basal cells (Oil-red O-positive); lipid droplets in horn cells, pilosebaceous epithelia and intraepidermal sweat ducts; monocytes (bone marrow) and peripheral granulocytes with pronounced lipid vacuoles; lipid accumulation in inner organs	Lipid vacuoles in monocytes, granulocytes, leukocytes, and epidermal cells (non-polar lipids); keratinosomes (lamellar or Odland bodies) accumulate lipid droplets between their normal polar lipid lamellae; both are co-discharged to intercellular spaces; impairment of corneocyte shedding?	Abnormality of intracellular triglyceride (neutral lipid/alkane) metabolism; enzyme deficiency of carnitine–palmityl-transferase?	LM demonstration of neutral lipid accumulation (Oil red O-positive) in peripheral granulocytes; EM demonstration of lipid droplets in abnormal keratinosomes discharged with polar lamellae to intercellular spaces in horny layer; very rare: 11 cases up to 1985

(Continued over)

Term	Inheritance	Clinical features	Histopathology	EM features	Biochemistry/basic defect	Diagnostically significant parameters
Ichthyosis congenita gravis (harlequin ichthyosis) type I (Buxman)[57]	AR	Most frequent genetic type; premature birth (weeks 32–36), premature rupture of fetal membranes; thick armour-like horn masses, deep fissures; pronounced ectropion and eclabium, absence of defined facial features; malformed ears; hands and feet fixed in flexed position; complete immobility; perinatal death in most cases; surviving cases with severe generalized scaling	Massive ortho- and hyperparakeratosis, acanthosis or normal thickness of epidermis; granular layer present or reduced; positive staining for neutral lipids in horn cells; massive follicular plugging	Massive compact horny layer, dense and compressed; specific abnormality of keratinosomes in granular and deep horn cells (vesicular structures, empty or with glycogen-like particles); keratohyalin present, reduced or absent; few tonofilaments, suppression of normal keratinization	Unknown; abnormality of keratinosome synthesis and function? Biochemical deviation of horn cell lipids: cholesterol and triglycerides elevated;[57] deviations in expression of filaggrin and cytokeratins[66]	Clinical features; demonstration of keratinosome abnormalities by EM; biochemical demonstration of lipid abnormalities, deviations in keratinization-specific proteins (possible further subtypes); prenatal diagnosis by EM of fetal skin biopsy after week 20
Ichthyosis congenita gravis (harlequin ichthyosis) type II	?	Less frequent and more severe than type I; premature birth (about week 34); thick armour-like horn masses, yellow-whitish colour, deep fissures into the dermis (more than 5 mm), no scaling; pronounced ectropion and eclabium, absence of facial features, malformed ears; flexion fixation of extremities, hands and feet, club feet; fatal course, death within hours or days	Massive hystrix-like hyperkeratosis with patent sweat duct openings; thinned epidermis, granular layer absent; papillomatosis; oedema of dermal connective tissue	Massive hystrix-like hyperkeratoses, no regular transformation to normal horn cells, stacking of densely attached flattened cells with marginal envelope, flocculent material and vesicular structures; some lipid droplets; keratin filaments few or absent; keratohyalin and abnormal keratinosomes as in type I only around sweat ducts; accumulation of lipid membranes (tubular or rolled-up) in suprabasal layers	Unknown	Clinical features; stacking of abnormally flattened cells with marginal envelope, lack of keratohyalin, complete suppression of keratinization; demonstration of lipid membranes in suprabasal cells

Hystrix-like ichthyoses					
Bullous congenital ichthyosiform erythroderma (Brocq)	AD	Newborns: 'burned baby' with blisters, erosions and erythroderma; never born as collodion baby; within few weeks development of grey-brown hyperkeratoses with accentuation of furrows and lichenification (elbows, wrists, dorsa of hands and feet, knees); severe involvement of great flexures, often hystrix-like; face, scalp skin, palms and soles spared or involved; distribution of hyperkeratoses variable; erythroderma present or lacking ('I. bullosa Siemens')	Acanthokeratolysis or epidermolytic hyperkeratosis: normal basal cells, suprabasal segregation and clumping of tonofilaments, large keratohyalin granules; acanthosis and hypergranulosis; hyperproliferation with increased mitotic rates; oedematization and destruction, subcorneal blister formation; massive hyperkeratotic horny layer, loose or compact; inflammatory infiltrate in erythrodermic cases	Suprabasal clumping of tonofilaments, increasing aggregations, perinuclear shells; increased synthesis of keratinization-specific proteins (keratins, keratohyalin) and keratinosomes; suprabasal blister formation via cytolysis (and acantholysis), mostly in high epidermal layers; same ultrastructural changes in nevus verrucosus acantho-keratolyticus and in Voerner-type palmo-plantar keratosis	Unknown; biochemical deviations in amino acid composition of keratins, and in the expression of keratin classes; increased formation of filaggrin
					Light and electron microscopic demonstration of suprabasal clumping of tonofilaments; cytolytic and acantholytic blister formation under mechanical stress or trauma; prenatal diagnosis (about weeks 19–21); cytolysis of suprabasal cells of unkeratinized interfollicular epidermis; tonofibrillar clumping only in areas of beginning keratinization (palms and soles)
Ichthyosis hystrix Curth–Macklin	AD	Born with white thickened skin; development of severe generalized hystrix-like dark hyperkeratoses including flexures, palms and soles; nails thickened, nipples hard; scalp skin spared; no blisters or superficial erosions	Granular degeneration, resembles mild changes of epidermolytic hyperkeratosis in paraffin sections; semithin sections: high numbers of binuclear cells, concentric perinuclear shells discernable; hyperproliferation, increased mitotic rates; thick horny layer	Suprabasal formation of binuclear cells (up to 30%) and concentric perinuclear shells of tonofilaments; oedematization in granular cells, keratohyalin attached to surface of shells; incomplete cornification	Unknown
					Ultrastructural demonstration of concentric perinuclear tonofilament shells, and of binuclear cells
Rare ichthyosiform dermatoses					
Congenital reticular ichthyosiform erythroderma[169]	?	Two solitary cases;[169,209] erythroderma and scaling since birth; gradual change to a reticulate skin pattern with normal areas enclosed by patch- and band-like confluent erythrokeratotic and pigmented skin; diffuse palmo-plantar keratosis, contractures of fingers, curved and thickened long nails	Band-like parakeratosis, irregular acanthosis with confluent rete pegs; increased basal and suprabasal mitotic rate; vacuolation of keratinocytes, many binuclear cells; papillary dermis with melanophages (pigmentary incontinence) and amyloid masses (PAS, congo-red, thioflavin-T-positive); perivascular lymphohistiocytic infiltrate	Suprabasal binuclear cells (reminiscent of I. hystrix Curth–Macklin) with perinuclear shells formed by a three-dimensional network of fine interlacing filaments (glycoproteins?); tonofilaments attached to outer surface of the shells; glycogen deposition; suppressed keratinization; oedema in upper epidermal cells; amyloid-like filaments of low diameter underneath basal lamina and in papillary dermis	Unknown
					Ultrastructural demonstration of binuclear cells and perinuclear shells formed by a three-dimensional network of fine interlacing filaments

(Continued over)

Term	Inheritance	Clinical features	Histopathology	EM features	Biochemistry/basic defect	Diagnostically significant parameters
Ichthyosis linearis circumflexa Comel (Netherton's syndrome)	AR	Netherton's syndrome: I. linearis circumflexa Comel, atopic diathesis, bamboo hairs (trichorrhexis invaginata); generalized erythroderma and scaling since birth (collodion skin?); migratory erythematous circinate or serpiginous skin lesions, centrifugal spreading, double-edged scaling border with eczematous changes; atopic diathesis (RAST, Prick test); seizures? oligophrenia? females predominantly affected	Parakeratosis and central orthohyperkeratosis; eczematous changes: moderate spongiosis and psoriasiform acanthosis at anterior scale margin; eosinophilic inclusions in granular and horny layer; dark ovoid granules in upper epidermis visible in semithin sections; exocytosis; moderate to pronounced inflammatory infiltrate	Specific changes at front of anterior scale margin: inclusions of dense, dark staining, round to ovoid granules of variable sizes in upper epidermal cells and in cornified layer, lack of keratohyalin and low amounts of tonofilaments; granular substances of moderate density in intercellular spaces (serum exudates?), suppression of keratinization, exocytosis of inflammatory cells, spongiosis and acanthosis; recovery stages: gradual changes to para- and orthohyperkeratosis	Unknown	Demonstration by EM of dense ovoid granular inclusions in upper epidermal and cornified cells at the anterior scale margin

(not shown, see Arnold et al[34]); and (3) vesicular complexes (distinct from multivesicular bodies) (Fig. 22.5, A and C) that are thought to represent aggregations of abnormal keratinosomes. Both elongated perinuclear membranes and vesicular complexes are retained in the lowermost horny cells (Fig. 22.5B). Some normal keratinosomes may be found together with the abnormal ones and with vesicular complexes. In the individual patient this pattern is highly stable and reproducible, even under oral retinoid treatment.[34] It should be noted, however, that a predominance of either membranes alone,[178] or mainly of vesicular complexes has been observed (unpublished). The underlying biochemical defect is as yet unknown, but abnormalities of keratinosome-related epidermal barrier lipids (glycosphingolipids such as ceramides) are likely to be involved. Possible further heterogeneity remains to be elucidated.

Ichthyosis congenita type IV. The frequency of this type of congenital ichthyosis is unknown as few cases have been identified. It may be assumed that perinatal death, often reported in cases of congenital ichthyosis other than of the harlequin ichthyosis type, may have been related to this type. Gruel-like amnion fluid filled with horn masses that may eventually lead to respiratory distress, was constantly found in all cases presently identified (to be published). Obviously, the overproduction of horn cells is accompanied by almost normal shedding as the amount of hyperkeratosis in surviving cases is low (Gedde-Dahl, personal communication). The characteristic feature — lentiform swollen paranuclear areas filled with masses of lipid membranes (Fig. 22.6, A and B) — clearly separates this type from type III.[10] Prenatal diagnosis has been performed by demonstration of these masses of lipid membranes in fetal epithelial cells of follicular orifices that had entered into keratinization (Fig. 22.6C and D).[10]

Ichthyosis congenita type V. A solitary case has been observed recently with severe erythroderma, scaling, growth retardation, hypospadias and hypogonadism that possibly represents a syndrome.[33] Complete suppression of keratinization-specific protein synthesis and lack of keratinosomes (i.e. of epidermal barrier lipid production) are associated with considerable hyperproliferation, high amounts of binuclear cells and abnormalities of nuclear morphology (Arnold et al, in preparation).

Autosomal dominant lamellar ichthyosis

This condition was reported by Traupe et al[224] in a family with three affected generations (Table 22.1). Clinically and histologically similar to recessive 'lamellar ichthyosis', distinction was made by abnormalities in the granular layer and an increase of the transit region.[156] Analysis of lipid composition of plantar scales revealed a decrease of free sterols and total ceramides together with increased amounts of free fatty acids, triglycerides and *n*-alkanes.[171] No analogous case has been identified as yet in the Heidelberg series.

A mother and two children with erythrodermic congenital ichthyosis[201] differed ultrastructurally from the above family and were indistinguishable from ichthyosis congenita type I.

Neutral lipid storage disease (Dorfman–Chanarin syndrome)

This represents an abnormality of intracellular triglyceride metabolism (see Table 22.1 for details). This type of systemic lipidosis with variable degrees of ichthyosiform scaling should be excluded in questionable cases of congenital ichthyosis by LM examination of peripheral granulocytes (blood smear) for lipid vacuoles (Oil red O) and by EM of keratinosomes; the latter reveal lipid droplets between their normal polar lipid lamellae, and both contents are co-discharged into, and are found within, the intercellular spaces at the granular–horny layer interface.[77,236]

Ichthyosis congenita gravis, harlequin ichthyosis

This is the severest form of keratinization disorder with armour-like hyperkeratoses, deep fissures, grossly abnormal facial appearance, and a lethal course within hours or days after delivery. Only a few exceptions with longer survival have been reported,[57,162] the latter case under successful oral retinoid therapy.

Collodion skin and harlequin ichthyosis[166] have often been confused; collodion skin describes the perinatal stage of various forms of congenital ichthyosis,[160] while harlequin ichthyosis is genetically a distinctive disorder.[166] Evidence for its heterogeneity is accumulating at present from biochemical studies.[66] Most cases reported in the literature were described merely clinically. The first ultrastructural characterization of the underlying abnormality was published by Buxman et al;[57] most cases studied so far — representing 'ichthyosis congenita gravis type I' — express this specific abnormality, with a complete lack of normal keratinosomes and an accumulation in the uppermost living and transitional epidermal cells of masses of defective keratinosomes (Fig. 22.7, A to C). Differences in the pattern of expression of cytokeratins, filaggrin[66], and other differentiation-specific markers (Anton-Lamprecht et al, in preparation) as well as in the amount of keratohyalin, indicate further heterogeneity of *type 1 harlequin ichthyosis*.

Prenatal diagnosis is possible in mid-pregnancy by the demonstration of defective keratinosomes (Fig. 22.7D) together with precocious hyperkeratinization and follicular plugging.[13,32,46]

Type II harlequin ichthyosis. This has been identified recently from a stillborn infant of 34 weeks' gestation with massive hystrix-like hyperkeratoses. In contrast to type I cases, keratinization-specific protein synthesis is more or less completely suppressed (Fig. 22.8, A and B). Abundant vesicular accumulations and some keratohyalin granules are found only around the sweat ducts (Fig. 22.8C); otherwise,

there is stacking of cells with mainly flocculent contents (Fig. 22.8, A and B). A feature not observed in the other cases of ichthyosis congenita gravis is lipid membrane accumulation in suprabasal cells (Fig. 22.8D), the nature of which is unknown (Anton-Lamprecht et al, in preparation).

Hystrix-like ichthyoses

This group comprises a series of unrelated, dominantly inherited keratinization disorders, the common feature of which is massive, often hystrix-like dark-coloured hyperkeratoses (Table 22.1).

Bullous congenital ichthyosiform erythroderma Brocq (bullous CIE; epidermolytic hyperkeratosis)

For a detailed description see Table 22.1. In contrast to the ichthyosis congenita group, children are never born as a 'collodion baby' but instead often present as a 'burnt baby'. Their blisters are frequently mistaken for epidermolysis bullosa (compare Figs. 22.9A & 22.21C with Fig. 22.21, A, B and D), since hyperkeratoses develop only gradually after birth, together with a decrease in the skin vulnerability.

It is noteworthy that the degree of severity varies largely among individual patients and families but is rather constant within the same kinship. The clinical spectrum includes generalized erythrodermic and non-erythrodermic cases (the latter corresponding to 'ichthyosis bullosa Siemens'[223]), cases with diffuse but more localized expression, naeviform variants and finally one type of palmoplantar keratoderma (Voerner type) that all share the same pathomorphogenesis and obviously the same basic underlying abnormality: suprabasal clumping of tonofilaments, followed by cytolysis and destruction, and leading to suprabasal blister formation (except in ridged skin where blisters normally are not clinically visible) (Figs 22.9, 22.11 and 22.16). These changes are termed acanthokeratolysis, granular degeneration, or epidermolytic hyperkeratosis by the histopathologist.

The mutation is transmitted as an autosomal dominant trait with full expression and penetrance. It seems that the respective normal allele has a high mutation rate: new mutations constitute a large part of all cases. Mutations do not only affect reproductive cells in the gonads but also somatic cells. The results are naevoid variants; those of larger extension follow the so-called 'Blaschko lines'.[121]

Prenatal diagnosis. Patients affected with bullous CIE have a 50% recurrence risk. Because of the usual severity, prenatal diagnosis is strongly demanded. In the fetus, cytolysis predominates at the developmental stages before the onset of keratinization (normally at about 24–26 weeks in the non-ridged skin) with low amounts of keratins (tonofilaments) per cell. Fetal tissue samples therefore may present with a wide range of changes (Fig. 22.10), and diagnosis demands a great deal of personal experience with normal and abnormal fetal skin and careful evaluation of possible artefacts.[6,12,13,14,17,137] Tonofibrillar clumps may be visible occasionally in part of the epithelial cells in amnion fluid samples,[137] but are normally restricted to a few cells around the keratinizing follicular orifices. Therefore, amnion fluid analysis alone does not allow safe exclusion of bullous CIE.

Ichthyosis hystrix Curth–Macklin

First described by Curth & Macklin in 1954,[65] this rare dominantly inherited disorder (Table 22.1) had been regarded as an unusual manifestation of bullous CIE because of 'granular degeneration', although blisters were never recorded. This genodermatosis is one example where EM finally allowed its separation as a distinctive nosologic entity.[7,12,20,180]

Most cases reported in the literature since then[7,109,148] are solitary cases due to dominant new mutations. The pathogenetic pattern common to them is so uniform and specific that it is almost impossible to distinguish separate patients morphologically: this includes tonofibrillar aggregations that do not form clumps as in bullous CIE, but form concentric perinuclear shells without increased keratin synthesis, and with a high percentage of binuclear cells in all suprabasal layers (Figs 22.12 and 22.14, A and B). In the shells, the different MW classes of keratin proteins may be distinguished by their contrast and electron-density.

A total of six cases, among them one of the original cases of Curth & Macklin[65] and the affected daughter,[180] and the case of Greither,[109] have been investigated by the author. These patients show an excellent response to treatment with retinoids; the specific abnormalities remain unchanged even following clinical clearing of the skin.[7,148]

Rare ichthyosiform dermatoses
Congenital reticular ichthyosiform erythroderma

The first case of this unusual keratinization disorder (Table 22.1) in a 57-year-old female was published by Marghescu et al.[169] A second case, in a male child, was reported recently.[209] The specific morphological abnormalities are confined to the hyperkeratotic skin areas that in the adult patient formed a reticular pattern encircling normally keratinizing skin on the trunk and extremities. The abnormal areas are rich in glycogen. Perinuclear shells and a high frequency of binuclear cells (Fig. 22.13) are reminiscent of the Curth–Macklin type. The shells are, however, formed by a tri-dimensional network of very fine interlacing filaments of unknown composition, with tonofilaments restricted to their periphery (Fig. 22.14C). Masses of amyloid deposits are found beneath the dermo-epidermal junction in the papillary dermis (see Ch. 5: legend to Fig. 5.6).

Ichthyosis linearis circumflexa Comel

This is the most characteristic skin manifestation of Neth-

erton's syndrome (Table 22.1), with the triad of ichthyosiform scaling, atopy, and bamboo hairs (trichorrhexis invaginata, see Fig. 22.47).[177,183]

The specific ultrastructural changes — inclusions of round to ovoid granules in the cells of the superficial epidermis and finely granular substances (serum exudates?) of similar density in the intercellar spaces (Fig. 22.15) — are exclusively demonstrable in front of the anterior margin of the migrating circinate scales[131] if the biopsy sites are properly chosen; many papers therefore deal with non-specific findings.

The inheritance is autosomal recessive, though females predominate; the reasons are unknown, but a higher degree of severity and perinatal mortality in males might be involved. We have identified ultrastructurally a male newborn who in fetal life (prenatal diagnosis) showed no abnormalities and developed eczematous skin lesions only gradually after birth, spreading slowly in a circinate fashion; at the same time hairs were still completely normal.[10] Very probably trichorrhexis invaginata develops not before birth and only in those hair shafts growing out concomitantly with eczematous aggravation in the skin. Prenatal diagnosis therefore does not seem to be possible during fetal development. Three other cases, two male siblings and one unrelated female, were born with generalized severely scaling erythroderma with merely non-specific eczematous changes of more or less acute dermatitis and without the specific ultrastructural markers in the skin. The diagnosis of Netherton's syndrome became clear with the demonstration of trichorrhexis invaginata three months (one male) and one year (female) after birth, respectively. In the literature, such cases have been described as combinations of congenital ichthyosiform erythroderma with bamboo hairs. The lack of hyperkeratoses and the predominance of eczematous changes separate these from typical cases of congenital ichthyosis.[16]

Palmo-plantar keratodermas

Palmo-plantar keratodermas (PPK) are a group of genodermatoses as large and heterogeneous as that of the ichthyoses but, in contrast, skin involvement is restricted to ridged skin, i.e. to the palms and soles.

In many dermatological disorders, palms and soles behave differently from the rest of the skin, with a specific clinical spectrum of changes. During fetal development, ridged skin is time-independent from the rest of the integument: the development of the dermal–epidermal interface (ridges) and of skin appendages (sweat glands), as well as the onset and completion of keratinization, occur weeks before that in non-ridged skin.[138,142,143] Nevertheless, the reasons for mutations affecting exclusively palms and soles (PPK Voerner type, see below), instead of the entire skin (bullous CIE), in spite of the same basic abnormality and dominant inheritance, are unknown.

The differential diagnosis of palmo-plantar keratodermas (PPK) is based on their distribution (diffuse or circumscript), their mode of inheritance (dominant or recessive), and on the presence or absence of associated symptoms (e.g. keratitis, periodontopathia, oesophageal carcinoma and others).[109]

Morphologically, most types of PPK show only non-specific quantitative changes by LM and EM. Only a few types are characterized by highly specific ultrastructural changes (to be discussed below in more detail). In an ultrastructural study on various types of PPK, Laurent et al[161] described composite keratohyalin granules as an abnormal feature of pathological hyperkeratinization of palms and soles. Composite keratohyalin granules are, however, a normal feature of the specific keratinization process in ridged skin[150,151] and are not distinctive of any type of PPK. In contrast, ridged skin (for instance at the transition to non-ridged skin at the dorsal aspects of hands and feet) can be identified immediately by the presence in the upper granular layer of composite keratohyalin granules in the interductal epidermis.

PPK type Voerner versus type Unna-Thost. Diffuse palmo-plantar keratosis with an erythematous borderline and with dominant transmission was generally diagnosed as PPK type Unna-Thost and regarded to be the most frequent type of PPK. In most instances, however, no biopsy samples for morphological control were taken. If controlled by LM and EM, most of these cases turn out to belong to the Voerner type (personal experience, and ref. 118).

PPK type Unna-Thost is characterized by hyperkeratosis, hypergranulosis, and acanthosis without specific structural abnormalities.[150,161] In contrast, the Voerner type reveals the same basic abnormality as bullous CIE (see Figs 22.9–22.11) with suprabasal clumps and aggregates of tonofilaments (Fig. 22.16; compare with Fig. 22.17). The higher density of these keratin aggregates corresponds to the higher amounts of tonofilaments in normal ridged skin. This, and the considerable amount of hyperkeratosis, render better protection to palms and soles in case of mechanical stress and trauma: in contrast to the non-ridged skin in bullous CIE, blisters do not develop in the Voerner type although superficial cytolysis may be found in skin sections.

Abnormalities are also seen in the form and deposition of keratohyalin (Fig. 22.18): the granules are more round than normal, often globular, and appear free in the cytoplasm or attached laterally to the keratin masses. These deviations are non-specific and are a consequence of the clumping of keratins[5] in bullous CIE (Fig. 22.18A and B), the Voerner type of PPK and the following type of PPK (Fig. 22.18C).

PPK with aggregation of tubular keratins (tonotubules) and dominant inheritance. This type of PPK, clinically appearing as a diffuse hyperkeratosis with a livid-red borderline as in the Unna-Thost type, was identified for the first time as an independent and distinct entity by the author[30] and later confirmed in additional patients (ref. 167; Anton-Lamprecht & Kastl, unpublished data). Patients

of three unrelated families with dominant transmission are presently known.

By LM, this type is either unremarkable (paraffin sections) or at the first view similar to the Voerner type (semithin sections), with suprabasal clumping of keratins. The tonotubular composition of these clumps is highly specific for this type of PPK. They originate as isolated groups of tonotubules in hexagonal array and increase steadily by the rolling up of newly formed tonofilaments in a supercoil fashion (Figs. 22.17 & Fig. 22.18C), with a fountain-like arrangement in the later stages (Fig. 22.17, C and E). Due to the segregation of the cytoplasm, actin filament bundles can be identified that normally remain obscured by the masses of keratins (Fig. 22.17E). Only little keratohyalin is deposited within the clumps of tonotubules; most of it is found adjacent to or in between them (not shown). The composite keratohyalin granules in the upper layers reveal larger differences of their constituents (Fig. 22.18C) than in normal plantar skin and in the Voerner type of PPK (Fig. 22.16, A and B). The keratin clumps formed by these tonotubules are still visible in the lower parts of the horny layer (not shown).

No tonotubular aggregates were present in the clinically normal non-ridged skin of our first patient; the keratinization pattern in skin regions other than palms and soles was normal.[30]

PPK Richner–Hanhart type, tyrosinaemia type II. This PPK with recessive inheritance and with associated symptoms is the only example of PPK where the underlying biochemical defect has been identified. Lack or abnormality of hepatic tyrosine aminotransferase leads to an accumulation of L-tyrosine in serum, urine and tissues. In the rat cornea after a high-tyrosine diet, tyrosine crystals have been shown to cause a severe inflammatory response leading to keratitis.[100,101] In humans, keratitis dendritica (pseudoherpetica) is normally the first clinical feature. Together with the demonstration of high L-tyrosine serum levels, this ocular manifestation is the basis of early diagnosis of Richner–Hanhart's syndrome.[106]

Hyperkeratoses develop gradually in relation to L-tyrosine levels and are most pronounced and painful on palms and soles. Excellent response may be achieved with a low tyrosine/low phenylalanine diet.[106] Ultrastructurally, the palmoplantar keratoses show mainly quantitative deviations, and tyrosine crystals are not deposited as in the cornea — probably prevented by the high amounts of proteins available to bind molecular tyrosine.[47]

Tubular keratins (tonotubules) were identified here for the first time[47] although they constitute only a small proportion of the overall keratins and are scattered in small groups in the periphery of the masses of densely arranged normal keratins — in contrast to the former dominant type of PPK, where tubular keratins are exclusively present in all suprabasal layers.

PPK type Meleda and related types. The palmo-plantar keratoses of the original cases from the isle of Meleda

(Yugoslavia) represent the severest of the PPK with tremendous hyperkeratoses on palms and soles, extending to the dorsal aspects of the hands and feet, wrists and heels, with distant keratoses on knees, elbows, face and elsewhere. Inheritance is autosomal recessive. The histological features are non-specific with orthohyperkeratosis, hypergranulosis, and acanthosis. Ultrastructurally, this type of PPK can be differentiated from others by its increased transition zone at the granular–horny layer interface and by the irregular arrangement of the tonofilaments.[150,152]

Several closely related types of recessive PPK with milder expression (see ref. 150) seem to constitute members of a series of allelic mutations of the Meleda gene; its chromosomal localization is still unknown. In the Gamborg-Nielsen type of PPK, differential diagnosis from the classical Meleda type is based especially on a much larger variation in the morphology (spongiosities) of the composite keratohyalin granules in ridged skin.[150,152]

Pachyonychia congenita.   This is a group of rare keratinization disorders with autosomal dominant inheritance, probably with high penetrance and variable expression, having pachyonychia (thickening of the nail plate associated with subungual keratoses in the nail bed) as a common feature. Differences in the presence or absence of associated symptoms such as leukokeratoses of oral and laryngeal mucosae, leukokeratoses of the cornea (corneal dystrophy), steatocystoma multiplex, and natal teeth, allow the distinction of three different subtypes.[210] Little is known of the pathogenesis of the lesions, and the basic defects are unknown. Skin lesions often start with periods of blistering before hyperkeratoses gradually develop. Blisters have been studied by LM and EM,[210,211] but their evolution remains questionable. In the hyperkeratotic lesions, often in spatial relationship to older blisters, dyskeratotic changes are seen in the epidermis[211] that are characterized by strictly unilaterally-oriented aggregates of tonofilaments (Fig. 22.19). This orientation seems to be the response to the presence of a gradient of diffusible factors produced, for instance, by granulocytes invading the blister cavity. Proof for this assumption is still lacking.

Although very characteristic, this type of unilateral dyskeratotic change is not specific for pachyonychia congenita and may be found in other comparable situations to a lesser extent. It is, however, distinctly different from the tonofibrillar aggregates in bullous CIE and from dyskeratosis in Darier's disease.

Dyskeratosis follicularis vegetans Darier

This disease is a dominantly inherited keratinization disorder preferentially localized in the seborrheic areas, on the chest and back, and in the axillae and groins, mostly restricted to the follicular regions. Generalized and segmentary manifestations are known; genetic counselling in the latter is problematical.

Pathomorphologically, Darier's disease is so characteristic by LM that EM is not required for the diagnosis. Ultrastructural investigations have, however, contributed to a better understanding of the pathogenetic process, although the underlying basic defect is unknown.[70,108,205,206] The first step in the development of the lesion is destruction of desmosomes, followed by suprabasal acantholysis in the centre of the lesions underneath the horn plugs. The isolated acantholytic cells in the centre undergo precocious keratinization to form the so-called 'grains' — dyskeratotic cells consisting mainly of keratin filaments that remain visible in the horny layer; they may be compared to the fibrillar or Civatte bodies formed by apoptosis and eliminated from the epidermis downwards into the papillary dermis. At the lateral border of the central acantholytic region or lacuna, individual isolated cells behave differently: their protein synthesis is enhanced[206] and they form the specific 'corps ronds', with concentrically arranged shells of tonofilaments, keratohyalin and peripheral cytoplasm, that are diagnostic of Darier's disease. No other keratinization disorder with dyskeratotic changes is known with this characteristic pattern.

Porokeratosis (PK) Mibelli

The classical form of this dominantly inherited keratinization disorder is generally not expressed before adulthood, and is most frequently found as circumscribed keratotic plaques with a double margin on the extremities and trunk. Various unusual clinical variants have been described,[168] including a more generalized form, so-called actinic porokeratosis.[204] PK Mibelli is characterized by the so-called cornoid lamella at the margin, and occasionally in the centre, of the lesion where a parakeratotic horn column piles up over an area of suppressed keratinization with the presence of: autophagocytic cells (Fig. 22.20A); isolated dyskeratoses (Fig. 22.20, A and B); and inflammatory infiltrates with ectasia of the capillary loops in the papillary dermis. Adjacent to these specific changes, non-specific disturbances with para- and ortho-hyperkeratosis are probably the consequence of the inflammatory reaction. Autophagocytic cells and vacuoles are of the highest diagnostic significance to identify PK Mibelli and its variants.

Erythrokeratodermias

This is a group of unusual sharply demarcated keratoses associated with erythema that develop from early childhood and are either stable or variable in their distribution. Most of the erythrokeratodermias (EKD) are inherited dominantly, including Mendes-da Costa's type (EKD figurata variabilis) and progressive EKD with hearing loss and keratitis[38,110,202] (mis-termed KID syndrome,[215] although keratitis is only secondary and not obligatory to the disorder, and the keratinization disturbance is not an ichthyosis[159]).

A solitary case of hystrix-like ichthyosis with inner ear

deafness (ichthyosis hystrix type Rheydt) reported by Gül-zow & Anton-Lamprecht[113] bears a striking similarity in facial appearance to patients suffering from progressive EKD with hearing loss and keratitis.[159] The hystrix-like hyper-keratoses were, however, generalized; they did not corre-spond to an erythrokeratodermia, and keratitis was lacking. The peculiar mucous granule-like cellular inclusions and mucus-like intercellular substances observed in skin samples of this patient,[4,113] have not been demonstrable in the cases of progressive EKD.[159] The inter-relationship between both types of keratinization disorder is still questionable.

Morphologically, the EKDs reveal only non-specific changes with various degrees of deviations or suppression of the normal keratinization process, and no specific ultrastruc-tural abnormalities are revealed to differentiate the various genetic types. Even the lack of keratinosomes, stressed for EKD figurata variabilis by Vandersteen & Muller[226] and in several consecutive papers, is not a constant feature[70] and may have been secondary to the disturbance of keratiniza-tion, perhaps in response to the underlying erythema. Because of this lack of specific changes, no detailed discus-sion of the EKDs is included here.

2. Ectodermal dysplasia (ED) syndromes

A highly heterogeneous group of mostly unrelated disorders[203] that share primary developmental abnormalities of skin, hair, teeth, nails and sweat glands (together with other related types of glands) is catalogued under this heading.[138] Associations with clefting (lip–jaw–palate) and other organ abnormalities are frequent. Freire-Maja & Pinheiro[89,90] have attempted a classification according to the involvement of only two, three, or all four of the adnexal ectodermally-derived structures.

Many of these disorders are extremely rare, and little is known about their pathogenesis and underlying biochemical and genetic abnormalities. The commonest and most fre-quent of all ED genotypes, Christ–Siemens–Touraine syn-drome, is closely linked to the centromeric region of the X-chromosome with the most important feature of anhidro-sis or hypohidrosis. Lack of sweat glands and a considerable reduction in the development of hair follicles in the skin of affected males and in localized areas in female carriers are taken as a basis for diagnosis, carrier detection, and prenatal diagnosis.[35,36] This is possible by LM. No ultrastructural abnormalities are revealed that would allow further cate-gorization. Molecular genetic technologies with X-DNA probes and cDNA are now available for early prenatal diagnosis.[244]

3. Epidermolysis bullosa (EB) — mechanobullous dermatoses

More than in all other groups of genodermatoses, EM has contributed significantly to the understanding of the patho-genesis, the identification of heterogeneities, and to the reliable classification of this large and heterogeneous group of disorders that share blister formation under mechanical stress and trauma as a common feature.[92] In all types of EB, blister formation occurs in the vicinity of the dermo-epidermal junction, the ultrastructure of which has been reviewed by Eady.[74]

According to the specific plane of initial blister formation, three main groups of EB are to be distinguished[93,95,96] (Figs 22.21 and 22.26):

a. EB simplex group with intra-epidermal blister formation via cytolysis of basal cells (Fig. 22.21, A, B and D; see also Figs 22.22–22.25)
b. The EB atrophicans group (or junctional EB) with junctional blister formation in the space of the lamina rara (Fig. 22.21E; see also Figs 22.27–22.31)
c. The EB dystrophica group (or scarring EB) with dermolytic blister formation underneath the basal lamina (Fig. 22.21 F; see also Figs 22.32–22.35).

The severity and sequelae depend on the plane of separation: intra-epidermal blisters normally heal without leaving scars but may induce post-bullous pigmentation. Repeated junctional blistering induces atrophy and pigmen-tation. Dermolytic blisters heal with scarring, atrophy and dyspigmentation.

Until recently only EB simplex and EB dystrophica (the latter with one dominant and one recessive type, and a lethal variant), had been distinguished on the basis of clinical features and routine histopathology. Nail dystrophies, haem-orrhagic blisters, and milia, that had been taken as a basis to diagnose dystrophic EB, turned out to be of almost no diagnostic reliability as they may be observed in each of the three main groups.[11] Especially in the newborn EB baby, the clinical features may be so non-specific that a proper diagnosis based on clinical symptoms alone is almost impossible without extensive expertise and personal experi-ence with many comparable cases. Skin biopsies are there-fore indispensable for a reliable diagnosis. By LM, no more than intra-epidermal and subepidermal blistering can be distinguished without a high risk of error. By immunofluor-escence, antigen mapping (using antibodies directed against specific structural constituents of the dermo–epidermal junction, such as bullous pemphigoid antigen, laminin, fibronectin, and collagen type IV) allows identification of intra-epidermal, junctional, and dermolytic separation,[134] but no further detailed diagnosis is possible within these three groups. More precise diagnosis may be expected from the application of specific monoclonal antibodies (such as LH 7-2, GB-3, 19-DEJ-1, AF-1 and AF-2, or collagen type VII).[53,54,75,79–81] In spite of these attempts, EM with a detailed ultrastructural analysis of skin biopsies is indispens-able for a clear and genetically reliable diagnosis of the more than 20 genetic types of EB.[11,96,115,154,187,188] Table 22.2

Table 22.2 Differential diagnosis of inherited epidermolysis bullosa types. (AD = autosomal dominant; AR = autosomal recessive)

Epidermolysis bullosa simplex group (EBS)

Term	Inheritance	Clinical features	Histopathology	Immunopathology	Ultrastructure	Remarks
EB simplex Köbner (D-EBS-K)	AD	Summer blistering; generalized; mucous membranes rarely affected; blisters serous and haemorrhagic; nails normal or disturbed; non-scarring; largely varying severity, many cases 'burnt out' at later age	Intra-epidermal blister formation, deep epidermis	Antigen mapping: bullous pemphigoid antigen, laminin, collagen IV, collagen VII at blister floor	Initial blister formation by cytolysis in subnuclear basal cell cytoplasm, no abnormalities of organelles, no persistent ultrastructural abnormalities; melanocytes uninvolved	Gene locus EBS 2? No linkage to GPT locus
EB simplex Weber–Cockayne (recurrent bullous eruptions of hands and feet) (D-EBS-WC)	AD	Summer blistering, localized (hands and feet or feet only), tardive onset; blisters form on volar and dorsal aspects of hands and feet; non-scarring	Intra-epidermal blister, often in high level or intracorneal (old!)	Same as in D-EBS-K	Initial blister formation by cytolysis in deep basal cell cytoplasm without preceding ultrastructural abnormalities; melanocytes uninvolved	Gene locus EBS 2; no linkage to GPT locus
EB simplex mottled pigmentation Fischer and Gedde-Dahl[83] (D-EBS-mottled)	AD	Non-scarring; mottled pigmentation pattern on trunk and extremities; nails thickened, curved or splitting; moderate skin atrophy	Intra-epidermal; blisters via cytolysis in basal cytoplasm of basal cells	Not done	Pigmented skin with hyperpigmentation of basal cells; cytolysis in basal parts of basal cells; multiplications of basal lamina	
EB simplex Ogna Gedde-Dahl (D-EBS-O)	AD	Non-scarring; easy bruising; blisters rarely developed; nails unaffected	Intra-epidermal blister	Not done	No primary ultrastructural abnormality before traumatic bruising or blistering	One large sibship in county of Ogna/Norway; EBS 1 gene; linkage to GPT (distance 2.6%, lods + 15.2) (on chromosome 18 or 16?)
EB simplex Barth (D-EBS-B)	AD	Non-scarring EB and localized absence of skin (lower extremities); nails in part affected, others normal; vulnerability and blistering only in first year of life	Probably intra-epidermal (original cases of Barth not investigated); many additional reports of questionable classification	Not done	Cytolytic blister formation in basal cells; no persistent ultrastructural abnormalities	One large (dominant) sibship published by Barth; later reports rely on 'localized absence of skin': other misclassified EB types included (e.g. EBD Hallopeau–Siemens type)
EB herpetiformis Dowling–Meara (D-EBH-DM)	AD	Severe blistering at birth and in first years of life, often generalized; mucous membranes involved; serous and haemorrhagic blisters; herpetiform spreading; milia possible; nails onychogryphotic, often severely affected; postbullous pigmentations; palmo-plantar keratoses; improvement at age 5–7 years; gangrene of lower extremities; lethal course and perinatal death possible	Subepidermal blister, invasion of eosinophilic leukocytes; intra-epidermal blister; non-specific	Direct immunofluorescence negative	Blister formation via cytolysis in basal cell cytoplasm; perilesional tonofilament clumping in basal (and suprabasal) cells is pathognomonic of D-EBH-DM; dyskeratotic cells in blister roof; aggregations of tonofilaments near dermo-epidermal junction at blister floor; severe inflammatory reaction	About 16–18% of all newborns with EB; prenatal diagnosis (about week 20) based on typical intrabasal blistering and tonofilament clumping

Epidermolysis bullosa atrophicans group (EBA)
(*Junctional epidermolysis bullosa*)

EB atrophicans generalisata gravis Herlitz (R-EBA-G)	AR	Blisters at birth or few hours later, pronounced at sites of mechanical stress and trauma; generalized, mucous membranes and internal organs involved; progressive lethal course; severe cases born with large epithelial defects (not aplasia cutis congenital) and pyloric obstruction (premature); serous blisters, later haemorrhagic; no scarring, but atrophy and postbullous pigmentation; nail plates elevated, early loss; nail bed granulation tissue; perioral and perinasal non-healing ulcers; milia possible	Antigen mapping: bullous pemphigoid antigen in blister roof; laminin, collagen IV and VII in blister floor: split in lamina rara; specific antibodies: lack of GB 3 and 19-DEJ-1 binding antigens	Junctional blister with basal lamina/anchoring fibrils at blister floor; split in space of lamina rara; fresh blisters clean; melanocytes in blister cavity; basal cells at fresh blister roof lack basal lamina and hemidesmosomes; rapid remodelling at blister roof; intact skin: severe hypoplasia of hemidesmosomes, low numbers, minute attachment plates, no sub-basal dense plates; most pronounced in cases with large epithelial defects and pyloric obstruction	Most frequent genetic type: about 45–50% of all newborns with EB; prenatal diagnosis about week 20 by EM of fetal skin: junctional separation, hemidesmosome hypoplasia, lack of sub-basal dense plates in intact regions; lack of GB 3 and 19-DEJ-1 binding antigens
EB atrophicans generalisata mitis Hashimoto (R-EBA-M)	AR	Blisters at birth or few hours later; symptoms as in Herlitz type; generalized, but milder course; in infancy many small facial blisters; diffuse alopecia, postbullous pigmentation, nevocellular nevi; nails thickened, elevated, granulation tissue in nail bed; palmar and plantar keratoses; enamel defects; milia possible	As in Herlitz type	Antigen mapping and reaction of GB 3 and 19-DEJ-1 antibodies as in Herlitz type	Hemidesmosome hypoplasia less pronounced than in Herlitz type: attachment plates more frequent and longer; lack of sub-basal dense plates	Less frequent than Herlitz type; prenatal diagnosis as in Herlitz type
EB atrophicans ulcerovegetans (R-EBA-UV)	AR	Severe non-healing facial ulcerations (granulation tissue)	As in Herlitz type	–	Regional variation in quality or abnormality of hemidesmosomes	Very rare
EB atrophicans inversa (R-EBA-I)	AR	Blistering and non-healing erosions most pronounced in inverse sites: neck, axillae, groins; corneal erosions, enamel defects	As in Herlitz type	–	Variations in abnormality of hemidesmosomes	Rare type
EB atrophicans localisata (R-EBA-L)	AR	Restricted to hands, feet, lower legs; enamel defects; nails elevated, dome-like	As in Herlitz type	–	As in mitis type	Very rare, mild variant

(Continued over)

Term	Inheritance	Clinical features	Histopathology	Immunopathology	Ultrastructure	Remarks
EB atrophicans cicatricans (R-EBA-C)	AR	Scar formation after blistering, syndactyly, contractures; loss of nails in early infancy; oral mucosa affected, dysphagia; stenosis of anterior nares; corneal opacities; cicatricial alopecia; no milia[114]	Subepidermal blister formation	Not done	Junctional blister formation in the lamina rara; basal lamina at blister floor; rudimentary hemidesmosomes lacking sub-basal dense plates in intact skin; blisters invaded by inflammatory cells[114]	Very rare, one family (4/11 siblings) and one solitary case reported; scarring secondary to inflammatory reaction and superinfection
EB progressiva Gedde-Dahl (R-EBP)	AR	Tardive EB with juvenile onset; nail dystrophy at 5–8 years, serous and haemorrhagic blisters on hands and feet a few years later; slow progression to diffuse skin atrophy, (hands, feet, knees, elbows), cigarette-paper skin; loss of dermatoglyphic ridge pattern; palmar keratoses and contractures; oral mucosa affected, loss of lingual papillae; enamel defective	Subepidermal blister; atrophy of papillary dermis, loss of papillae, amorphous matrix; loss of elastic fibres in superficial dermis	Not done	Widening of lamina rara with deposits of amorphous material; hemidesmosomes normal; junctional separation?	Genetic linkage to hypoacusis in three families; to red hair in one family; very rare

Epidermolysis bullosa dystrophica group (EBD)

Term	Inheritance	Clinical features	Histopathology	Immunopathology	Ultrastructure	Remarks
EB dystrophica Hallopeau–Siemens type (R-EBD-HS)	AR	Scarring EB with predominance in acral regions; localized, generalized and severely mutilating variants; mild cases with gradual development of blisters and scarring, no mucous membrane involvement; severe cases born with large epithelial defects (legs); cigarette-paper scars and milia; nails dystrophic or complete loss; synechiae and mutilations; involvement of mucous membranes; oesophageal stenosis; teeth dystrophic; corneal erosions, scarring, and symblepharon; scarring alopecia; renal disturbances; glomerulonephritis; amyloidosis; risk of scar carcinomas	Subepidermal blistering; epidermis atrophic, loss of normal dermal architecture, scar tissue; severe inflammatory reaction	Antigen mapping: bullous pemphigoid antigen, laminin, and collagen IV in blister roof, dermolytic separation; variable expression of collagen type VII: antigenic domains of anchoring fibrils; absent binding of KF-1 and LH7:2 monoclonal antibodies	Dermolytic blister formation below basal lamina; severe cases have few hypoplastic anchoring fibrils in intact regions; milder cases show intralesional variation from normal to absence; initial changes by focal collagenolysis, sparing basal lamina, anchoring fibrils, and elastic microfibrils (oxytalan); rapid secondary changes at blister roof: remodelling and translocation of basal lamina to higher levels at blister roof: lack at undersurface in older blister roofs!	Frequency high: about 30% of all newborns with EB; true homozygotes and compound heterozygotes of various allelic mutants in EBR 1 locus assumed; basic defect: genetically abnormal enzyme collagenase produced in excessive amounts;[43] gene locus for collagenase: CLG locus on chromosome 11 cDNA available; identical with EBR 1 locus? Therapy with phenytoins; prenatal diagnosis (week 20) by EM of fetal skin: dermolytic separation; prenatal and postnatal changes identical

Disease	Inheritance	Clinical features	Histopathology	Antigen mapping	Ultrastructural features	Genetics/comments
EB dystrophica inversa Gedde-Dahl (R-EBD-I)	AR	Scarring EB with predominance in inverse regions: neck, axillae, groins and sacral region most severely affected; no synechiae or mutilations; nails dystrophic; milia occasionally present; mucous membranes involved; oesophageal stenosis; teeth, eyes and scarring alopecia similar to R-EBD-HS	Histopathology similar to R-EBD-HS: dermolytic blistering	Type VII collagen expressed[245]	Ultrastructural features similar to R-EBD-HS: dermolytic blistering, focal collagenolysis; variation in amount and quality of anchoring fibrils	Rare genetic type; probably allelic mutation to R-EBD-HS, collagenase abnormality in CLG locus on chromosome 11, abnormality of anchoring fibrils
EB dystrophica dominans Pasini (D-EBD-P)	AD	Scarring EB with predominance of lesions on acral locations: hands and feet, elbows and knees; palms and soles also affected, but dorsal aspects more pronounced; lesions on neck and sacral region; milia in children on back of hands; albopapuloid spots in 2nd decade; nails dystrophic or partly normal; mucous membrane involvement; no oesophageal stenosis; no synechiae or mutilations	Subepidermal blister formation; loss of elastic fibres in scars	Antigen mapping: same distribution as in R-EBD-HS; some cases lack collagen type VII antigen[54]	Dermolytic blister formation below basal lamina; intact regions either lack anchoring fibrils completely or have ±normal anchoring fibrils; no intra-individual variation as in R-EBD-HS; same amount of AF hypoplasia whether in sites of predilection or not	Genetic linkage with secretor locus (chromosome 19)? Gene locus EBD 1; prenatal diagnosis is not yet done; possible by evaluation of anchoring fibrils in fetal skin in families with AF hypoplasia
EB dystrophica dominans Cockayne–Touraine (D-EBD-CT)	AD	Mildest localized scarring type of EB, blisters mainly on hands and feet, ankles; scars; infants milia with multiple milia; no mucous membrane involvement; no albopapules	As in the Pasini type (predilection sites)	Antigen mapping: same distribution as in R-EBD-HS; normal expression of LH7:2 monoclonal AB in postnatal and fetal skin; reduced binding of KF-1 monoclonal antibody	Dermolytic blister formation; normal anchoring fibrils in non-predilection sites, hypoplasia in predilection sites	Prenatal diagnosis about week 20 by EM (and immunology)
Pretibial EB dystrophica Kuske–Portugal (D-EBD-KP)	AD	Onset with very mild involvement; mainly small serous blisters, no severe scarring; very slow progression; generalized tendency to blistering; nails normal or dystrophic; milia; in adults very slow and gradual development of hypertrophic scars on lower legs, mainly pretibial, with sharp demarcation from 'normal' skin, centripetal spreading;[82] no synechiae or mutilations, no oesophageal stenosis	Subepidermal blister	Antigen mapping: bullous pemphigoid antigen, laminin and collagen IV at blister roof;[82] KF-1 monoclonal antibody (lamina densa) as in R-EBD-HS; very faint binding[82]	Dermolytic blister formation; basal lamina without or with many long anchoring fibrils at blister roof; inter-individual variation in quality of anchoring fibrils	Rare genetic type; dominant inheritance; isolated cases have been regarded as recessive variants of scarring EB; risk for scar carcinoma; amputation of lower leg in one case because of carcinoma in scarred skin

lists the most important clinical, morphological, biochemical and genetic criteria for the identification of the specific type of EB, including prenatal diagnosis.

The proper selection of the biopsy site, and of the respective skin lesion, the careful evaluation of semithin sections, and the critical selection of optimal sites for subsequent ultrathin sectioning are of the highest significance for reliable diagnostic statements in EB. Tissue samples should always include clinically and morphologically intact pre-lesional skin and skin with initial stages of blister formation (Fig. 22.21, A to F). Most pre-existing blisters are too old, with predominance of secondary changes. Most patients are not able to delineate the age of a lesion exactly. Initial changes and fresh blisters can be induced experimentally by friction. Sites of predilection and of non-predilection as well as the special conditions in the pathogenetic events preceding the clinical appearance of blisters, such as the temperature threshold in EB simplex Köbner and Weber–Cockayne ('summer blistering') should be considered. Time intervals after friction necessary to induce the primary changes are to be kept in mind: in junctional EB, especially of the Herlitz type, friction will immediately lead to the separation of the epidermis from the papillary dermis, while a time interval depending on the actual activity of the disease (at least 30–60 min) is required after friction to allow collagenolysis to proceed to visible changes in recessive dystrophic EB (Hallopeau–Siemens and inversa types). Friction should be performed as gently as possible, using a small firm cotton swab and never by whirling a pencil eraser on the skin surface; the latter generally destroys the tissue, especially the epidermis, to a degree that prevents correct identification of the specific primary abnormalities because of overlap with secondary destruction.

Many controversies and discrepancies in the literature concerning the pathogenetic events in EB have been due to the selection of lesions that were too old, and to mechanical artefacts in taking the biopsies.

Secondary changes begin soon after separation of the epidermis from the dermal connective tissue and include:

a. Remodelling of the blister roof with formation of an ectoplasm (Fig. 22.23 B) and translocation of hypoplastic hemidesmosomes in cases of junctional EB (Fig. 22.31); stepwise infolding of the basal lamina and its translocation to higher cellular layers within the blister roof in cases of dystrophic EB (Fig. 22.35).
b. Destruction of the undersurface of the blister roof with gaps in the basal lamina, deposition of fibrin, debris and serum proteins, obscurity or complete destruction of the basal lamina in cases of dystrophic EB (Fig. 22.35).
c. Destruction of the blister floor by (non-specific) activation of enzymes in full-blown blister with loss of basal lamina in cases of junctional EB, and destruction of cytoplasmic remnants of basal cells in cases of the EB simplex group ('pseudojunctional blister') (not shown).
d. Invasion of inflammatory cells (granulocytes, lymphocytes, macrophages) into the blister cavity (Fig. 22.35A).
e. Formation of granulation tissue in older erosions in junctional EB.
f. Wound repair with invasion and proliferation of keratinocytes at the blister floor, to be differentiated from intra-epidermal blistering in cases of junctional EB.

As a rule, blisters older than 2 to 8 hours and haemorrhagic blisters are unsuitable for diagnostic purposes.

Tissue samples in EB should never be taken by a punch; full-skin knife biopsies are best suited, and are superior to shave biopsies, the larger parts of which do not consist of the whole tissue. Healing after knife biopsy is normally uncomplicated in EB.

Proper diagnosis is not possible from the blister roof or blister floor alone; if separated under the sampling procedure, blister roofs should be prepared together with the remaining tissue.

EB skin samples should not be subdivided before the tissue is sufficiently fixed (2 hours at minimum) to avoid mechanical artefacts. Mailing of tissue samples to the EM laboratory is best done in toto, without subdivision, to ensure optimal preparation.

Epidermolysis bullosa simplex group
EB simplex Köbner and EB simplex Weber–Cockayne

Summer blistering, absence of nail dystrophies (exceptions possible), and lack of scarring, together with intra-epidermal blister formation in basal cells, are distinctive of both types of EB simplex with generalized or localized involvement, respectively (Table 22.2). The Köbner type generally manifests at birth or soon after. Most cases of the Weber–Cockayne type are recognized only with crawling and walking, or in adulthood. The frequency of the latter type may be underestimated. The Köbner type was regarded as the most frequent type of EB until recently; this estimate was based mostly on clinical features alone, and sometimes including LM. In the more than 460 unselected, ultrastructurally investigated cases of EB in the Heidelberg series that include the Norwegian cases collected by Gedde-Dahl,[92] the Köbner type accounts for only about 4% of all newborn EB babies.

The pathomorphogenesis is the same in both types of EB simplex. Initial changes become visible as fluid accumulation in the subnuclear region of basal cells (Fig. 22.21A), followed by cytolysis via focal dissolution of the cytoplasm,[217] while organelles, membranes, cytoskeleton and nuclei are spared (Figs 22.21A and 22.22). Epidermal keratinocytes are affected selectively, as shown by non-involvement of melanocytes and Langerhans' cells.[119]

In the Weber–Cockayne type, blisters are often found high in the epidermis, including intra-corneal splits.[119,187,188] In ridged skin many fresh blisters seem to remain subclinical under the protection of the thick horny layers of palms and soles; experimental friction or physiological stress therefore disclose old blisters at high levels, as shown by the surrounding tissue ultrastructure. For diagnostic purposes, friction blisters are better provoked on non-ridged skin of the foot instep (base of the toes); in these cases fresh intra-basal blisters are obtained.

Prenatal diagnosis might be demanded for risk of severe Köbner cases (50% recurrence risk). Because of the lack of persistent ultrastructural abnormalities, the chances of identifying affected fetuses are uncertain,[8] and have not yet been recorded.

EB herpetiformis Dowling–Meara

This dominant type of EB was misclassified until recently because of the large spectrum of clinical symptoms in individual patients, during development and in the course of the disease, and because of the many possible variations in the LM and EM changes (Table 22.2). First described by Dowling & Meara[72], this EB resembled dermatitis herpetiformis Duhring and was thought to be a recessive, subepidermal bullous disorder. Gedde-Dahl[93] was the first to prove the dominant inheritance, and the specific ultrastructural changes were first delineated by the author.[21,29,55,116,179] More than 60 cases have been identified in the Heidelberg series; among newborns with EB, the Dowling–Meara type accounts for about 16–18%, thus being one of the most frequent genetic types of EB.[8]

Many of the patients are isolated cases (dominant new mutations). Families with large pedigrees have been observed (Anton-Lamprecht, personal experience; also ref. 116). The degree of severity is highly variable. Clinical and ultrastructural findings are most pronounced in early childhood (at the age of about 2–3 years). Because of the centrifugal spreading and rapid central healing of the lesions, with many small fresh blisters forming at the periphery, the term EB herpetiformis has been coined.[21,29]

Tonofibrillar clumps and aggregates in basal (and partly suprabasal) cells are pathognomonic of the Dowling–Meara type. They are not persistently expressed in clinically uninvolved skin and are found predominantly in perilesional skin (Figs 22.21D, 22.23 and 22.24) preceding blister formation (Figs 22.21D and 22.25). In cases of exaggerated cytolysis (Fig. 22.21B) this clumping may not be expressed similarly. The selection of the biopsy site is therefore of utmost importance.[11] Demonstration of clumping proves EB herpetiformis, whereas its absence does not disprove the diagnosis. The degree and amount of clumping is highly variable among patients and within the same tissue sample (Figs 22.23 and 22.24). Rapid spreading and high repair activity are responsible for the large variation in findings

during the progression of the blisters (Fig. 22.25). Prenatal diagnosis has successfully been performed in one case with demonstration of tonofilament clumps in fetal skin.[19]

Curled strands of tonofibrils may be seen occasionally during blister formation in EB simplex Weber–Cockayne[119] because of the higher amounts of tonofilaments in ridged skin; true clumps are never formed.

Epidermolysis bullosa atrophicans (EBA) group

Differentiation of genetic subtypes within this group refers mainly to clinical symptoms, severity, course of the disease and prognosis (Table 22.2). They all share junctional blister formation in the plane of the lamina rara (Figs 22.21E, 22.26, 22.30 and 22.31), with the basal lamina covering the blister floor. In the Heidelberg series, the EBA group accounts for about one-third of all EB cases investigated by EM; the (lethal) Herlitz type is by far the most frequent, occurring in about 45–50% of all newborn EB babies.[8,11]

All genetic subtypes of EBA reveal the same underlying basic defect: a more or less severe hypoplasia of hemidesmosomes with lack of the sub-basal dense plates in the lamina rara[4,11,12,28] (Figs 22.26, 22.27 and 22.29). Immunologically, this defect is expressed by the lack of hemidesmosome-associated antigenic epitopes 19-DEJ-1 and others.[75,79,81] The degree of hypoplasia corresponds to the degree of clinical severity. Cases of 'epidermolysis bullosa with pyloric atresia'[189] that represent the severest manifestation of the Herlitz type, mostly born premature and with large epithelial defects, reveal the severest degree of hemidesmosome hypoplasia[10,173] (Fig. 22.27). Milder, non-lethal, benign variants[11,127,136] (Table 22.2) may show a better structural development of the attachment plates but no sub-basal dense plates (Fig. 22.29).

Prenatal diagnosis of the junctional epidermolyses[6,8,10,12–15] is based on the demonstration of hemidesmosome hypoplasia with lack of sub-basal dense plates (Fig. 22.28B) and junctional separation, whereas normally developed hemidesmosomes[6,8,165] (Fig. 22.28A) permit safe exclusion in fetuses at risk.

Post-bullous pigmentations and large naevus cell naevi are frequent in patients with junctional EB:[28,111,127] during blister formation, melanocytes (and naevus cells) lose their normal support in the basal layer and are found dropping into or floating in the blister cavity (Fig. 22.30C) or seated on the blister floor, where naevus cells may spread freely.

Hypoplasia of hemidesmosomes is not only responsible for junctional separation in the skin, but also in mucous membranes of the oral cavity and in many inner organs (unpublished data), and it causes enamel defects of decidual and permanent teeth in junctional EB patients as shown recently for the enamel organ of the developing tooth buds of Herlitz fetuses.[208]

Epidermolysis bullosa dystrophica group

This group comprises dominant (3) and recessive (2) types of EB, all characterized by nail dystrophy and pronounced scarring (Table 22.2). Split formation in all of them is dermolytic, immediately below the basal lamina or in close proximity to the papillary dermis (Fig. 22.26).

The typical aspect of dermolytic blisters with the basal lamina at the blister roof is found only in initial and in very fresh blisters (Figs 22.21F, 22.32 and 22.33), as rapid changes take place as soon as the separation has occurred. Remodelling of the blister roof with infolding of the basal lamina (Fig. 22.35, C to E) and its gradual translocation to central layers of the roof lead to lack of the basal lamina and formation of an ectoplasm-like undersurface (Fig. 22.35B), with the risk of misinterpretation and erroneous diagnosis. If the blister cavity is filled with fibrin, cells and debris, the basal lamina may be obscured (Fig. 22.35A) or destroyed. Therefore, fresh blisters, blister roof and blister floor, *and* intact dermo–epidermal junction areas have to be analysed for reliable diagnosis.

The differential diagnosis of the EB dystrophica group is especially difficult. As a rule, in the recessive types focal collagenolysis is demonstrable as the first step of (enzymatic) destruction adjacent to blisters and in intact skin regions; in the dominant types the split lies immediately below the basal lamina in the region of the anchoring fibrils (AF) which possess collagen type VII as a major structural protein.[53,54] In the dominant Pasini type, a few very thin and faint hypoplastic AF are demonstrable in any location; in the milder Cockayne–Touraine type, AF hypoplasia is restricted to the sites of predilection of blister formation.[22,125,126] Patients with the dominant pretibial Kuske–Portugal type may reveal long AF at the basal lamina in the blister roof, and variations in their amount and quality in intact skin (Anton-Lamprecht, unpublished). The most pronounced variation in the presence or absence and quality of AF is found in intact junctional areas of the recessive types, especially the Hallopeau–Siemens type. Newborns and infants have pronounced suppression of AF or total lack in mutilating cases (Fig. 22.34, A and B), while in adults AF are more variable. Heterozygotes do not express any ultrastructural abnormality (Fig. 22.34C).

The Hallopeau–Siemens type belongs to the most frequent types of EB. Among newborns with EB this type accounts for about 27–30%[8,11] and there is a high risk of the disorder in all children born to 'at-risk' parents. Prenatal diagnosis is strongly demanded because of this high risk and the general severity, especially in mutilating cases. Affected fetuses show the same dermolytic blister formation as found in postnatal cases, areas of focal collagenolysis, and lack of normal anchoring fibrils in intact junction areas.[6,8,13,15,25] Prenatal exclusion is based on the ultrastructural normality of the constituents of the dermo–epidermal junction of at-risk fetuses.[8]

4. Connective tissue disorders

The diagnostic ultrastructural features of several important connective tissue disorders, such as the Ehlers–Danlos syndrome,[58,59,94,139,140,191] scleroedema adultorum Buschke,[129] scleromyxoedema Arndt-Gottron,[123,218] cutis laxa[59,67,70,88,128,139,140,176,225,228] and pseudoxanthoma elasticum,[68,70,88,192,193,200,207,225,230] are discussed in Chapter 5, together with the ultrastructural, functional and biochemical properties, and recent molecular genetic aspects of the normal dermal connective tissue and its non-cellular constituents.[53,56,59,62,88,94,140,143,199,214,216]

5. Pigmentary disorders

Disorders of the human pigment cell system are manifold because of the occurrence of melanocytes not only in skin, hairs and eyes, but also in the inner ear, nervous system (pia-arachnoid), genital and other mucous membranes. They include genetic, acquired (e.g. post-bullous or post-inflammatory), immunological and malignant disturbances of pigmentation.

Most genetic pigmentary disorders present as hypopigmentations. Referred to as albinism, they result from interference of gene mutations with the normal multistep metabolic pathway of melanin synthesis, or from disturbances in the migration of melanocytes to the skin, eyes or inner ear from the neural crest (Klein–Waardenburg syndromes, BADS syndrome, i.e. black lock, oculocutaneous albinism, and deafness of the sensorineural type). The various types of albinism are distinguished on the basis of clinical, genetic, biochemical and ultrastructural criteria.[238,239]

Ultrastructural investigations are important in distinguishing the various forms. Tyrosinase-negative (tyr –) and tyrosinase-positive (tyr +) albinism are differentiated by EM demonstration of tyrosinase activity in melanocytes of hair bulbs and skin (Fig. 22.36). The Hermansky–Pudlak syndrome, a combination of tyr + albinism with haemorrhagic diathesis, may be identified by the demonstration of storage material resembling ceroid and lipofuscin, phospholipids and neutral lipids — in macrophages, in peripheral monocytes or neutrophils, in cells of the reticulo-endothelial system or of oral mucosa, in the bone marrow and in urinary sediment — and by demonstrating platelet abnormalities with virtual absence of dense bodies (reviewed by Witkop et al[239]). The Chediak–Higashi syndrome is characterized by pigment dilution, the presence of giant granules in melanocytes, (interfering with pigmentation) and in leucocytes (interfering with chemotaxis and degranulation) and by marked susceptibility to infection (reviewed by Witkop et al[239]) (see also Ch. 30).

Oculocutaneous albinism

The two major forms, tyr – and tyr + albinism, occur with similar frequency, and both are recessively inherited. They are *not* allelic: mating of tyr + and tyr − albino individuals produces normally pigmented offspring.[238]

Tyr − melanocytes are fully functional except for their enzyme deficiency that blocks the melanin pathway at the level of stage II melanosomes, even after successful cellular stimulation (Fig. 22.36, A and B).[147] Tyr + albinism shows a larger range of phenotypic expression, depending on the age, racial and family background, and possibly also on heterogeneity (ref. 238; Hausser & Anton-Lamprecht, unpublished data). The enzyme tyrosinase exists in several isoenzyme forms. Tyrosinase (isoenzyme T_3) is synthesized in the RER and is transported in soluble form to the Golgi apparatus where it becomes demonstrable ultrastructurally in the outermost Golgi cisterna after glycosylation by addition of neutral sugars and sialic acid (isoenzyme T_1). Synthetic activity of tyrosinase is probably blocked by a tyrosinase inhibitor until the enzyme has been bound to the melanosomal matrix (insoluble isoenzyme T_4). Further factors cooperate in the sequence of melanogenesis after initial DOPA formation from tyrosine by T_4 tyrosinase (reviewed by Witkop et al[239]). Transport of the soluble isoenzymes T_3 and T_1 to the Golgi apparatus and to the melanosomes, absence or defects of post-tyrosinase regulation, or disturbed binding of tyrosinase to (defective?) melanosomes are among possible reasons for lack of melanin formation — in spite of the presence of tyrosinase in tyr + albinism.

Although tyrosinase activity is demonstrable in the outermost Golgi cisterna, DOPA is converted to melanin in only a few of the small melanosomes of patients with tyr + albinism (Fig. 22.36, C and D). Most melanosomes (stages I and II) fail to form melanin in the DOPA reaction (Hausser, unpublished data).

Prenatal diagnosis of oculocutaneous albinism (unclassified) has been performed using melanocytes of fetal scalp hair bulbs by ultrastructural evaluation of the hair bulb melanosomes[73] that are normally more developed than skin melanosomes in neighbouring fetal skin (see discussion in ref. 14).

Klein–Waardenburg syndrome

The classical type (I) is now referred to as Waardenburg's syndrome and is characterized by: partial albinism; white forelock or premature greying; dilute pigmentation or heterochromia of the irides; unilateral or bilateral inner ear deafness or hearing loss; a peculiar centrofacial appearance with lateral displacement of the inner canthi, epicanthus, hypertelorism and synophrys, broad nasal bridge and hypoplastic alae nasi; cupid-bow form of the upper lip; full lower lip; deep-set ears and occasional helical abnormalities; and possible further malformations such as clefting or CNS involvement. The expression is highly variable, and many formes frustes exist.

Recently the syndrome was further differentiated.[107,117]

Types I and II are dominantly inherited, differing mainly in the incidence of deafness (25% in type I, with severe deafness if present; about 50% in type II, with milder hypoacusis) and in the expression of the centrofacial abnormalities. Hypertelorism and lateral displacement of the inner canthi are pronounced in type I and mild or lacking in type II. Type III[155] is a rare, recessively inherited disorder combining features of type I with severe bone abnormalities, especially of the upper extremities and the shoulder girdle.[107]

Hypopigmentation: variable frequencies of melanocytes in combination with suppression of melanin synthetic activity have been found in type I cases, pointing to disturbances of the migration of melanocytes to the skin from the neural crest. DOPA reaction of the melanocytes in hypopigmented skin areas shows suppression of the melanogenic activity in all stages of melanosomes, in contrast to oculocutaneous albinism (Hausser et al, in preparation).

Partial albinism in type III (original case of Klein[155]) was combined with hyperpigmentation. Low numbers of melanocytes with completely suppressed melanogenic activity but intact, undamaged cytoplasm are demonstrable in hypopigmented skin. Melanocytes of hyperpigmented areas are present in low concentration as well; the cells are, however, large and hypertrophic (possibly polyploid) with prominent RER and Golgi apparatus, and excessive numbers of melanosomes of all stages, with their prominent dendrites filled with fully melanized melanosomes (ref. 24; Anton-Lamprecht, unpublished). Abnormalities of melanocyte migration combined with disturbed regulation of melanogenic activity may be assumed.

Tuberous sclerosis Bourneville–Pringle

Tuberous sclerosis (TS) is an autosomal dominant neurocutaneous disorder combining mental retardation, convulsions, and calcification of the brain with characteristic skin manifestations such as: adenoma sebaceum in the face; cobble stone naevi (connective tissue naevi) on the trunk; subungual fibromas (Koenen tumours) of the toes; and gingival fibromas. Eye, bone, and cardiac involvement may be present. TS belongs to the phakomatoses[196] that are all caused by dominant genes with highly variable expression and often incomplete penetrance.

Hypopigmented spots, so-called white leaf-shaped macules, are most often the first visible sign of TS, appearing in early childhood before other more severe clinical manifestations. Their identification therefore is important for the early detection of TS[84,222] and an important aid in carrier detection and genetic counselling.[130]

TS hypopigmented macules may be differentiated from vitiligo by the presence of melanocytes in normal densities, by their normal ultrastructure and apparent lack of visible cell and organelle damage, and by suppression of melanogenesis with only stage I and II melanosomes (Fig. 22.37A) and intralesional variation in the expression of tyrosinase activity (DOPA reactivity; Fig. 22.37, B to D).[130]

Hypopigmented vitiligo spots lack melanocytes centrally or in long-standing lesions, and they show variably reduced melanocyte densities and signs of melanocyte damage at the margins of fresh, spreading vitiligo lesions (probably immunologically caused); active normal melanocytes in normal density are present in the surrounding tissue.[130]

Incontinentia pigmenti Bloch–Sulzberger

This disorder is an X-linked dominant trait (mapped to Xp 11 close to the centromere on the short arm of the X-chromosome[94]) with lethality in the hemizygous male, that is viable only as a functional mosaic.[122] Due to random X-inactivation (Lyonization) early in embryonal development, heterozygous females represent functional mosaics of two kinds of cell lines carrying either the normal or the mutant X-chromosome. The severity and extent of the disease, including convulsions, severe CNS abnormalities, or clefting, depend on how many cell lines carry the mutant X in an active state.

In the skin these cell lines follow the Blaschko lines.[121] The initial stage, present at or soon after birth, is a linear vesicular rash with exocytosis of granulocytes, mainly eosinophils, which develops to form small micro-abscesses, pustules and small to large vesicles high in the epidermis. These lesions heal within weeks or some months passing through a verrucous hyperkeratotic stage, in which isolated dyskeratotic cells are found in the epidermis. The final stage is characterized by hyperpigmentation due to pigmentary incontinence in dermal melanophages that vanishes with time, and sometimes with hypopigmented scars.

Incontinentia pigmenti Bloch–Sulzberger is easily diagnosed clinically and by light microscopy: EM is not required for its identification.

BULLOUS SKIN DISEASES OF IMMUNOLOGICAL ORIGIN

This group of disorders, with localized or generalized blister formation on skin and partly also on mucous membranes, may be regarded as non-hereditary counterparts and phenocopies of the inherited epidermolyses. They are all autoimmune disorders that result from the generation of autoantibodies against antigenic sites in the epidermis (pemphigus; herpes gestationis) or along the dermoepidermal junction (bullous pemphigoid; cicatricial pemphigoid; dermatitis herpetiformis Duhring; linear IgA bullous dermatosis; EB acquisita).[153]

Considerable progress has been achieved in recent years in the understanding and differentiation of these disorders. In addition to the classical types — pemphigus, bullous pemphigoid (BP), and dermatitis herpetiformis Duhring

(DHD) — new and unusual types have been identified. All of them occur not only in adults but also in children.

Linear IgA bullous dermatosis combines features of BP and DHD by immunology, plane of splitting, and response to steroid versus sulfone therapy. Conventional EM and immuno-EM have shown two distinctive types with linear IgA patterns: a lamina lucida type (with junctional splitting as in BP and junctional EB) and a lamina densa type (with dermolytic splitting as in DHD and dystrophic epidermolysis bullosa).

Cicatricial pemphigoid (CP) exists in several clinically different forms and with different immunological reaction patterns;[79] their cleavage plane by EM is below the basal lamina, sometimes also junctional.

Acquired epidermolysis bullosa (AEB) with scarring, milia, and nail dystrophies, is a phenocopy of scarring or dystrophic EB. Proof for AEB being a separate nosologic entity and not a manifestation of CP (as claimed by some authors) came from EM and from the identification of the EB acquisita and CP antigens at different sites of the dermo–epidermal junction (see refs 79 and 240). The AEB antigen detected by patient sera and by monoclonal antibodies, has been shown to be part of the anchoring fibrils, namely type VII procollagen.[240,241,243] The CP antigen is assumed to reside in the lamina lucida; however, the clinical and EM diversity of CP cases points to possible heterogeneity of these antigens too (for further details see ref. 79).

The BP antigen is localized in the uppermost lamina rara, associated with the basal cell plasma membrane; it seems that various types of BP antigens exist in the skin.[79]

These bullous dermatoses are normally diagnosed by means of direct and indirect immunofluorescence methods, in part by immuno-EM.[153] Patients with AEB often fail to show circulating antibodies; the same is true for milder cases of BP, and skin samples of DHD may be negative unless repeated biopsies are investigated. Immunological patterns often do not allow a clear distinction between BP, CP and AEB cases.

In such doubtful cases, normal transmission EM can help to identify the specific type of bullous dermatosis (Fig. 22.38). Bullous pemphigoid is identified by the cleavage plane in the lamina rara (l. lucida), by *normal* hemidesmosomes outside the blister areas (in contrast to junctional EB with hypoplasia of hemidesmosomes), and by migration of inflammatory cells into the blister cavity and perilesional epidermis (Fig. 22.38A). Cicatricial pemphigoid — disseminated variant — shows a characteristic pattern of initial blister formation (Fig. 22.38B) by the coalescence of microvesicles below the basal lamina by which it may be identified and distinguished from other types of dermolytic blister formation.[132] Acquired EB may be identified by EM without immunological aids by its band-like granular deposits (immune complexes) below the basal lamina in intact skin and in split areas at the blister roof, obscuring the anchoring fibrils (Fig. 22.38, C and D).[132]

DISORDERS WITH DEPOSITION OF PATHOLOGICAL SUBSTANCES

Amyloidoses

The ultrastructural characteristics of the cutaneous deposits seen in the amyloidoses[49,50,52,102,104,129,135,158,164,228] are considered in detail in Chapter 5.

Erythropoietic protoporphyria and hyalinosis cutis et mucosae

Both of these diseases are genetically determined and share clinical and morphological features, although the underlying basic abnormalities are completely different. Both become manifest in infancy with blistering episodes, leaving small linear (vermicular) scars on the face and back of hands, and gradually proceed to a thickening and coarsening of the involved skin (pachydermia).

Erythropoietic protoporphyria (EPP)

This disease, first described in 1953 by Kosenow & Treibs,[157] is caused by a dominantly transmitted defect in porphyrin metabolism, probably of haem synthetase (ferrochelatase) activity, that leads to an accumulation of protoporphyrin in circulating erythrocytes (demonstrable by unstable red autofluorescence), as well as to an increase of coproporphyrin in the blood (with no increase of porphyrins in the urine and faeces). Absorption of UV (λ = 400–460 mμ) by protoporphyrin in light-exposed peripheral skin regions provokes vascular damage with partial destruction and subsequent repair of the endothelia.[18,112] Series of basal laminae formed during such phases of repair are concentrically arranged around the small vessels and capillaries in the outermost dermal connective tissue.[18] Leakage of serum proteins, together with exocytosis of erythrocytes, further contributes to the PAS-positive deposits in the perivascular spaces (tryptophan). Degenerating collagen is enclosed in these masses (Fig. 22.39A). The basal lamina at the dermo–epidermal junction is uninvolved; a small layer of the superficial papillary connective tissue remains unaltered in EPP.

Restriction to light-exposed skin areas ('persistent light urticaria'), mainly perivascular deposits formed by basal lamina multiplication and serum exudates in the superficial dermis, and a normal dermo–epidermal junction characterize EPP.

Hyalinosis cutis et mucosae (HCM) Urbach–Wiethe (lipoid proteinosis)

First described by Urbach and Wiethe in 1929, this autosomal recessive disorder affects the entire skin and mucous membranes without relation to light exposure. One of the first clinical signs is hoarseness that is evident in the newborn or develops in infancy. This hoarseness, as well as gradually developing pachydermia, are due to the increasing deposition of PAS- and Hale–PAS-positive substances in the perivascular connective tissue of skin and mucous membranes, from the epidermis down to the subcutis. Ultrastructurally, frequent focal calcifications (Fig. 22.39B) distinguish HCM from EPP, while the amount of concentrically arranged perivascular basal laminae may exceed that of EPP. The application of antibodies has demonstrated basal lamina constituents, namely collagen type IV and laminin, throughout the deposits,[85,86] pointing to their origin from a hyperproliferation of epithelial and endothelial basement membranes, with progressive gradual destruction of the normal connective tissue architecture and mechanical properties. Cultured HCM cells produce collagen type IV-specific mRNA in amounts up to four-fold greater than that produced by normal cells,[181] indicating that the respective genes are expressed at an increased rate; it is as yet unknown whether defective gene regulation, or gene amplification of collagen type IV sequences are the reason.

Porphyria cutanea tarda (PCT)

PCT also shows multiplications of basal lamina of the cutaneous vasculature, comparable to EPP, but there is no additional deposition of perivascular substances as in EPP or HCM. Blistering is more pronounced in manifest cases of PCT. The extension of these blisters, including the superficial reticular and papillary dermis, dermo–epidermal junction, and basal epidermis,[124] points to toxic effects in their origin.

PCT is another genetically determined inborn error of porphyrin metabolism, with a defect of uroporphyrinogen decarboxylase, linked to chromosome 1 (1p34),[94] and an abnormal feed-back inhibition of other enzymes of the porphyrin pathway, resulting in a dominant mode of inheritance.[227] The disorder becomes manifest only with additional factors that lead to hepatic damage (viral hepatitis; alcohol; hormonal contraception; hepatotoxic medications), with an increase of porphyrins and predominance of uroporphyrin 1 in the urine. The diagnosis is made on clinical and biochemical criteria. EM is not required.

LYSOSOMAL STORAGE DISEASES

Lysosomal storage diseases are inborn errors of metabolism that, because of catabolic (lysosomal) enzyme deficiency, accumulate degradation products of metabolic pathways in membrane-bound lysosomal compartments (see Ch. 6). Most of them are not primarily dermatological disorders. The neurolipidoses, gangliosidoses, mucopolysaccharidoses or mucolipidoses are degenerative metabolic disorders of infancy or childhood with major central nervous system involvement (amaurosis) and often with only mild skin involvement.[87,212]

Those lysosomal storage disorders in which the basic defect has been identified are usually diagnosed biochemically. EM is a useful aid for the demonstration of storage substances,[231] often of characteristic ultrastructure, in tissue biopsies, cultured cells such as fibroblasts, or in amnion fluid cells prenatally.[64,227,242]

Formerly, CNS biopsy was performed in order to determine the type of a neurodegenerative disorder. This was then substituted by rectal biopsy as a less invasive and less risky procedure.[103] In recent years it has been shown that even in cases of clinically normal-appearing skin, the specific storage products can be demonstrated in skin samples.[170,231] This is of particular importance in those (neurodegenerative) disorders where the biochemical defect is still unknown. The various clinical types of ceroid lipofuscinosis (juvenile, late infantile and infantile) are examples with characteristic lysosomal storage substances (fingerprint profiles; curvilinear profiles), the origin, nature, and biochemical composition of which are unknown. In such instances EM is the only means for establishing the diagnosis[231] and has been used for prenatal diagnosis in at-risk pregnancies.[64] Skin samples are readily accessible and may serve as a useful source to check for specific storage products and may obviate the need for more invasive procedures, such as renal biopsy, to verify a diagnosis. Cells which are involved — mostly in the dermal connective tissue — may include nerves and Schwann cells, vasculature, macrophages and fibroblasts, muscle cells and epithelia of the epidermal appendages, especially sweat glands. Sweat ducts are much more numerous in infant skin than in adult skin. Their periluminal cells contain membrane-bound vesicle complexes filled with lamellated contents (probably polar or glycolipids) as a normal differentiation product, analogous to keratinosomes of the upper interductal epidermis. This should be kept in mind when examining skin for abnormal storage substances.

Angiokeratoma corporis diffusum Fabry

Angiokeratomas are small, bluish-red vascular tumours that result from ectasias of superficial skin capillaries covered by an orthohyperkeratotic, and later atrophic epidermis. In Fabry's disease multiple pin-head-sized angiokeratomas are scattered on the skin, with predominance on abdomen, buttocks and scrotum.

Fabry's disease is a sphingolipidosis. The underlying basic defect — deficiency of alpha-galactosidase A (a ceramide trihexosidase) — leads to the accumulation of ceramide trihexosides in lysosomes (see refs. 70 and 129) of endothelial cells in skin, heart, kidneys, CNS and many other inner organs. The storage products (Fig. 22.40) may increase to exceed nuclear size, fill the endothelia and cause loss of their plasticity. The clinical symptoms are due mainly to func-

tional impairment of the vascular walls. Though skin symptoms are of only minor clinical relevance, angiokeratomas may give the first hint to the diagnosis in doubtful cases.

The disorder is inherited as an X-linked recessive trait that is fully expressed in hemizygous males and shows mild symptoms depending on Lyonization in heterozygous female carriers. The gene has been mapped to the long arm of the X-chromosome (Xq 22[71,227]). The ultrastructural demonstration of ceramide accumulation in skin — even if clinically uninvolved — is an important means for diagnosis, carrier detection,[48] and (using amniotic fluid cells) for prenatal diagnosis.[242] Biochemical verification is necessary, as fucosidosis (another lysosomal storage disease) may induce angiokeratomas and leads to similar laminated storage products.[78]

For the electronmicroscopist, ceramide accumulations in endothelial or other cells may serve as a useful tool to test the efficacy and potency of goniometer stages in high resolution EM (see Fig. 22.40C). (See also Ch. 6 and 17).

'HISTIOCYTIC DISORDERS': DISORDERS OF THE PHAGOCYTIC MONOCYTE SERIES

A series of skin eruptions, in part with systemic involvement, that are caused by proliferation of phagocytic monocytes or 'histiocytes'[133] is placed in this group. Histiocytic disorders occur in children and in adults. They differ from each other in their extent, localization, degree of cellular differentiation, course, and prognosis. Clinically and histopathologically they may closely resemble each other.

The lesions occur as infiltrates, papular nodules, or granulomatous eruptions in which lymphocytes, granulocytes, and macrophages may form inflammatory reaction patterns in response to, and depending on, the kind and stage of the proliferation of the specific histiocytic/phagocytic cells.

By immunopathology it is not yet possible to differentiate and classify these disorders. In contrast to the subtle identification of the various subtypes of lymphocytes and their different functional stages with monoclonal antibodies, relatively few antibodies are available to identify cells of the phagocytic monocyte series (eg. MAC 387, CD1, S100). No subtyping of phagocytic cells is possible.

On the other hand, the various types of proliferating histiocytic cells[99] are characterized by specific subcellular markers.[60] Histiocytic disorders are best classified by means of EM. Some of the most important of them will be discussed here. Table 22.3 has been reproduced from Caputo[60] (with permission).

Histiocytosis X

Histiocytosis X was the first dermatological disorder recognized to demand ultrastructural analysis for verification of the diagnosis. Its nature — whether merely hyperproliferative and thus reactive, or whether a true neoplasm with more or less pronounced malignant potential — is still under debate (see also Chs. 13 and 29). Undoubtedly this condition represents a disorder of the Langerhans' cells (LC), a member of the phagocytic monocyte series.[219] LC are CD 1 (OKT 6)[+] and S-100[+].[175] They normally reside within the epidermis (Fig. 22.41A) and are recognized as specialized macrophage-related dendritic cells capable of antigen presentation to immune-competent lymphocytes, credited with the function of a first outpost of cellular immune response to foreign antigens and in the development of contact sensitivity.[51,219]

Normal LC are able to undergo mitosis within the epidermis and to traffic and pass through the dermo-epidermal junction (Fig. 22.41A). Their specific markers are the LC (Birbeck) granules (Fig. 22.41B).

LC form the major cell type of the dermal infiltrate in lesions of histiocytosis X[42]; their uniformity (size and form of nuclei, amount of cytoplasm, cellular activity) points to probable clonal proliferation. Lymphocytes, mast cells and granulocytes (neutrophils and eosinophils) accompany the proliferating LC that show considerable epidermotropism.[60]

Histiocytosis X occurs in three distinctive clinical forms:[99] Abt–Letterer–Siwe disease, Hand–Schüller–Christian disease,[97] and eosinophilic granuloma. They differ with respect to distribution, age of onset, and prognosis from each other. EM (LC granules) and immunopathology (CD 1[+], S-100[+]) are used for their identification.

Non-Langerhans' cell histiocytoses (non X-histiocytoses)

Juvenile xanthogranuloma (naevoxanthoendothelioma)

This benign, spontaneously regressing disorder of infants and children[60,99] is one of the most frequent differential diagnoses in cases suspected to be histiocytosis X. The granulomatous infiltrate is almost exclusively composed of densely packed 'histiocytic' macrophages (Fig. 22.42), but Langerhans' cells are not encountered. Their ultrastructure depends on the age and progression of the individual lesion. In the prexanthomatous stage, cells contain characteristic dense lysosomal bodies. In later stages, foam cells filled with lipid droplets develop (Fig. 22.42A); during further progression, increasing numbers of heterolysosomes containing myelin-like material and products of breakdown are found in the cells (Fig. 22.42B); foreign-body giant cells and Touton-type giant cells appear in the granulomatous infiltrate; they contain lipid droplets, cholesterol clefts and heterolysosomes in addition to lobulated nuclei.

Benign cephalic histiocytosis

This papulonodular histiocytic eruption of childhood was first described by Gianotti & Caputo.[98] Lesions appear in

Table 22.3 Cytoplasmic markers in histiocytic proliferations of the skin*

	Langerhans' granules	Comma-shaped bodies	Pleomorphic cytoplasmic inclusions	Dense bodies[a]	Regularly laminated bodies[a]	Myelinoid bodies[a]	Coated vesicles	Fatty droplets without limiting membranes
Histiocytosis X	+++	+	-	+	+	+	+	+
Multicentric reticulo-histiocytosis	-	-	+++	++	-	+++	++	+
Congenital self-healing histiocytosis	++	+	-	+++	++	+	+	-
Generalized eruptive histiocytoma	-	+	-	+++	++	+	+	-
Benign cephalic histiocytosis	-	+++	-	+	-	+	+++	-
Juvenile xanthogranuloma	-	+	-	++	-	+	+	++
Papular xanthoma	-	-	+	++	- -	++	++	+++
Unclassified nodular histiocytosis	-	-	+++	++	-	+	+	+

*Reproduced from Caputo 1985,[60] with permission.
[a]Lysosomes.

the first year of life, spread over the head and neck, but spare mucous membranes; visceral involvement has not been observed. Spontaneous regression leaves atrophic pigmented macules.[60] Ultrastructurally, the specific histiocytes are characterized by three cytoplasmic markers: (1) comma-shaped or vermiform bodies (see Fig. 22.44B) with mean diameters of about 20 nm, that are thought to represent particular modifications of the RER; (2) two populations of coated vesicles — small Golgi-related, and large endocytosis-related forms covered by a typical clathrin coat; and (3) incomplete desmosome-like junctions between the densely interdigitating cells. The specific cells lack lipid inclusions, myelin-like laminated bodies, or Langerhans' cell granules.[60]

Eruptive cephalic xanthomas

H. Arnold & colleagues have encountered an unusual case of nodular, eruptive cephalic xanthomas developing rapidly on the face and later extending to scalp and neck of a 67-year-old female being treated with cytostatic drugs for a T-cell lymphoma. The predominantly histiocytic cellular infiltrate (Fig. 22.43) showed similarities to the cells seen in benign cephalic histiocytosis, and generalized eruptive histiocytoma (compare with Fig. 22.44), but it differed by virtue of the presence of foam cells containing lipid droplets and cholesterol, and multinucleated giant cells, features more typical of xanthoma (unpublished data).

The relationship between cephalic eruptions is unknown. One may speculate whether benign cephalic histiocytosis can evolve to a xanthomatous stage before final regression, or whether age and special circumstances such as cytostatic treatment can induce the storage of various lipids in residual bodies of the specific histiocytic cells.

Generalized eruptive histiocytomas

Winkelmann & Muller[237] described 'generalized eruptive histiocytoma, a benign papular histiocytic reticulosis' that is preferentially found in males, that may last for some years without progressing to systemic involvement, and which shows spontaneous regression.[37]

The infiltrate is formed by densely packed histiocytic cells, occasionally multinucleated or binuclear, without formation of typical giant cells, and scattered fibroblasts and mast cells. There is variable lipid storage with some cases lacking lipid in the histiocytes,[61,174] whereas others[37] report the presence of lipid droplets, cholesterol clefts and residual bodies (Fig. 22.44). Generalized eruptive histiocytoma is specifically characterized by histiocytes displaying pronounced surface membrane proliferating activity with multiple microvillous-like processes (Fig. 22.44A), and by vermiform or comma-shaped bodies in relation to RER areas[37,60,99] (Fig. 22.44B). Table 22.4, adapted from Arnold

et al[37], shows the ultrastructural differences from multinodular and multicentric reticulohistiocytosis (see below).

Multicentric reticulohistiocytosis (MCR) (or lipoidarthrosis)

This rare disorder affecting adults (beyond 40 years of age) is characterized by a papulonodular eruption of skin and mucous membranes associated with severe polyarthritis.[39,60,99] Specific infiltrative cells with a ground-glass appearance are intermingled with macrophages and lymphocytes. Langerhans' cells are constantly absent. The ground-glass appearance of the specific mononuclear or multinucleated histiocytic cells is due to their abundant cytoplasm, filled with often dilated cisternae of ER, and to a proliferation of the plasma membrane resulting in a highly vesiculated, irregularly shaped cell periphery with many fine cell processes. These cells have therefore been called 'spider cells' by some authors. Close interdigitations between neighbouring histiocytes are a characteristic finding. Complex heterolysosomes may be found in these cells; moreover, about 40% of them exhibit a multitude of so-called 'pleomorphic cytoplasmic inclusions' (not shown). Macrophages actively engulf and degrade collagen fibrils.

The relationship between MCR and multinodular reticulohistiocytosis (MNR) is as yet unclear. The latter disorder lacks internal involvement and polyarthritis but may be regarded as an initial stage that may eventually progress into multicentric histiocytosis (see Arnold et al[37]). Both disorders overlap in a series of features (Table 22.4). MCR lacks vermiform granules that are found in MNR. Both are distinguished from generalized eruptive histiocytoma by the presence of firm interdigitations and variable expression of intercellular contacts.[37]

DISORDERS WITH HAIR SHAFT ABNORMALITIES

Hair shaft abnormalities are of special interest among the multi-fold disturbances that may affect hair.[9,129,144,182,194] Hair shaft abnormalities may represent isolated, sometimes heritable disorders such as monilethrix[44] and pili anulati[195] with a periodic banding pattern of unusual light reflection, due to a finely pleated surface texture.[9,232] Idiopathic trichoclasia is another example of an isolated but much more severe abnormality of the hair shafts[232] (see Fig. 22.48).

Hair shaft abnormalities may occur as a part of syndromes such as ectodermal dysplasias (see Fig. 22.46), Björnstad syndrome (pili torti and deafness)[9,229] or Netherton's syndrome (Trichorrhexis invaginata, ichthyosis linearis circumflexa Comel, and atopic diathesis;[9,131,177,183] see Figs 22.15 and 22.47). They may be further associated with often severe inborn errors of metabolism, such as Menkes' kinky hair syndrome,[9,69,172] (see Fig. 22.45), trichothiodystrophy, arginosuccinic aciduria, and other metabolic

Table 22.4 Ultrastructural differential diagnosis of reticulohistiocytic disorders*

	Generalized eruptive histiocytoma	Multinodular reticulohistiocytosis	Multicentric reticulohistiocytosis
Histiocytes			
Nuclei: round/oval	– / +	+ +	+ +
indented	+ +	+ +	+ +
Cell membrane			
specializations:			
interdigitations	–	+ +	+ +
intercellular contacts	–	– / +	+ / –
cell processes	+ +		– / +
Organelles:			
distended ER	+		+ +
osmiophilic granules	+ +	+ +	+ +
vermiform granules	+ +	+ +	–
laminated granules	+ / –		–
pinocytotic vesicles	–		+
Storage products:			
lipids (neutral lipids)	– / + +	+ +	+ / –
phospholipids	– / + +	+ +	+ +
cholesterol	– / + +	+ + / –	–
Foam cells	– / +	+	–
Giant cells	–	+ +	+ +
Fibroblasts	+		+ +
Mast cells	+		+
Langerhans' cells	–	–	–

*Adapted from Arnold et al.[37]

abnormalities.[63,105,194] In such instances the abnormal hair pattern may give important clues to possibly severe underlying basic disorders.[182]

On the other hand, hair shaft disturbances may also result from the effect of exogenous factors[186] — such as hair styling — and may thus be avoidable.

Therefore, the knowledge and distinction of specific patterns of hair shaft abnormalities — in many cases disclosed only at the scanning EM level — may be invaluable in identifying much more important internal changes (e.g. Menkes' syndrome) or in clarifying the genetic nature of severe neonatal exfoliations with high mortality (Netherton's syndrome[16]).

Menkes' kinky hair syndrome

This X-linked recessive neurodegenerative disorder is probably caused by a defect of copper transport across cell membranes resulting in a metabolic disturbance of intestinal copper absorption and utilization with decrease of serum copper levels and functional deficiency of many copper-dependent enzyme systems.[63,69,172,194,225] The gene is linked to Xcen and has been mapped to the centromeric region Xp11-q11 of the X-chromosome.[94] Progressive psychomotor and growth retardation, convulsions and death in early infancy, mostly before the age of 4 years, are the clinical consequences. Arterial degeneration, bone abnormalities, cutis laxa, micrognathia and arched gothic palate are frequently associated. Leading symptoms of high diag-

nostic significance are the low degree of pigmentation and the hair shaft abnormalities.[9]

Arterial degeneration and cutis laxa are due to abnormalities of elastic fibres.[69] Lysyloxidase, a copper-dependent enzyme, is markedly reduced in Menkes' syndrome. Therefore, connective tissue manifestations of Menkes' syndrome could be the consequence of defective cross-linking of elastin and collagen[225] (see also Ehlers–Danlos syndrome V and IX in Ch. 5).

The hair is blond and fine, wire-like and extremely brittle. Torsions of highly regular pitch and dimension (true pili torti) are regularly present over long distances of the hair shaft. No other type of contorted or twisted hair displays a similar degree of regularity. Longitudinal and transverse breaks (trichoschisis) are frequent (Fig. 22.45A). The typical 'kinky' appearance is due to multiple breaks (Fig. 22.45, B and C) with node formation (trichorrhexis nodosa; Fig. 22.45, B to E) by which Menkes' syndrome is identified in doubtful cases.

Trichorrhexis nodosa in anhidrotic ectodermal dysplasia (AED)

Severe hair shaft abnormalities resulting in so-called 'uncombable hair', stiff and brittle hair, characterize various different syndromes, including some types of ectodermal dysplasias.[9,26] The patterns of hair shaft abnormalities in the group of ectodermal dysplasia syndromes cover a broad range of abnormalities.[120] Twisted hair shafts may reveal longitudinal impressions, infoldings or flattened portions and irregular torsions with a high pitch (Fig. 22.46A). Irregularities and disturbances of the cuticular scales with subsequent loss of the cuticle (Fig. 22.46B) are initial stages of multiple breaks (trichorrhexis nodosa; Fig. 22.46C). Morphologically these cases of trichorrhexis nodosa are completely different from those observed in Menkes' kinky hair syndrome where the cuticle is spared (see Fig. 22.45, B and C), while in autosomal recessive AED the cuticle is more or less completely lost, pointing to more fundamental abnormalities of hair growth and keratinization.

Netherton's syndrome (trichorrhexis invaginata)

Netherton's syndrome[177] is an autosomal-recessive keratinization disorder with skin and hair shaft disturbances. Ichthyosis linearis circumflexa Comel describes the skin manifestation of this syndrome (see Fig. 22.15). The hair shaft disturbances are highly specific and permit a safe diagnosis by the demonstration of the bamboo-hairs (trichorrhexis invaginata) that are pathognomonic of Netherton's syndrome (Fig. 22.47).[9,129,183,194]

Torsions of the hair shaft are a regular though less specific finding (Fig. 22.47). Almost every hair displays some amount of twisting, while most bamboo nodes break readily and are thus mostly incomplete and located at the tip of short hair shaft rudiments. Trichorrhexis invaginata is probably induced by periodic disturbances concomitant with the inflammatory changes preceding the para- and hyperkeratotic circumscript skin lesions. In the hair, incomplete keratinization in the keratogenous zone of the growing hair shaft results in circumscribed segments with weak cortical keratin that is compressed and twisted under the mechanical pressure of the surrounding follicle during further growth and transport to the skin surface. As a result, the distal shaft 'intussuscepts' into the proximal portion producing the 'bamboo-like' node.

Idiopathic trichoclasia

Idiopathic trichoclasia is distinguished from other types of hair shaft abnormalities by its specific cuticular and cortex abnormalities and different mode of fracture: in many hairs, cuticular cells are partly elevated from the surface with their irregular free cell border (Fig. 22.48A), and shafts readily break off and expose the cortex fibres (Fig. 22.48B). Fractures do not produce trichorrhexis nodosa (compare Fig. 22.45B to D, with Fig. 22.46C), but result in long drawn-out tips of cortex fibres (Fig. 22.48C). By ultrastructural examination of cross sections, increased amounts of matrix substances and of paracortex configuration in the cortex (Fig. 22.48D) are revealed[232] when compared with normal hair cortex.[185]

REFERENCES

1. Anton-Lamprecht I 1972 Zur Ultrastruktur hereditärer Verhornungsstörungen. I. Ichthyosis congenita. Archiv für Dermatologische Forschung 243: 88–100
2. Anton-Lamprecht I 1973 Zur Ultrastruktur hereditärer Verhornungsstörungen. III. Autosomal-dominante Ichthyosis vulgaris. Archiv für Dermatologische Forschung 248: 149–172
3. Anton-Lamprecht I 1974 Zur Ultrastruktur hereditärer Verhornungsstörungen. IV. X-chromosomal-rezessive Ichthyosis. Archiv für Dermatologische Forschung 248: 361–378
4. Anton-Lamprecht I 1978 Electron microscopy in the early diagnosis of genetic disorders of the skin. Dermatologica 157: 65–85
5. Anton-Lamprecht I 1981 Disturbances of tonofilament and keratohyalin structure and arrangement in inborn errors of keratinization. In: Marks R, Christophers E (eds) The epidermis in disease (Proceedings of the ESDR Symposium). MTP Press, Lancaster, pp 61–77
6. Anton-Lamprecht I 1981 Prenatal diagnosis of genetic disorders of the skin by means of electron microscopy. Human Genetics 59: 392–405
7. Anton-Lamprecht I 1983 Genetically induced abnormalities of epidermal differentiation and ultrastructure in ichthyoses and epidermolyses: pathogenesis, heterogeneity, fetal manifestation, and prenatal diagnosis. Journal of Investigative Dermatology 81: 149s–156s
8. Anton-Lamprecht I 1984 Prenatal diagnosis of epidermolysis bullosa hereditaria: a review. Seminars in Dermatology 3: 229–240
9. Anton-Lamprecht I 1985 Erkrankungen und Entwicklungsstörungen des Haarschaftes. Swiss Medicine 7/5b: 41–50
10. Anton-Lamprecht I 1988 Pränatale Diagnostik von Genodermatosen. Hautarzt 39 (suppl VIII): 16–20
11. Anton-Lamprecht I 1989 Epidermolysis bullosa. In: Altmeyer P, Schultz-Ehrenburg U, Luther H (eds) Handsymposium. Dermatologische Erkrankungen der Hände und Füsse. Editiones Roche, Basel, pp 129–155
12. Anton-Lamprecht I 1989 Pathomorphogenese von Genodermatosen. Möglichkeiten der Identifizierung und Charakterisierung von Genodermatosen mit Hilfe elektronenmikroskopischer Untersuchungen und deren praktische Anwendung in der frühen postnatalen sowie in der pränatalen Diagnostik schwerer erblicher Hautkrankheiten. Ulmensien 2, Universitätsverlag Ulm pp 129–159
13. Anton-Lamprecht I, Arnold M-L 1987 Pränatale Diagnostik von erblichen Hautkrankheiten. In: Murken J (ed) Pränatale Diagnostik und Therapie. Enke, Stuttgart, pp 184–214
14. Anton-Lamprecht I, Arnold M-L 1987 Prenatal diagnosis of severe genetic disorders of the skin. In: Happle R, Grosshans E (eds) Pediatric dermatology. Advances in diagnosis and treatment. (Proceedings of the First Congress of the European Society of Pediatric Dermatology.) Springer, Berlin, pp 3–22
15. Anton-Lamprecht I, Arnold M-L 1987 Prenatal diagnosis of inherited epidermolyses. Current Problems in Dermatology 16: 146–157
16. Anton-Lamprecht I, Arnold M-L 1989 The skin of the newborn under normal and pathological conditions. Symposium Neonatal Dermatology. In: Proceedings of the 5th International Congress of Pediatric Dermatology, Milan 1989
17. Anton-Lamprecht I, Arnold M-L, Holbrook K A 1984 Methodology in sampling of fetal skin and pitfalls in the interpretation of fetal skin biopsy specimens. Seminars in Dermatology 3: 203–215
18. Anton-Lamprecht I, Bersch A 1971 Histopathologie und Ultrastruktur der Haut bei Protoporphyrinämie. Virchows Archiv, Abteilung A, Pathologische Anatomie 352: 75–89

19. Anton-Lamprecht I, Blanchet-Bardon C, Holbrook K A 1988 Prenatal diagnosis of genodermatoses. In: Orfanos C E, Stadler R, Gollnick H (eds) Dermatology in five continents. Proceedings of the XVII World Congress of Dermatology, Berlin, May 24–29, 1977. Springer, Berlin, pp 838–843

20. Anton-Lamprecht I, Curth H O, Schnyder U W 1973 Ultrastructure of inborn errors of keratinization. II. Ichthyosis hystrix type Curth–Macklin. Archiv für Dermatologische Forschung 246: 77–91

21. Anton-Lamprecht I, Gedde-Dahl T Jr, Schnyder U W 1979 Ultrastructural characterization of a new dominant epidermolysis bullosa. Journal of Investigative Dermatology 72: 280

22. Anton-Lamprecht I, Hashimoto I 1976 Epidermolysis bullosa dystrophica dominans (Pasini) — a primary structural defect of the anchoring fibrils. Human Genetics 32: 69–76

23. Anton-Lamprecht I, Kahlke W 1974 Zur Ultrastruktur hereditärer Verhornungsstörungen. V. Ichthyosis beim Refsum-Syndrom (Heredopathia atactica polyneuritiformis). Archiv für Dermatologische Forschung 250: 185–206

24. Anton-Lamprecht I, Klein D, Goos M 1972 Zur Ultrastruktur der Haut beim Klein–Waardenburg-Syndrom. Hautarzt 23: 462–473

25. Anton-Lamprecht I, Rauskolb R, Jovanovic V, Kern B, Arnold M-L, Schenck W 1981 Prenatal diagnosis of epidermolysis bullosa dystrophica Hallopeau–Siemens with electron microscopy of fetal skin. Lancet ii: 1077–1079

26. Anton-Lamprecht I, Schleiermacher E, Wolf M 1988 Autosomal recessive anhidrotic ectodermal dysplasia: report of a case and discrimination of diagnostic features. In: Salinas C F, Opitz J M, Paul N W (eds) March of Dimes Birth Defects Foundation. Birth defects: original article series, vol. 24, number 2. Recent advances in ectodermal dysplasias. (Proceedings of the VIII Annual Symposium of the Society of Craniofacial Genetics.) Alan R Liss, New York, pp 183–195

27. Anton-Lamprecht I, Schnyder U W 1974 Ultrastructure of inborn errors of keratinization. VI. Inherited ichthyoses — a model system for heterogeneities in keratinization disturbances. Archiv für Dermatologische Forschung 250: 207–227

28. Anton-Lamprecht I, Schnyder U W 1979 Zur Ultrastruktur der Epidermolysen mit junktionaler Blasenbildung. Dermatologica 159: 377–382

29. Anton-Lamprecht I, Schnyder U W 1982 Epidermolysis bullosa herpetiformis Dowling–Meara. Report of a case and pathomorphogenesis. Dermatologica 164: 221–235

30. Anton-Lamprecht I, Werner I 1985 Palmoplantar keratosis (PPK) with dominant transmission and unusual tubulo-fibrillar aggregations. 12th Society for Cutaneous Ultrastructure Research Meeting, Florence 1985

31. Arnold M-L, Anton-Lamprecht I 1985 Problems in prenatal diagnosis of the ichthyosis congenita group. Human Genetics 71: 301–311

32. Arnold M-L, Anton-Lamprecht I 1987 Prenatal diagnosis of epidermal disorders. Current Problems in Dermatology 16: 120–128

33. Arnold M-L, Anton-Lamprecht I, Albrecht-Nebe H 1989 Ultrastructural evidence of a new type of nonbullous congenital ichthyosiform erythroderma. Society of Cutaneous Ultrastructural Research 16th Annual Meeting, Köln

34. Arnold M-L, Anton-Lamprecht I, Melz-Rothfuss B, Hartschuh, W 1988 Ichthyosis congenita type III. Clinical and ultrastructural characteristics and distinction within the heterogeneous ichthyosis congenita group. Archives of Dermatological Research 280: 268–278

35. Arnold M-L, Anton-Lamprecht I, Rauskolb R 1984 Prenatal diagnosis of ectodermal dysplasias. Seminars in Dermatology 3: 247–252

36. Arnold M-L, Rauskolb R, Anton-Lamprecht I, Schinzel A, Schmid W 1984 Prenatal diagnosis of anhidrotic ectodermal dysplasia. Prenatal Diagnosis 4: 85–98

37. Arnold M-L, Wirth H, Anton-Lamprecht I, Petzoldt D 1982 Generalisierte eruptive histiocytome. Hautarzt 33: 428–437

38. Baden H P, Alper J C 1977 Ichthyosiform dermatoses, keratitis and deafness. Archives of Dermatology 113: 1701–1704

39. Bahmer F, Liebe D, Anton-Lamprecht I 1980 Unusual type of multicentric reticulohistiocytosis. Giornale Italiano Dermatologia e Venerologia 115: 153–154

40. Ballabio A, Parenti G, Carrozzo R, Sebastio G, Andria G, Buckle V, Fraser N, Craig I, Rocchi M, Romeo G, Jobsis A C, Persico M G 1987 Isolation and characterization of a steroid sulfatase cDNA clone: genomic deletions in patients with X-chromosome-linked ichthyosis. Proceedings of the National Academy of Sciences of the USA 84: 4519–4523

41. Ballabio A, Sebastio G, Carrozzo R, Parenti G, Piccirillo A, Persico M G, Andria G 1987 Deletions of the steroid sulphatase gene in 'classical' X-linked ichthyosis and in X-linked ichthyosis associated with Kallmann syndrome. Human Genetics 77: 338–341

42. Basset F, Nezelof C 1969 L'histiocytose X. Microscopie électronique, culture 'in vitro' et histo-enzymologie. Discussion à propos de 21 cas. Revue française des études cliniques et biologiques 14: 31–45

43. Bauer E A, Tabas M 1988 A perspective on the role of collagenase in recessive dystrophic epidermolysis bullosa. Archives of Dermatology 124: 734–736

44. Bentley-Phillips B 1979 Monilethrix und Pseudomonilethrix. In: Orfanos C E (ed) Haar und Haarkrankheiten. Fischer, Stuttgart, New York pp 447–465

45. Bick D, Curry C J R, McGill J R, Schorderet D F, Bux R C, Moove C M 1989 Male infant with ichthyosis, Kallmann syndrome, chondrodysplasia punctata, and an Xp chromosome deletion. American Journal of Medical Genetics 33: 100–107

46. Blanchet-Bardon C, Dumez Y 1984 Prenatal diagnosis of a harlequin fetus. Seminars in Dermatology 3: 225–228

47. Bohnert A, Anton-Lamprecht I 1982 Richner–Hanhart's syndrome — ultrastructural abnormalities of epidermal keratinization indicating a causal relationship to high intracellular tyrosine levels. Journal of Investigative Dermatology 79: 68–74

48. Brady R O, Johnson W G, Uhlendorf B W 1971 Identification of heterozygous carriers of lipid storage diseases. American Journal of Medicine 1971: 423–431

49. Breathnach S M 1985 The cutaneous amyloidoses. Pathogenesis and therapy. Archives of Dermatology 121: 470–475

50. Breathnach S M 1988 Amyloid and amyloidosis. Journal of the American Academy of Dermatology 18: 1–16

51. Breathnach S M 1988 The Langerhans' cell. British Journal of Dermatology 119: 463–469

52. Breathnach S M, Bhogal B, Dyck R F, DeBeer F C, Black M M, Pepys M B 1981 Immunohistochemical demonstration of amyloid P component in skin of normal subjects and patients with cutaneous amyloidosis. British Journal of Dermatology 105: 115–124

53. Bruckner-Tuderman L, Mitsuhashi Y, Schnyder U W, Bruckner P 1989 Anchoring fibrils and type VII collagen are absent from skin in severe recessive dystrophic epidermolysis bullosa. Journal of Investigative Dermatology 93: 3–9

54. Bruckner-Tuderman L, Schnyder U W 1989 Type VII collagen as a probe for heterogeneity of dystrophic epidermolysis bullosa. Archives of Dermatological Research 281: 121

55. Buchbinder L H, Lucky A W, Ballard E, Stanley J R, Stolar E, Tabas M, Bauer E A, Paller A S 1986 Severe infantile epidermolysis bullosa simplex. Dowling–Meara type. Archives of Dermatology 122: 190–198

56. Burgeson R E 1987 The collagens of skin. Current Problems in Dermatology 17: 61–75

57. Buxman M M, Goodkin P E, Fahrenbach W H, Dimond R L 1979 Harlequin ichthyosis with epidermal lipid abnormality. Archives of Dermatology 115: 189–193

58. Byers P H, Wenstrup R J 1984 Prenatal diagnosis of inherited connective tissue disorders. Seminars in Dermatology 3: 257–264

59. Byers P H, Wenstrup R J, Bonadio J F, Starman B, Cohn D H 1987 Molecular basis of inherited disorders of collagen biosynthesis: implications for prenatal diagnosis. Current Problems in Dermatology 16: 158–174

60. Caputo R 1985 Histiocytic syndromes. In: Johannessen V, Hashimoto K (eds) Electron microscopy in human medicine, vol. 11a, The skin. McGraw-Hill, New York, pp 65–86

61. Caputo R, Alessi E, Allegra F 1981 Generalized eruptive histiocytoma. A clinical, histologic, and ultrastructural study. Archives of Dermatology 117: 216–221

62. Caterson B, Baker J R, Christens J E, Couchman J R 1982 Immunologic methods for the detection and determination of

connective tissue proteoglycans. Journal of Investigative Dermatology 79 (suppl 1): 45s–50s

63. Comaish J S 1979 Allgemeinzustand, Stoffwechsel und Haarkrankheiten. In: Orfanos C E (ed) Haar und Haarkrankheiten. Fischer, Stuttgart, New York, pp 321–342

64. Conradi N G, Uvebrant P, Hökegard K-H, Wahlström J, Mellqvist L 1989 First-trimester diagnosis of juvenile neuronal ceroid lipofuscinosis by demonstration of fingerprint inclusions in chorionic villi. Prenatal Diagnosis 9: 283–287

65. Curth H O, Macklin M T 1954 The genetic basis of various types of ichthyosis in a family group. American Journal of Human Genetics 6: 371–382

66. Dale B A, Holbrook K A, Fleckman P, Kimball J R, Sybert V P 1989 Classification of harlequin ichthyosis into three genetically distinct types. Journal of Investigative Dermatology 92: 416

67. Dallaire L, Cantin M, Melançon S B, Perreault G, Potier M 1976 A syndrome of generalized elastic fiber deficiency with leprechaunoid features: a distinct genetic disease with an autosomal recessive mode of inheritance. Clinical Genetics 10: 1–11

68. Danielsen L 1979 Morphological changes in peudoxanthoma elasticum and senile skin. Acta Dermato-Venereologica suppl 83

69. Danks D M, Campbell P E, Stevens B J, Mayne V, Cartwright E 1972 Menkes' kinky hair syndrome: inherited defect in copper absorption with widespread effects. Pediatrics 50: 188–200

70. Daróczy J, Rácz I 1987 Diagnostic electron microscopy in practical dermatology. Akademiai Kiado, Budapest

71. de la Chapelle A 1982 The map of the human X chromosome. In: Crosignani P G, Rubin B L (eds) Genetic control of gamete production and function. Academic Press, London, pp 33–48

72. Dowling G B, Meara R H 1954 Epidermolysis bullosa resembling juvenile dermatitis herpetiformis. British Journal of Dermatology 66: 139–143

73. Eady R A J 1984 Prenatal diagnosis of oculocutaneous albinism: implications for other hereditary disorders of pigmentation. Seminars in Dermatology 3: 241–246

74. Eady R A J 1988 The basement membrane. Interface between the epithelium and the dermis: structural features. Archives of Dermatology 124: 709–712

75. Eady R A J, Tidman M J, Heagerty A H M, Kennedy A R 1987 Approaches to the study of epidermolysis bullosa. Current problems in dermatology 17: 127–141

76. Elias P M 1981 Epidermal lipids, membranes, and keratinization. International Journal of Dermatology 20: 1–19

77. Elias P M, Williams M L 1985 Neutral lipid storage disease with ichthyosis. Defective lamellar body contents and intracellular dispersion. Archives of Dermatology 121: 1000–1008

78. Epinette W W, Norins A L, Drew A L, Zeman W, Patel V 1973 Angiokeratoma corporis diffusum with alfa-fucosidase deficiency. Archives of Dermatology 107: 754–757

79. Fine J D 1987 Altered skin basement membrane antigenicity in epidermolysis bullosa. Current Problems in Dermatology 17: 111–126

80. Fine J D 1988 Antigenic features and structural correlates of basement membranes. Archives of Dermatology 124: 713–717

81. Fine D J, Couchman J 1988 19-DEJ-1, a hemidesmosome-anchoring filament complex-associated monoclonal antibody, defines a new skin basement membrane antigenic defect in junctional and dystrophic epidermolysis bullosa. Clinical Research 36: 375 A

82. Fine J-D, Osment L S, Gay S 1985 Dystrophic epidermolysis bullosa. A new variant characterized by progressive symmetrical centripetal involvement with scarring. Archives of Dermatology 121: 1014–1017

83. Fischer T, Gedde-Dahl T Jr 1979 Epidermolysis bullosa simplex and mottled pigmentation: a new dominant syndrome. I. Clinical and histological features. Clinical Genetics 15: 228–238

84. Fitzpatrick T B, Szabo G, Hori Y, Simone A, Reed W B, Greenberg M H 1968 White leaf-shaped macules. Earliest visible sign of tuberous sclerosis. Archives of Dermatology 98: 1–6

85. Fleischmajer R, Krieg T H, Dziadek M, Altchek D, Timpl R 1984 Ultrastructure and composition of connective tissue in hyalinosis cutis et mucosae skin. Journal of Investigative Dermatology 82: 252–258

86. Fleischmajer R, Timpl R, Graves P, Perlish J S, Raisher L, Altchek D 1981 Hyalinosis cutis et mucosae. A basal lamina disease. Journal

of Investigative Dermatology 76: 314–315

87. Fluharty A L 1982 The mucopolysaccharidoses: a synergism between clinical and basic investigation. Journal of Investigative Dermatology 79 (suppl 1): 38s–44s

88. Frances C, Robert L 1984 Elastin and elastic fibers in normal and pathologic skin. International Journal of Dermatology 23: 166–179

89. Freire-Maia N, Pinheiro M 1984 Ectodermal dysplasias: a clinical and genetic study. Alan R Liss, New York

90. Freire-Maia N, Pinheiro M 1988 Ectodermal dysplasias — some recollections and a classification. Birth defects: original article series, vol. 24, no. 2. March of Dimes Birth Defects Foundation, Alan R Liss, New York, pp 3–14

91. Frenk E, Mevorah B 1977 The keratinization disorder in collodion babies evolving into lamellar ichthyosis. Its possible relevance for determining the primary defect in lamellar ichthyosis. Journal of Cutaneous Pathology 4: 329–337

92. Gedde-Dahl T Jr 1970 Epidermolysis bullosa. A clinical, genetic and epidemiological study. Universitetsforlaget, Oslo (1970), and Johns Hopkins Press, Baltimore (1971)

93. Gedde-Dahl T Jr 1981 Sixteen types of epidermolysis bullosa. On the clinical discrimination, therapy and prenatal diagnosis. Acta Dermato-venereologica (suppl 95): 74–87

94. Gedde-Dahl T Jr 1987 The human gene map and genes expressed in the skin. Current Problems in Dermatology 16: 45–64

95. Gedde-Dahl T Jr 1987 Epidermolysis bullosa syndromes. Current Problems in Dermatology 16: 129–145

96. Gedde-Dahl T Jr, Anton-Lamprecht I 1990 Epidermolysis bullosa. In: Emery A E H, Rimoin D L (eds) The principles and practice of medical genetics. Churchill Livingstone, Edinburgh, 2nd ed, pp 855–876

97. Gianotti F, Caputo R 1969 Skin ultrastructure in Hand-Schüller–Christian disease. Report on abnormal Langerhans' cells. Archives of Dermatology 100: 342–349

98. Gianotti F, Caputo R 1972 Unknown histiocytosis with intracytoplasmic worm-like particles in two children. Excerpta Medica Congress Series 289: 47

99. Gianotti F, Caputo R 1985 Histiocytic syndromes: a review. Journal of the American Academy of Dermatology 13: 383–404

100. Gibson I K, Anderson R A 1977 Response of the lysosomal system of the corneal epithelium to tyrosine-induced cell injury. Journal of Histochemistry and Cytochemistry 125: 1351–1362

101. Gibson I K, Burns R P, Wolfe-Lande J D 1975 Crystals in corneal epithelial lesions of tyrosine fed rats. Investigative Ophthalmology 14: 937–941

102. Glenner G G, Terry W D, Isersky C 1973 Amyloidosis: its nature and pathogenesis. Seminars in Hematology 10: 65–86

103. Goebel H H, Kohlschütter A, Schulte F J 1980 Rectal biopsy findings in infantile neuroaxonal dystrophy. Neuropediatrics 11: 388–392

104. Goerttler E, Anton-Lamprecht I, Kotzur B 1976 Amyloidosis cutis nodularis. Klinische, histopathologische und ultrastrukturelle Befunde. Hautarzt 27: 16–25

105. Goldsmith L A 1979 Molekularmechanismen der genetisch bedingten Haarkrankheiten. In: Orfanos C E (ed) Haar und Haarkrankheiten. Fischer, Stuttgart, New York, pp 343–369

106. Goldsmith L A 1983 Other genetic disorders of the skin. In: Emery A E H, Rimoin D L (eds) The principles and practice of medical genetics, vol 1. Churchill Livingstone, Edinburgh, pp 688–702

107. Goodman R M, Levital I, Solomon A, Klein D 1981 A survey of the Klein–Waardenburg syndrome in Israel with emphasis on upper extremity involvement: evidence for further genetic heterogeneity — type III. In: Huber A, Klein D (eds) Neurogenetics and neuro-ophthalmology. Developments in neurology, vol. 5. Elsevier, North-Holland, pp 393–406

108. Gottlieb S K, Lutzner M A 1973 Darier's disease. An electron microscopic study. Archives of Dermatology 107: 225–230

109. Greither A 1969 Systemische Keratosen. Ichthyosen, follikuläre Keratosen, Palmo-Plantar-Keratosen, Erythrokeratodermien, Dyskeratosen (einschließlich Morbus Darier) und keratotische Dysplasien. In: Jadassohn J (ed) Handbuch der Haut- und Geschlechtskrankheiten, Ergänzungswerk III/2. Springer, Berlin, pp 1–306

110. Grob J J, Breton A, Bonafe J L, Sauvan-Ferdani M, Bonerandi J J 1987 Keratitis, ichthyosis, and deafness (KID) syndrome. Archives

of Dermatology 123: 777–782

111. Grubauer G, Hintner H, Klein G, Fritsch P 1989 Erworbene, flächige Riesen-Nävuszellnävi bei generalisierter, atrophisierender, benigner Epidermolysis bullosa. Hautarzt 40: 523–526

112. Gschnait F, Wolff K, Konrad K 1975 Erythropoietic protoporphyria – submicroscopic events during the acute photosensitivity flare. British Journal of Dermatology 92: 545–557

113. Gülzow J, Anton-Lamprecht I 1977 Ichthyosis hystrix gravior Typus Rheydt: Ein otologisch-dermatologisches Syndrom. Laryngologie, Rhinologie, Otologie 56: 949–955

114. Haber R M, Hanna W, Ramsay C A, Boxall L B H 1985 Cicatricial junctional epidermolysis bullosa. Journal of the American Academy of Dermatology 12: 836–844

115. Haber R M, Hanna W, Ramsay C A, Boxall L B H 1985 Hereditary epidermolysis bullosa. Journal of the American Academy of Dermatology 13: 252–278

116. Hacham-Zadeh S, Rappersberger K, Livshin R, Konrad K 1988 Epidermolysis bullosa herpetiformis Dowling–Meara in a large family. Journal of the American Academy of Dermatology 18: 702–706

117. Hagemann M J, Dellemann J M 1977 Heterogeneity in Waardenburg syndrome. American Journal of Human Genetics 29: 468–485

118. Hamm H, Happle R, Butterfass T, Traupe H 1988 Epidermolytic palmoplantar keratoderma of Voerner: is it the most frequent type of palmoplantar keratoderma? Dermatologica 177: 138–145

119. Haneke E, Anton-Lamprecht I 1982 Ultrastructure of blister formation in epidermolysis bullosa hereditaria: V. Epidermolysis bullosa simplex localisata type Weber–Cockayne. Journal of Investigative Dermatology 78: 219–223

120. Haneke E, Wilsch L 1981 Scanning electron microscopic investigations of the hair in ectodermal dysplasia syndromes. In: Orfanos C E, Montagna W, Stüttgen G (eds) Hair research. Status and future aspects. Proceedings 1st International Congress on Hair Research, Hamburg 1979. Springer, Berlin, pp 433–435

121. Happle R 1987 The lines of Blaschko: a developmental pattern visualizing functional X-chromosome mosaicism. Current problems in dermatology 17: 5–18

122. Happle R 1987 Lethal genes surviving by mosaicism: a possible explanation for sporadic birth defects involving the skin. Journal of the American Academy of Dermatology 16: 899–906

123. Hardmeier T, Vogel A 1970 Electron microscopic lesions in scleromyxedema Arndt-Gottron. Archiv für klinische und experimentelle Dermatologie 237: 722–736

124. Hartschuh W, Voigtländer V, Anton-Lamprecht I 1979 Porphyria cutanea tarda hereditaria – Ultrastrukturelle Untersuchungen. Zeitschrift für Hautkrankheiten 54: 501–508

125. Hashimoto I, Anton-Lamprecht I, Gedde-Dahl T Jr, Schnyder U W 1975 Ultrastructural studies in epidermolysis bullosa hereditaria. I. Dominant dystrophic type of Pasini. Archiv für Dermatologische Forschung 252: 167–178

126. Hashimoto I, Gedde-Dahl T Jr, Schnyder U W, Anton-Lamprecht I 1976 Ultrastructural studies in epidermolysis bullosa hereditaria. II. Dominant dystrophic type of Cockayne and Touraine. Archives of Dermatological Research 255: 285–295

127. Hashimoto I, Schnyder U W, Anton-Lamprecht I 1976 Epidermolysis bullosa hereditaria with junctional blistering in an adult. Dermatologica 152: 72–86

128. Hashimoto K, Kanzaki T 1975 Cutis laxa. Ultrastructural and biochemical studies. Archives of Dermatology 111: 861–873

129. Hashimoto K, Niizuma K 1983 Skin pathology by light and electron microscopy. Igaku-Shoin, New York

130. Hausser I, Anton-Lamprecht I 1987 Electron microscopy as a means for carrier detection and genetic counselling in families at risk of tuberous sclerosis Bourneville–Pringle. Human Genetics 76: 73–80

131. Hausser I, Anton-Lamprecht I, Hartschuh W, Petzoldt D 1989 Netherton's syndrome: ultrastructure of the active lesion under retinoid therapy. Archives of Dermatological Research 281: 165–172

132. Hausser I, Fartasch M, Schleiermacher E, Anton-Lamprecht I 1987 Disseminated cicatricial pemphigoid in a child and in an adult. Ultrastructural diagnostic criteria and differential diagnosis with special reference to acquired epidermolysis bullosa. Archives of Dermatological Research 279: 357–365

133. Headington J T 1986 The histiocyte. In memoriam. Archives of Dermatology 122: 532–533

134. Hintner H, Stingl G, Schuler G, Fritsch P, Stanley J, Katz S, Wolff K 1981 Immunofluorescence mapping of antigenic determinants within the dermal-epidermal junction in mechanobullous diseases. Journal of Investigative Dermatology 76: 113–118

135. Hintner H, Stoessl H, Hoepfl R, Grubauer G, Fritsch P 1988 Amyloid K. Hautarzt 39: 419–425

136. Hintner H, Wolff K 1982 Generalized atrophic benign epidermolysis bullosa. Archives of Dermatology 118: 375–384

137. Holbrook K A 1984 Progress in prenatal diagnosis of bullous congenital ichthyosiform erythroderma (epidermolytic hyperkeratosis). Seminars in Dermatology 3: 216–220

138. Holbrook K A 1988 Structural abnormalities of the epidermally derived appendages in skin from patients with ectodermal dysplasia: insight into developmental errors. Birth defects: original article series vol. 24, no. 2. March of Dimes Birth Defects Foundation. Alan R Liss, New York, pp 15–44

139. Holbrook K A, Byers P 1982 Structural abnormalities in the dermal collagen and elastic matrix from the skin of patients with inherited connective tissue disorders. Journal of Investigative Dermatology 79: 7s–16s

140. Holbrook K A, Byers P H 1989 Skin is a window on heritable disorders of connective tissue. American Journal of Medical Genetics 34: 105–121

141. Holbrook K A, Dale B A, Williams M L, Perry T B, Hoff M S, Hamilton E F, Fisher C, Senikas V 1988 The expression of congenital ichthyosiform erythroderma in second trimester fetuses of the same family: morphologic and biochemical studies. Journal of Investigative Dermatology 91: 521–531

142. Holbrook K A, Hoff M S 1984 Structure of the developing human embryonic and fetal skin. Seminars of Dermatology 3: 185–202

143. Holbrook K A, Smith L T 1981 Ultrastructural aspects of human skin during the embryonic, fetal, premature, neonatal, and adult periods of life. Birth defects: original article series vol. 17, no 2. March of Dimes Birth Defects Foundation. Alan R Liss, New York, pp 9–13

144. lto M, Hashimoto K 1985 Hair abnormalities. In: Johannessen J V, Hashimoto K (eds) Electron microscopy in human medicine, vol. 11a, The skin. McGraw-Hill, New York, pp 229–273

145. Jagell S 1981 Sjögren–Larsson syndrome in Sweden. An epidemiological, genetic, clinical and biochemical study. Umeå University Medical Dissertations, New series no. 68

146. Johannessen J V, Hashimoto K 1985 Electron microscopy in human medicine, vol. 11a, The skin. McGraw-Hill, New York

147. Jung E G, Anton-Lamprecht I 1971 Investigation of a case of oculocutaneous albinism. Birth defects: original article series, vol. VII, no. 8. March of Dimes Birth Defects Foundation. Wiliams & Wilkins, Baltimore, pp 26–30

148. Kanerva L, Karvonen J, Oikarinen A, Lauharanta J, Ruokonen A, Niemi K-M 1984 Ichthyosis hystrix (Curth–Macklin). Light and electron microscopic studies performed before and after etretinate treatment. Archives of Dermatology 120: 1218–1223

149. Kanerva L, Lauharanta J, Niemi K-K, Lassus A 1983 New observations on the fine structure of lamellar ichthyosis and the effect of treatment with etretinate. American Journal of Dermatopathology 5: 555–568

150. Kastl I 1989 Zur normalen und pathologischen Keratinisierung der Leistenhaut (Palmae und Plantae). Elektronenmikroskopische Charakterisierung und Abgrenzung einer neuen Palmoplantarkeratose mit autosomal-rezessivem Erbgang. Dissertation Heidelberg

151. Kastl I, Anton-Lamprecht I 1990 Bicomponent keratohyalin in normal human ridged skin. Archives of Dermatological Research 282: 71–75

152. Kastl I, Anton-Lamprecht I, Gamborg Nielsen P 1990 Hereditary palmoplantar keratosis of the Gamborg Nielsen type: clinical and ultrastructural characteristics of a new type of autosomal recessive palmoplantar keratosis. Archives of Dermatological Research 282: 363–370

153. Katz S 1984 The epidermal basement membrane zone — structure, ontogeny, and role in disease. Journal of the American Academy of Dermatology 11: 1025–1037

154. Kero M, Niemi K-M 1986 Epidermolysis bullosa. International Journal of Dermatology 25: 75–82
155. Klein D 1950 Albinisme partiel (leucisme) avec surdi-mutité, blépharophimosis et dysplasie myo-ostéo-articulaire. Helvetica Paediatrica Acta 5: 38–58
156. Kolde G, Happle R, Traupe H 1985 Autosomal-dominant lamellar ichthyosis: ultrastructural characteristics of a new type of congenital ichthyosis. Archives of Dermatological Research 278: 1–5
157. Kosenow W E, Treibs A 1953 Lichtüberempfindlichkeit und Porphyrinaemie. Zeitschrift für Kinderheilkunde 73: 82–92
158. Kumakiri M, Hashimoto K 1979 Histogenesis of primary localized cutaneous amyloidosis: sequential change of epidermal keratinocytes to amyloid via filamentous degeneration. Journal of Investigative Dermatology 73: 150–162
159. Lamprecht A, Goecke T, Anton-Lamprecht I, Kuester W 1988 Progressive erythrokeratodermia and cochlear hearing impairment. A case report and review of the literature. International Journal of Pediatric Otorhinolaryngology 15: 279–289
160. Larrègue M, Gharbi R, Daniel J, Le Marec Y, Civatte J 1976 Le bébé collodion. Évolution à propos de 29 cas. Annales de Dermatologie et de Syphiligraphie 103: 31–56
161. Laurent R, Prost O, Nicollier M, Coumes Marquet S, Balzer M M, Adessi G 1985 Composite keratohyalin granules in palmoplantar keratoderma: an ultrastructural study. Archives of Dermatological Research 277: 384–394
162. Lawlor F, Peiris S 1985 Harlequin fetus successfully treated with etretinate. British Journal of Dermatology 112: 585–590
163. Liden S, Jagell S 1984 The Sjögren–Larsson syndrome. International Journal of Dermatology 23: 247–253
164. Linke R P, Nathrath W B J, Wilson P D 1983 Immuno-electron microscopic identification and classification of amyloid in tissue sections by postembedding protein-A gold method. Ultrastructural Pathology 4: 1–7
165. Löfberg L, Anton-Lamprecht I, Michaelsson G, Gustavii B 1983 Prenatal exclusion of Herlitz syndrome by electron microscopy of fetal skin biopsies obtained at fetoscopy. Acta Dermato-venereologica 63: 185–189
166. Luderschmidt C, Dorn M, Bassermann R, Linderkamp O 1980 Kollodiumbaby und Harlekinfetus. Gegenüberstellung zweier Beobachtungen. Hautarzt 31: 154–158
167. Mahrle G, Küchmeister B 1986 Voerner and Voerner-like palmoplantar keratosis. 13th Society for Cutaneous Ultrastructure Research Meeting, Paris 1986
168. Marghescu S, Anton-Lamprecht I, Melz-Rothfuss B 1987 Disseminated bilateral hyperkeratotic variant of porokeratosis Mibelli. Archives of Dermatological Research 279 (suppl): 38–47
169. Marghescu S, Anton-Lamprecht I, Rudolph P-O, Kaste R 1984 Kongenitale retikuläre ichthyosiforme Erythrodermie. Hautarzt 35: 522–529
170. Martin J J, Ceuterick C 1978 Morphological study of skin biopsy specimens: a contribution to the diagnosis of metabolic disorders with involvement of the nervous system. Journal of Neurology, Neurosurgery and Psychiatry 41: 232–248
171. Melnik B, Kuester W, Hollmann J, Plewig G, Traupe H 1989 Autosomal dominant lamellar ichthyosis exhibits an abnormal scale lipid pattern. Clinical Genetics 35: 152–156
172. Menkes J H 1972 Kinky hair disease. Pediatrics 50: 181–183
173. Müller H, Bode H, Krone C, Anton-Lamprecht I, Orlowska M 1988 Herlitz-Syndrom und 'Pylorusatresie'. Helvetica Paediatrica Acta 43: 457–466
174. Muller S A, Wolff K, Winkelmann R K 1967 Generalized eruptive histiocytoma. Enzyme histochemistry and electron microscopy. Archives of Dermatology 96: 11–17
175. Murphy G F, Bhan A K, Sato S, Harrist T J, Mihm M C 1981 Characterization of Langerhans' cells by the use of monoclonal antibodies. Laboratory Investigation 45: 465–468
176. Nanko H, Voss Jepsen L, Zachariae H, Soegaard H 1979 Acquired cutis laxa (generalized elastolysis): light and electron microscopic studies. Acta Dermato-venereologica 59: 315–324
177. Netherton E W 1958 A unique case of trichorrhexis nodosa — 'bamboo hairs'. Archives of Dermatology 78: 483–487
178. Niemi K-M, Kanerva L 1989 Ichthyosis with laminated membrane structures. American Journal of Dermatopathology 11: 149–156
179. Niemi K-M, Kero M, Kanerva L, Mattila R 1983 Epidermolysis bullosa simplex. A new histologic subgroup. Archives of Dermatology 119: 138–141
180. Ollendorff-Curth H, Allen F H, Schnyder U W, Anton-Lamprecht I 1972 Follow-up of a family group suffering from ichthyosis hystrix type Curth–Macklin. Humangenetik 17: 37–48
181. Olsen D R, Chu M L, Uitto J 1988 Expression of basement membrane zone genes coding for type IV procollagen and laminin by human skin fibroblasts in vitro: elevated alpha 1 (IV) collagen mRNA levels in lipoid proteinosis. Journal of Investigative Dermatology 90: 734–738
182. Orfanos C E (ed) 1979 Haar und Haarkrankheiten. Fischer, Stuttgart, New York
183. Orfanos C E, Mahrle G, Salamon T 1971 Netherton-Syndrom. Ichthyosiforme Hautveränderungen und Trichorrhexis invaginata. Nachweis eines krankhäft veränderten Cortexkeratins im Haar. Hautarzt 22: 397–409
184. Orfanos C E, Montagna W, Stüttgen G (eds) 1981 Hair research. Status and future aspects. Proceedings of the 1st International Congress on Hair Research, Hamburg, 1979. Springer, Berlin
185. Orfanos C E, Ruska H 1968 Die Feinstruktur des menschlichen Haares. II. Der Haar-Cortex. Archiv für klinische und experimentelle Dermatologie 231: 264–278
186. Orfanos C E, Sterry W, Leventer T 1979 Haar und haarkosmetische Massnahmen. In: Orfanos C E (ed) Haar und Haarkrankheiten. Fischer, Stuttgart, New York, pp 853–885
187. Pearson R W 1962 Studies on the pathogenesis of epidermolysis bullosa. Journal of Investigative Dermatology 39: 551–575
188. Pearson R W 1988 Clinicopathologic types of epidermolysis bullosa and their non-dermatological complications. Archives of Dermatology 124: 718–725
189. Peltier F A, Tschen E H, Raimer S S, Kuo T 1981 Epidermolysis bullosa letalis associated with congenital pyloric atresia. Archives of Dermatology 117: 728–731
190. Peracchia C, Mittler B S 1972 Fixation by means of glutaraldehyde-hydrogen peroxide reaction products. Journal of Cell Biology 53: 234–238
191. Pinnell S R 1982 Molecular defects in Ehlers–Danlos syndrome. Journal of Investigative Dermatology 79 (suppl 1): 90s–92s
192. Pope F M 1974 Two types of autosomal recessive pseudoxanthoma elasticum. Archives of Dermatology 110: 209–212
193. Pope F M 1975 Historical evidence for the genetic heterogeneity of pseudoxanthoma elasticum. British Journal of Dermatology 92: 493–509
194. Price V H 1979 Strukturanomalien des Haarschaftes. In: Orfanos C E (ed) Haar und Haarkrankheiten. Fischer, Stuttgart, New York, pp 387–446
195. Price V H, Thomas R S, Jones F T 1968 Pili anulati. Optical and electron microscopic studies. Archives of Dermatology 98: 640–647
196. Riccardi V M 1983 The phakomatoses. In: Emery A E H, Rimoin D L (eds) The principles and practice of medical genetics, vol. 1. Churchill Livingstone, Edinburgh, pp 313–319
197. Rizzo W B, Dammann A L, Craft D A 1988 Sjögren–Larsson syndrome. Impaired fatty alcohol oxidation in cultured fibroblasts due to deficient fatty alcohol:nicotinamide adenine dinucleotide oxidoreductase activity. American Society for Clinical Investigation 81: 738–744
198. Ross J B, Allderdice P W, Shapiro L J, Aveling J, Eales B A, Simms D 1985 Familial X-linked ichthyosis, steroid sulfatase deficiency, mental retardation, and nullisomy for Xp22.3-pter. Archives of Dermatology 121: 1524–1528
199. Ross R 1973 The elastic fiber; a review. Journal of Histochemistry and Cytochemistry 21: 199–208
200. Ross R, Fialkow P J, Altman L K 1978 Fine structure alterations of elastic fibers in pseudoxanthoma elasticum. Clinical Genetics 13: 213–223
201. Rossmann-Ringdahl I, Anton-Lamprecht I, Swanbeck G 1986 A mother and two children with nonbullous congenital ichthyosiform erythroderma. Archives of Dermatology (Chicago) 122: 559–564
202. Rycroft R J G, Moynahan E J, Wells R S 1976 Atypical ichthyosiform erythroderma, deafness and keratitis. A report of two cases. British Journal of Dermatology 94: 211–217
203. Salinas C F, Opitz J M, Paul N W (eds) 1988 Recent advances in

ectodermal dysplasias. Birth defects: original article series vol. 24, no. 2. March of Dimes Birth Defects Foundation, Alan R Liss, New York

204. Sato A, Anton-Lamprecht I, Schnyder U W 1976 Ultrastructure of inborn errors of keratinization. VII. Porokeratosis Mibelli and disseminated superficial actinic porokeratosis. Archives of Dermatological Research 255: 271–284

205. Sato A, Anton-Lamprecht I, Schnyder U W 1977 Ultrastructure of dyskeratosis in Darier's disease. Journal of Cutaneous Pathology 4: 173–184

206. Sato A, Anton-Lamprecht I, Schnyder U W 1979 RNA and protein synthesis of dyskeratotic cells in morbus Darier. An autoradiographic study. Dermatologica 158: 221–228

207. Schärer K, Hausser I, Anton-Lamprecht I, Tilgen W 1990 Clinical Quiz (Pseudoxanthoma elasticum). Pediatric Nephrology 4: 97–99

208. Schmidt W 1987 Schmelzhypoplasien — Eine Manifestation des Gendefektes der Epidermolysis bullosa atrophicans? Vergleichende licht-und elektronenmikroskopische Untersuchung von Zahnkeimen bei Feten mit hereditären junktionalen Epidermolysen und Feten mit normaler Zahnentwicklung. Dissertation Heidelberg

209. Schneider B V, Rufli Th, Schnyder U W 1988 Ichthyosis with perinuclear filamentous shells — a special type of nonbullous congenital ichthyosiform erythroderma? Society for Cutaneous Ultrastructure Research Meeting, Nice, May 1988

210. Schoenfeld P H I R 1980 The pachyonychia congenita syndrome. Acta Dermato-venereologica 60: 45–49

211. Schoenfeld P H I R, Woerdeman M J 1984 Pachyonychia congenita syndrome: electron microscopic, histological and clinical findings of an unusual case. British Journal of Dermatology 111: 477–497

212. Shapiro L J 1981 The mucopolysaccharidoses and mucolipidoses as model systems for the investigation of genetic disorders. Birth defects: original article series vol. 17, no. 2. March of Dimes Birth Defects Foundation. Alan R. Liss, New York, pp 191–203

213. Shapiro L J 1984 Steroid sulfatase deficiency and the genetics of the short arm of the human X chromosome. Advances in Human Genetics 14: 331–389

214. Silbert J E 1982 Structure and metabolism of proteoglycans and glycosaminoglycans. Journal of Investigative Dermatology 79 (suppl 1): 31s–37s

215. Skinner B A, Greist M C, Norins A L 1981 The keratitis, ichthyosis and deafness (KID) syndrome. Archives of Dermatology 117: 285–289

216. Smith L T, Holbrook K A, Byers P H 1982 Structure of the dermal matrix during development and in the adult. Journal of Investigative Dermatology 79 (suppl 1): 93s–104s

217. Steuhl K P, Anton-Lamprecht I, Arnold M-L, Thiel H-J 1988 Recurrent bilateral corneal erosions due to an association of epidermolysis bullosa simplex Köbner and X-linked ichthyosis with steroid sulfatase deficiency. Graefe's Archive of Clinical and Experimental Ophthalmology 226: 216–233

218. Stiefel A, Hausser I 1988 Skleromyxödem Arndt-Gottron. Hautarzt 39: 478–479

219. Stingl G, Tamaki K, Katz S L 1980 Origin and function of epidermal Langerhans' cells. Immunological Reviews 53: 149–174

220. Sybert V P, Dale B A, Holbrook K A 1985 Ichthyosis vulgaris: identification of a defect in synthesis of filaggrin correlated with an absence of keratohyalin granules. Journal of Investigative Dermatology 84: 191–194

221. Theile U 1974 Sjögren–Larsson syndrome. Oligophrenia — ichthyosis — di/tetraplegia. Humangenetik 22: 91–118

222. Tilgen W 1973 Zur Ultrastruktur der sogenannten white leaf-shaped macules bei der tuberösen Hirnsklerose Bourneville–Pringle. Archiv für Dermatologische Forschung 248: 13–27

223. Traupe H, Kolde G, Hamm H, Happle R 1986 Ichthyosis bullosa of Siemens: a unique type of epidermolytic hyperkeratosis. Journal of the American Academy of Dermatology 14: 1000–1005

224. Traupe H, Kolde G, Happle R 1984 Autosomal dominant lamellar ichthyosis: a new skin disorder. Clinical Genetics 26: 457–461

225. Uitto J, Ryhänen L, Abraham P A, Perejda A J 1982 Elastin in diseases. Journal of Investigative Dermatology 79 (suppl 1): 160s–168s

226. Vandersteen P R, Muller S A 1971 Erythrokeratodermia variabilis.

An enzyme, histochemical and ultrastructural study. Archives of Dermatology 103: 362–370

227. Vogel F, Motulsky A G 1986 Human genetics. Problems and Approaches, 2nd edn. Springer, Berlin

228. Voigtländer V, Arnold M-L, Neu P, Anton-Lamprecht I, Jung E G 1985 Cutis laxa acquise avec amyloidose cutanée et paraprotéinémie (IgG kappa). Annales de Dermatologie et Vénéréologie 112: 779–780

229. Voigtländer V, Tilgen W, Anton-Lamprecht I, Haneke E 1981 Bjoernstad-Syndrome (pili torti with deafness): clinical, genetic, and ultrastructural findings. In: Orfanos C E, Montagna W, Stüttgen G (eds) Hair research. Status and future aspects. Proceedings of the 1st International Congress on Hair Research, Hamburg, 1979. Springer, Berlin, pp 430–432

230. Walker E R, Frederickson R G, Mayes M D 1989 The mineralization of elastic fibers and alterations of extracellular matrix in pseudoxanthoma elasticum. Archives of Dermatology 125: 70–76

231. Walter S, Goebel H H 1988 Ultrastructural pathology of dermal axons and Schwann cells in lysosomal diseases. Acta Neuropathologica 76: 489–495

232. Wiest L G, Anton-Lamprecht I 1976 Haarschaftanomalie und Bruchmechanismus bei einer Form von idiopathischer Trichoklasie. Ärztliche Kosmetologie 6: 153–158

233. Williams M L 1983 The ichthyoses — pathogenesis and prenatal diagnosis: a review of recent advances. Pediatric Dermatology 1: 1–24

234. Williams M L, Elias P M 1984 Elevated n-alkanes in congenital ichthyosiform erythroderma. Phenotypic differentiation of two types of autosomal recessive ichthyosis. Journal of Clinical Investigation 74: 296–300

235. Williams M L, Elias P M 1985 Heterogeneity in autosomal recessive ichthyosis. Clinical and biochemical differentiation of lamellar ichthyosis and nonbullous ichthyosiform erythroderma. Archives of Dermatology 121: 477–488

236. Williams M L, Koch T K, O'Donnell J J, Frost P H, Epstein L B, Sanderson Grizzard W, Epstein C J 1985 Ichthyosis and neutral lipid storage disease. American Journal of Medical Genetics 20: 711–726

237. Winkelmann R K, Muller S A 1963 Generalized eruptive histiocytoma. A benign papular histiocytic reticulosis. Archives of Dermatology 88: 586–596

238. Witkop C J 1983 Abnormalities in pigmentation. In: Emery A E H, Rimoin D L (eds) The principles and practice of medical genetics, vol. 1. Churchill Livingstone, Edinburgh, pp 622–652

239. Witkop C J, Quevedo W C, Fitzpatrick T B 1983 Albinism and other disorders of pigment metabolism. In: Stanbury J B, Wyngaarden J B, Frederickson D S, Goldstein J L, Brown M S (eds) The metabolic basis of inherited disease, 5th edn. McGraw-Hill, New York, pp 301–346

240. Woodley D T, Briggaman R A, O'Keefe E J, Inman A O, Queen L L, Gammon W R 1984 Identification of the skin basement-membrane autoantigen in epidermolysis bullosa acquisita. New England Journal of Medicine 310: 1007–1013

241. Woodley D T, Burgeson R E, Lunstrum G P, Reese M J, Bruckner-Tuderman L, Gammon W R, Briggaman R A 1987 The epidermolysis bullosa acquisita antigen is type VII procollagen. Journal of Investigative Dermatology 88: 525

242. Wyatt P R, Cox D M 1977 Utilization of electron microscopy in the prenatal diagnosis of genetic disease. Human Heredity 27: 22–37

243. Yoshiike T, Woodley D T, Briggaman R A 1988 Epidermolysis bullosa acquisita antigen: relationship between the collagenase-sensitive and -insensitive domains. Journal of Investigative Dermatology 90: 127–130

244. Zonana J, Schinzel A, Upadhyaya M, Thomas N S T, Anton-Lamprecht I, Harper P S 1990 Prenatal diagnosis of X-linked hypohidrotic ectodermal dysplasia by linkage analysis. American Journal of Medical Genetics 35: 132–135

245. Bruckner-Tuderman L, Niemi K-M, Kero M, Schnyder U W, Reunala T 1990 Type VII collagen is expressed but anchoring fibrils are defective in dystrophic epidermolysis bullosa inversa. British Journal of Dermatology 122: 383–390

Appendix I. List of abbreviations

A	= actin filaments	IS	= intercellular spaces
ADI	= autosomal dominant ichthyosis vulgaris	K	= keratinosomes
AEB	= acquired epidermolysis bullosa	KH	= keratohyalin
AED	= anhidrotic ectodermal dysplasia	L	= lipid droplets
AF	= anchoring fibrils	LC	= Langerhans' cell
AP	= autophagic vacuoles	LG	= Langerhans' cell granule
BL	= basal lamina	LU	= lumen
BP	= bullous pemphigoid	LY	= lysosomes and heterolysosomes
C	= centriole/cilium	LYM	= lymphocyte
CB	= Civatte body, fibrillar or colloid body, dyskeratotic keratin mass	M	= mitochondria
		MC	= melanocyte
CIE	= congenital ichthyosiform erythroderma	ME	= marginal envelope of horn cells
CO	= collagen fibrils	MG	= melanin granules
CP	= cicatricial pemphigoid	MP	= macrophage
CRIE	= congenital reticular ichthyosiform erythroderma	MT	= microtubule
		MW	= molecular weight
CV	= coated vesicle	N	= nucleus
D	= desmosome	NA	= axons of unmyelinated nerve
E	= elastic microfibrils (elastotubules, oxytalan fibrils)	NG	= neutrophil granulocyte
		P	= peridermal cell
EB	= epidermolysis bullosa	PL	= primary lysosome
EBA	= epidermolysis bullosa atrophicans	PPK	= palmo-plantar keratosis
EBD	= epidermolysis bullosa dystrophica	PV	= pinocytotic vesicle
EBH	= epidermolysis bullosa herpetiformis	R	= ribosomes
EBP	= epidermolysis bullosa progressiva	RER	= granular endoplasmic reticulum
EBS	= epidermolysis bullosa simplex	SB	= stratum basale, basal cells
EC	= erythrocyte	SC	= stratum corneum, horny layer
EP	= pores of eccrine sweat ducts	SG	= stratum granulosum, granular layer
EPL	= ectoplasm	SP	= sweat gland primordium
EPP	= erythropoietic protoporphyria	SS	= stratum spinosum
ER	= endoplasmic reticulum	T	= tonofilaments
F	= fibroblast	TT	= tonotubules
FD	= fibrin deposit	V	= vimentin
G	= glycogen	VC	= vesicular complexes
GA	= gestational age	X	= X-linked inheritance
GAG	= glycosaminoglycans	XRI	= X-linked ichthyosis
GEH	= generalized eruptive histiocytoma		
GO	= Golgi apparatus		
HCM	= hyalinosis cutis et mucosae		
HD	= hemidesmosomes		

Appendix II. Technical considerations

Many different methods of tissue fixation and processing for EM have been developed. Some have found broad application and are widely and often exclusively used for tissue preparation in routine EM (e.g. Karnovsky solution, now mostly used half-strength). It is well appreciated, however, that each organ tissue has its own needs for modifications of preparation methods. Skin is a complex organ with three very different major compartments: (1) the cellular epidermis, (2) its compact and poorly penetrable horny layer (often increased or hyperkeratotic), and (3) the predominantly fibrous connective tissue, with high water-binding capacity, interspersed with adnexal, nervous and vascular tissue elements. Pathological events affecting one or the other of these compartments may further influence and modify the normal tissue reaction to fixation and embedding procedures.

Keratinocytes react with high sensitivity to osmotic imbalance, mechanical stress and trauma. 'Dark' and 'light' cells in the germinative basal cell layer of the epidermis are the result of concomitant shrinkage and swelling of neighbouring basal cells via fluid translocation due to osmotic imbalance during the initial fixation, or because of hyperosmolarity of the fixatives. In the author's laboratories, the best results have been achieved by the application of a fixation procedure modified after Peracchia & Mittler.[190] Partial oxidation of the glutaraldehyde (GA) to glutaric acid by hydrogen peroxide is thought to enhance tissue penetration and to supplement for increased oxygen demand. Dark and light cells do not occur in the basal layer with this fixation mode.

Cacodylate buffer was found to be superior to phosphate buffer with respect to general tissue preservation of skin samples (except for the excellent preservation of ribosomes with the latter). Fixation at room temperature yields better preservation than it does at low temperatures (4–8°C).

Skin biopsy and sample dissection mean considerable mechanical stress and trauma to living tissue, especially to the epidermis. Keratinocytes possess actin filaments in addition to their keratin cytoskeleton. These may be visualized under special circumstances (see Fig. 22.17E) and are especially expressed during tissue remodelling and wound repair (see Figs 22.23B and 22.38A). Basal keratinocytes react to mechanical stress by pronounced contractures,

resulting in widened intercellular spaces and the formation of long slender microvilli. Knife biopsy instead of punch biopsy, and avoidance of any mechanical stress, are prerequisites for avoidance of these artefacts. Most importantly, dissection and subdivision of the tissue samples should be performed only after sufficient fixation of the tissue (at least 1–2 h). Penetration of undissected skin samples by cacodylate-buffered, partially oxidized GA is excellent. If tissue is to be mailed to an EM laboratory, it should be mailed *in toto* in GA fixation solution.

Fixation procedure used in the author's laboratories at Heidelberg

GA stock solution

3% GA in 0.1 M cacodylate buffer solution, pH 7.4
100 ml (12 ml GA 25% + 88 ml cacodylate buffer)

First fixation solution

Add 6 drops of hydrogen peroxide (30%) with a Pasteur (capillary) pipette to 25 ml GA stock solution.
Stir for 10 min (magnet stirrer and teflon sticks) to ensure that the oxidation reaction proceeds.

Fixation and embedding procedure

Fix undissected tissue samples *in toto* for 2 h in first fixation solution (3% GA + H_2O_2) at room temperature. Tissue can be subdivided after at least 1 h. Change fixative and continue fixation in GA stock solution (without H_2O_2) overnight, or store in a refrigerator until further preparation. Mailing is possible at this stage at room temperature. Rinse carefully in cacodylate buffer (depending on previous time of GA fixation). Postfix in cacodylate-buffered 1% osmic acid. Dehydrate in graded ethanols.

Embedding media affects contrast, stainability, and preservation of the tissue (see Figs 22.1, 22.2 and 22.16). Araldite or Epon epoxy resins often penetrate poorly into and within hyperkeratotic horny layers. Improvement of horny layer preservation may be achieved by the use of low-viscosity epoxy resins (Spurr medium; see Fig. 22.2E).

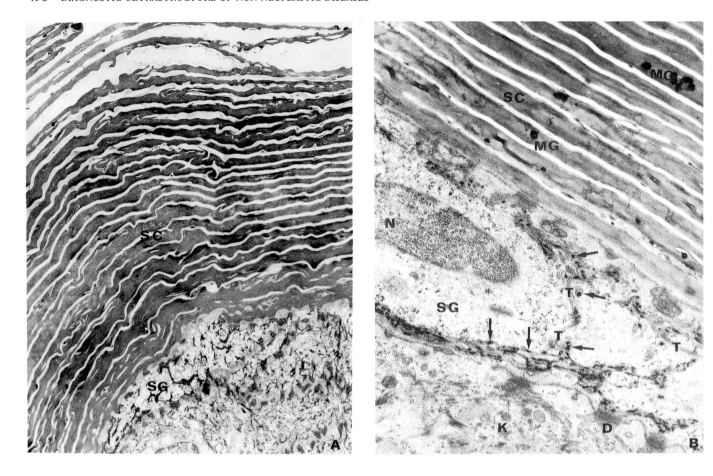

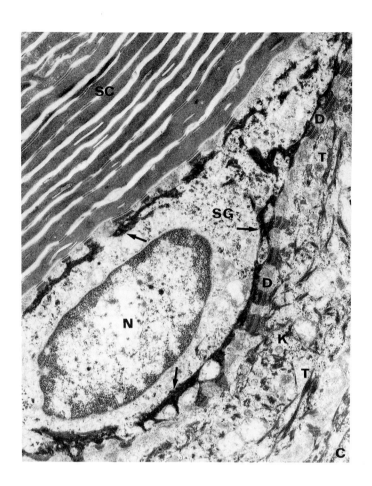

Fig. 22.1 Autosomal dominant ichthyosis vulgaris. **A** A compact orthohyperkeratotic horny layer composed of smooth flattened horn cells covers the interfollicular epidermis. Granular cells containing only small amounts of minute keratohyalin granules occur sporadically beneath the lowermost horn cells. (× 5750) **B** and **C** The abnormal ultrastructure and mode of deposition of keratohyalin granules is better demonstrated by fixation with osmic acid in potassium dichromate solution (**B**), than with glutaraldehyde–osmic acid double fixation (**C**), due to the lower contrast of the tonofilaments after fixation with osmic acid alone (Epon embedding). Minute keratohyalin granules (arrows) line the tonofilaments and do not become confluent as in normal skin and in all other types of inherited ichthyoses. (B, × 19 200; C, × 11 370)

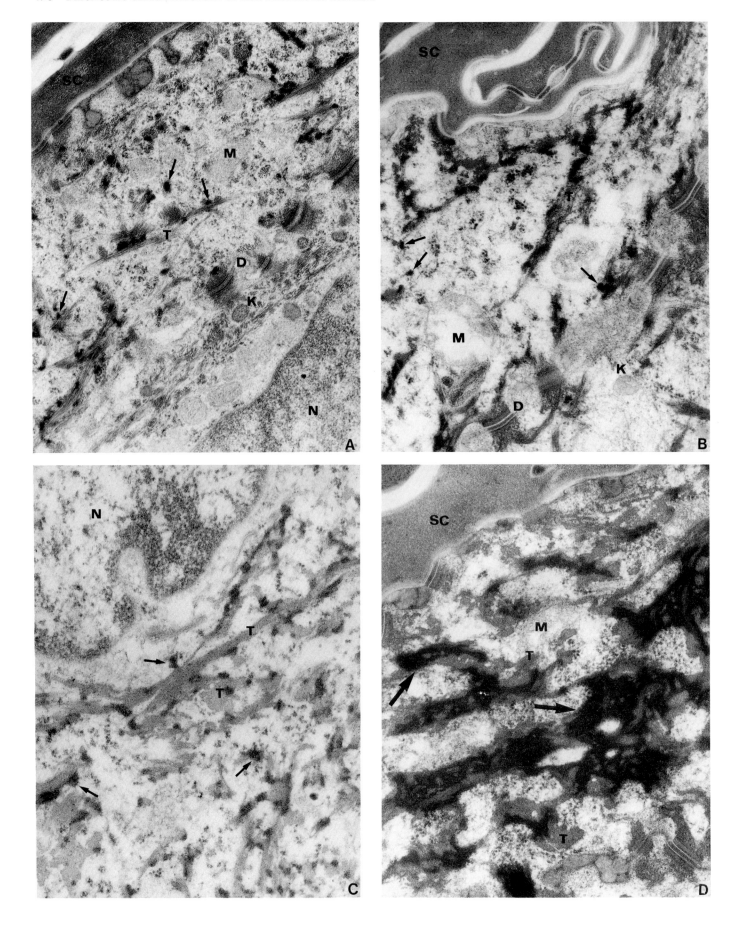

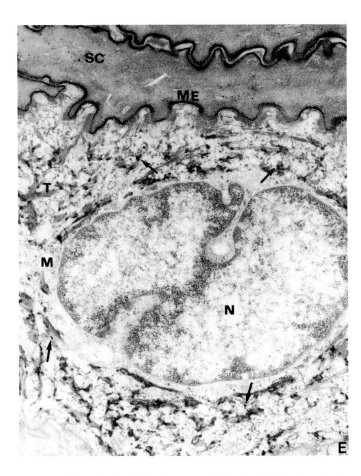

Fig. 22.2 Keratohyalin defect in autosomal dominant ichthyosis vulgaris (ADI). Technical variations which demonstrate the defective nature of keratohyalin (arrows) in ADI (**A**, **B**, **C** and **E**), when compared to normal keratohyalin in congenital ichthyosis (**D**). **A** Fixation in osmic acid/potassium dichromate solution, epon embedding. **B–E** Glutaraldehyde/osmic acid double fixation. **B** and **D** Epon embedding. **C** and **E** Low viscosity epoxy resin. (A, × 31 420; B, × 31 920; C, × 41 600; D, × 40 300; E, × 13 200)

Fig. 22.3 (Overleaf, left) Autosomal recessive congenital ichthyosis; ichthyosis congenita type I (non-bullous congenital ichthyosiform erythroderma). Hyperproliferative acanthotic epidermis, with a granular layer composed of up to six layers of incompletely flattened cells containing small amounts of keratinization-specific proteins, namely keratin (tonofilaments) and keratohyalin. Massive compact orthokeratotic horny layer with numerous lipid vacuoles indicating storage of neutral lipids such as triglycerides or alkanes. (× 4970) Electron micrograph: Dr M-L. Arnold.

Fig. 22.4 (Overleaf, right) Autosomal recessive congenital ichthyosis; ichthyosis congenita type II, cholesterol type. **A** and **B** Moderate to pronounced hyperproliferation with acanthosis and compact orthokeratotic horny layer of varying degree. Groups of cholesterol clefts (★) and smaller amounts of lipid droplets in comparison to type I, are significant diagnostic markers. Keratins (tonofilaments) and keratohyalin are in near normal amounts, and granular cells are flattened. (A, × 3450; B, × 8890). **C** and **D** Prenatal diagnosis of ichthyosis congenita type II. Irregularly arranged membrane inclusions in horn cells of follicular plugs in a boy aged 2.5 years (**C**) and in the horn cells of the follicular openings in an affected fetus at 20 weeks (**D**). There is no keratinization of the interfollicular epidermis and no hyperkeratosis, whereas cholesterol crystals are not demonstrable in fetal skin samples at that age. (C and D, × 40 300) Electron micrographs: Dr M-L Arnold.

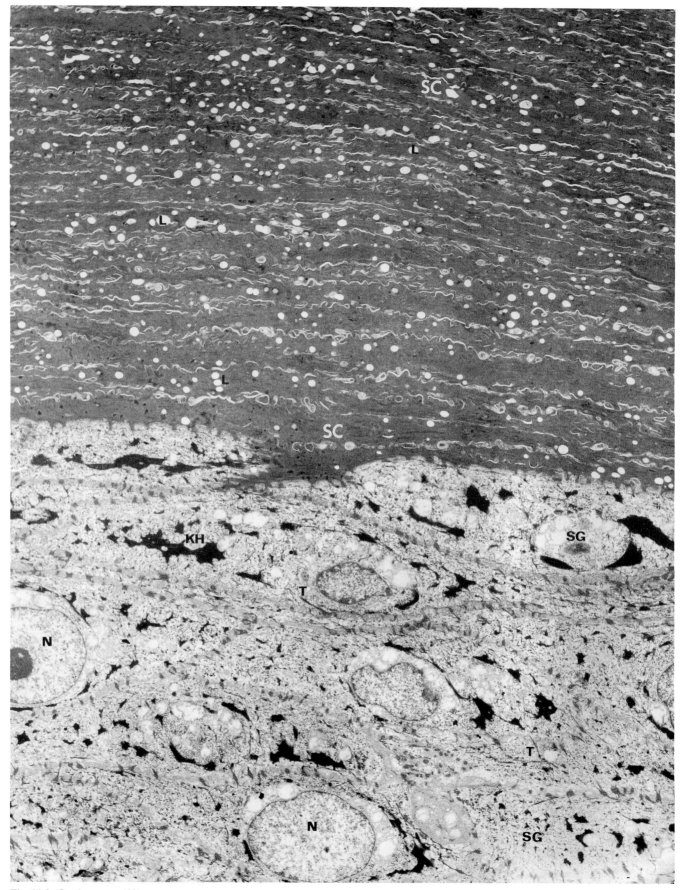

Fig. 22.3 (Caption on p. 499)

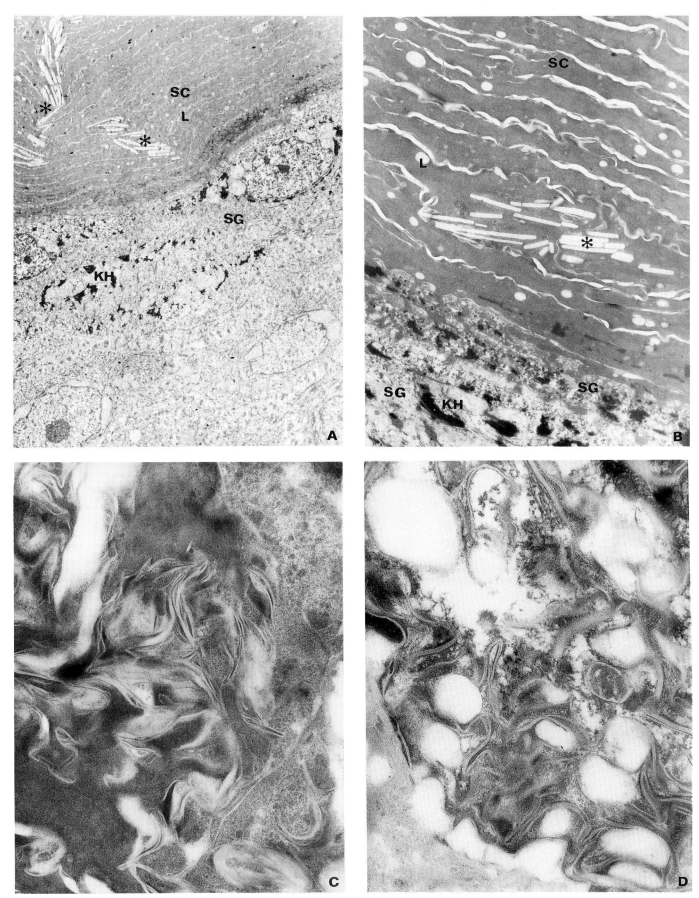

Fig. 22.4 (Caption on p. 499)

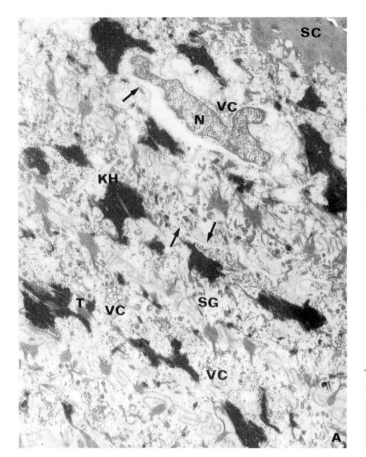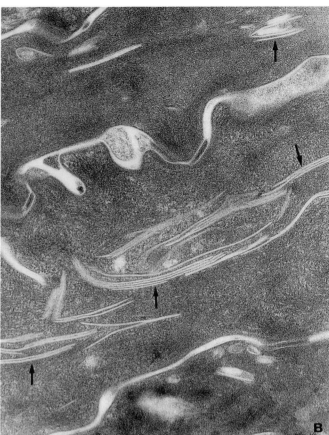

Fig. 22.5   Autosomal recessive congenital ichthyosis; ichthyosis
congenita type III. **A–D** Diagnostic markers in the granular and horny
layer consist of elongated, mostly perinuclear membranes (**A**, **B** and **D**,
arrows) and vesicular complexes of abnormal keratinosomes (**A** and **C**),
both of which are retained in the horny layer (**B**, shows membranes only)
— this indicates disturbance in the synthesis or metabolism of polar
lipids. Keratinization-specific proteins (keratins or tonofilaments, and
keratohyalin), are found in normal amounts (**A**, **C** and **D**). Females aged
30 years (**A**), 12 years (**B**, **C**) and 1.5 years (**D**). (A, × 11 370; B,
× 45 000; C and D, × 40 300) Electron micrographs: Dr M-L Arnold.

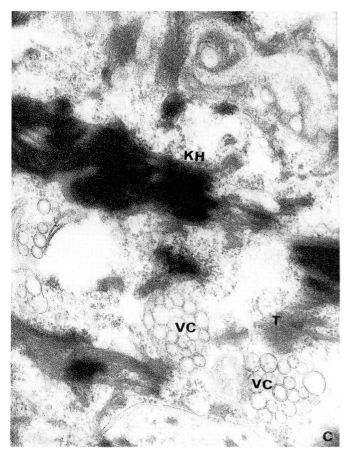

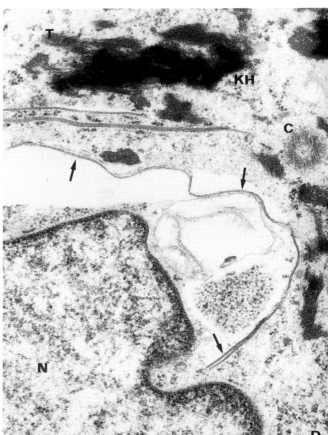

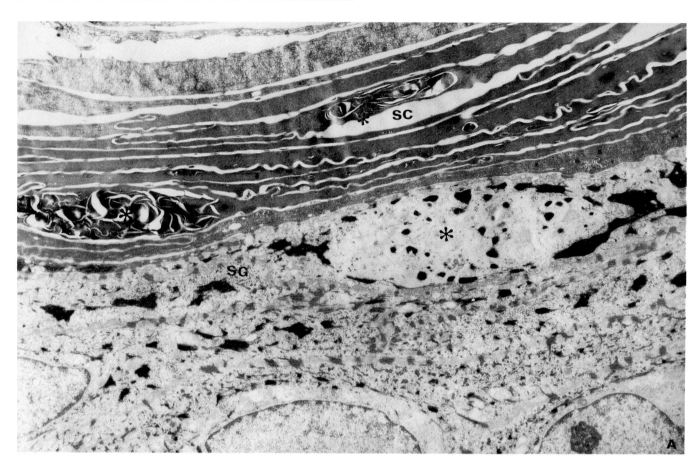

Fig. 22.6 Autosomal recessive congenital ichthyosis; ichthyosis congenita type IV. **A–B** Characteristic accumulated masses of long, irregularly arranged membranes in lenticularly swollen paranuclear cell regions (⋆) in the uppermost granular cells (**A**), where keratohyalin granules may attach to them (**D**). They remain undegraded in the horny layer, appearing as irregular small clefts (**A** and **B**), and are demonstrable even after re-embedding of paraffin material for EM (**B**); **A** and **B** Postnatal skin (A, × 6670; B, × 33 800) **C** and **D** Prenatal diagnosis of ichthyosis congenita type IV by demonstration of membrane accumulations in granular (**D**) and horny cells (**C**) lining the hair follicle openings of an affected fetus at 22 weeks GA. (C, × 19 500; D, × 15 300) Electron micrographs: A, Dr I Hausser; C, Dr M-L Arnold.

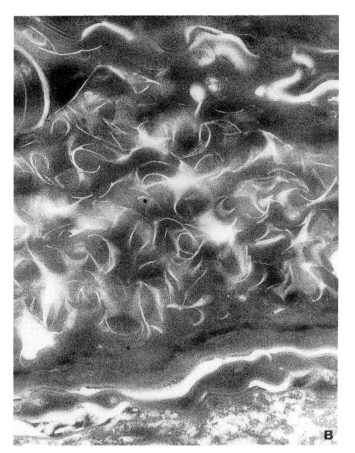

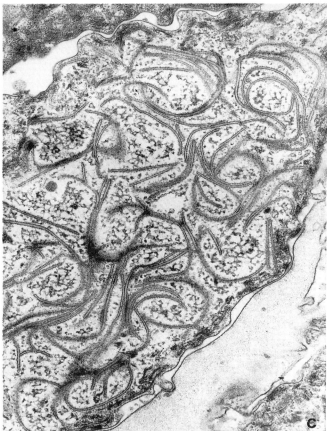

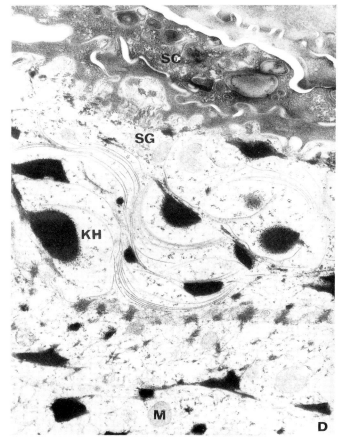

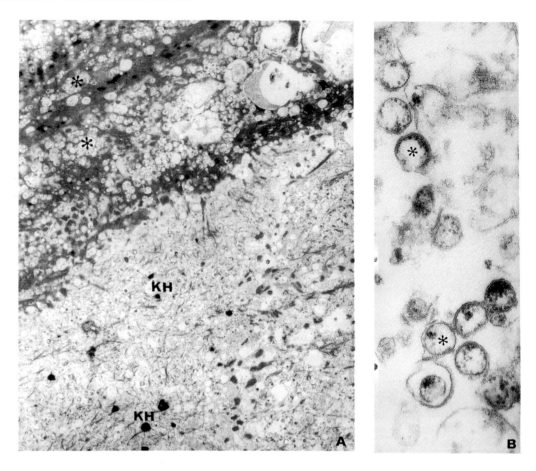

Fig. 22.7   Ichthyosis congenita gravis; harlequin ichthyosis type I. **A–C** Accumulations of groups of membrane-bound vesicles (*) in the massive compact horny layer are combined with suppression of normal keratinization products. Vesicles are empty or contain varying numbers of small granules resembling glycogen (**B** and **C**) and are first demonstrable in cells in the uppermost spinous cell layer; they represent severely defective keratinosomes. (A, × 7700; B, × 51 670; C, × 40 930) **D** Prenatal diagnosis of harlequin ichthyosis type I. Demonstration of the same abnormality of keratinosomes (arrows) in an affected fetus at 23 weeks' GA. (× 40 950)

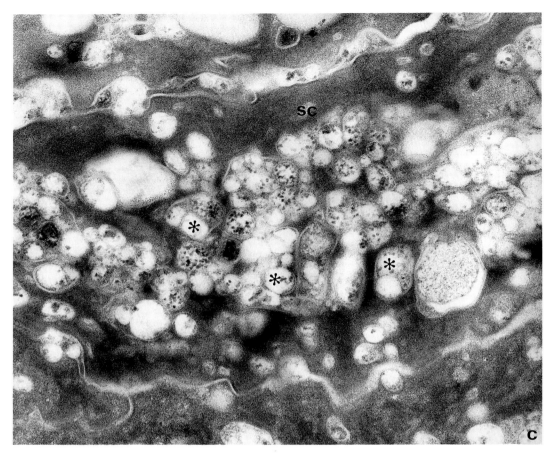

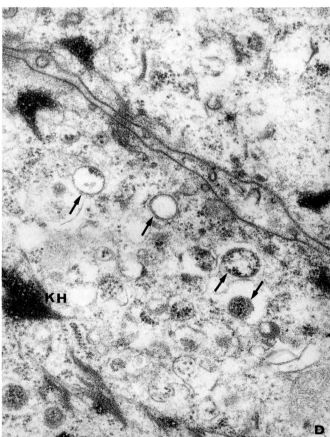

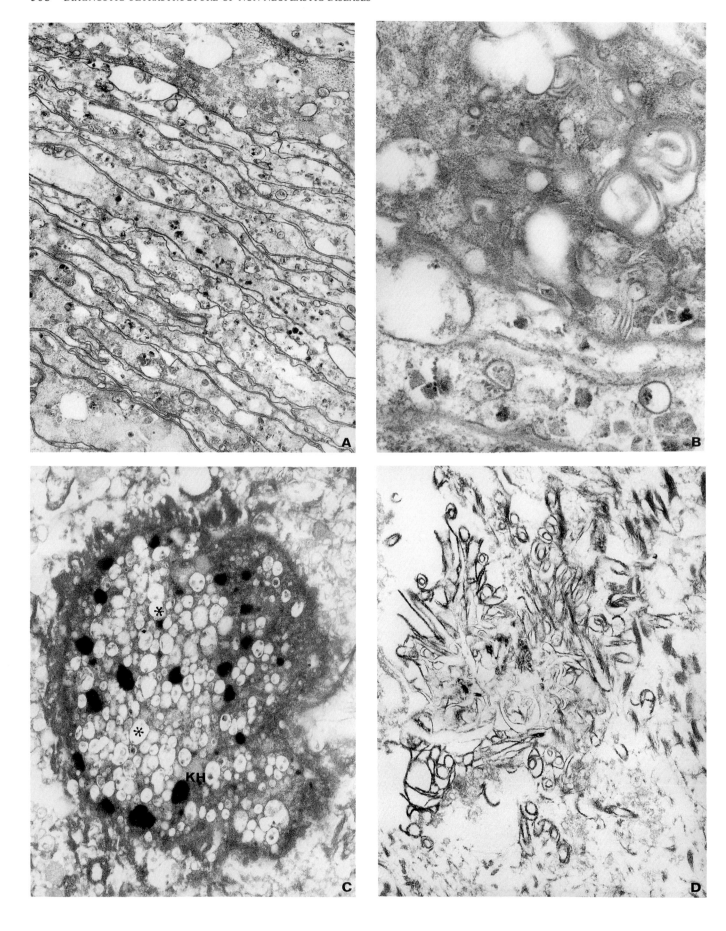

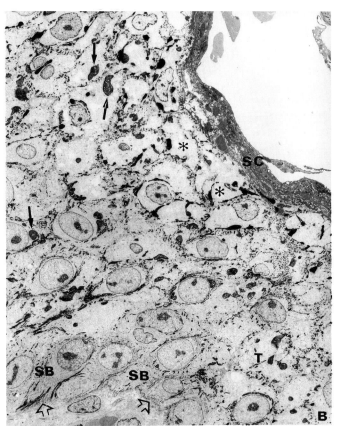

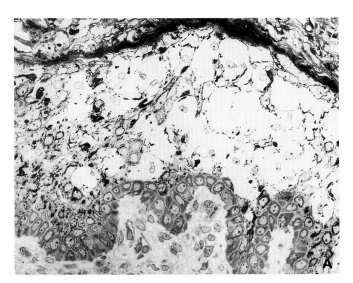

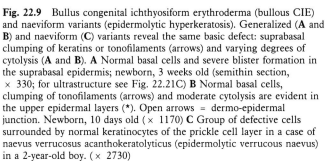

Fig. 22.9 Bullus congenital ichthyosiform erythroderma (bullous CIE) and naeviform variants (epidermolytic hyperkeratosis). Generalized (**A** and **B**) and naeviform (**C**) variants reveal the same basic defect: suprabasal clumping of keratins or tonofilaments (arrows) and varying degrees of cytolysis (**A** and **B**). **A** Normal basal cells and severe blister formation in the suprabasal epidermis; newborn, 3 weeks old (semithin section, × 330; for ultrastructure see Fig. 22.21C) **B** Normal basal cells, clumping of tonofilaments (arrows) and moderate cytolysis are evident in the upper epidermal layers (*). Open arrows = dermo-epidermal junction. Newborn, 10 days old (× 1170) **C** Group of defective cells surrounded by normal keratinocytes of the prickle cell layer in a case of naevus verrucosus acanthokeratolyticus (epidermolytic verrucous naevus) in a 2-year-old boy. (× 2730)

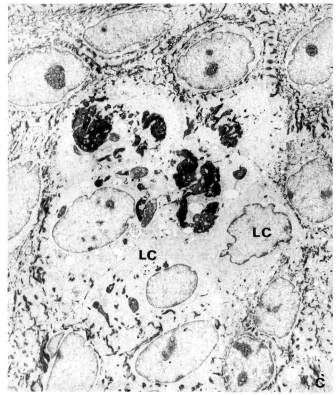

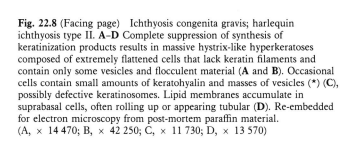

Fig. 22.8 (Facing page) Ichthyosis congenita gravis; harlequin ichthyosis type II. **A–D** Complete suppression of synthesis of keratinization products results in massive hystrix-like hyperkeratoses composed of extremely flattened cells that lack keratin filaments and contain only some vesicles and flocculent material (**A** and **B**). Occasional cells contain small amounts of keratohyalin and masses of vesicles (*) (**C**), possibly defective keratinosomes. Lipid membranes accumulate in suprabasal cells, often rolling up or appearing tubular (**D**). Re-embedded for electron microscopy from post-mortem paraffin material. (A, × 14 470; B, × 42 250; C, × 11 730; D, × 13 570)

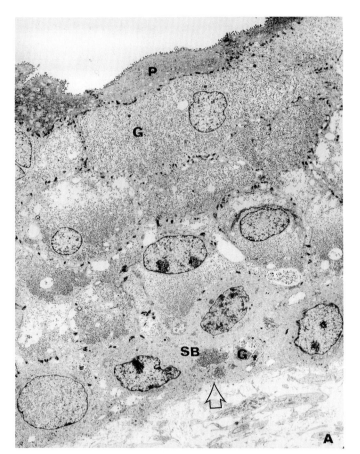

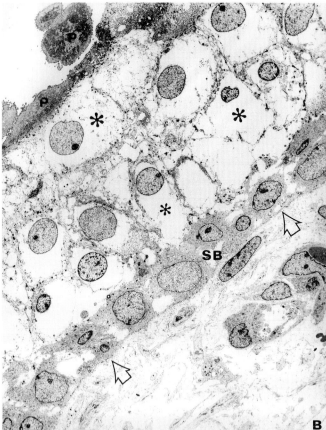

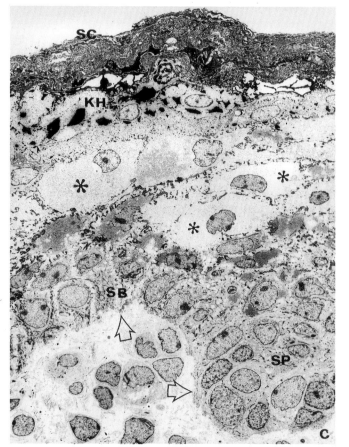

Fig. 22.10 Fetal manifestations of bullous CIE and prenatal diagnosis. Cytolysis predominates in affected fetuses before the onset of keratinization (after 24–26 weeks in non-ridged skin regions), whereas clumping of tonofilaments is only occasionally demonstrable. **A** and **B** Affected fetus at 19 weeks' GA, scalp skin sample: keratinization is restricted to the follicular openings, the basal cell layer is normal but considerable variation in the degree of cytolysis (★) of suprabasal cells occurs. **A** = normal cells (× 2490); **B** = severe cytolysis of intermediate cells, normal peridermal cells; open arrows = dermo-epidermal junction. (× 1450) **C** Affected fetus after termination at 22 weeks' GA (sibling of fetus in A and B), showing hyperkeratosis and pronounced suprabasal cytolysis (★); palmar skin sample; open arrows = dermo-epidermal junction. (× 1450)

Fig. 22.11 (Facing page) Ultrastructure of tonofibrillar clumping; bullous CIE and naevus verrucosus acanthokeratolyticus. **A–D** Variation in the diameter of the tonofilaments, as well as their contrast, density and degree of aggregation, reflect the range of molecular weights (MW) of the keratin protein family sequentially synthesized in the keratinizing epidermis — such variations are not distinguishable in normal keratinocytes. Low-MW keratins of moderate electron-density form round to oval clumps with smooth surfaces (**A, B, D**). Higher-MW keratins with increasing electron-density aggregate at the periphery of the clumps (**A**, arrows) forming curled strands and loosely aggregated perinuclear shells (**A**) or large dyskeratotic clumps (**D**). Only a few clumps or aggregates maintain contact with desmosomes (**A, B, C, D**). **A** and **B** = bullous CIE, postnatal skin; **C** = bullous CIE, fetal palmar skin, 22 weeks' GA, after termination; clumping tonofilaments of uniform diameters, contrast and density, **D** = naevus verrucosus, postnatal skin. (A, × 5170; B, × 27 360; C, × 43 330; D, × 11 670); Electron micrograph A: B Melz-Rothfuss.

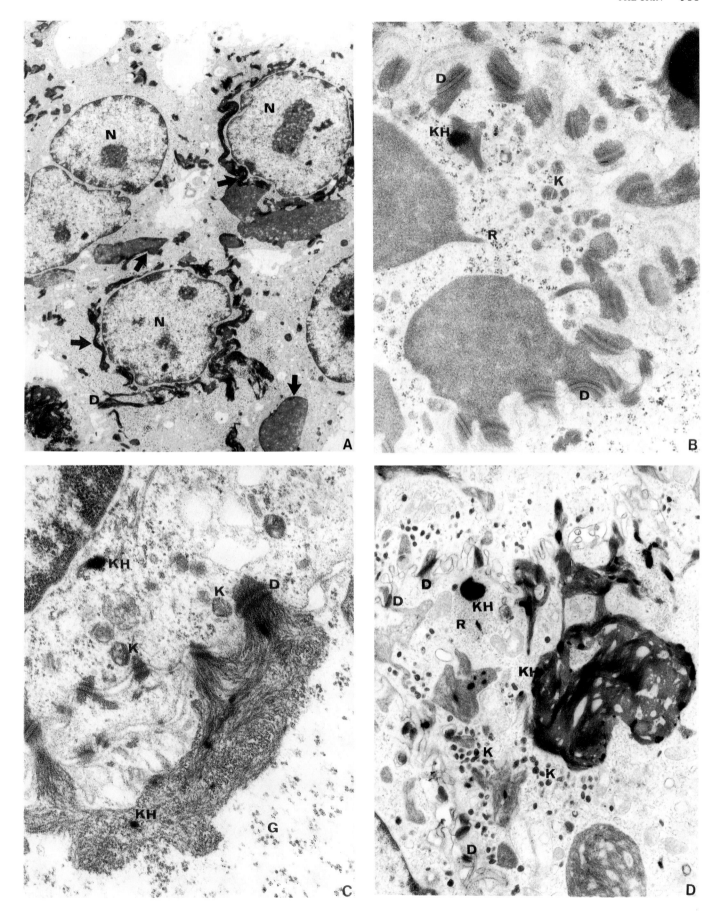

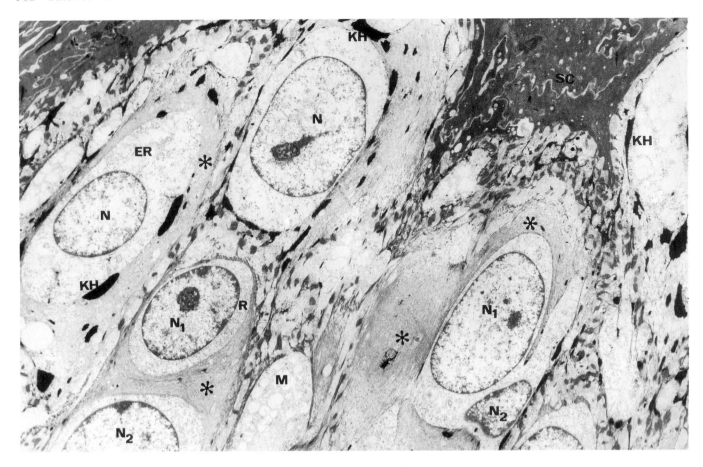

Fig. 22.12 Ichthyosis hystrix Curth-Macklin. Concentric shells of tonofilaments (*) surround and enclose nuclei and perinuclear cytoplasm containing polyribosomes, mitochondria and endoplasmic reticulum. Shells are in contact with desmosomes and have a smooth inner surface; keratohyalin is predominantly deposited on the inner surface of the shells. Binuclear cells are frequent (compare with Figs 22.9 and 22.13). (× 4160)

Fig. 22.13 (Facing page) Congenital reticular ichthyosiform erythroderma. **A** and **B** At low magnification the concentric shells (*) encircling nuclei and perinuclear cytoplasm resemble those of ichthyosis hystrix Curth–Macklin (see Fig. 22.12). Their different ultrastructure is disclosed at high magnification (see Fig. 22.14). Keratins (tonofilaments) are arrayed mainly at the periphery of the shells (**B**); keratohyalin is deposited at their inner surface (**A**). Binuclear cells are frequent. A = granular layer; B = spinous cell layer. (× 4680)

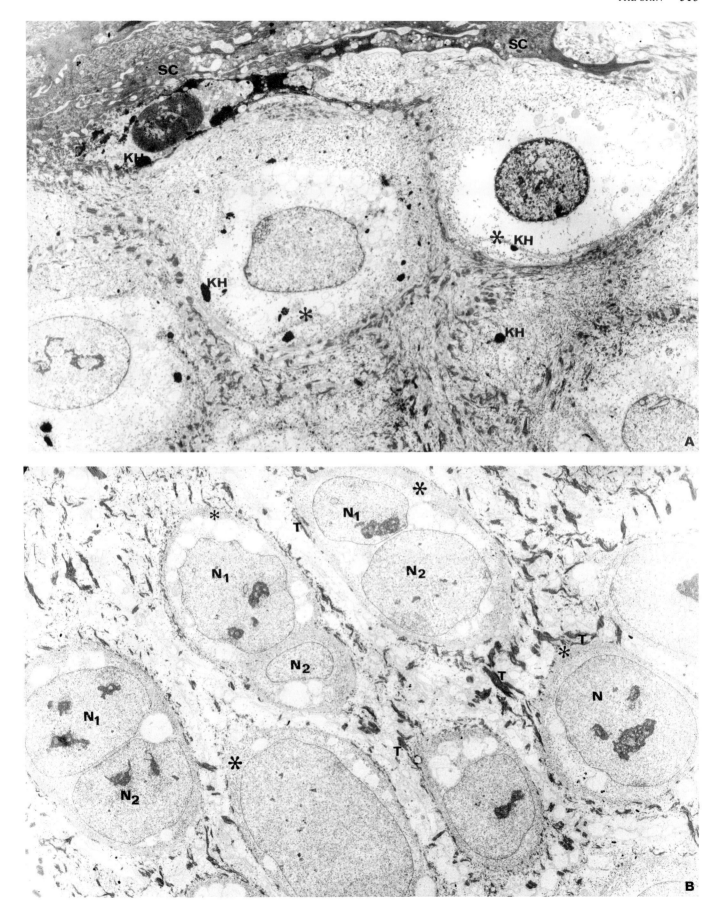

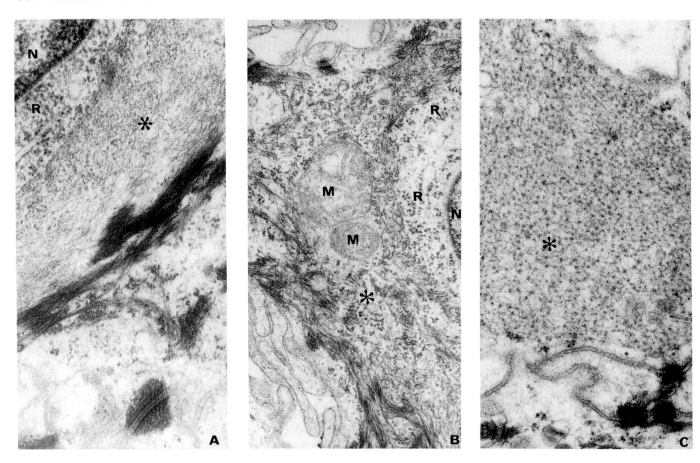

Fig. 22.14 Ultrastructural differential diagnosis of ichthyosis hystrix Curth–Macklin and congenital reticular ichthyosiform erythroderma (CRIE). **A–C** High magnification reveals the significant differences between the filaments forming the concentric shells (★). Tonofilaments often showing the increasing density and diameters of the keratin family (**A**) constitute the shells in the Curth–Macklin type (**A** and **B**), whereas a three-dimensional network of much finer filaments of unknown biochemical nature (glycoproteins?) forms the shells in CRIE (**C**). (A, × 41 600; B, × 32 430; C, × 40 300)

Fig. 22.15 (Facing page) Ichthyosis linearis circumflexa Comel (Netherton's syndrome). Specific abnormalities are exclusively demonstrable at the edge of the actively progressing lesional margin and underneath the border of the thick anterior horn scale. Keratinocytes in the upper Malpighian layer accumulate round to oval membrane-bound granules of varying density and increasing sizes (arrows). They resemble lysosomes but probably represent material phagocytozed from intercellular spaces that are filled with similar substances (*) (serum exudates?). Keratinization-specific protein synthesis is suppressed, and keratohyalin is entirely lacking. (× 6240; inset, × 19 200) Electron micrographs: Dr M-L Arnold.

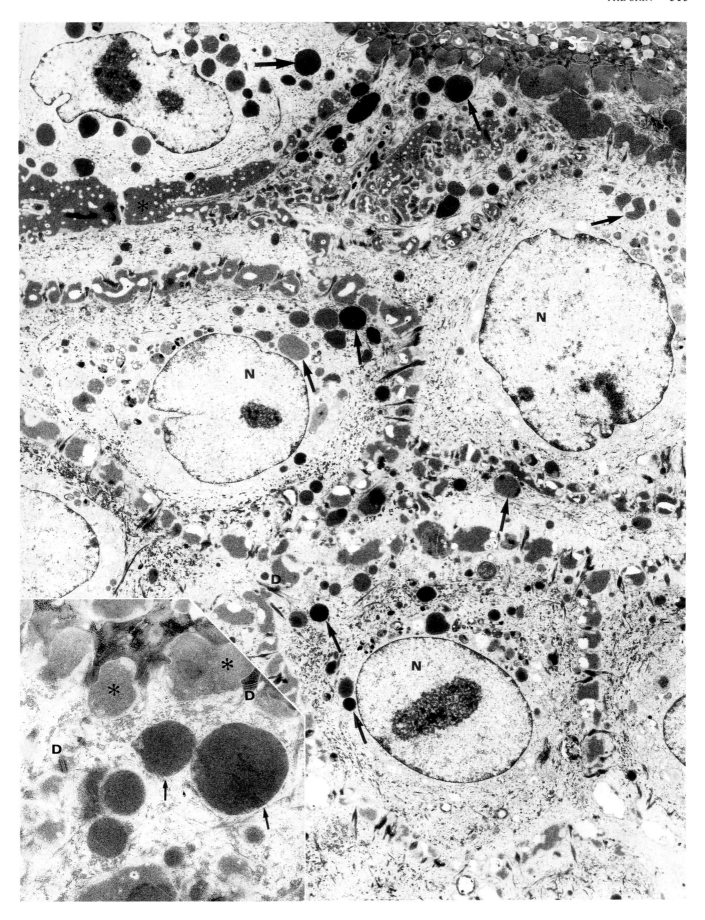

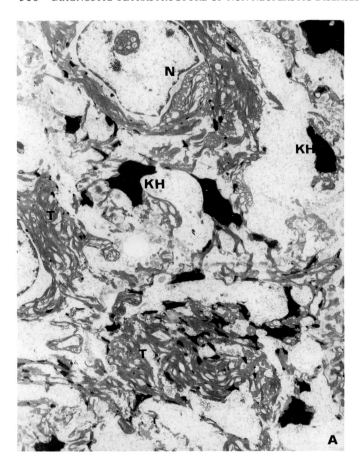

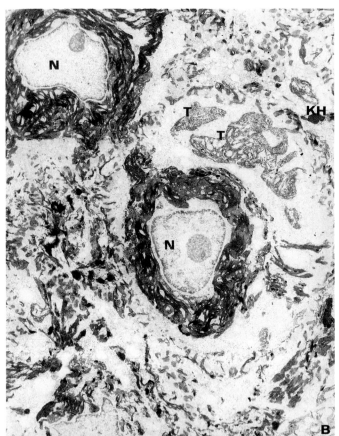

Fig. 22.16 (Above) Palmo-plantar hyperkeratosis with acanthokeratolysis (so-called 'granular degeneration'), Voerner type. **A** and **B** The basic defect is the same as in bullous CIE and its naeviform variants (see Figs 22.9–22.11), namely increased clumping of keratin proteins in suprabasal layers. Amounts of tonofilaments are due to the anatomical location (ridged skin). The mode of embedding influences the contrast of keratins and keratohyalin. (A = epoxy resin Epon 812, × 4170; B = low viscosity epoxy resin, × 3510) Electron micrographs: B. Melz-Rothfuss.

Fig. 22.17 (Right and facing page) Palmo-plantar hyperkeratosis with aggregation of tonotubules (tubular keratins) and dominant inheritance (first identified by the author). **A–E** Very similar to the Voerner type (see Fig. 22.16) at low magnification (**A** = lower spinous layer; **B** = upper spinous layer). The increasing aggregation of keratins into round to oval dense clumps, with a unique abnormality of the keratins, separates this PPK as a distinct nosologic entity. Clumps are irregularly arranged in the cells (**B**) and do not form perinuclear shells (compare with Figs 22.16 and 22.11A); they consist of masses of tubular elements (**C**) arranged in fountain-like arrays (**C**, **E**, arrows) and originate from tonofilaments rolling up in a supercoil fashion; tonotubules first appear in hexagonal arrays in suprabasal cells (**D**) and are synthesized in increasing amounts in the later differentiation stages (**A**, **E**). With segregation of the cytoplasmic constituents, actin filament bundles become discernible among the tonotubules (**E**). (A, × 3380; B, × 1730; C, × 11 370; D, × 40 300; E, × 32 500)

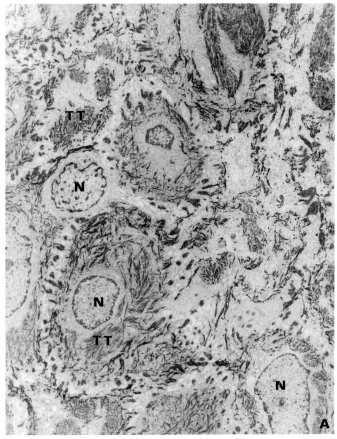

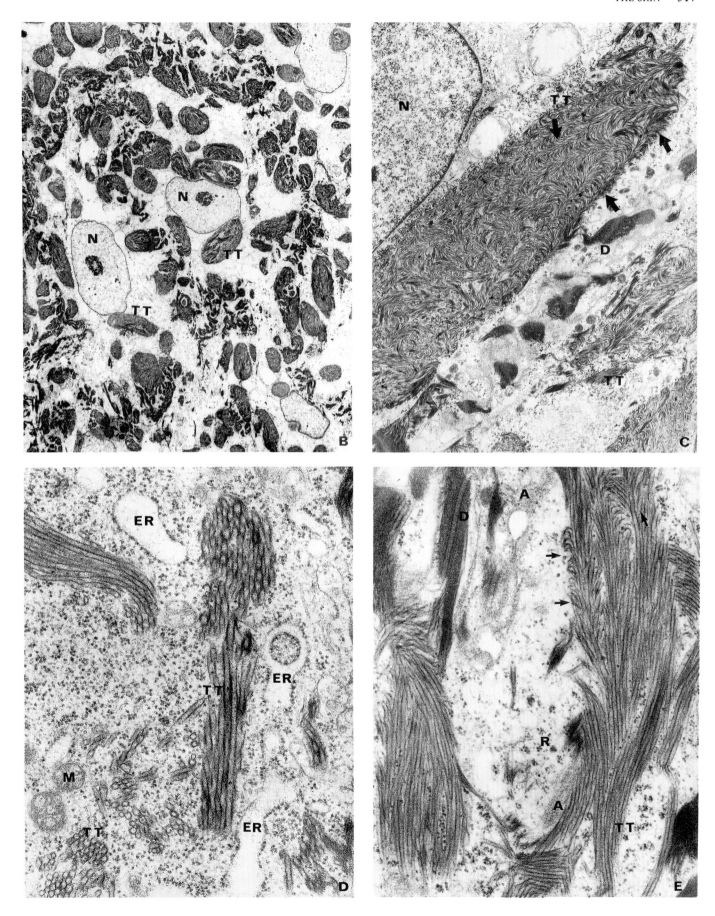

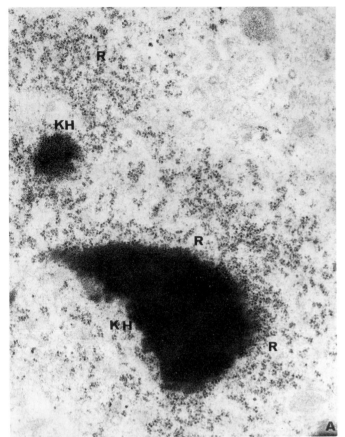

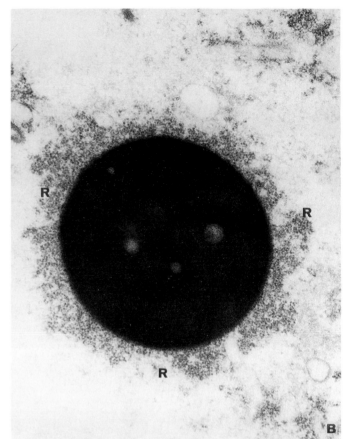

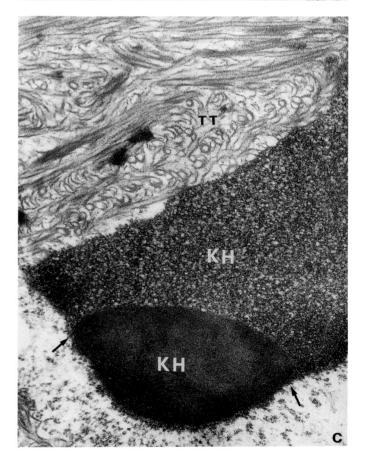

Fig. 22.18   Keratohyalin synthesis in disorders with tonofibrillar (or keratin) aggregation. **A–C** Due to early aggregation and clumping of keratins and the resulting cytoplasmic segregation, keratohyalin is synthesized free within the cytoplasm (**A**), often in globular form (**B**), (**A** and **B**, bullous CIE) or at the lateral surface of keratin clumps or aggregates (**C**), (PPK with tonotubular aggregates). Masses of polyribosomes concentrating around keratohyalin granules (**A** and **B**) indicate active protein synthesis. In ridged skin, KH is composed of two distinctive proteins that are very similar in contrast and density in both normal ridged skin and in the Voerner type of PPK. In PPK with tonotubules the main component has a spongy appearance (**C**, arrows) reflecting differences in KH composition (note tonotubular supercoils in **C**). (A, × 36 400; B, × 28 930; C, × 40 300)

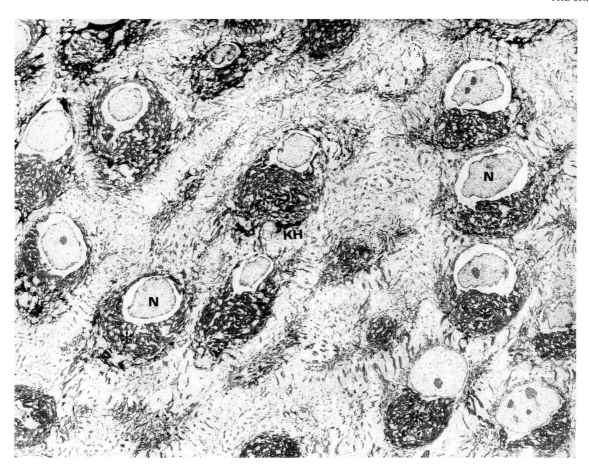

Fig. 22.19 Pachyonychia congenita. Following blister formation and in close proximity to the initial foci of disturbance, dyskeratotic changes with loose aggregations of tonofilaments (*) occur in lesional skin. Keratohyalin is deposited preferentially in the periphery of these aggregates, as in the previous examples of tonofilamentous aggregation (see Figs 22.9, 22.12, 22.13 and 22.18). Diagnostically significant is the unilateral orientation of the dyskeratotic keratin masses instead of the perinuclear or irregular arrangement seen in the previous disorders. Lesional skin from the knee. (× 1450)

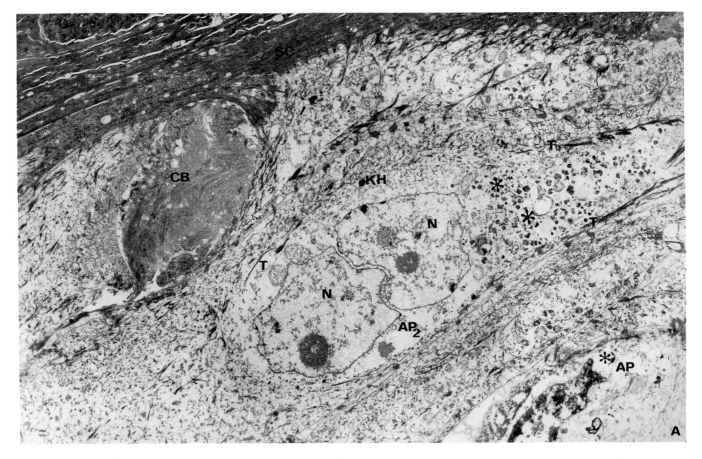

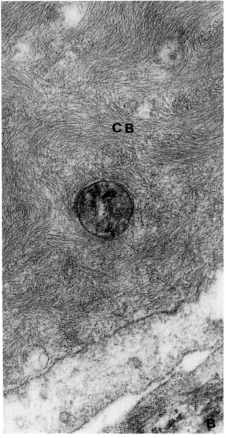

Fig. 22.20 Porokeratosis Mibelli. **A** and **B** Specific abnormalities of the keratinization process are restricted to areas of the so-called 'cornoid lamella' (**A**), localized regions of parakeratotic horn cell columns at the margin, and, occasionally, in the centre of the Mibelli lesion. Autophagocytic cells, occasionally binuclear (**A**), with perinuclear oedema, displacement of tonofilaments to the cell periphery and paranuclear accumulation of autophagic vacuoles (★) are seen. Synthesis of keratinization-specific proteins (high-MW keratins and KH) is suppressed, although low amounts of KH can be formed even in the autophagocytic cells. Isolated cells undergo dyskeratotic changes resembling those in Darier's disease, to become transformed to fibrillar or Civatte bodies composed of masses of keratin filaments (**A** and **B**). (A, × 4810; B, × 40 300) A: reproduced from Marghescu et al [168] with permission.

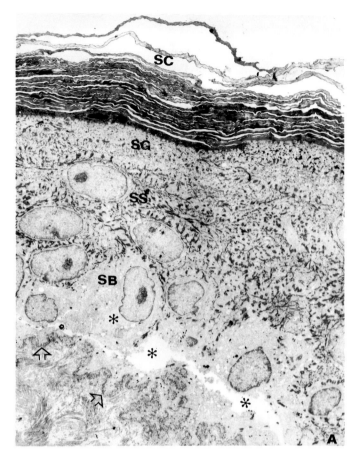

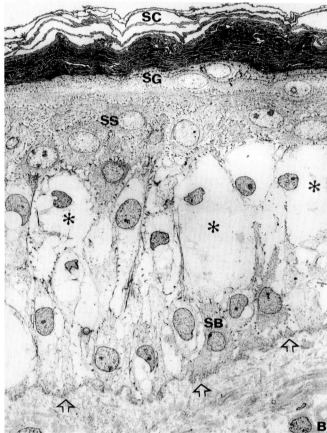

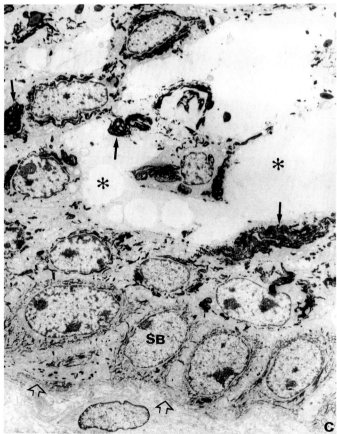

Fig. 22.21 (This page and overleaf)   Differential diagnosis of blister formation in epidermolysis bullosa (EB), initial stages (see also Fig. 22.26). **A** EB simplex, Köbner type. Basal cell oedema, focal cytolysis and intrabasal split formation (★) parallel to the dermo-epidermal junction (open arrows) are evident, mostly below basal cell nuclei. The ultrastructure of all suprabasal layers is normal. Adult male. (× 2420) **B** EB herpetiformis Dowling–Meara. Oedema and cytolysis (★) of individual basal and suprabasal cells, still showing normal ultrastructure of cell constituents, is the first step to compartmentalized blisters — one of the initial changes preceding clinical blisters. Newborn male, 3 days old (see also Fig. 22.25, A–C). (× 1170) **C** Bullous congenital ichthyosiform erythroderma. Suprabasal blister formation due to cytolysis (★) occurs following tonofibrillar clumping (arrows) and segregation of cytoplasm. The ultrastructure of basal cells and dermo-epidermal junction (open arrows) is normal. Newborn male, 3 weeks old (same case as in Fig. 22.9A — clinical diagnosis: epidermolysis bullosa). (× 2420)

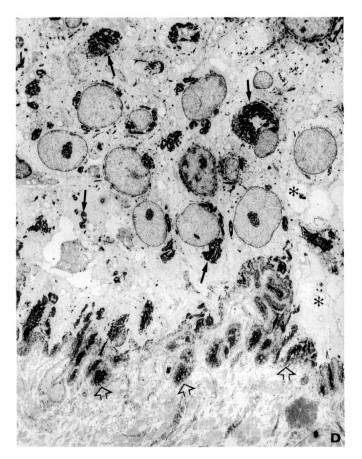

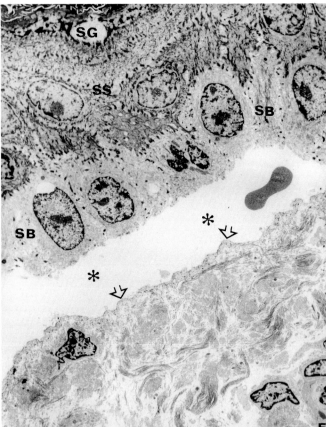

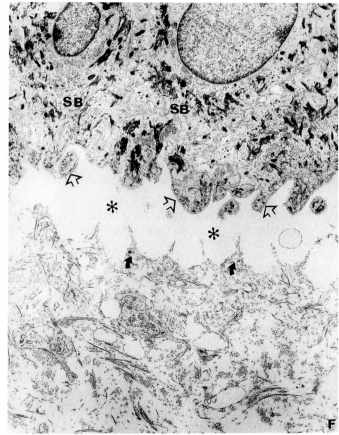

Fig. 22.21 (*cont'd*) **D** Epidermolysis bullosa herpetiformis Dowling–Meara. Pronounced clumping of tonofilaments (arrows) in basal and suprabasal cells, tonofibrillar aggregation along the dermo-epidermal junction (open arrows), segregation of cytoplasm and focal early cytolysis (*). Male child, 8.5 years old — same case as in Fig. 22.23C (see also Figs 22.23 and 22.25C). (× 2490) **E** Epidermolysis bullosa atrophicans, Herlitz type. Junctional separation of entire epidermis including normal-appearing basal cells from dermal connective tissue in the space of the lamina rara (*) of the dermo-epidermal junction. Basal lamina overlies the floor of the split (open arrows). Five days-old premature newborn male of 33 weeks' GA, with pyloric obstruction and large epithelial defects of the lower extremities (see also Figs 22.30 and 22.31). (× 2420) **F** Epidermolysis bullosa dystrophica, recessive Hallopeau–Siemens type. Dermolytic split formation (*) occurs below the dermo-epidermal junction. Basal lamina (open arrows) remains at the blister roof while the basal cells appear normal. The superficial relief of the blister floor with projections of small tips (curved arrows) indicates initial focal collagenolysis; the composition of the underlying connective tissue depends on previous phases of possible blistering. Newborn male, 2 months old (see also Figs 22.32–22.35). (× 5470) Electron micrographs: D, Dr M-L. Arnold; E, Dr I Hausser; F, J Deimel-Hatzenbühler; B and F reproduced from Anton-Lamprecht[12] (with permission).

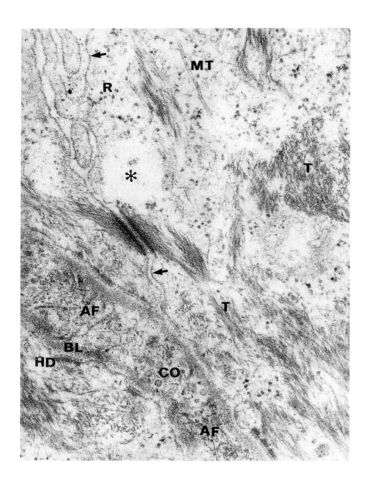

Fig. 22.22 Epidermolysis bullosa simplex Weber–Cockayne. Initial stages of blister formation are the same as in the generalized Köbner type (see Fig. 22.21A): focal cytolysis (⋆) of the basal cell cytoplasm above the dermo-epidermal junction (see Fig. 22.26), initially sparing cell organelles such as mitochondria, microtubules, ribosomes, desmosomes and plasma membranes (arrows), coated vesicles and tonofilaments. Melanocytes are generally uninvolved. Adult female. (× 53 330) Reproduced from Haneke and Anton-Lamprecht,[119] with permission.

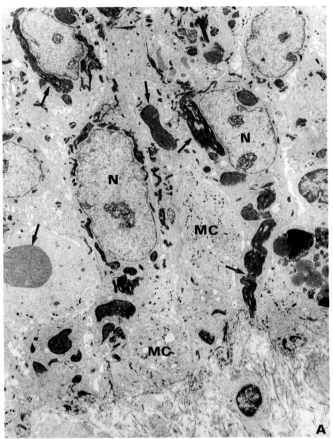

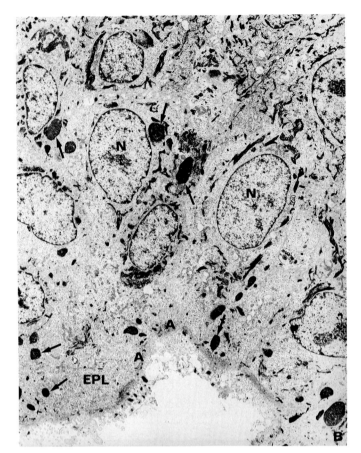

Fig. 22.23 Epidermolysis bullosa herpetiformis Dowling–Meara.
Specific ultrastructural markers. Clumping of tonofilaments (arrows) in
basal (and suprabasal) cells is pathognomonic of the Dowling–Meara type
and does not occur in other genetic types of EB. Most pronounced in
perilesional skin and in the erythematous margin of spreading
herpetiform blisters, clumping of keratins and segregation of cytoplasm
precede blister formation. Most easily demonstrable in infants up to 2
years of age (see text). **A** Varying density and contrast of tonofilament
clumps (arrows) reflect the different MW classes of the keratin protein
family coexisting in the epidermal keratinocytes (see also Fig. 22.11).
Female, 2 months old. (× 3250) **B** Tonofibrillar clumps (arrows) are
retained in the blister roof. Basal cells after separation undergo
remodelling and reorganization of their cytoplasm at the undersurface of
the blister roof forming multiple cell projections into the blister cavity
and an 'ectoplasm-like' region of cytoplasm that is rich in ribosomes but
lacks most other cell organelles — except actin filament bundles that run
parallel to the plasma membrane. Newborn male, 11 days old; same case
as in Fig. 22.24B. (× 3190) **C** Tonofibrillar clumps and curled strands
(arrows) occurring close to regions with initial stages of cytolysis (★),
oedema of basal cell cytoplasm, and formation of compartmentalized
blisters (compare Fig. 22.21B and 22.25, A and B). Aggregation of
tonofilaments in rootlets of basal cells along the dermo-epidermal
junction (open arrows) is highly — specific for the Dowling–Meara type.
C = male, 8.5 years old, same case as in Fig. 22.21D. (× 2530) Electron
micrographs: A, B Melz-Rothfuss, reproduced from Anton-Lamprecht[11]
with permission; C, Dr M-L Arnold.

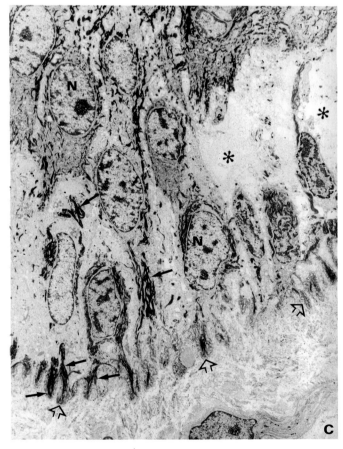

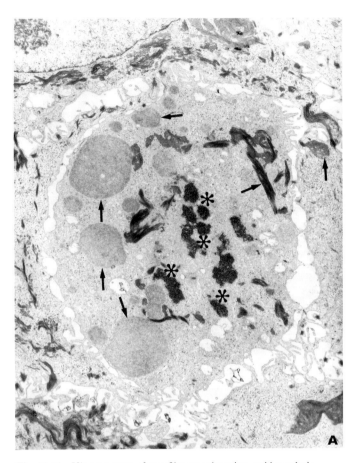

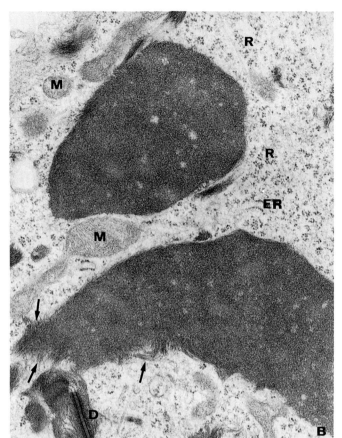

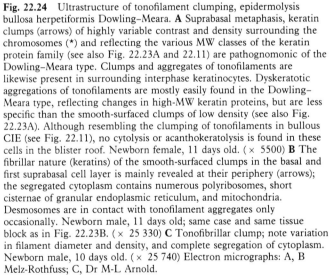

Fig. 22.24   Ultrastructure of tonofilament clumping, epidermolysis
bullosa herpetiformis Dowling–Meara. **A** Suprabasal metaphasis, keratin
clumps (arrows) of highly variable contrast and density surrounding the
chromosomes (*) and reflecting the various MW classes of the keratin
protein family (see also Fig. 22.23A and 22.11) are pathognomonic of the
Dowling–Meara type. Clumps and aggregates of tonofilaments are
likewise present in surrounding interphase keratinocytes. Dyskeratotic
aggregations of tonofilaments are mostly easily found in the Dowling–
Meara type, reflecting changes in high-MW keratin proteins, but are less
specific than the smooth-surfaced clumps of low density (see also Fig.
22.23A). Although resembling the clumping of tonofilaments in bullous
CIE (see Fig. 22.11), no cytolysis or acanthokeratolysis is found in these
cells in the blister roof. Newborn female, 11 days old. (× 5500) **B** The
fibrillar nature (keratins) of the smooth-surfaced clumps in the basal and
first suprabasal cell layer is mainly revealed at their periphery (arrows);
the segregated cytoplasm contains numerous polyribosomes, short
cisternae of granular endoplasmic reticulum, and mitochondria.
Desmosomes are in contact with tonofilament aggregates only
occasionally. Newborn male, 11 days old; same case and same tissue
block as in Fig. 22.23B. (× 25 330) **C** Tonofibrillar clump; note variation
in filament diameter and density, and complete segregation of cytoplasm.
Newborn male, 10 days old. (× 25 740) Electron micrographs: A, B
Melz-Rothfuss; C, Dr M-L Arnold.

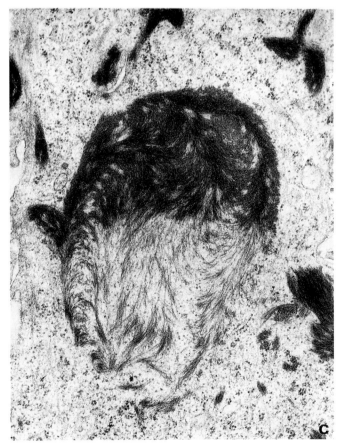

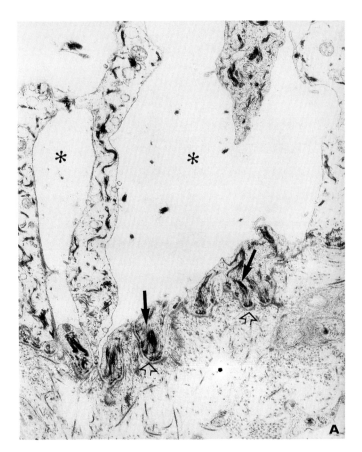

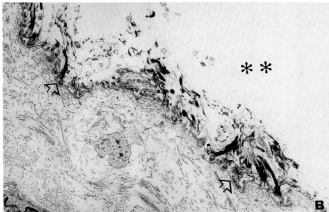

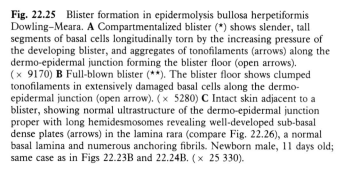

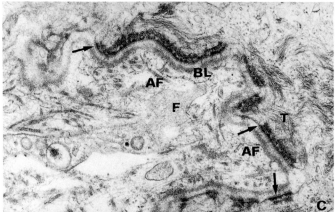

Fig. 22.25   Blister formation in epidermolysis bullosa herpetiformis Dowling–Meara. **A** Compartmentalized blister (*) shows slender, tall segments of basal cells longitudinally torn by the increasing pressure of the developing blister, and aggregates of tonofilaments (arrows) along the dermo-epidermal junction forming the blister floor (open arrows). (× 9170) **B** Full-blown blister (**). The blister floor shows clumped tonofilaments in extensively damaged basal cells along the dermo-epidermal junction (open arrow). (× 5280) **C** Intact skin adjacent to a blister, showing normal ultrastructure of the dermo-epidermal junction proper with long hemidesmosomes revealing well-developed sub-basal dense plates (arrows) in the lamina rara (compare Fig. 22.26), a normal basal lamina and numerous anchoring fibrils. Newborn male, 11 days old; same case as in Figs 22.23B and 22.24B. (× 25 330).

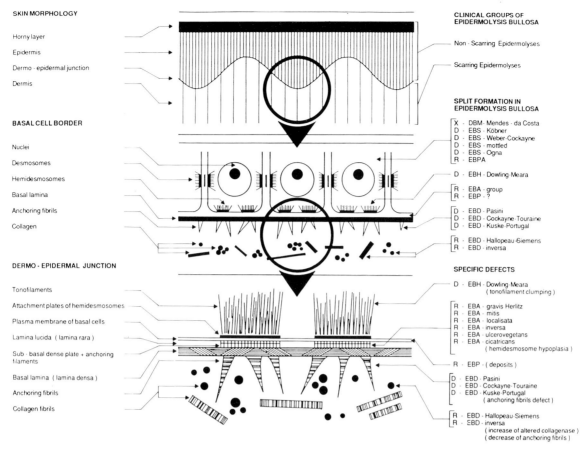

SKIN MORPHOLOGY

Horny layer

Epidermis

Dermo - epidermal junction

Dermis

BASAL CELL BORDER

Nuclei

Desmosomes

Hemidesmosomes

Basal lamina

Anchoring fibrils

Collagen

DERMO - EPIDERMAL JUNCTION

Tonofilaments

Attachment plates of hemidesmosomes

Plasma membrane of basal cells

Lamina lucida (lamina rara)

Sub - basal dense plate + anchoring filaments

Basal lamina (lamina densa)

Anchoring fibrils

Collagen fibrils

CLINICAL GROUPS OF EPIDERMOLYSIS BULLOSA

Non - Scarring Epidermolyses

Scarring Epidermolyses

SPLIT FORMATION IN EPIDERMOLYSIS BULLOSA

X - DBM- Mendes - da Costa
D - EBS - Köbner
D - EBS - Weber-Cockayne
D - EBS - mottled
D - EBS - Ogna
R - EBPA

D - EBH - Dowling-Meara

R - EBA - group
R - EBP - ?

D - EBD - Pasini
D - EBD - Cockayne-Touraine
D - EBD - Kuske-Portugal

R - EBD - Hallopeau-Siemens
R - EBD - inversa

SPECIFIC DEFECTS

D - EBH - Dowling-Meara
(tonofilament clumping)

R - EBA - gravis Herlitz
R - EBA - mitis
R - EBA - localisata
R - EBA - inversa
R - EBA - ulcerovegetans
R - EBA - cicatricans
(hemidesmosome hypoplasia)

R - EBP - (deposits)

D - EBD - Pasini
D - EBD - Cockayne-Touraine
D - EBD - Kuske-Portugal
(anchoring fibrils defect)

R - EBD - Hallopeau-Siemens
R - EBD - inversa
(increase of altered collagenase)
(decrease of anchoring fibrils)

A

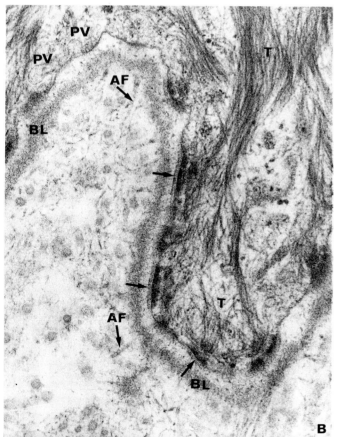

B

Fig. 22.26 Pathomorphogenesis of blister formation in epidermolysis bullosa. **A** (**left**) Architecture of skin (top), basal cell border (middle) and dermo- epidermal junction (lowermost). **A** (**right**) Main groups of epidermolysis bullosa (top) in old classification by histopathology; middle and lowermost parts: specific planes of split formation and specific defects in epidermolysis bullosa as recognized by EM. Adapted from Gedde-Dahl & Anton-Lamprecht.[96] **B** Ultrastructure of dermo-epidermal junction of normal interfollicular epidermis (non-ridged skin), with hemidesmosomes, tonofilaments, pinocytotic vesicles along plasma membrane of basal cell, basal lamina and many anchoring fibrils revealing a non-periodic banding pattern. Arrows point to sub-basal dense plates of hemidesmosomes in the plane of the lamina rara. (see also Figs 22.27–22.31) Adult male. (× 68 200)

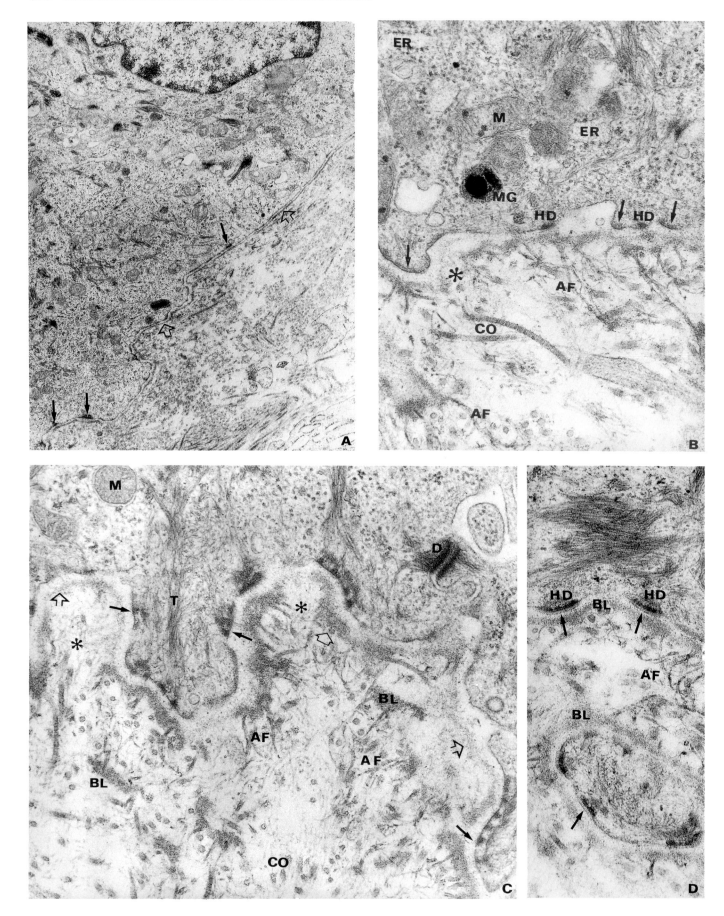

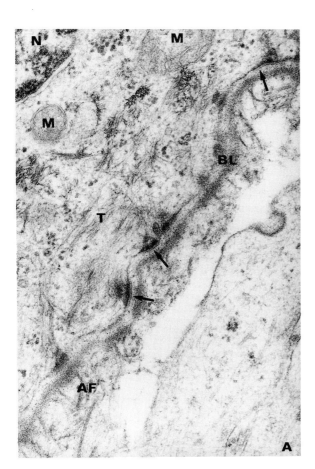
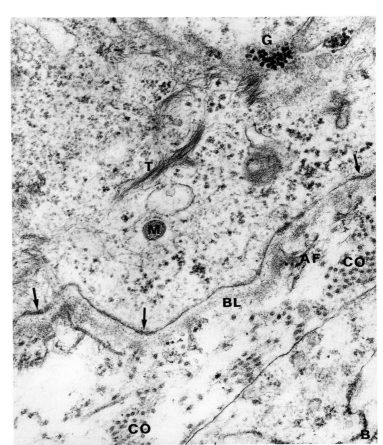

Fig. 22.28 Fetal manifestation and prenatal diagnosis of the Herlitz type and EBA group. **A** Hemidesmosomes start to develop about the 12th gestational week and are present in a focal patchy distribution in sufficient numbers at about 20 weeks. They have the same ultrastructural features as in postnatal skin with well-defined sub-basal dense plates (arrows). Basal lamina shows focal thickening below hemidesmosomes, while anchoring fibrils concentrate in these regions. Fetus at risk of EBA, Herlitz type, prenatal exclusion at 19 weeks' gestation. (× 40 930) **B** Fetus at risk of EBA, Herlitz type, affected, showing severe hypoplasia of hemidesmosomes, their epitopes recognizable by focal deposition of granular material on the plasma membrane (arrows) and focal thickenings of basal lamina. Herlitz fetus, prenatal diagnosis at week 20 GA. (× 40 330)

Fig. 22.27 (Facing page)   Epidermolysis bullosa atrophicans group; hemidesmosome hypoplasia (e.g. Herlitz type; EB atrophicans generalisata gravis). If mechanical stress is avoided in taking tissue samples of intact skin, unseparated and undamaged basal cell/dermo-epidermal junction areas can be obtained that reveal a single abnormality in otherwise normal-appearing skin, viz. severe hypoplasia of hemidesmosomes (**A–C**), the degree determining prognosis. **A** Only a few extremely small and incomplete attachment plates of hemidesmosomes (arrows) are present along the plasma membrane. The basal cytoplasm has a normal organelle composition, with no other abnormality (open arrows mark the dermo-epidermal junction); premature newborn male of 34 weeks' GA with large epithelial defects of lower legs and pyloric obstruction. Biopsy performed at the age of 9 days; the infant died within 34 days (see Müller et al[173]). (× 11 330) **B** A few extremely hypoplastic attachment plates of hemidesmosomes and focal deposition of granular material on the plasma membrane (arrows) indicating sites where hemidesmosomes should be formed. Basal lamina is partly interrupted with beginning repair (*). Anchoring fibrils are unusually long, broad and well-developed in Herlitz cases. There are no other signs of destruction or abnormality in the basal cells. (× 5330) **C** Even when hemidesmosomes are numerous, their special connections to the basal lamina in the lamina rara, the sub-basal dense plates, are totally and constantly missing (arrows). In contrast, desmosomes appear normal as is the remainder of the basal cell cytoplasm. The basal lamina shows breakage (*) and repair by new, very thin and immature parts (open arrows). Fragments of basal lamina with numerous large anchoring fibrils are scattered around in the papillary dermis. Newborn female, 3 weeks old. (× 53 330) **D** Normal hemidesmosomes with sub-basal dense plates (arrows) at similar magnification. Adult female (see also Figs 22.25C and 22.26). (× 52 530) Electron micrograph A: B Melz-Rothfuss.

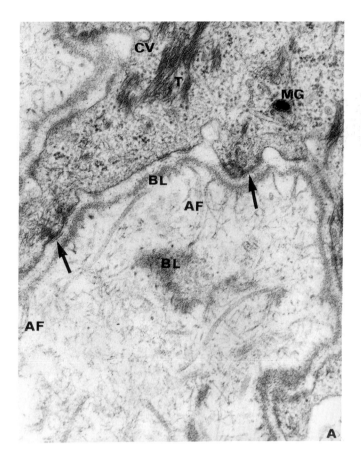

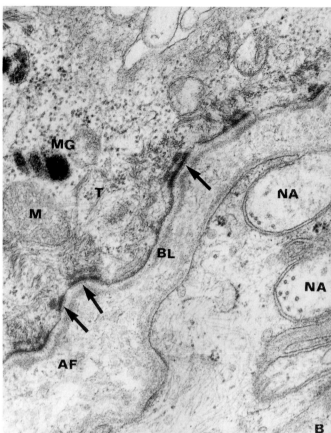

Fig. 22.29 Epidermolysis bullosa atrophicans, mitis type (benign adult EBA); hemidesmosome hypoplasia. **A** and **B** Hypoplasia of hemidesmosomes is less extreme than in the Herlitz type (see Figs 22.27, A–C). The hemidesmosomes are larger in diameter but are highly variable in number; few are to be found in most areas (**A**), but groups of hemidesmosomes (**B**) may occur here and there. Some material in the lamina rara (arrows) is present, but the normal ultrastructure of sub-basal dense plates is not evident. **A** = newborn male, 6 weeks old (× 38 330); **B** = newborn female with pyloric obstruction at birth, 6 weeks old at biopsy; minimal blister formation in later life; now 3 years old (same case as in Fig. 22.31C). (× 40 330) Electron micrographs: B Melz-Rothfuss.

Fig. 22.30 (Facing page) Epidermolysis bullosa atrophicans group, junctional separation and blister floor. The split forms in the plane of the main basic defect: in the lamina rara, where the defective hemidesmosomes lack sub-basal dense plates (junctional separation). **A** Basal cells easily detach (★) from the basal lamina under minimal mechanical trauma, often re-attaching and repairing small breaks (curved arrows) before blisters become clinically manifest. Fragments of basal lamina are scattered in the papillary dermis (see also Fig. 22.27C). Anchoring fibrils are unusually large, broad and numerous, with a well-developed banding pattern (arrows); EBA Herlitz type, newborn male, 20 days old (same case as in Fig. 22.31E). (× 32 530) **B** Floor of junctional blisters (★) is covered by basal lamina (open arrows) to which numerous anchoring fibrils are attached; they are especially well-formed in the EBA group. Fragments of basal lamina are scattered in the papillary dermis. Note the convex surface profile of the blister floor (see also Fig. 22.21E), which is very typical of junctional blisters due to the maintenance of the profile of the basal cell rootlets. The thickness of basal lamina depends on the age of the patient. Benign adult mitis type; female, 50 years old. Compare samples of fetal (Fig. 22.28), premature newborn (Fig. 22.27A), and newborn skin (A, and Fig. 22,27C). (× 32 530) **C** Melanocytes in blister cavity. After junctional separation, melanocytes often lose contact with surrounding keratinocytes and float in the blister cavity. Melanocytes (and naevus cells) are also often found at the blister floor, keeping contact with the basal lamina. Newborn female, Herlitz type, 3 weeks old — same case as in Fig. 22.27, B and C and Fig. 22.31D. (× 6270)

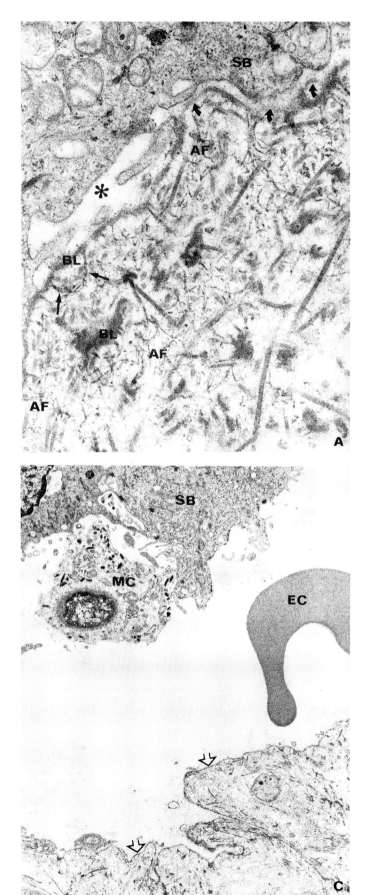

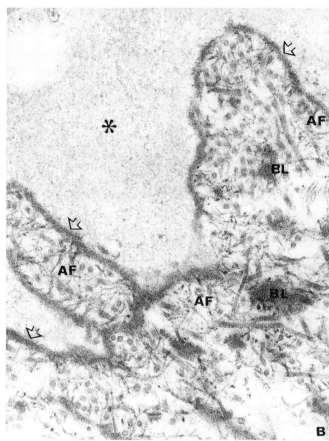

Fig. 22.31 (Overleaf)   Epidermolysis bullosa atrophicans group; junctional separation and blister roof (e.g. Herlitz type). The blister roof lacks basal lamina and undergoes rapid remodelling and reorganization of its undersurface after detachment from the basal lamina. **A** Fresh junctional blister (★): small cytoplasmic processes project into the blister cavity (arrows). Basal cells still have normal ultrastructure and distribution of cell organelles. **B–E** Progressive stages of remodelling with ingestion and translocation of remnants of hypoplastic hemidesmosomes into the inner cytoplasm of basal cells, where they are then rapidly degraded; all stages less than 1–2 hours after detachment. **B** Only small deposits of granular material indicate epitopes for hemidesmosome formation. Severe hypoplasia with separation due to skin biopsy procedure, and no sign of remodelling. **C** Remnants of hypoplastic hemidesmosomes (arrows) in small infoldings of basal cell undersurface, beginning ingestion. **D** Translocation of hemidesmosome remnants to the interior of basal cell (arrows). **E** Hypoplastic hemidesmosomes in the interior of a basal cell engulfed within small vesicles (derived from the plasma membrane) prior to complete degradation. **A** and **B** Newborn female, 15 days old. (A, × 6800; B, × 39 000). **C** = Newborn female, EBA mitis with pyloric obstruction — same case as in Fig. 22.29B; 6 weeks old at biopsy. (× 40 330) **D** = Newborn female, Herlitz type, 3 weeks old — same case as in Fig. 22.30C (× 24 600) **E** = Newborn male, 20 days old — same case as in Fig. 22.30A. (× 40 930) Electron micrographs: B, J. Deimel-Hatzenbühler; C, B Melz-Rothfuss.

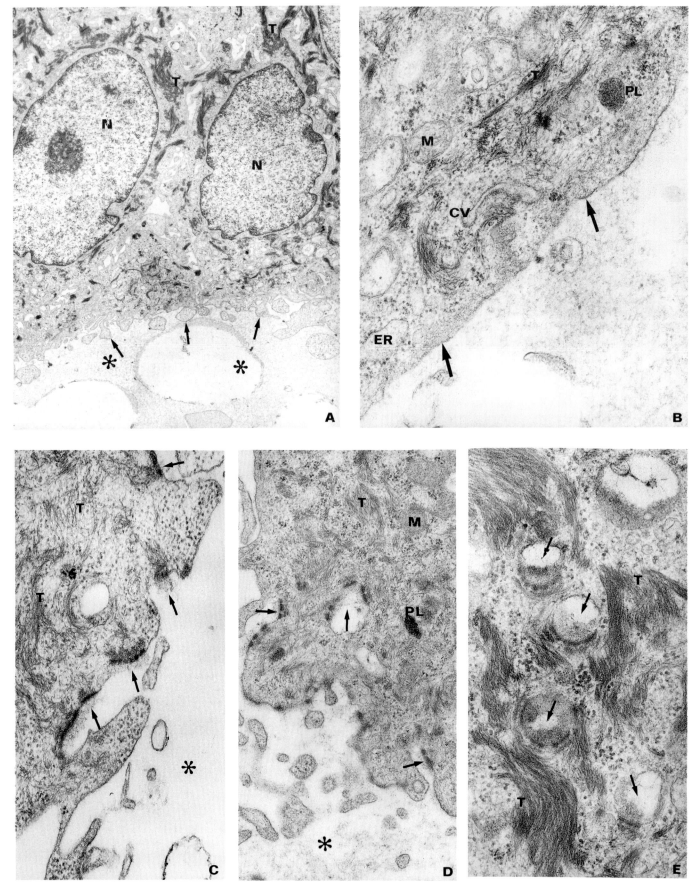

Fig. 22.31 (Caption on p. 531)

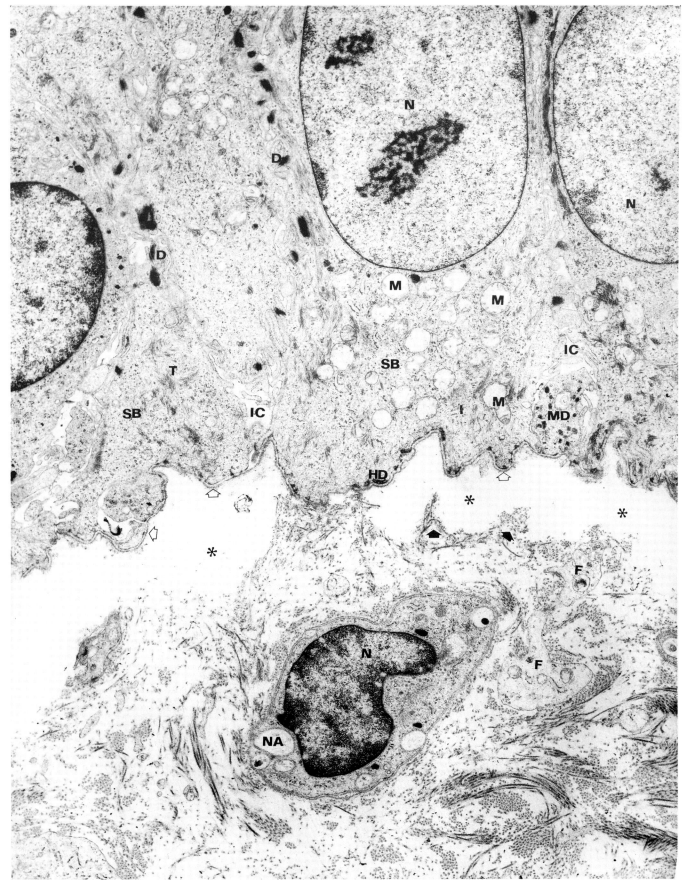

Fig. 22.32 (Caption on p. 534)

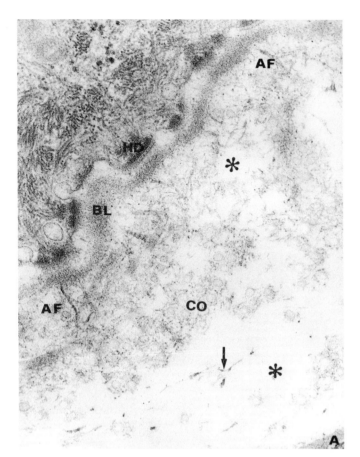

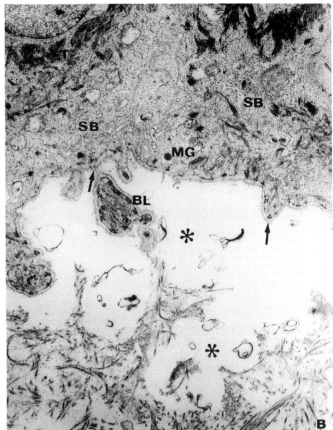

Fig. 22.33 Epidermolysis bullosa dystrophica recessiva; Hallopeau–Siemens type. Stages of initial blister formation via focal collagenolysis. **A** As a rule, the split in adults forms somewhat deeper in the dermal connective tissue than in the newborn and young infants (**B,C**). Focal collagenolysis (*) with partial dissolution of collagen is evident, sparing the proteoglycans and glycosaminoglycans of the ground substance (arrow). Initially, anchoring fibrils and basal lamina as well as hemidesmosomes with prominent sub-basal dense plates are also maintained. 32 year-old male with severe scarring but only moderate mutilation tendency. (× 68 200) **B, C** Collagenolysis (*) is evident in the uppermost papillary dermis with clean split below basal lamina of the basal cells which possesses normal hemidesmosomes, tonofilaments, and, melanin granules. Note the impressive signs of focal collagenolysis in (**B**). Many anchoring fibrils are visible in the adult (**A**), but only few remnants in the severely affected child (**B** and **C**, arrows). **B** and **C** Male infant with pronounced scarring and mutilation tendency, aged 13 months. (B, × 9170; C, × 23 790)

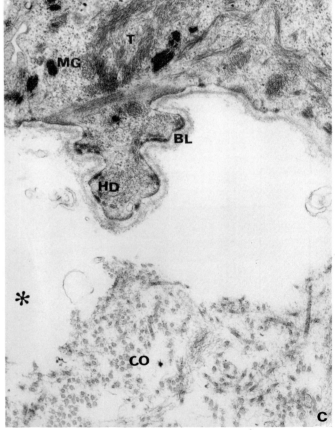

Fig. 22.32 (Preceding page) Epidermolysis bullosa dystrophica recessiva; Hallopeau–Siemens type. Typical ultrastructural appearance of a fresh blister (*) with dermolytic separation immediately beneath the basal lamina (open arrows) in a newborn. Note the tip-like projections of the connective tissue at the floor of the split (solid arrows), indicating focal collagenolysis (see also Fig. 22.21F), and remnants of dermal tissue at the undersurface of the blister roof. Basal cells are undisturbed except for swollen mitochondria. Newborn female, 4 days old — same case as in Figs 22.34A and 22.35C and E. (× 11 000)

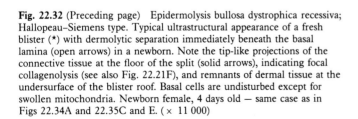

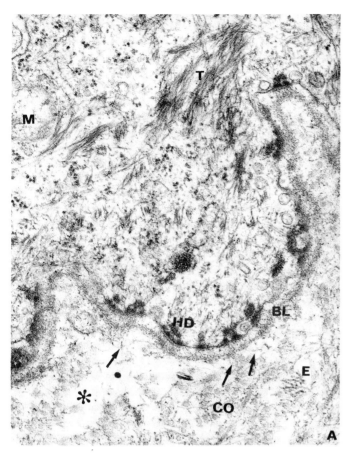

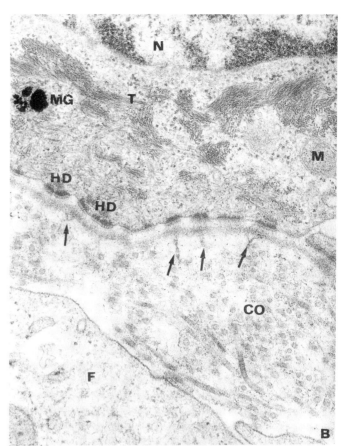

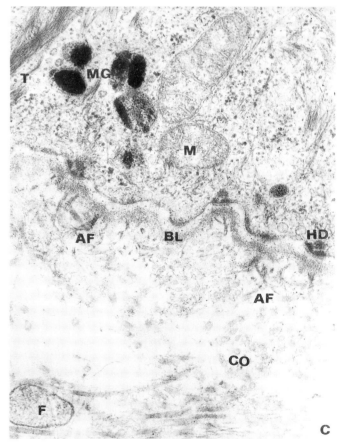

Fig. 22.34 Epidermolysis bullosa dystrophica recessiva, Hallopeau–
Siemens type. Ultrastructure of intact skin. Completely normal
ultrastructure of the epidermis is found in non-traumatized, intact skin —
even in newborns with the mutilating variety of the recessive scarring
Hallopeau–Siemens type. **A** Details of intact skin adjacent to blister edge,
demonstrating normal ultrastructure of hemidesmosomes, thin basal
lamina and few remnants of small, faint anchoring fibrils (arrows). Initial
focal collagenolysis (*) has occurred beneath the dermo-epidermal
junction. Newborn female 4 days old with large epithelial defects and
generalized blistering — same case as in Figs. 22.32 and 22.35 C and E
(× 40 300) **B** Intact dermo-epidermal junction in the adult displays
varying numbers of anchoring fibrils (arrows) that are not uniform in
length and diameter as seen normally, most probably reflecting the effect
of collagenolysis. Note the normal ultrastructure of hemidesmosomes and
distinct sub-basal dense plates in the lamina rara. Adult male with
moderate mutilation tendency, but pronounced scarring and oesophageal
stenosis; submutilating variety of Hallopeau–Siemens type. (× 51 670) **C**
Normal dermo-epidermal junction with well-developed hemidesmosomes,
a prominent basal lamina and groups of broad, typically banded
anchoring fibrils in the (normal) skin of an obligatory heterozygous
carrier of the Hallopeau–Siemens type. Father of a female baby with
severe mutilations and oesophageal stenosis. Tests for heterozygozity by
EM are impossible. (× 40 300)

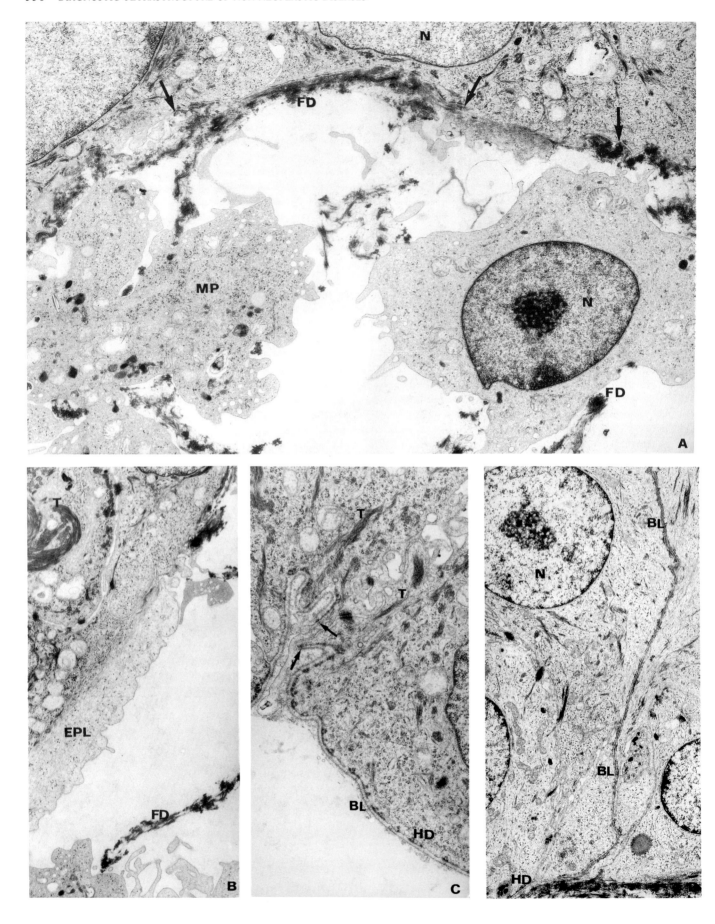

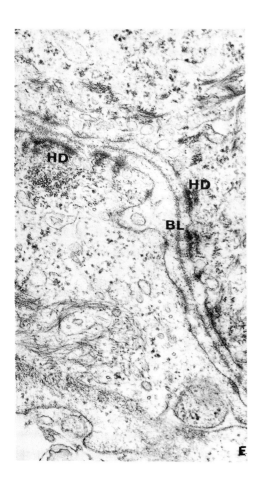

Fig. 22.35 Epidermolysis bullosa dystrophica recessiva, Hallopeau–Siemens type. Modification of blister roof after separation. Rapid changes occur following dermolytic separation of the epidermis and dermal connective tissue (compare fresh blisters in Figs 22.32 and 22.33) — including haemorrhage and fibrin deposition at the surface of the blister cavity, gradually obscuring the basal lamina at the blister roof (**A**, arrows) — and secondary invasion of the blister by inflammatory cells such as (neutrophil) granulocytes, macrophages (**A**), and lymphocytes. Older blisters are unsuitable for diagnostic purposes. **A** Basal lamina, though covered with fibrin deposits, is still visible at the blister roof and shows occasional gaps (arrows) with basal cell protrusions into the blister cavity. Female infant with severe mutilating variety of Hallopeau-Siemens type, 1 month old. (× 8580) **B–E** Changes at the blister roof after dermo-epidermal separation that may result in possible misinterpretation. **B** Remodelling of the undersurface of basal cells with formation of 'ectoplasm-like' cytoplasm. Lack of basal lamina (gradual lytic destruction in the secondary course of blister evolution) might erroneously indicate junctional splitting; same case and same tissue block as in (**A**). (× 6820) **C–E** Various steps of infolding of the basal lamina at the undersurface of the blister roof due to remodelling and movement of basal cells. **C** Small invagination and pouch-like infolding with small gap (arrows) in the basal lamina. **D** and **E** Basal lamina extends upwards into the blister roof over long distances. The one basal lamina is faced by hemidesmosomes on either side (**E**). **C** and **E** Newborn female with severe mutilating variety, 4 days old; same case as in Figs 22.32 and 22.34A. (C, × 14 470; E, × 40 950). **D** Male infant with generalized, non-mutilating variety, 3 weeks old. (× 7260) Electron micrographs A, B: J. Deimel-Hatzenbühler.

In the blister roof of a full-blown blister (even if not yet haemorrhagic and filled with fibrin and erythrocytes), the basal lamina is often completely absent from the undersurface of basal cells. Hence, if only the blister roof is available for evaluation, such samples might be mistaken as indicating junctional separation with the basal lamina having remained at the blister floor (see Figs 22.21E and 22.30–22.31). Careful control of the entire thickness of the blister roof will disclose the basal lamina in the central parts of the epidermis, faced by hemidesmosomes on either side, and sometimes, islands of collagen fibrils may remain as evidence of the previous translocation.

Fig. 22.36 (Overleaf) Oculocutaneous albinism. **A** and **B** Tyrosinase-negative type. Epidermal melanocyte after stimulation by 32 days' UV irradiation, combined with oral application of alpha-methyl-DOPA and I-DOPA. Response similar to that of control melanocytes with activation of protein synthesis systems (endoplasmic reticulum and Golgi apparatus), and production of numerous melanosomes in the peripheral cytoplasm. In the albino patient melanosomes do not develop beyond stage II — with cross-striated cores (**B**, arrows) — in spite of stimulation, because of the enzyme deficiency and the resultant block in the initial steps of melanin synthesis. No melanin deposition occurs in these melanosomes. Male patient, 20 years old — tissue sample from anterior aspect of upper arm, fixation by osmic acid/potassium dichromate; embedding in polyester resin (Vestopal). (A, × 11 730; B, × 41 330) **C** and **D** Tyrosinase-positive type. In spite of the presence of enzyme activity as revealed by the DOPA reaction (**D**), melanocytes produce mainly stage I, and few stage II melanosomes (**C**, arrows), the latter with a central laminated/cross-striated core. By the DOPA reaction, tyrosinase activity is restricted to the outermost cisternae of Golgi bodies and demonstrated only in a few melanosomes (**D**, arrows). **C** Female patient, 29 years old. Tissue sample from inguinal skin; fixation by glutaraldehyde and osmic acid; embedding in epoxy resin (Epon 812). **D** Female patient, 25 years old. Tissue sample from sacral region; fixation and embedding as in (C), I-DOPA-incubation *en bloc*. (C, × 31 410; D, × 19 800) Electron micrographs C and D: Dr I Hausser.

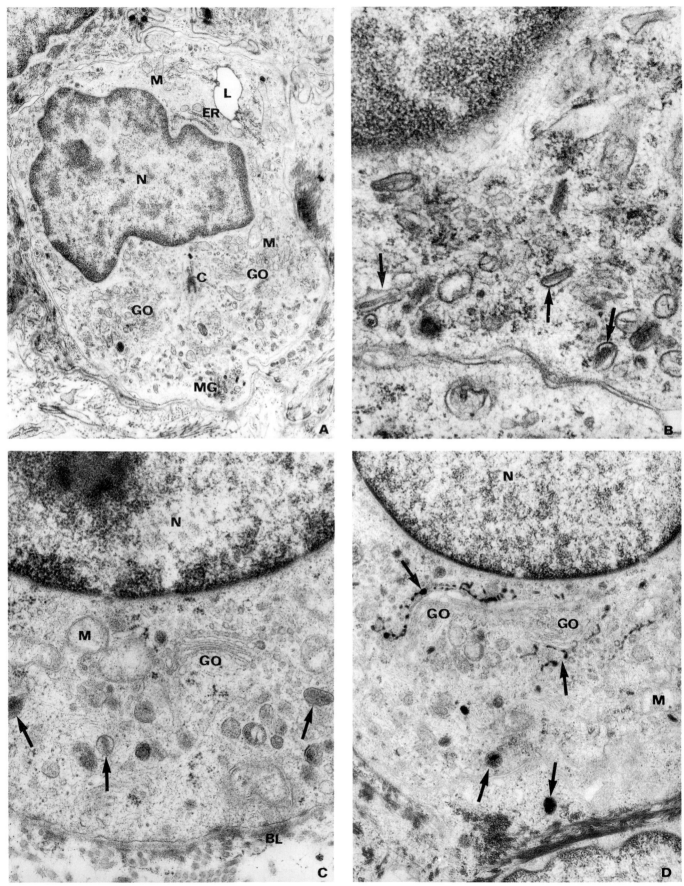

Fig. 22.36 (Caption on p. 537)

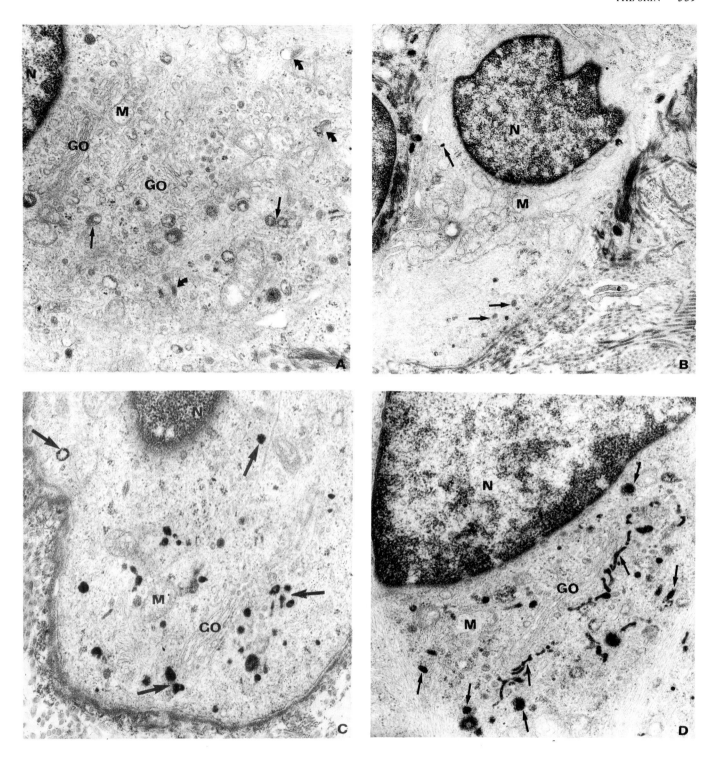

Fig. 22.37 White leaf-shaped macules in tuberous sclerosis (TS) Bourneville–Pringle. Hypopigmented macules of TS may be differentiated from other hypomelanotic skin lesions by their characteristic DOPA reaction pattern. **A** Golgi region of a melanocyte surrounded by stage I (arrows) and stage II melanosomes, the latter with typical cross-striated cores (curved arrows). **B–D** DOPA reaction: almost completely negative melanocyte (**B**). Melanocyte with almost complete conversion of pre-existing melanosomes to fully melanized stage IV (arrows); terminal cisternae of Golgi bodies, however, are unstained, (i.e. lacking tyrosinase activity; **C**). Melanocyte with DOPA-positive outermost Golgi cisternae and DOPA-positive melanosomes (arrows, **D**). **A, B, D** Female carrier, 27 years old; mother of severely affected child; hypopigmented macule on calf. **C** Female carrier, 31 years old; mother of affected child; hypopigmented macule on abdominal skin. (A, × 25 330; B, × 15 000; C, 24 180; D, × 25 330) Electron micrographs: Dr I Hausser. Reproduced from Hausser & Anton-Lamprecht,[130] with permission.

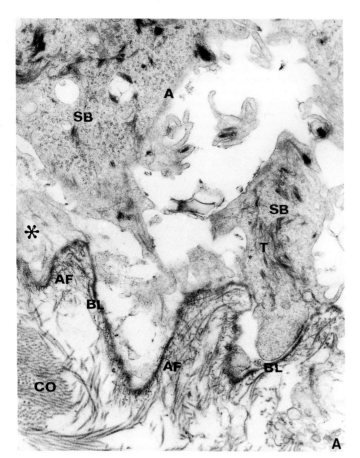

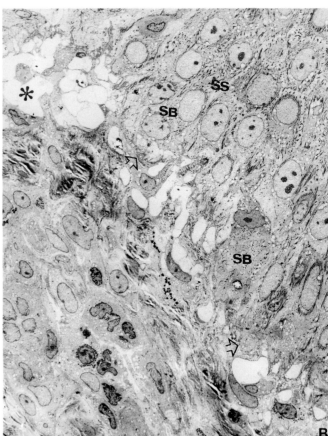

Fig. 22.38 Bullous skin diseases of immunological origin. As in the inherited epidermolyses, initial ultrastructural changes may give the best differential diagnostic criteria in those cases which are not classifiable by means of immunological techniques. **A** Bullous pemphigoid, characterized by junctional blister formation. Full-blown blisters reveal the same ultrastructure of blister floor as shown in Fig. 22.30B for the junctional epidermolyses (EB atrophicans group). In contrast to these, BP has **normal** hemidesmosomes within the intact uninvolved skin (not shown) and lacks hemidesmosomes in pre-blistered and blister regions. Inflammatory changes and migration of lymphocytes, macrophages, and granulocytes, with partial destruction of perilesional basal cells are typical findings. Electron micrograph from perilesional skin shows junctional separation of basal cell cytoplasm, lack of hemidesmosomes, areas of focal repair (*) of basal lamina to which anchoring fibrils are attached, and actin filaments parallel to the plasma membrane. Adult male, 65 years old; tissue sample from lower leg. (× 11 670) **B** Cicatricial pemphigoid, disseminated variant, is characterized by dermolytic blister formation below the basal lamina. Differential diagnosis from AEB may be difficult by clinical and immunofluorescence features. Initial stages are distinctly different from BP and AEB: coalescence of microvesicles below the basal

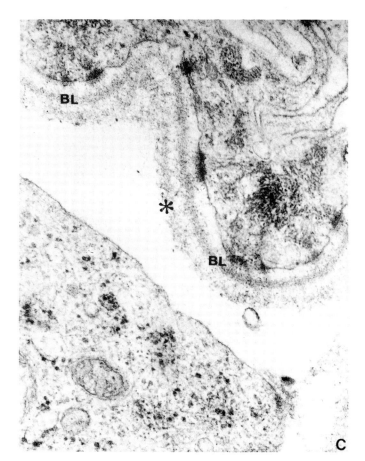

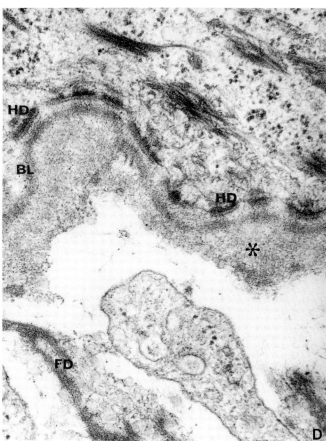

lamina (open arrows), originating from lysis of cells and non-cellular components of the superficial papillary dermis ('micro-oedema'), gives rise to nascent blisters. Low-magnification electron micrograph of papillary dermis, dermo-epidermal junction at edge of nascent blister (⋆) with basal and suprabasal epidermal cells. Female infant, 5 years old (case published by Hausser et al;[132] tissue sample from lower leg (band-like immunofluorescence for IgG and C_3 and focal IgM). (× 1100) **C** and **D** Acquired epidermolysis bullosa; (EB acquisita). In the dermo-epidermal junction, band-like granular deposits (⋆) are demonstrable in lesional and perilesional skin, representing immune complexes (IgG, C_3d), directed

against the recently identified AEB antigen that seems to be associated with the anchoring fibrils. The amount of deposit parallels the quantity of immunoreaction. The band-like deposits in **C** run strictly parallel to the basal lamina, just covering and obscuring the area of the anchoring fibrils; **D** reveals heavier deposition. **C** Male patient, 33 years old; tissue sample from forearm; IgG^{++}, C_3d^{++}. (× 43 330); D Male patient, 24 years old; tissue sample from finger; IgG^{+++}, IgA^+, C_3d^{++}, C_3b^+, C_9^+. (× 43 330) Electron micrographs A, B: Dr I Hausser; C, D: E Schleiermacher; C, D reproduced from Hausser et al.[132]

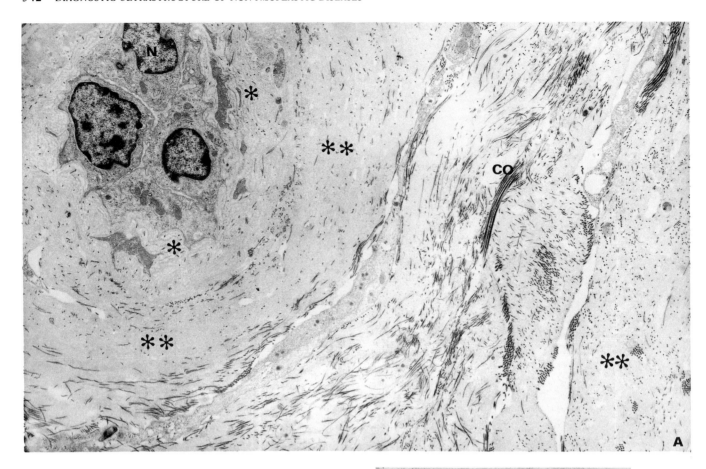

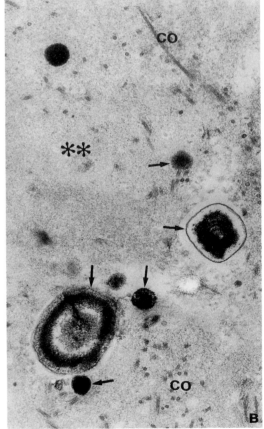

Fig. 22.39 Erythropoietic protoporphyria (EPP) and hyalinosis cutis et mucosae (HCM) Urbach–Wiethe. Morphological changes in both disorders are strikingly similar although of completely different aetiology and pathogenesis. In EPP, changes are restricted to light-exposed skin and spare mucous membranes, whereas in HCM changes are present in skin and mucous membranes in a systemic distribution. **A** Erythropoietic protoporphyria: small vessels of the papillary dermis of light-exposed skin are surrounded by concentric layers of homogenous, finely filamentous material (**), about 6–7 nm in diameter (PAS-positive, Congo red-negative), intermingled with very thin collagen fibrils, some of which are in small bundles. Multiplication of basal lamina of the capillary endothelia is evident (*). Adolescent male, 18 years old: pachydermic skin from back of the hand; protoporphyrin blood level 1716 μg% (normal range 20–50 μg%); coproporphyrin 5.23 μg% (normal range 0.5–2.0 μg%) ($\times$ 6330) Reproduced from Anton-Lamprecht and Bersch,[18] with permission. **B** Hyalinosis cutis et mucosae (or lipoid proteinosis): multiplication of endothelial basal lamina and perivascular deposition of a finely filamentous material occurs as in EPP (**A**) but is found throughout the skin and in mucous membranes. However, distinction from EPP is made by finding focal mineralization (calcification) which is regularly present in HCM (arrows) but lacking in EPP. Female, 38 years old; skin from elbow. ($\times$ 31 200) Electron micrograph B: I Werner.

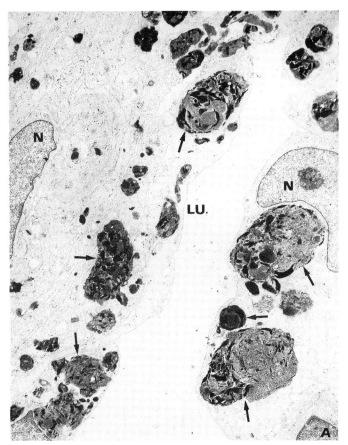

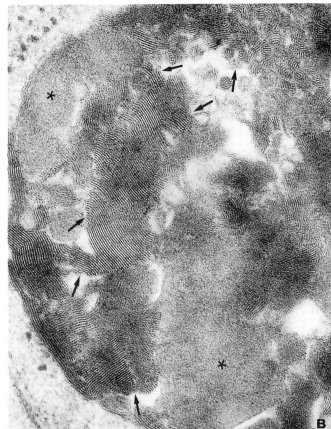

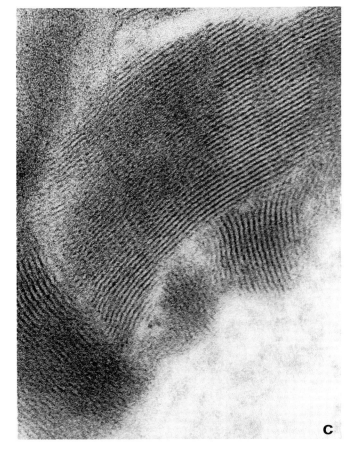

Fig. 22.40 Angiokeratoma corporis diffusum Fabry. In the skin, ceramides accumulate not only in endothelia of angiokeratomas and dilated capillaries, but also in clinically uninvolved skin. Storage material is also deposited in fibroblasts, macrophages, Schwann cells and adipocytes of subcutaneous fat tissue (not shown). **A** Endothelial cells of small skin vessels are laden with irregularly shaped heterolysosomes (arrows) filled with masses of densely staining material that may reach the size of nuclei. (× 5670) **B** High magnification of this storage material discloses randomly arranged stacks of strictly parallel lamellae; only those stacks that are cut exactly perpendicular to the plane of the lamellae disclose their regular periodicity (arrows). In stacks with an oblique plane of sectioning (*) the underlying lamellar pattern remains obscure, but may be visualized by tilting in a goniometer stage (see **C**). (× 93 330) **C** Part of a ceramide storage body at high magnification tilted by means of goniometer stage (+ 42°) to reveal the lamellar pattern: the periodicity is about 4 nm. Storage material may occasionally appear 'myelin-like' at low magnification. At high magnification, however, the specific lamellar arrangement and periodicity of the ceramides is found to be perpendicular to the plane of the 'myelin-like lamellae'. (× 32 400) Adult male, 48 years old (X-linked pedigree).

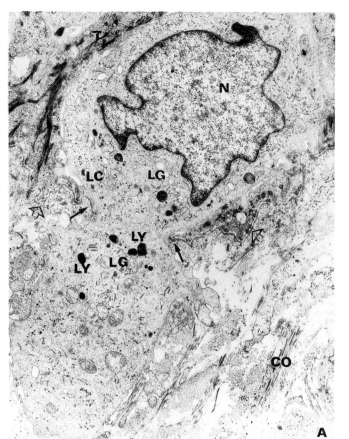 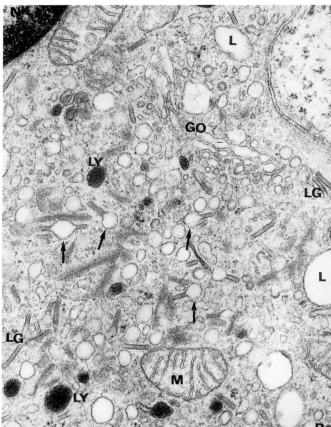

Fig. 22.41 Histiocytosis X. **A** Normal Langerhans' cell (LC) passing through the dermo-epidermal junction (open arrows). Newborn male, 7 days old. (× 7170) **B** The specific markers are the LC granules, flat disks of about 30 nm in diameter and 0.1–0.5 μm in length, with a paracrystalline intermembrane particle arrangement and often with a vesicular swelling (arrows) that reflects their endocytotic origin by infolding of the plasma membrane. Their function is still unresolved, although it has been demonstrated that they are able to transport endocytotic material (ferritin, lanthanum or other tracers) to the interior of the cell and to the Golgi region. Newborn male, 9 days old. (× 32 430) Refer also to Chapters 13 and 29.

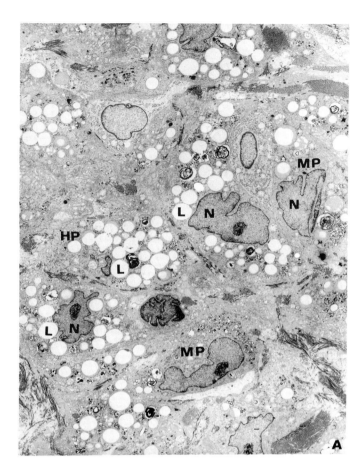

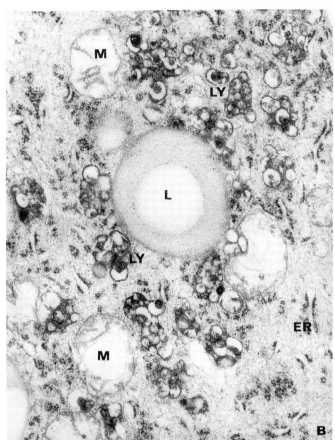

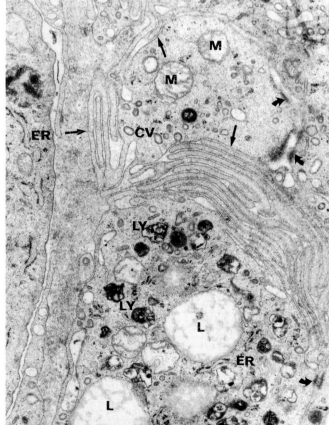

Fig. 22.42 (Above and above right) Juvenile xanthogranuloma. **A** and **B** Macrophage-like histiocytic cells with deeply indented nuclei, and filled with lipid droplets (foam cells) constitute the granulomatous infiltrate. During progression, lipid droplets are gradually replaced by heterolysosomes containing myelin-like material and products of breakdown, forming residual bodies (**B**). Touton-type giant cells with multiple deeply indented nuclei appear in the infiltrate, and similarly contain lipid droplets, cholesterol clefts, and residual bodies. Male infant, 14 months old; tissue sample from inguinal region. (A, × 2490; B, × 24 500) Electron micrographs: J Deimel-Hatzenbühler.

Fig. 22.43 (Right) Eruptive cephalic xanthoma. Densely packed histiocytic cells in the infiltrate display features of those in xanthomas possessing lipid droplets, cholesterol clefts (not shown) and residual bodies, combined with features of benign cephalic histiocytosis: close interdigitations formed by long microvillous processes between the cells (arrows), desmosome-like membrane specializations (curved arrows), coated vesicles of varying sizes thought to be involved in the formation of the desmosome-like junctions,[60] and groups of worm-like (vermiform or comma-shaped) bodies (not shown; compare with Fig. 22.40B). Langerhans' cells are not present in the infiltrate. Adult female, 67 years old, with T cell lymphoma; tissue sample from the cheek for ultrastructural exclusion of histiocytosis X. (× 14 930) Electron micrograph: Dr M-L Arnold.

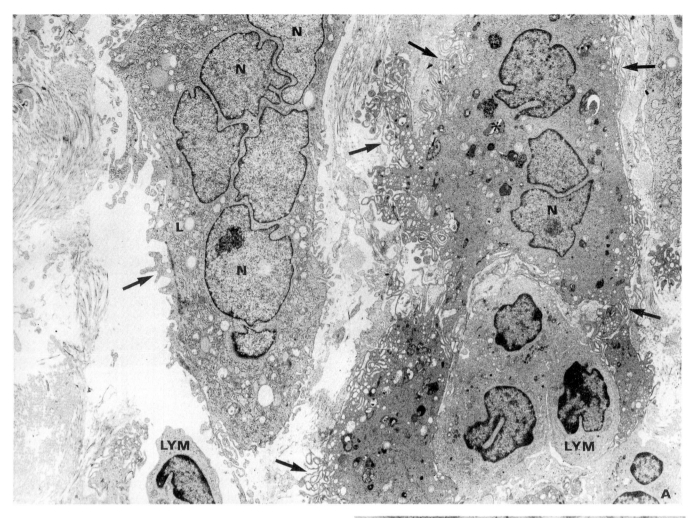

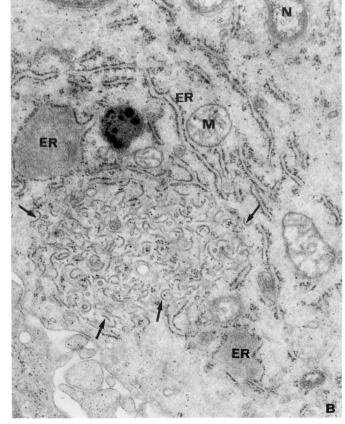

Fig. 22.44 Generalized eruptive histiocytoma (GEH). **A** and **B** The infiltrate of this benign, spontaneously regressing histiocytic disorder of adults is composed of histiocytic cells, fibroblasts, lymphocytes, few mast cells, and some eosinophilic and neutrophilic granulocytes. Langerhans' cells are not encountered in GEH. Specific histiocytic cells (**A**) possess irregularly shaped nuclei, are often multinucleated, and have multiple small microvillus-like processes (arrows) protruding from the cell surface. Interdigitations are rather moderate. Some lipid droplets, cholesterol clefts and heterolysosomes are found in these histiocytes (**A**). A characteristic finding in GEH, and in some other histiocytic disorders, is the presence of vermiform or comma-shaped bodies in close relation to RER (**B**; arrows). Adult male, 52 years old; skin biopsy sample from the axilla; case published by Arnold et al.[37] (A, × 4050; B, × 24 960) Electron micrographs: Dr M-L Arnold.

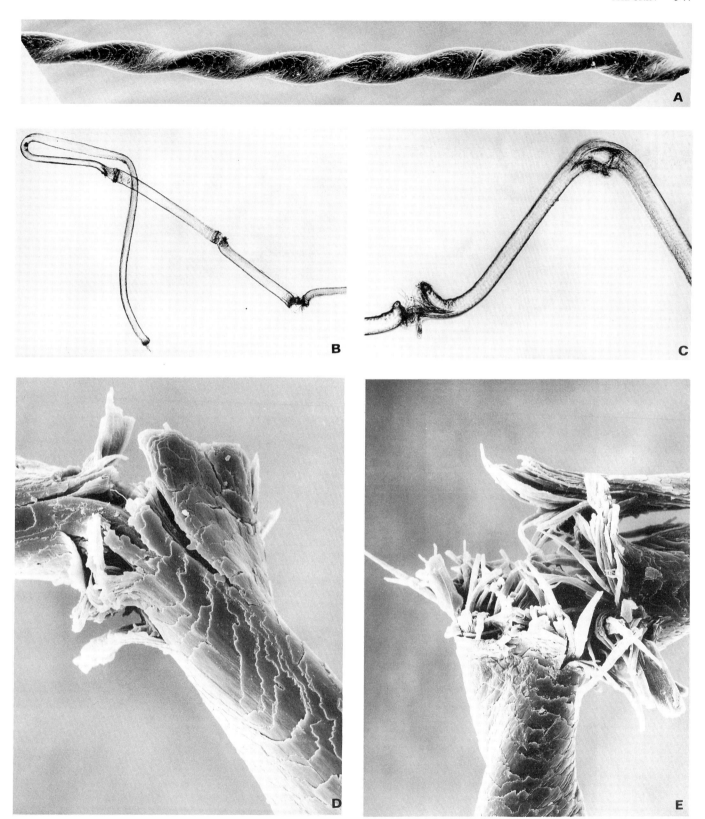

Fig. 22.45 Menkes' kinky hair syndrome — pili torti. **A–E** Torsions of highly regular pitch and dimension (true pili torti) are present over long distances of the hair shaft (**A**), with longitudinal and transverse breaks (trichoschisis). The typical 'kinky' appearance is due to multiple breaks (**B, C**) with different stages of node formation (trichorrhexis nodosa) (**B–E**) revealing cortical cell elements (**D, E**). Note the presence of the cuticle and the torsions of the hair shaft close to the fracture (**E**). Severely affected male infant, 10 months old. (B and C light micrographs: B, × 63; C, × 157; A, D and E scanning electron micrographs: A, × 196; D, × 810; E, × 536)

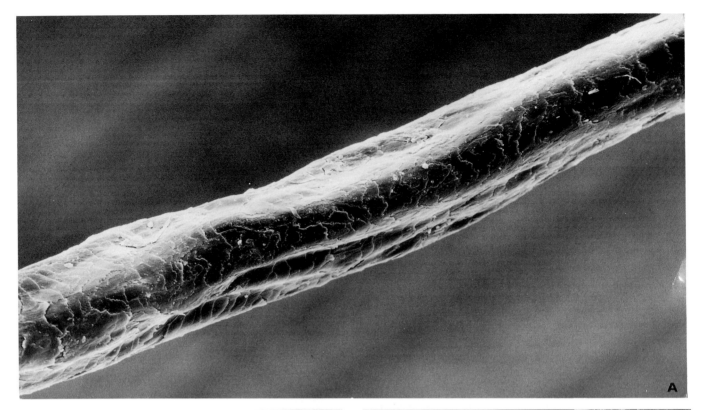

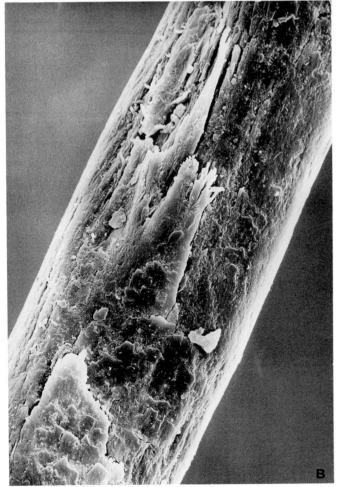

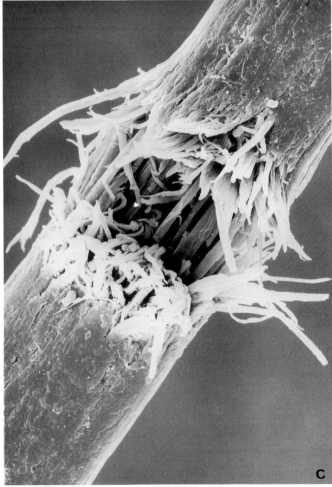

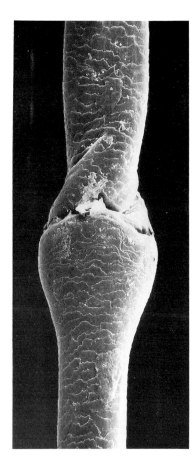

Fig. 22.47 Trichorrhexis invaginata in Netherton's syndrome. Bamboo-hairs (trichorrhexis invaginata) are pathognomonic of Netherton's syndrome (see text). Torsions of the hair shaft are a regular although less specific finding. They may be incomplete or may have a high pitch. Female, 15 years old; case published by Hausser et al.[131] (× 252)

Fig. 22.46 (Facing page) Trichorrhexis nodosa in anhidrotic ectodermal dysplasia (AED). **A–C** Severe hair shaft abnormalities in a child with autosomal recessive type of AED with extremely brittle hair keratin, subsequent loss of cuticle (**B**) and multiple breaks (trichorrhexis nodosa) in all stages of development (**C**). Twisted hair shafts have longitudinal impressions, infoldings or flattened portions and irregular torsions with a high pitch (**A**). Note irregularities and disturbances in the cuticle. Female child, 4.5 years old; case published by Anton-Lamprecht et al.[26] (A, × 545; B, × 930; C, × 890)

Fig. 22.48 (Overleaf) Idiopathic trichoclasia. **A–D** The cuticular cells are partly elevated from the surface (**A**) exposing the cortex fibres (**B**). Fractures produce long drawn-out tips of cortex fibres (**C**). Cross sections reveal increased amounts of matrix substances and paracortex configuration in the cortex (**D**). Adult female, 25 years old; no associated abnormalities; amino acid analysis and laboratory values in the normal range. Case published by Wiest and Anton-Lamprecht;[232] Figs A–C reproduced from Anton-Lamprecht.[9] (A, × 920; B, × 2750; C, × 480; D, × 64 000)

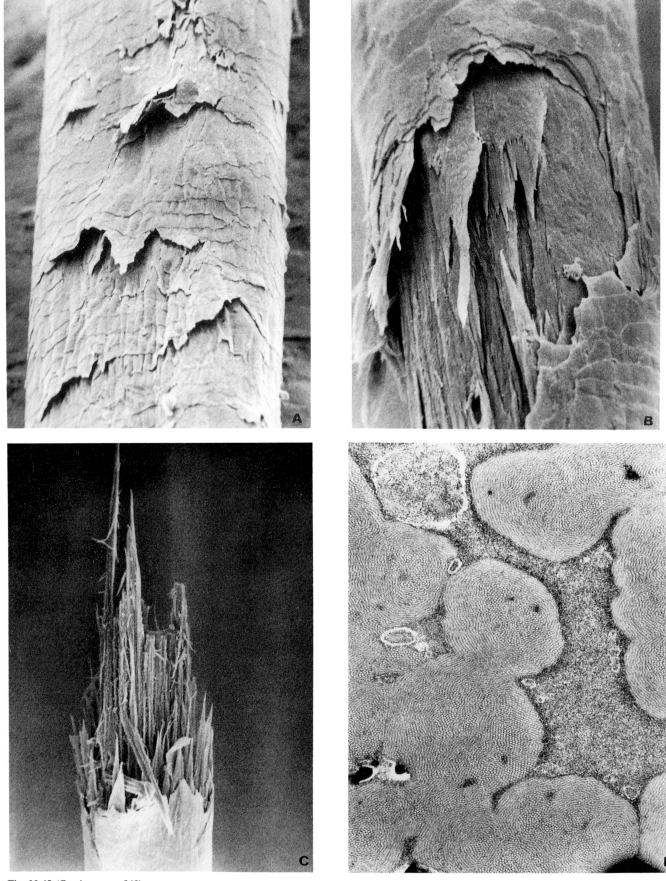

Fig. 22.48 (Caption on p. 549)

23. The central nervous system

A. Hirano

INTRODUCTION

Under normal circumstances the central nervous system consists almost entirely of neurons, astrocytes, oligodendrocytes and ependyma, in addition to blood vessels and their components. Parenchymal extracellular spaces are generally narrow and inconspicuous.

It is useful to view the pathological changes in terms of alterations of the normal cellular constituents, the appearance of apparently new components, or the widening of the extracellular space.

Because of space limitation some ultrastructural features of the pathological central nervous system have been omitted. These include some storage diseases, most features of inflammatory changes and vascular pathology. For the most part these changes are similar to those seen in other tissues and are covered in other chapters.

More comprehensive descriptions of the fine-structural aspects of central nervous system pathology are covered in other publications.[9,33,63,70,81]

NEURONS

The neuron is the principal cell of the central nervous system. It is characterized by the presence of well-formed cell processes which consist of an axon and dendrites. The perikaryon contains stacks of well-developed rough endoplasmic reticulum (RER) known as Nissl substance, Golgi apparatus, mitochondria, lysosomes, lipofuscin and prominent fibrillary structures consisting of 10-nm neurofilaments, microfilaments and microtubules. Neurofilaments are intermediate filaments unique to the neuron. Abnormal accumulation of 10-nm neurofilaments (Figs 23.1 and 23.2), the neurofibrillary changes in Alzheimer's disease (Fig. 23.3) and the appearance of Hirano bodies (Fig. 23.4), Lewy bodies (Fig. 23.5), Lafora bodies and polyglucosan bodies (Fig. 23.6), have been described in the soma as well as in neuronal processes in various pathological conditions. The fine-structural characteristics of these changes are all well documented and serve as diagnostic hallmarks for certain disease entities.

Accumulation of 10-nm neurofilaments

Abnormal accumulation of 10-nm neurofilaments may be observed in neurons in various pathological conditions (Figs 23.1 and 23.2). Involvement of the soma and proximal neurites are observed in experimental aluminium,[92] maytansine,[14] colchicine, or vinca alkaloid intoxication.[46] Accumulation of 10-nm neurofilaments in the proximal portion of the axon, on the other hand, is observed after the administration of β-β' iminodiproprionitrile (IDPN).[7] Focal accumulation of 10-nm neurofilaments in the axons or soma of anterior horn cells is observed in patients with amyotrophic lateral sclerosis,[42,58] and in normal individuals. In the former, the filamentous masses are often larger than 20 μm (spheroids), while in the latter they are usually smaller than 20 μm (globules) and confined mostly to a certain area of the lumbar cord.[5] In both spheroids and globules, bundles of 10-nm neurofilaments are irregularly interwoven (Fig. 23.1) while mitochondria, elements of smooth endoplasmic reticulum (SER), and vesicles are intermingled with the filaments. A prominent accumulation of 10-nm neurofilaments in motor neurons is also observed in various hereditary and sporadic diseases of the central nervous system of several animal species.[8,43]

Alzheimer's neurofibrillary changes

Alzheimer's neurofibrillary changes consist of abnormal accumulations of filaments which differ from the normal 10-nm neurofilaments or microtubules.[50] They reveal a characteristic morphology possessing regular constrictions at 80-nm intervals (Fig. 23.3).[65,90] Some authors consider that the fundamental elements actually consist of paired helical filaments.[101] Straight tubules with a diameter of 15-nm may coexist with the abnormal filaments, or they may sometimes constitute the entire tangle.[35,50,76,86,102]

Alzheimer's neurofibrillary tangles have so far been observed only in humans and only in certain neurons. These changes were originally observed in Alzheimer's disease, but they have since been observed in a number of other conditions including postencephalitic parkinsonism,

parkinsonism–dementia complex of Guam, subacute sclerosing panencephalitis, Down's syndrome, in the brains of prize-fighters, and in apparently normal elderly individuals.[27,36]

Eosinophilic rod-like structures (Hirano bodies)

Eosinophilic rod-like structures may be found in both the normal aged brain and in a variety of degenerative diseases including Alzheimer's disease, Pick's disease, parkinsonism-dementia complex of Guam and Creutzfeldt–Jakob disease. For the most part, this alteration is confined to Sommer's sector and immediately adjacent zones, but on rare occasions it has been seen in other areas of the brain.

By LM, Hirano bodies are rod-like in shape and of variable length, and they appear strongly eosinophilic and refractile. As revealed by EM (Fig. 23.4), these structures are intracytoplasmic and consist of a layered arrangement of electron-dense lines, about 10–15-nm thick, interspersed with layers of regularly arranged circular densities about 6–10-nm in diameter.[24] In some sections, the structures display a herringbone-like pattern or lattice-like structure. These bodies react with anti-actin antisera.[15]

Fine-structural study has allowed the detection of Hirano bodies in various parts of the nervous system, and they have been identified not only in neurons but also in glial cells and Schwann cells, both in humans and in various experimental animals.[29,41,85,93]

Lewy bodies

Lewy bodies, a histological hallmark of Parkinson's disease, may also be observed in a small fraction of apparently normal elderly individuals. They appear most prominently in pigmented neurons of the brain stem and nucleus basalis of Meynert, but may also appear in certain other areas of the nervous system. Lewy bodies are composed of filamentous structures admixed with granular and vesicular material (Fig. 23.5).[10,72,73,83] The filaments are radially oriented at the periphery, while they are random and more tightly packed in the core. The diameter of the filaments is approximately 10-nm, but thicker linear structures associated with granular material are also observed. Despite the clear demarcation between the halo and the core, and between the halo and the cytoplasm seen by LM, no membrane separates these structures. In general, Lewy bodies in the cerebral cortex lack formation of the core,[60,103] while Lewy bodies in the autonomic ganglia display a more distinct core which contains highly electron-dense granular amorphous material.[11] Observations of the co-existence of Alzheimer's neurofibrillary tangles and Lewy bodies within a single neuron have also been reported.[95] Recent studies indicate that Lewy bodies contain neurofilamentous antigens.[12,16]

Lewy body-like hyaline inclusions in the anterior horn cells have been observed in some patients with familial amyotrophic lateral sclerosis.[59] There are many neurofilaments and scattered, ill-defined, coarse linear structures which are similar to those reported in a sporadic case of juvenile amyotrophic lateral sclerosis.[74]

Certain other inclusions are composed of electron-dense granular material rather than fibrillary structures. These include granulovacuolar degeneration (Fig. 23.7) and Bunina bodies (Fig. 23.8).

Granulovacuolar degeneration

Granulovacuolar degeneration, first described by Simchowicz is frequently encountered in apparently normal aged brains, Alzheimer's disease, Pick's disease, parkinsonism-dementia complex of Guam, and Down's syndrome, among other conditions. Usually this alteration is confined to the pyramidal cells of Sommer's sector and adjacent areas of Ammon's horn. The spherical bodies characteristic of this phenomenon (often referred to as Simchowicz bodies) are 3–4 μm in diameter and contain a dense, haematoxylinophilic, argentophilic core within an empty-appearing halo.

Electron-microscopic study has revealed that the granulovacuolar bodies consist of a membrane-bound vacuole containing a highly osmiophilic granular core (Fig. 23.7).[50] Except for the core, the vacuole appears empty. The nature and origin of these bodies, as well as their role in disease and ageing processes, is still obscure. Recently, tubulin-like immunoreactivity has been reported to be present within such granules.[78]

Bunina bodies

Bunina bodies, first described by Bunina in 1962, are small, eosinophilic granules in the soma of anterior horn cells of patients with amyotrophic lateral sclerosis. The granules are several micrometres wide; they may be single or multiple and are sometimes arranged in a chain. Their fine structure consists of irregularly shaped, dense, granular material whose poorly defined border is associated with vesicles, cisterns and other nearby organelles (Fig. 23.8). Small islands of scattered neurofilaments are sometimes found in their interior.[22,34,94,96]

While originally suspected to be viral in nature, viral particles have not been demonstrated by fine-structural studies. It is noteworthy that a number of other small eosinophilic inclusions have been reported in anterior horn cells in patients with or without amyotrophic lateral sclerosis, but the fine structure of these inclusions is distinct from that of Bunina bodies.

Synapses

The synapse is a highly specialized cell junction and is the characteristic hallmark of the neuron. The synapse consists of two distinct elements: the presynaptic and the postsynaptic terminals separated by the synaptic cleft — an extracellular space which contains an electron-dense material (Fig. 23.9).[31] The presynaptic terminal is characterized by the presence of synaptic vesicles and the presynaptic density subjacent to the synaptic cleft. The postsynaptic terminal is also characterized by the presence of an osmiophilic submembranous density. The postsynaptic terminal may be either at the surface of a protrusion (spine) or on a flat portion of the neuronal plasma membrane.

Pathological changes of the synapse vary a great deal according to the underlying disease, stage of illness, and so forth. Swelling of synaptic terminals is seen in anoxia or in Creutzfeldt–Jakob disease (Fig. 23.10). In axonal dystrophy (Fig. 23.11), diseases characterized by senile plaques (Figs 23.12 and 23.13), and in other conditions, accumulations of various organelles, including tubulo-vesicular bodies (Fig. 23.11) and synaptic vesicles are found (Fig. 23.12).

Neuro-axonal dystrophy

Pronounced swelling of axonal presynaptic terminals is characteristic of neuro-axonal dystrophy. The distended terminals are filled with various normal as well as abnormal axonal organelles. Among them, the tubulo-vesicular structure illustrated in Fig. 23.11 is the most characteristic feature. The changes are observed in the cerebral cortex and other areas in infantile neuro-axonal dystrophy (Seitelberger disease)[48] and in certain other diseases.[17,18,48,62,82] The presynaptic terminal in the nucleus gracilis is one of the most conspicuous areas to show these changes in ageing brains,[13] and in children with long-standing mucoviscidosis[88] or congenital biliary atresia.[89] Dystrophic axons can also be induced experimentally in vitamin E-deficient rats.[67]

Senile plaques

Senile plaques are well-known ageing changes and are especially prominent in Alzheimer's disease. They are easily identifiable by their argentophilia and congophilia. They are usually found in the cerebral cortex, but they may be seen in other areas of subcortical grey matter, brain stem and cerebellar cortex. They consist of an amyloid core (Fig. 23.12) surrounded by argentophilic material, the latter being composed of swollen neuronal processes, reactive astrocytic processes and microglia (Fig. 23.13). The neuronal processes may contain accumulations of neurofilaments, microtubules, mitochondria, dense bodies, synaptic vesicles, tubulo-vesicular structures, Alzheimer's neurofibrillary tangles, Hirano bodies and other abnormal organelles.[20,64,91,100]

Abnormal synaptic development

There are at least two pathological conditions leading to abnormal synaptic development of the Purkinje cells of the human cerebellum. The first is the granular cell type of cerebellar degeneration in which only small numbers of granular cells are observed in contrast to a relatively well preserved Purkinje cell population. This is accompanied by a pronounced abnormality of dendritic arborization in which numerous dendritic spines are found. These spines are unattached to their usual presynaptic mates, the parallel fibres of the granular cells. Instead, the unattached spines are covered by voluminous astrocytic processes (Fig. 23.14). In spite of the absence of presynaptic elements, the unattached dendritic spines are identical to their normal counterparts. These changes are observed not only in patients with granular cell type cerebellar degeneration,[56] but also have been reported in patients with 'kinky hair' disease,[57] and in animals as a result of genetic defects,[21,38,39] intoxication,[54] infection or X-irradiation.[23] In these experimental animals, large numbers of granular cells are destroyed before their descent into the internal granular cell layer. The Purkinje cell is, however, able to form dendritic spines, apparently without the one-to-one influence of presynaptic elements.[31,32]

A similar ability for independent development of presynaptic terminals has been indicated in fine-structural studies of neuroblastoma. Many of the tumour cell processes show synaptic vesicles floating within the axons (Fig. 23.15). In addition, there are aggregates of synaptic vesicles at the periphery of the axon where a submembranous density, virtually identical to that seen in normally developing presynaptic terminals, is seen (Fig. 23.15). Postsynaptic elements are not observed in the immediate vicinity of the unattached presynaptic element.[32,45] Similar findings have been reported in certain experimental animals.[87]

ASTROCYTES

Astrocytes and oligodendrocytes are the two major glial cells of the central nervous system. The basic configuration of the astrocyte is star-like with processes radiating from the cell body. Almost the entire surface of the central nervous system is covered by a layer of astrocytic processes interposed between the parenchyma and the pial membrane. Similarly, the surface of the blood vessels within the central nervous system is virtually covered by a layer of astrocytic foot processes. In both of these locations, adjacent astrocytic processes are joined by punctate adhesions and occasional gap junctions. A continuous basal lamina separates the astrocytic processes from the subarachnoid and perivascular spaces. In addition, astrocytic processes are also found at neuronal surfaces. For example, the soma, as well as the dendritic arborizations of the Purkinje cells are almost completely covered by astrocytic processes. Only the synapses penetrate between the astrocytic processes, and the synapse itself is closely invested by astrocytic processes (Fig. 23.9). When one considers the extreme convolution of the central nervous system, and the richness of its vascular bed and neuronal population, one must be impressed by the extent of the peripheral astrocytic expansion.[30]

The protoplasmic astrocytes reside in the grey matter, while fibrillary astrocytes are found in the white matter. Fibrillary astrocytes have long, relatively straight processes, and contain far more glial fibrils than do protoplasmic astrocytes.

Under various pathological conditions astrocytes demonstrate conspicuous alterations. These include nuclear changes, watery swelling of the cytoplasm, hypertrophy, and fibrillary gliosis. Glial bundles, first reported in the spinal roots of patients with Werdnig–Hoffmann disease, are a special form of fibrillary gliosis.[6] They are, for the most part, confined to the proximal portion of anterior roots, but are occasionally seen in posterior roots. They consists of large accumulations of filament-containing astrocytic processes (Figs 23.16–23.18). Since their original description, glial bundles have been seen in a variety of human diseases and in experimental conditions affecting the spinal roots.[34]

Intracytoplasmic inclusions are frequently observed under both normal and pathological conditions. Lipofuscin is common, and various degenerated tissue products may be observed as a result of phagocytic activity. Among astrocytic inclusions two structures — corpora amylacea[80] and Rosenthal fibres[84] — deserve special mention. Corpora amylacea (Fig. 23.18) are invariably present in the astrocytes of aged individuals. It should be noted that structures identical to corpora amylacea in astrocytes are also observed in many neurons and their processes in Lafora disease in children, in axons in polyglucosan body disease,[75] in patients with amyotrophic lateral sclerosis (Fig. 23.6), and occasionally in the axons of the spinal cord of 'normal' aged individuals. Rosenthal fibres (Fig. 23.19) may appear in long-standing lesions and are also characteristic features of Alexander's disease. Descriptions of these inclusions are found in the captions to the illustrations.

Under normal conditions the astrocytic process has certain anatomical and functional domains. Under pathological conditions both the domain and the shape may change.[30] In some cases, such as in certain astrocytic neoplasms or in immature astrocytes, the processes are short, sometimes of only microvillous or filopodial proportions, and no clear-cut domain is apparent.[61] Under other pathological conditions, such as in granular cell-type cerebellar degeneration, the astrocytic processes in the cerebellar cortex assume voluminous, balloon-like configurations (Fig. 23.14). The tendency toward sheet-like expansion becomes more exaggerated in certain gliotic conditions (Figs 23.20 and 23.21). This process may result in the formation of whorls of concentric lamellae of extremely flattened astrocytic processes.[40] Finally, one may often observe cylindrically-shaped astrocytic processes filled with many glial fibrils. Examples of such changes are seen in glial scars, in demyelinated white matter lesions or in glial bundles in the spinal nerve roots in Werdnig–Hoffmann disease (Figs 23.16–23.18).

OLIGODENDROGLIA

The oligodendroglial cells are the myelin-forming cells of the central nervous system. For the most part, the cell bodies are found within the white matter, arranged in chains between myelinated nerve fibres where they are referred to as the interfascicular oligodendroglia. The dense nucleus of the oligodendrocyte is surrounded by a narrow rim of dark cytoplasm. The oligodendroglial processes are attached to myelin sheaths, but due to their length it is very difficult to trace a single process from its origin in the cell body to the myelin sheath in normal adult tissue. Direct continuities between the oligodendroglial cell body and the myelin sheath have, however, been illustrated in developing[4,77] or remyelinating[25] tissue. The myelin sheath (Fig. 23.22) consists of a sheet-like membrane of compacted oligodendroglial plasma membrane.[37]

Lesions of the myelin sheath are the most conspicuous changes occurring in pathologically altered oligodendroglia. Various inborn metabolic errors are known to affect the oligodendroglial cell. Metachromatic leucodystrophy, Krabbe's disease, and other lipidoses result in defects of myelin formation (dysmyelination)[53] (Fig. 23.23). Certain toxic substances, such as triethyltin,[2,52,97] produce alterations of the myelin (Fig. 23.24), and certain viral infections induce changes of both the oligodendrocyte and the myelin sheath. Subacute sclerosing panencephalitis and progressive multifocal leucoencephalopathy are good examples. The demonstration of viral particles within oligodendroglia is diagnostic for these conditions. Alteration of the myelin sheath may also be the result of axonal pathology as in Wallerian degeneration. Alteration of myelin with apparent preservation of the axon, such as in multiple sclerosis and experimental allergic encephalomyelitis, is termed demyelination.[28,66,68] Remyelination also occurs in the central nervous system to a limited extent.[47,51] The various fine-structural alterations of the myelin sheath are complex and readers are referred to specific texts dealing with these subjects.[1,71,79,98,99,104]

BRAIN OEDEMA

Brain oedema is associated with virtually any expanding intracranial lesion. In vasogenic oedema, fluid originates from blood plasma, traverses the vascular wall and perivascular astrocytic foot processes, and appears in the extracellular space of the brain parenchyma.[26,44,49] The extracellular space is severely distended in the white matter and is filled with electron-dense material (Figs 23.25 and 23.26). Swelling of astrocytes also contributes to the increase in volume of the brain. These changes are most conspicuous in ischaemic lesions. In contrast to vasogenic oedema the white matter swelling in triethyltin intoxication is electron-lucent. The blood–brain barrier remains intact and there is no alteration of the extracellular space.

REFERENCES

1. Adachi M, Hirano A, Aronson S M 1985 The pathology of the myelinated axon. Igaku-Shoin, New York, pp 1–406
2. Aleu F P, Katzman R, Terry R D 1963 Fine structure and electrolyte analysis of cerebral edema induced by alkyltin intoxication. Journal of Neuropathology and Experimental Neurology 22: 403–413
3. Bignami A, Forno L S 1970 Status spongiosus in Jakob–Creutzfeldt disease. Electron microscopic study of a cortical biopsy. Brain 93: 89–94
4. Bunge M B, Bunge R P, Pappas G D 1962 Electron microscopic demonstration of connections between glia and myelin sheaths in the developing mammalian central nervous system. Journal of Cell Biology 12: 448–453
5. Carpenter S 1968 Proximal axonal enlargement in motor neuron disease. Neurology 18: 841–851
6. Chou S M, Fakadej A V 1971 Ultrastructure of chromatolytic motoneurons and anterior spinal roots in a case of Werdnig–Hoffmann disease. Journal of Neuropathology and Experimental Neurology 30: 368–379
7. Chou S M, Hartman H A 1964 Axonal lesions and waltzing syndrome after IDPN administration in rats. With a concept 'Axostasis'. Acta Neuropathologica (Berlin) 3: 428–450
8. Cork L C, Griffin J W, Munnell J F, Lorenz M D, Adams R J, Price D L 1979 Hereditary canine spinal muscular atrophy. Journal of Neuropathology and Experimental Neurology 38: 209–221
9. Davis R L, Robertson D M 1985 Textbook of neuropathology. Williams & Wilkins, Baltimore
10. Duffy P O, Tennyson V M 1965 Phase and electron microscopic observations of Lewy bodies and melanin granules in the substantia nigra and locus ceruleus in Parkinson's disease. Journal of Neuropathology and Experimental Neurology 24: 398–414
11. Forno L S, Norville R L 1976 Ultrastructure of Lewy bodies in the stellate ganglion. Acta Neuropathologica (Berlin) 34: 183–197
12. Forno L S, Strefling A M, Sternberger L A, Sternberger N H, Eng L F 1983 Immunocytochemical staining of neurofibrillary tangles and of the periphery of Lewy bodies with monoclonal antibody to neurofilaments (abstract). Journal of Neuropathology and Experimental Neurology 42: 342
13. Fujisawa K, Shiraki H 1978 Study of axonal dystrophy. l. Pathology of the neuropil of the gracile and the cuneate nuclei in ageing and old rats. A steriological study. Neuropathology and Applied Neurobiology 4: 1–20
14. Ghetti B 1979 Induction of neurofibrillary degeneration following treatment with maytansine in vivo. Brain Research 163: 9–19
15. Goldman J E 1983 The association of actin with Hirano bodies. Journal of Neuropathology and Experimental Neurology 42: 146–152
16. Goldman J E, Yes S-H, Chin F C, Peress N S 1983 Lewy bodies of Parkinson's disease contain neurofilament antigens. Science 221: 1082–1084
17. Gonatas N K, Goldensohn E S 1965 Unusual neocortical presynaptic terminals in a patient with convulsions, mental retardation and cortical blindness. An electron microscopic study. Journal of Neuropathology and Experimental Neurology 24: 539–562
18. Gonatas N K, Moss A 1975 Pathologic axons and synapses in human neuropsychiatric disorders. Human Pathology 6: 571–582
19. Gonatas N K, Terry R D, Weiss M 1965 Electron microscopy study in two cases of Jakob–Creutzfeldt disease. Journal of Neuropathology and Experimental Neurology 24: 575–598
20. Gonatas N K, Anderson W, Evangelista I 1967 The contribution of altered synapses in the senile plaque: an electron microscopic study in Alzheimer dementia. Journal of Neuropathology and Experimental Neurology 26: 25–39
21. Hanna R B, Hirano A, Pappas G D 1976 Membrane specializations of dendritic spines and glia in the weaver mouse cerebellum. A freeze fracture study. Journal of Cell Biology 68: 403–410
22. Hart M N, Cancilla P A, Frommes S, Hirano A 1977 Anterior horn cell degeneration and Bunina-type inclusions associated with dementia. Acta Neuropathologica (Berlin) 38: 225–228
23. Herndon R M, Margolis G, Kilham L 1971 The synaptic organization of the malformed cerebellum induced by perinatal infection with the feline panleukopenia virus (PLV). II. The Purkinje cell and its afferents. Journal of Neuropathology and Experimental Neurology 30: 557–580
24. Hirano A 1965 Pathology of amyotrophic lateral sclerosis. In: Gajdusek D C, Gibbs C J Jr (eds) Slow latent and temperate virus infections. NINDB monograph no. 2, National Institutes of Health, Washington, pp 23–37
25. Hirano A 1968 A confirmation of the oligodendroglial origin of myelin in the adult rat. Journal of Cell Biology 38: 637–640
26. Hirano A 1969 The fine structure of brain edema. In: Bourne G H (ed) The structure and function of nervous tissue. Academic Press, New York, pp 69–135
27. Hirano A 1970 Neurofibrillary changes in conditions related to Alzheimer's diseases. In: Wolstenholme G E W, O'Connor M (eds) Ciba foundation symposium. Alzheimer's disease and related conditions. Churchill Livingstone, London, pp 185–201
28. Hirano A 1972 The pathology of the central myelinated axon. In: Bourne G H (ed) The structure and function of nervous tissue, vol. 5. Academic Press, New York, pp 73–162
29. Hirano A 1972 Progress in the pathology of motor neuron disease. In: Zimmerman H M (ed) Progress in neuropathology, vol. 2. Grune & Stratton, New York, pp 181–227
30. Hirano A 1978 Neuronal and glial processes in neuropathology. Journal of Neuropathology and Experimental Neurology 37: 365–374
31. Hirano A 1978 Aberrant synapses in the cerebellum. Progress in Brain Research (Tokyo) 22: 1281–1297
32. Hirano A 1979 On the independent development of the pre- and postsynaptic terminals. In: Zimmerman H M (ed) Progress in neuropathology, vol. 4. Raven Press, New York, pp 79–99
33. Hirano A 1981 A guide to neuropathology. Igaku-Shoin, New York, pp 1–350
34. Hirano A 1982 Aspects of the ultrastructure of amyotrophic lateral sclerosis. In: Rowland L P (ed) Human motor neuron diseases. Raven Press, New York, pp 75–88
35. Hirano A 1983 Some aspects of the neuropathological hallmarks of neuropsychiatric disorders in the elderly. In: Hirano A, Miyoshi K (eds) Neuropsychiatric disorders in the elderly. Igaku-Shoin, New York, pp 3–15
36. Hirano A 1985 Neurons, astrocytes, and ependyma. In: Davis R L, Robertson D M (eds) Textbook of neuropathology. Williams & Wilkins, Baltimore, pp 1–91
37. Hirano A, Dembitzer H M 1967 A structural analysis of the myelin sheath in the central nervous system. Journal of Cell Biology 34: 555–567
38. Hirano A, Dembitzer H M 1974 Observations on the development of the weaver mouse cerebellum. Journal of Neuropathology and Experimental Neurology 33: 354–364
39. Hirano A, Dembitzer H M 1975 The fine structure of staggerer cerebellum. Journal of Neuropathology and Experimental Neurology 34: 1–11
40. Hirano A, Dembitzer H M 1976 The fine structure of astrocytes in the adult staggerer. Journal of Neuropathology and Experimental Neurology 35: 63–74
41. Hirano A, Dembitzer H M 1976 Eosinophilic rod-like structures in myelinated fibers of hamster spinal roots. Neuropathology and Applied Neurobiology 2: 225–232
42. Hirano A, Inoue K 1980 Early pathological changes of amyotrophic lateral sclerosis. Electron microscopic study of chromatolysis, spheroids and Bunina bodies. Neurological Medicine (Tokyo) 13: 148–160
43. Hirano A, Iwata M 1979 Pathology of motor neurons with special reference to amyotrophic lateral sclerosis. In: Tsubaki T, Toykura Y (eds) Amyotrophic lateral sclerosis. University of Tokyo Press, Tokyo, pp 107–133
44. Hirano A, Llena J F 1983 Morphological aspects of brain edema. In: Federoff S, Hertz L (eds) Advances in cellular neurobiology, vol. 40. Academic Press, New York, pp 223–247
45. Hirano A, Shin Y Y 1979 Unattached presynaptic terminals in a cerebellar neuroblastoma in the human. Neuropathology and Applied Neurobiology 5: 63–70
46. Hirano A, Zimmerman H M 1970 Some effects of vinblastine

implantation in the cerebral white matter. Laboratory Investigation 23: 358–367

47. Hirano A, Zimmerman H M 1971 Some new pathological findings in the central myelinated axon. Journal of Neuropathology and Experimental Neurology 30: 325–336

48. Hirano A, Zimmerman H M 1973 Aberrant synaptic development. Archives of Neurology 28: 359–366

49. Hirano A, Zimmerman H M, Levine S 1964 Fine structure of cerebral fluid accumulation. III. Extracellular spread of cryptococcal polysaccharide in acute stage. American Journal of Pathology 45: 1–19

50. Hirano A, Dembitzer H M, Kurland L T, Zimmerman H M 1968 The fine structure of some intraganglionic alterations. Journal of Neuropathology and Experimental Neurology 27: 167–182

51. Hirano A, Levine S, Zimmerman H M 1968 Remyelination in the central nervous system after cyanide intoxication. Journal of Neuropathology and Experimental Neurology 27: 234–245

52. Hirano A, Zimmerman H M, Levine S 1968 Intramyelinic and extracellular spaces in triethyltin intoxication. Journal of Neuropathology and Experimental Neurology 27: 571–580

53. Hirano A, Sax D, Zimmerman H M 1969 The fine structure of the cerebellar of jimpy mice and their 'normal' litter mates. Journal of Neuropathology and Experimental Neurology 28: 388–400

54. Hirano A, Dembitzer H M, Jones M 1972 An electron microscopic study of cycasin-induced cerebellar alterations. Journal of Neuropathology and Experimental Neurology 31: 113–125

55. Hirano A, Ghatak N P, Johnson A B, Partnow M J, Gomori A J 1972 Argentophilic plaques in Creutzfeldt–Jakob disease. Archives of Neurology 26: 530–542

56. Hirano A, Dembitzer H M, Ghatak N R, Fan K-J, Zimmerman H M 1973 On the relationship between human and experimental granule cell type cerebellar degeneration. Journal of Neuropathology and Experimental Neurology 32: 493–502

57. Hirano A, Llena J F, French J H, Ghatak N R 1977 Fine structure of the cerebellar cortex in Menkes' kinky hair disease. X-chromosome-linked copper malabsorption. Archives of Neurology 34: 52–56

58. Hirano A, Donnenfeld H, Sasaki S, Nakano I 1984 Fine structural observations of neurofilamentous changes in amyotrophic lateral sclerosis. Journal of Neuropathology and Experimental Neurology 43: 461–470

59. Hirano A, Nakano I, Kurland L T, Mulder D W, Holley P W, Saccomanno G 1984 Fine structural study of neurofibrillary changes in a family with amyotrophic lateral sclerosis. Journal of Neuropathology and Experimental Neurology 43: 471–480

60. Ikeda K, Ikeda S, Yoshimura T, Kato H, Namba M 1978 Idiopathic parkinsonism with Lewy-type inclusions in cerebral cortex. A case report. Acta Neuropathologica (Berlin) 41: 165–168

61. Ikuta F, Ohama E, Yamazaki K, Takeda S, Egawa S, Ichikawa T 1979 Morphology of migrating glial cells in normal development, neoplasia and other disorders. Progress in Neuropathology 4: 377–405

62. Jellinger K 1973 Neuroaxonal dystrophy: its natural history and related disorders. In: Zimmerman H M (ed) Progress in neuropathology, vol. 2. Grune & Stratton, New York, pp 129–180

63. Johannessen J V (ed) 1979 Electron microscopy in human medicine, vol. 6, Nervous system, sensory organs, and respiratory tract. McGraw-Hill, New York

64. Katzman R, Terry R D, Bick K L (eds) 1978 Alzheimer's disease: senile dementia and related disorder (aging, vol. 1). Raven Press, New York

65. Kidd M 1963 Paired helical filaments in electron microscopy in Alzheimer's disease. Nature 197: 192–193

66. Lampert P W 1965 Demyelination and remyelination in experimental allergic encephalomyelitis. Journal of Neuropathology and Experimental Neurology 24: 371–385

67. Lampert P W 1967 A comparative electron microscopic study of reactive degeneration, regenerative and dystrophic axons. Journal of Neuropathology and Experimental Neurology 26: 345–368

68. Lampert P W 1968 Fine structural changes of myelin sheaths in the central nervous system. In: Bourne G H (ed) The structure and function of nervous tissue, vol. 1. Academic Press, New York, pp 187–204

69. Lampert P W, Gajdusek D C, Gibbs C J Jr 1971 Experimental spongiform encephalopathy (Creutzfeldt–Jakob disease) in chimpanzees. Journal of Neuropathology and Experimental Neurology 30: 20–32

70. Malamud N, Hirano A 1975 Atlas of neuropathology, 2nd edn. University of California Press, Berkeley

71. Morell P 1984 Myelin, 2nd edn. Plenum Press, New York

72. Morimura Y, Hirano A 1985 Circular profile in Lewy bodies. Neurological Medicine (Tokyo) 23: 91–93

73. Morimura Y, Hirano A 1986 Fine structural observations of Lewy bodies in the nucleus basalis of Meynert. Neurological Medicine (Tokyo) 24: 370–378

74. Oda M, Akagawa N, Tabuchi Y, Tanabe H 1978 A sporadic juvenile case of the amyotrophic lateral sclerosis with neuronal intracytoplasmic inclusions. Acta Neuropathologica (Berlin) 44: 211–216

75. Okamoto K, Llena J F, Hirano A 1982 A type of adult polyglucosan body disease. Acta Neuropathologica (Berlin) 58: 73–77

76. Oyanagi S 1974 An electron microscopic observation on senile dementia, with special references to transformation of neurofilaments to twisted tubules and a structural connection of Pick bodies to Alzheimer's neurofibrillary changes. Advances in Neurological Science (Tokyo) 18: 77–88

77. Peters A 1964 Observations on the connections between myelin sheaths and glial cells in the optic nerves of young rats. Journal of Anatomy 98: 125–134

78. Price D L, Struble R G, Altschuler R J, Casanova M F, Cork L C, Murphy D B 1985 Aggregation of tubulin in neurons in Alzheimer's disease. Journal of Neuropathology and Experimental Neurology 44: 366

79. Raine C S 1985 Oligodendrocytes and central nervous system myelin. In: Davis R L, Robertson D M (eds) Textbook of neuropathology. Williams & Wilkins, Baltimore, pp 92–116

80. Ramsey H J 1965 Ultrastructure of corpora amylacea. Journal of Neuropathology and Experimental Neurology 24: 25–39

81. Rosenberg R N, Schochet S S Jr (eds) 1983 The clinical neuro-sciences, 3, Neuropathology. Churchill Livingstone, New York

82. Sandbank U 1965 Infantile neuroaxonal dystrophy. Archives of Neurology 12: 155–159

83. Schochet S S Jr 1972 Neuronal inclusions. In: Bourne G H (ed) The structure and function of nervous tissue, vol. 4. Academic Press, New York, pp 129–177

84. Schochet S S Jr, Lampert P W, Earle K M 1968 Alexander's disease. A case report with electron microscopic observations. Neurology 18: 543–549

85. Schochet S S Jr, Lampert P W, Lindenberg R 1968 Fine structure of the Pick and Hirano bodies in a case of Pick's disease. Acta Neuropathologica (Berlin) 11: 330–337

86. Shibayama H, Kitoh J 1978 Electron microscopic structure of the Alzheimer's neurofibrillary changes in a case of atypical senile dementia. Acta Neuropathologica (Berlin) 41: 229–234

87. Sotelo C 1973 Permanence and fate of paramembranous synaptic specialization in 'mutant' and experimental animals. Brain Research 62: 345–351

88. Sung J H 1964 Neuroaxonal dystrophy in mucoviscidosis. Journal of Neuropathology and Experimental Neurology 23: 567–583

89. Sung J H, Stadlan E M 1966 Neuroaxonal dystrophy in congenital biliary atresia. Journal of Neuropathology and Experimental Neurology 25: 341–361

90. Terry R D 1963 The fine structure of neurofibrillary tangles in Alzheimer's disease. Journal of Neuropathology and Experimental Neurology 22: 629–642

91. Terry R D, Gonatas N K, Weiss M 1964 Ultrastructural studies in Alzheimer's presenile dementia. American Journal of Pathology 44: 269–297

92. Terry R D, Pena C 1965 Experimental production of neurofibrillary degeneration. Journal of Neuropathology and Experimental Neurology 24: 200–210

93. Tomonaga M 1974 Ultrastructure of Hirano bodies. Acta Neuropathologica (Berlin) 28: 365–366

94. Tomonaga M 1980 Selective appearance of Bunina bodies in amyotrophic lateral sclerosis. A study of the distribution in midbrain and sacral cord. Journal of Neurology 223: 959–967

95. Tomonaga M 1981 Neurofibrillary tangles and Lewy bodies in the locus ceruleus neurons of the aged brain. Acta Neuropathologica (Berlin) 53: 165–168
96. Tomonaga M, Saito M, Yoshimura M, Shimada H, Tohgi H 1978 Ultrastructure of the Bunina bodies in anterior horn cells of amyotrophic lateral sclerosis. Acta Neuropathologica (Berlin) 42: 81–86
97. Towfighi J, Gonatas N K, McCree L 1973 Hexachlorophene neuropathy in rats. Laboratory Investigation 29: 428–436
98. Waxman S G 1978 Physiology and pathobiology of axons. Raven Press, New York
99. Waxman S G, Ritchie J M 1981 Advances in Neurology, vol. 31, Demyelinating diseases, basic and clinical electrophysiology. Raven Press, New York
100. Wiśniewski H M, Terry R D 1973 Re-examination of the

pathogenesis of the senile plaque. In: Zimmerman H M (ed) Progress in neuropathology, vol. 2. Grune & Stratton, New York, pp 1–26
101. Wiśniewski H M, Terry R D, Hirano A 1970 A neurofibrillary pathology. Journal of Neuropathology and Experimental Neurology 29: 163–176
102. Yagishita S, Ito Y, Nan W, Amano N 1981 Reappraisal of the fine structure of Alzheimer's neurofibrillary tangles. Acta Neuropathologica (Berlin) 54: 239–246
103. Yoshimura M 1983 Cortical changes in parkinsonian brain. A contribution to the delineation of 'diffuse Lewy body disease'. Journal of Neurology 229: 17–32
104. Zagoren J C, Fedoroff S 1984 The node of Ranvier. Academic Press, New York

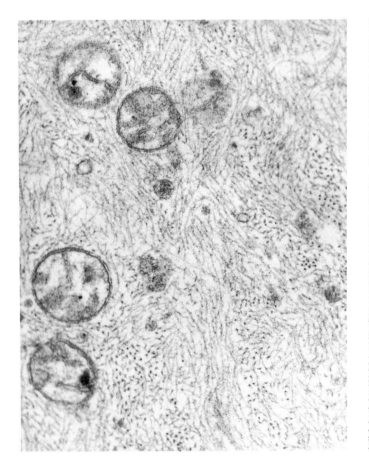

Fig. 23.1 Amyotrophic lateral sclerosis: portion of a spheroid with prominent 10-nm neurofilament accumulation in an anterior horn. Mitochondria and small vesicles are intermingled with filaments. (× 60 000) References: 42 and 58.

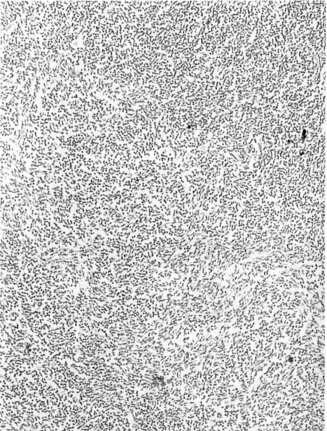

Fig. 23.2 Familial amyotrophic lateral sclerosis: cross section of a uniformly enlarged myelinated axon in an anterior horn. Compactly arranged parallel neurofilaments are present. (× 36 000) Reference: 59.

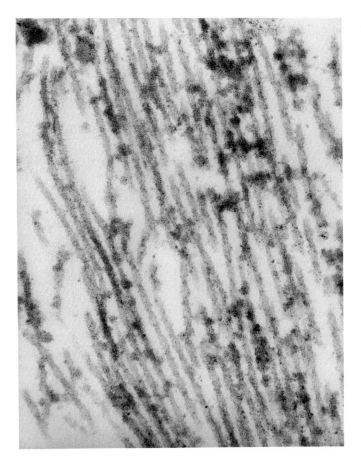

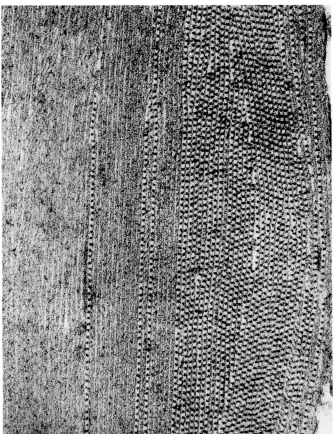

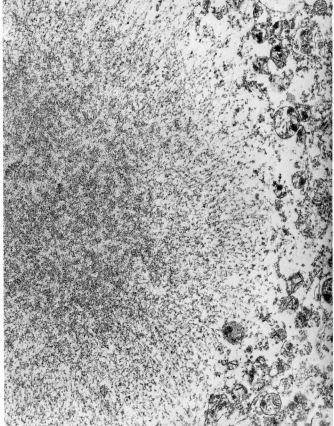

Fig. 23.3 (Above) Alzheimer's disease: high magnification of a longitudinal section of an Alzheimer's neurofibrillary tangle in a neuron in Sommer's sector. The regular constrictions usually occur at 8-nm intervals, but these may vary. At the constrictions, the fibrils appear 10-nm wide and they are 20-nm wide midway between the constrictions. (× 137 000) References: 27, 36, 50, 65, 90 and 101.

Fig. 23.4 (Above right) Neuron: Hirano body. The various components of this inclusion are readily apparent. (× 142 000) (Reproduced with permission from Hirano et al.[50]) References: 15, 24, 29, 41, 50, 85 and 93.

Fig. 23.5 (Right) Parkinson's disease: Lewy body in the substantia nigra. References: 10–12, 16, 60, 72, 73, 83, 95 and 103.

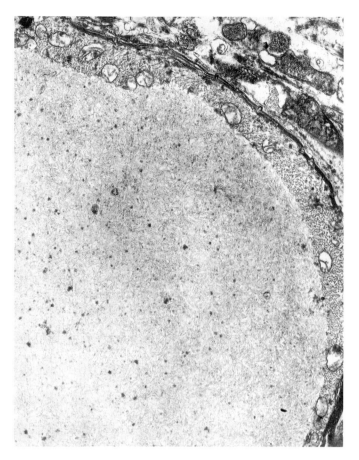

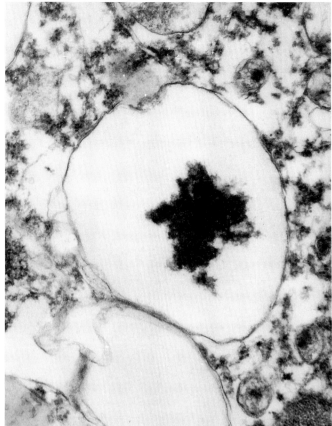

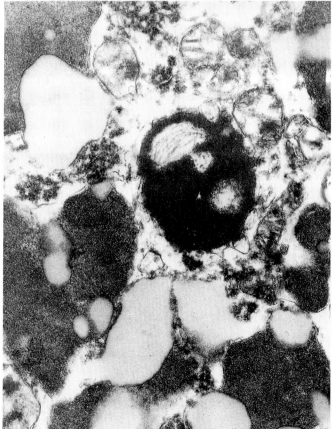

Fig. 23.6 (Above)   Amyotrophic lateral sclerosis: polyglucosan body in a myelinated axon in an anterior horn. The centre of a distended axon is occupied by a fibrillary structure identical to the corpora amylacea seen in astrocytes and to Lafora bodies in neuronal soma in myoclonic epilepsy. This axonal inclusion body is, however, surrounded by neuronal organelles, especially 10-nm neurofilaments. The axon is surrounded by several layers of myelin lamellae. (× 17 000) References: 42, 58 and 75.

Fig. 23.7 (Above right)   Neuron: granulovacuolar degeneration. Membrane-bound vacuoles and osmiophilic granular cores are present. (× 45 000) (Reproduced with permission from Hirano et al.[50]) References 50 and 78.

Fig. 23.8 (Right)   Amyotrophic lateral sclerosis: a Bunina body surrounded by lipofuscin in an anterior horn cell. Electron-dense material associated with vesicles characterize the inclusion. (× 38 000) References: 22, 34, 94 and 96.

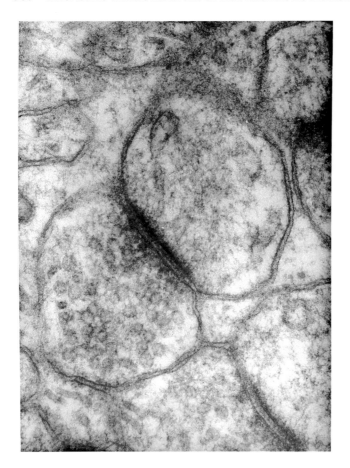

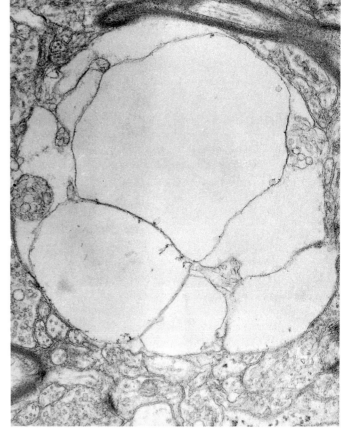

Fig. 23.9 (Above)   Cerebellum: a synapse between a pre-synaptic bouton of parallel fibre and a dendritic spine of Purkinje cell. A pre-synaptic element with synaptic vesicles and a post-synaptic element with a prominent post-membranous thickening are visible. The synapse is invested by astrocytic cytoplasm. (× 107 000) (Reproduced with permission from Malamud et al.[70]) References: 21, 31, 38, 54 and 70.

Fig. 23.10 (Above right)   Creutzfeldt–Jakob disease: spongy change. Membrane-bound vacuoles in the cerebral cortex are seen. Many of these vacuoles are composed of distended synaptic terminals. (× 40 000) (Reproduced with permission from Malamud & Hirano.[70]) References: 3, 19, 55, 69 and 70.

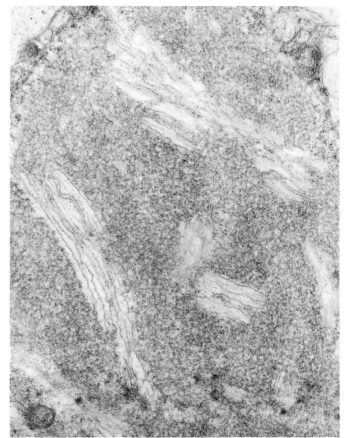

Fig. 23.11 (Right)   Infantile neuroaxonal dystrophy: tubulovesicular structure. Tubulovesicular structures are readily apparent within the distended pre-synaptic terminals in the cerebral cortex. (× 30 000) References: 17, 48, 62 and 82.

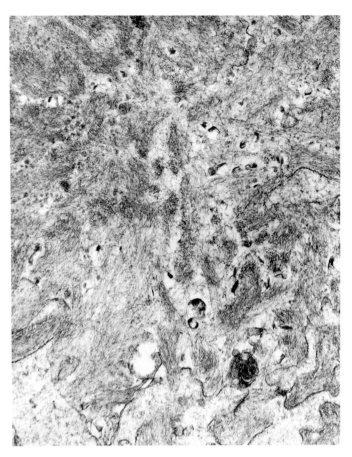

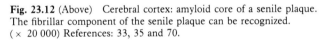

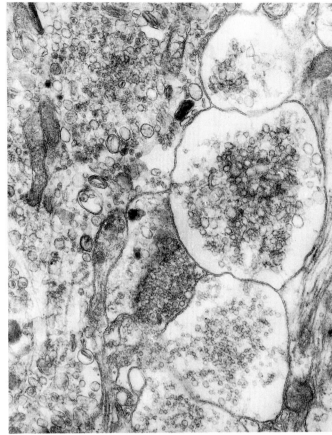

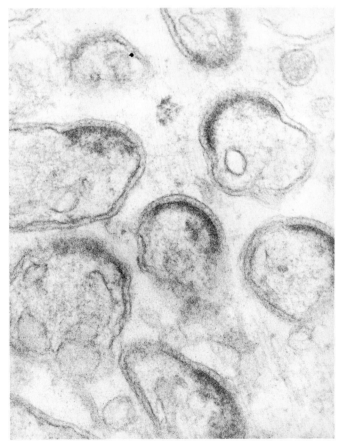

Fig. 23.12 (Above) Cerebral cortex: amyloid core of a senile plaque. The fibrillar component of the senile plaque can be recognized. (× 20 000) References: 33, 35 and 70.

Fig. 23.13 (Above right) Senile plaque: swollen neuronal processes containing many synaptic vesicles in the periphery. (× 37 000) (Reproduced with permission from Hirano.[33])

Fig. 23.14 (Right) Purkinje cell: unattached dendritic spines. Molecular layer of the cerebellar cortex of a cycasin-treated mouse. Several unattached dendritic spines of a Purkinje cell are embedded in astrocytic cytoplasm. (× 120 000) (Reproduced with permission from Hirano.[31]) References: 21, 23, 31, 32, 38, 39, 54, 56, 57 and 87.

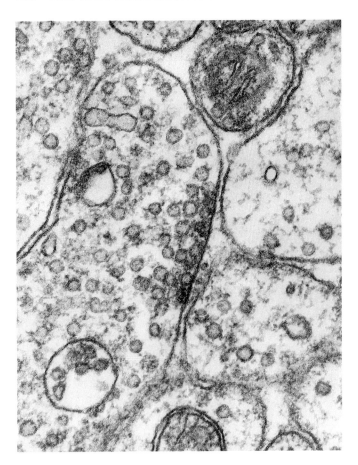

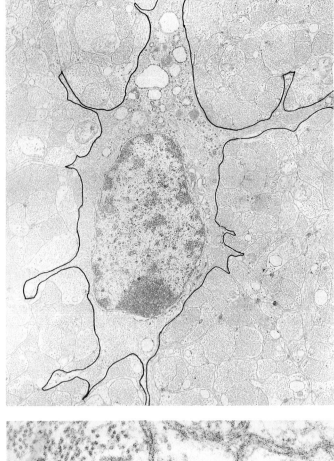

Fig. 23.15 (Above)   Cerebellar neuroblastoma: unattached pre-synaptic terminal. An unattached presynaptic terminal is seen near other cell processes. The post-synaptic element is not visible. (× 133 000) References: 31–33 and 45.

Fig. 23.16 (Above right)   Werdnig-Hoffmann disease: a fibrillary astrocyte in a glial bundle. A section through a glial bundle in the proximal portion of the anterior root in a patient with Werdnig–Hoffmann disease. An astrocytic cell body is seen in the centre of the micrograph. It is surrounded by bundles of astrocytic processes (outlined). Glial filaments fill the processes as well as the cell body. (× 12 000) (Reproduced with permission from Hirano.[36]) References: 6, 34 and 36.

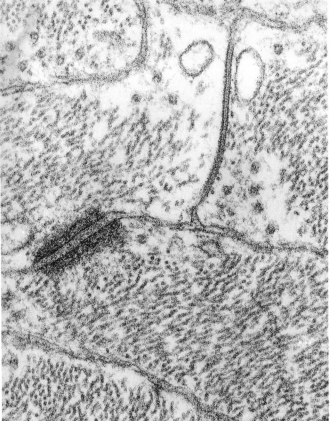

Fig. 23.17 (Right)   Fibrillary gliosis: junctions. A desmosome-like junction and a gap junction are present between astrocytic processes within a glial bundle. Glial filaments and scattered microtubules are seen. (× 1 200 000) (Reproduced with permission from Hirano.[36]) References: 34 and 36.

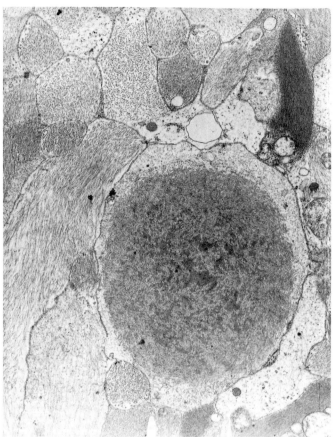

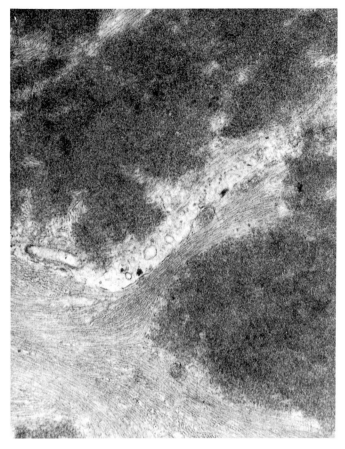

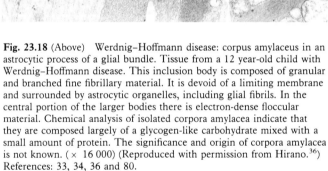

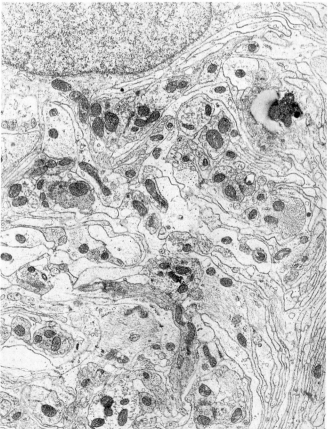

Fig. 23.18 (Above) Werdnig–Hoffmann disease: corpus amylaceus in an astrocytic process of a glial bundle. Tissue from a 12 year-old child with Werdnig–Hoffmann disease. This inclusion body is composed of granular and branched fine fibrillary material. It is devoid of a limiting membrane and surrounded by astrocytic organelles, including glial fibrils. In the central portion of the larger bodies there is electron-dense floccular material. Chemical analysis of isolated corpora amylacea indicate that they are composed largely of a glycogen-like carbohydrate mixed with a small amount of protein. The significance and origin of corpora amylacea is not known. (× 16 000) (Reproduced with permission from Hirano.[36]) References: 33, 34, 36 and 80.

Fig. 23.19 (Above right) Reactive astrocytic gliosis: Rosenthal fibres. Rosenthal fibres in gliotic area adjacent to a craniopharyngioma. They consist of electron-dense granular material, often permeated by condensed glial filaments. (× 40 000) References: 33, 70 and 84.

Fig. 23.20 (Above) Gliosis: lamellar arrangement of astrocytic processes. Several sheet-like processes arising from a filament-filled astrocytic trunk in the cerebellum of a six-month-old staggerer mutant mouse. (× 30 000) References: 31, 33 and 40.

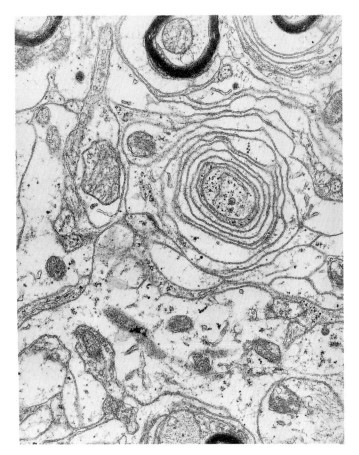

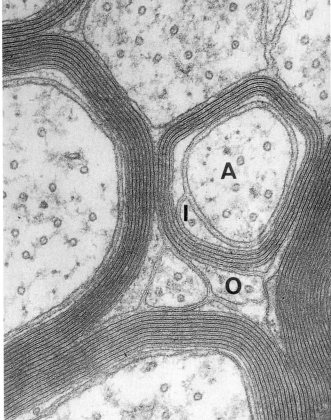

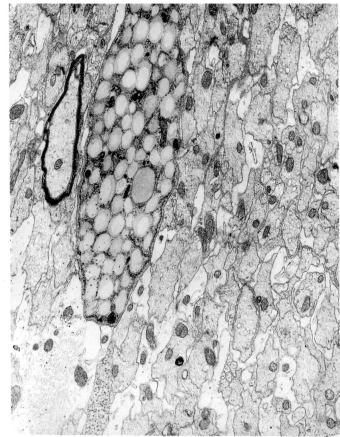

Fig. 23.21 (Above) Gliosis: concentric arrangement of astrocytic processes. A cell process and two myelinated axons are surrounded by sheet-like astrocytic processes in the cerebellum of a seven month old staggerer mutant mouse. (× 18 000) (Reproduced with permission from Hiranoet et al.[40]) References: 31, 33 and 40.

Fig. 23.22 (Above right) Central myelinated nerve fibres: cross section. An axon (A) in the centre of the myelinated fibre is surrounded by the myelin sheath. The myelin is formed by a single spirally arranged compressed plasma membrane derived from an oligodendrocyte. The periodicity of the lamellae is approximately 12 nm. The innermost end of the myelin widens to form the inner cytoplasmic loop (I) and at the outer surface of the sheath it forms the outer loop (O). Extracellular space is very narrow. (× 150 000) (Reproduced with permission from Hirano.[33]) Reference: 33.

Fig. 23.23 (Right) White matter of the cerebellum of a mutant mouse ('Jimpy'): dysmyelination. A single myelinated axon is visible adjacent to a macrophage filled with lipid granules. Most of the other axons are devoid of myelin, although some of the axons are surrounded by a narrow oligodendroglial process. (× 14 000) (Reproduced with permission from Hirano et al.[53]) Reference: 53.

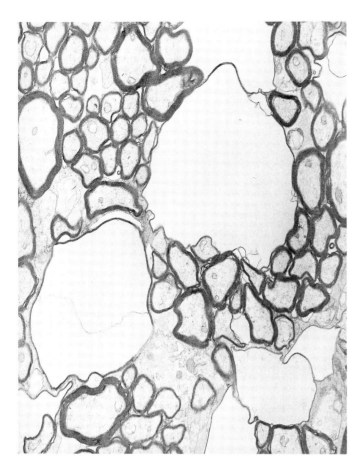

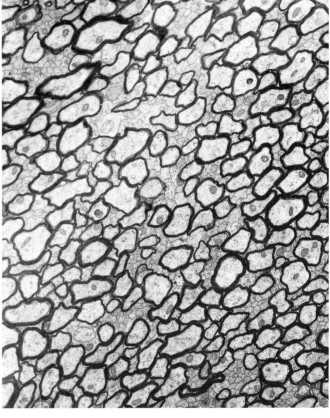

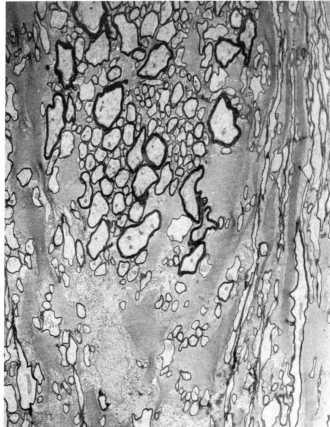

Fig. 23.24 (Above)   Optic nerve of a rat after triethyltin intoxication: intralamellar split. Intralamellar splits of the myelin sheath form large or small vacuole-like spaces in the white matter. Similar changes are also induced in experimental animals by other chemicals such as isonicotinic acid hydrazide of hexachlorophene. They are also seen in a variety of human diseases such a Canavan's disease. (× 9000) References: 26 and 52.

Fig. 23.25 (Above right)   Normal rat: cerebral white matter. Myelinated and unmyelinated processes are compactly arranged. (× 12 000) References: 28 and 49.

Fig. 23.26 (Right)   Rat brain 24 hours after intracerebral implantation of cryptococcal polysaccharide: oedematous cerebral white matter. Streaks of electron-dense haematogenous oedema fluid admixed with polysaccharide occupy the extracellular spaces. (× 7500) (Reproduced with permission from Hirano et al.[49]) References: 28 and 49.

24. The eye

A. D. Proia   G. K. Klintworth

INTRODUCTION

Electron microscopy has been used to study a wide variety of ocular diseases (Tables 24.1–24.4) and has made major contributions to our understanding of the pathophysiology of the eye and its adnexa. However, the role of electron microscopy as a diagnostic modality in ocular pathology is limited. Aside from tumours, the technique has proven to be useful in the diagnosis of ocular infections, several uncommon corneal disorders, and a number of metabolic disorders (Table 24.5). In addition, energy dispersive X-ray microanal-

Table 24.1 Disorders of the conjunctiva, eyelid, and orbit studied by electron microscopy

Disorder	References
Conjunctiva	
Amyloidosis	91 200
Argyrosis	255
Conjunctivitis:	
Giant papillary	129
Ligneous	92
Prickly pear-induced	406
Vernal	50,82
Cysts	240 357
Herpes zoster ophthalmicus	221
Keratoconjunctivitis, superior limbic	343
Nodules, allergic granulomatous	15
Pemphigoid, cicatricial	284
Practolol toxicity	294
Pterygium	38
Rhinosporidosis	332
Sicca syndrome	245 373
Storage diseases, lysosomal	See Table 24.8
Trachoma	389 390
Eyelid	
Ectropion, involutional	359
Lupus erythematosis, discoid	153
Nodules, allergic granulomatous	15
Xanthelasmata	4,73
Xeroderma pigmentosum	111
Orbit	
Amyloidosis	91 200
Muscles:	
Myotonic dystrophy	207
Overacting extra-ocular	219 244

ysis is useful in confirming the composition of certain ocular foreign bodies.

INFECTIOUS DISEASES

A variety of viruses produce ocular lesions in humans (Table 24.6), with adenoviruses and herpes simplex being the organisms most frequently encountered.[407] Most ocular viral infections are self-limiting, non-specific conjunctivitides which resolve without sequelae;[59] therefore, positive identification of the viral agent is not required in most cases.

Adenoviruses cause epidemic keratoconjunctivitis and pharyngoconjunctival fever. Both of these adenoviral infections are highly contagious, and rapid positive identification of the virus can help to minimize spread of the disease. Herpes simplex is a common cause of corneal blindness, but in the early stage of primary ocular infection there may be conjunctivitis or keratoconjunctivitis without typical corneal lesions.[394] Rapid diagnosis of herpes simplex virus allows initiation of antiviral therapy with the potential to prevent serious sequelae of infection.

In both adenovirus and herpes simplex ocular infections, electron microscopy of tears and/or eye scrapings have been used to identify the offending organisms which otherwise require long periods in cell culture before they can be identified.[28,322,387,407,408] In one study, EM aided in the identification of adenoviral particles in 7/13 culture-positive and 2/21 culture-negative patients suspected clinically of having adenoviral conjunctivitis.[28] In the same study, herpes simplex virus particles were identified by transmission EM in two-thirds of the patients whose tears were culture-positive for virus.[28] The usefulness of EM for the diagnosis of ocular adenovirus and herpes simplex will undoubtedly decrease as fluorescent antibody techniques become more advanced[407] and rapid viral culture procedures are developed.[394]

EM is a useful adjunct in the diagnosis of several other ocular infections. *Toxoplasma gondii* is the most important

Table 24.2 Corneal disorders studied by electron microscopy

Disorder	References	Disorder	References
Corneal amyloidoses		*Infections*	
Amyloidosis (secondary)	184, 336	Bacterial colonization of grafts	123, 237
Amyloidosis, familial subepithelial		Keratitis:	
(gelatinous drop-like dystrophy)	267, 366	Fusarium	155
Lattice corneal dystrophy	122, 192, 194, 286, 421	Herpetic	144, 151, 175, 242, 347
Polymorphic amyloid degeneration	224	Syphilitic	175, 333
		Varicella	259
Drug-induced keratopathies		Measles	71
Amiodarone	45, 58	Nosematosis	275
Amodiaquine	147		
Argyrosis	355	*Miscellaneous keratopathies/disorders*	
Perhixilene maleate	118	Bleb dystrophy	60
Thimerosal, effects on endothelium	386	Blood staining	233
		Foreign bodies	197, 223
Familial corneal dystrophies		Keratopathy:	
Crystalline stromal dystrophy	405	Aphakic bullous	166, 177
Fuchs' dystrophy	3, 31, 149, 277, 414	Calcific band	62, 303
Granular dystrophy	156, 165, 307, 317, 361	Chronic actinic	167, 199
Hereditary fleck dystrophy	181, 261	Lipid	54
Macular dystrophy	152, 185, 187, 188, 196, 282, 416	Keloids	209
		Keratitis, Thygeson's punctate	65
Meesmann's dystrophy	254, 374	Keratoconus	1, 11, 263, 414
Posterior polymorphous dystrophy	30, 125, 143, 164, 280, 310, 313, 319, 320	Pellucid marginal corneal degeneration	309
		Peters' anomaly	205, 281
Reis–Bücklers dystrophy	418	Sclerocornea	397
		Siderosis bulbi	367
Disorders of endothelium and Descemet's membrane		Ulceration:	
Chandler's sydrome	266, 272	Non-infectious	27, 423
Congenital epithelialization of posterior cornea	163	Xerophthalmic	352
Descemet's membrane detachment	279	*Systemic disorders*	
Endothelial:		Acrodermatitis enteropathica	400
Disorders (review)	16, 396, 399	Cystinosis	329, 413
Overgrowth of angle	139	Fabry's disease	95, 104, 300, 382, 403
Pigment deposits	140, 173, 350	Glycogen storage diseases	23
Essential iris atrophy	346	Lecithin cholesterol acyl transferase deficiency	26
Pseudoguttata	201	Mucolipidoses	25
Retrocorneal membranes	364, 395	Mucopolysaccharidoses	115, 189, 232
		Multiple myeloma and monoclonal gammopathy	44, 193
Epithelial disorders		Ochronosis	174
Defects:		Sphingolipidoses	24
Adhesion defects	93, 108, 240, 335	Vitamin A deficiency	351
Persistent	42	Wilson's disease	381
Superficial unwettable	198		
Downgrowth	348, 424	*Effects of treatment*	
Oedema	217	Histoacrylic glue	283
Erosion, recurrent	241	Keratomileusis	417
'Dystrophies':		Laser effects on endothelium	178
Fingerprint	32, 306	Radial keratotomy	154
Microcystic	49, 61, 63	Tattoo	268
		Ultrasound	269

protozoal parasite of the eye and characteristically causes a focal necrotizing retinitis or retinochoroiditis.[265] The proliferating parasites are crescent-shaped and measure approximately 3 by 7.5 μm.[265] Cysts of the parasite are much easier to identify in tissue sections since they are large (approximately 15–20 μm in diameter) and contain hundreds of dormant organisms. Immunofluorescence studies or EM may aid in identifying the causative parasite in cases where toxoplasmic retinochoroiditis is suspected clinically but routine histological sections do not reveal any organisms[295] (see also Ch. 10). Members of the protozoal genus *Nosema* have been identified in two cases of corneal ulceration.[275]

The organisms are 2.5 to 3 μm wide and 4.5 to 5.0 μm long, and stain with the acid-fast technique and Grocott's methenamine silver.[275] Ultrastructurally, this protozoan has characteristic polar filaments with 11 to 13 tubular coils.[275]

Ophthalmomyiasis is an infestation of ocular tissues by larvae of certain diptera and is classified according to whether the larvae reside external to the globe (ophthalmomyiasis externa) or within the globe (ophthalmomyiasis interna).[56] Entomological classification of the offending parasite depends on distinctive external morphological features; scanning EM has proven to be particularly useful for this purpose.[56]

Table 24.3   Disorders of the trabecular meshwork, lens, and iris studied by electron microscopy

Disorder	References	Disorder	References
Anterior chamber angle		*Contact lenses/prosthetic lenses*	
Axenfeld–Rieger syndrome	344, 345	Contact lens deposits	76, 100–103
Chandler's syndrome	272, 318	Prosthetic intra-ocular lenses	6, 7, 77, 78, 202, 238, 252, 349, 363
Glaucoma	5, 6, 30, 43, 72, 120, 121, 130, 146, 220, 222, 230, 257, 287, 316, 323, 328, 338, 340, 354, 369, 376, 401	*Iris*	
		Gyrate atrophy of choroid/retina	388
		Iris neovascularization (rubeosis iridis)	161, 162, 301
Crystalline lens		Iris nevus (Cogan–Reese) syndrome	79, 179, 262, 291
Capsular cyst	327	Laser effects	314, 315, 384, 385, 412
Cataracts	34, 52, 53, 83–86, 94, 114, 128, 136, 137, 141, 142, 150, 160, 231, 234, 264, 292, 293, 341, 378	Pigmentary dispersion	39, 40, 131, 171, 302
		Siderosis bulbi	367
Delamination of the lens capsule (true exfoliation syndrome)	33, 117, 221		
Ectopic lens	88		
Pseudo-exfoliation syndrome	20, 21, 64, 66–69, 74, 75, 138, 243, 339, 342, 362		

Table 24.4   Disorders of the choroid, optic nerve, retina and vitreous studied by electron microscopy

Disorder	References	Disorder	References
Choroid		Toxoplasma gondii	422
Neovascularization	10	Kawasaki disease	97
Choroideremia	116, 304	Laser effects	87, 225, 305, 402
Sympathetic ophthalmia	96, 158	Light damage	235
		Lipidosis, ophthalmoplegic	368
Optic nerve		Lipoprotein disorders	206
Atrophy	182	Macrophage infiltration	212
Corpora amylacea	415	Macular lesions, miscellaneous	17, 19, 106, 273, 297, 330, 375, 379, 404
Drusen	285		
Glaucoma	288–290, 324	Membranes:	
Inflammation, idiopathic	326	Epiretinal	126, 135, 148, 170, 172, 216, 247, 311
Krabbe's disease (globoid leukodystrophy	35	Preretinal	19, 48, 134, 260, 297, 365, 393
Mucopolysaccharidosis type II (Hunter)	18	Myelin artefact	425
Papilloedema	380	Neovascularization:	
		Retinal	8, 9
Other		Subretinal	331
Endophthalmitis:		Pigment epithelium disorders	37, 391, 411
Due to caterpillar setae	358	Pseudoxanthoma elasticum	159
Endogenous	258	Retinitis pigmentosa	29, 246, 308, 365
		Retinopathy:	
Retina		Diabetic	14, 145, 180, 229, 251, 392
Angioid streaks	159	Pigmentary	29, 80, 208, 218, 246, 296, 308, 365
Bodies, cytoid	253		
Bruch's membrane:		Prematurity	110, 203, 204
Calcification	70	Retinoschisis	124
Drusen	331	Syndromes:	
Cellular bands, subretinal	89	Acute retinal necrosis	55
Degenerations:		Alstrom	337
Peripheral cystoid	124	Kearns–Sayre	80, 236
Photoreceptor	36	Telangiectasis	127
Detachment	57, 168	Uveitis/retinitis	98
Drugs:		Vascular abnormalities, miscellaneous	109
Tamoxifen retinopathy	169		
Thioridazine retinopathy	249		
Chloroquine toxicity	119	*Vitreous*	
Dystrophies:		Asteroid hyalosis	250, 360, 372
Best's macular	106, 404	Ophthalmomyiasis	56
Foveomacular vitelliform	273	Cylinders	325
Oedema, cystoid macular	379, 420	Cysticercus cellulose (Taenia solium)	107
Fluid, subretinal	90		
Fundus flavimaculatus	81	Cysts, pigmented	270
Incontinentia pigmenti	239	Gas compression	371
Infections:		Haemorrhage	99, 183
Cytomegalovirus	312	Membranes/fibrosis	170, 370
Herpes simplex	46, 271		
Measles	133		

Table 24.5 Ophthalmic disorders in which electron microscopy is diagnostically useful

Disorder	Reference
Infections	28, 322, 387, 407
Herpes simplex	28, 322, 407
Nosematosis	275
Ophthalmomyiasis	56
Toxoplasmosis	265, 295
Cornea	
Crystal deposition:	
Central crystalline dystrophy	188, 277, 398, 410
Cystinosis	329, 413
Infectious keratopathy	123, 237
Multiple myeloma/monoclonal gammopathy	44, 192
Meesmann's dystrophy	188, 254, 277, 321, 398
Reis–Bücklers dystrophy	188, 274, 277, 321, 398
Metabolic disorders	
Neuronal ceroid lipofuscinosis	41, 132
Mucolipidosis type IV	51, 210, 299, 426
Infantile neuro-axonal dystrophy	2, 12, 13, 227
Foreign bodies	197, 298

Table 24.6 Lesions of the eye and its adnexa produced by viruses

Virus	Lesions
Adenovirus, type 3	Pharyngoconjunctival fever
Adenovirus, type 8	Epidemic keratoconjunctivitis
Adenovirus, types 1–11, 14–17, 20, 22, 26 and 27	Follicular conjunctivitis, keratoconjunctivitis
Bovine foot and mouth	Keratoconjunctivitis
Coxsackie	Conjunctivitis
Cytomegalovirus	Uveitis, retinitis
Epstein–Barr	Conjunctivitis
Herpes simplex	Conjunctivitis, keratitis, uveitis
Influenza	Follicular conjunctivitis
Marburg virus	Uveitis
Molluscum contagiosum	Eyelid papules, blepharoconjunctivitis, keratoconjunctivitis
Mumps	Conjunctivitis, episcleritis, keratitis
Newcastle disease	Conjunctivitis
Papovavirus	Eyelid warts, verrucose keratitis, conjunctivitis
Rubella	Conjunctivitis, keratitis
Rubeola	Mucopurulent conjunctivitis, punctate keratitis
Sandfly fever	Conjunctivitis
Vaccinia	Blepharoconjunctivitis, purulent conjunctivitis, keratitis
Varicella-zoster	Conjunctivitis, keratitis, scleritis, iridocyclitis, optic neuritis
Variola (smallpox)	Catarrhal conjunctivitis, keratitis
Yellow fever	Conjunctivitis, conjunctival haemorrhage

CORNEAL DYSTROPHIES

Dystrophies

While numerous corneal dystrophies are recognized and have characteristic ultrastructural features, most of them can be diagnosed histopathologically by light microscopy with the aid of special stains (Table 24.7). In two rare corneal dystrophies, Meesmann's dystrophy and Reis–Bücklers dystrophy, however, transmission EM is of paramount diagnostic importance.

Meesmann's dystrophy (juvenile familial epithelial dystrophy) is an autosomal dominant disorder confined to the corneal epithelium.[186,254,278,321,398] The dystrophy is bilateral and is manifested by numerous punctate epithelial opacities which usually appear in the first year or two of life. There may be blurred vision or irregular astigmatism as well as intermittent irritation and photophobia.[186,321] Patients with Meesmann's dystrophy rarely require corneal transplantation. Histopathologically, the major abnormalities are the presence of abundant intra-epithelial microcysts (diameters range from 10 to 120 μm) which contain degenerated epithelial cells. These cysts stain with periodic acid–Schiff reagent and with Hale's colloidal iron technique. The characteristic ultrastructural feature of Meesmann's dystro-

Table 24.7 Corneal dystrophies

Disorder	Ultrastructural features	Characteristics with other techniques	References
Granular dystrophy	Aggregates of discrete rod-shaped bodies in stroma, especially superficial stroma	Stromal deposits: intensely eosinophilic, brilliant red with Masson trichrome	156, 165, 188, 195, 278, 307, 317, 361, 398
Lattice dystrophy	Extracellular deposits of amyloid fibrils	Amyloid deposits in stroma and sometimes subepithelial; deposits stain with Congo red	122, 194, 278, 286, 398, 421
Macular dystrophy	Fibrillogranular material in cytoplasmic vacuoles of corneal fibroblasts and endothelial cells	Extracellular and intracellular (fibroblasts and endothelial cells) material stains with Alcian blue and colloidal iron techniques	152, 185–188, 196, 278, 282, 398, 416
Meesmann's dystrophy	Fibrillogranular 'peculiar substance' in cytoplasm of epithelial cells	Intra-epithelial microcysts stain with periodic acid–Schiff and colloidal iron procedures	188, 254, 278, 374, 398
Posterior polymorphous dystrophy	Endothelium replaced by cells with features of squamous epithelium (tonofilaments, desmosomes)	'Endothelium' multilayered; cytokeratin positive	30, 125, 143, 163, 280, 310, 313, 319, 320
Reis–Bücklers dystrophy	Curly fibrils in superficial stroma	Fibrous tissue beneath epithelium	188, 278, 321, 398, 418

phy is electron-dense fibrillogranular material (termed 'peculiar substance') within the cytoplasm of epithelial cells (Fig. 24.1).[186,321,374] The nature of this 'peculiar substance' is unknown.

Reis–Bücklers dystrophy is a bilaterally symmetrical, central corneal dystrophy with reticular superficial corneal opacification which progressively evolves into a central ring-shaped pattern.[186,278,321,398] There is an autosomal dominant mode of inheritance and the condition becomes clinically manifest within the first few years of life. Visual acuity is impaired by corneal opacification and irregular astigmatism, and superficial keratectomy or keratoplasty may be necessary to restore vision. Histopathologically, corneas from patients with Reis–Bücklers dystrophy have epithelium that varies in thickness. The basal corneal epithelium, the epithelial basement membrane, and Bowman's layer have variable degrees of degeneration and irregular fibrous tissue is present beneath the epithelium. Transmission EM shows the irregular fibrous tissue replacing Bowman's layer to consist of disoriented regular collagen fibres (20–25 nm in diameter) interspersed with electron-dense fibrils having diameters of 8–10 nm.[186,278,321,398] Perry et al[274] drew attention to masses of short curly filaments, with diameters of approximately 10 nm, located among the collagen fibres replacing Bowman's layer. Curly filaments (Fig. 24.2) have not been observed in any other corneal dystrophy and thus appear to be specific for Reis–Bücklers dystrophy.

Crystal deposition

Crystals are observed in the cornea in patients with central crystalline corneal dystrophy[186,278,398,410] and cystinosis[190,329,413] and may also be observed in cases of multiple myeloma or monoclonal gammopathy[44,192] and

in certain corneas with bacterial colonization in the absence of inflammation (infectious keratopathy).[123,237]

Central crystalline corneal dystrophy (Schnyder's dystrophy) is an uncommon autosomal dominant disorder which presents in early infancy.[186,278,398,410] Clinical features are usually limited to the cornea where the anterior stroma contains numerous fine needle-like crystals. The crystals have the morphological, solubility, and histochemical characteristics of cholesterol.[186,398,410] Ultrastructurally, the cornea has intra- and extra-cellular rectangular or needle-like electron-lucent spaces in the stroma caused by dissolved cholesterol crystals.[186,278,398] Clumps of electron-dense material are often observed adjacent to the crystals.

Cystinosis occurs as childhood, juvenile, and adult forms; all are characterized by the presence of delicate scintillating cystine crystals in the cornea, conjunctiva and iris.[190,329,413] The cystine crystals are soluble in aqueous solutions but are insoluble in absolute ethanol and may be easily seen with polarized light.[190] EM demonstrates needle-, rectangular-, or hexagonal-shaped crystals within membrane-bound intracytoplasmic vacuoles which have been identified as lysosomes by the presence of acid phosphatase.[190]

The presence of crystals within the cornea, and sometimes also in the conjunctiva and lens, is a rare manifestation of hypergammaglobulinaemia.[44,193] The crystals may be throughout the corneal stromal or may be predominantly in certain locations, such as the corneal epithelium.[193] The crystals are eosinophilic and stain brilliant red with Masson's trichrome stain.[193] Ultrastructurally, the crystals are electron-dense hexagons and have a fine internal periodicity; 10–11 nm spacings between linear electron densities have been observed in some crystals.[193]

Branching, needle-like, white crystalline stromal opacities have been rarely observed in corneal grafts of patients treated with topical corticosteroids.[123,237] These crystalline opacities increase in size slowly and correspond to bacterial colonies without an associated inflammatory reaction histologically.[123,237] Ultrastructural examination has confirmed the bacterial composition of the opacities in this unusual condition.[123,237] Mason et al[228] reported clinical observations on five patients with intrastromal crystalline deposits following corneal graft rejection and speculated that immune globulin or immune complex deposition may provide an alternative mechanism for crystal formation.

METABOLIC DISORDERS

Ocular manifestations are associated with metabolic disorders that involve amino acids,[22,190] collagen,[215] glycogen,[22,23] glycolipids,[22,25] lipids,[410] metals,[112] monosaccharides,[409] glycosaminoglycans(mucopolysaccharides),[22,105,189] sphingolipids,[22,24,113] and vitamins.[191] Ocular tissues have been examined by EM in many of these conditions (see refs 18, 22, 176, 377 and 383 for reviews).

A wide variety of inborn errors of metabolism such as mucopolysaccharidoses,[232,383,419] lipidoses,[13,213,214,383,419] mucolipidoses,[47,385,419] oligosaccharidoses,[383] cystinosis,[329,413] and adrenoleukodystrophy[13,226,256,419] exhibit their characteristic ultrastructural lesions in conjunctival biopsies (Table 24.8; see also Ch. 6). In most of these diseases, however, there are biochemical abnormalities which may allow a diagnosis without the necessity of conjunctival biopsy. Arsénio-Nunes et al[13] reviewed 127 skin and 59 conjunctival biopsies performed on 136 children with chronic neurological disorders and noted that in all children with a skin or conjunctival biopsy having diagnostic changes, the clinical and ultrastructural diagnoses were in agreement. They also observed that ultrastructural abnormalities in the conjunctiva (and skin) were never observed in patients with nonprogressive encephalopathies and hence they recommended

Table 24.8 Electron microscopy of conjunctiva biopsies in lysosomal[a] storage diseases

Disease	Conjunctival ultrastructural lesions			
	Epithelium	Fibroblasts	Capillary endothelium	Schwann cells
Mucopolysaccharidoses				
Type IH (Hurler)	+ + +	+ + +	±	+
Type IS (Scheie)	+ +	+ +	−	+
Type II (Hunter)	+ + +	+ + +	±	+
Types III A and B (Sanfilippo)	+ +	+ +	−	+
Type IV (Morquio)	±	+	−	−
Type V (Marteaux–Lamy)	+ +	+ +	−	−
Oligosaccharidoses				
Fucosidosis	+ + +	+ + +	+ + +	±
Mannosidosis	−	+ + +	+	+
Mucolipidosis				
Type II	−	+ + +	+	+
Type IV	+ + +	+ +	+	*
Mucosulphatidosis	+ +	+ +	−	+ +
Lipidoses				
GM$_1$ gangliosidosis	+ + +	+ + +	+ + +	+ + +
GM$_2$ gangliosidosis type I (Tay–Sachs)	−	+	−	+ + +
GM$_2$ gangliosidosis type II (Sandhoff)	+ + +	+ +	+ +	+ + +
Niemann–Pick A	+ +	+ + +	+ + +	+ + +
Niemann–Pick B	+	+	+	−
Niemann–Pick C	+	+ +	+	−
Fabry's disease	+ + +	+ +	+ + +	±
Metachromatic leukodystrophy	−	−	−	+ + +
Krabbe's disease	−	−	−	+ + +
Ceroid–lipofuscinoses				
Infantile type	+	+	+ +	+
Late infantile type	+	+	+ +	+
Juvenile type	+	+	+ +	+
Adult type (Kufs)	−	−	−	−
Glycogenosis type II				
Infantile (Pompe)	+ + +	+ + +	+ + +	+ +
Adult form	−	−	−	−

[a] Adapted from Van Hoof et al.[383] The number of crosses indicates the relative abundance of lesions.
* Not specified.

that conjunctival and/or skin biopsy be reserved for patients with progressive neurological disorders in which biochemical diagnosis is not feasible. This section will review only those metabolic disorders for which EM of conjunctival biopsies has been shown to be of critical diagnostic significance.

Neuronal ceroid lipofuscinosis

Neuronal ceroid lipofuscinosis (also known as Batten's disease or Batten–Vogt's disease) is characterized by the intracellular accumulation of abnormal autofluorescent material which has histochemical properties similar to normal lipofuscin.[24,41,132,157,248,353] A consistent biochemical abnormality has not been identified, and in all forms of neuronal ceroid lipofuscinosis the diagnosis is based on clinical and morphological findings. The disease can be divided into four groups on the basis of clinical and ultrastructural findings. The infantile form of neuronal ceroid lipofuscinosis (Haltia–Santavuori type) has an onset of rapid developmental regression (loss of speech, severe visual failure, secondary microcephaly) starting at about one year of age; electron microscopy shows granular osmiophilic deposits.[41,132] The late infantile variant (Jansky–Bielschowsky) presents at 2–4 years of age with seizures followed by rapid intellectual, visual and motor deterioration;[248,334] ultrastructurally there are cytosomes filled with curvilinear or fingerprint profiles.[41,334] The juvenile form (Spielmeyer–Sjögrem) starts with visual loss followed by intellectual and motor decline beginning at 6–8 years of age;[248,353] fingerprint profiles or granular osmiophilic deposits are found ultrastructurally.[41] The so-called adult form of the disease (Kufs') is very rare, may not have blindness or seizures, and begins in adolescence or adulthood;[41,353] cytosomes contain fingerprint profiles or granular osmiophilic deposits.[41] Studies by Van Hoof et al[383] and Arsénio-Nunes et al[13] have clearly established the feasibility of diagnosing neuronal ceroid lipofuscinosis by ultrastructural examination of conjunctival biopsies. The characteristic ultrastructural lesions are present in conjunctival epithelial cells, fibroblasts, capillary endothelium and Schwann cells.[383]

Mucolipidosis type IV

Mucolipidosis type IV (see also Ch. 6) is distinguished from mucolipidosis types I, II and III by its milder clinical manifestations and lack of an identifiable lysosomal enzyme defect.[51] This rare storage disease has its onset in infancy,[51] affects both males and females, and is manifest by slowly progressive neurological abnormalities (increased deep tendon reflexes, hypotonia, dystonia, impaired psychomotor development) and bilateral corneal clouding.[51,210,299,426] Strabismus and corneal clouding are frequently the first signs of this disorder.[51] Currently, the diagnosis of mucolipidosis type IV rests on the clinical history and the ultrastructural finding of membrane-bound fibrillogranular inclusions (glycosaminoglycan) and concentric lamellar bodies (complex lipids) in fibroblasts and other tissues.[51,210,299,426] Many studies have documented the presence of characteristic inclusions within the conjunctiva.[12,51,210,299,426] The inclusions are most abundant in the epithelial cells but are also seen in stromal fibroblasts, macrophages, leukocytes, and the endothelial cells of capillaries and lymphatics.[426]

Infantile neuro-axonal dystrophy

Infantile neuro-axonal dystrophy becomes clinically manifest at the end of the first or during the second year of life and is marked by slowing and then loss of motor and mental milestones, marked hypotonia, visual disturbances, symmetrical pyramidal tract signs, and peripheral motor involvement.[2] Death usually occurs before ten years of age.[2] The diagnosis of infantile neuro-axonal dystrophy is established by finding ballooned axons containing spheroid bodies (collections of packed membranous and tubular structures); specific biochemical abnormalities have not been described. Several studies have shown that conjunctival biopsies can be used to diagnose infantile neuro-axonal dystrophy since the conjunctival nerves contain the ultrastructural hallmarks of the disease[2,12,13,227] (See also Ch. 23).

FOREIGN BODIES

The applications of energy-dispersive microprobe analysis in ophthalmic pathology has recently been reviewed by Klintworth et al.[197] This technique has been used to study contact lens deposits, prosthetic intra-ocular lenses, foreign bodies, and a variety of ocular disorders such as Wilson's disease, calcific band keratopathy, corneal blood staining, corneal dystrophies, cataracts, asteroid hyalosis, and calcification of Bruch's membrane.[197] Energy-dispersive microprobe analysis is diagnostically important for precise identification of the elemental composition of certain foreign bodies, which can be particularly critical in medico-legal disputes.[197]

REFERENCES

1. Abelson M B, Collin H B, Gillette T E, Dohlman C H 1980 Recurrent keratoconus after keratoplasty. American Journal of Ophthalmology 90: 672–676
2. Aicardi J, Castelein P 1979 Infantile neuroaxonal dystrophy. Brain 102: 727–748
3. Alexander R A, Grierson I, Garner A 1981 Oxytalan fibers in Fuchs' endothelial dystrophy. Archives of Ophthalmology 99: 1622–1627
4. Anderson D R 1969 Ultrastructure of xanthelasma. Archives of Ophthalmology 81: 692–694
5. Anderson D R 1981 The development of the trabecular meshwork and its abnormality in primary infantile glaucoma. Transactions of the American Ophthalmological Society 79: 458–485
6. Apple D J, Craythorn J M, Olson R J, Little L E, Lyman J B, Reidy J J, Loftfield K 1984 Anterior segment complications and neovascular glaucoma following implantation of a posterior chamber intraocular lens. Ophthalmology 91: 403–419
7. Apple D J, Reidy J J, Googe J M, Mamalis N, Novak L C, Loftfield K, Olson R J 1985 A comparison of ciliary sulcus and capsular bag fixation of posterior chamber intraocular lenses. Journal of the American Intraocular Implant Society 11: 44–63
8. Archer D B 1976 Neovascularization of the retina. Transactions of the Ophthalmological Society of the United Kingdom 46: 471–493
9. Archer D B 1983 Retinal neovascularization. Transactions of the Opthalmological Society of the United Kingdom 103: 2–27
10. Archer D B, Gardiner T A 1983 Experimental choroidal neovascularization. International Ophthalmology 6: 171–177
11. Arentsen J J, Rodrigues M M, Laibson P R 1977 Histopathologic changes after thermokeratoplasty for keratoconus. Investigative Ophthalmology and Visual Science 16: 32–38
12. Arsénio-Nunes M L, Goutiéres F 1978 Diagnosis of infantile neuroaxonal dystrophy by conjunctival biopsy. Journal of Neurology, Neurosurgery and Psychiatry 41: 511–515
13. Arsénio-Nunes M L, Goutiéres F, Aicardi J 1981 An ultramicroscopic study of skin and conjunctival biopsies in chronic neurological disorders of childhood. Annals of Neurology 9: 163–173
14. Ashton N 1974 Vascular basement membrane changes in diabetic retinopathy. Montgomery lecture, 1973. British Journal of Ophthalmology 58: 344–366
15. Ashton N, Cook C 1979 Allergic granulomatous nodules of the eyelid and conjunctiva. The XXXV Edward Jackson Memorial Lecture. American Journal of Ophthalmology 87: 1–28
16. Bahn C F, Falls H F, Varley G A, Meyer R F, Edelhauser H F, Bourne W M 1984 Classification of corneal endothelial disorders based on neural crest origin. Ophthalmology 91: 558–563
17. Basu P K 1983 A new look at some macular lesions. Topography of the human pathological retinas using scanning electron microscopy. Indian Journal of Ophthalmology 31: 143–148
18. Beck M, Cole G 1984 Disc oedema in association with Hunter's syndrome: ocular histopathological findings. British Journal of Ophthalmology 68: 590–594
19. Bellhorn M B, Friedman A H, Wise G N, Henkind P 1975 Ultrastructure and clinicopathologic correlation of idiopathic preretinal macular fibrosis. American Journal of Ophthalmology 79: 366–373
20. Benedikt O, Roll P 1979 The trabecular meshwork of a non-glaucomatous eye with the exfoliation syndrome. Electron microscopic study. Virchows Archiv A, Pathological Anatomy and Histopathology 384: 347–355
21. Bergmanson J P, Jones W L, Chu L W F 1984 Ultrastructural observations on (pseudo-) exfoliation of the lens capsule: a re-examination of the involvement of the lens epithelium. British Journal of Ophthalmology 68: 118–123
22. Berman E R 1982 Lysosomal storage diseases. In: Garner A, Klintworth G K (eds) Pathobiology of ocular disease. A dynamic approach. Marcel Dekker, New York pp 845–855
23. Berman E R 1982 Glycogen storage diseases. In: Garner A, Klintworth G K (eds) Pathobiology of ocular disease. Marcel Dekker, New York, pp 857–861
24. Berman E R 1982 Sphingolipidoses and neuronal ceroid-lipofuscinosis. In: Garner A, Klintworth G K (eds) Pathobiology of

ocular disease. A dynamic approach. Marcel Dekker, New York, pp 897–929
25. Berman E R 1982 Mucolipidoses. In: Garner A, Klintworth G K (eds) Pathobiology of ocular disease. A dynamic approach. Marcel Dekker, New York, pp 931–946
26. Bethell W, McCullough C, Ghosh M 1975 Lecithin cholesterol acyl transferase deficiency. Light and electron microscopic finding from two corneas. Canadian Journal of Ophthalmology 10: 494–501
27. Binder P S, Zavala E Y, Stainer G A 1982 Non-infectious peripheral corneal ulceration: Mooren's ulcer or Terrien's marginal degeneration? Annals of Ophthalmology 14: 425–426, 428–429, 432–435
28. Boerner C F, Lee F K, Wickliffe C L, Nahmias A J, Cavanagh H D, Strauss S E 1981 Electron microscopy for the diagnosis of ocular viral infections. Ophthalmology 88: 1377–1381
29. Boulton M, Marshall J, Mellerio J 1984 Retinitis pigmentosa: a quantitative study of the apical membrane of normal and dystrophic human retinal pigment epithelial cells in tissue culture in relation to phagocytosis. Graefes Archive for Clinical and Experimental Ophthalmology 221: 214–229
30. Bourgeois J, Shields M B, Thresher R 1984 Open-angle glaucoma associated with posterior polymorphous dystrophy. A clinicopathologic study. Ophthalmology 91: 420–423
31. Bourne W M, Johnson D H, Campbell R J 1982 The ultrastructure of Descemet's membrane. III. Fuchs' dystrophy. Archives of Ophthalmology 100: 1952–1955
32. Brodrick J D, Dark A J, Peace G W 1974 Fingerprint dystrophy of the cornea. A histologic study. Archives of Ophthalmology 92: 483–489
33. Brodrick J D, Tate G W Jr 1979 Capsular delamination (true exfoliation) of the lens. Report of a case. Archives of Ophthalmology 97: 1693–1698
34. Bron A J, Habgood J O 1976 Morgagnian cataract. Transactions of the Ophthalmological Society of the United Kingdom 96: 265–277
35. Brownstein S, Meagher-Villemure K, Polomeno R C, Little J M 1978 Optic nerve in globoid leukodystrophy (Krabbe's disease). Ultrastructural changes. Archives of Ophthalmology 96: 864–870
36. Buchanan T A, Gardiner T A, Archer D B 1984 An ultrastructural study of retinal photoreceptor degeneration associated with bronchial carcinoma. American Journal of Ophthalmology 97: 277–287
37. Buettner H 1974 Congenital hypertrophy of the retinal pigment epithelium (RPE). A nontumorous lesion. Modern Problems in Ophthalmology 12: 528–535
38. Cameron M E 1983 Histology of pterygium: an electron microscopic study. British Journal of Ophthalmology 67: 604–608
39. Campbell D G 1979 Pigmentary dispersion and glaucoma. A new theory. Archives of Ophthalmology 97: 1667–1672
40. Campbell D G, Jeffrey C P 1979 Pigmentary dispersion in the human eye, SEM. Scanning Electron Microscopy 3: 329–333
41. Carpenter S, Karpati G, Andermann F, Jacob J C, Anderman E 1977 The ultrastructural characteristics of the abnormal cytosomes in Batten — Kufs' disease. Brain 100: 137–156
42. Cavanagh H D, Pihlaja D, Thoft R A, Dohlman C H 1976 The pathogenesis and treatment of persistent epithelial defects. Transactions of the American Academy of Ophthalmology and Otolaryngology 81: 754–769
43. Chaudhry H A, Dueker D K, Simmons R J, Bellows A R, Grant W M 1979 Scanning electron microscopy of trabeculectomy specimens in open-angle glaucoma. American Journal of Ophthalmology 88: 78–92
44. Cherry P M H, Kraft S, McGowan H, Ghosh M, Shenken E 1983 Corneal and conjunctival deposits in monoclonal gammopathy. Canadian Journal of Ophthalmology 3: 143–149
45. Chew E, Ghosh M, McCullough C 1982 Amiodarone-induced cornea verticillata. Canadian Journal of Ophthalmology 3: 96–99
46. Cibis G W, Flynn J T, Davis E B 1978 Herpes simplex retinitis. Archives of Ophthalmology 96: 299–302
47. Cibis G W, Tripathi R C, Harris D J 1982 Mucolipidosis I. Birth Defects 18: 359–380
48. Clarkson J G, Green W R, Massof D 1977 A histopathologic review

of 168 cases of preretinal membrane. American Journal of Ophthalmology 84: 1–17

49. Cogan D G, Kuwabara T, Donaldson D D, Collins E 1974 Microcystic dystrophy of the cornea. A partial explanation for its pathogenesis. Archives of Ophthalmology 92: 470–474

50. Collin H B, Allansmith M R 1977 Basophils in vernal conjunctivitis in humans: an electron microscopic study. Investigative Ophthalmology and Visual Science 16: 858–864

51. Crandall B F, Philippart M, Brown W J, Bluestone D A 1982 Review article: mucolipidosis IV. American Journal of Medical Genetics 12: 301–308

52. Creighton M O, Trevithick J R, Mousa G Y, Percy D H, McKinna A J, Dyson C, Maisel H, Bradley R 1978 Globular bodies: a primary cause of the opacity in senile and diabetic posterior cortical subcapsular cataracts? Canadian Journal of Ophthalmology 13: 166–181

53. Creighton M O, Trevithick J R, Sanford S E, Dukes T W 1982 Modelling cortical cataractogenesis. IV. Induction by hygromycin B in vivo (swine) and in vitro (rat lens). Experimental Eye Research 34: 467–476

54. Croxatto J O, Dodds C M, Dodds R 1985 Bilateral and massive lipoidal infiltration of the cornea (secondary lipoidal degeneration). Ophthalmology 92: 1686–1690

55. Culbertson W W, Blumenkranz M S, Haines H, Gass D M, Mitchell K B, Norton E W 1982 The acute retinal necrosis syndrome. Part 2. Histopathology and etiology. Ophthalmology 89: 1317–1325

56. Custis P H, Pakalnis V A, Klintworth G K, Anderson W B, Machemer R 1983 Posterior internal ophthalmomyiasis. Identification of a surgically removed cuterebra larva by scanning electron microscopy. Ophthalmology 90: 1583–1590

57. Daicker B 1985 Constricting retroretinal membranes associated with traumatic retinal detachments. Graefes Archive for Clinical and Experimental Ophthalmology 222: 147–153

58. D'Amico D J, Kenyon H R, Ruskin J N 1981 Amiodarone keratopathy: drug-induced lipid storage disease. Archives of Ophthalmology 99: 257–261

59. Daniels C A 1982 Viral and rickettsial infections. In: Garner A, Klintworth G K (eds) Pathobiology of ocular disease. A dynamic approach. Marcel Dekker, New York, pp 249–279

60. Dark A J 1977 Bleb dystrophy of the cornea: histochemistry and ultrastructure. British Journal of Ophthalmology 61: 65–69

61. Dark A J 1978 Cogan's microcystic dystrophy of the cornea: ultrastructure and photomicroscopy. British Journal of Ophthalmology 62: 821–830

62. Dark A J, Proctor J 1982 Atypical band-shaped calcific keratopathy with keratocyte changes. British Journal of Ophthalmology 66: 309–316

63. Dark A J, Proctor J 1983 Blue fleck corneal iridescence: an occasional feature of Cogan's microcystic corneal dystrophy. British Journal of Ophthalmology 67: 799–803

64. Dark A J, Streeten B W, Cornwall C C 1977 Pseudoexfoliative disease of the lens: a study in electron microscopy and histochemistry. British Journal of Ophthalmology 61: 462–472

65. Darrell R W 1981 Thygeson's superficial punctate keratitis: natural history and association with HLA DR3. Transactions of the American Ophthalmological Society 79: 486–516

66. Davanger M 1980 Pseudo-exfoliation material. Electron microscopy after the application of lanthanum as tracer particles and ionic stain. Acta Ophthalmologica (Copenhagen) 58: 512–519

67. Davanger M 1980 On the ultrastructure and the formation of pseudo-exfoliation material. Acta Ophthalmologica (Copenhagen) 58: 520–527

68. Davanger M, Hovig T 1978 Pseudo-exfoliation fibrils examined by negative staining. Acta Ophthalmologica (Copenhagen) 56: 226–232

69. Davanger M, Pederson O O 1975 Pseudo-exfoliation material on the anterior lens surface. Demonstration and examination of an interfibrillar ground substance. Acta Ophthalmologica (Copenhagen) 53: 3–18

70. Davis W L, Jones R G, Hagler H K 1981 An electron microscopic histochemical and analytical X-ray microprobe study of calcification in Bruch's membrane from human eyes. Journal of Histochemistry and Cytochemistry 29: 601–608

71. Dekkers N W 1981 The cornea in measles. Documenta Ophthalmologica 52: 1–119

72. deLuise V P, Anderson D R 1983 Primary infantile glaucoma (congenital glaucoma). Survey of Ophthalmology 28: 1–19

73. Depot M J, Jakobiec F A, Dodick J M, Iwamoto T 1984 Bilateral and extensive xanthelasma palpebrarum in a young man. Ophthalmology 91: 522–527

74. Dickson D H, Ramsey M S 1979 Fibrillopathia epitheliocapsularis: review of the nature and origin of pseudoexfoliative deposits. Transactions of the Ophthalmological Society of the United Kingdom 99: 284–292

75. Dickson D H, Ramsey M S 1975 Fibrillopathia epitheliocapsularis (pseudoexfoliation): a clinical and electron microscope study. Canadian Journal of Ophthalmology 10: 148–161

76. Doughman D J, Mobilia E, Drago D, Havener V, Gavin M 1975 The nature of 'spots' on soft lenses. Annals of Ophthalmology 7: 345–348, 351–353

77. Drews R C 1982 The Barraquer experience with intraocular lenses. 20 years later. Ophthalmology 89: 386–393

78. Drews R C, Smith M E, Okun N 1978 Scanning electron microscopy of intraocular lenses. Ophthalmology 85: 415–424

79. Eagle R C Jr, Font R L, Yanoff M, Fine B S 1980 The iris naevus (Cogan–Reese) syndrome: light and electron microscopic observations. British Journal of Ophthalmology 64: 446–452

80. Eagle R C Jr, Hedges T R, Yanoff M 1982 The atypical pigmentary retinopathy of Kearns-Sayre syndrome. A light and electron microscopic study. Ophthalmology 89: 1433–1440

81. Eagle R C Jr, Lucier A C, Bernardino V B Jr, Yanoff M 1980 Retinal pigment epithelial abnormalities in fundus flavimaculatus: a light and electron microscopic study. Ophthalmology 87: 1189–1200

82. Easty D L, Birkenshaw M, Merrett T, Merrett J, Entwhistle C, Amer B 1980 Immunological investigations in vernal eye disease. Transactions of the Ophthalmological Society of the United Kingdom 100: 98–107

83. Eshaghian J, Rafferty N S, Goossens W 1980 Ultrastructure of human cataract in retinitis pigmentosa. Archives of Ophthalmology 98: 2227–2230

84. Fagerholm P, Palmquist B M, Philipson B 1984 Atopic cataract: changes in the lens epithelium and subcapsular cortex. Graefes Archive for Clinical and Experimental Ophthalmology 221: 149–152

85. Fagerholm P P, Philipson B T 1979 Human traumatic cataract. A quantitative microradiographic and electron microscopic study. Acta Ophthalmologica (Copenhagen) 57: 20–32

86. Fagerholm P, Philipson B, Carlströmm D 1981–82 Calcification in the human lens. Current Topics in Eye Research 11: 629–633

87. Fankhauser F, Van der Zypen E, Kwasniewska S, Loertscher H 1985 The effect of thermal mode Nd:YAG laser radiation on vessels and ocular tissue. Experimental and clinical findings. Ophthalmology 92: 419–426

88. Farnsworth P N, Burke P A, Blanco J, Maltzman B 1978 Ultrastructural abnormalities in a microspherical ectopic lens. Experimental Eye Research 27: 399–408

89. Federman J L, Folberg R, Ridley M, Arbizo V A 1983 Subretinal cellular bands. Transactions of the American Ophthalmological Society 81: 172–181

90. Feeney L, Burns R P, Mixon R M 1975 Human subretinal fluid. Its cellular and subcellular components. Archives of Ophthalmology 93: 62–69

91. Finlay K R, Rootman J, Dimmick J 1980 Optic neuropathy in primary orbital amyloidosis. Canadian Journal of Ophthalmology 15: 189–192

92. Firat T 1974 Ligneous conjunctivitis. American Journal of Ophthalmology 78: 679–688

93. Fogle J A, Kenyon K R, Stark W J, Green W R 1975 Defective epithelial adhesion in anterior corneal dystrophies. American Journal of Ophthalmology 79: 925–940

94. Font R L, Brownstein S 1974 A light and electron microscopic study of anterior subcapsular cataracts. American Journal of Ophthalmology 78: 972–984

95. Font R L, Fine B S 1972 Ocular pathology in Fabry's disease. Histochemical and electron microscopic observations. American Journal of Ophthalmology 73: 419–430

96. Font R L, Fine B S, Messmer E, Rowsey J F 1983 Light and

electron microscopic study of Dalén–Fuchs nodules in sympathetic ophthalmia. Ophthalmology 90: 66–75

97. Font R L, Mehta R S, Streusand S B, O'Boyle T E, Kretzer F L 1983 Bilateral retinal ischemia in Kawasaki disease. Postmortem findings and electron microscopic observations. Ophthalmology 90: 569–577

98. Forrester J V, Borthwick G M 1983 Clinical relevance of S-antigen induced experimental uveoretinitis. Transactions of the Ophthalmological Society of the United Kingdom 103: 497–502

99. Forrester J V, Lee W R 1981 Cellular composition of post-haemorrhagic opacities in the human vitreous. Albrecht Von Graefes Archiv für Klinische und Experimentalle Ophthalmologie 215: 279–295

100. Fowler S A, Allansmith M R 1980 The surface of the continuously worn contact lenses. Archives of Ophthalmology 98: 1233–1236

101. Fowler S A, Allansmith M R 1980 Evolution of soft contact lens coatings. Archives of Ophthalmology 98: 95–99

102. Fowler S A, Greiner J V, Allansmith M R 1979 Soft contact lenses from patients with giant papillary conjunctivitis. American Journal of Ophthalmology 88: 1056–1061

103. Fowler S A, Korb D R, Finnemore V M, Allansmith M R 1984 Surface deposits on worn hard contact lenses. Archives of Ophthalmology 102: 757–759

104. Francois J, Hanssens M, Teuchy H 1977 Corneal ultrastructural changes in Fabry's disease. Bulletin de la Societe Belge d'Ophtalmologie 179: 7–23

105. Francois J 1974 Ocular manifestations of the mucopolysaccharidoses. Ophthalmologica 169: 345–361

106. Frangieh G T, Green W R, Fine S L 1982 A histopathologic study of Best's macular dystrophy. Archives of Ophthalmology 100: 1115–1121

107. Friedman A H, Pokorny K S, Suhan J, Ritch R, Zinn K M 1980 Electron microscopic observations of intravitreal cysticercus cellulose (Taenia solium). Ophthalmologica 180: 267–273

108. Friend J, Ishii Y, Thoft R A 1982 Corneal epithelial changes in diabetic rats. Ophthalmic Research 14: 269–278

109. Fryczkowski A W, Grimson B S, Peiffer R L 1985 Vascular casting and scanning electron microscopy of human ocular vascular abnormalities. Archives of Ophthalmology 103: 118–120

110. Fryczkowski A W, Peiffer R L, Merritt J C, Kraybill E H, Eifrig D E 1985 Scanning electron microscopy of the ocular vasculature in retinopathy of prematurity. Archives of Ophthalmology 103: 224–228

111. Gaasterland D E, Rodrigues M M, Moshell A N 1982 Ocular involvement in xeroderma pigmentosum. Ophthalmology 89: 980–986

112. Garner A 1982 Metabolic disorders involving metals. In: Garner A, Klintworth G K (eds) Pathobiology of ocular disease. A dynamic approach. Marcel Dekker, New York, pp 1097–1105

113. Garner A 1973 Ocular pathology of GM_2 gangliosidosis – type 2 (Sandhoff's disease). British Journal of Ophthalmology 57: 514–520

114. Ghosh M, McCulloch C 1975 Anterior subcapsular cataract. An electron microscopic study. Canadian Journal of Ophthalmology 10: 502–510

115. Ghosh M, McCulloch C 1974 The Morquio syndrome — light and electron microscopic findings from two corneas. Canadian Journal of Ophthalmology 9: 445–452

116. Ghosh M, McCulloch J C 1980 Pathological findings from two cases of choroideremia. Canadian Journal of Ophthalmology 15: 147–153

117. Ghosh M, Speakman J S 1983 The origin of senile lens exfoliation. Canadian Journal of Ophthalmology 18: 340–343

118. Gibson J M, Fielder A R, Garner A, Millac P 1984 Severe ocular side effects of perhexilene maleate: case report. British Journal of Ophthalmology 68: 553–560

119. Gleiser C A, Dukes T W, Zanwill T, Read W K, Bay W W, Brown R S 1969 Ocular changes in swine associated with chloroquine toxicity. American Journal of Ophthalmology 67: 399–405

120. Goldberg M R, Tso M O 1978 Rubeosis iridis and glaucoma associated with sickle cell retinopathy: a light and electron microscopic study. Ophthalmology 85: 1028–1041

121. Goldberg M F, Tso M O 1979 Sickled erythrocytes, hyphema, and secondary glaucoma. VII. The passage of sickled erythrocytes out of

the anterior chamber of the human and monkey eye: light and electron microscopic studies. Ophthalmic Surgery 10: 89–123

122. Gorevic P D, Rodrigues M M, Krachmer J H, Green C, Fujihara S, Glenner G G 1984 Lack of evidence for protein AA reactivity in amyloid deposits of lattice corneal dystrophy and amyloid corneal degeneration. American Journal of Ophthalmology 98: 216–224

123. Gorovoy M S, Stern G A, Hood C I, Allen C 1983 Intrastromal noninflammatory bacterial colonization of a corneal graft. Archives of Ophthalmology 101: 1749–1752

124. Göttinger W 1981 Formation of basement membranes and collagenous fibrils in peripheral cystoid degeneration and retinoschisis. Developmental Ophthalmology 2: 363–368

125. Grayson M 1974 The nature of hereditary deep polymorphous dystrophy of the cornea: its association with iris and anterior chamber dygenesis. Transactions of the American Ophthalmological Society 72: 516–559

126. Green W R, Kenyon K R, Michels R G, Gilbert H D, de la Cruz Z 1979 Ultrastructure of epiretinal membranes causing macular pucker after retinal re-attachment surgery. Transactions of the Ophthalmological Society of the United Kingdom 99: 65–77

127. Green W R, Quigley H A, de la Cruz Z, Cohen B 1980 Parafoveal retinal telangiectasis. Light and electron microscopy studies. Transactions of the Ophthalmological Society of the United Kingdom 100: 162–170

128. Greiner J V, Chylack L T Jr 1979 Posterior subcapsular cataracts: histopathologic study of steroid-associated cataracts. Archives of Ophthalmology 97: 135–144

129. Greiner J V, Covington H I, Allansmith M R 1978 Surface morphology of giant papillary conjunctivitis in contact lens wearers. American Journal of Ophthalmology 85: 242–252

130. Grierson I, Lee W R, Moseley H, Abraham S 1979 The trabecular wall of Schlemm's canal: a study of the effects of pilocarpine by scanning electron microscopy. British Journal of Ophthalmology 63: 9–16

131. Haddad R, Strasser G, Heilig P, Jurecka W 1981 Decompensation of chronic open-angle glaucoma following mydriasis-induced pigmentary dispersion into the aqueous humour: a light and electron microscopic study. British Journal of Ophthalmology 65: 252–257

132. Hagberg B, Haltia M, Sourander P, Svennerholm L, Eeg-Olofsson O 1974 Polyunsaturated fatty acid lipidosis. Infantile form of so-called neuronal ceroid lipofuscinosis. I. Clinical and morphological aspects. Acta Pediatrica Scandinavica 63: 753–763

133. Haltia M, Tarkkanen A, Vaheri A, Paetau A, Kaakinen K, Erkkilä H 1978 Measles retinopathy during immunosuppression. British Journal of Ophthalmology 62: 356–360

134. Hamilton C W, Chandler D, Klintworth G K, Machemer R 1982 A transmission and scanning electron microscopic study of surgically excised preretinal membrane proliferations in diabetes mellitus. American Journal of Ophthalmology 94: 473–488

135. Harada T, Chauvaud D, Pouliquen Y 1981 An electron microscopic study of the epiretinal membrane of human eyes. Albrecht Von Graefes Archiv für Klinische und Experimentalle Ophthalmologie 215: 327–339

136. Harding C V, Chylack L T Jr, Susan S R, Lo W K, Bobrowski W F 1982 Elemental and ultrastructural analysis of specific human lens opacities. Investigative Ophthalmology and Visual Science 23: 1–13

137. Harding C V, Chylack L T Jr, Susan S R, Lo W H, Bobrowski W E 1983 Calcium-containing opacities in the human lens. Investigative Ophthalmology and Visual Science 24: 1194–1202

138. Harnisch J P, Barrach H J, Hassell J R, Sinha P K 1981 Identification of a basement membrane proteoglycan in exfoliation material. Albrecht Von Graefes Archiv für Klinische und Experimentalle Ophthalmologie 215: 273–278

139. Harris M, Tso A Y, Kaba F W, Green W R, de la Cruz Z C 1984 Corneal endothelial overgrowth of angle and iris. Evidence of myoblastic differentiation in three cases. Ophthalmology 91: 1154–1160

140. Hartmann C 1982 Studies on the development of extra-endothelial and intra-endothelial pigment deposits by means of direct and indirect contact specular microscopy of the cornea. Graefes Archive for Clinical and Experimental Ophthalmology 218: 75–82

141. Hayes B P, Fisher R F 1979 Influence of a prolonged period of

low-dosage X-rays on the optic and ultrastructural appearances of cataract of the human lens. British Journal of Ophthalmology 63: 457–464

142. Hayes B P, Fisher R F 1984 Ultrastructural appearances of a lens with marked polychromatic lustre: evidence for diffraction as a cause. British Journal of Ophthalmology 68: 553–560

143. Henriquez A S, Kenyon K R, Dohlman C H, Boruchoff S A, Forstot S L, Meyer R F, Hanninen L A 1984 Morphologic characteristics of posterior polymorphous dystrophy. A study of nine corneas and review of the literature. Survey of Ophthalmology 29: 139–147

144. Henson D, Helmsen R, Becker K E, Strano A J, Sullivan M, Harris D 1974 Ultrastructural localization of herpes simplex virus antigens on rabbit corneal cells using sheep antihuman IgG antihorse ferritin hybrid antibodies. Investigative Ophthalmology 13: 819–827

145. Hersch P S, Green W R, Thomas J V 1981 Tractional venous loops in diabetic retinopathy. American Journal of Ophthalmology 92: 661–671

146. Herschler J, Davis E B 1980 Modified goniotomy for inflammatory glaucoma. Histologic evidence for the mechanism of pressure reduction. Archives of Ophthalmology 98: 688–696

147. Hirst L W, Sanborn G, Green W R, Miller N R, Heath W D 1982 Amodiaquine ocular changes. Archives of Ophthalmology 100: 1300–1304

148. Hiscott P S, Grierson I, Hitchins C A, Rahi A H, McLeod D 1983 Epiretinal membranes in vitro. Transactions of the Ophthalmological Society of the United Kingdom 103: 89–102

149. Hogan M J, Wood I, Fine M 1974 Fuchs' endothelial dystrophy of the cornea. 29th Sanford Gifford Memorial lecture. American Journal of Ophthalmology 78: 363–383

150. Holladay J T, Bishop J E, Lewis J W 1985 Diagnosis and treatment of mysterious light streaks seen by patients following extracapsular cataract extraction. Journal of the American Intraocular Implant Society 11: 21–23

151. Hollenberg M J, Wilkie J S, Hudson J B, Lewis B J 1976 Lesions produced by human herpes viruses 1 and 2. Morphologic features in rabbit corneal epithelium. Archives of Ophthalmology 94: 127–134

152. Hori S, Tanishima T 1982 Transmission and scanning electron microscopic studies on endothelial cells in macular corneal dystrophy. Japanese Journal of Ophthalmology 26: 190–198

153. Huey C, Jakobiec F A, Iwamoto T, Kennedy R, Farmer E R, Green W R 1983 Discoid lupus erythematosus of the eyelids. Ophthalmology 90: 1389–1398

154. Ingraham H J, Guber D, Green W R 1985 Radial keratotomy. Clinicopathologic case report. Archives of Ophthalmology 103: 683–688

155. Ishida N, Brown A C, Rao G N, Aquavella J V, del Cerro M 1984 Recurrent Fusarium keratomycosis: a light and electron microscopic study. Annals of Ophthalmology 16: 354–356, 358–360, 362–366

156. Iwamoto T, Stuart J C, Srinivasan B D, Mund M L, Farris R L, Donn A, DeVoe A G 1975 Ultrastructural variation in granular dystrophy of the cornea. Albrecht Von Graefes Archiv für Klinische und Experimentalle Ophthalmologie 194: 1–9

157. Jaben S L, Flynn J T, Parker J C 1983 Neuronal ceroid lipofuscinosis. Diagnosis from peripheral blood smear. Ophthalmology 90: 1373–1377

158. Jakobiec F A, Marboe C C, Knowles D M II, Iwamoto T, Harrison W, Chang S, Coleman D J 1983 Human sympathetic ophthalmia. An analysis of the inflammatory infiltrate by hybridoma-monoclonal antibodies, immunochemistry, and correlative electron microscopy. Ophthalmology 90: 76–95

159. Jensen O A 1977 Bruch's membrane in pseudoxanthoma elasticum. Histochemical, ultrastructural, and X-ray microanalytical study of the membrane and angioid streak areas. Albrecht Von Graefes Archiv für Klinische und Experimentalle Ophthalmologie 203: 311–320

160. Jensen O A, Laursen A B 1980 Human senile cataract. Light and electron microscopic studies of the morphology of the anterior lens structures, with special reference of anterior capsular/subcapsular opacity. Acta Ophthalmologica (Copenhagen) 58: 481–495

161. John T, Sassani J W, Eagle R C Jr 1982 Scanning electron microscopy of rubeosis iridis. Transactions of the Pennsylvania Academy of Ophthalmology and Otolaryngology 35: 119–121

162. John T, Sassani J W, Eagle R C Jr 1983 The myofibroblastic component of rubeosis iridis. Ophthalmology 90: 721–728

163. Johnson B L, Brown S I 1976 Congenital epithelialization of the posterior cornea. American Journal of Ophthalmology 82: 83–89

164. Johnson B L, Brown S I 1978 Posterior polymorphous dystrophy: a light and electron microscopic study. British Journal of Ophthalmology 62: 89–96

165. Johnson B L, Brown S I, Zaidman G W 1981 A light and electron microscopic study of recurrent granular dystrophy of the cornea. American Journal of Ophthalmology 92: 49–58

166. Johnson D H, Bourne W M, Campbell R J 1982 The ultrastructure of Descemet's membrane. II. Aphakic bullous keratopathy. Archives of Ophthalmology 100: 1948–1951

167. Johnson G J, Ghosh M 1975 Labrador keratopathy: clinical and pathological findings. Canadian Journal of Ophthalmology 10: 119–135

168. Johnson N F 1977 Distribution of acid mucopolysaccharides in normal and detached retinae. A study by electron microscopy. Transactions of the Ophthalmology Society of the United Kingdom 97: 557–564

169. Kaiser-Kupfer M I, Kupfer C, Rodrigues M M 1981 Tamoxifen retinopathy. A clinicopathologic report. Ophthalmology 88: 89–93

170. Kampik A, Green W R, Michels R G, Nase P K 1980 Ultrastructural features of progressive idiopathic epiretinal membrane removed by vitreous surgery. American Journal of Ophthalmology 90: 797–809

171. Kampik A, Green W R, Quigley H A, Pierce L H 1981 Scanning and transmission electron microscopic studies of two cases of pigment dispersion syndrome. American Journal of Ophthalmology 91: 573–587

172. Kampik A, Kenyon K R, Michels R G, Green W R, de la Cruz Z C 1981 Epiretinal and vitreous membranes. Comparative study of 56 cases. Archives of Ophthalmology 99: 1445–1454

173. Kampik A, Patrinely J R, Green W R 1982 Morphologic and clinical features of retrocorneal melanin pigmentation and pigmented pupillary membranes: review of 225 cases. Survey of Ophthalmology 27: 161–180

174. Kampik A, Sani J N, Green W R 1980 Ocular ochronosis. Clinicopathological, histochemical, and ultrastructural studies. Archives of Ophthalmology 98: 1441–1447

175. Kanai A, Kaufman H E 1982 The retrocorneal ridge in syphilitic and herpetic interstitial keratitis: an electron-microscopic study. Annals of Ophthalmology 14: 120–124

176. Kenyon K R, Green W R 1979 Inborn lysosomal diseases. In: Johannessen J V (ed) Electron microscopy in human medicine, vol. 6. McGraw-Hill, New York, pp 267–283

177. Kenyon K R, Van Horn D L, Edelhauser H F 1978 Endothelial degeneration and posterior collagenous proliferation in aphakic bullous keratopathy. American Journal of Ophthalmology 85: 329–336

178. Kerr Muir M G, Sherrard E S 1985 Damage to the corneal endothelium during Nd/YAG photodisruption. British Journal of Ophthalmology 65: 77–85

179. Khalil M K, Finlayson M H 1980 Electron microscopy in iris nevus syndrome. Canadian Journal of Ophthalmology 15: 44–48

180. Kishi S, Numaga T, Yamazaki S 1982 Structure of the inner retinal surface in simple diabetic retinopathy. Japanese Journal of Ophthalmology 26: 141–149

181. Kiskaddon B M, Campbell R J, Waller R R, Bourne W M 1980 Fleck dystrophy of the cornea: case report. Annals of Ophthalmology 12: 700–704

182. Kjer P, Jensen O A, Klinken L 1983 Histopathology of eye, optic nerve and brain in a case of dominant optic atrophy. Acta Ophthalmologica (Copenhagen) 61: 300–312

183. Klemen U M, Freyler H, Kulnig W 1980 Electron microscopical studies on the resorption of vitreous hemorrhages. Albrecht Von Graefes Archiv für Klinische und Experimentalle Ophthalmologie 214: 245–251

184. Klemen U M, Kulnig W, Radda T M 1983 Secondary corneal amyloidosis: clinical and pathohistological examinations. Graefes Archive for Clinical and Experimental Ophthalmology 220: 130–138

185. Klintworth G K 1980 Research into the pathogenesis of macular

corneal dystrophy. Transactions of the Ophthalmological Society of the United Kingdom 100: 186–194

186. Klintworth G K 1980 Corneal dystrophies. In: Nicholson E H (ed) Ocular pathology update. Masson, New York, pp 23–54

187. Klintworth G K 1982 Macular corneal dystrophy — a localized disorder of mucopolysaccharides metabolism? Progress in Clinical and Biological Research 82: 69–101

188. Klintworth G K 1982 Current concept of macular corneal dystrophy. Birth Defects 18: 463–477

189. Klintworth G K 1982 Disorders of glycosaminoglycans (mucopolysaccharides) and proteoglycans. In: Garner A, Klintworth G K (eds) Pathobiology of ocular disease. A dynamic approach. Marcel Dekker, New York, pp 863–895

190. Klintworth G K 1982 Disorders of amino acid metabolism in ocular disease. In: Garner A, Klintworth G K (eds) Pathobiology of ocular disease. A dynamic approach. Marcel Dekker, New York, pp 947–964

191. Klintworth G K 1982 Vitamin deficiencies and excesses. In: Garner A, Klintworth G K (eds) Pathobiology of ocular disease. A dynamic approach. Marcel Dekker, New York, pp 1107–1123

192. Klintworth G K 1982 Proteins in ocular disease. In: Garner A, Klintworth G K (eds) Pathobiology of ocular disease. A dynamic approach. Marcel Dekker, New York, pp 965–1008

193. Klintworth G K, Bredehoeft S J, Reed J W 1978 Analysis of corneal crystalline deposits in multiple myeloma. American Journal of Ophthalmology 86: 303–313

194. Klintworth G K, Ferry A P, Sugar A, Reed J 1982 Recurrence of lattice corneal dystrophy type I in corneal grafts of two siblings. American Journal of Ophthalmology 94: 540–546

195. Klintworth G K, McCracken J S 1979 Corneal diseases. In: Johannessen J V (ed) Electron microscopy in human medicine. McGraw-Hill, New York, pp 239–266

196. Klintworth G K, Reed J, Stainer G A, Binder P S 1983 Recurrence of macular corneal dystrophy within grafts. American Journal of Ophthalmology 95: 60–72

197. Klintworth G K, Streeten B W, Eagle R C 1989 Applications of energy dispersive microprobe analysis in ophthalmic pathology. In: Ingram P, Shelburne J, Roggli V L (eds) Microprobe analysis in medicine. Hemisphere Publishing Corporation, New York, pp 253–290

198. Kloucek F 1975 Corneal superficial unwettable defect. II. Electron microscopic study. Albrecht Von Graefes Archiv für Klinische und Experimentalle Ophthalmologie 194: 23–38

199. Kloucek F 1977 Familial band-shaped keratopathy and spheroidal degeneration. Clinical and electron microscopic study. Albrecht Von Graefes Archiv für Klinische und Experimentalle Ophthalmologie 205: 47–59

200. Knowles D M, Jakobiec F A, Rosen M, Howard G 1975 Amyloidosis of the orbit and adnexae. Survey of Ophthalmology 19: 367–384

201. Krachmer J H, Schnitzer J I, Fratkin J 1981 Cornea pseudoguttata: a clinical and histopathologic description of endothelial cell edema. Archives of Ophthalmology 99: 1377–1381

202. Kraff M C, Sanders D R, Lieberman H L, Peyman G A, Levine R A 1980 Membrane formation after implantation of polyvinyl alcohol-coated intraocular lenses. Journal of the American Intraocular Implant Society 6: 129–136

203. Kretzer F L, Hittner H M, Johnson A T, Mehta R S, Godio L B 1982 Vitamin E and retrolental fibroplasia ultrastructural support of clinical efficacy. Annals of the New York Academy of Sciences 393: 145–166

204. Kretzer F L, Mehta R S, Johnson A T, Hunter D G, Brown E S, Hittner H M 1984 Vitamin E protects against retinopathy of prematurity through action on spindle cells. Nature 309: 793–795

205. Kupfer C, Kuwabara T, Stark W J 1975 The histopathology of Peters' anomaly. American Journal of Ophthalmology 80: 653–660

206. Kurz G H, Shakib M, Sohmer K K, Friedman A H 1976 The retina in type 5 hyperlipoproteinemia. American Journal of Ophthalmology 82: 32–43

207. Kuwabara T, Lessell S 1976 Electron microscopic study of extraocular muscles in myotonic dystrophy. American Journal of Ophthalmology 82: 303–309

208. Lahav M, Albert D M, Buyukmihci N, Jampol L, McLean E B, Howard R, Craft J 1977 Ocular changes in Lawrence Moon Bardet Biedl Syndrome: a clinical and histopathologic study of a case. Advances in Experimental Medicine and Biology 77: 51–84

209. Lahav M, Cadet J C, Chirambo M, Rehani U, Ishii Y 1982 Corneal keloids — a histopathological study. Graefes Archive for Clinical and Experimental Ophthalmology 218: 256–261

210. Lake B D, Milla P J, Taylor D S, Young E P 1982 A mild variant of mucolipidosis type 4 (ML4). Birth Defects 18: 391–404

211. Layden W E, Shaffer R N 1974 Exfoliation syndrome. American Journal of Ophthalmology 78: 835–841

212. Lee W R, Grierson I 1977 Macrophage infiltration in the human retina. Albrecht Von Graefes Archiv für Klinische und Experimentalle Ophthalmologie 203: 293–309

213. Libert J, Danis P 1979 Differential diagnosis of type A, B, and C Niemann–Pick disease by conjunctival biopsy. An ultrastructural study of 16 cases. Journal of Submicroscopic Cytology 11: 143–157

214. Libert J, Tondeur M, Van Hoof F 1976 The use of conjunctival biopsy and enzyme analysis in tears for the diagnosis of homozygotes and heterozygotes with Fabry disease. Birth Defects 12: 221–239

215. Lindberg K A, Pinnell S R 1982 Collagen and its disorders. In: Garner A, Klintworth G K (eds) Pathobiology of ocular disease. A dynamic approach. Marcel Dekker, New York, pp 1009–1031

216. Lindsey P S, Michels R G, Luckenbach M, Green W R 1983 Ultrastructure of epiretinal membrane causing retinal starfold. Ophthalmology 90: 578–583

217. Lohman L E, Rao G N, Tripathi R C, Tripathi B J, Aquavella J V 1982 In vivo specular microscopy of edematous human corneal epithelium with light and scanning electron microscopic correlation. Ophthalmology 89: 621–629

218. Luckenbach M W, Green W R, Miller N R, Moser H W, Clark A W, Tennekoon G 1983 Ocular clinicopathologic correlation of Hallervorden–Spatz syndrome with acanthocytosis and pigmentary retinopathy. American Journal of Ophthalmology 95: 369–382

219. Ludatscher R M, Meyer E, Zonis S, Lichtig C 1984 Capillaries of human overacting extraocular muscles. Investigative Ophthalmology and Visual Science 25: 1441–1447

220. Lütjen-Drecoll E, Futa R, Rohen J W 1981 Ultrahistochemical studies on tangential sections of the trabecular meshwork in normal and glaucomatous eyes. Investigative Ophthalmology and Visual Science 21: 563–773

221. MacLeod C, Murphy A 1982 Herpes zoster: complications, pathogenesis and pathology. The specialist view. Australian Family Physician 11: 173–177

222. Maglio M, McMahon C, Hoskins D, Alvarado J 1980 Potential artifacts in scanning electron microscopy of the trabecular meshwork in glaucoma. American Journal of Ophthalmology 90: 645–653

223. Mannis M J, Fiori C E, Krachmer J R, Rodrigues M M, Pardos G 1981 Keratopathy associated with intracorneal glass. Archives of Ophthalmology 99: 850–852

224. Mannis M J, Krachemer J H, Rodrigues M M, Pardos G J 1981 Polymorphic amyloid degeneration of the cornea. A clinical and histopathological study. Archives of Ophthalmology 99: 1217–1233

225. Marshall J, Bird A C 1979 A comparative histopathologic study of argon and krypton laser irradiations of the human retina. British Journal of Ophthalmology 63: 657–668

226. Martin J J, Ceuterick C, Martin L, Libert J 1977 Skin and conjunctival biopsies in adrenoleukodystrophy. Acta Neuropathologica (Berlin) 38: 247–250

227. Martin J J, Leroy J G, Libert J, van Eygen M, Logghe N 1979 Skin and conjunctival biopsies in an infantile neuroaxonal dystrophy. Acta Neuropathologica (Berlin) 45: 247–451

228. Mason C M, Sugar A, Meyer R F 1984 Intrastromal crystalline deposits following corneal graft rejection. Cornea 3: 89–94

229. Matsuura H, Setogawa T, Tamai A 1976 Electron microscopic studies on retinal capillaries in human diabetic retinopathy. Yonago Acta Medica 20: 7–10

230. Maul E, Strozzi L, Muñoz C, Reyes C 1980 The outflow pathway in congenital glaucoma. American Journal of Ophthalmology 89: 667–673

231. McDonald J E, Roy F H, Hanna C 1974 Mechanism of formation of lentoid of Thiel. Annals of Ophthalmology 6: 899–901, 903–904

232. McDonnell J M, Green W R, Maumenee I H 1985 Ocular histopathology of systemic mucopolysaccharidosis, type II-A (Hunter syndrome, severe). Ophthalmology 92: 1772–1779
233. McDonnell P J, Green W R, Stevens R E, Bargeron C B, Riquelme J L 1985 Blood staining of the cornea. Light microscopic and ultrastructural features. Ophthalmology 92: 1668–1674
234. McDonnell P J, Zarbin M A, Green W R 1983 Posterior capsule opacification in pseudophakic eyes. Ophthalmology 90: 1548–1553
235. McKechnie N M, Ghafour I M 1982 Potential retinal light damage from the use of therapeutic instruments. Transactions of the Ophthalmological Society of the United Kingdom 102: 140–146
236. McKechnie N M, King M, Lee W R 1985 Retinal pathology in the Kearns–Sayre syndrome. British Journal of Ophthalmology 69: 63–75
237. Meisler D M, Langston R H S, Naab T J, Aaby A A, McMahon J T, Tubbs R R 1984 Infectious crystalline keratopathy. American Journal of Ophthalmology 97: 337–343
238. Meltzer D W 1980 Sterile hypopyon following intraocular lens surgery. Archives of Ophthalmology 98: 100–104
239. Mensheha-Manhart O, Rodrigues M M, Shields J A, Shannon G M, Mirabelli R P 1975 Retinal pigment epithelium in incontinentia pigmenti. American Journal of Ophthalmology 79: 571–577
240. Messmer E, Font R L, Sheldon G, Murphy D 1983 Pigmented conjunctival cysts following tetracycline/minocycline therapy. Histochemical and electron microscopic observations. Ophthalmology 90: 1462–1468
241. Messmer G, Isakow I, Dabush S, Romem M 1983 Post-traumatic recurrent corneal erosion, #2. Ultrastructural findings in epithelium and stroma. Metabolic, Pediatric and Systemic Ophthalmology 7: 59–66
242. Metcalf J E, Helmsen R 1977 Immunoelectron microscopic localization of herpes simplex virus antigens in rabbit cornea with antihuman IgG–antiferritin hybrid antibodies. Investigative Ophthalmology and Visual Science 16: 779–786
243. Meyer E, Haim T, Zonis S, Gidoni O, Gitay H, Levanon D, Nir I 1984 Pseudoexfoliation: epidemiology, clinical and scanning electron microscopic study. Ophthalmologica 188: 141–147
244. Meyer E, Ludatscher R M, Zonis S 1984 Primary and secondary overacting inferior oblique muscles: an ultrastructural study. British Journal of Ophthalmology 68: 416–420
245. Meyer E, Scharf Y, Schechner R, Zonis S, Scharf Y, Nahir M 1985 Light and electron microscopical study of the conjunctiva in sicca syndrome. Ophthalmologica 190: 45–51
246. Meyer K T, Heckenlively J R, Sptiznas M, Foos R Y 1982 Dominant retinitis pigmentosa. A clinicopathologic correlation. Ophthalmology 89: 1414–1424
247. Michels R G 1982 A clinical and histopathologic study of epiretinal membranes affecting the macula and removed by vitreous surgery. Transactions of the American Ophthalmological Society 80: 580–656
248. Miley C E, Gilbert E F, France T D, O'Brien J F, Chun R W M 1978 Clinical and extraneural histologic diagnosis of neuronal ceroid-lipofuscinosis. Neurology 28: 1008–1012
249. Miller F S III, Bunt-Milam A H, Kalina R E 1982 Clinical-ultrastructural study of thioridazine retinopathy. Ophthalmology 89: 1478–1488
250. Miller H, Miller B, Rabinowitz H, Zonis S, Nir I 1983 Asteroid bodies – an ultrastructural study. Investigative Ophthalmology and Visual Science 24: 133–136
251. Miller H, Miller B, Zonis S, Nir I 1984 Diabetic neovascularization: permeability and ultrastructure. Investigative Ophthalmology and Visual Science 25: 1338–1342
252. Munton C G, Tandon M K 1983 Optiflex angle fixation lens. Journal of the American Intraocular Implant Society 9: 171–175
253. Murata M, Yoshimoto H 1983 Morphological study of the pathogenesis of retinal cotton wool spot. Japanese Journal of Ophthalmology 27: 362–379 (in Japanese)
254. Nakanishi I, Brown S I 1975 Ultrastructure of the epithelial dystrophy of Meesman. Archives of Ophthalmology 93: 259–263
255. Neetens A, Dockx P, Smets R M, Jacob W 1979 Fate of conjunctival argyrosis. Bulletin de la Societe Belge d'Ophtalmologie 186: 101–107
256. Neetens A, Martin J J 1983 Superior oblique myokymia in a case of hereditary metabolic neurodegenerative disease (adrenoleucodystrophy). Bulletin de la Societe Belge d'Ophtalmologie 208: 219–223
257. Neetens A, Rubbens M C 1977 Hyperproduction glaucoma. Transactions of the Ophthalmological Society of the United Kingdom 97: 701–708
258. Neetens A, Verschueren C, De Smet N, Delgadillo R 1981 Bilateral endogenous endophthalmitis. Bulletin de la Societe Belge d'Ophtalmologie 193: 123–130
259. Nesburn A B, Borit A, Pentelei-Molnar J, Lazaro R 1974 Varicella dendritic keratitis. Investigative Ophthalmology 13: 764–770
260. Newsome D A, Rodrigues M M, Machemer R 1981 Human massive periretinal proliferation. *In vitro* characteristics of cellular components. Archives of Ophthalmology 99: 873–880
261. Nicholson D H, Green W R, Cross H E, Kenyon H R, Massof D 1977 A clinical and histopathological study of Francois–Neetens speckled corneal dystrophy. American Journal of Ophthalmology 83: 554–560
262. Nik N A, Hidayat A, Zimmerman L E, Fine B S 1981 Diffuse iris nevus manifested by unilateral open angle glaucoma. Archives of Ophthalmology 99: 125–127
263. Nirankari V S, Karesh J, Bastion F, Lakhanpal V, Billings E 1983 Recurrence of keratoconus in donor cornea 22 years after successful keratoplasty. British Journal of Ophthalmology 67: 23–28
264. Novotny G E, Pau H 1984 Myofibroblast-like cells in human anterior capsular cataract. Virchows Archiv A, Pathological Anatomy and Histopathology 404: 393–401
265. O'Conner G R 1982 Protozoal infections. In: Garner A, Klintworth G K (eds) Pathobiology of ocular disease. A dynamic approach. Marcel Dekker, New York, pp 345–358
266. Offret H, Saraux H 1981 Corneal decompensation in Chandler's syndrome. Clinical, histopathologic and ultrastructural study. Ophthalmologica 182: 130–135
267. Ohnishi Y, Shinoda Y, Ishibashi T, Taniguchi Y 1982–83 The origin of amyloid in gelatinous drop-like corneal dystrophy. Current Eye Research 2: 225–231
268. Olander K, Kanai A, Kaufman H E 1983 An analytical electron microscopic study of a corneal tattoo. Annals of Ophthalmology 15: 1046–1049
269. Olson L E, Marshall J, Rice N S, Andrews R 1978 Effects of ultrasound on the corneal endothelium: I. The acute lesion. British Journal of Ophthalmology 62: 134–144
270. Orellana J, O'Malley R E, McPherson A R, Font R L 1985 Pigmented free-floating vitreous cysts in two young adults. Electron microscopic observations. Ophthalmology 92: 297–302
271. Partamian L G, Morse P H, Klein H Z 1981 Herpes simplex type 1 retinitis in an adult with systemic herpes zoster. American Journal of Ophthalmology 92: 215–220
272. Patel A, Kenyon K R, Hirst L W, Quigley H A, Stark W J, Meyer R F, Green W R 1983 Clinicopathologic features of Chandler's syndrome. Survey of Ophthalmology 27: 327–344
273. Patrinely J R, Lewis R A, Font R L 1985 Foveomacular vitelliform dystrophy, adult type. A clinicopathologic study including electron microscopic observations. Ophthalmology 92: 1712–1718
274. Perry H D, Fine B S, Caldwell D R 1979 Reis–Bückler's dystrophy. A study of eight cases. Archives of Ophthalmology 97: 664–670
275. Pinnolis M, Egbert P R, Font R L, Winter F C 1981 Nosematosis of the cornea. Case report, including electron microscopic studies. Archives of Ophthalmology 99: 1044–1047
276. Pokorny K S, Ritch R, Friedman A H, Desnick R J 1982 Ultrastructure of the eye in fetal type II glycogenosis (Pompe's disease). Investigative Ophthalmology and Visual Science 22: 25–31
277. Polack F M 1974 The posterior corneal surface in Fuchs' dystrophy. Scanning electron microscope study. Investigative Ophthalmology 13: 913–922
278. Polack F M 1976 Contributions of electron microscopy to the study of corneal pathology. Survey of Ophthalmology 20: 375–414
279. Polack F M, Binder P S 1975 Detachment of Descemet's membrane from grafts following wound separation: light and electron microscopic study. Annals of Ophthalmology 7: 47–54
280. Polack F M, Bourne W M, Forstot S L, Yamaguchi T 1980 Scanning electron microscopy of posterior polymorphous corneal dystrophy. American Journal of Ophthalmology 89: 575–584

281. Polack F M, Graue E L 1979 Scanning electron microscopy of congenital corneal leukomas (Peters' anomaly). American Journal of Ophthalmology 88: 169–178
282. Pouliquen Y, Dhermy P, Renard G, Giraud J P, Savoldelli M 1980 Combined macular dystrophy and cornea guttata: an electron microscopic study. Albrecht Von Graefes Archiv für Klinische und Experimentalle Ophthalmologie 212: 149–158
283. Prause J U, Jensen O A 1981 Studies on human corneal ulcers treated with histoacrylic glue. Morphological studies of a successful and unsuccessful membrane. Acta Ophthalmologica (Copenhagen) 59: 674–682
284. Proia A D, Foulks G N, Sanfilippo F P 1985 Ocular cicatricial pemphigoid with granular IgA and complement deposition. Archives of Ophthalmology 103: 1669–1672
285. Puck A, Tso M O, Fishman G A 1985 Drusen of the optic nerve associated with retinitis pigmentosa. Archives of Ophthalmology 103: 231–234
286. Purcell J J Jr, Rodrigues M, Chisti M I, Riner R N, Dooley J M 1983 Lattice corneal dystrophy associated with familial systemic amyloidosis (Meretoja's syndrome). Ophthalmology 90: 1512–1517
287. Quigley H A, Addicks E M 1980 Scanning electron microscopy of trabeculectomy specimens from eyes with open-angle glaucoma. American Journal of Ophthalmology 90: 854–857
288. Quigley H A, Addicks E M 1981 Regional differences in the structure of the lamina cribrosa and their relation to glaucomatous optic nerve damage. Archives of Ophthalmology 99: 137–143
289. Quigley H A, Addicks E M, Green W R, Maumenee A E 1981 Optic nerve damage in human glaucoma. II. The site of injury and susceptibility to damage. Archives of Ophthalmology 99: 635–649
290. Quigley H A, Green W R 1979 The histology of human glaucoma cupping and optic nerve damage: clinicopathologic correlation in 21 eyes. Ophthalmology 86: 1803–1830
291. Radius R L, Herschler J 1980 Histopathology in the iris–nevus (Cogan–Reese) syndrome. American Journal of Ophthalmology 89: 780–786
292. Rafferty N S, Gossens W 1977 Ultrastructure of traumatic cataractogenesis in the frog: a comparison with mouse and human lens. American Journal of Anatomy 148: 385–407
293. Rafferty N S, Gossens W, March W F 1974 Ultrastructure of human traumatic cataract. American Journal of Ophthalmology 78: 985–995
294. Rahi A H, Chapman C M, Garner A, Wright P 1976 Pathology of practolol-induced ocular toxicity. British Journal of Ophthalmology 60: 312–323
295. Rao N A, Font R L 1977 Toxoplasmic retinochoroiditis. Electron-microscopic and immunofluorescence studies of formalin-fixed tissue. Archives of Ophthalmology 95: 273–277
296. Rayborn M E, Moorhead L C, Hollyfield J G 1982 A dominantly inherited chorioretinal degeneration resembling sectoral retinitis pigmentosa. Ophthalmology 89: 1441–1452
297. Rentsch F J 1977 The ultrastructure of preretinal macular fibrosis. Albrecht Von Graefes Archiv für Klinische und Experimentalle Ophthalmologie 203: 321–337
298. Riddle P J, Font R L, Johnson F B, McLean I W 1981 Silica granuloma of eyelid and ocular adnexa. Archives of Ophthalmology 99: 683–687
299. Riedel K G, Zwaan J, Kenyon K R, Kolodny E H, Hanninen L, Albert D M 1985 Ocular abnormalities in mucolipidosis IV. American Journal of Ophthalmology 99: 125–136
300. Riegel E M, Pokorny K S, Friedman A H, Suhan J, Ritch R H, Desnick R J 1982 Ocular pathology of Fabry's disease in a hemizygous male following renal transplantation. Survey of Ophthalmology 26: 247–252
301. Ringvold A, Davanger M 1981 Iris neovascularization in eyes with pseudoexfoliation syndrome. British Journal of Ophthalmology 65: 138–141
302. Robinson C H Jr, Nopanitaya W, McPherson S D Jr 1982 Pigmentary glaucoma: an ultrastructural study. Annals of Ophthalmology 100: 1635–1640
303. Robinson M R, Streeten B W 1984 Energy dispersive X-ray analysis of the cornea. Application to paraffin sections of normal and diseased corneas. Archives of Ophthalmology 102: 1678–1682
304. Rodrigues M M, Ballintine E J, Wiggert B N, Lee L, Fletcher R T,

305. Chader G J 1984 Choroideremia: a clinical, electron microscopic, and biochemical report. Ophthalmology 91: 873–883
305. Rodrigues M M, Currier C A 1983 Histopathology of argon laser photocoagulation in juvenile diabetic retinopathy. Ophthalmology 90: 1023–1027
306. Rodrigues M M, Fine B S, Laibson P R, Zimmerman L E 1974 Disorders of the corneal epithelium. A clinicopathologic study of dot, geographic, and fingerprint patterns. Archives of Ophthalmology 92: 475–482
307. Rodrigues M M, Gaster R N, Pratt M V 1983 Unusual superficial confluent form of granular corneal dystrophy. Ophthalmology 90: 1507–1511
308. Rodrigues M M, Newsome D 1982 Retinitis pigmentosa: electron microscopy and cell culture studies. Birth Defects 18: 81–94
309. Rodrigues M M, Newsome D A, Krachmer J H, Eiferman R A 1981 Pellucid marginal corneal degeneration: a clinicopathologic study of two cases. Experimental Eye Research 33: 277–288
310. Rodrigues M M, Newsome D A, Krachmer J H, Sun T T 1981 Posterior polymorphous dystrophy of the cornea: cell culture studies. Experimental Eye Research 33: 535–544
311. Rodrigues M M, Newsome D A, Machemer R 1981 Further characterization of epiretinal membranes in human massive periretinal proliferation. Current Eye Research 1: 311–315
312. Rodrigues M M, Palestine A, Nussenblatt R, Masur H, Macher A M 1983 Unilateral cytomegalovirus retinochoroiditis and bilateral cytoid bodies in a bisexual man with the acquired immunodeficiency syndrome. Ophthalmology 90: 1577–1582
313. Rodrigues M M, Phelps C D, Krachmer J H, Cibis G W, Weingeist T A 1980 Glaucoma due to endothelialization of the anterior chamber angle. A comparison of posterior polymorphous dystrophy of the cornea and Chandler's syndrome. Archives of Ophthalmology 98: 688–696
314. Rodrigues M M, Spaeth G L, Donohoo P 1982 Electron microscopy of argon laser therapy in phakic open-angle glaucoma. Ophthalmology 89: 198–210
315. Rodrigues M M, Spaeth G L, Moster M, Thomas G, Hackett J 1985 Histopathology of neodymium:YAG laser iridectomy in humans. Ophthalmology 92: 1696–1700
316. Rodrigues M M, Spaeth G L, Sivalingam E, Weinreb S 1976 Histopathology of 150 trabeculectomy specimens in glaucoma. Transactions of the Ophthalmological Society of the United Kingdom 96: 245–255
317. Rodrigues M M, Streeten B W, Krachmer J H, Laibson P R, Salem N Jr, Passonneau J, Chock S 1983 Microfibrillar protein and phospholipid in granular corneal dystrophy. Archives of Ophthalmology 101: 802–810
318. Rodrigues M M, Streeten B, Spaeth G L 1978 Chandler's syndrome as a variant of essential iris atrophy. A clinicopathologic study. Archives of Ophthalmology 96: 643–652
319. Rodrigues M M, Sun T, Krachmer J, Newsome D 1980 Epithelialization of the corneal endothelium in posterior polymorphous dystrophy. Investigative Ophthalmology and Visual Science 19: 832–835
320. Rodrigues M M, Sun T, Krachmer J, Newsome D 1982 Posterior polymorphous corneal dystrophy: recent developments. Birth Defects 18: 479–491
321. Rodrigues M M, Waring G O 1982 Anterior and posterior corneal dystrophies. In: Garner A, Klintworth G K (eds) Pathobiology of ocular disease. A dynamic approach. Marcel Dekker, New York, pp 1153–1166
322. Rodrigues M M, Lennette D A, Arentsen J J, Thompson C 1979 Methods for rapid detection of human ocular viral infections. Ophthalmology 86: 452–464
323. Rohen J W 1982 Presence of matrix vesicles in the trabecular meshwork of glaucomatous eyes. Graefes Archive for Clinical and Experimental Ophthalmology 218: 171–176
324. Rohen J W, Futa R, Lütjen-Drecoll E 1981 The fine structure of the cribiform meshwork in normal and glaucomatous eyes as seen in tangential sections. Investigative Ophthalmology and Visual Science 21: 574–585
325. Roizenblatt J, Grant S, Foos R Y 1980 Vitreous cylinders. Archives of Ophthalmology 98: 734–739
326. Rush J A, Kennerdell J S, Martinez A J 1982 Primary idiopathic

inflammation of the optic nerve. American Journal of Ophthalmology 93: 312–316

327. Salisbury J A, Foulks G N, Klintworth G K 1980 Lens capsular cyst. American Journal of Ophthalmology 90: 229–233

328. Sampaolesi R, Argento C 1977 Scanning electron microscopy of the trabecular meshwork in normal and glaucomatous eyes. Investigative Ophthalmology and Visual Science 16: 302–314

329. Sanderson P O, Kuwabara T, Stark W J, Wong V G, Collins E M 1974 Cystinosis: a clinical, histopathologic and ultrastructural study. Archives of Ophthalmology 91: 270–274

330. Sarks S H 1976 Ageing and degeneration in the macular region: a clinicopathological study. British Journal of Ophthalmology 60: 324–341

331. Sarks S H, Van Driel D, Maxwell L, Killingsworth M 1980 Softening of drusen and subretinal neovascularization. Transactions of the Ophthalmological Society of the United Kingdom 100: 414–422

332. Savino D E, Margo C E 1983 Conjunctival rhinosporidiosis. Light and electron microscopic study. Ophthalmology 90: 1482–1489

333. Scattergood K D, Green W R, Hirst L W 1983 Scrolls in Descemet's membrane in healed syphilitic interstitial keratitis. Ophthalmology 90: 1518–1523

334. Schochet S S, Font R L, Morris H H 1980 Jansky–Bielschowsky form of neuronal ceroid-lipofuscinosis. Ocular pathology of the Batten–Vogt syndrome. Archives of Ophthalmology 98: 1083–1088

335. Schultz R O, Van Horn D L, Peters M A, Klewin K M, Schutten W H 1981 Diabetic keratopathy. Transactions of the American Ophthalmological Society 79: 180–199

336. Schwartz M F, Green W R, Michels R G, Kincaid M C, Fogle J 1982 An unusual case of ocular involvement in primary systemic nonfamilial amyloidosis. Ophthalmology 89: 394–401

337. Sebag J, Albert D M, Craft J L 1984 The Alström syndrome: ophthalmic histopathology and retinal ultrastructure. British Journal of Ophthalmology 68: 494–501

338. Segawa K 1979 Electron microscopic changes of the trabecular tissue in primary open-angle glaucoma. Annals of Ophthalmology 11: 49–54

339. Seland J H 1978 The ultrastructure of the deep layer of the lens capsule in fibrillopathia epitheliocapsularis (FEC), so-called senile exfoliation or pseudoexfoliation. A scanning electron microscopic study. Acta Ophthalmologica 56: 335–348

340. Seland J H 1978 The ultrastructure of the human lens capsule. I. Cataractous lenses from eyes with simple glaucoma. A transmission electron microscopic study. Acta Ophthalmologica 56: 715–722

341. Seland J H 1978 The ultrastructure of the human lens capsule. II. Cataracta complicata. A transmission electron microscopic study. Acta Ophthalmologica 56: 723–734

342. Seland J H 1979 Histopathology of the lens capsule in fibrillopathia epitheliocapsularis (FEC) or so-called senile exfoliation or pseudoexfoliation. An electron microscopic study. Acta Ophthalmologica 57: 477–499

343. Sendele D D, Kenyon K R, Mobilia E F, Rosenthal P, Steinert R, Hanninen L A 1983 Superior limbic keratoconjunctivitis in contact lens wearers. Ophthalmology 90: 616–622

344. Shields M B 1983 Axenfeld–Rieger syndrome: a theory of mechanism and distinctions from their iridocorneal endothelial syndrome. Transactions of the American Ophthalmological Society 81: 736–784

345. Shields M B, Buckley E, Klintworth G K, Thresher R 1985 Axenfeld–Rieger syndrome: a spectrum of developmental disorders. Survey of Ophthalmology 29: 387–409

346. Shields M B, McCracken J S, Klintworth G K, Campbell D G 1979 Corneal edema in essential iris atrophy. Ophthalmology 86: 1533–1548

347. Shimeld C, Tullo A B, Easty D L, Thomsitt J 1982 Isolation of herpes simplex virus from the cornea in chronic stromal keratitis. British Journal of Ophthalmology 66: 643–647

348. Sidrys L A, Demong T 1982 Epithelial downgrowth after penetrating keratoplasty. Canadian Journal of Ophthalmology 17: 29–31

349. Siepser S B, Kline O R Jr 1983 Scanning electron microscopy of removed intraocular lenses. Journal of the American Intraocular Implant Society 9: 176–183

350. Snip R C, Green W R, Kreutzer E W, Hirst L W, Kenyon K R 1981 Posterior corneal pigmentation and fibrous proliferation by iris melanocytes. Archives of Ophthalmology 99: 1232–1238

351. Sommer A 1983 Effects of vitamin A deficiency on the ocular surface. Ophthalmology 90: 592–600

352. Sommer A, Green W R, Kenyon K R 1982 Clinicohistopathologic correlations in xerophthalmic ulceration and necrosis. Archives of Ophthalmology 100: 953–963

353. Spalton D J, Taylor D S I, Sanders M D 1980 Juvenile Batten's disease: an ophthalmological assessment of 26 patients. British Journal of Ophthalmology 64: 726–732

354. Spellacy E, Bankes J L, Crow J, Dourmashkin R, Shah D, Watts R W 1980 Glaucoma in a case of Hurler disease. British Journal of Ophthalmology 64: 773–778

355. Spencer W H, Garron L K, Contreras F, Hayes T L, Lai C 1980 Endogenous and exogenous ocular and systemic silver deposition. Transaction of the Ophthalmological Society of the United Kingdom 100: 171–178

356. Spitznas M, Luciano L, Reale E 1981 Occluding junctions surrounding cystoid spaces in the human peripheral retina. A thin-section and freeze-fracture study. Albrecht Von Graefes Archiv für Klinische und Experimentalle Ophthalmologie 217: 155–165

357. Srinivasan B D, Jakobiec F A, Iwamoto T, DeVoe A G 1978 Epibulbar mucogenic subconjunctival cysts. Archives of Ophthalmology 96: 857–859

358. Steele C, Lucas D R, Ridgway A E 1984 Endophthalmitis due to caterpillar setae: surgical removal and electron microscopic appearances of the setae. British Journal of Ophthalmology 68: 284–288

359. Stefanyszyn M A, Hidayat A A, Flanagan J C 1985 The histopathology of involutional ectropion. Ophthalmology 92: 120–127

360. Streeten B W 1982 Vitreous asteroid bodies. Ultrastructural characteristics and composition. Archives of Ophthalmology 100: 969–975

361. Stuart J C, Mund M L, Iwamoto T, Troutman R C, White H, DeVoe A G 1975 Recurrent granular corneal dystrophy. American Journal of Ophthalmology 79: 18–24

362. Sugar H S 1982 The pseudoexfoliation syndrome. Metabolic, Pediatric and Systemic Ophthalmology 6: 227–235

363. Sugar J, Burnett J, Forstot S L 1978 Scanning electron microscopy of intraocular lens and endothelial cell interaction. American Journal of Ophthalmology 86: 157–161

364. Sutton D P, Green W R, Luckenbach M, Goldberg H K 1983 Retrocorneal smooth-muscle proliferation on rejected corneal dystrophy. Archives of Ophthalmology 101: 429–433

365. Szamier R B 1981 Ultrastructure of the preretinal membrane in retinitis pigmentosa. Investigative Ophthalmology and Visual Science 21: 227–236

366. Takahasi M, Yokota T, Yamashita Y, Ishihara T, Uchino F, Imada N, Matsumoto N 1985 Unusual inclusions in stromal macrophages in a case of gelatinous drop-like corneal dystrophy. American Journal of Ophthalmology 99: 312–316

367. Talamo J H, Topping T M, Maumenee A E, Green W R 1985 Ultrastructural studies of cornea, iris, and lens in a case of siderosis bulbi. Ophthalmology 92: 1675–1680

368. Taylor D, Lake B D, Marshall J, Garner A 1981 Retinal abnormalities in ophthalmoplegic lipidosis. British Journal of Ophthalmology 65: 484–488

369. Taylor H R 1976 A histologic survey of trabeculectomy. American Journal of Ophthalmology 82: 733–735

370. Thomas E L, Michels R G, Rice T A, Green W R, Malouf G 1982 Idiopathic progressive unilateral vitreous fibrosis and secondary traction retinal detachment. Retina 2: 134–144

371. Thresher R J, Ehrenberg M, Machemer R 1984 Gas-mediated vitreous compression: an experimental alternative to mechanized vitrectomy. Graefes Archive for Clinical and Experimental Ophthalmology 221: 192–198

372. Topilow H W, Kenyon K R, Takahasi M, Freeman H M, Tolentino F I, Hanninen L A 1982 Asteroid hyalosis. Biomicroscopy, ultrastructure and composition. Archives of Ophthalmology 100: 964–968

373. Török M, Süveges I 1982 Morphological changes in 'dry eye

syndrome'. Graefes Archive for Clinical and Experimental Ophthalmology 219: 24–28

374. Tremblay M, Dubé I 1982 Meesmann's corneal dystrophy: ultrastructural features. Canadian Journal of Ophthalmology 17: 24–28

375. Trese M, Chandler D B, Machemer R 1983 Macular pucker. II. Ultrastructure. Graefes Archive for Clinical and Experimental Ophthalmology 221: 16–26

376. Tripathi R C 1977 Pathologic anatomy in the outflow pathway of aqueous humour in chronic simple glaucoma. Experimental Eye Research 25: 403–407

377. Tripathi R C, Ashton N 1976 Application of electron microscopy to the study of ocular inborn errors of metabolism. Birth Defects 12: 69–104

378. Tripathi R C, Tripathi B J 1983 Lens morphology, aging, and cataract. Journal of Gerontology 38: 258–270

379. Tso M O 1982 Pathology of cystoid macular edema. Ophthalmology 89: 902–915

380. Tso M O, Fine B S 1976 Electron microscopic study of human papilledema. American Journal of Ophthalmology 82: 424–434

381. Tso M O, Fine B S, Thorpe H E 1975 Kayser–Fleischer ring and associated cataract in Wilson's disease. American Journal of Ophthalmology 79: 479–488

382. Tuppurainen K, Collan Y, Rantanen T, Hollman A 1981 Fabry's disease and cornea verticillata. A report of 3 cases. Acta Ophthalmologica 59: 674–682

383. Van Hoof F, Libert J, Aubert-Tulkens G, Serra M V 1977 The assay of lacrymal enzymes and the ultrastructural analysis of conjunctival biopsies: new techniques for the study of inborn lysosomal diseases. Metabolic Ophthalmology 1: 165–171

384. Van der Zypen E, Fankhauser F 1979 The ultrastructural features of laser trabeculopuncture and cyclodialysis. Problems related to successful treatment of chronic simple glaucoma. Ophthalmologica 179: 189–200

385. Van der Zypen E, Fankhauser F 1982 Lasers in the treatment of chronic simple glaucoma. Transactions of the Ophthalmological Society of the United Kingdom 102: 147–153

386. Van Horn D L, Edelhauser H F, Prodanovich G, Eiferman R, Pederson H F 1977 Effect of the ophthalmic preservative thimerosal on rabbit and human corneal endothelium. Investigative Ophthalmology and Visual Science 16: 273–280

387. Van Rij G, Klepper L, Peperkamp E, Schaap G J 1982 Immune electron microscopy and a cultural test in the diagnosis of adenovirus ocular infection. British Journal of Ophthalmology 66: 317–319

388. Vannas-Sulonen K, Vannas A, O'Donnell J J, Sipila I, Wood I 1983 Pathology of iridectomy specimens in gyrate atrophy of the retina and choroid. Acta Ophthalmologica (Copenhagen) 61: 9–19

389. Vérin P, Gendre P, Maitrot C, Nguyen D T, Nguyen D H 1984 Recent data on trachomatous pannus. Revue Internationale du Trachome et de Pathologie Oculaire Tropicale et Subtropicale et de Sante Publique 61: 61–71

390. Vérin P, Gendre P, Vildy A 1976 Ultrastructural study of trachoma and inclusion conjunctivitis. Differences and Similarities. Revue Internationale du Trachome et de Pathologie Oculaire Tropicale et Subtropicale et de Sante Publique 53: 91–104

391. Vidaurri-Leal J, Hohman R, Glaser B M 1984 Effect of vitreous on morphologic characteristics of retinal pigment epithelial cells. A new approach to the study of proliferative vitreoretinopathy. Archives of Ophthalmology 102: 1220–1223

392. Wallow I H, Geldner P S 1980 Endothelial fenestrae in proliferative diabetic retinopathy. Investigative Ophthalmology and Visual Science 19: 1176–1183

393. Wallow I H, Stevens T S, Greaser M L, Bindley C, Wilson R 1984 Actin filaments in contracting preretinal membranes. Archives of Ophthalmology 102: 1370–1375

394. Walpita P, Darougar S, Thaker U 1985 A rapid and sensitive culture test for detecting Herpes simplex from the eye. British Journal of Ophthalmology 69: 637–639

395. Waring G O III 1982 Posterior collagenous layer of the cornea. Ultrastructural classification of abnormal collagenous tissue posterior to Descemet's membrane in 30 cases. Archives of Ophthalmology 100: 122–134

396. Waring G O III, Bourne W M, Edelhauser H F, Kenyon K R 1982 The corneal endothelium. Normal and pathologic structure and function. Ophthalmology 89: 531–590

397. Waring G O III, Rodrigues M M 1980 Ultrastructure and successful keratoplasty of sclerocornea in Mietens' syndrome. American Journal of Ophthalmology 90: 492–502

398. Waring G O, Rodrigues M M, Laibson P R 1978 Corneal dystrophies. I. Dystrophies of the epithelium, Bowman's layer and stroma. Survey of Ophthalmology 23: 71–122

399. Waring G O III, Rodrigues M M, Laibson P R 1978 Corneal dystrophies. II. Endothelial dystrophies. Survey of Ophthalmology 23: 147–168

400. Warshawsky R S, Hill C W, Doughman D J, Harris J E 1975 Acrodermatitis enteropathica. Corneal involvement with histochemical and electron micrographic studies. Archives of Ophthalmology 93: 194–197

401. Watson P G, Grierson I 1981 The place of trabeculectomy in the treatment of glaucoma. Ophthalmology 88: 175–196

402. Weingeist T A 1974 Argon laser photocoagulation of the human retina. I. Histopathologic correlation of chorioretinal lesions in the region of the maculopapillar bundle. Investigative Ophthalmology 13: 1024–1032

403. Weingeist T A, Blodi F C 1971 Fabry's disease: ocular findings in a female carrier. A light and electron microscopic study. Archives of Ophthalmology 85: 169–176

404. Weingeist T A, Kobrin J L, Watzke R C 1982 Histopathology of Best's macular dystrophy. Archives of Ophthalmology 100: 969–975

405. Weller R O, Rodger F C 1980 Crystalline stromal dystrophy: histochemistry and ultrastructure of the cornea. British Journal of Ophthalmology 64: 46–52

406. Whiting D A, Bristow J H 1975 Dermatitis and keratoconjunctivitis caused by prickly pear (Opuntia microdasys). South African Medical Journal 49:1445–1448

407. WHO Scientific Group 1981 Rapid laboratory techniques for the diagnosis of viral infections. World Health Organization Technical Report Series 661: 1–60

408. Wigand R, Gelderblom H, Ozel M, Distler H, Adrian T 1983 Characteristics of mastadenovirus h 8, the causative agent of epidemic keratoconjunctivitis. Archives of Virology 76: 307–319

409. Winder A F 1982 Disorders of monosaccharide metabolism. In: Garner A, Klintworth G K (eds) Pathobiology of ocular disease. A dynamic approach. Marcel Dekker, New York, pp 1033–1045

410. Winder A F 1982 Disorders of lipid and lipoprotein metabolism. In: Garner A, Klintworth G K (eds) Pathobiology of ocular disease. A dynamic approach. Marcel Dekker, New York, pp 1047–1075

411. Wirz K, Lee W R, Coaker T 1982 Progressive changes in congenital hypertrophy of the retinal pigment epithelium. Graefes Archive for Clinical and Experimental Ophthalmology 219: 214–221

412. Wise J B 1981 Long-term control of adult open angle glaucoma by argon laser treatment. Ophthalmology 88: 89–93

413. Wong V G, Kuwabara T, Brubaker P, Olson W, Schulman J, Seegmiller J E 1970 Intralysosomal cystine crystals in cystinosis. Investigative Ophthalmology 9: 83–88

414. Wong S, Rodrigues M M, Blackman H J, Guimaraes R, Lemp M A 1984 Color specular microscopy of disorders involving the corneal epithelium. Ophthalmology 91: 1176–1183

415. Woodford B, Tso M O 1980 An ultrastructural study of the corpora amylacea of the optic nerve head and retina. American Journal of Ophthalmology 90: 492–502

416. Woog J J, Kenyon K R, Gonder J R, Pavan-Langston D, Hettinger M E, Hamniner L A, Alberg D M, Klintworth G K 1986 Macular corneal dystrophy with clinical features of posterior polymorphous dystrophy. (in preparation)

417. Yamaguchi T, Friedlander M H, Kimura T, Koenig S B, Kaufman H E 1983 The ultrastructure of well-healed lenticules in keratomileusis. Ophthalmology 90: 1495–1506

418. Yamaguchi T, Polack F M, Valenti J 1980 Electron microscopic study of recurrent Reis–Bücklers' corneal dystrophy. American Journal of Ophthalmology 90: 95–101

419. Yamano T, Shimada M, Okada S, Yutaka T, Yabuuchi H, Nakao Y 1979 Electron microscopic examination of skin and conjunctival

biopsy specimens in neuronal storage diseases. Brain and Development 1: 16–25

420. Yanoff M, Fine B S, Brucker A J, Eagle R C Jr 1984 Pathology of human cystoid macular edema. Survey of Ophthalmology 28: 505–511

421. Yanoff M, Fine B S, Colosi N J, Katowitz J A 1977 Lattice corneal dystrophy. Report of an unusual case. Archives of Ophthalmology 95: 651–655

422. Yeo J H, Jakobiec F A, Iwamoto T, Richard G, Kreissig I 1983 Opportunistic toxoplasmic retinochoroiditis following chemotherapy for systemic lymphoma. A light and electron microscopic study. Ophthalmology 90: 885–898

423. Young R D, Watson P G 1982 Light and electron microscopy of corneal melting syndrome (Mooren's ulcer). British Journal of Ophthalmology 66: 341–346

424. Zavala E Y, Binder P S 1980 The pathologic findings of epithelial ingrowth. Archives of Ophthalmology 98: 2007–2014

425. Zimmerman L E, Fine B S 1965 Myelin artifacts in the optic disc and retina. Archives of Ophthalmology 74: 394–398

426. Zwaan J, Kenyon K R 1982 Two brothers with presumed mucolipidosis IV. Birth Defects 18: 381–390

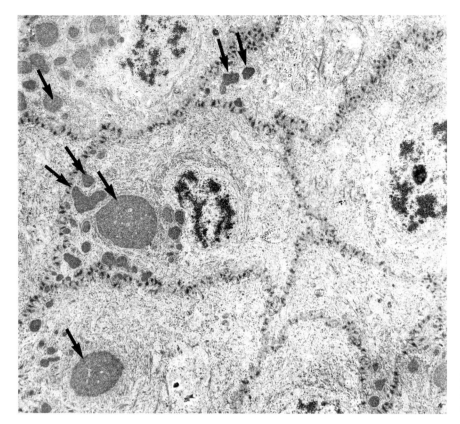

Fig. 24.1 Cornea: Meesmann's dystrophy. Epithelial cells contain variable amounts of electron-dense fibrillogranular material termed 'peculiar substance' (arrows). (× 5800)

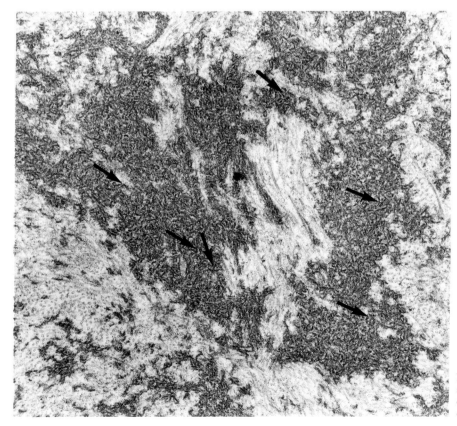

Fig. 24.2 Cornea: Reis–Bücklers dystrophy. The superficial corneal stroma contains characteristic curly fibrils as shown here (arrows) amongst collagen fibres. (× 41 000)

25. The peripheral nervous system

C. Vital

INTRODUCTION

Diseases of the peripheral nervous system, or peripheral neuropathies (PN) are frequent but their aetiology remains unknown in almost 13% of cases.[8] Routine examination of paraffin-embedded sections accounts for only five definitive diagnoses: amyloidosis, lepromatous lesions, vasculitides, sarcoidosis and lymphomatous infiltrates — the three latter entities producing lesions which are visible mainly in the epineurium. Direct immunopathological examination (IPE) provides conclusive information in many cases of IgM monoclonal gammopathy (MG) and in cases of amyloidosis which are secondary to dysglobulinaemia. In many patients the aetiology of a PN is established by the familial background or by metabolic, toxic and immunological data. Light microscopy examination of teased fibres and semithin sections of plastic-embedded fragments — associated with a histogram of the dimensions of myelinated fibres — provides important evidence of the severity of lesions that alter myelinated fibres and of their pathogenesis. However, electron microscopy (EM) is invaluable for elucidating these lesions and for disclosing the aetiology in certain cases, such as intoxications and storage disorders. Post-mortem fragments, however, suffer rapid and dramatic autolytic modifications in axons and myelin sheaths; EM is therefore carried out on biopsies, particularly from sural or superficial peroneal nerves.

ELEMENTARY LESIONS

Experimental pathology had already shown in the 19th century that the two main lesions were Wallerian degeneration resulting from the section of the nerve fibres, and segmental demyelination. These lesions have been studied in detail for the past 25 years and have been correlated with modifications seen on human biopsies;[1-4,13,16,19,23] they now appear more varied and complex. As in other parenchymas, biopsy provides only a 'still-shot' of evolving lesions, and careful attention must be paid to patterns of progression. A particular problem with nerve biopsy is that only two or three centimetres of a very thin one-metre-long axon may be

visible. The status of this axon depends on nutrition from its distant neuronal cytoplasm, by way of axoplasmic flows. It also depends on the state of the myelin sheath surrounding it, with regular internodal wrapping. In fact, the axon and its myelin sheath are very dependent on each other, and the primary site of their injury may be difficult to assess.

Axonal lesions

Wallerian degeneration

Within four days of section or crush of the nerve tract, the myelinated fibres in the distal part are transformed into ovoids and arrayed in a row on longitudinal section. By EM these ovoids appear as entangled myelinic and axonal debris within a Schwann cell (SC) (Fig. 25.1A). These ovoids are then transformed into the bands of Büngner which appear as bands of altered SC cytoplasm enclosed within a basement membrane (Fig. 25.1B). These bands are then penetrated by small axonal sprouts, which grow and form distinct clusters. These clusters appear as closely packed axons, some of which are ensheathed by myelin of varying thickness (Fig. 25.1C) and are easily seen on semithin sections. In human pathology, Wallerian degeneration is seen mainly in cases presenting as focal or multifocal PN due to vasculitides, amyloid deposits or cellular infiltrates.

Neuronopathies

These lesions are due to damage of the neuronal cell body. Wallerian-like lesions may result when such damage is severe.

Distal axonopathies or dying-back neuropathies

These lesions correspond to symmetrical generalized PN; they are probably secondary to a metabolic impairment of the whole axon, but first appear at its distal portions. In experimental conditions such as acrylamide intoxication,[1,13,15] there is intra-axonal filament accumulation at the very distal part of the fibres, and also in some preterminal nodes of Ranvier. A centripetal axonopathy then develops with axonal enlargement due to filament accumulation and thinning of the myelin sheath. Such lesions have been reported in human PN due to industrial agents such as acrylamide and *n*-hexane.[1,15] Similar axonal modifications have been described in the giant axonal neuropathy observed in children, which is probably an autosomal recessive illness.[1]

Other axonal lesions

a. Permanent axotomy has been thoroughly studied by Dyck et al[4] on amputated cats. The axon volume is progressively reduced, and the myelin undergoes progressive modifications: crenations, infoldings and wrinkling. Dyck et al[4] concluded that there is a similarity between these lesions and those observed in uraemic neuropathy.
b. Enlarged axons, which are also crowded with vesicular bodies, abnormal mitochondria and bundles of filaments, are sometimes observed in vascular disorders (Fig. 25.1D), and this has been reproduced in experimental conditions.
c. Polyglucosan bodies and/or rounded vesicles full of glycogen accumulate only rarely in human neuropathies, but without any specificity.[19]

Myelinated nerve fibre loss

This can be estimated from histograms of nerve fibre dimensions made from transversely-cut semithin sections. The loss may be homogeneous or may predominantly affect large or small fibres, thereby altering the normal bimodal distribution.[4]

Unmyelinated fibres

These can be validly studied and counted only by EM. In cases of acute degeneration the axons are enlarged with a watery appearance. In chronic PN some axons are flattened, or have even disappeared.[9] Occasionally, there are enlarged axons crowded with tubular and vesicular structures. There are numerous collagen pockets in certain fibres (Fig. 25.1E), but these formations can be seen in normal nerves. Regenerating fibres appear as miniature axonal sprouts located at the periphery of SC cytoplasm rich in organelles. It may be difficult to distinguish altered unmyelinated fibres from certain bands of Büngner.

Primary myelin modifications

Myelin is a very frail structure and its modifications have to be cautiously considered at ultrastructural examination. It must be established, firstly, that myelin alterations are not secondary to technical artefacts and, secondly, that they are

not due to primary axonal damage, as has been emphasized by Dyck et al.[4] Indeed, the best feature indicating primary demyelination is the presence of a naked intact axon, or of an axon wrapped in a myelin sheath which is too thin for its diameter; the latter points to a remyelinating process following prior demyelination. Such a fibre should be well isolated and not belong to a cluster of regenerating fibres; this pitfall is more frequent on examination of semithin sections, and can be avoided by the combined interpretation of teased fibres and careful electron microscopy. At times, this problem is more difficult when SC processes containing small axons without myelin are present around such a demyelinated fibre.

Non-inflammatory segmental demyelination

This can be observed in certain metabolic and hereditary PN (Fig. 25.2A). Primary myelinic modifications are present in certain leukodystrophies and are associated with intralysosomal accumulation of specific inclusions.[1,2,4,6,14,16,19,20]

Inflammatory demyelination

This was first studied in experimental allergic neuritis and Marek's disease.[6] Biopsies from cases of inflammatory demyelinating PN — the Guillain–Barré syndrome and allied conditions — exhibit certain of these lesions.[11,19] The most frequent and prominent lesion is a macrophage invading the SC cytoplasm and peeling away myelin lamellae by clear elongated processes (Fig. 25.2B); however, the axon remains almost normal. This phenomenon is also called active demyelination. Other myelin modifications observed in experimental conditions are occasionally observed in human cases. Vesicular disruption of some myelin sheaths (VDMS) was present only in seven biopsies from 65 cases of the Guillain–Barré syndrome studied in our laboratory in the past 13 years. Moreover, less than 1% of the myelinated fibres were affected in these seven biopsies. It is likely that most of the VDMS reported on post-mortem peripheral nerves and spinal roots was of autolytic origin. Yet this particular mode of myelin disruption was present in 22% of myelinated fibres in one biopsy from a diabetic patient with the Guillain-Barré syndrome[20] (Fig. 25.2C).

Atypical myelin organizations

These are known in experimental conditions[5] and especially in cultures of peripheral myelin treated with serum from animals with experimental allergic neuritis.[12] In human pathology the following two distinct conditions exist:

1. Widening of some myelin lamellae (WML) — consisting of increased spacing of some lamellae which are usually joined to each other and to the normal portion of the

myelin sheaths (Fig. 25.2, D and E). It has been described by Sluga[14] in a case of myeloma, and subsequently in cases of Waldenström's macroglobulinaemia. Until now, it has been almost exclusively reported in cases of Waldenström's macroglobulinaemia, and of benign IgM monoclonal gammopathy.[16,18,19] Almost all these cases exhibited a typical fixation of anti-IgM serum on myelin sheaths at direct immunopathological examination. King & Thomas[5] have carefully analysed this characteristic spacing and have estimated that the distance between the separated leaflets of the intermediate line is 23 nm. This spacing can be seen in the outer mesaxon and is sometimes limited to the outermost lamella of the myelin sheath or of an additional loop. Such a restricted widening must not be confused with the peeling away of a myelin lamella by an elongated macrophage process. Curiously, until now, WML has not been reported in experimental dysglobulinaemic PN.

2. Uncompacted myelin lamellae (UML) — a distinctive myelin modification where some lamellae are neither flattened nor joined together (Fig. 25.3A). Unlike widened myelin lamellae, they are frequently located in the inner part of the myelin sheath. Raine & Bornstein have reproduced the typical features of both UML and WML in their outstanding experimental work.[12] In human pathology, uncompacted myelin lamellae have been described by Ohnishi & Hirano.[10] They are not as specific as the widened lamellae but are mainly observed in patients with POEMS syndrome[19] (polyneuropathy osteosclerotic lesions, endocrinopathy, M protein and skin lesions) and in both acute and chronic cases of inflammatory demyelinating PN.[5,19] Uncompacted lamellae were present in 11 out of 65 patients with the Guillain–Barré syndrome studied in the laboratory, but in less than 1% of myelinated fibres.

Hypermyelination

This has mainly been reported in cases of PN with liability to pressure palsy.[7] The lamellae are much too numerous for the size of the axon and are frequently irregularly arrayed, looking like sausages on teased fibre examination, and this alteration has also been observed occasionally in a few cases of various hereditary PN. In certain cases of peripheral neuropathy with IgM MG, hypermyelination is a prominent feature (Fig. 25.3B) and is combined in certain fibres with the typical spacing visible in the outermost lamellae[19].

Schwann cell pathology

Schwann cell hyperplasia

The nature of the classical onion-bulb formations was debated for several decades until EM easily demonstrated that these concentric elongated processes were of Schwan-

nian origin. Indeed, these are flattened cytoplasmic processes bordered by the characteristic basal lamina (Fig. 25.3C). Small non-myelinated axons are encased in certain of these processes. EM has also revealed in some cases of early infantile polyneuropathy that most or all processes are very thin Schwann cell debris appearing as paired and/or unpaired membranes (Fig. 25.2A). Experimental pathology has highlighted the prominent role of successive episodes of demyelination and remyelination in the development of onion-bulb formation which also accounts for the central fibre of the formations sometimes being totally demyelinated, or at various stages of remyelination. The problem, however, is that some of the 'onion-bulbs' probably correspond to a primitive axonal degeneration (Fig. 25.3B), as had already been suggested on experimental grounds. EM may show that certain onion-bulb formations correspond to clusters of regenerating fibres when a large nerve fibre is surrounded by concentric processes containing one or two thinly myelinated axons. Formations which exhibit only small non-myelinated axons scattered among flattened Schwannian processes are, however, difficult to interpret. These are encountered mainly in cases of hereditary sensory-motor PN and also in cases of PN associated with diabetes mellitus or monoclonal gammopathy. Nerve fibre loss is often associated, and two explanations may be offered: all the modifications may be secondary to axonal damage, or, alternatively, axonal degeneration and primary myelin damage may develop independently.

Schwann cell inclusions

Besides their role in remodelling the myelin in regenerating sheaths, Schwann cells can contain various inclusions of lysosomal origin. Pi granules contain periodically arrayed lamellae and are considered to be normal structures of myelinated fibres (Fig. 25.4A). They are another pitfall of ultrastructural examination, and some have been reported as 'zebra' bodies. Characteristic inclusions are well known in various leukodystrophies, especially metachromatic leukodystrophy (Fig. 25.4B) and Krabbe's disease (Fig. 25.4C). In such cases, EM of peripheral nerve biopsy makes correct diagnosis possible. Inclusions of adrenoleukodystrophy are more difficult to find in peripheral nerve biopsies. In certain forms of medicamentous intoxication, features very similar to those of storage diseases may be seen (Fig. 25.4D).[2,19]

Endoneurial and perineurial modifications

Some of these are quite visible on semithin sections. Renaut's bodies appear as subperineurial rounded structures and are considered as a normal component of the endoneurium. At times, they have been confused with softening or amyloid deposits at ultrastructural examination.[1] This problem can be resolved because the centre of Renaut bodies appears to contain large amounts of fibrillar material mixed with a few collagen fibres. The capillaries must be carefully examined, and EM makes it possible to assess the duplication of basal lamina in diabetic microangiopathy. Capillary modifications are probably responsible for nerve fibre damage, particularly in a few but clear-cut cases of PN with IgM monoclonal gammopathy (Fig. 25.5A). In such cases, granular deposits of IgM are scattered in the endoneurium and some encroach on the basal lamina of nearby Schwann cells. These modifications, which are similar to those described in the light-chain deposits disease, must not be confused with amyloidosis, whose fibrillar components are sometimes arrayed like sunflowers (Fig. 25.5B). Such deposits are also not to be confused with small amounts of short fibrils which are normally present in some endoneurial areas, especially subperineurial ones, and with tubular aggregates reported in a case of cryoglobulinaemic neuropathy[17] (Fig. 25.5C). Cellular infiltrates of the endoneurium are rarely seen on paraffin-embedded fragments but can be properly analysed by EM. In some cases of dysglobulinaemic PN, atypical plasma cells are scattered in the endoneurium. The multilayered perineurial cells can be separated by cellular infiltrates which sometimes also invade the neighbouring endoneurium in cases of PN due to sarcoidosis or malignant lymphoma. Hyperplasia of perineurial cells has been reported in various cases of PN, as well as the presence of rounded calcified deposits.

AETIOLOGICAL DIAGNOSIS

In this section the different aetiological conditions which may be confirmed or revealed by ultrastructural examination of a peripheral nerve biopsy are outlined.

Toxic

Drugs

Chloroquine and amiodarone are responsible for lysosomal deposits in the cytoplasm of Schwann cells, vessel walls, macrophages and perineurial cells. There are rounded deposits composed of paracrystalline or concentrically lamellated structures. Vincristine therapy can be followed by severe axonal modifications.[19]

Organic components

Acrylamide and hexacarbons may be responsible for typical 'dying-back' PN with large intra-axonal filamentous accumulations.[1,13,15]

Metabolic

Metabolic impairment often gives rise to axonopathies having no specific features (hypothyroidism, alcoholism, porphyria).

Genetic

Hereditary motor and sensory PN

These neuropathies, as now classified,[4] provide examples of onion-bulb formation which are sometimes difficult to assess as being secondary to axonal or myelinic impairment.

Various types of hereditary sensory PN

These neuropathies exhibit severe modifications of unmyelinated fibres.[9]

Neurolipidosis

Cases of metachromatic leukodystrophy and Krabbe's disease show characteristic inclusions in the cytoplasm of some Schwann cells. Cases of Fabry's disease display characteristic lamellated inclusions in some perineurial cells and vessel walls (Fig. 25.5D). In Tangier disease there is accumulation of rounded lipid droplets in the cytoplasm of altered nerve fibres.[4] Certain cases of ceroid–lipofuscinoses exhibit accumulation of fingerprint and/or curvilinear bodies in vessel walls and in the SC cytoplasm of a few myelinated fibres.[6,19]

Amyloidosis

Amyloidosis can be occasionally disclosed by EM when deposits are very small, invisible on semithin sections and absent on paraffin-embedded sections. However, entangled fibrils which are characteristic of amyloid deposits must not be confused with other fibrillar deposits, as has already been emphasized.

Immunological disorders

Inflammatory demyelinating peripheral neuropathies

Paraffin-embedded fragments rarely exhibit cellular infiltrates, contrary to a widely accepted opinion. Small endoneurial infiltrates were seen in only five biopsies from patients with the Guillain–Barré syndrome examined in our laboratory; EM makes it possible to see scattered macrophages in almost all cases of this disorder, and some of these cause active demyelination — which is highly characteristic, at least in human pathology. Though not observed in all cases of the Guillain–Barré syndrome, this is a very prominent finding in certain cases of subacute or chronic PN which would otherwise be difficult to classify on clinical and biological grounds.

Monoclonal gammopathies

These provide clear-cut examples of myelin impairment. Other cases display endoneurial deposits. Besides this diagnostic contribution, EM has shed new light on the mechanisms of PN with plasma cell dyscrasia.[18]

Vascular diseases

Apart from very exceptional examples,[1] vascular disorders never give rise to true infarcts, but to severe lesions, varying in intensity from one fascicle to another and sometimes occurring predominantly in central fascicular areas. Here, there are Wallerian-like degenerations, and enlarged axons crowded with abnormal mitochondria and vesicular structures[19].

REFERENCES

1. Asbury A D Johnson R C 1978 Pathology of peripheral nerve. Saunders, Philadelphia
2. Bischoff A J 1979 The peripheral nerves. In: Johannessen J V (ed) Electron microscopy in human medicine, vol 6, McGraw-Hill, pp 137–236
3. Bradley W G 1974 Disorders of peripheral nerves. Blackwell, Oxford
4. Dyck P J, Karnes J, Lais A, Lofgren E P, Stevens J C 1984 Pathologic alterations of the peripheral nervous system of humans. In: Dyck P J, Thomas P K, Lambert E G, Bunge R (eds) Peripheral neuropathy I. Saunders, Philadelphia, pp 760–870
5. King R H M, Thomas P K 1984 The occurrence and significance of myelin with unusually large periodicity. Acta Neuropathologica 63: 319–329
6. Lampert P W, Schochet S S 1979 Ultrastructural changes of peripheral nerve. In: Trump B (ed) Diagnostic electron microscopy, vol. 2. Wiley, New York, pp 309–350
7. Madrid R, Bradley W G 1975 The pathology of neuropathies with focal thickening of the myelin sheath (tomaculous neuropathy). Studies on the formation of the abnormal myelin sheath. Journal of the Neurological Sciences 25: 415–448
8. McLeod J G, Tuck R R, Pollard J D, Cameron J, Walsh J C 1984 Chronic polyneuropathy of undetermined cause. Journal of Neurology, Neurosurgery and Psychiatry 47: 530–535
9. Ochoa J 1978 Recognition of unmyelinated nerve fiber disease. Morphologic criteria. Muscle and Nerve 1: 375–387
10. Ohnishi A, Hirano A 1981 Uncompacted myelin lamellae in dysglobulinemic neuropathy. Journal of the Neurological Sciences 51: 131–140
11. Prineas J W 1981 Pathology of the Guillain–Barré syndrome. Annals of Neurology 9 (Suppl 9): 6–19
12. Raine S, Bornstein M B 1979 Experimental allergic neuritis: ultrastructure of serum induced myelin aberrations in peripheral nervous system cultures. Laboratory Investigation 40: 423–432
13. Schaumburg H H, Spencer P S, Thomas P K 1983 Disorders of peripheral nerves. F.A. Davis, Philadelphia
14. Sluga E 1970 Entmarkungserkrankungen: untersuchungen an peripheren nerven. In: Proceedings of the VIth International Congress of Neuropathology. Masson, Paris, pp 654–663
15. Spencer P S, Schaumburg H H 1976 Central–peripheral distal axonopathy. The pathology of dying-back polyneuropathies. In: Zimmerman H M (ed) Progress in neuropathology III. Grune and Stratton, New York, pp 253–395
16. Thomas P K, Landon D N, King R H M 1984 Diseases of the peripheral nerves. In: Adams J H, Corsellis J A N, Duchen L W (eds) Greenfield's neuropathology. Arnold, London, pp 807–920
17. Vallat J M, Desproges–Gotteron R, Leboutet M J, Loubet A, Gualde N, Treves R 1980 Cryoglobulinemic neuropathology. A pathological study. Annals of Neurology 8: 179–185
18. Vital C, Vallat J M, Deminiere C, Brechenmacher C, Vital A 1984 Peripheral nerve damage during monoclonal gammopathy and plasma cell dyscrasia (36 cases). In: Sobue I (ed) Proceedings of the International Symposium on Peripheral Neuropathy, Nagoya. Excerpta Medica, Amsterdam pp 341–352
19. Vital C, Vallat J M 1987 Ultrastructural study of the human diseased peripheral nerve. Elsevier, New York
20. Vital C, Brechenmacher C, Cardinaud J P, Manier G, Vital A, Mora B 1985 Acute inflammatory demyelinating polyneuropathy in a diabetic patient: predominance of vesicular disruption in myelin sheaths. Acta Neuropathologica 67: 337–340
21. Vital C, Henry P, Loiseau P, Julien J, Vallat J M, Tignol J, Bonnaud E 1975 Les neuropathies peripheriques de la maladie de Waldenstrom. Etude histologique et ultrastructurale de 5 cas. Annales d'Anatomie Pathologique (Paris) 20: 93–108
22. Vital A, Vital C 1984 Amyloid neuropathy: relationship between amyloid fibrils and macrophages. Ultrastructural Pathology 7: 21–24
23. Weller R O, Cervos-Navarro J 1977 Pathology of peripheral nerves. Butterworths, London

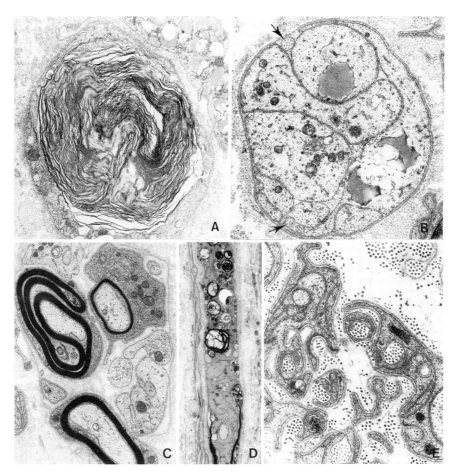

Fig. 25.1 Axonal modifications: major lesions. **A** An ovoid and a macrophage overloaded with lipid droplets. (× 11 600) **B** This band of Büngner exhibits a few axonal sprouts at its periphery (arrows). (× 16 000) **C** This typical cluster is made up of three myelinated axons and a few non-myelinated ones. (× 11 900) **D** In longitudinal section, this fibre is enlarged and the myelin sheath is visible only in the paranodal area. (× 2900) **E** Typical features of collagen pockets. (× 20 000)

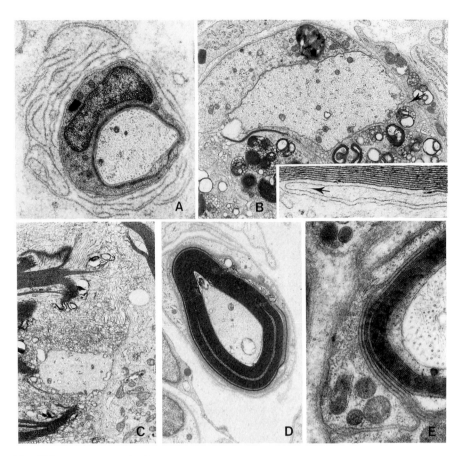

Fig. 25.2 Myelinic modifications: common features. **A** This isolated remyelinating fibre is surrounded by elongated debris from Schwann cell basement membranes. (× 16 000) **B** Inflammatory demyelinating polyneuropathy: a macrophage has penetrated through the basement membrane of this fibre (arrow). The myelin sheath is disrupted and the axon remains intact. (× 11 900) *Inset* Another elongated macrophage process peeling away the outermost lamella (arrow). (× 58 000) **C** This fibre shows typical features of vesicular disruption of the myelin sheath into rounded and elongated structures. The axon remains intact. Reprinted with permission from Vital et al.[20] (× 10 500) **D** IgM MG: the outermost lamellae are widened and joined together. (× 10 500) **E** The outer mesaxon and the outermost lamellae are widened. Reprinted, with permission, from Vital et al.[21] (× 25 000)

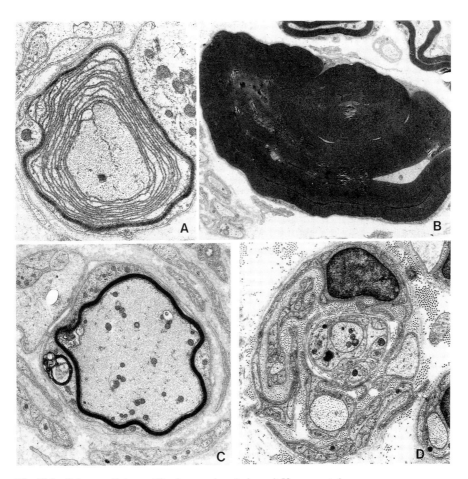

Fig. 25.3 Other myelinic modifications: various lesions. **A** Uncompacted myelin lamellae are present in the inner part of this myelin sheath. (× 18 200) **B** A myelinated fibre has a myelin sheath which is too large and some lamellae are irregularly arrayed. (× 6700) **C** A remyelinating fibre is surrounded by flattened Schwann cell processes. (× 11 600) **D** A cluster of regenerating fibres is surrounded by flattened Schwann cell processes. (× 11 600)

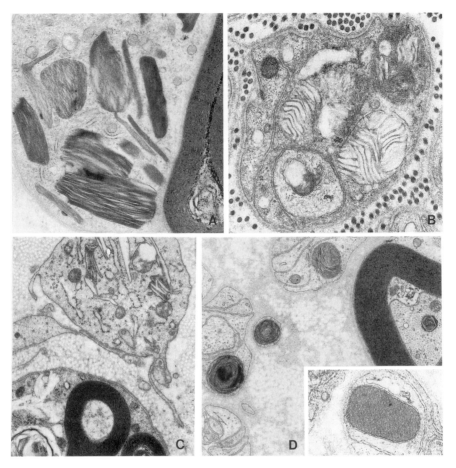

Fig. 25.4 Schwann cell modifications: various features. **A** Pi granules are seen in the Schwannian cytoplasm. (× 18 200) **B** Metachromatic leukodystrophy: this unmyelinated fibre exhibits two 'zebra' bodies. (× 34 200) **C** Krabbe's disease: typical inclusions are present in a Schwannian cell cytoplasm of a myelinated fibre and in a nearby macrophage. (× 14 400) **D** Chloroquine intoxication: three rounded and lamellated inclusions are present in unmyelinated fibres, and another is located in the axon of a myelinated fibre. (× 21 500) **Inset** Another drug intoxication: a paracrystalline inclusion is seen in an unmyelinated fibre. (× 33 000)

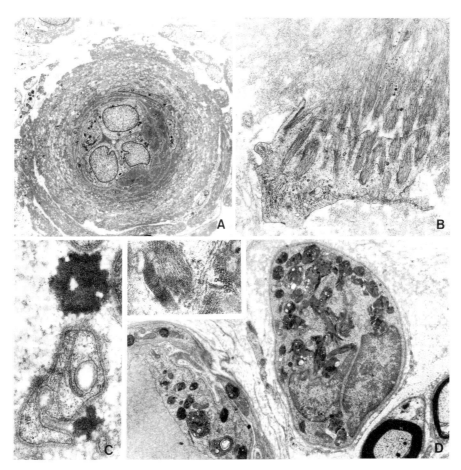

Fig. 25.5 Endoneurial modifications: various lesions. **A** IgM monoclonal gammopathy: immunoglobulin deposits dissociate the basement membrane of a capillary and are present also in the endoneurium. (× 3500) **B** A few tufts of amyloid fibrils are seen in the cytoplasm of this macrophage. Reprinted with permission from Vital & Vital.[23] (× 16 500) **C** Tubular aggregates are seen in the vicinity of an unmyelinated fibre. (× 30 800) (Courtesy of Professor J. M. Vallat.) **D** Fabry's disease: typical inclusions are present in a capillary wall and in the cytoplasm, which is probably of Schwannian origin. (× 8300) *Inset* Lamellar and circular structures are present in an endothelial cell. (× 87 000)

26. Skeletal muscle

J. M. Papadimitriou   D. W. Henderson   D. V. Spagnolo

INTRODUCTION

A range of ultrastructural lesions occurs in the muscle fibres of patients with primary muscular diseases as well as those secondary to various neurological disorders. Few of these lesions are specific for a particular disease, but in many instances the patterns of ultrastructural abnormality are sufficiently distinctive to be of diagnostic significance. In this chapter the various structural anomalies in the nuclei and cytoplasm of diseased human muscle fibres will be considered and their relevance discussed. Unfortunately, the biochemical abnormalities responsible for the ultrastructural lesions are often ill understood, but it is possible that the electron-microscopic findings will provide useful leads to the underlying biochemical defects in at least a few disorders. It should be emphasized, however, that ultrastructural assessment is most informative in the context of the relevant clinical, light-microscopic, immunocytochemical and histochemical findings. Moreover, the assessment of anomalies by electron microscopy demands a detailed knowledge of the fine structure of normal human muscle. This is the subject of many excellent reviews[35,66,98,159,160,172,208] and the reader is referred to them for descriptions of the range of structural appearances in normal muscle fibres.

SATELLITE CELLS

Satellite cells (Fig. 26.1) are generally uncommon in normal muscle but they are frequently encountered in fibres when regeneration is established or when denervation has occurred.[66,168,169,199] Increased numbers have also been reported in polymyositis,[29] Duchenne muscular dystrophy,[222] congenital myotonic dystrophy,[173] Werdnig–Hoffmann disease[221] and Kugelberg–Welander syndrome.[121] They may display evidence of activation and myogenic differentiation with increased amounts of euchromatin, prominent nucleoli, many ribosomal rosettes, strands of rough endoplasmic reticulum (RER), scattered mitochondria and obvious myofilaments. These features are significantly more prominent in polymyositis than in Duchenne muscular dystrophy or myo-

tonic dystrophy.[93] In instances where inflammatory cells have invaded a muscle fibre they may be confused with satellite cells — especially when viewed at relatively low magnification.

NUCLEI

Crowding of the normally well dispersed nuclei occurs in atrophic fibres,[122] while the nuclear contours become convoluted in atrophy and nemaline myopathy.[122] Internal nuclei, on the other hand, are seen in various myopathic and neurogenic disorders and are especially numerous in myotonic dystrophy[44] as well as being a distinctive feature of centronuclear (myotubular) myopathy[33,89,174,185,206,226] including the rare X-linked recessive form.[6,7]

Augmentation of nuclear euchromatin and prominent nucleoli is seen in regenerating myofibres[104,121,155] as well as those in Werdnig–Hoffmann disease and congenital myotonic dystrophy,[173] while apoptotic changes have been observed in AIDS-associated myopathy.[153] Intranuclear inclusions resembling myxovirus nucleocapsids have been seen in polymyositis[23,28,176] and in a case of chronic distal myopathy,[20] but a viral nature has remained unproven. Tubular inclusions, 8.5 nm in diameter, have been reported in oculopharyngeal dystrophy,[215] while filamentous intranuclear inclusions (Fig. 26.2) have been observed in polymyositis,[28] in inclusion body myositis[23,182,230] (Fig. 26.3) and in a carrier of Duchenne muscular dystrophy.[91] Intranuclear nemaline bodies have been observed in a few cases of polymyositis,[176] in occasional patients with late onset rod disease[57] and in one instance of childhood nemaline myopathy.[94] Vacuoles and nuclear pseudo-inclusions consisting of invaginating sarcoplasm have also been encountered in a wide range of disorders.[117,121]

Annulate lamellae (Fig. 26.4) are occasionally seen in diseased muscle fibres. They have been reported in polymyositis[26] and in the muscles of patients with polyarteritis nodosa and arteritis associated with rheumatoid arthritis.[127]

THE GOLGI APPARATUS

In normal fibres the Golgi apparatus is generally small and inconspicuous. In regenerating or denervated myofibres, however, the organelle becomes enlarged and prominent.[121] The Golgi apparatus is probably involved in autophagosome formation,[50,51] while structural continuity with elements of the T-system have been observed (vide infra).

MYOFIBRILS

A common observation in diseased muscle fibres is the presence of hypercontracted myofibrils. This is a non-specific finding and can also be induced artefactually, in which case the affected fibres tend to be grouped at the periphery of the sample where handling tends to be maximal.[37] The areas of hypercontraction may be localized or widespread, and, although non-specific, the phenomenon is often encountered in patients with Duchenne muscular dystrophy[34] in which it may be of some pathogenetic significance.

Aberrant bundles of normal fibrils spiralling or encircling the long axis of myofibres are seen in ring fibres. Such profiles are frequent in myotonic dystrophy[156,187,193] but have also been observed in Duchenne muscular dystrophy,[186] congenital fibre disproportion,[143] hypothyroid myopathy[4] and periarteritis.[117]

A frequent finding in diseased myocytes is the disorganization of the orderly sarcomeric pattern of myofibrils. Focal disruption of a few sarcomeres occurs in a variety of disorders and lacks specificity. Such disruptions are, however, common in the muscle fibres (both type 1 and 2) of children with certain congenital myopathies termed multicore and minicore diseases[52,80,209] (Fig. 26.5) — the focal myofibrillar lesions corresponding with the cores within the affected cells. Rarely, nemaline rods[67] or centrally located nuclei[217] are other significant lesions in these two myopathies.

Extensive disorganization of the central region of type 1 myofibres is the major lesion in 'target' and 'core-targetoid' fibres.[122,152] In the former a central region of complete disruption of the sarcomeric pattern is separated from an outer layer of normal myofibrils by a zone in which the myofibrillar disarray is only mild (Fig. 26.6), while in the latter this intermediate zone is absent (Fig. 26.7). In the region of complete disorganization all other sarcoplasmic organelles are conspicuously infrequent. Target fibres occur in recent denervation,[110] during re-innervation[42] and in polymyositis and familial periodic paralysis.[122] Core-targetoid fibres are seen in denervating and myopathic conditions[59] as well as in the aged.[177] Core-targetoid lesions displaying a significant proportion of distinct sarcomeric patterns, correspond to the cross-striated cores which are usually seen in central core disease.[58,79,144,203] These cores are usually central, but on occasions they are somewhat eccentric, rarely peripheral, and more than one per fibre may be present. Not only are many sarcomeres preserved but they are also in register. The sarcomeres in the cores, however, are shorter than those of peripheral myofibrils while the Z-discs exhibit a zigzag appearance. In addition, Z-disc streaming and even nemaline rod formation may be present.[10,152] Core-targetoid fibres are also seen in the myopathy associated with malignant hyperthermia, but in this instance they are not limited to type 1 fibres.[81]

In one rare congenital neuromuscular disease, 15% of the myofibres exhibited three concentric zones.[170] The innermost zone contained mitochondria, single filaments, electron-dense material and glycogen granules. The middle region consisted of myofibrils with Z-disc streaming, and the outer of disorganized myofibrils and sarcoplasm.

Peripheral subsarcolemmal aggregates (subsarcolemmal masses) of disorganized myofibrils and sarcoplasm (Fig. 26.8) are also seen in a variety of conditions but are particularly characteristic of myotonic dystrophy.[107,187,193] They have also been observed in limb girdle muscular dystrophy and hypothyroid myopathy.[62]

Rarely, loss of the myofilaments in A bands has been observed. This change has been reported in polymyositis,[23] congenital hypotonia,[228] and in a case of polyradiculopathy.[229]

It has been suggested that all these various myofibrillar lesions are related and reflect a continuous spectrum of structural damage.[180] The pathogenetic mechanisms are, however, obscure and it is unclear whether the damage represents degradation of normally assembled myofibrils or is the result of disorganized myofibril assembly.

Z-DISCS

Ultrastructural abnormalities of Z-discs are very frequent in diseased skeletal muscle. Streaming of Z-disc material together with Z-disc duplication and zigzag irregularities are the three most common lesions.[47,143,161] When streaming occurs, the electron-dense material may extend along the full length of the sarcomere (Fig. 26.9) and is accompanied by varying degrees of myofibrillar disarray. Z-disc streaming is often observed in type 1 fibres and is associated with focal mitochondrial loss; it has been reported in neurogenic atrophy,[110,164,186,198] polymyositis,[121,176] ageing myofibres,[177] Duchenne muscular dystrophy,[62,134,182] myotonic dystrophy,[107,187] central core disease,[143] multicore disease,[52] a range of metabolic and toxic myopathies,[4,43,143,185] and after intense eccentric exercise.[68] Some degree of Z-disc streaming, however, occurs in muscle fibres from healthy subjects. Fischman and his colleagues[66] have concluded that if streaming covers more than four sarcomere lengths in four adjacent myofibrils in more than 2% of fibres then it should be considered abnormal.

Elongated rod-shaped electron-dense bodies 6–7 μm in length and somewhat similar to Z-discs in structure are the major feature of nemaline myopathy[78,86,143,163,204] (Figs

26.10–26.12). They consist of closely parallel filaments with periodic cross-striations (Fig. 26.11) while cross-sections reveal a quadratic lattice configuration resembling that of the normal Z-disc (Fig. 26.12). The transverse striations have a periodicity of 15–17 nm while the sides of the latticed square measure 9–10 nm. Moreover they have been shown to contain both actin and alpha-actinin.[227] Although they characterize nemaline myopathy they are found sporadically in polymyositis,[19,167,176] ageing myofibres,[177] Duchenne muscular dystrophy,[62] central core disease,[2,143] distal myopathy[184] and centronuclear myopathy.[185]

Widespread loss of Z-disc material has been described in several disease states. Together with some loss of Z-band filaments it occurs in denervation atrophy,[100] central core disease,[75] myotonic dystrophy[100] and is prominent in ischaemic myofibres.[104,124,211]

Cytoplasmic bodies are osmiophilic, discrete but unbounded structures of variable size (Fig. 26.13). They have been observed in a variety of diseased myofibres, but because of their electron-density and topography they are thought to be related to Z-discs.[114] They consist of a central mass of granular osmiophilic material and a peripheral halo of radiating filaments most of which have a diameter of 6 nm. In some instances they connect with A bands or are associated with thick filaments. They have been reported in neurogenic atrophy,[199] polymyositis,[114,230] Duchenne muscular dystrophy,[114] myotonic dystrophy,[193] periodic paralysis,[83,116,149] inclusion body myositis,[23] Werdnig–Hoffmann disease,[133] perhexiline maleate-induced myopathy[63] and various other metabolic myopathies.[16,38] In addition they appear to be the predominant structural lesion of a rare myopathy.[31,76,99,155,224]

MITOCHONDRIA

Non-specific swelling of mitochondria followed by deposition of osmiophilic material in the inner chamber or the formation of myelin figures is a common feature in a variety of muscle diseases.[104,117,168,169,217] In denervation[208] and ischaemia[104] their long axis coincides with that of myofibrils — while their numbers are reduced in target and core-targetoid fibres,[42,110] in areas of Z-disc streaming,[47] and in central core disease[144] and multicore disease.[52] On the other hand, focal mitochondrial proliferation, especially in the subsarcolemmal region, has been reported in corticosteroid myopathy,[46] facioscapulohumeral muscular dystrophy,[41,122] thyrotoxic myopathy[109] and the periodic paralyses.[116]

Structurally abnormal mitochondria, which are often conspicuous in the subsarcolemmal region, have been observed in a range of muscle disorders including the so-called 'mitochondrial myopathies'[41,140,197] and 'mitochondrial encephalomyopathies'.[141,156,175] It must be emphasized, however, that not all biochemically defined mitochondrial deficiencies show significant alterations in mitochondrial structure.[41,140] Except for one rare congenital

neuromuscular disorder,[64] they are invariably observed in type 1 fibres. Such mitochondria are often enlarged, sometimes irregular, and they may possess tubular or lamellar cristae[183] (Figs 26.14–26.16). The cristae may be increased in number and irregularly arranged or they may form concentric whorls.[41] In some instances there is a reduction in the concentration of cristae resulting in a vacuolated appearance.[41] Enlarged, structurally abnormal mitochondria have also been reported in patients with AIDS-associated myopathy who have been treated with zidovudine.[153]

Prominent electron-dense granules (Fig. 26.17) have been observed in the inner chamber of mitochondria in muscle from patients with hypothyroid myopathy,[122] glycogen storage diseases,[49] Luft's disease,[113] and occasionally in other myopathies,[144,195,208] including the childhood myopathic syndrome associated with lactic acidosis.[108] Glycogen[33,41,143,193] and triglyceride[41] globule accumulation has also been described, but the exact significance of this is unclear.

Crystalline inclusions in the outer mitochondrial chamber, especially within the cristae (Figs 26.18 and 26.19), and seen mainly in the subsarcolemmal mitochondrial clusters, have been reported in a variety of conditions; in some of which biochemical defects have been demonstrated. They are the characteristic lesion in Luft's syndrome,[3,113] in which there is uncoupling of oxidative phosphorylation, as well as in the Kearns–Sayre syndrome,[1,40,90,103,151] where lack of respiratory control using a glycerophosphate as the substrate has been demonstrated in one case.[40] They have also been reported in mitochondria shown to possess defects of cytochromes,[137,138,165,207,219] NADH-coenzyme Q reductase,[139] or mitochondrial ATPase[137,190] — or with abnormalities of the pyruvate–dehydrogenase complex,[102] or the carnitine–acyl carnitine system.[39,56,92,105,137] In addition to their occurrence in the various 'mitochondrial myopathies' listed above, these inclusions have also been seen in polymyositis,[27,176,199] neurogenic atrophy,[199,200] Duchenne muscular dystrophy,[117] thyrotoxic periodic paralysis,[195,210] lipid storage myopathy,[87,143,202,204] late onset glycogenoses,[50,216] and a few other poorly defined myopathies.[89,143,202,204] The inclusions appear as sets of parallel lines, usually four in number, measuring some 5 nm in width and separated by an electron-lucent zone measuring 6 nm. In addition, Mukherjee et al[142] have shown that these crystalloids are composed of 8-nm particles arranged in a somewhat unique array. It has been suggested that all such inclusion-containing mitochondria have deficient respiratory control.[101]

Recently, abnormal mitochondrial genomes have been identified in patients with the clinical presentation of the Kearns–Sayre syndrome and related disorders.[83,136,160,231] Thus far, both mitochondrial DNA deletions[83,136,231] and mitochondrial DNA reduplications have been reported.[160] It will not be surprising if other such abnormalities are to be found.

TRANSVERSE TUBULAR SYSTEM

Displacement, distortion and reduplication of triads are common in injured or atrophic fibres.[143] Dilatation of T-system tubules has been reported in polymyositis, Duchenne muscular dystrophy,[122] and in the periodic paralyses,[48,49] but the possibility of artefact always needs to be excluded. Honeycomb patterns of membrane are produced by a regular three-dimensional array of coalescing T-system tubules (Figs 26.20–26.22), the tubular component measuring between 30 and 40 nm in diameter. A connection with the T-system (Fig. 26.21) and the extracellular space (Fig. 26.22) can be demonstrated by using electron-dense tracers,[187] while structural continuity with the Golgi lamellae has also been observed (Fig. 26.20). Such honeycomb profiles have been observed in neurogenic atrophy,[198] polymyositis,[27,121] myotonic dystrophy,[187,193] the periodic paralyses,[48,116,195] Duchenne muscular dystrophy,[62] hypothyroid myopathy,[4] autophagic glycogenosis,[50] chloroquine myopathy,[62] Cushing's syndrome,[95] alcoholic neuropathy,[214] distal myopathy,[119] perhexiline maleate-induced myopathy,[63] reducing body myopathy[143] and idiopathic myoglobinuria.[195]

SARCOPLASMIC RETICULUM

Dilation of sarcoplasmic cisternae is especially prominent in the periodic paralyses[48,51,84,116,195] (Fig. 26.23) , but it has also been seen after denervation,[178] in regenerating fibres,[51] in the various types of hereditary myotonia[25,187,194] and in Duchenne muscular dystrophy,[134] where it appears to be one of the earliest changes in this disorder.[34] It has also been reported in distal myopathy,[119] alcoholic myopathy,[171] myopathy with hyperaldosteronism,[71] and in AIDS-associated myopathy.[153]

Elongated tubular aggregates which are thought to be derived from the sarcoplasmic reticulum are found in the subsarcolemmal region of type 2 fibres, often near the poles of nuclei (Fig. 26.24). Occasionally direct connections between a tubular and a lateral sac have been demonstrated,[183] while the cytoplasm surrounding the tubular aggregates is often inundated with glycogen granules. They have been reported in the myofibres of patients with the periodic paralyses,[9,14,60,132,194] the exertional muscle cramp syndrome,[18] hereditary myotonia[194] and alcoholic myopathy.[30] The tubules range from 60 to 80 nm in diameter and may contain rod shaped cores (Figs 26.25–26.26), columns of spheroids or coaxial inner tubules, while their osmiophilia is somewhat similar to that of lateral sacs.

Cylindrical structures consisting of paired membranes arranged in a spiral pattern and enclosing a core of glycogen have been observed at the periphery of myofibres in a number of diverse conditions.[13,24,74,129] Their origin is unclear but it is possible that they are derived from elements of the sarcoplasmic reticulum.

AUTOPHAGIC VACUOLES

Autophagic vacuoles (Fig. 26.27) may occur in almost any myopathic state but they are particularly prominent and frequent in chloroquine and vincristine myopathy and in acid maltase deficiency.[50,115,116] They have also been observed in polymyositis,[121] Duchenne muscular dystrophy,[134,143] myotonic dystrophy,[117] juvenile Batten's disease, distal myopathy,[119,212] inclusion body myositis[23] and in various other metabolic and toxic myopathies.[84,167] They invariably contain sequestered sarcoplasmic organelles and are bound by single, double or even multiple membranes which are probably derived from the T-tubular system, sarcoplasmic reticulum and Golgi complex.[36,51]

In some instances autophagic vacuoles have been found to consist mainly of multilaminated membranes (Fig. 26.28) together with glycogen, dense bodies and amorphous granular and fibrillar material.[25,44,70] They correspond to the rimmed vacuoles described by Dubowitz & Brooke,[44] and although they are the predominant lesion in an unusual distal myopathy[111,148] they do not appear to have any specificity in most instances. The contents of the autophagosomes possess acid phosphatase activity but the primary lysosomes have not been positively identified.[36]

GLYCOGEN

Large quantities of glycogen (Fig. 26.29) are present in regenerating fibres,[8] as well as in the muscles of patients with glycogen storage disease, especially types II and III.[17,50,55,73,88,188] Generally, membrane-bound glycogen particles are seen frequently in type II glycogenosis[55,128,188] (Fig. 26.30), but they can occur in the other glycogenoses, albeit to a lesser degree,[54,73,88,128,188] as well as contributing to the contents of autophagic vacuoles.

Moderate amounts of glycogen are seen in neurogenic atrophy,[117] Duchenne muscular dystrophy,[62,134,143] the periodic paralyses[9,14,84,132,210] and myopathies associated with mitochondrial abnormalities.[40,131,164]

Accumulations of polyglucosan are seen as granular and fibrillar material. Such deposits are found in type IV glycogenosis,[181] hypothyroidism[61] and Lafora's disease.[22,32,145]

LIPID

Excessive accumulation of neutral lipid spherules occurs in the myopathies associated with mitochondrial abnormalities,[15,40,90,103,143,151,164,205] in carnitine deficiency,[53,105,118,220] disorders of carbohydrate metabolism,[11,95] steroid myopathy,[82] in a rare syndrome associated with cleft palate, club foot, scoliosis and arthrogryposis multiplex,[147] and in a wide variety of other muscle diseases,[143] including the so-called lipid storage myopathies.[87,145,202,205]

LIPOPIGMENTS

In muscle from elderly patients lipofuscin bodies (Fig. 26.31) are numerous, but they are also frequent in chronic neurogenic muscular atrophy,[199,200] myotonic dystrophy,[193] thyrotoxic myopathy,[109] distal myopathy[212] and complicating occlusive vascular diseases.[143]

Membrane-bound aggregates of small curvilinear bodies (see Ch. 6) are a feature of patients with certain types of neuronal ceroid–lipofuscinosis[21,75] but they have also been observed in chloroquine-induced myopathy.[125,146]

SARCOPLASMIC INCLUSIONS

Filamentous bodies

These consist of masses of thin filaments 6–7 nm in diameter (Fig. 26.32). They are invariably found in the subsarcolemmal region and often in a paranuclear position. They have been observed in neurogenic atrophy,[117] Duchenne muscular dystrophy,[117] myotonic dystrophy,[117] the periodic paralyses,[116,184] nemaline myopathy,[201] intermittent claudication[211] and perhexiline maleate-induced myopathy[63] — but they have also been found in normal muscle.[117]

Concentric laminated bodies

These are cylindrical subsarcolemmal structures which possess walls that are formed by 5–20 concentric fibrillar lamellae (Fig. 26.33). Their interior may be empty or may contain vesicles, glycogen granules or amorphous material.[183] They are often restricted to type 2 fibres, and actin contributes significantly to their formation.[157] They have been reported in neurogenic atrophy,[117] polymyositis,[36] the periodic paralyses,[195] congenital fibre disproportion,[143] central core disease,[43] nemaline myopathy,[201] hypothyroid myopathy,[130] infantile neuro-axonal dystrophy,[213] cerebral hypotonia,[157] Luft's disease,[113] Canavan's disease,[72] Krabbe's disease,[183] neuronal ceroid–lipofuscinosis,[183] and a few other non-specific muscle disorders.[65]

Zebra-striped bodies

These consist of fine filaments that are traversed by bands of electron dense material (Fig. 26.34). They are seen in normal extra-ocular muscles, near myotendinous junctions and in intrafusal fibres.[117] They have been described in the muscles of a patient with slowly progressive congenital myopathy,[112] and in one instance of hypothyroid myopathy.[122]

Fingerprint bodies

These are composed of aggregates of serrated curvilinear lamellae separated from each other by a 30–36-nm space (Fig. 26.35). They are found predominantly in type 1 fibres[158] and they have been reported in myotonic dystrophy,[214] benign congenital myopathy,[54] dermatomyositis,[214] and oculopharyngeal muscular dystrophy.[101]

Paracrystalline arrays

Aggregates of 20–30-nm particles in orderly paracrystalline arrays (Fig. 26.36) have been reported in idiopathic scoliosis,[223] dermatomyositis,[121] Reye's syndrome[5] and malignant hyperthermia.[179] It had been thought that they represented glycogen but Fukuhara[69] has shown they contain nucleic acids and postulated that they may represent an RNA virus.

Reducing bodies

These subsarcolemmal masses are composed mainly of osmiophilic granules which measure 12–16 nm in diameter, but mitochondria, triads and glycogen granules are also present. They are regarded as the characteristic feature of a rare form of lethal congenital myopathy,[16,85] but they have also been described in a benign variant of the disorder.[150]

Spheroidal bodies

These inclusions consist of finely fibrillar and amorphous granular components that have been reported in the members of a family with a slowly progressive autosomal dominant neuromuscular disease.[76]

THE FIBRE SURFACE

Surface contours

Small papillary projections are common in normal fibres that are fixed in a contracted state, the hollows of the scalloped contour being maximal at the level of the Z-discs. They are also prominent in atrophic fibres,[121,143] or in those in which exocytosis is a feature,[51] while deep infoldings are often present in myotonic dystrophy.[25,192]

The external lamina

Folding and redundancy of the external lamina (Fig. 26.37) are features of muscle atrophy,[121,143] while reduplication occurs in the muscular dystrophies and other necrotizing myopathies in which muscle fibre regeneration has occurred.[104,143] Thickening, however, is seen in a wide variety of disorders and is of no diagnostic significance,[120] although it may be prominent in myotonic dystrophy,[117] vascular insufficiency[211] and rheumatoid arthritis.[225]

Plasmalemma

Focal breaks in the cell membrane of muscle fibres have been reported in injury induced by cold[162] or ischaemia,[143] as well as in Duchenne muscular dystrophy.[135] In the latter they are associated with localized regions of myofibrillar hypercontraction. It is most unlikely, however, that they represent the fundamental defect in this disorder and they are probably secondary lesions. On the other hand, freeze-fracture studies have demonstrated depletion of intramembranous particles in the plasmalemma of myofibres in patients with Duchenne muscular dystrophy,[106,191] together with a significant increase in the concentration of caveolae.[12,106] An increased frequency of pinocytic vesicles has, however, been observed in various disorders and has little specificity.

REFERENCES

1. Adachi M, Torii J, Volk B W, Briet P, Wolintz S, Scheck L 1973 Electron microscopic and enzyme histochemical studies of cerebellum ocular and skeletal muscles in chronic progressive ophthalmoplegia with cerebellar ataxia. Acta Neuropathologica (Berlin) 23: 300–312
2. Afifi A K, Smith J W, Zellweger H 1965 Congenital non-progressive myopathy. Central core disease and nemaline myopathy in one family. Neurology (Minneapolis) 15: 371–381
3. Afifi A K, Ibrahim M Z M, Bergman R A, Abuhaydar N, Mire J, Bahuth N, Kailani F 1972 Morphologic features of hypermetabolic mitochondrial disease. Journal of the Neurological Sciences 15: 271–290
4. Afifi A K, Najjar S S, Mire-Salman J, Bergman R A 1974 The myopathology of the Kocher–Debre–Semelaign Syndrome. Electromyography, light and electron microscopic study. Journal of the Neurological Sciences 22: 445–470
5. Alvira M M, Mendoza M 1975 Letter: Reye's Syndrome: a viral myopathy. New England Journal of Medicine 292: 1297
6. Ambler M W, Neave C, Tutschka B G, Pueschel S M, Orson J M, Singer D B 1984 X-linked recessive myotubular myopathy. I. Clinical and pathologic findings in a family. Human Pathology 15: 566–574
7. Ambler M W, Neave C, Singer D B 1984 X-linked recessive myotubular myopathy. II. Muscle morphology and human myogenesis. Human Pathology 15: 1107–1120
8. Baloh R, Cancilla P A, Kalyanaraman K, Munsat T, Pearson C M, Rich R 1972 Regeneration of human muscle: a morphologic and histochemical study of normal and dystrophic muscle after injury. Laboratory Investigation 26: 319–328
9. Bergman R A, Afifi A K, Dunkle L M, Johns R T 1970 Muscle pathology in hypokalemic periodic paralysis with hyperthyroidism. Annals of the New York Academy of Science 126: 100–118
10. Bethlem J, Arts W F, Dingemans K P 1978 Common origin of rods, cores, miniature cores and total loss of cross striations. Archives of Neurology (Chicago) 35: 555–566
11. Blass J P, Kark R A P, Engel W K 1971 Clinical studies of a patient with pyruvate decarboxylase deficiency. Archives of Neurology 25: 449–460
12. Bonilla E, Fischbeck K, Schotland D L 1981 Freeze fracture studies of muscle caveolae in human muscular dystrophy. American Journal of Pathology 104: 167–173
13. Bove K E, Iannaccone S T, Hilton P K, Samaha F 1980 Cylindrical spirals in a familial neuromuscular disorder. Annals of Neurology 7: 550–556
14. Bradley W G 1969 Ultrastructural changes in adynamia episodica hereditaria and normakalaemic familial periodic paralysis. Brain 92: 379–390
15. Bradley W G, Jenkinson M, Park D C, Hudgson E, Gardner-Medwin D, Pennington R J T, Walton J N 1972 A myopathy associated with lipid storage. Journal of the Neurological Sciences 16: 137–154
16. Brooke M H, Neville H E 1972 Reducing body myopathy. Neurology (Minneapolis) 22: 829–840
17. Brunberg J A, McCormick W F, Schochet S S Jr 1971 Type III glycogenosis: an adult with diffuse weakness and muscle wasting. Archives of Neurology (Chicago) 25: 171–178
18. Brumback R A, Staton R D, Susag M E 1981 Exercise induced pain, stiffness and tubular aggregation in skeletal muscle. Journal of Neurology, Neurosurgery and Psychiatry 44: 250–254
19. Cape C A, Johnson W M, Pitner S E 1970 Nemaline structures in polymyositis. Neurology (Minneapolis) 20: 494–502
20. Carpenter S, Karpati G, Wolfe L 1970 Virus like filaments and phospholipid accumulation in skeletal muscle. Neurology (Minneapolis) 20: 889–903
21. Carpenter S, Karpati G, Andermann F 1972 Specific involvement of muscle nerve and skin in late infantile and juvenile amaurotic idiocy. Neurology (Minneapolis) 22: 170–186
22. Carpenter S, Karpati G, Andermann F, Andermann E 1974 Lafora's disease: peroxisomal storage in skeletal muscle. Neurology (Minneapolis) 24: 531–538
23. Carpenter S, Karpati G, Heller I, Eisen A 1978 Inclusion body myositis: a distinct variety of idiopathic inflammatory myopathy. Neurology (Minneapolis) 28: 8–17
24. Carpenter S, Karpati G, Lobitaille Y, Melmed C 1979 Cylindrical spirals in human skeletal muscle. Muscle and Nerve 2: 282–287
25. Casanova G, Jerusalem F 1979 Myopathology of myotonic dystrophy. Acta Neuropathologica (Berlin) 45: 231–240
26. Chou S M 1968 Myxovirus-like particles and accompanying nuclear changes in chronic polymyositis. Archives of Pathology (Chicago) 86: 649–658
27. Chou S M 1969 Megaconial mitochondria observed in a case of chronic polymyositis. Acta Neuropathologica (Berlin) 12: 68–89
28. Chou S M 1973 Prospects of viral aetiology in polymyositis. In: Kakulas B A (ed) Clinical studies in myology. Excerpta Medica, Amsterdam, pp 17–28
29. Chou S M, Nonaka I 1977 Satellite cells and muscle regeneration in diseased human skeletal muscle. Journal of the Neurological Sciences 34: 131–145
30. Chui L A, Nerstein H, Munsat T L 1975 Tubular aggregates in subclinical alcoholic myopathy. American Journal of Neurology 25: 405–412
31. Clark J R, D'Agostino A N, Wilson J, Brooks R R, Cole G C 1978 Autosomal dominant myofibrillar inclusion body myopathy–clinical, histologic, histochemical and ultrastructural characteristics. Neurology (Minneapolis) 28: 309–310
32. Coleman D L, Gambetti P, Di Mauro S, Blume R E 1974 Muscle in Lafora disease. Archives of Neurology (Chicago) 31: 396–406
33. Collins J E, Collins A, Radford M R, Weller R O 1983 Perinatal diagnosis of myotubular (centronuclear) myopathy: a case report. Clinical Neuropathology 2: 79–82
34. Cullen M J, Fulthorpe J J 1975 Stages in fibre breakdown in Duchenne muscular dystrophy. Journal of the Neurological Sciences 24: 179–200
35. Cullen M J, Weightman D 1975 The ultrastructure of normal human muscle in relation to fibre type. Journal of the Neurological Sciences 25: 43–56
36. Cullen M J, Appleyard S T, Bindoff L 1978 Morphologic aspects of muscle breakdown and lysosomal activation. Annals of the New York Academy of Science 317: 440–464
37. Cullen M J, Mastaglia F L 1982 Pathological reactions of skeletal muscle. In: Mastaglia F L, Walton J (eds) Skeletal muscle pathology. Churchill Livingstone, Edinburgh, pp 88–139
38. D'Agostino A N, Ziter F A, Rallison M L, Bray P F 1968 Familial myopathy with abnormal muscle mitochondria. Archives of Neurology (Chicago) 18: 388–401
39. Di Donato, S, Cornelio F, Balestrini M R, Bertagnolio B, Peluchetti D 1978 Mitochondria-lipid-glycogen myopathy, hyperlactic acidaemia and carnitine deficiency. Neurology (Minneapolis) 28: 1110–1116

40. Di Mauro S, Schotland P L, Bonilla E, Lee C P, Gambetti P, Rowland L P 1973 Progressive ophthalmoplegia, glycogen storage disease and abnormal mitochondria. Archives of Neurology (Chicago) 29: 170–179

41. Di Mauro S, Bonilla E, Zevianni M, Nagakawa M, De Vivo D C 1985 Mitochondrial myopathies. Annals of Neurology 17: 521–538

42. Dubowitz V 1967 Pathology of experimentally reinnervated skeletal muscle. Journal of Neurology, Neurosurgery and Psychiatry 30: 99–110

43. Dubowitz V, Roy S 1970 Central core disease of muscle: clinical, histochemical and electron microscopic studies of an affected mother and child. Brain 93: 133–146

44. Dubowitz V, Brooke M H 1973 Muscle biopsy: a modern approach. W B Saunders, London and Philadelphia, pp 1–475

45. Edström L, Wróblewski R, Mair W G P 1982 Genuine myotubular myopathy. Muscle and Nerve 5: 604–613

46. Engel A G 1966 Thyrotoxic and corticosteroid induced myopathies. Mayo Clinic Proceedings 41: 785–796

47. Engel A G 1967 Pathological reactions of the Z disk. In: Milhorat A T (ed) Exploratory concepts in muscular dystrophy and related disorders. Excerpta Medica, Amsterdam, pp 398–412

48. Engel A G 1970 Evolution and content of vacuoles in primary hypokalaemic periodic paralysis. Mayo Clinic Proceedings 45: 774–814

49. Engel A G 1973 Vacuolar myopathies etiologies and sequential structural studies. In: Peason C M, Mostofi F K (eds) The striated muscle. Williams & Wilkins, Baltimore, pp 301–341

50. Engel A G, Dale A J D 1968 Autophagic glycogenosis of late onset with mitochondrial abnormalities: light and electron microscopic observations. Mayo Clinic Proceedings 43: 233–279

51. Engel A G, MacDonald R D 1970 Ultrastructural reactions in muscle disease and their light microscopic correlates. In: Walton J N, Canal N, Scarlato G (eds) Muscle diseases. Excerpta Medica, Amsterdam, pp 1–89

52. Engel A G, Gomez M R, Groover R V 1971 Multicore disease. A recently recognized congenital myopathy associated with multifocal degeneration of muscle fibers. Mayo Clinic Proceedings 46: 666–681

53. Engel A G, Siekert R G 1972 Lipid storage myopathy responsive to prednisone. Archives of Neurology (Chicago) 27: 174–181

54. Engel A G, Angelini C, Gomez M R 1972 Fingerprint body myopathy. Mayo Clinic Proceedings 47: 377–388

55. Engel A G, Gomez M R, Seybold M E, Lambert E H 1973 The spectrum and diagnosis of acid maltase deficiency. Neurology (Minneapolis) 23: 95–106

56. Engel A G, Barker B Q, Eiben R M 1977 Carnitine deficiency: clinical, morphological and biochemical observations in a fatal case. Journal of Neurology, Neurosurgery and Psychiatry 40: 313–322

57. Engel W K, Oberc M A 1975 Abundant nuclear rods in adult-onset rod disease. Journal of Neuropathology and Experimental Neurology 34: 119–132

58. Engel W K, Foster J B, Hughes B P, Huxley H E, Mahler R 1961 Central core disease: an investigation of a rare muscle abnormality. Brain 84: 167–185

59. Engel W K, Brooke M H, Nelson P G 1966 Histochemical studies of denervated or tenotomized cat muscle illustrating difficulties in relating experimental animal conditions to human neuromuscular diseases. Annals of the New York Academy of Science 138: 160–185

60. Engel W K, Bishop D W, Cunningham G C 1970 Tubular aggregates in type II muscle fibers: ultrastructural and histochemical correlation. Journal of Ultrastructure Research 31: 507–525

61. Ewing S L, Rosai J 1974 Basophilic (mucoid) degeneration of skeletal muscle. Archives of Pathology (Chicago) 97: 60–62

62. Fardeau M 1970 Ultrastructural lesions in progressive muscular dystrophies. A critical study of their specificity. In: Walton J N, Canal N, Scarlato G (eds) Muscle diseases. Excerpta Medica, Amsterdam, pp 98–108

63. Fardeau M, Tomé F M S, Simon P 1979 Muscle and nerve changes induced by perhexiline maleate in man and mice. Muscle and Nerve 2: 24–36

64. Fardeau M, Tomé F M S, Rolland J C 1981 Congenital neuromuscular disorder with predominant mitochondrial changes in type II muscle fibers. Acta Neuropathologica (Berlin) Supplement 8: 279–281

65. Fisher E R, Gonzalez A R, Khurana R C, Danowski T S 1972 Unique concentric laminated membranous inclusions in myofibers. American Journal of Clinical Pathology 48: 329–244

66. Fischman D A, Meltzer H Y, Poppei R W 1973 The ultrastructure of human skeletal muscle: variations from archetypal morphology. In: Pearson C M, Mostofi F K (eds) The striated muscle. Williams & Wilkins, Baltimore, pp 58–76

67. Fitzsimons R B, McLeod J G 1982 Myopathy with pathological features of both centronuclear myopathy and multicore disease. Journal of the Neurological Sciences 57: 395–405

68. Fridén J, Sjöström M, Ekblom B 1983 Myofibrillar damage following intense eccentric exercise in man. International Journal of Sports Medicine 4: 170–176

69. Fukuhara N 1979 Electron microscopical demonstration of nucleic acids in virus like particles in the skeletal muscle of a traffic accident victim. Acta Neuropathologica (Berlin) 47: 55–59

70. Fukuhara N, Kumamoto T, Tsubaki T 1980 Rimmed vacuoles. Acta Neuropathologica (Berlin) 51: 229–235

71. Gallai M 1977 Myopathy with hyperaldosteronism — an electron microscopic study. Journal of the Neurological Sciences 32: 337–345

72. Gambetti P, Mellman W J, Gonatas N K 1969 Familial spongy degeneration of the central nervous system (van Bogaert–Bertrand disease). An ultrastructural study. Acta Neuropathologica (Berlin) 12: 103–115

73. Garancis J C 1968 Type II glycogenosis: biochemical and electron microscopic study. American Journal of Medicine 44: 289–300

74. Gibbels E, Henke U, Schädlich H-J, Haupt W F, Fiehn W 1983 Cylindrical spirals in skeletal muscle: a further observation with clinical, morphological, and biochemical analysis. Muscle and Nerve 6: 646–655

75. Goebel H H, Zeman W, Pilz H 1975 Significance of muscle biopsies in neuronal ceroid lipofuscinosis. Journal of Neurology, Neurosurgery and Psychiatry 38: 985–993

76. Goebel H H, Muller J, Gillen H W, Merritt A D 1978 Autosomal dominant spheroid body myopathy. Muscle and Nerve 1: 14–26

77. Goebel H H, Schloom H, Lenard H G 1981 Congenital myopathy with cytoplasmic bodies. Neuropediatrics 12: 166–180

78. Gonatas N K 1966 The fine structure of the rod like bodies in nemaline myopathy and their relation to the Z discs. Journal of Neuropathology and Experimental Neurology 25: 409–421

79. Gonatas N K, Perez M C, Shy L M, Evangelista I 1965 Central 'core' disease of skeletal muscle. Ultrastructural and cytochemical observations in two cases. American Journal of Pathology 47: 503–524

80. Gullotta F, Pavone L, La Rosa M, Grasso A 1982 Minicore myopathy. Klinische Wochenschrift 60: 1351–1355

81. Harriman D G 1982 The pathology of malignant hyperpyrexia. In: Mastaglia F L, Walton J (eds) Skeletal muscle pathology. Churchill Livingstone, Edinburgh, pp 575–591

82. Harriman D G F, Reed R 1972 The incidence of lipid droplets in human skeletal muscle in neuromuscular disorders. Journal of Pathology 106: 1–24

83. Holt I J, Harding A E, Morgan-Hughes J A 1988 Deletions of muscle mitochondrial DNA in patients with mitochondrial myopathies. Nature 331: 717–719

84. Howes E L, Price H M, Pearson C M, Blumberg J M 1966 Hypokalemic periodic paralysis: electron microscopic changes in the sarcoplasm. Neurology (Minneapolis) 16: 242–256

85. Hübner G, Pongratz D 1981 Granularkörpermyopathie (sog. reducing body myopathy). Virchows Archiv A 392: 97–104

86. Hudgson P, Gardner-Medwin D, Fulthorpe J J, Walton J N 1967 Nemaline myopathy. Neurology (Minneapolis) 17: 1125–1142

87. Hudgson P, Bradley W G, Jenkinson M 1972 Familial mitochondrial myopathy: a myopathy associated with disordered oxidative metabolism in muscle fibres. Journal of the Neurological Sciences 16: 343–370

88. Hug G, Garancis J C, Schubert W K, Kaplan S 1966 Glycogen storage disease types II, III, VIII and IX: a biochemical and electron microscopic analysis. American Journal of Diseases of Children 111: 457–474

89. Hülsmann N, Gullotta F, Okur H 1981 Cytopathology of an unusual case of centronuclear myopathy. Journal of the Neurological Sciences 50: 311–333

90. Iannaccone S T, Griggs R C, Markesbery W R, Joynt R J 1972 Familial progressive external ophthalmoplegia and ragged-red fibers. Neurology (Minneapolis) 24: 1033–1038

91. Ionasescu V, Radu H, Nicholescu P 1975 Identification of Duchenne muscular dystrophy carriers. Archives of Pathology (Chicago) 99: 436–441

92. Isaacs H, Heffron J J A, Badenhorst M, Pickering A 1976 Weakness associated with the pathological presence of lipid in skeletal muscle: a detailed study of a patient with carnitine deficiency. Journal of Neurology, Neurosurgery and Psychiatry 39: 1114–1123

93. Ishimoto S, Goto I, Ohta M, Kuroiwa Y 1983 A quantitative study of the muscle satellite cells in various neuromuscular disorders. Journal of the Neurological Sciences 62: 303–314

94. Jenis E H, Lindquist R R, Lister R C 1969 New congenital myopathy with crystalline intranuclear inclusions. Archives of Neurology (Chicago) 20: 281–287

95. Jerusalem F 1970 Bioptische befunde des T-systems und tubulare strukturcomplexe bei neoplasticher cortisonmyopathie. Acta Neuropathologica (Berlin) 14: 338–344

96. Jerusalem F, Angelini C, Engel A G, Groover R V 1973 Mitochondrial lipid glycogen (MLG) disease of muscle. A morphologically regressive congenital myopathy. Archives of the Neurological Association 98: 89–93

97. Jerusalem F, Engel A G, Gomez M R 1973 Sarcotubular myopathy. A newly recognized, benign, congenital familial muscle disease. Neurology (Minneapolis) 23: 897–906

98. Jerusalem F, Engel A G, Peterson H A 1975 Human muscle fiber fine structure: morphometric data on controls. Neurology (Minneapolis) 25: 127–134

99. Jerusalem F, Ludin H, Bischoff A, Hartmann G 1979 Cytoplasmic body neuromyopathy presenting as respiratory failure and weight loss. Journal of the Neurological Sciences 41: 1–9

100. Johnson A G 1969 Alterations of the Z-lines and I-band myofilaments in human skeletal muscle. Acta Neuropathologica (Berlin) 12: 218–226

101. Julien J, Vital C L, Vallat J M, Vallat M, Le Blanc M 1974 Oculopharyngeal muscular dystrophy — a case with abnormal mitochondria and fingerprint inclusions. Journal of the Neurological Sciences 21: 165–169

102. Kark R A P, Rodriguez-Budelli M 1979 Pyruvate dehydrogenase deficiency in spinocerebellar degeneration. Neurology (Minneapolis) 29: 126–131

103. Karpati G, Carpenter S, Labrisseau A, Lafontaine R 1973 The Kearns–Sayre syndrome — a multisystem disease with mitochondrial abnormality demonstrated in skeletal muscle and skin. Journal of the Neurological Sciences 19: 133–151

104. Karpati G, Carpenter S, Melmed C, Eisen A A 1974 Experimental ischaemic myopathy. Journal of the Neurological Sciences 23: 129–161

105. Karpati G, Carpenter S, Engel A G, Watters G, Allen J, Rothman S, Kassen G, Mamer O A 1975 The syndrome of systemic carnitine deficiency. Clinical morphologic, biochemical and pathophysiologic features. Neurology (Minneapolis) 25: 16–24

106. Ketelsen U P 1980 Quantitative freeze fracture studies of human skeletal muscle cell membranes under normal and pathological conditions. In: Angelini C, Danielli G A, Fontanari D (eds) Muscular dystrophy research: advances and new trends. Excerpta Medica, Amsterdam, pp 79–87

107. Klinkerfuss G H 1967 An electron microscopic study of myotonic dystrophy Archives of Neurology (Chicago) 16: 181–193

108. Kobayashi Y, Miyabayashi S, Takada G, Narisawa K, Tada K, Yamamoto T Y 1982 Ultrastructural study of the childhood mitochondrial myopathic syndrome associated with lactic acidosis. European Journal of Pediatrics 139: 25–30

109. Korényi-Both A, Korényi-Both I, Kayes B C 1981 Thyrotoxic myopathy: pathomorphological observations of human material and experimentally induced thyrotoxicosis in rats. Acta Neuropathologica (Berlin) 53: 237–248

110. Kovarsky J, Schochet S C Jr, McCormick W F 1973 The significance of target fibres: a clinicopathological review of 100 patients with neurogenic atrophy. American Journal of Clinical Pathology 59: 790–797

111. Kuzuhara S, Nakanishi T 1984 Tubulomembranous and finger-print like inclusions in biopsied muscle of distal myopathy with rimmed vacuoles. Acta Neuropathologica (Berlin) 62: 194–200

112. Lake B D, Wilson J 1975 Zebra body myopathy. Clinical, histochemical and ultrastructural studies. Journal of the Neurological Sciences 24: 437–446

113. Luft R, Ikkos D, Palmieri G, Ernster L, Afzelius B 1962 A case of severe hypermetabolism of non-thyroid origin with a defect in the maintenance of mitochondrial respiratory control: a correlated clinical, biochemical and morphological study. Journal of Clinical Investigation 41: 1776–1804

114. MacDonald R D, Engel A G 1969 The cytoplasmic body: another structural anomaly of the Z discs. Acta Neuropathologica (Berlin) 14: 99–107

115. MacDonald R D, Engel A G 1970 Experimental chloroquine myopathy. Journal of Neuropathology and Experimental Neurology 29: 479–499

116. MacDonald R D, Rewcastle N B, Humphrey J G 1969 Myopathy of hypokalaemic periodic paralysis. An electron microscopic study. Archives of Neurology (Chicago) 20: 565–585

117. Mair W G P, Tóme F M S 1972 Atlas of the ultrastructure of diseased muscle. Churchill Livingstone, Edinburgh and London, pp 1–243

118. Markesbery W R, McQuillen M P, Procopis P Q, Harrison A R, Engel A G 1974 Muscle carnitine deficiency. Association with lipid myopathy, vacuolar neuropathy and vacuolated leukocytes. Archives of Neurology (Chicago) 31: 320–324

119. Markesbery W R, Griggs R C, Herr B 1977 Distal myopathy: electron microscopic and histochemical studies. Neurology (Minneapolis) 27: 727–735

120. Mastaglia F L, Walton J N 1970 Coxsackie virus-like particles in skeletal muscle from a case of polymyositis. Journal of the Neurological Sciences 11: 593–599

121. Mastaglia F L, Walton J N 1971 An ultrastructural study of skeletal muscle in polymyositis. Journal of the Neurological Sciences 12: 473–504

122. Mastaglia F L, Hudson P 1981 Ultrastructural studies of diseased muscle. In: Walton J N (ed) Disorders of voluntary muscle. Churchill Livingstone, Edinburgh and London, pp 296–355

123. Mastaglia F L, McCollum J P K, Larson P F, Hudgson P 1970 Steroid myopathy complicating McArdle's disease. Journal of Neurology, Neurosurgery and Psychiatry 33: 111–120

124. Mastaglia F L, Dawkins R L, Papadimitriou J M 1975 Morphological changes in skeletal muscle after transplantation: a light and electron microscopic study of the initial phase of degeneration and regeneration. Journal of the Neurological Sciences 25: 227–247

125. Mastaglia F L, Papadimitriou J M, Dawkins R L, Beveridge B 1977 Vacuolar myopathy associated with chloroquine, lupus erythematosus and thymoma. Journal of the Neurological Sciences 34: 315–328

126. Matsubara S 1980 Ultrastructural changes in granulomatous myopathy. Acta Neuropathologica (Berlin) 50: 91–96

127. Matsubara S, Mair W G 1980 Ultrastructural changes of skeletal muscle in polyarteritis nodosa and in arteritis associated with rheumatoid arthritis. Acta Neuropathologica (Berlin) 50: 169–174

128. McAdams A J, Hug G, Bove K E 1974 Glycogen storage disease type I to X. Criteria for morphologic diagnosis. Human Pathology 5: 463–486

129. McDougall J, Wiles C M, Edwards R H T 1980 Spiral membrane cylinders in the skeletal muscle of a patient with melorheostosis. Neuropathology and Applied Neurobiology 6: 69–74

130. McKeran R O, Slavin G, Ward P, Paul E, Mair W G P 1980 Hypothyroid myopathy. A clinical and pathological study. Journal of Pathology 132: 35–54

131. McLeod J G, Baker W De C, Shorey C D, Kerr C B 1975 Mitochondrial myopathy with multisystem abnormalities and normal ocular movements. Journal of the Neurological Sciences 24: 39–52

132. Meyers K R, Gilden D H, Rinaldi C F, Hansen J L 1972 Periodic muscle weakness normokalemia and tubular aggregates. Neurology (Minneapolis) 22: 269–279

133. Miike T, Tamari H, Ohtani Y, Kondo Y 1983 Intracytoplasmic

inclusions in the atrophic muscle fibers in Werdnig–Hoffman disease. Brain Development 5: 315–319

134. Milhorat A T, Shafiq S A, Goldstone L 1966 Changes in muscle structure in dystrophic patients, carriers and normal siblings seen by electron microscopy: correlation with levels of serum creatinephosphokinase (CPK). Annals of the New York Academy of Science 138: 246–292

135. Mokri B G, Engel A G 1975 Duchenne dystrophy: electron microscopic findings pointing to a basic or early abnormality in the plasma membrane of the muscle fibres. Neurology (Minneapolis) 256: 1111–1120

136. Moraes C T, Di Mauro S, Zeviani M, Lombes A, Shanske S, Miranda A F, Nakase H, Bonilla E, Werneck L C, Servidei S, Nonaka I, Koga Y, Spiro A J, Brownell K W, Schmidt B, Schotland D L, Zupanc M, De Vivo D, Schon E A, Rowland L P 1989 Mitochondrial DNA deletions in progressive external ophthalmoplegia and Kearns–Sayre syndrome. New England Journal of Medicine 320: 1293–1299

137. Morgan-Hughes J A 1982 Defects of the energy pathways of skeletal muscle. In: Matthews W B, Glasser G H (eds) Recent advances in clinical neurology, vol. 3. Churchill Livingstone, Edinburgh, p 146

138. Morgan-Hughes J A, Darveniza P, Kahn S N, Landon D N, Sherrat R M, Land J M, Clark J B 1977 A mitochondrial myopathy characterised by a deficiency in reducible cytochrome b. Brain 100: 617–640

139. Morgan-Hughes J A, Darveniza P, Landon E N, Land J M, Clark J B 1979 A mitochondrial myopathy with deficiency of respiratory chain NADH-CoQ reductase activity. Journal of the Neurological Sciences 45: 27–46

140. Morgan-Hughes J A 1982 Mitochondrial myopathies. In: Mastaglia F L, Walton J (eds) Skeletal muscle pathology. Churchill Livingstone, Edinburgh, pp 309–339

141. Morgan-Hughes J A, Hayes D J, Clark J B, Landon D N, Swash M, Stark R J, Rudge P 1982 Mitochondrial encephalomyopathies. Biochemical studies in two cases revealing defects in the respiratory chain. Brain 105: 553–582

142. Mukherjee T M, Dixon B R, Blumbergs P C, Swift J G, Hallpike J F 1986 The fine structure of the intramitochondrial crystalloids in mitochondrial myopathy. Journal of Submicroscopic Cytology 18: 595–604

143. Neville H E 1973 Ultrastructural changes in muscle disease. In: Dubowitz V, Brooke M H (eds) Muscle biopsy: a modern approach. Saunders, London and Philadelphia, pp 383–470

144. Neville H E, Brooke M H 1973 Central core fibres: structured and unstructured. In: Kakulas B A (ed) Basic research in myology. Excerpta Medica, Amsterdam, pp 497–511

145. Neville H E, Brooke M H, Austin J H 1974 Studies in myoclonus epilepsy (Lafora body form). IV. Skeletal muscle abnormalities. Archives of Neurology (Chicago) 30: 466–474

146. Neville H E, Maunder-Sewry C A, McDougall J, Sewell J R, Dubowitz V 1979 Chloroquine-induced cytosomes with curvilinear profiles in muscle. Muscle and Nerve 2: 376–381

147. Nogami H, Ogasawara N, Kasai T, Oki T, Murachi S 1983 Lipid storage myopathy associated with scoliosis and multiple joint contractures. Acta Neuropathologica (Berlin) 61: 305–310

148. Nokana I, Sunohara N, Ishiura S, Satoyoshi E 1981 Familial distal myopathy with rimmed vacuoles and lamellar myeloid body formation. Journal of the Neurological Sciences 51: 141–155

149. Odor D L, Patel A N, Pearce L A 1967 Familial hypokalemic periodic paralysis with permanent myopathy. A clinical and ultrastructural study. Journal of Neuropathology and Experimental Neurology 26: 98–114

150. Oh S, Meyers G J, Wilson E R, Alexander C B 1983 A benign form of reducing body myopathy. Muscle and Nerve 6: 278–282

151. Olson W, Engel W K, Walsh G O, Einaugler R 1972 Oculocraniosomatic neuromuscular disease with 'ragged-red' fibres. Archives of Neurology (Chicago) 26: 193–211

152. Palmucci L, Bertolotto A, Monga G, Andizzone G, Schiffer D 1978 Histochemical and ultrastructural findings in a case of centronuclear myopathy. European Neurology 17: 327–332

153. Panegyres P K, Papadimitriou J M, Hollingsworth P N, Armstrong J A, Kakulas B A 1990 Vesicular changes in the myopathies of AIDS. Ultrastructural observations and their relationship to Zidovudine treatment. Journal of Neurology, Neurosurgery and Psychiatry 53: 649–655

154. Papadimitriou J M, Mastaglia F L 1982 Ultrastructural changes in human muscle fibres in disease. Journal of Submicroscopic Cytology 14: 525–551

155. Patel H, Berry K, MacLeod P, Dunn H G 1983 Cytoplasmic body myopathy. Report of a family and review of the literature. Journal of the Neurological Sciences 60: 281–292

156. Pavlakis S G, Phillips P C, Di Mauro S, De Vivo D C, Rowland L P 1984 Mitochondrial myopathy, encephalopathy, lactic acidosis and stroke like episodes: a distinctive clinical syndrome. Annals of Neurology 16: 481–488

157. Payne C M, Curless R G 1976 Concentric laminated bodies — ultrastructural demonstration of fibre type specificity. Journal of the Neurological Sciences 29: 311–322

158. Payne C M, Curless R G 1977 Fingerprint inclusions. Ultrastructural demonstration of muscle fiber type specificity. Journal of the Neurological Sciences 31: 379–386

159. Payne C M, Stern L Z, Curless R G, Hanapel L K 1975 Ultrastructural fibre typing in normal and diseased human muscle. Journal of the Neurological Sciences 25: 99–108

160. Poulton J, Deadman M E, Gardiner R M 1989 Duplications of mitochondrial DNA in mitochondrial myopathy. Lancet 1: 236–239

161. Price H M 1974 Ultrastructure of the skeletal muscle fibre. In: Walton J N (ed) Disorders of voluntary muscle. Churchill Livingstone, Edinburgh and London, pp 31–67

162. Price H M, Howes E L, Blumberg J M 1964 Ultrastructural alterations in skeletal muscle fibres injured by cold. I. The acute degenerative changes. Laboratory Investigation 13: 1264–1278

163. Price H M, Gordon G B, Pearson C M, Munsat T L, Blumberg J M 1965 New evidence for accumulation of excessive Z band material in nemaline myopathy. Proceedings of the National Academy of Science of the USA 64: 1398–1406

164. Price H M, Gordon G B, Munsat T L, Pearson C M 1967 Myopathy with atypical mitochondria in type I skeletal muscle fibres. A histochemical and ultrastructural study. Journal of Neuropathology and Experimental Neurology 26: 475–497

165. Prick M J J, Gabreels F J M, Trijbels J M F, Janssen A J M, le Coultre R, van Dam K, Jaspar H H J, Ebels E J, Op A A W 1983 Progressive poliodystrophy (Alpers' disease) with a defect in cytochrome aa_3 in muscle: a report of two unrelated patients. Clinical Neurology and Neurosurgery 85: 57–70

166. Resnick J S, Engel W K 1967 Target fibres — structural and cytochemical characteristics and their relationship to neurogenic muscle disease and fiber type. In: Milhorat A T (ed) Exploratory concepts in muscular dystrophy and related disorders. Excerpta Medica, Amsterdam, pp 255–267

167. Rewcastle N B, Humphrey J G 1965 Vacuolar myopathy: clinical histochemical and microscopic study. Archives of Neurology (Chicago) 12: 570–582

168. Reznik M 1969 Origin of myoblasts during skeletal muscle regeneration. Electron microscopic observations. Laboratory Investigation 20: 353–363

169. Reznik M 1973 Current concepts of skeletal muscle regeneration. In: Pearson C M, Mostofi F K (eds) The striated muscle. Williams & Wilkins, Baltimore, pp 185–225

170. Ringel S P, Neville H E, Durster M C, Carroll J E 1978 A new congenital neuromuscular disease with trilaminar muscle fibres. Neurology (Minneapolis) 28: 282–289

171. Rubin E, Katz A M, Lieber C S, Stein E P, Purzkin S 1976 Muscle damage produced by chronic alcohol consumption. American Journal of Pathology 83: 499–515

172. Saltis L M, Mendell J R 1974 The fine structural differences in human muscle fibres based on peroxidatic activity. Journal of Neuropathology and Experimental Neurology 33: 632–640

173. Sarnat H B, Silbert S W 1976 Maturational arrest of fetal muscle in neonatal myotonic dystrophy. Archives of Neurology (Chicago) 33: 466–474

174. Sarnat H B, Roth S I, Jimenez J F 1981 Neonatal myotubular myopathy: neuropathy and failure of postnatal maturation of fetal muscle. Journal Canadien des Sciences Neurologiques 8: 313–320

175. Sarnat H B, Machin S, Danvish H Z, Rubin S Z 1983 Mitochondrial myopathy of cerebro-hepato-renal (Zellweger) syndrome. Canadian Journal of Neurological Sciences 10: 170–177

176. Sato T, Walker D L, Peters H A, Reese H N, Chou S M 1971 Chronic polymyositis and myxovirus-like inclusions. Electron microscopic and viral studies. Archives of Neurology (Chicago) 24: 409–418

177. Scelsi R, Marchetti C, Poggi P 1980 Histochemical and ultrastructural aspects of m. vastus lateralis in sedentary old people (age 65–89 years). Acta Neuropathologica (Berlin) 51: 99–105

178. Schiaffino S, Settembrini P 1970 Studies on the effect of degeneration in developing muscle. Virchows Archiv A 4: 345–356

179. Schiller H H, Mair W G P 1974 Ultrastructural changes of muscle in malignant hyperthermia. Journal of the Neurological Sciences 21: 93–100

180. Schmitt H P, Volk B 1975 The relationship between target, targetoid and targetoid core fibres in severe neurogenic muscular atrophy. Journal of Neurology 210: 167–181

181. Schochet S S Jr, McCormick W F, Kovarsky J L 1971 Light and electron microscopy of skeletal muscle in type IV glycogenosis. Acta Neuropathologica (Berlin) 19: 137–144

182. Schochet S S Jr, McCormick W F 1973 Polymyositis with intranuclear inclusions. Archives of Neurology (Chicago) 28: 280–283

183. Schochet S S Jr, Lampert P W 1978 Diagnostic electron microscopy of skeletal muscle. In: Trump B F, Jones R T (eds) Diagnostic electron microscopy, vol. 1. John Wiley and Sons, New York, pp 209–253

184. Schochet S S Jr, McCormick W F, Kovarsky J L 1971 Light and electron microscopy of skeletal muscle in type IV glycogenosis. Acta Neuropathologica (Berlin) 19: 137–144

185. Schochet S S Jr, Zellweger H, Ionasescu V, McCormick W F 1972 Centronuclear myopathy: disease entity or a syndrome? Journal of the Neurological Sciences 16: 215–228

186. Schotland D L 1969 An electron microscopic study of target fibres, target-like fibres and related abnormalities in human muscle. Journal of Neuropathology and Experimental Neurology 28: 214–228

187. Schotland D L 1970 An electron microscopic investigation of myotonic dystrophy. Journal of Neuropathology and Experimental Neurology 29: 241–253

188. Schotland D L 1973 Ultrastructure of muscle in glycogen storage diseases. In: Pearson C M, Mostofi F K (eds) The striated muscle. Williams & Wilkins, Baltimore, pp 410–426

189. Schotland D L, Spiro D, Carmel P 1966 Ultrastructural studies of ring fibres in human muscle disease. Journal of Neuropathology and Experimental Neurology 25: 431–442

190. Schotland D L, Di Mauro S, Bonilla E, Scarpa A, Lee C P 1976 Neuromuscular disorders associated with a defect in mitochondrial energy supply. Archives of Neurology (Chicago) 33: 475–479

191. Schotland D L, Bonilla E, Wakayama Y 1980 Application of the freeze fracture technique to the study of human neuromuscular disease. Muscle and Nerve 3: 21–27

192. Schroder J M 1970 Sarcolemmal indentations resembling junctional folds in myotonic dystrophy. In: Walton J N, Canal N, Scarlato G (eds) Muscle diseases. Excerpta Medica, Amsterdam, pp 109–122

193. Schroder J M, Adams R D 1968 Ultrastructural morphology of the muscle fibre in myotonic dystrophy. Acta Neuropathologica (Berlin) 10: 218–241

194. Schroder J M, Becker P E 1972 Anomalien des T-systems und des sarkoplasmatischen reticulums bei der myotonic, paramyotonic und adynamic. Virchows Archiv A 357: 319–344

195. Schutta H S Armitage J L 1969 Thyrotoxic hypokalaemic periodic paralysis: a fine structure study. Journal of Neuropathology and Experimental Neurology 28: 321–336

196. Schutta H S, Kelly A M, Zacks S I 1969 Necrosis and regeneration of muscle in paroxysmal idiopathic myoglobinuria. Electron microscopic observation. Brain 92: 191–202

197. Sengers R C A, Stadhouders A M Trijbels J M F 1984 Mitochondrial myopathies. Clinical, morphological and biochemical aspects. European Journal of Pediatrics 141: 192–207

198. Shafiq S A, Milhorat A T 1967 Some comments on the specificity of alterations in the fine structure in muscle disease. In: Milhorat A T (ed) Exploratory concepts in muscular dystrophy and related disorders. Excerpta Medica, Amsterdam, pp 268–273

199. Shafiq S A, Goricki M A, Milhorat A T 1967 An electron microscopic study of regeneration and satellite cells in human muscle. Neurology (Minneapolis) 17: 567–574

200. Shafiq S A, Milhorat A T, Gorycki M A 1967 Giant mitochondria in human muscle with inclusions. Archives of Neurology (Chicago) 17: 666–671

201. Shafiq S A, Dubowitz V, Peterson H de C, Milhorat A T 1967 Nemaline myopathy: report of a fatal case with histochemical and electron microscopic studies. Brain 90: 817–828

202. Shibasaki H, Santa T, Kuroiwa T 1973 Late onset mitochondrial myopathy. Journal of the Neurological Sciences 18: 301–310

203. Shy G M, Magee K R 1956 A new non-progressive myopathy. Brain 79: 610–621

204. Shy G M, Engel W K, Somers J E, Wanko T 1963 Nemaline myopathy: a new congenital myopathy. Brain 86: 793–810

205. Shy G M, Gonatas N K, Perez M 1966 Two childhood myopathies with abnormal mitochondria. I. Megaconial myopathy. II. Pleoconial myopathy. Brain 89: 133–158

206. Spiro A J, Shy G M, Gonatas N K 1966 Myotubular myopathy. Persistence of fetal muscle in an adolescent boy. Archives of Neurology (Chicago) 14: 1–14

207. Spiro A J, Moore C L, Prineas J W, Strasberg P M, Rapin I 1970 A cytochrome-related inherited disorder of the nervous system and muscle. Archives of Neurology (Chicago) 23: 103–112

208. Stonnington H H, Engel A G 1973 Normal and denervated muscle: a morphometric study of fine structure. Neurology (Minneapolis) 23: 714–724

209. Swash M, Schwartz M S 1981 Familial multicore disease with focal loss of cross striations and ophthalmoplegia. Journal of the Neurological Sciences 52: 1–10

210. Takagi A, Schotland D L, Di Mauro S, Rowland L P 1973 Thyrotoxic periodic paralysis. Function of sarcoplasmic reticulum and muscle glycogen. Neurology (Minneapolis) 23: 1008–1016

211. Teräväinen H, Mäkitie J 1977 Striated muscle ultrastructure in intermittent claudication. Archives of Pathology and Laboratory Medicine 101: 230–235

212. Thornell LE, Edström L, Billeter R, Butler-Browne G S, Kjorell V, Whalen R G 1984 Muscle fibre type composition in distal myopapthy (Welander). Journal of the Neurological Sciences 65: 269–292

213. Toga M, Berard-Badier M, Gambarelli D, Pinsard N, Hassoun J 1971 Un cas de dystrophie neuroaxonale infantile on maladie de Seitelberger. III. Etude ultrastructurale du muscle strie. Acta Neuropathologica (Berlin) 18: 327–341

214. Tomé F M S, Fardeau M 1973 'Fingerprint inclusions' in muscle fibres in dystrophia myotonica. Acta Neuropathologica (Berlin) 24: 62–67

215. Tomé F M S, Fardeau M 1980 Nuclear inclusions in oculopharyngeal dystrophy. Acta Neuropathologica (Berlin) 49: 85–87

216. Torvik A, Dietrichson P, Svaar H, Hudgson P 1974 Myopathy with tremor and dementia: a metabolic disorder? Journal of the Neurological Sciences 21: 181–190

217. Trump B F, Valigorsky J M, Dees J H, Mergner W J, Kim K K, Jones R T, Pendergrass R E, Garbus J, Cowley R A 1973 Cellular change in human diseases. A new method of pathological analysis. Human Pathology 4: 89–109

218. Vallat J M, de Lumley L, Loubet A, Leboutet M J, Corvisier N, Umdenstock R 1982 Coexistence of minicores, cores, and rods in the same muscle biopsy. Acta Neuropathologica (Berlin) 58: 229–232

219. van Biervliet J P G M, Bruinvis L, Ketting D, de Bree P K, van der Heiden C, Wadnan S K, Willems J L, Bookelman H, van Haelst V, Monnens A H 1977 Hereditary mitochondrial myopathy with lactic acidaemia, a De Toni–Fanconi–Debre syndrome and a defective respiratory chain in voluntary striated muscles. Pediatric Research 11: 1088–1093

220. van Dyke D H, Griggs R C, Markesbery W, di Mauro S 1975 Hereditary carnitine deficiency of muscle. Neurology (Minneapolis) 25: 154–159

221. van Haelst V 1970 An electron microscopic study of muscle in

Werdnig–Hoffmann's disease. Virchows Archiv A 351: 291–305

222. Wakayama Y, Schotland D L, Bonilla E, Orecchio E 1979 Quantitative ultrastructural study of muscle satellite cells in Duchenne dystrophy. Neurology (Minneapolis) 29: 401–407

223. Webb J N, Gillespie W J 1976 Virus-like particles in paraspinal muscles in scoliosis. British Medical Journal 4: 912–913

224. Wolburg H, Schlote W, Langohr H D, Pieffer J, Reiher K H, Heckl R W 1982 Slowly progressive congenital myopathy with cytoplasmic bodies — report of two cases and a review of the literature. Clinical Neuropathology 1: 55–66

225. Wróblewski R, Nordemar R 1975 Ultrastructural and histochemical stuidies of muscle in rheumatoid arthritis. Scandinavian Journal of Rheumatology 4: 197–204

226. Wróblewski R, Edström L, Mair W G P 1982 Five different types of centrally nucleated muscle fibres in man: elemental composition and morphologic criteria. Journal of Submicroscopic Cytology 14: 377–387

227. Yamaguchi M, Robson R M, Stromer M H, Dahl D S, Oda T 1978 Actin filaments form the backbone of nemaline myopathy rods. Nature 271: 265–267

228. Yarom R, Shapira Y 1977 Myosin degeneration in a congenital myopathy. Archives of Neurology (Chicago) 34: 114–115

229. Yarom R, Reaches A 1980 Thick filament degeneration in a case of acute quadriplegia. Journal of the Neurological Sciences 45: 13–22

230. Yunis E J, Samaha F J 1971 Inclusion body myositis. Laboratory Investigation 25: 240–248

231. Zeviani M, Moraes C T, Di Mauro S, Nakase H, Bonilla E, Schon E A, Rowland L P 1988 Deletions of mitochondrial DNA in Kearns–Sayre syndrome. Neurology (Minneapolis) 38: 1339–1346

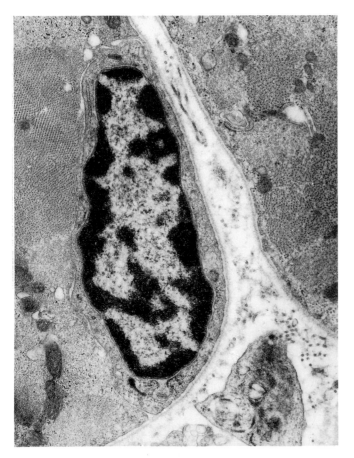

Fig. 26.1 Polymyositis: satellite cell. The satellite cell possesses a nucleus with much heterochromatin, scant cytoplasm, and is enclosed within the external lamina that envelopes the fibre. (× 20 500)

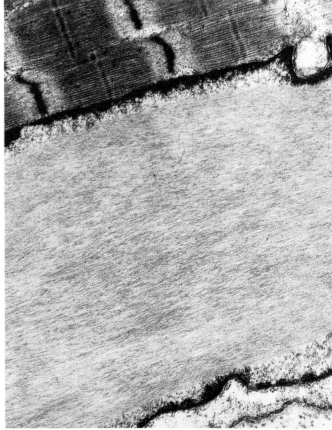

Fig. 26.2 Polymyositis: fibrillar nuclear inclusion. Most of the nuclear mass is replaced by fine filaments. (× 18 500)

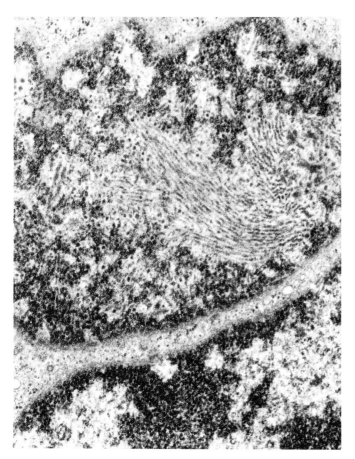

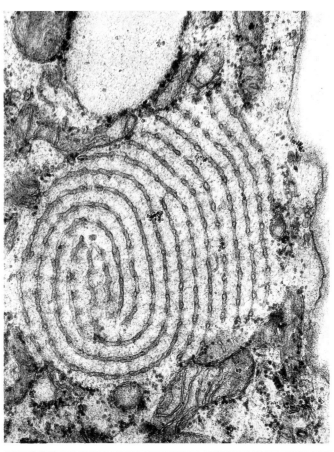

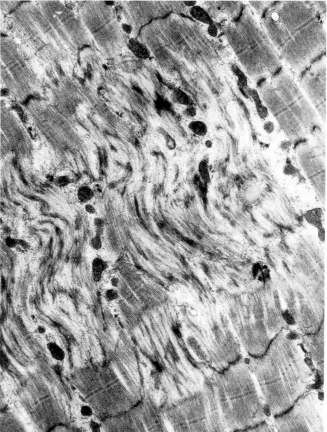

Fig. 26.3 (Above)   Inclusion body myositis: fibrillar nuclear inclusion. Filaments, measuring 18 nm in diameter, occupy the central regions of a muscle fibre nucleus. Similar filaments may also be present in the sarcoplasm, often near autophagic vacuoles. (× 40 000)

Fig. 26.4 (Above right)   Polymyositis: annulate lamellae. Stacks of annulate lamellae are seen in the paranuclear region of the muscle fibre. (× 36 100)

Fig. 26.5 (Right)   Multicore disease: myofibrillar lesion. Focal disruption of a few sarcomeres is seen in this field. (× 10 300)

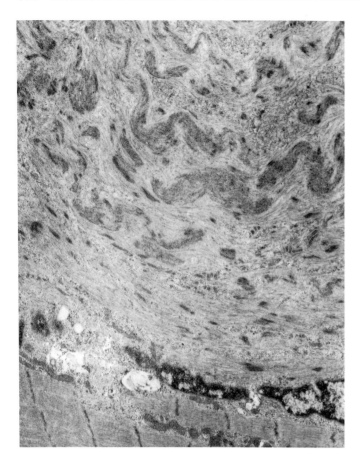

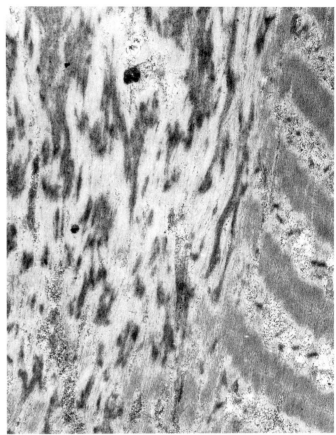

Fig. 26.6 Muscle denervation: target fibre. A region of complete disruption of the sarcomeric pattern is separated from a peripheral normal zone by a layer where the damage is only moderate. (× 8300)

Fig. 26.7 Senile atrophy: core-targetoid fibre. A zone of complete sarcomeric disruption abuts directly onto a region where damage is absent. (× 9000)

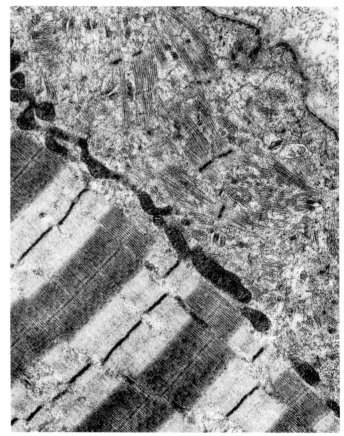

Fig. 26.8 Myotonic dystrophy: subsarcolemmal masses. Aggregates of disorganized sarcomeres and myofibrils are present in the subsarcolemmal region of this fibre. (× 13 300)

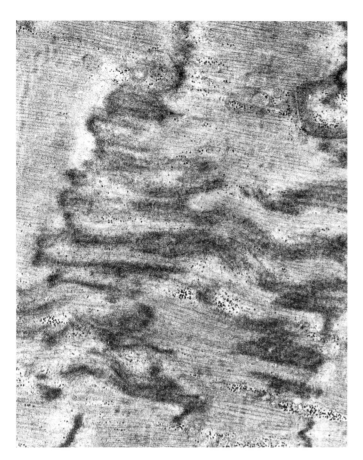

Fig. 26.9 Neurogenic atrophy: Z-disc streaming. Streaming of the osmiophilic material of Z-discs is present in a few sarcomeres. (× 19 400)

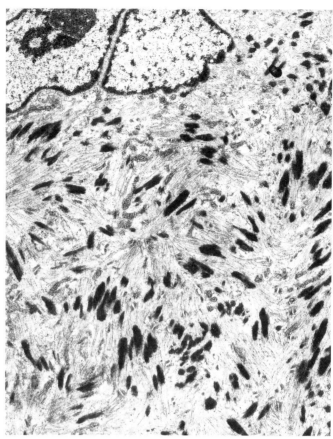

Fig. 26.10 Nemaline myopathy: survey. Many nemaline rods are present in the periphery of this muscle fibre. (× 7200)

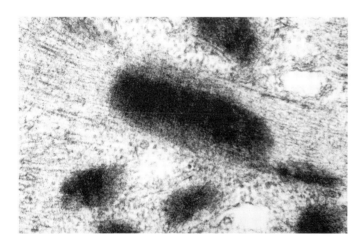

Fig. 26.11 Nemaline myopathy: nemaline rod. The periodic cross striations of a nemaline rod can be seen. (× 54 600)

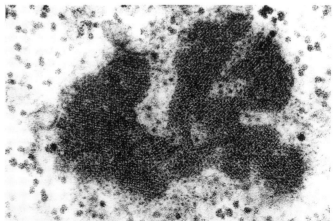

Fig. 26.12 Nemaline myopathy: cross-section of a nemaline rod. Nemaline rods when cross-sectioned display a quadratic lattice configuration. (× 74 200)

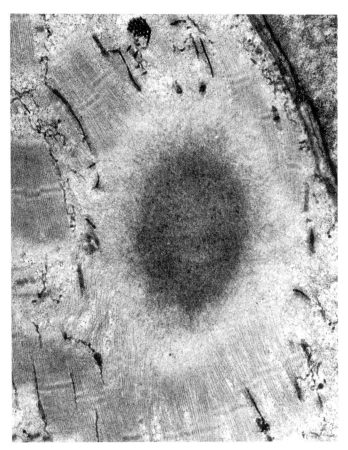

Fig. 26.13 Neurogenic atrophy: cytoplasmic body. Cytoplasmic bodies consist of a central osmiophilic mass and a halo of radiating filaments. In this particular instance the T-system has been stained with Karnovsky's potassium ferrocyanide technique. (× 18 500)

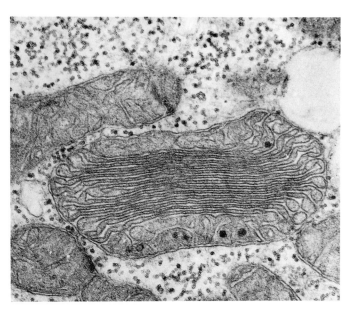

Fig. 26.14 Mitochondrial myopathy: large mitochondria. This enlarged mitochondrion displays parallel stacks of cristae mitochondriales and prominent matrical granules. (× 50 400)

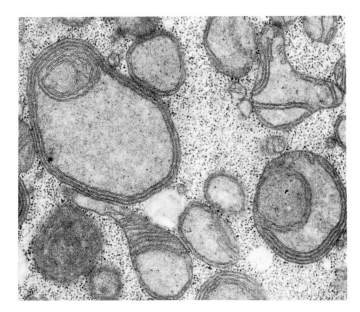

Fig. 26.15 Mitochondrial myopathy: enlarged mitochondria. Many mitochondria are enlarged, distorted and possess concentrically arrayed cristae mitochondriales. (× 23 500)

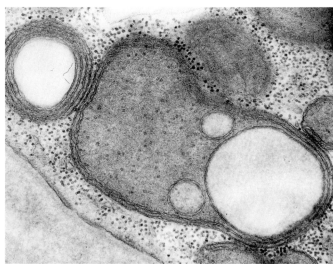

Fig. 26.16 Mitochondrial myopathy: enlarged mitochondria. Enlarged, distorted mitochondria are seen containing concentrically arranged cristae mitochondriales. (× 23 300)

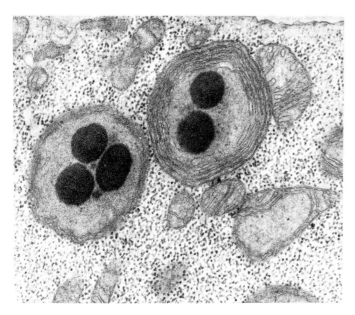

Fig. 26.17 Mitochondrial myopathy: large matrix granules. Large electron-dense granules are present in the inner chamber of enlarged mitochondria. (× 31 700)

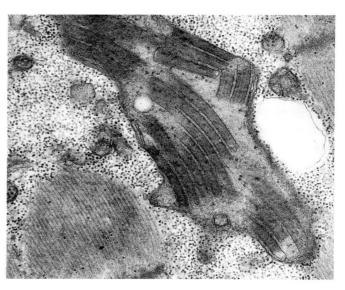

Fig. 26.18 Mitochondrial myopathy: crystalline inclusions. Many crystalline inclusions are present within the cristae mitochondriales of this enlarged mitochondrion. (× 23 300)

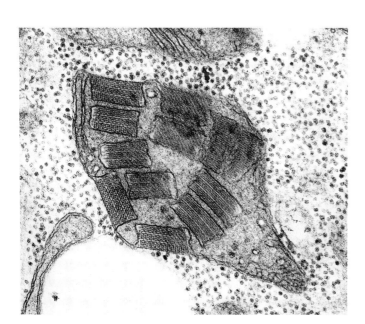

Fig. 26.19 Mitochondrial myopathy: crystalline inclusion. The substructure of the crystalline inclusions which are situated within the cristae mitochondriales can be seen. (× 50 400)

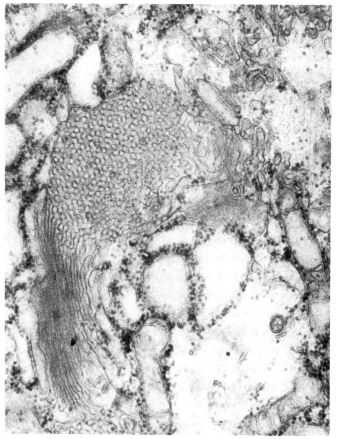

Fig. 26.20 Periodic paralysis: transverse tubular system. The honeycomb arrays of transverse tubules are in continuity with the lamellae of the Golgi apparatus. (× 38 300)

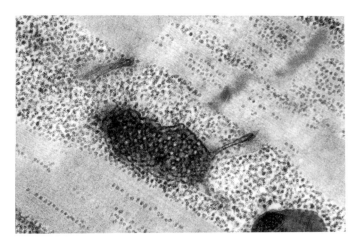

Fig. 26.21 Periodic paralysis: transverse tubular system. The T-tubule of a triad connects with a small honeycomb array. (× 39 200)

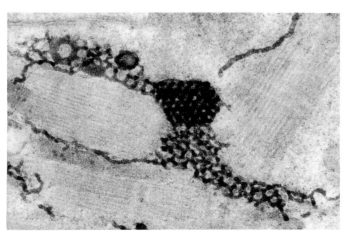

Fig. 26.22 Periodic paralysis: transverse tubular system. Staining with Karnovsky's potassium ferrocyanide technique enhances the detection of the contents of the transverse tubular system. (× 32 800)

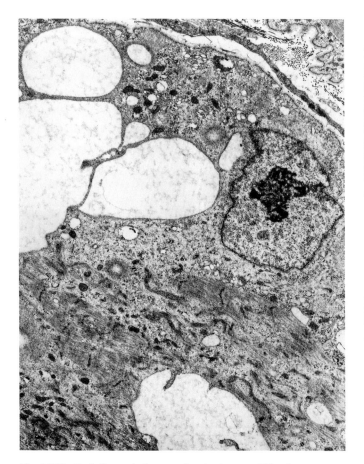

Fig. 26.23 Periodic paralysis: sarcoplasmic cisternae. Dilated sarcoplasmic cisternae are scattered throughout the fibre. (× 6000)

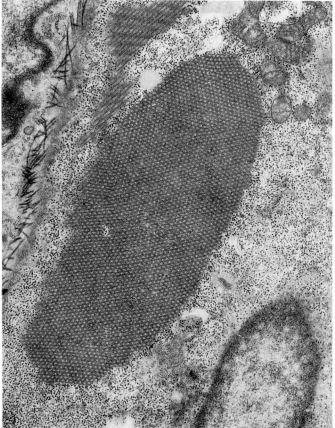

Fig. 26.24 Exertional muscle cramp syndrome: sarcoplasmic reticulum. Tubular aggregates are present in the paranuclear region of this muscle fibre. (× 16 500)

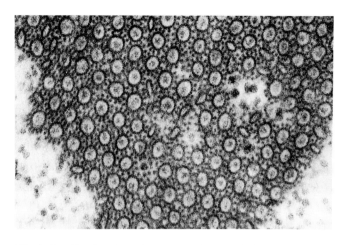

Fig. 26.25 Exertional muscle cramp syndrome: tubular aggregates. The tubules possess an inner core while granules adorn their outer surface. (× 98 800)

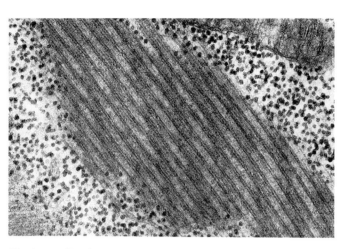

Fig. 26.26 Exertional muscle cramp syndrome: tubular aggregates. Central cores can be discerned within the tubules that comprise this aggregate. (× 43 900)

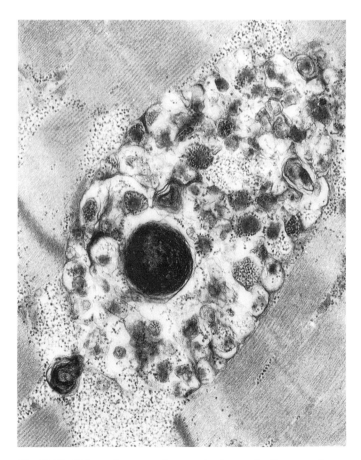

Fig. 26.27 Chloroquine myopathy: autophagic vacuole. Sequestered fragments of sarcoplasmic organelles are seen within an autophagic vacuole. (× 28 900)

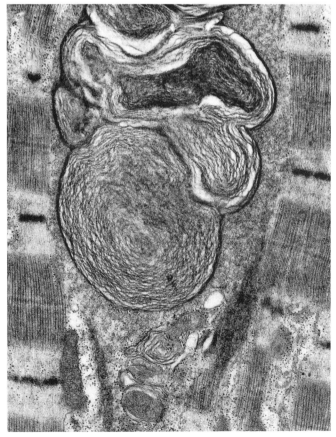

Fig. 26.28 Chloroquine myopathy: multilaminated membrane. This autophagic vacuole consists of tightly packed membranes. (× 21 300)

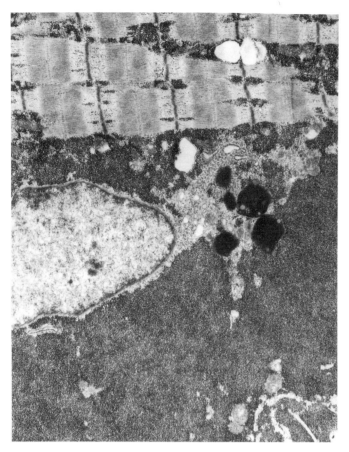

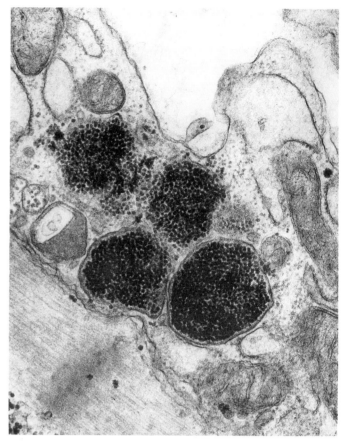

Fig. 26.29 (Above) Glycogen storage disease: glycogen aggregates. Large masses of tightly packed glycogen granules are seen, especially at the periphery of the muscle fibre. (× 9000)

Fig. 26.30 (Above right) Glycogen storage disease: lysosomes. Accumulation of glycogen granules within lysosomes in a patient with type II glycogenosis. (× 15 200)

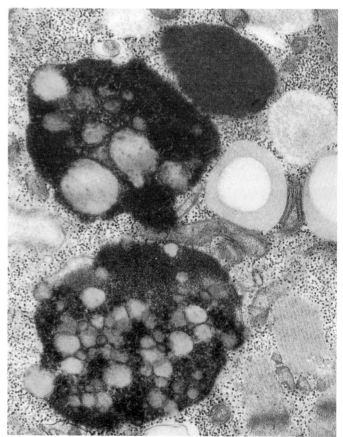

Fig. 26.31 (Above right) Senile atrophy: lipofuscin bodies. Large lipofuscin bodies containing lipidic globules and granular osmiophilic material are present. (× 24 800)

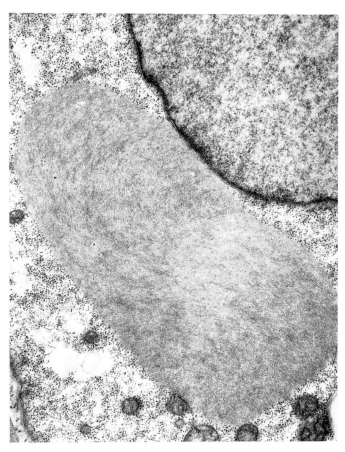

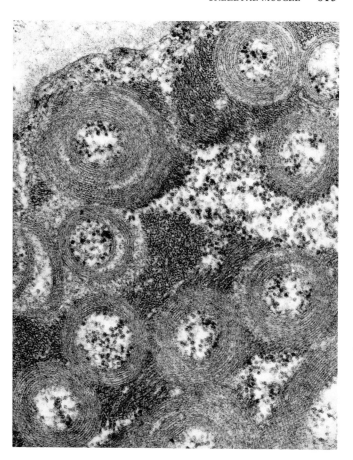

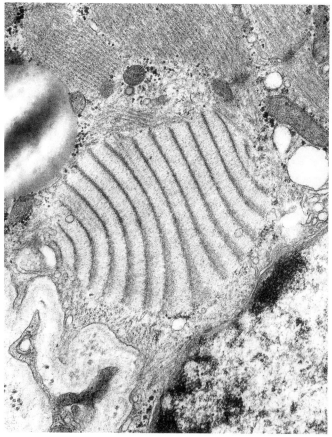

Fig. 26.32 (Above)   Neurogenic atrophy: filamentous body. A structure composed of tightly packed fine filaments is present in the paranuclear region of a muscle fibre. (× 16 600)

Fig. 26.33 (Above right)   Polymyositis: concentric laminated bodies. Aggregates of cylindrical structures composed of concentric lamellae are seen. Glycogen granules are seen in their core while intermediate filaments are present at their periphery. (× 46 600)

Fig. 26.34 (Right)   Hypothyroid myopathy: zebra-striped body. Fine filaments traversed by osmiophilic bands characterize this inclusion. (× 27 100)

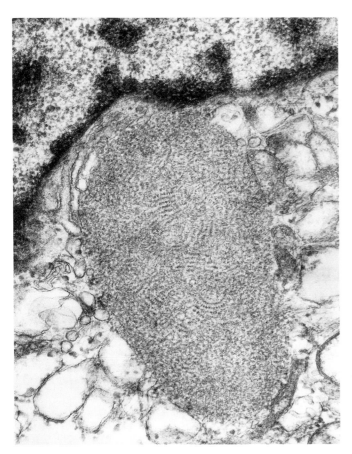

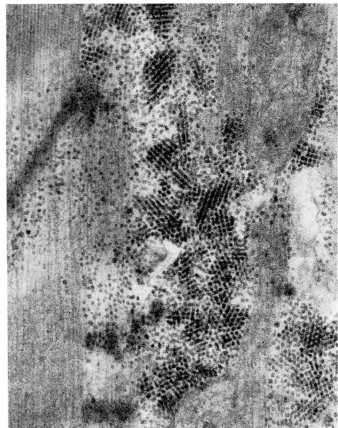

Fig. 26.35 (Above)   Myotonic dystrophy: fingerprint body. Aggregates of serrated curvilinear lamellae are embedded in an osmiophilic matrix. (× 41 100)

Fig. 26.36 (Above right)   Idiopathic scoliosis: paracrystalline arrays. Particles measuring 20–30 nm are arranged in paracrystalline arrays between adjacent myofibrils. (× 54 600)

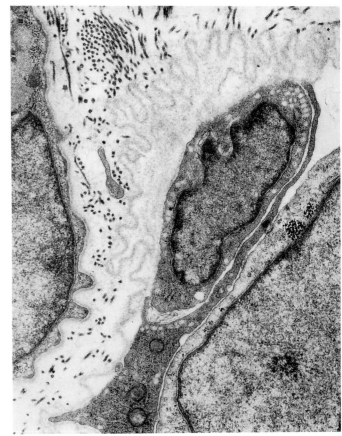

Fig. 26.37 (Right)   Muscle atrophy: folded external lamina. Folding and redundancy of the external lamina are prominent in this field. (× 16 600)

27. Bones

G. C. Steiner

INTRODUCTION

Non-neoplastic diseases of bone include a variety of disorders which can be diagnosed in the majority of cases by light microscopy in correlation with the clinical and radiological manifestations. With few exceptions, the use of electron microscopy for diagnostic purposes is of limited value. EM is more useful when it is applied to the study of the pathogenesis and aetiology of these disorders. In osteopetrosis for example, absence of ruffled borders on the osteoclasts explains the decrease in bone resorption observed in this condition. The finding of intranuclear filaments in the osteoclasts of Paget's disease has stimulated research into its possible viral aetiology. The bone diseases to be illustrated in this chapter represent conditions that the writer thought would be of interest to the general pathologist. Tumour-like conditions of soft tissue such as tumoural calcinosis and myositis ossificans are also included here because they are related to the mechanisms of mineralization and bone formation.

PAGET'S DISEASE

Paget's disease of bone is a disorder characterized by active bone turnover with increased osteoclastic activity. The osteoclasts are large, with a substantial increase in the number of nuclei. The cell membranes show numerous infoldings which are probably a reflection of their increased surface activity and motility.[35] The ruffled border in contact with the bone matrix demonstrates numerous deep folds of the cell membrane with finger-like projections of the cytoplasm. The presence of large calcified fragments of bone matrix incorporated into the cytoplasm suggests that the degree of bone resorption is abnormal.[35] Studies by scanning electron microscopy indicate that, in addition to osteoclastic changes, there is probably also a dysfunction of the osteoblasts.[6] The most important specific abnormality of this disorder is the presence of intranuclear inclusions in the osteoclasts. They consist of microtubular filamentous structures measuring approximately 12–15 nm in diameter, and

in cross-section they contain a clear centre about 5 nm in diameter[15,19,35] (Fig. 27.1). Recently, similar intranuclear inclusions were identified in the cells of an osteosarcoma arising in Paget's disease,[50] and in osteoclast-like cells of giant cell tumours also arising in Paget's disease.[10,29] It has been suggested that the frequency of intranuclear inclusions is related to the histological severity of the disease and the number of osteoclasts.[15] The similarity of these filaments to measles virus and respiratory syncytial virus has led to the suggestion that Paget's disease is a slow viral disorder.[19,35,43] Recent investigations using immunofluorescence and immunohistochemistry on tissue and cell cultures give further support to a possible viral aetiology.[28,34] However, no virus has been isolated or transferred in this condition. The presence in osteoclasts of intranuclear inclusions similar to the ones described above is characteristic of Paget's disease and is consistent with this diagnosis. They are not found in normal osteoclasts or in osteoclasts of any other bone disorder.[43] The only exceptions are rare cases of giant cell tumour of bone, where similar structures have been identified in a few multinucleated giant cells.[39,51] Occasional tumour cells of osteosarcoma may contain filamentous structures, but they are larger than those of Paget's disease.[11,20]

OSTEOPETROSIS

Osteopetrosis is a rare inherited disorder of the skeletal system characterized by a decrease in the rate of bone and cartilage resorption.[26,41] Although the osteoclasts are often increased in number, and are normally located on the surface of the bone and cartilage, their cell membrane is smooth and lacks the typical foldings characteristic of the ruffled borders (Figs 27.2 and 27.3); in addition, some authors have found increased numbers of nuclei and mitochondria containing calcium crystals.[3] Like others, we have found vacuoles in the cytoplasm adjacent to the bone surface, some containing calcium crystals. Because of the lack of osteoclastic resorption, the surface of the adjacent bone and cartilage remains calcified, as manifested by the persistence of the lamina limitans.[41] This organic structure disappears during resorption. Scanning EM studies of osteopetrotic bone have shown disorganized bone architecture with the presence of cartilaginous matrix, and areas of abnormal ossification with absence of well organized lamellar bone.[22] In a study of osteopetrosis fetalis, Bonucci et al[3] found evidence of degeneration and vacuolization of chondrocytes in areas of endochondral ossification, in addition to the osteoclastic abnormalities. The absence of ruffled borders in osteopetrotic osteoclasts is a diagnostic feature of this condition[40,41] (Figs 27.2 and 27.3). The nature of the osteoclast defect is not known; it may be due to inability to synthesize factors involved in bone resorption, or inability to respond to stimuli of bone resorption.[26]

Osteoclast defects similar to those of human osteopetrosis have been observed in osteopetrosis in animals.[25] In osteopetrotic rats, some authors have found increased levels of intracellular acid phosphatase[25] and an absence of extracellular lysosomal enzymes.[41]

OSTEOGENESIS IMPERFECTA

Osteogenesis imperfecta is a genetic disorder characterized by skeletal abnormalities and increased bone fragility.[5] Ultrastructural studies of osteoblasts and osteocytes have shown evidence of increased metabolic activity with dilatation of the rough endoplasmic reticulum (RER)[1] in some cells. The cartilage cells also have dilated RER, and in some cells the RER forms concentric rings.[5] The extracellular matrix of the cartilage shows depletion of collagen fibres (Fig. 27.4). Cultured fibroblasts and skin fibroblasts in this condition have dilated RER. Scanning EM studies have shown that there is an abnormality of collagen formation. The collagen fibres are thin, and they fail to aggregate in bundles as occurs in normal bone.[49] The aetiology of this condition is unknown. There is apparently a quantitative deficiency of collagen production in the bone.[5,49]

OSTEOCHONDRODYSPLASIAS

Osteochondrodysplasias are constitutional disorders of the skeletal system characterized by abnormalities of growth and development of cartilage and/or bone. Classification of these diseases is based particularly on clinical, genetic, and radiographic abnormalities.[37,42] The pathogenesis of these conditions is poorly understood; however, specific morphological and biochemical abnormalities have been found in several of those disorders suggesting a particular biochemical defect.[45] It is possible that a pathogenetic classification of osteochondrodysplasias will be available in the future after further research in this area.[45]

Pseudoachondroplasia

In this condition the growth plate is somewhat disorganized, while the cartilage cells are larger than normal. They contain cytoplasmic inclusions[45] which consist of markedly dilated RER containing dense material, disposed in the form of dense lamellae or parallel sheets alternating with electronlucent areas. The lamellae measure approximately 45 nm in thickness, and the lucent areas approximately 90 nm.[7] The RER surrounding the inclusions is covered by ribosomes and sometimes projects into the interior of the inclusions (Figs 27.5 and 27.6). Abundant glycogen is seen in the cartilage cells containing the inclusions; otherwise they appear normal. The extracellular matrix is normal and the process of calcification and ossification is not particularly abnormal. Other ultrastructural abnormalities observed in osteochondrodysplasias are listed in Table 27.1.

BROWN TUMOUR OF HYPERPARATHYROIDISM

Brown tumour is a tumour-like reaction which appears in hyperparathyroidism and is characterized by the presence of large numbers of multinucleated giant cells and mononu-

Table 27.1 Ultrastructural abnormalities of the cartilage growth plate in osteochondrodysplasias*

Kniest dysplasia	Dilated RER with fibrillogranular material; abundant microtubules in some cells; long-spacing collagen (one patient)[42]
Spondylometaphyseal dysplasia (Koslowsky type)	Large intracellular vacuoles containing spiral filaments formed by granules[45]
Diastrophic dysplasia	Abnormal organization and thickening of collagen; degenerating cells encircled by collagen, vesicles and granules; intracellular lipid;[30] increased proteoglycans[30]
Spondylo-epiphyseal dysplasia	Dilated RER containing homogeneous fine material
Achondroplasia	Increased number of necrotic cells; large collagen fibrils; intracellular lipid;[30] increased proteoglycans[30]
Metatrophic dysplasia	Intracellular vacuolation of chondrocytes
Asphyxiating thoracic dysplasia	Intracellular lipid inclusions in chondrocytes; increased proteoglycans[30]
Multiple epiphyseal dysplasia	Intracellular vacuoles with dilated RER
Pseudo-achondroplasia	Dilated RER containing alternating layers of electon-dense and electron-lucent material
Metaphyseal dysplasia	Dilated RER containing granular material[8]
Pyknodysostosis	Intracellular inclusions containing lamellar structures[45]

* References: 7, 8, 27, 30, 32, 36, 37, 42 and 45.

clear stromal cells. Generally the ultrastructural features of brown tumour are non specific. The giant cells have abundant mitochondria and sparse RER. The increased number of giant cells in brown tumour is probably the result of hypersecretion of parathyroid hormone, and we would therefore expect them to resemble the osteoclasts induced experimentally by PTH stimulation.[14,17,18] However, the giant cells are not located adjacent to bone, and they differ from osteoclasts (Fig. 27.7). It is known that parathyroid hormone stimulates osteoclast precursor cells, presumably of the mononuclear phagocytic system, increasing their rate of maturation into osteoclasts.[14,26] However, in two cases of brown tumor studied by us, most of the mononuclear cells appeared to be fibroblasts rather than histiocytes (Fig. 27.8). Rare cell junctions were observed. A few cells appear more primitive, with scanty cytoplasm. Brown tumour should be differentiated ultrastructurally from bone tumours containing giant cells. In giant cell tumour of bone, although the giant cells are basically similar to those of brown tumour, the mononuclear cells are ovoid or rounded, and some have histiocytic features.[46] In non-ossifying fibroma, although the mononuclear cells are predominantly fibroblastic, they demonstrate histiocytic and myofibroblastic differentiation.[46] The cells of aneurysmal bone cyst and giant cell reparative granuloma may be indistinguishable from brown tumour.[24,46]

TUMOURAL CALCINOSIS

In this rare disorder there is accumulation of large masses of calcified material in the peri-articular soft tissues. The mineral deposits are of variable size, usually rounded, and composed of solid aggregates of needle-shaped crystals. They vary in density, and this is related to the degree of removal or dissolution of crystals during processing of the tissue. The crystals have no special orientation, but at the periphery of the aggregates they tend to be arranged radially. In our experience, the mineral deposits are localized mainly extracellularly and less frequently intracellularly.[4,9] In the extracellular spaces they are not associated with or related to collagen fibres. The deposits are frequently adjacent to and surrounded by large mononuclear and multinucleated giant cells containing abundant lipid material and often showing changes of degeneration. Small vesicular structures are seen associated with the extracellular deposits (Fig. 27.9). Intracellularly, the crystals are seen in the cytoplasm of degenerating cells and rarely within dilated endoplasmic reticulum (Fig. 27.10). X-ray diffraction, electron diffraction and X-ray microanalysis have demonstrated that the mineral deposits represent hydroxyapatite[4] (Fig. 27.11). The crystals are large and/or more perfect than those present in bone.[4] The aetiology of this disorder is unknown, and the mechanism of mineral deposition is not clearly established. Some

Table 27.2 Non-neoplastic conditions associated with pathological calcification (hydroxyapatite) in tissue*

Tumoral calcinosis
Calcinosis cutis
Idiopathic calcification of the scrotum
Calcific tendinitis
Ageing human aortic valve
Atherosclerosis
Hyperparathyroidism
Severe renal disease (haemodialysis)
Sarcoidosis
Hypervitaminosis D
Milk–alkali syndrome
Osteo-arthritis

* References: 2, 4, 9, 21, 38, 47 and 48.

authors believe that calcification begins intracellularly.[2] Others consider it to be extracellular[9,31] and to be related to collagen;[9] additional experience is necessary to clarify this point. Table 27.2 lists different disorders associated with pathological calcification.

MYOSITIS OSSIFICANS

Myositis ossificans is a non-neoplastic process characterized by a cellular reaction of the soft tissue which undergoes bone differentiation at the periphery. Tissue examined from the centre of the lesion reveals a proliferation of cells with fibroblastic features (see also Ch. 11). They have varying amounts of RER and glycogen, and often possess slender cell processes; they are frequently in close apposition, and rare primitive cell junctions are seen (see Ch. 11). In addition, some cells demonstrate myofibroblastic differentiation (Fig. 27.12), while others represent less differentiated mononuclear cells. Sparse multinucleated giant cells are also seen with many mitochondria and sparse RER. Tissue examined from the periphery of the lesion exhibits osteoblastic differentiation with bone formation (Fig. 27.13). There is abundant osteoid deposition between the cells, with extensive calcification. A few cells show evidence of cartilaginous differentiation (Fig. 27.14). Myositis ossificans is a reactive disorder. Myofibroblasts have been documented previously in this condition.[33] Some authors have also found macrophages and have interpreted this finding as an indication of a different histogenesis of myositis ossificans from the group of fibromatosis and nodular fasciitis, where macrophages are rare[13,33,52] (see Ch. 11). The osteoblastic differentiation at the periphery (zonal phenomenon) favours a reactive rather than a neoplastic process. The osteoblasts resemble their normal counterparts; however, sometimes it is not possible on purely morphological grounds to differentiate between normal and neoplastic osteoblasts.[46]

REFERENCES

1. Albright J P, Albright J A, Grelin E S 1975 Osteogenesis imperfecta tarda. The morphology of rib biopsies. Clinical Orthopaedics and Related Research 108: 204–213
2. Anderson H C 1980 Calcification process. Pathology Annual 15: 45–75
3. Bonucci E, Sartori E, Spina M 1975 Osteopetrosis fetalis. Report on a case with special reference to ultrastructure. Virchows Archiv A, Pathological Anatomy and Histopathology 368: 109–121
4. Boskey A L, Vigorita V J, Sencer O, Stuchin S A, Lane J M 1983 Chemical, microscopic and ultrastructural characterization of the mineral deposits in tumoral calcinosis. Clinical Orthopaedics and Related Research 178: 258–269
5. Bullough P G, Davidson D D, Lorenzo J C 1981 The morbid anatomy of the skeleton in osteogenesis imperfecta. Clinical Orthopaedics and Related Research 159: 42–57
6. Chappard D, Alexandre C, Laborier J C, Robert J M, Riffat G 1984 Paget's disease of bone. A scanning electron microscopic study. Journal of Submicroscopic Cytology 16: 341–348
7. Cooper R R, Ponseti I V, Maynard J A 1973 Pseudoachondroplastic dwarfism. A rough surfaced endoplasmic reticulum storage disorder. Journal of Bone and Joint Surgery 55(A): 475–484
8. Cooper R R, Ponseti I V 1973 Metaphyseal dysostosis: description of an ultrastructural defect in the epiphyseal plate of chondrocytes. Case report. Journal of Bone and Joint Surgery 55(A): 485–495
9. Cornelius C E, Tenenhouse A, Weber J C 1968 Calcinosis cutis. Metabolic, sweat, histochemical, X-ray diffraction and electron microscopic study. Archives of Dermatology 98: 219–229
10. El-Labban N G 1984 Ultrastructural study of intranuclear tubulo-filaments in a giant cell tumor of bone in a patient with Paget's disease. Journal of Oral Pathology 13: 650–660
11. Ferguson R J, Yunis E J 1978 The ultrastructure of human osteosarcoma. Clinical Orthopaedics and Related Research 131: 234–246
12. Gherardi G, Lo Cascio V, Bonucci E 1980 Fine structure of nuclei and cytoplasm of osteoclasts in Paget's disease of bone. Histopathology 4: 63–74
13. Goellner J R, Soule E H 1980 Desmoid tumour: an ultrastructural study of eight cases. Human Pathology 11: 43–50
14. Gothlin G, Ericsson J L E 1976 The osteoclast. Review of ultrastructure, origin and structure–function relationship. Clinical Orthopaedics and Related Research 120: 201–231
15. Harvey L, Gray T, Beneton M N C, Douglas D L, Kanis J A, Russell R G G 1982 Ultrastructural features of the osteoclasts from Paget's disease of bone in relation to a viral aetiology. Journal of Clinical Pathology 35: 771–779
16. Henderson D W, Papadimitriou J M Coleman M 1986 Ultrastructural appearances of tumours. Diagnosis and classification of human neoplasia by electron microscopy. Churchill Livingstone, Edinburgh
17. Holtrop M E, Raisz L G, Simmons H A 1974 The effects of parathyroid hormone, colchicine and calcitonin on the ultrastructure and the activity of osteoclasts in organ culture. The Journal of Cell Biology 60: 346–355
18. Holtrop M E, King G J 1977 The ultrastructure of the osteoclast and its functional implications. Clinical Orthopaedics and Related Research 123: 177–196
19. Howatson A F, Fornasier V L 1982 Microfilaments associated with Paget's disease of bone: comparison with nucleocapsids of measles virus and respiratory syncytial virus. Intervirology 18: 150–159
20. Jenson A B, Spjut H J, Smith M N, Rapp F 1971 Intracellular branched tubular structures in osteosarcoma. Cancer 27: 1440–1448
21. Kim K M, Valigorsky J M, Mergner W J, Jones R T, Pendergrass R F, Trump B F 1976 Aging changes in the human aortic valve in relation to dystrophic calcification. Human Pathology 7: 47–60
22. Kuo T T, Davis C P 1981 Osteopetrosis: a scanning electron microscopic study. Human Pathology 12: 376–379
23. Lafferty F W, Reynolds E S, Pearson O H 1965 Tumoral calcinosis. A metabolic disease of obscure etiology. American Journal of Medicine 38: 105–118
24. Lorenzo J C, Dorfman H D 1980 Giant cell reparative granuloma of short tubular bones of the hands and feet. American Journal of Surgical Pathology 4: 551–563

25. Marks S C 1973 Pathogenesis of osteopetrosis in the rat: reduced bone resorption due to reduced osteoclast function. American Journal of Anatomy 13: 165–190
26. Marks S C 1984 Congenital osteopetrotic mutations as probes of the origin, structures and function of osteoclasts. Clinical Orthopaedics and Related Research 189: 239–263
27. Maynard J A, Ippolito E G, Ponseti I V, Mickelson M R 1981 Histochemistry and ultrastructure of the growth plate in achondroplasia. Journal of Bone and Joint Surgery 63(A): 969–979
28. Mills B A, Singer F R, Weiner L P, Holst P A 1980 Cell cultures from bone affected by Paget's disease. Arthritis and Rheumatism 23: 1115–1120
29. Mirra J M, Bauer F C H, Grant T T 1981 Giant cell tumor with viral-like intranuclear inclusions associated with Paget's disease. Clinical Orthopaedics and Related Research 158: 243–251
30. Nogami H, Oohira A, Ozeki K, Oki T, Ogino T, Murachi S 1979 Ultrastructure of cartilage in heritable disorders of connective tissue. Clinical Orthopaedics and Related Research 143: 251–259
31. Paegle R D 1966 Ultrastructure of mineral deposits in calcinosis cutis. Archives of Pathology 82: 474–482
32. Phillips S J, Magsamen B F, Punnett H H, Kistenmacher M L, Campo R D 1974 Fine structures of skeletal dysplasia as seen in pseudochondroplastic spondyloepiphyseal dysplasia and asphyxiating thoracic dystrophy. Birth Defects 10: 314–326
33. Povysil G, Matejovsky Z 1979 Ultrastructural evidence of myofibroblasts in pseudomalignant myositis ossificans. Virchows Archiv A, Pathological Anatomy and Histopathology 381: 189–203
34. Rebel A, Basle M, Pouplard A, Malkani K, Filmon R, Lepatezour A 1980 Bone tissue in Paget's disease of bone. Arthritis and Rheumatism 23: 1104–1114
35. Rebel A, Malkani K, Basle M, Bregeon C H 1976 Osteoclast ultrastructure in Paget's disease. Calcified Tissue Research 20: 187–199
36. Rimoin D L, Silberberg R, Hollister D W 1976 Chondro-osseous pathology in the chondrodystrophies. Clinical Orthopaedics and Related Research 114: 137–152
37. Rimoin D L 1978 International nomenclature of constitutional diseases of bone. Journal of Pediatrics 93: 614–616
38. Sarkar K, Uhthoff H K 1978 Ultrastructural localization of calcium in calcifying tendinitis. Archives of Pathology 102: 266–269
39. Schajowicz F, Ubios A M, Santini-Araujo E, Cabrini R L 1985 Viral-like intranuclear inclusions in giant cell tumors of bone. Clinical Orthopaedics and Related Research 201: 247–250
40. Shapiro F 1982 Ultrastructural abnormalities of osteoclasts in malignant-recessive osteopetrosis. Archives of Pathology and Laboratory Medicine 106: 425
41. Shapiro F, Glimcher M J, Holtrop M E, Tashjian A H, Brickley-Parson D, Kenzora J E 1980 Human osteopetrosis: a histological, ultrastructural and biochemical study. Journal of Bone and Joint Surgery 62(A): 384–399
42. Sillence D O, Horton W A, Rimoin D L 1979 Morphologic studies in the skeletal dysplasias. American Journal of Pathology 96: 813–870
43. Singer F R, Mills B G 1977 The etiology of Paget's disease of bone. Clinical Orthopaedics and Related Research 127: 37–42
44. Singer F R, Mills B G 1983 Evidence of a viral etiology of Paget's disease of bone. Clinical Orthopaedics and Related Research 178: 245–251
45. Stanescu V, Stanescu R, Maroteaux P 1984 Pathogenic mechanisms in osteochondrodysplasia. Journal of Bone and Joint Surgery 66(A): 817–836
46. Steiner G C 1981 Tumors and tumor-like conditions of bone. In: Johannessen J V (ed) Electron microscopy in human medicine. McGraw-Hill, New York, vol. 4, pp 54–140
47. Suzuki K, Takahashi S, Ito K, Tanska Y, Sezai Y 1979 Tumoral calcinosis in a patient undergoing hemodialysis. Acta Orthopaedica Scandinavica 50: 27–31
48. Takayama H, Pak K, Tomoyoshi T 1982 Electron microscopic study in mineral deposits in idiopathic calcinosis of the scrotum. Journal of Urology 127: 915–918
49. Teitelbaum S L, Kraft W J, Lang R, Avioli L V 1974 Bone collagen aggregation abnormalities in osteogenesis imperfecta. Calcified Tissue Research 17: 75–79

50. Viola M V, Eilon G, Lazarus M 1982 Virus-like inclusions in osteosarcoma cells arising in Paget's disease. Lancet i: 848

51. Welsh R A, Meyer A T 1970 Nuclear fragmentations and associated fibrils in giant cell tumor of bone. Laboratory Investigation 22: 63–72

52. Wirman J A 1976 Nodular fasciitis, a lesion of myofibroblasts. An ultrastructural study. Cancer 38: 2378–2389

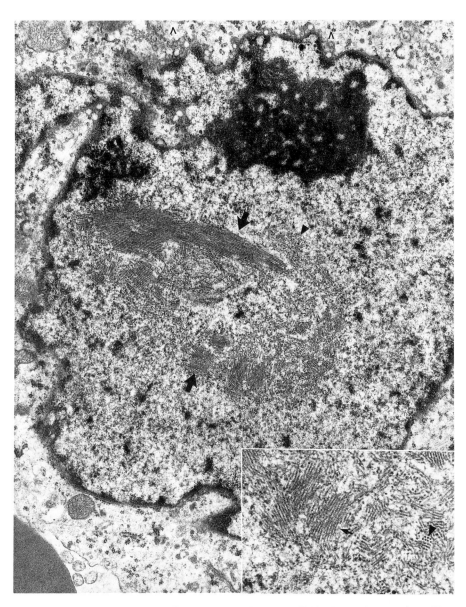

Fig. 27.1 Paget's osteoclast: nuclear filamentous inclusions. The nucleus contains multiple filamentous inclusions measuring approximately 12–15 nm. They form dense groups seen in longitudinal section (arrows) and cross section (arrowhead). Some filaments are disposed in parallel and paracrystalline arrays. In other cells they are seen at random. Intranuclear filamentous inclusions of different morphology have been observed in many neoplastic and non-neoplastic tissues (see Tables 21.1 and 21.2, ref. 16). The osteoclast nucleus shows also the presence of small perinuclear vesicles (v). They have been described in this condition. (× 19 800) *Inset* High power of the intranuclear inclusions seen in this figure. They are seen in longitudinal section (arrow) and cross section (arrowhead). (× 33 000) References: 15, 16, 18, 19 and 35.

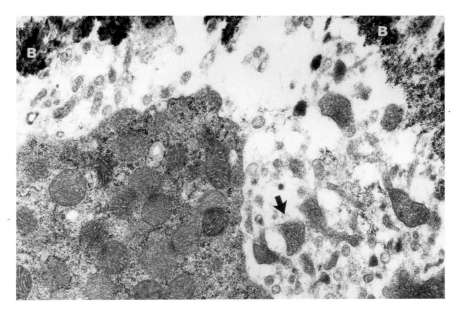

Fig. 27.2   Osteopetrosis: osteoclast adjacent to bone. The cell membrane lacks the deep infoldings typical of the ruffled borders. Only cell processes (arrow) are seen projecting towards the bone (B). The mitochondria appear normal. Compare with the normal osteoclast seen in Fig. 27.3.

The decrease in bone resorption in this condition is due to absence of ruffled borders in the osteoclasts. Clear zones, which are components of the normal osteoclasts, are occasionally seen adjacent to bone. (× 17 800) References: 3 and 41.

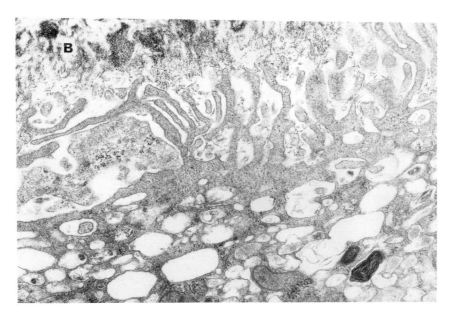

Fig. 27.3   Normal human osteoclast: ruffled border. A well-developed ruffled border composed of numerous folds and cell projections is seen in close relationship to bone (B). Numerous clear vacuoles are also evident in the cytoplasm adjacent to the ruffled border. They are seen in normal osteoclasts. Compare to the osteopetrotic osteoclast seen in Fig. 27.2. (× 17 800) Reference: 18.

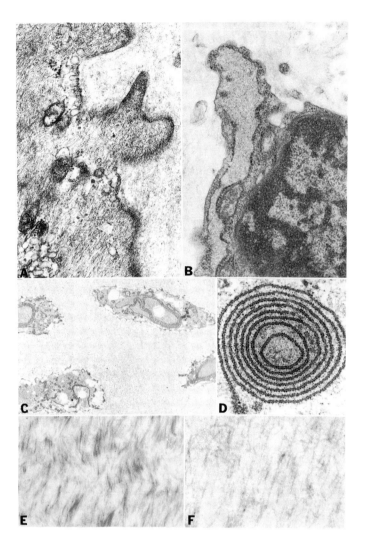

Fig. 27.4 Osteogenesis imperfecta: fibroblasts and chondrocytes. **A** Portion of skin fibroblast showing abundant intracytoplasmic filaments. (× 27 500) **B** Portion of skin fibroblast with dilated RER. (× 19 900) **C** Chondrocytes from the proliferative zone of the growth plate showing whorled appearance of the RER. (× 8600) **D** Chondrocyte cytoplasm containing concentric rings. (× 14 100) **E** Normal cartilage matrix from iliac crest in an 18-month-old girl. Bundles of collagen fibres are identified. (× 25 100) **F** Cartilage matrix from the iliac crest of a 3-month-old girl with osteogenesis imperfecta. There is a decreased amount of collagen fibres. Compare with **E**. (× 25 100) References: 1 and 5.

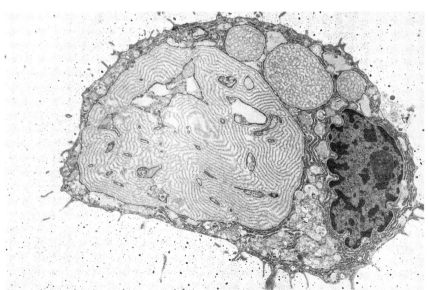

Fig. 27.5 Pseudoachondroplasia: chondrocytes from growth plate. Chondrocytes from an iliac crest biopsy of a 5-year-old girl. The nucleus is eccentric and the cytoplasm shows dilated cisternae of RER containing alternating electron-dense and electron-lucent layers. They form a pattern similar to that seen in a fingerprint or in moiré figures in watered silk.[32] They are characteristic of this condition. Proteoglycan granules are seen in the matrix. (× 5500) References: 32, 42 and 45.

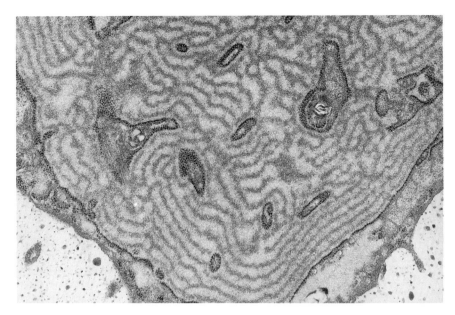

Fig. 27.6 Pseudoachondroplasia: cytoplasm of chondrocytes. Detail of cell shown in Fig. 27.5. Parallel layers of electron-lucent and electron-dense lamellae are seen within dilated RER. Some authors believe that the inclusions represent abnormal proteoglycans stored in the RER and not transported to the Golgi apparatus. (× 20 800) Reference: 45.

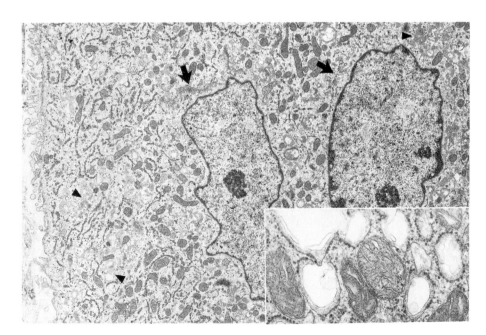

Fig. 27.7 Brown tumour of hyperparathyroidism: multinucleated giant cell. Tissue from the phalanx of the finger of a 38-year-old male with primary hyperparathyroidism. The cytoplasm contains many mitochondria and the Golgi apparatus is disposed as usual (but not always) around the nuclei (arrow). The lysosomal system is well developed and consists of electron-dense vacuoles and tubular structures (arrowheads). Most of the giant cells are indistinguishable from the giant cells seen in other bone conditions such as giant cell tumour, non-ossifying fibromas, giant cell reparative granuloma and aneurysmal bone cyst. (× 5300) *Inset* Giant cell cytoplasm showing RER with dilated lucent spaces surrounded by a membrane. This finding was observed in some giant cells. (× 33 000) References: 24 and 46.

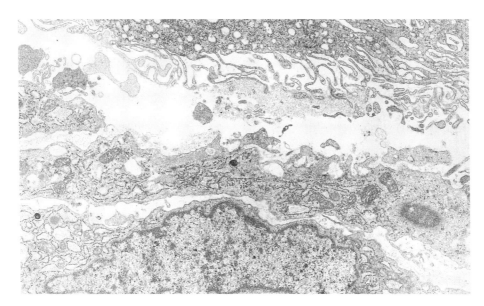

Fig. 27.8 Brown tumour: stromal cells and giant cell. The same case as in Fig. 27.7. The stromal cells (lower part) have fibroblastic features, with focally dilated RER. In other areas they contain a few intracytoplasmic filaments and glycogen granules. No myofibroblastic cells were seen. Part of the giant cell (upper part) contains dilated RER which is seen at higher magnification in the inset of Fig. 27.7. The giant cell contains numerous cell projections suggestive of a ruffled border. This is an uncommon finding. The giant cells of brown tumour differ from osteoclasts in that they lack a well developed ruffled border and fail to show evidence of resorption activity. (× 6900) References: 14 and 18.

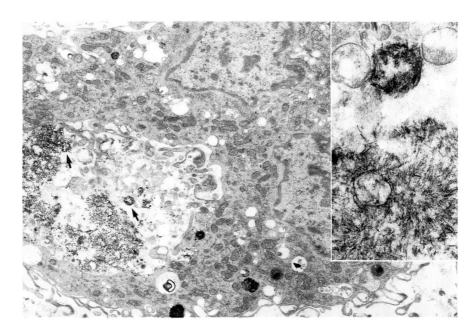

Fig. 27.9 Extracellular calcification: tumoural calcinosis. Tissue obtained from the knee region of an 18-month-old boy. A multinucleated giant cell surrounds deposits of extracellular calcification (arrows). Numerous vesicles are seen in this area, probably derived from the giant cell. (× 8250) *Inset* High-power view of extracellular calcification, showing needle-like crystal aggregates, some of which are associated with vesicular structures. In some aggregates the crystals show a suggestion of radial orientation. (× 33 000) In pathological calcification in general, the process of mineralization may involve intracellular (mitochondria) or extracellular (matrix vesicle-like structures) mechanisms, or both.[9] References: 2 and 4.

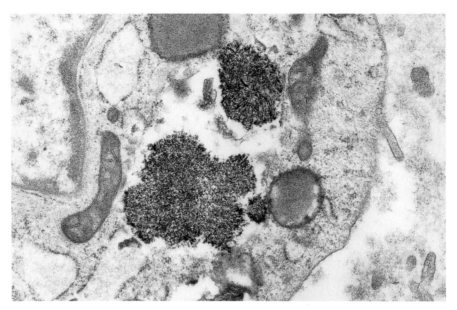

Fig. 27.10 Tumoral calcinosis: part of a mononuclear cell. Tissue obtained from the same case as in Fig. 27.9. Round aggregates of hydroxyapatite crystals are seen within dilated spaces, most probably representing RER. This appears to be a real finding and not an artefact. Several lipid droplets are also seen. Calcification was seen also in degenerated cells and some authors have found it in mitochondria.[2] Lead stain only. (× 29 700) References: 2, 4 and 31.

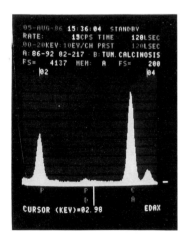

Fig. 27.11 Tumoural calcinosis: X-ray microanalysis. Energy-dispersive X-ray spectrum of crystal deposits from the same case shown in Figs 27.9 and 27.10. The calcium (CA) and phosphorus (P) peaks are consistent with hydroxyapatite. Reference: 4.

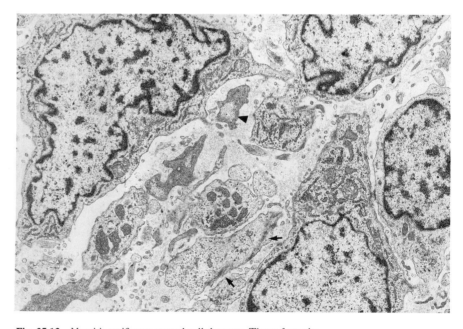

Fig. 27.12 Myositis ossificans: central cellular area. Tissue from the thigh of a 31-year-old female. There are several cells with fibroblastic features, some showing abundant RER. Peripheral aggregates of intracytoplasmic filaments with dense bodies (arrows) are seen, consistent with myofibroblastic differentiation. They have also been described in reactive lesions such as nodular fasciitis, fibromatosis, and benign and malignant neoplasms. Glycogen is also noted (arrowhead). (× 5400) References: 13, 16, 33 and 52. See also Ch. 11.

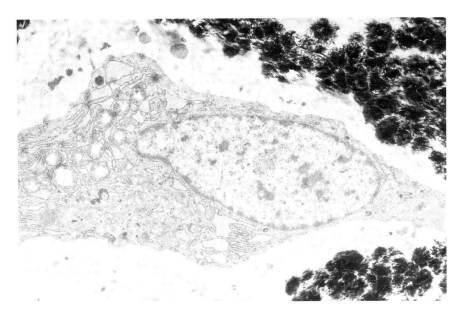

Fig. 27.13 Myositis ossificans: osteocyte from peripheral area. Tissue from the same case as in Fig. 27.12. The osteocyte has a small amount of cytoplasm with sparse organelles. The pericellular matrix consists of osteoid, and mineralization is seen surrounding part of the entire cell. Lead stain only. (× 5900)

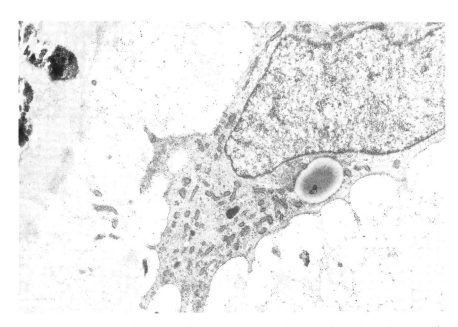

Fig. 27.14 Myositis ossificans: chondrocyte from peripheral area. Tissue from the same area as in Fig. 27.12. The chondrocyte is well developed with scalloping of the cell membrane and small cell processes. The pericellular matrix (lacuna) contains sparse fine proteoglycan granules. Matrix calcification is seen in the right upper corner. (× 9000)

28. Joints

G. C. Steiner

INTRODUCTION

The application of electron microscopy to the diagnosis of joint disorders is of limited value. The joint abnormalities of the group of rheumatic diseases show a wide range of inflammatory changes which are usually not pathognomonic or specific. Some of these changes can also occur up to a certain degree in synovial reactions secondary to injury. In only very rare instances (i.e. Whipple's disease)[26] does electron microscopy help to establish a specific diagnosis. In crystal-induced synovitis, electron microscopy may play a role in the diagnosis in those cases where the crystals in the synovial fluid are sparse and difficult to identify by light microscopy. The combined use of TEM, SEM and — particularly — electron dispersive X-ray analysis is often necessary to determine the specific nature of the crystals.

RHEUMATOID ARTHRITIS

The earliest synovial changes in rheumatoid arthritis consist of some hyperplasia of the lining cells involving particularly types A and AB cells.[44] There is rare perivascular infiltration of lymphocytes and plasma cells.[44] When viewed with the scanning electron microscope, the earliest synovial lesions show a fine pebbled appearance of the surface, and in the chronic stages of the disease hyperplastic villi develop in large numbers — increasing substantially the area of the synovial surface (Fig. 28.1).[19,25] In well-established chronic rheumatoid arthritis, transmission electron microscopy reveals increased thickness of the synovial lining cells, with overall hyperplasia and some degree of hypertrophy of the individual cells as well. With a few exceptions,[55] type B or AB cells appear to be the predominant cells in the synovial surface (Fig. 28.2).[22,25] The type A (macrophage-like) cells seem to differ from normal type A cells because they have increased lysosomes, fewer filopodia and smaller Golgi apparatus (Fig. 28.3).[6,53] The secondary lysosomes represent heterolysosomes produced by active endocytosis of fibrin and necrotic cells.[22] Fibrinoid material is often seen on the synovial surface and is also present between the cells (Fig.

28.4).[22,53] Large numbers of lymphocytes and plasma cells are seen in the subsynovial tissues (Fig. 28.5). The presence of reduplication of the basement membrane in the capillaries is not a specific finding because it can be found in reactive synovial disorders.[22] Also, the presence of lymphocytes within the lumen and wall of small blood vessels is non-specific for rheumatoid arthritis.[20] Although the synovial inflammatory changes described above are typical of rheumatoid arthritis they are not necessarily specific for this disease. There are other inflammatory joint disorders that may have synovial changes resembling rheumatoid arthritis (see Table 28.1). In juvenile rheumatoid arthritis some authors find a preponderance of type A synovial cells[55] while others find no significant difference from adult rheumatoid arthritis.[35] In psoriatic arthritis there is no significant synovial hyperplasia,[17,19] but the vascular changes are more prominent than they are in rheumatoid arthritis.[17] The synovitis of Reiter's syndrome shows vascular plugging with platelets and neutrophils, and inclusions are found in mononuclear cells.[34]

SYNOVIAL CHANGES SECONDARY TO JOINT TRAUMA AND OSTEO-ARTHRITIS

In traumatic synovitis (resulting from torn meniscus, or joint trauma) there is a mild synovial hyperplasia (Fig. 28.6) and, with progression of time after the trauma, an increase in collagen deposition on the lining surface[47] (see Table 28.1). There is also apparently increased phagocytic activity in the synovial cells, with an abundance of lysosomes, and siderosomes are noted resulting from previous haemorrhage.[22]

In osteo-arthritis, scanning electron microscopy shows changes varying from villous proliferation to synovial atrophy.[19] At the transmission EM level, the synovial changes are basically similar to traumatic synovitis (Fig. 28.7). The subsynovial tissue usually shows a small degree of chronic inflammation, but in some cases the inflammatory infiltration may be significant (Fig. 28.8) (see Table 28.1).

Table 28.1 Comparative ultrastructure of synovial pathology in different joint disorders*

Synovial lining cells	Normal human synovium[5,14,22,54]	Traumatic synovitis (TS) and osteo-arthritis (O)	Rheumatoid arthritis	Psoriatic arthritis[17]	Pigmented villonodular synovitis
Predominant cell type	Type A cells (in adults);[22] type B cells;[14] type AB (intermediate, C) cells are also present[22]	TS: Types A, B and AB are frequent[22] O: Types AB[40] and B[47] Some degree of synovial hyperplasia	Types B or AB cells;[22] prominent hyperplasia of all synovial cells	No abnormalities of types A and B cells	Types B and AB cells;[23,45] synovial hyperplasia
Lysosomes	Several in type A cells	TS: Increased in types B and AB cells[22] O: Increased	Increased in size and number Rare siderosomes		Increased siderosomes
Golgi apparatus	Prominent in type A cells	O: Decreased[40]	Small in type A cells		
Mitochondria	Normal	O: Abnormal cristae and giant mitochondria[40]	Often swollen and large		Normal
Rough endoplasmic reticulum	Well developed in type B cells	O: Increased and often dilated[40]	Increased in type B cells		Well developed
Intermediate filaments	Rare	TS: Sparse[22]	Prominent		Prominent in type B cells[23]
Cell junctions	Absent in humans;[22] present in animals[22]	TS: Rare desmosome-like junctions[22]	Few desmosome-like structures[22]		Rare desmosome-like structures[23]
Nuclear fibrous lamina	Thin (up to 20 nm)[22]	Thin	Thick (mean thickness 40.7 nm)[22]		Thin
Fibrinoid material in synovial surface	Rare	Present in a few cases	Abundant		Rare
Subsynovial tissue	Fat, collagen, fibroblasts and macrophages	TS and O: Fibrosis may be prominent;[47] few lymphocytes and plasma cells; occasionally they are numerous (O)	Many lymphocytes and plasma cells	Perivascular infiltration of lymphocytes; abundant collagen[9]	Marked proliferation of fibroblast-like cells and histiocytes;[52] iron and lipid accumulation; erythrophagocytosis[23]
Capillary vessels	Continuous, fenestrated and discontinuous endothelium	O: Stasis and dilatation[4] TS: Swelling of endothelial cell[22] TS and O: Vascular fibrosis	Re-duplication of basement membrane, endothelial swelling, necrosis, inflammation	Prominent endothelial swelling, dilatation of RER; increased perivascular collagen, re-duplication of membrane	Re-depulication of basement membrane; swollen endothelial cells; endothelial gaps
Remarks	Dendritic cells have been[14] identified in synovium; type A and B cells are variants of cells whose morphology depends on their functional activity	O: Synovial cell atrophy in some cases[47] TS: Lipid droplets in some synovial cells[22]	Multinucleated giant cells may be present;[7,24] lipid droplets are observed (particularly in the chronic cases)[35]	Main difference from RA: no significant hyperplasia of synovial cells and more prominent vascular changes	Numerous multinucleated giant cells in synovial and subsynovial tissue;[45] lipid in synovial lining cells[45]

*References: 1, 2, 4–9, 14, 17, 20, 22–25, 27, 29, 34, 35, 40, 44, 45, 47, 48, 52, 53 and 55.

PIGMENTED VILLONODULAR SYNOVITIS

This synovial disorder (see also Ch. 11) is characterized by villous and nodular proliferation with hyperplasia of synovial lining cells (Fig. 28.9) (Table 28.1). The features that distinguish this condition from other types of inflammatory synovitis is the marked cellular proliferation of the sub-synovial tissue, composed of fibroblast-like cells and histiocytes. Iron deposition, in the form of siderosomes, and lipid droplets are seen in the synovial lining cells but particularly in the sub-synovial cells (Fig. 28.10).[23,45] Another characteristic feature of this disorder is the presence of multinucleated osteoclast-like giant cells in the deep synovial tissue, presumably derived from the mononuclear stromal cells. These cells contain numerous mitochondria (Fig. 28.11) and differ from the giant cells of rheumatoid arthritis in that the latter resemble macrophages and contain numerous lysosome-like bodies.[24]

OSTEO-ARTHRITIS

Osteo-arthritis is a disorder characterized by progressive degenerative changes of the articular cartilage associated with abortive attempts at repair and regeneration. The earliest osteo-arthritis changes consist of surface irregularities and loss of the fine fibrils covering the articular surface (Fig. 28.12) (see Table 28.2). These irregularities progress to fibrillation involving the superficial layers, and as the disease advances the fibrillation extends to the intermediate and deeper layers, with formation of deep clefts (Fig. 28.13).[50,51] When observed with the SEM, the fibrillated cartilage surface shows torn and disrupted collagen bundles (Fig. 28.14).[32] The matrix alterations and cell degeneration are probably secondary to the release of enzymes by injured chondrocytes.[22] The collagen fibres in osteo-arthritis apparently have a composition and orientation different to those of normal cartilage. As the degenerative changes take place, a reparative reaction develops in the cartilage with proliferation of chondrocytes and increase in matrix proteoglycans.[50,51] Clusters of chondrocytes progressively enlarge as the osteo-arthritis advances in severity (Fig. 28.15). Eventually, the regenerative response is inadequate to compensate for the loss of tissue, and the cartilage undergoes complete degradation of its matrix and disintegration of its cells.[50,51]

GOUT

The recognition and diagnosis of gouty arthritis is established by the presence of monosodium urate crystals (MSU) in the synovial fluid by the use of compensated polarized light microscopy. If the crystals are very small in size or if they are present in small numbers in the joint, identification by light microscopy is not possible.

Ultrastructural studies of centrifuged synovial fluid show the presence of crystals within large mononuclear cells and polymorphonuclear leukocytes in the form of electron-

Table 28.2 Ultrastructural (TEM) differences between normal and osteo-arthritic cartilage*

	Normal human adult articular cartilage	Osteo-arthritis
Zone I (superficial)		
Matrix:	A thin layer of fine fibrils–lamina splendens–covers the articular surface;[50] closely packed collagen fibres with scanty ground substance that runs parallel to the surface	Surface irregularities; progressive fibrillation; infoldings of surface layer; clefts[51]
Cells:	Elongated chondrocytes resembling fibroblasts[50]	Chondrocytes are larger than their normal counterparts with increased organelles; degenerated cells; a few chondrocyte clusters
Zone II (intermediate)		
Matrix:	Collagenous fibres arranged randomly; fibres are widely spread with more ground substances than in Zone I; lipid debris (derived from cell necrosis)	Deep cleft formation; collagen fibres arranged perpendicular to joint surface; decreased proteoglycan granules; frequent lipid debris (derived from cell necrosis)
Cells:	Oval and rounded chondrocytes with prominent RER and Golgi apparatus;[22] small amounts of glycogen and intracytoplasmic filaments	Clusters of proliferating chondrocytes with increased RER and Golgi apparatus; abundant intracytoplasmic filaments (degenerative changes);[22] degeneration and necrosis
Zone III (deeper)		
Matrix:	Similar to Zone II, although fibres have thicker diameter (40–100 nm);[50] occasional unusually wide fibres (150 nm or more in diameter)	Changes basically similar to those in Zone II; increased diameter of collagen fibres; occasional giant (amianthoid) fibres[22]
Zone IV (calcified)		
Matrix:	Calcified	No studies available
Cells:	Progressive degeneration and necrosis[22]	

*References: 22, 31, 32, 38, 46 and 49–51.

lucent, elongated crystal-shaped spaces within phagosomes (Fig. 28.16).[1,43] In a tophus, the crystals are longer and are mostly needle-shaped (Fig. 28.17). If the crystals are embedded directly in Epon, they appear as elongated rods of variable electron density, depending on the exposure to the electron beam.[37] By SEM the crystals from the synovial fluid (Fig. 28.18) are basically similar to those from the tophus, although in the latter the crystals appear to be longer with a smaller amount of coating material.[18,19,37] Recently, immunoglobulins were identified, by EM, forming a coating on the surface of the MSU crystals, and it is thought that this binding may influence the ability of the crystals to induce synovial inflammation.[16] Electron microscopy is useful in the diagnosis of gout in those cases where the crystals are not identified by light microscopy and where ultrastructural investigation of centrifuged synovial fluid is required.[28] It is important to know that MSU and calcium pyrophosphate crystals may have a similar morphology by SEM, and that both may be present in the same joint.[18,37] Also, there are other types of water-soluble crystals that may resemble urates.[43] Therefore, accurate identification of the MSU crystals may be necessary by means of X-ray diffraction.[18,37]

CALCIUM PYROPHOSPHATE CRYSTAL DEPOSITION DISEASE (CPPD)

In calcium pyrophosphate crystal deposition disease (CPPD) the crystals, like those of gout, are soluble in water-based fixatives for electron microscopy, and most of them are dissolved.[42] They usually appear as rod-like rhombic or irregular spaces within synovial cells and polymorphonuclear leukocytes of synovial fluid.[15,30,42] In cartilage and meniscal tissue the crystals are seen extracellularly (Fig. 28.19).[3,12,33,39] If CPPD crystals are embedded directly in resins they have rod-like shape and demonstrate a 'bubbled' appearance (Fig. 28.20).[30] Some authors believe that the electron-lucent spaces represent the glycosaminoglycan areas around which the crystals precipitate.[36] At SEM, the crystals usually have parallelepiped, rod-like rhomboid shapes with variations in size from 1 to 10 μm (Fig. 28.21).[11,19,36] It is possible that the crystals originate in the cartilage matrix[12] due to abnormal metabolic disturbances.

Electron microscopy is useful in the diagnosis of those cases of CPPD in which the crystals in the synovial fluid are too small to be identified by compensated polarized light microscopy.[11,15] In centrifuged synovial fluid the crystals can be identified within the cells of the synovial fluid[42] or directly on the coated EM grid.[11] Crystallographic identification of crystals is necessary in order to avoid misinterpretation of their morphology. This is usually accomplished by electron dispersive X-ray analysis (Fig. 28.22).[11,21,36] This latter method is also useful to identify other types of crystals such as apatite crystals, which can be the cause of arthropathies and should be differentiated from other types of crystal deposition diseases.[15]

REFERENCES

1. Agudelo C A, Schumacher H R 1973 The synovitis of acute gouty arthritis. A light and electron microscopic study. Human Pathology 4: 265–279
2. Alguacil-Garcia A, Unni K K, Goellner J R 1978 Giant cell tumor of tendon sheath and pigmented villonodular synovitis. An ultrastructural study. American Journal of Clinical Pathology 69: 6–17
3. Ali S Y, Griffiths M T, Bayliss M T, Dieppe P A 1974 Ultrastructural studies of pyrophosphate crystal deposition in articular cartilage. Annals of the Rheumatic Diseases (abstr suppl) pp 97–98
4. Arnoldi C C, Reimann I, Bretlau P 1980 The synovial membrane in human coxarthrosis: light and electron microscopic studies. Clinical Orthopaedics and Related Research 148: 213–220
5. Barland P, Novikoff A B, Hamerman D 1962 Electron microscopy of the human synovial membrane. Journal of Cell Biology 14: 207–220
6. Barland P, Novikoff A B, Hamerman D 1964 Fine structure and cytochemistry of the rheumatoid synovial membrane, with special reference to lysosomes. American Journal of Pathology 44: 853–866
7. Bhan A K, Roy S 1971 Synovial giant cell in rheumatoid arthritis and other joint diseases. Annals of the Rheumatic Diseases 30: 294–298
8. Bhawan J, Joris I, Cohen N, Majno G 1980 Microcirculatory changes in post-traumatic pigmented villonodular synovitis. Archives of Pathology and Laboratory Medicine 104: 328–332
9. Bierther V M, Streit W, Wessinghage D 1973 Feinstrukturelle veränderungen der synovialis bei arthropathia psoriatica. Zeitschrift für Rheumaforschung 32: 202–211
10. Bjelle A 1972 Morphological study of articular cartilage in pyrophosphate arthropathy (chondrocalcinosis articularis or calcium pyrophosphate dihydrate crystal deposition disease). Annals of the Rheumatic Diseases 31: 449–456
11. Bjelle A, Crocker P, Willoughby D 1980 Ultra-microcrystals in pyrophosphate arthropathy: crystal identification and case report. Acta Medica Scandinavica 207: 89–92
12. Boivin G, Lagier R 1983 An ultrastructural study of articular chondrocalcinosis in cases of knee osteoarthritis. Virchows Archiv, Pathology Anatomy and Histopathology 400: 13–29
13. Cameron H, Fornasier V L, Macnab I 1975 Pyrophosphate arthropathy. American Journal of Clinical Pathology 63(2): 192–198
14. Carson D A, Fox R 1985 Structure and function of synoviocytes. In: McCarty D (ed) Arthritis and allied conditions, 10th edn. Lea & Febiger, Philadelphia, pp 257–269
15. Cherian P V, Schumacher H R 1982 Diagnostic potential of rapid electron microscopic analysis of joint effusions. Arthritis and Rheumatism 25: 98–100
16. Cherian P V, Schumacher H R 1986 Immunochemical and ultrastructural characterization of serum proteins associated with monosodium urate crystals (MSU) in synovial fluid cells from patients with gout. Ultrastructural Pathology 10: 209–219
17. Espinoza L R, Vasey F B, Espinoza C G, Bocanegra T S, Germain B F 1982 Vascular changes in psoriatic synovium. Arthritis and Rheumatism 25: 677–684
18. Faure G, Netter P 1978 Urate crystals in gout. Correspondence. Journal of Rheumatology 5: 353–355
19. Faure G, Netter P, Gaucher A 1979 Microscopic electronique a balayage et pathologie articulaire. Etude de la membrane synoviale humaine. Published by Merck-Sharp and Dohme-Chibret, 3, Avenue Hoche 75008, Paris
20. Freemont A J, Jones C J P, Bromley M, Andrew P 1983 Changes in vascular endothelium related to lymphocyte collections in diseased synovia. Arthritis and Rheumatism 26: 1427–1433
21. Gaucher A, Faure G, Netter P, Malaman B, Steinmetz J 1977

Identification of microcrystals in synovial fluids by combined scanning electron microscopy and X-ray diffraction. Application of triclinic calcium pyrophosphate dihydrate. Biomedicine 27: 242–244

22. Ghadially F N 1983 Fine structure of synovial joints. A text and atlas of the ultrastructure of normal and pathological articular tissues. Butterworths, London

23. Ghadially F N, Lalonde J M A, Dick C E 1979 Ultrastructure of pigmented villonodular synovitis. Journal of Pathology 127: 19–26

24. Grimley P M, Sokoloff L 1966 Synovial giant cells in rheumatoid arthritis. American Journal of Pathology 49: 931–954

25. Harris E D 1985 Pathogenesis of rheumatoid arthritis. In: Kelley W N, Harris E D, Ruddy S, Sledge C B (eds) Textbook of rheumatology, 2nd edn. Saunders, Philadelphia, pp 886–915

26. Hawkins C F, Farr M, Morris C J, Hoare A M, Williamson N 1976 Detection by electron microscope of rod-shaped organisms in synovial membrane from a patient with the arthritis of Whipple's disease. Annals of the Rheumatic Diseases 35: 502–509

27. Hirohata K 1968 Light microscopic and electron microscopic studies of individual cells in pigmented villonodular synovitis and bursitis. (Jaffe) Kobe Journal of Medical Sciences 14: 251–279

28. Honig S, Gorevic P, Hoffstein S, Weissman G 1977 Crystal deposition disease. Diagnostic by electron microscopy. The American Journal of Medicine 63: 161–164

29. Kobayashi I, Ziff M 1973 Electron microscopic studies of lymphoid cells in the rheumatoid synovial membrane. Arthritis and Rheumatism 16: 471–486

30. Laschi R, Govoni E, Cenacchi G, Trotta F 1986 Calcium pyrophosphate dihydrate microcrystal-associated arthropathy. Case 2. Ultrastructural Pathology 10: 395–400

31. Meachim G, Stockwell R A 1979 The matrix. In: Freeman M A R (ed) Adult articular cartilage. 2nd edn. Pitman Medical Publishing, London, pp 1–68

32. Minns R J, Stevens P S, Hardinge K 1977 Osteoarthrotic articular cartilage lesions of the femoral head observed in the scanning electron microscope. Journal of Pathology 122: 63–70

33. Mitrovic D R 1983 Pathology of articular deposition of calcium salts and their relationship to osteoarthritis. Annals of the Rheumatic Diseases 42 (Supplement): 19–26

34. Norton W L, Lewis D, Ziff M 1966 Light and electron microscopic observation on the synovitis of Reiter's disease. Arthritis and Rheumatism 9: 747–757

35. Norton W L, Ziff M 1966 Electron microscopic observation on the rheumatoid synovial membrane. Arthritis and Rheumatism 9: 589–610

36. Pritzker K P H, Phillips H, Luk S C, Koven I H, Kiss A, Houpt J B 1976 Pseudotumor of temporomandibular joint; destructive calcium pyrophosphate dihydrate arthropathy. Journal of Rheumatology 3: 70–81

37. Pritzker K P H, Zahn C E, Nyburg S C, Luk S C, Houpt J B 1978 The ultrastructure of urate crystals in gout. Journal of Rheumatology 5: 7–18

38. Redler O 1974 A scanning electron microscopic study of human normal and osteoarthritis articular cartilage. Clinical Orthopaedics 103: 261–268

39. Reginato A J, Schumacher H R, Martinez V A 1974 The articular cartilage in familial chondrocalcinosis: light and electron microscopic study. Arthritis and Rheumatism 17: 977–992

40. Roy S 1967 Ultrastructure of synovial membrane in osteoarthritis. Annals of Rheumatic Diseases 26: 517–527

41. Ryan L M, McCarthy D J 1985 Calcium pyrophosphate crystal deposition disease: pseudogout, articular chondrocalcinosis. In: McCarthy D J (ed) Arthritis and allied conditions. Lea & Febiger, Philadelphia, pp 1515–1529

42. Schumacher H R 1968 The synovitis of pseudogout: electron microscopic observation. Arthritis and Rheumatism 11: 426–435

43. Schumacher H R 1975 Pathology of the synovial membrane in gout. Light and electron microscopic studies. Interpretation of crystals in electron micrographs. Arthritis and Rheumatism 18: 771–782

44. Schumacher H R, Kitridou R C 1972 Synovitis of recent onset: a clinicopathologic study during the first month of disease. Arthritis and Rheumatism 15: 465–484

45. Schumacher H R, Lotke P, Athreya B, Rothfuss S 1982 Pigmented villonodular synovitis: light and electron microscopic studies. Seminars in Arthritis and Rheumatism 12: 32–43

46. Silberberg B 1968 Ultrastructure of articular cartilage in health and disease. Clinical Orthopaedics and Related Research 57: 233–257

47. Soren A, Klein W, Huth F 1978 The synovial changes in post-traumatic synovitis and osteoarthritis. Rheumatology and Rehabilitation 17: 38–45

48. Steiner G C 1981 Tumor and tumor-like conditions of bone and joints. In: Johannnessen J V (ed) Electron microscopy in human medicine. McGraw-Hill, New York, vol. 4, pp 54–140

49. Stockwell R A, Meachim G 1979 The chondrocytes. In: Freeman., M A R (ed) Adult cartilage, 2nd edn. Pitman Medical Publishing, London, pp 69–144

50. Weiss C 1979 Normal and osteoarthritic articular cartilage. Orthopaedic Clinics of North America 10: 175–189

51. Weiss C, Mirow S 1972 Ultrastructural study of osteoarthritic changes in the articular cartilage of human knees. Journal of Bone and Joint Surgery 54(A): 954–972

52. Wyllie J C 1969 The stromal cell reaction of pigmented villonodular synovitis: an electron microscopic study. Arthritis and Rheumatism 12: 205–214

53. Wyllie J C, Haust M D, More R H 1966 The fine structure of synovial lining cells in rheumatoid arthritis. Laboratory Investigation 15: 519–529

54. Wynee-Roberts C R, Anderson C 1978 Light and electron microscopic studies of normal juvenile human synovium. Seminars in Arthritis and Rheumatism 7: 279–286

55. Wynne-Roberts C R, Anderson C H, Turano A M, Baron N 1978 Light and electron microscopic findings of juvenile rheumatoid arthritis synovium. Comparison with normal juvenile synovium. Seminars in Arthritis and Rheumatism 7: 287–302

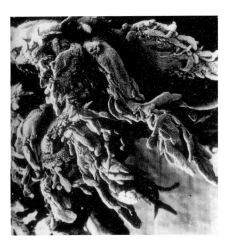

Fig. 28.1 Rheumatoid arthritis: synovial tissue. SEM of the synovium in the chronic, well-established disease, showing numerous proliferating villi with marked increase of the surface area. (× 23) References: 19 and 25.

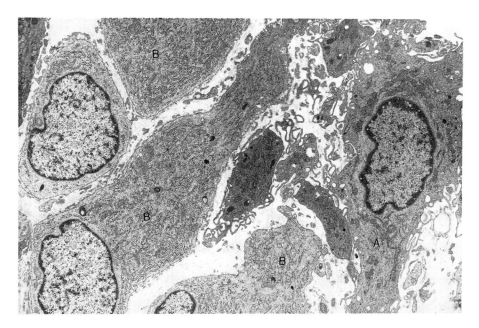

Fig. 28.2 Rheumatoid arthritis: synovial lining cells. There are several type B synovial cells (B) with abundant rough endoplasmic reticulum and occasional lysosomes. The type A cell (A) has sparse rough endoplasmic reticulum, several lysosomes and vacuoles and numerous filopodia. The joint cavity (J) is in the right upper corner. In some cases the rough endoplasmic reticulum of the type B cells is dilated and contains dense proteinaceous material.[22] In those instances where the synovial cells are closely packed, desmosome-like structures may be found.[22] (× 4300) References: 14, 22, 25 and 53.

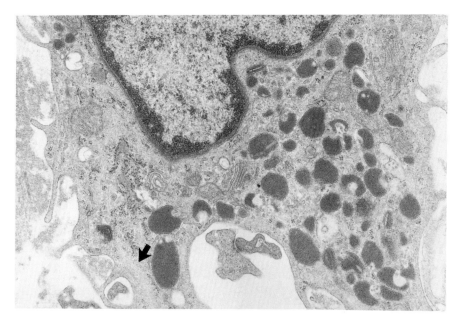

Fig. 28.3 Rheumatoid arthritis: type A cell. Large numbers of lysosomes are seen as well as intermediate-type filaments (arrow). The increased number of lysosomes and the presence of hydrolytic enzymes in the synovial cells[6] is probably related to the active role that they play in the pathogenesis of this disease and the degradation of the cartilage.[22] The presence of abundant cytoplasmic filaments has been interpreted as a regressive or degenerative change.[22] (× 12 100) References: 6, 22 and 53.

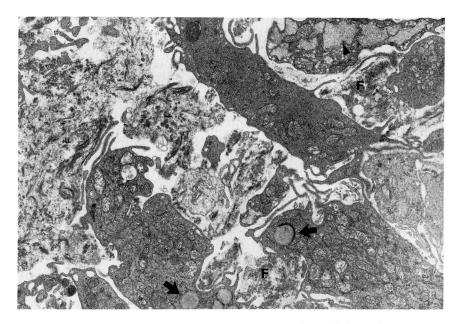

Fig. 28.4 Rheumatoid arthritis: surface cells and fibrinoid material. Deposits of fibrin-like filamentous material (F) are seen located adjacent to the surface cells. Fibrin accumulation is a frequent feature of this condition; it is present to a lesser degree in other synovial disorders (see Table 28.1). Several lipid droplets (arrows) are observed in the synovial cells, as well as dilated rough endoplasmic reticulum (arrow head). (× 4700) References: 22 and 35.

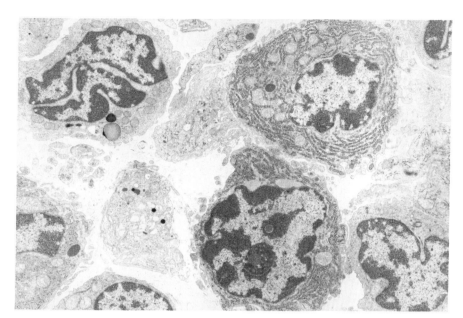

Fig. 28.5 Rheumatoid arthritis: subsynovial tissue. Several inflammatory cells including plasma cells and lymphocytes are seen. The presence of many chronic inflammatory cells in the subsynovial tissue is characteristic of this condition. Most of the lymphocytes are T cells although B lymphocytes are also seen.[14,25,29] Both B lymphocytes and plasma cells synthesize immunoglobulins and the rheumatoid factor.[25] (× 3600) References: 14, 22, 25 and 29.

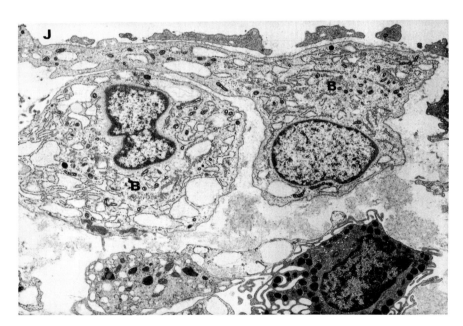

Fig. 28.6 Traumatic synovitis: synovial surface. The patient is a 51-year-old male with a torn meniscus. There are two type B cells (B) with dilated rough endoplasmic reticulum. The increase in rough endoplasmic reticulum in this condition is thought to indicate heightened protein secretory activity which is released into the joint.[22] A mast cell is also noted. The joint space is at the top (J). (× 3100) References: 22 and 47.

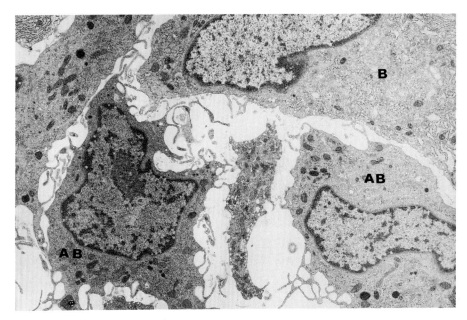

Fig. 28.7 Osteoarthritis: synovial lining surface of the hip. The patient is a 62-year-old female with osteoarthritis. Predominantly type AB (AB) and B (B) cells are seen. Some authors found that the rough endoplasmic reticulum is often dilated and the number of lysosomes is more frequent than in normal synovium.[40] In some cases the synovium of the hip joint may show atrophic lining cells with fibrosis.[47] (× 3700) References: 22, 40 and 47.

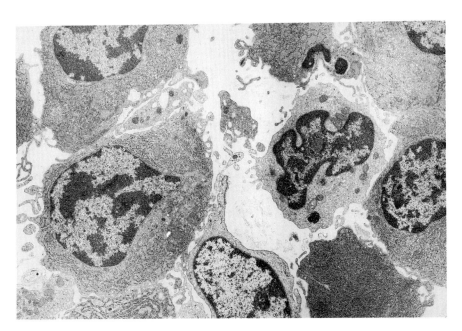

Fig. 28.8 Osteoarthritis: subsynovial tissue. Focal chronic inflammation in the hip joint of the same patient from the preceding illustration. There are several plasma cells and a lymphocyte. In this particular area, the inflammation resembles that of rheumatoid arthritis. In most cases of osteoarthritis, however, the inflammatory infiltration is sparse. (× 3600) Reference: 47.

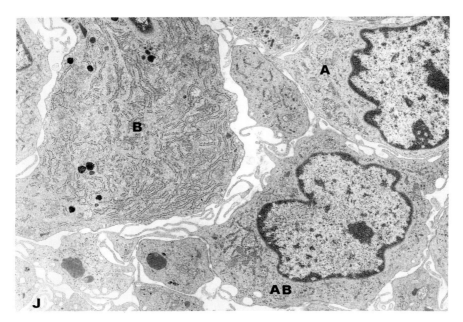

Fig. 28.9 Pigmented villonodular synovitis: synovial lining cells. The lesion was present in the shoulder joint of a 37-year-old female. A type B cell (B) is seen with abundant rough endoplasmic reticulum and siderosomes; an intermediate cell (AB) and an A cell (A) are also seen. The joint space (J) is covered by numerous cell projections. Type B cell hyperplasia is usually common in this condition, and lipid droplets and siderosomes may be observed in the lining cells. (× 3700) References: 23 and 45. See also Ch. 11, Figs 11.9–11.14.

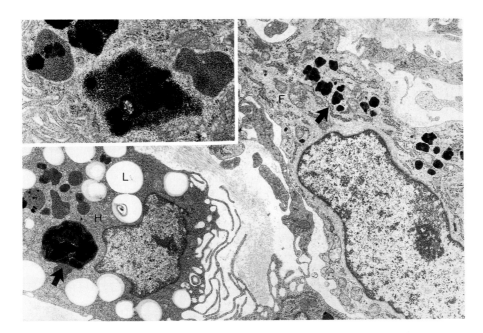

Fig. 28.10 Pigmented villonodular synovitis: subsynovial cells. Fibroblastic (F) and histiocytic (H) stromal cells are seen. Numerous siderosomes (arrows) are observed in both fibroblasts and histiocytes, and lipid droplets (L) are seen in the histiocytes. Iron deposition is a common finding in this condition; the iron is found in the siderosomes but may also be scattered in the cytoplasm. Lipid droplets are also noted in both fibroblasts and histiocytes.[45] In some instances 'foam cells' with large amounts of lipid material are seen.[52] *Inset* High magnification of siderosomes (S) containing fine electron-dense iron-containing particles. (× 5400) *Inset* (× 16 500) References: 23, 45 and 52.

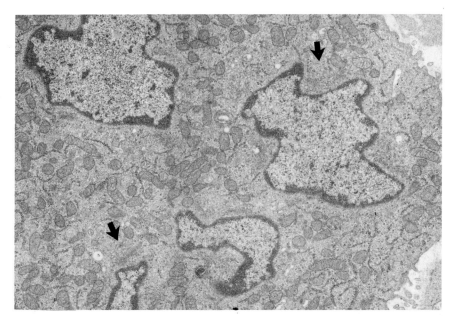

Fig. 28.11 Pigmented villonodular synovitis: multinucleated giant cell. Part of a giant cell with several nuclei and numerous mitochondria. The Golgi apparatus (arrows) is perinuclear in location. These cells are frequently found in this condition and they usually lack evidence of phagocytic activity, iron and lipid droplets. This giant cell resembles the multinucleated giant cells seen in other bone lesions (i.e., giant cell tumour, non-ossifying fibroma).[48] (× 4800) References: 23, 45 and 48.

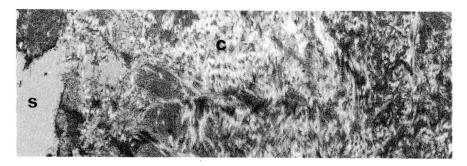

Fig. 28.12 Early osteoarthritis: articular surface of knee. Early degenerative changes are seen on the cartilage surface (S) with disruption of the filamentous surface layer (lamina splendens).[51] The bundles of mature collagen fibres of the superficial layer (C) of the cartilage are running for the most part parallel to the articular surface. (× 7300) References: 19, 22, 50 and 51.

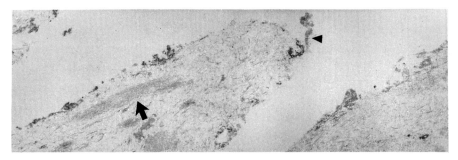

Fig. 28.13 Osteoarthritis: fibrillated cartilage of knee. There is cleft formation extending into the deeper layer of the cartilage. In some areas (arrow) fine collagen fibres are seen running parallel to the cleft. Small amounts of amorphous material (arrowhead) are present on the surface. In severe osteoarthritis, all layers of the cartilage show extensive degeneration of the matrix and chondrocytes. (× 5400) References: 19, 50 and 51.

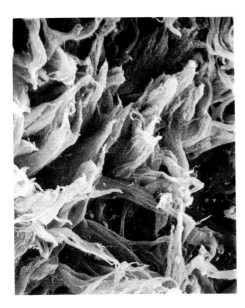

Fig. 28.14 Osteoarthritis: articular surface of hip. SEM showing the tapered and frayed collagen bundles exposed on the surface of the degenerated cartilage. The tissue was pretreated with H_2O_2 and trypsin in order to remove the embedded matrix and reveal the collagen.[32] In normal cartilage the articular surface is slightly undulated and contains fine collagen fibrils and ridges.[38] ($\times$ 130) References: 19, 32 and 38.

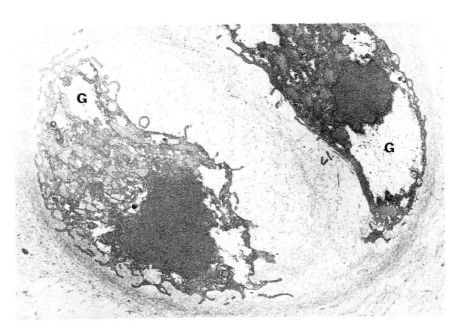

Fig. 28.15 Osteoarthritis: chondrocytes. Group of two chondrocytes seen in the intermediate zone of the cartilage. The pericellular matrix contains fine filamentous structures and small proteoglycan granules. Glycogen (G) is present in the chondrocyte cytoplasm. Chondrocyte proliferation with dilatation of their RER and formation of clusters is common in osteoarthritis, and represents a reparative attempt at regeneration of the articular cartilage. ($\times$ 3600) References: 22, 50 and 51.

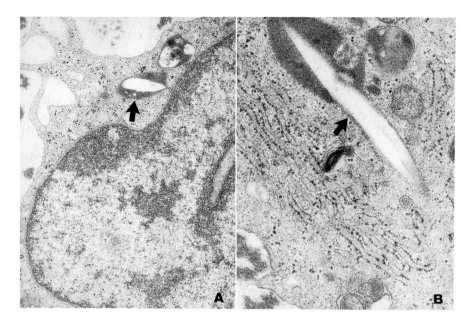

Fig. 28.16 Gout: urate crystals in synovial fluid cells. The patient was a 28-year-old man with gouty arthritis of the knee. The specimen represents the synovial cells obtained from the pellet of centrifuged joint fluid; it was processed for TEM in a routine fashion and double-stained. **A** The phagosome contains an electron-lucent, elongated space (arrow) which represents the dissolved urate crystal. (× 9 200) **B** High-power view of another cell showing a urate crystal projecting out of the phagosome (arrow). (× 17 200) MSU crystals are water-soluble and are usually dissolved by the common fixatives used for electron microscopy as well as by the liquids used for staining. References: 37 and 43.

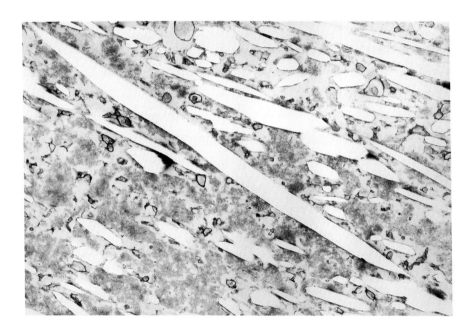

Fig. 28.17 Gout: tophus from hand. Seventy-two-year-old male with chronic gout. There are many electron-lucent, elongated acicular spaces consistent with dissolved MSU crystals. Other spaces are smaller and probably also represent MSU crystals; however, the possibility of being CPPD crystals cannot be entirely ruled out. (× 8300) Both MSU and CPPD crystals may be present in a tophus, and proper crystallographic identification is necessary. The specimen was processed for TEM in a routine fashion and double-stained. References: 11, 18, 21, 36 and 37.

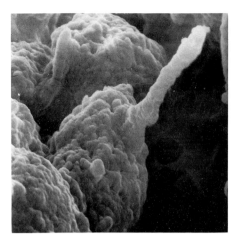

Fig. 28.18 Gout: synovial fluid cell. SEM of an elongated MSU crystal contained in part within a synovial fluid cell. There is amorphous material adherent to the crystal surface. (× 6600) References: 18 and 19.

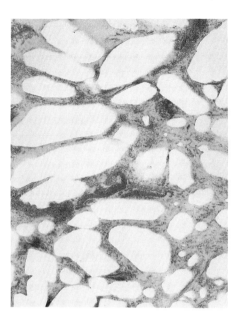

Fig. 28.19 Crystal pyrophosphate deposition disease: meniscal tissue. The crystals have been dissolved, and the spaces are rhomboid and rod-like in shape. There is some distortion and enlargement of the spaces due to exposure to the electron beam. In our experience and that of others, most of the crystals found in the meniscus and cartilage in CPPD are extracellular and are apparently not related to collagen fibres. Section stained with uranyl acetate and lead citrate. (× 21 500) References: 3, 12, 39 and 41.

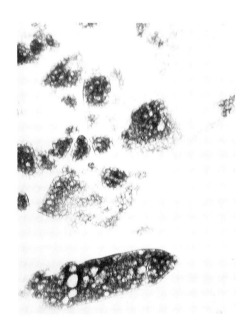

Fig. 28.20 Crystal pyrophosphate deposition disease: meniscal tissue. TEM of the crystals examined at 80 kv showing irregular shapes and a 'bubbled' appearance. It is not certain whether this electron-lucent appearance is a real finding[30,36] or an artefact.[10] (× 54 500) References: 10, 11, 30 and 36.

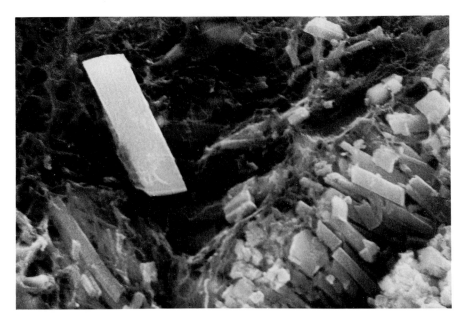

Fig. 28.21 Crystal pyrophosphate deposition disease: meniscal tissue. SEM showing one large and many small crystals, the latter partially fragmented and arranged in a parallel fashion. Many of the crystals are rhomboid in shape. CPPD crystals may vary in shape and size, and giant crystals can be observed.[13,19] (× 4800) References: 13, 19, 21 and 36.

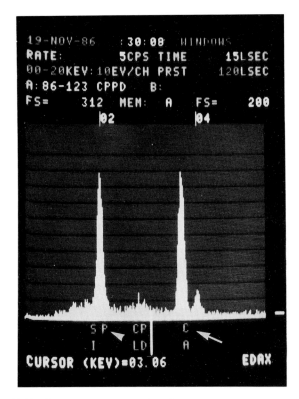

Fig. 28.22 Crystal pyrophosphate deposition disease: electron dispersive X-ray analysis. X-ray microanalysis from the same area as illustrated in Fig. 28.21. It shows almost equal values for calcium (arrow) and phosphorous (arrowhead): this is compatible with calcium pyrophosphate dihydrate crystals. References: 11, 21 and 36.

29. Lymphoid system, including immunopathology

D. V. Spagnolo   J. A. Armstrong   J. M. Papadimitriou
D. W. Henderson

INTRODUCTION

Accurate diagnosis of non-neoplastic disorders of the lymphoid system can almost always be made by thorough scrutiny of technically adequate histological sections, supplemented by appropriate immunophenotypic or even immunogenotypic studies in some instances. Electron microscopy (EM) is not essential for diagnosis of non-neoplastic conditions, but familiarity with the normal structure and cellular constituents of the lymphoid organs, and the range of appearances in various reactive states, is essential in order to avoid misinterpretation when pathologically altered lymphoid tissues are examined. Furthermore, ultrastructural studies of reactive lymph node and thymus have contributed greatly to an understanding of the nature and pathogenesis of many non-neoplastic conditions affecting these organs.

In this chapter the normal ultrastructure of lymph nodes and thymus gland is presented, followed by the changes in selected reactive, or borderline, conditions. Any relevant immunological perturbations are also considered where appropriate. By necessity, coverage cannot be encyclopaedic, and the interested reader should consult the bibliography for additional information.

LYMPH NODE

NORMAL STRUCTURE

The lymph node is organized into different anatomical and functional compartments. Traditionally, three zones are recognized: the B-dependent superficial cortex, containing primary and secondary lymphoid follicles; the T-dependent para-cortex where T and B lymphocyte traffic occurs; and the medulla, where, in addition to lymphocytes, there are developing and mature plasma cells. Intralymphatic and intravascular compartments course through these parenchymal zones, which are important for cellular and molecular traffic.

The structure of the lymphatic sinuses, high endothelial venules, and the various cellular constituents of the lymph node will be considered briefly.

Sinuses

The intralymphatic space includes the subcapsular (marginal) sinus, cortical and deep cortical (intermediate) sinuses, and the medullary sinuses. The sinus wall is discontinuous, and — although it shows some regional structural variation[91,165,182,213] — it consists essentially of a layer of endothelial cells resting on basement membrane of varying thickness and continuity, and surrounding stroma (Fig. 29.1).

Endothelial cells are weakly phagocytic, show strong non-specific esterase activity, weak to strong acid phosphatase activity depending on their location, and no alkaline phosphatase activity[92] (in contrast to blood vascular endothelium which contains alkaline phosphatase).

High endothelial venules (HEV)

The specialized HEV (postcapillary venules) important in lymphocyte recirculation are found in the paracortex. The tissue distributions of functionally distinct lymphocyte subpopulations[299] are thought to be directed through the interaction of HEV receptors with complementary lymphocyte receptors. The development of monoclonal antibodies specific for HE cell differentiation antigens will enable study of the role of HEV in mediating lymphocyte traffic in various immunological conditions.[79]

The HEV are lined by distinctive endothelial cells (Fig. 29.2),[92,97,182,213] which show high beta-glucuronidase, non-specific esterase, ATPase and acid-phosphatase activity, but no alkaline phosphatase activity (cf. capillary and arteriolar endothelium which do show alkaline phosphatase activity).[92,97] Apart from the specialized HEV, other blood vessels in the lymph node have the same structure as in other organs.

Cellular constituents

The main cellular elements are lymphocytes with varying morphology, phenotype and function, and accessory or supporting cells which are important in antigen presentation to lymphocytes.

Table 29.1 Ultrastructural characteristics of lymphoid cells*

Morphology	Mantle zone or primary follicle	Germinal centre (gc) lymphocytes			Paracortical lymphocytes	Plasma cell
		Cleaved lymphocyte	Large non-cleaved lymphocyte	Immunoblast		
Size and shape	Small, round 5–7 μm diameter	Small–medium; ovoid or irregular; up to 10 μm diameter	Medium–large, round 12–14 μm diameter	Large, >15 μm diameter	Small and round in non-stimulated node	Ovoid; approx. 10 μm; sites: medulla > paracortex > gc
Nucleus	Round or slightly irregular	Irregular, notched; nuclear pockets	Round, but may be deeply indented; nuclear pockets	Large, round or slightly irregular	Round or slightly irregular; some may show lobulated, deeply indented contours	Round; eccentric
chromatin	Clumped	Moderately clumped; condensed at nuclear membrane	More dispersed; small clumps at nuclear membrane	Dispersed; very narrow condensed nuclear rim	Coarse in unstimulated cells; larger, activated nuclei have chromatin clearing	Coarse; large peripheral clumps
nucleoli	Small, usually single and chromatin-associated	Single, medium size, usually central	1–3 round, large, central or peripheral	2–3 very large, central or paracentral; prominent nucleolonema	Inconspicuous, unless activated	Medium-szied, central
Cytoplasm	Scant	Scant	Moderate	Abundant, pale	Scant to moderate	Abundant
monoribosomes	+ +	+ +	+	+	+	+
polyribosomes	+	+	+ + +	+ + + +	+	+
RER	Scant	Few short profiles	+ Long strands	+ + Long strands	Scant	+ + + Parallel cisternae; may be distended with secretory product forming dense Russell bodies or crystalline patterns
Golgi	Small	Medium sized	Well developed	Very well-developed	Small	Very well-developed with prominent smooth vesicles
mitochondria	Few; dense matrices	Few	Several, often at one side of nucleus	Moderate number; randomly distributed	Few; may be aggregated near Golgi	Large, globular, surrounded by lamellae of RER
glycogen	Sparse	Sparse	Sparse	Small deposits	Sparse	Sparse
lysosomes	None, or rare	+	+	+ near Golgi	+ often clustered near Golgi, with mitochondria	Rare; near Golgi; may contain large lipid droplet ('lipochondrion')

See Figs 29.5, 29.6 and 29.18.

Comments

1. Immature plasma cell precursors (plasmablasts and proplasmacytes) show a spectrum of appearances between the immunoblast and the mature plasma cell. They are larger than mature plasma cells, their nuclei have less chromatin clumping and larger nucleoli; the more abundant cytoplasm contains less, and more randomly arranged, RER, and relatively more polyribosomes and monoribosomes.
2. Rarely, B-cells with convoluted nuclei and expressing surface B-differentiation antigens immuno-ultrastructurally are found in reactive germinal centres;[304] this may explain the origin of those uncommon B-lymphomas having markedly irregular nuclei, mimicking T-lymphomas morphologically.[206,235,242,387]
3. Morphometric light- and electron-microscopic, and immuno-ultrastructural studies, of reactive follicles and follicular lymphomas have been performed, assessing parameters such as nuclear contour index and nuclear form factor.[66,67,71,304,349] Results vary, possibly as a consequence of some workers using cell suspensions as opposed to tissue sections, and differences in morphometric methods.
4. NK cells and plasmacytoid T cells — see text.

*References: 180, 182, 213 and 244.

Lymphoid cells

The salient structural, enzyme-histochemical and immunophenotypic features of lymphocytes in their different functional compartments appear in Tables 29.1 and 29.2, and a schematic representation of B-cell and T-cell differentiation is presented in Figs 29.3 and 29.4. Natural killer cells and plasmacytoid T-cells are not included in the tables, but are briefly considered in the text which follows.

The B-cell compartment is typified by the reactive follicle (Fig. 29.5) composed of a small lymphocytic mantle or corona surrounding a germinal centre. Stromal fibroblasts and myofibroblasts occur at the interface between mantle and germinal centre. The latter is composed of B-lymphocytes in various stages of development, dendritic reticulum cells (DRC), tingible body macrophages, and fewer T-cells (mainly helper cells and some natural killer cells).[150,274,298] There is good evidence that lymph nodes also contain lymphocytes analogous to splenic marginal zone lymphocytes.[368,371a]

The T-zone or paracortex contains mainly small lymphocytes in the non- stimulated node. Interdigitating reticulum cells (IDRC), histiocytes and HEV are also essential constituents of the paracortex. In the stimulated node, this area often has a nodular appearance, more noticeable in superficial lymph nodes, variously referred to as tertiary nodules, tertiary follicles or T-nodules.[182] In T-zone reactions, increased numbers of large lymphoid cells and immunoblasts are present, along with varying numbers of plasma cells (Fig. 29.6), pale-staining histiocytes and IDRC in varying numbers. Van den Oord et al[367] describe a 'composite nodule' in reactive nodes made up of two functional domains, the B-follicle and the adjacent T-nodule, surrounded by a rim of HEV. They hypothesize that this nodule may represent a flexible basic structural and functional unit of the reactive node: either compartment may enlarge at the expense of the other.

Natural killer (NK) cells are specialized lymphocytes that mediate cytotoxic reactions independent of class I or II MHC molecule expression on target cells. A better understanding of the biology of these cells has led to a proposed clearer nomenclature for lymphocytes having such cytolytic activity,[129a] and at least two populations of lymphocytes are now recognized.

The major cell type, to which the term 'NK cell' should be restricted, consists of large granular lymphocytes (LGL) which exhibit characteristic azurophilic granules in peripheral blood. They are CD3⁻ and T-cell receptor⁻ (there is no productive rearrangement of their T-cell receptor genes), and they exhibit characteristic surface markers such as CD16, CD56 and CD57. They are non-adherent, have avid receptors for the Fc portion of IgG, do not phagocytize inert or opsonized particles, and contain various acid hydrolases.[33,89,129,351] The ultrastructural features of granular lymphocytes in the blood are well-described,[16,115,225,259]

but less so in solid tissues.[373] In the blood they measure 10–13 μm in diameter, have a low N/C ratio, an eccentric nucleus with highly condensed chromatin, and they often possess a uropod[225] in which the organelles are concentrated. Round or ovoid dense granules 200–800 nm in diameter are present in the cytoplasm, some of which contain highly distinctive parallel tubular arrays.[259] Ultrastructural cytochemical studies have localized various acid hydrolases to these dense granules, as well as within vacuoles and coated vesicles.[16,115]

The second cell type comprises a small proportion of CD3⁺ T-lymphocytes which may exhibit similar NK activity, particularly upon activation. It is proposed that they be referred to as T-lymphocytes displaying 'NK-like activity' or 'non-MHC requiring' cytolysis.[129a] In the peripheral blood most T-lymphocytes with NK activity express CD8. In lymph nodes, CD57⁺ cells have been found mainly in germinal centres where most co-express CD4; very few cells are seen in the mantle zone or interfollicular tissues.[18,204,212,268,275,319,336,373] They account for 1–10% of germinal centre cells,[212] and constitute 10–20% of the T cells in the germinal centre.[268]

Lymphocytes in either of these two groups which exhibit cytolytic activity upon activation by interleukin-2 are referred to as lymphokine-activated killer cells (LAK).[129a]

Plasmacytoid T-cells (PTC) are distinguishable from other T-zone cells and plasma cells only in high-quality Giemsa-stained, or B5-fixed H & E sections. They are medium-sized cells, seen relatively frequently as focal clusters in the marginal areas of hyperplastic T-regions, close to epithelioid venules, in non-specific lymphadenitides,[182,184,376] and also in some specific reactive conditions.[85a,86,127] IDRC are frequently seen in these clusters. The cells have well-developed parallel cisternae of RER circumferentially disposed around the nucleus; prominent Golgi apparatus with many small vesicles and smooth tubules; scarce or absent lysosomes; few mitochondria; ribosomes and few polyribosomes; relatively abundant glycogen; and cytoplasmic microfilaments.[26,84a,222] Tubuloreticular inclusions may be seen in some RER cisternae.[84a] Nuclei are round to ovoid and sometimes indented; they have a marginal rim of heterochromatin, and one or two small nucleoli. The cells show little or no mitotic activity. Pyknotic and degenerate forms are frequent, and they are phagocytozed by large macrophages.[184]

The lineage of these cells has yet to be clarified, and their unique phenotype suggests either T-lineage or a relationship to myelomonocytic cells. The cells lack pan-B markers, SIg or CIg, or C3bR. They also lack pan-T markers, but express CD4, an antigen expressed by both T-helper cells and macrophages,[86,127,184,253] are CD45⁺ CD38⁻ (unlike B-lineage plasma cells),[127] and express the transferrin receptor[134,277] and HLA-class II antigens.[222] In paraffin sections they are MT1⁺ (CD43) LN2⁺ (CD74).[84,84a] Most cells do not express the nuclear proliferation antigen

Table 29.2 Histochemical and immunophenotypic characteristics of lymphoid cells*

	Mantle zone or primary follicle	Germinal centre lymphocytes	Paracortical lymphocytes	Plasma cells
Enzyme histochemistry				
Non-specific esterase	–	–	–	
Acid phosphatase	–	–	+ focal, dot-like	
Acidic ANAE	–	–	+ focal, dot-like	
s Alkaline phosphatase	+ outer cells only	–	–	
s ATPase	+	–	–	
s 5'-nucleotidase	+	–	–	
Immunohistochemistry				
cIg + J chain	–	+ variable number of cells	– (T cells) + (any B-blast cells)	+
sIg M	+	Weak, or no lymphoid staining (some sIgM/D on centroblasts may occur in early germinal centre reaction); dendritic staining in FS due to AgAb complexes on DRC cell processes	– (T cells) + (variable number of large B-blast cells)	–
G	–			–
A	–			–
D	+			–
Ig light chains	–	As for heavy chains	–	+ cytoplasmic
C3 receptors (C3R)	+ strong staining	+ / –	–	–
HLA-DR	+ strong	+ strong	–	–
B-differentiation antigens				
CD10 (J5; CALLA)	–	+	–	–
CD19 (B4)	+	+ dendritic (probably DRC staining)	–	–
CD20 (B1)	+ strong	+ strong	–	–
CD21 (B2)	+	+ dendritic (probably DRC staining)	–	–
CD24 (BA 1)	+	+ / – (10–20% cells)	–	–
BA 2	+ / – (10–20% cells)	+	–	–
T-differentiation antigens				
CD1a (T6)	–	–	–	–
CD2 (T11)	–	–	+	–
CD3 (OKT3, Leu4)	–	as for CD4	+	–
CD4 (OKT4, Leu3a)	–	– most; up to 20% positive	+	–
CD5(T101, Leu1)	–	–	+	–
CD8 (OKT8, Leu2a)	–	– (rare positive cell)	– (less than CD4)	–
CD38 (OKT10)	–	+ / –	–	– cytoplasmic
CD57 (Leu7)	–	– most, but some positive cells	–	–
Plasma cell antigens PC-1 and PCA-1	–	–	–	+

Abbreviations: ANAE = alpha naphthyl acetate esterase; c = cytoplasmic; s = surface; Ig = immunoglobulin; FS = frozen section; DRC = dendritic reticulum cell; + / – = weak staining.

Comment

Immunophenotypic profiles have been obtained from studies done on frozen tissue sections and cell suspensions. The results of enzyme-histochemical and immunophenotypic profiles in the table are not quantitative but merely reflect the staining pattern obtained for most, but not necessarily all, lymphocytes in each anatomical compartment. For example, while most lymphocytes in the follicular mantle are B cells, occasional T cells are also seen. Similarly, in the paracortex, most cells are T cells, but B cells also occur there in varying numbers and stages of maturity, depending on the functional state of the lymph node.

References: (enzyme histochemistry) 65, 182, 183, 219 and 250.

        (immunohistochemistry) B-Cells: 7, 133, 136, 138, 139, 173a, 196, 214, 227–229, 240, 328–330; 371;

               T-Cells: 81, 133, 136, 140, 150, 173a, 214, 274, 275, 282, 297, 298, 330, 371 and 410.

See also Figs 29.3 and 29.4.

Ki-67,[26,222] are in the G_0/G_1 phase of the cell cycle,[26] and resist stimulation in vitro, suggesting that they may be terminally differentiated cells.[26,222] An analogy to plasma cells of the B-series has been suggested, with a postulated secretory function (possibly lymphokines). More recently, PTC have been found to express certain myelomonocytic antigens.[22,85,134] The development of myelomonocytic leukaemia in all cases of malignant lymphomas of PTC so far reported[25,222,277] underscores the likely relationship of PTC to cells of the myelomonocytic series. Accordingly, the less committal terms 'plasmacytoid T-zone cell',[26] or 'plasmacytoid monocytes',[85] has been proposed for these cells, which probably play a role in T-cell-mediated immune responses.

Accessory or supporting cells

The main supporting or accessory lymph node cells are histiocytic reticulum cells, fibroblastic reticulum cells, DRC and IDRC.[182] To these can be added the intralymphatic veiled cells and Langerhans' cells (LC). The DRC, IDRC and LC (along with indeterminate cells in skin) form a system of cells which have important accessory antigen-presenting functions in the immune system. They have characteristic dendritic morphology, little phagocytic capability, contain low levels of lysosomal enzymes and express HLA-DR.[132,276,326,347] The ultrastructural, enzyme-histochemical and immunophenotypic features of the accessory cells are presented in Tables 29.3 and 29.4 (see Figs 29.7, 29.8 and 29.9). Veiled cells, so-called because of their prominent cytoplasmic 'veils' or lamellipodia, are present in small numbers in the afferent lymph and subcapsular sinus.[17,167] They are thought to be the circulatory precursors of IDRC in the lymph node, and of indeterminate cells and LC in the skin, maturing into the latter cell types under the influence of the specific tissue environment.[132,276]

Scanning electron microscopy (SEM)

The SEM appearances of leukocytes are well described.[70,271,272] It is important to note that lymphocyte surface morphology can alter markedly, depending on how the cells are prepared[4,238,287] and whether the cells are studied in suspension or in a tissue matrix, where the local microenvironment may affect the surface morphology.[271] SEM has not found application in the routine investigation of non-neoplastic disorders of the reticulo-endothelial system.

REACTIVE LYMPHADENOPATHY

Histological scrutiny of the abnormal but non-neoplastic lymph node is usually sufficient to arrive at a diagnosis. Most often, ultrastructural examination is not needed as a first-line ancillary diagnostic technique. Nevertheless, in conjunction with immunohistochemistry, EM provides valuable differen-

tial diagnostic information in difficult cases. In selected instances (e.g. AIDS-related lymphadenopathy), ultrastructural examination is often of diagnostic importance.

Lymph nodes may be involved by virtually any non-neoplastic disorder including specific infections, metabolic disorders, systemic collagen–vascular disorders and so on. These are covered elsewhere and will not be considered further. Rather, various reactive lymphadenopathies will be considered with discussion of essential clinico-pathological features in addition to ultrastructural and immunological alterations.

It is established histological practice, according to the scheme popularized by Dorfman & Warnke,[76] to group reactive lymphadenopathies according to the predominant pattern of reaction resulting in the lymph node (Table 29.5). Not all of the conditions listed in the table will be considered in detail.

Follicular patterns of reaction

Reactive follicular hyperplasia

The cellular composition of the secondary follicle in non-specific follicular hyperplasia is detailed in Table 29.1 (Fig. 29.5). The relative number of the various cell types varies, reflecting the stage of germinal centre development following antigenic stimulation.[180,182,183,188] Quantitative ultrastructural studies have shown some differences between reactive and neoplastic follicles.[261,279] In the latter, histiocytic reticulum cells are sparse, smaller and possess fewer but larger phagolysosomes. DRC are fewer; their cell processes are broader rather than labyrinthine, and they lack surface electron-dense coating; binucleation is less frequent, and nuclear outlines are more regular; and, overall, organelles are fewer in number. These features suggest that neoplastic follicles are functionally less active than reactive ones.[279]

AIDS-related lymphadenopathy

There is a substantial and growing literature describing the histological,[37,116,146,199,202,203] ultrastructural[10,11,175,176,185,187,246,247,267,320,321,345,379] and immunohistological[13,109,151,193,207,303,355,396,400] alterations in lymphoid tissues, especially lymph nodes, of patients with persistent generalized lymphadenopathy (PGL) or the acquired immunodeficiency syndrome (AIDS), evidently caused by infection with retroviral agent HIV (human immunodeficiency virus). Some recent studies have tried to correlate the distinctive patterns of pathology with the clinical course of the disease, with a view to gaining an improved understanding of the underlying pathogenetic mechanisms.[29,45,54a,73,88,152,264,278]

Histology. Various classifications of the histopathological changes in lymph nodes from PGL and AIDS patients

Table 29.3 Ultrastructural features of lymph nodal accessory cells*

	Histiocytic reticulum cell[a] (HRC)	Fibroblastic reticulum cell[b] (FRC)	Dendritic reticulum cell[c] (DRC)	Interdigitating reticulum cell (IDRC)	Langerhans' cell[d] (LC)
Location	In all areas of lymph node	Mainly at margins of germinal centres and T zones; perisinusoidal; perivascular; single cells may be seen anywhere	Specific for B-zones; in germinal centres especially in the pale 'dendritic cap' zone	Exclusively in the T-cell region i.e. paracortex	In paracortex and occasionally in sinuses; uncommon in nodes but markedly increased in dermatopathic lymphadenopathy
Structure					
Nucleus	Round, oval, or indented	Oblong, often serrated border; sphaeridia common	Ovoid or angular; may be binucleate or multinucleate; sphaeridia frequent	Very irregular, indented or tortuous	Markedly convoluted and deeply cleft
nucleolus	Medium-sized, eccentric; coarse nucleolonema	Central or peripheral; may be ring-shaped	Central, solitary; coarse nucleolonema	Small to medium-sized; often peripheral	Medium-sized, central or peripheral
chromatin	Fine, dispersed, with a thin marginated rim	Finely granular to coarse, with marginal condensation	Moderately coarse; narrow condensed rim	Fine, dispersed, with thin marginated rim	Fine, with thin marginated rim
Cytoplasm	Abundant, pale; broad cell processes extend between lymphocytes	Long, tapering cytoplasmic extension; electron-dense	Narrow perikaryon; complex ramifying and interdigitating long processes insinuate between lymphoid cells	Abundant, pale; broad villous cytoplasmic processes interdigitate with other IDRC and lymphocytes; organelles concentrated in cytocentre; cell processes are organelle-poor	Pale; irregular dendritic cytoplasmic processes
Golgi	One or more well-developed fields, with surrounding vesicles	Poorly developed in most cells	May be small, or well-developed	Well-developed	Well-developed; often multiple fields; numerous vesicles
smooth ER	Short, branched profiles	Little	Well developed	Well developed, tubular and vesicular	Moderate amount
rough ER	Variable, may be abundant; short cisterns	Moderately to well-developed; may be dilated	Usually sparse but may be prominent	Moderate amount; flat profiles	Variable; may be well-developed
ribosomes	Free	Free	Free; some polyribosomes	Free	
mitochondria	Usually many	Few or moderate numbers	Few	Moderate numbers	Moderate numbers or many
lysosomes	Prominent; variable size and density	Rare	Rare	Few	Variable
phagolysosomes	May be numerous, large and heterogeneous; in germinal centre chiefly contain degraded lymphocytes; in paracortex may contain melanin, ceroid, haemosiderin and lipid	None, or rare	None	None usually, but may show selective phagocytosis	None or rare

[a] Epithelioid histiocytes are immunologically stimulated histiocytes, derived from phagocytic macrophages, but which show little phagocytic capability. They are secretory cells possessing large amounts of RER, multiple well-developed Golgi zones, cytoplasmic secretory vesicles and many mitochondria. They are large cells, have one or more nuclei, often eccentric, and show prominent filopodial interdigitations with other cells.[182,352] See Fig. 29.23.

[b] FRC show features of fibroblasts, myofibroblasts or myoid cells, and are closely associated with reticular fibres. They often contain bundles of 4–7 nm filaments with fusiform densities, which converge on cell surface attachment plaques surrounded by patchy external lamina. They contain smooth muscle actin and myosin.[221] Intermediate junctions may form between cell processes.

[c] Cell processes of DRC are joined by desmosomes into which insert fine cytoplasmic filaments. Hemidesmosomes are not formed. Intracytoplasmic desmosomes may occur.[261] Electron-dense granular material, probably antigen–antibody complexes, is present between cell processes in later stages of germinal centre formation. Fibrin and collagen fibrils may be seen between cytoplasmic processes. There is good evidence from frozen section, touch imprint and cell suspension studies that DRC may occur as multinucleate giant cells, analogous to thymic nurse cells;[111] further, they may contain B-cells within their cytoplasm, but this needs verification. Multinucleated cells are difficult to discern in routine histology or ultrastructure because of their intimate admixture with lymphocytes. Studies of isolated murine DRC indicate that DRC are structurally heterogeneous, possibly representing different stages of maturation.[338]

[d] LC are distinguishable morphologically from IDRC only by the presence of the Birbeck granule in LC. These granules are flat or discoid structures approximately 50-nm wide and up to 1 μm in diameter. Their appearance varies depending on the plane of section; they are most commonly seen as a membrane-bound rod with a central lamella (composed of granules 5–6 nm apart), and a vesicular expansion at one end. High-resolution microscopy of the internal structure in fact reveals four rows of granules, two lining the inner aspect of the limiting membrane while two closely-apposed rows constitute the central lamella. Viewed *en face*, each row of granules consists of a 2-D sheet of particles. The Birbeck granules are concentrated in the region of the Golgi, and may be continuous with elements of the smooth ER, or may be fused with the cell membrane.

*References: general: 92, 182, 213, 244 and 305; HRC: 92, 182, 279 and 352; FRC: 221, 265, 348 and 356; IDRC: 111, 188, 221, 261, 279 and 338; IDRC: 92, 162 and 163; LC: 30, 291, 301 and 390–392.

Table 29.4 Histochemical and immunophenotypic features of lymph nodal accessory cells*

	Histiocytic reticulum cell[a]	Fibroblastic reticulum cell	Dendritic reticulum cell[e]	Interdigitating reticulum cell	Langerhans' cell
Enzyme histochemistry					
NS esterase[b]	+ diffuse, cytoplasmic	+ / –	+	+ / – diffuse	+ / –
AcPh	+ diffuse, cytoplasmic	+ / –	–	+ / – focal	+ / –
AlkPh	–	+ strong, surface	–	–	–
5'-nucleotidase	–	–	+ surface	–	–
ATPase	–	–	–	+	+
β Gluc	+ strong	–	+ / –	–	–
Immunohistochemistry					
α_1-AT; α_1-ACT	+	– (may be + in imprints or suspensions)	–	–	–
Muramidase	+	–	–	–	–
Cathepsin B	+	–	–		
Lectin receptors[c]	+	+ / –	–	+	+
HLA–A,B,C	+ strong		+ strong	+ strong	+
HLA–DR	+ strong		+ / –	+ strong	+
CD45(LCA)	+	–	+	+	+
C3bR	– (sinus histiocytes +)	–	+	+ / –	+
S-100[d]	+ (α subunit only)	–	+ (α and β subunits)	+ (predominantly β subunit)	+ (β subunit only)
CD1a (T6; NA1/34)	–		–	–	+
CD11b(OKMI)	+ (paracortical and sinus cells only)	+ (portion only)	+	–	–
CD14(LeuM3)	+	–	+	+ / –	+
KiM1	+	–	–	–	+
-2	–	–	–	+	+
-3	+	+	+	+	–
-4	–	–	+	–	–
-6 (CD68)	+	–	–	–	–
R4/23	–		+	–	–
RFD1	–		–	+	–
-2	+		–	–	–
-3	–		+	–	–
CD4 (Leu3a)	+		+	+	+

Abbreviations: NS esterase = non-specific esterase; AcPh = acid phosphatase; AlkPh = alkaline phosphatase; α_1AT = α_1-antitrypsin; α_1-ACT = α_1-antichymotrypsin; LCA–leucocyte common antigen; C3R = C3 receptor; FS = frozen section; + / – = weak staining reaction.

[a] Macrophages in different locations in the lymph node exhibit varying immunophenotypes (for example, they show site-specific heterogeneity in expression of α_1-AT, α_1-ACT and muramidase), possibly reflecting different functional states due to specific micro-environmental influences, or response to varying antigenic stimulation.[21,92,141,395] Epithelioid histiocytes show strong ATPase activity, while NS esterase and AcPh activity vary from weak to strong (but not as strong as in phagocytic macrophages).[182,352]

[b] Ultrastructural demonstration of NS esterase, using α-naphthyl acetate or 2-naphthyl thiol acetate as substrates has also been used to identify histiocytes, and may find particular use in identifying neoplastic histiocytic proliferations, which may not demonstrate diagnostic ultrastructural features.[170,258]

[c] Histiocytes show cytoplasmic staining for various lectin receptors, in contrast to membranous or cap-like staining on lymphoid cells.[137] Different patterns of reaction may be obtained in different cells with the same lectin; for example, with peanut agglutinin (PNA) there is diffuse or globular cytoplasmic staining in tingible-body macrophages and sinus histiocytes, while cell surface and paranuclear staining occurs in IDRC and Langerhans' cells, but lymphocytes do not bind PNA at all.[137,285,286,292,334]

[d] S-100 protein has been demonstrated in histiocytes, DRC, IDRC and Langerhans' cells, using polyclonal antisera to S-100.[46,47,233,276,339,341,357,395] With antisera monospecific for the α or β subunits of S-100 protein, it is apparent that there is differential tissue distribution of these subunits.[119] Thus, germinal centre macrophages and sinus histiocytes contain S-100 α but not S-100 β,[119,339,341] DRC express both α and β subunits,[46,47,119,343] IDRC express predominantly the β subunit, and Langerhans' cells apparently exclusively express the β subunit.[119] S-100 protein has also been demonstrated in small lymphocyte-like cells (probably T cells) light microscopically and immuno-ultrastructurally in lymph node paracortex, thymic medulla and in the splenic peri-arteriolar lymphoid sheath.[119,342,357] Their numbers increase in the T-zone of lymph nodes showing non-specific T-zone hyperplasia.[357]

[e] Anti-DRC antibodies such as R4/23 can be used only on frozen sections, but DRC can be demonstrated in routinely processed tissue using antibodies to acid cysteine-proteinase inhibitor which is expressed by DRC.[1,289] Recent in situ immunophenotypic studies using antibodies reactive with different cell lineages, reveal immunophenotypic heterogeneity of DRC within their micro-environment, possibly reflecting differing stages of maturation and/or function.[50]

*References: (*enzyme histochemistry*) 24, 65, 68, 69, 98, 162, 170, 182, 183, 219, 221, 258 and 352.
(*immunohistochemistry*) α_1-AT, α_1-ACT: 147, 215, 252, 292, 293; muramidase: 65, 98, 147, 195; cathepsin: 68; lectins: 135, 137, 285, 286, 292, 334; HLA: 111, 276, 282, 283, 300, 371, 395; CD45: 24, 210, 282, 283, 393, 395; C3R: 24, 110, 111, 210, 276, 282, 283, 288, 333, 360, 371, 395; S-100: 24, 46, 47, 119, 144, 233, 276, 339, 341–343, 357, 395; CD1: 21, 24, 224, 276, 282, 283, 393, 395; CD11b, CD14: 21, 24, 98, 111, 141, 360, 371, 395; KiM: 256, 257, 280, 281; R4/23: 111, 232, 282, 283, 395; RFD: 276; CD4: 282, 283, 360, 395.

Table 29.5 Non-neoplastic lymphadenopathy*

Follicular pattern
Reactive follicular hyperplasia
  non-specific
  associated with rheumatoid arthritis or syphilis
  AIDS-related lymphadenopathy
Progressive transformation of germinal centres
Angiofollicular lymph node hyperplasia (Castleman's disease)

Sinus pattern
Sinus histiocytosis
Monocytoid B-cell reaction (immature sinus histiocytosis)
Sinus histiocytosis with massive lymphadenopathy
Lymphangiogram effect
Polyvinylpyrrolidone storage[340]
Infection-associated haemophagocytic syndromes

Diffuse pattern
Postvaccinial lymphadenopathy
Diphenyl hydantoin and other drug-associated lymphadenopathy[12,306,398]
Viral lymphadenitis (Herpes zoster)
Dermatopathic lymphadenopathy
Angio-immunoblastic lymphadenopathy
Necrotizing lymphadenitis
Systemic lupus erythematosus

Mixed pattern
Infectious mononucleosis
Toxoplasmosis
Granulomatous disorders
  Sarcoidosis
  Silicone lymphadenopathy[172,350]
  Cat-scratch disease
Tuberculosis

*Based on the scheme popularized by Dorfman & Warnke.[76]

have been proposed.[41,83,88,199,313,354] Regular changes, particularly as revealed in sequential biopsy specimens, point to a dynamic process, with evolution from a state of florid follicular hyperplasia through to one of eventual atrophy with follicle destruction and lymphocyte depletion. Three main patterns of reactive lymphadenopathy have been widely recognized:

a. Florid follicular hyperplasia, with variably increased interfollicular and paracortical cellularity

b. A mixed pattern, comprising follicular hyperplasia and commencing follicle involution in the same node

c. Severe follicular involution, and generalized lymphocyte depletion.

The first pattern is found typically in markedly enlarged nodes. Germinal centres are large and often irregular, and contain a high proportion of centroblasts and tingible body macrophages. Mantle zones are attenuated or even absent, and from them small lymphocytes may penetrate the germinal centres giving rise to an appearance described as 'follicle lysis'.[41,396]

Additional changes in other areas of the node include sinus-related clusters of pale 'monocytoid' cells; focal dermatopathic features; occasional polykaryocytes resembling Warthin–Finkeldey giant cells;[49] and hypervascularity with

proliferating immunoblasts. A distinct but less common presentation is one of hypervascular follicular hyperplasia with extra-follicular plasmacytosis resembling the plasma cell variant of Castleman's disease, and said to be prone to the development of lymphadenopathic Kaposi's sarcoma.[125,178]

In nodes exhibiting the mixed follicular pattern, hyperplastic follicles co-exist with others that are disorganized, fragmented, or reduced to 'burned-out' remnants. Interfollicular changes are comparable to those already described, but hypervascularity with focal fibrosis or hyalinization, and sinus histiocytosis are more common. Focal signs of lymphocyte depletion may foreshadow end-stage lymphadenopathy.[278]

The third pattern of generalized lymphocyte depletion is usually found in nodes of only moderate or reduced size, in association with clinically established AIDS, and is common in AIDS autopsy specimens. It is characterized by follicular atrophy and profoundly reduced cellularity of remaining tissue. In some cases an angio-immunoblastic lymphadenopathy-like pattern may develop. Patients whose nodes show generalized lymphocyte depletion are at greatest risk of developing opportunistic infections, lymphoma or Kaposi's sarcoma.

These various patterns of reactive lymphadenopathy, although sufficiently unusual to be highly suggestive of HIV infection, are not in themselves diagnostic.[179,245,327] Their diagnostic significance and role in staging of the disease are substantially enhanced by recourse to immunohistological and ultrastructural studies.

Immunohistology. Lymph nodes from PGL and early AIDS cases consistently reveal a modified pattern of T-lymphocyte subset distribution in both follicular and paracortical microenvironments.[13,109,151,193,207,303,355,396,400] Marked quantitative reduction or reversal of the CD_4^+/CD_8^+ lymphocyte ratio is usual, due both to an absolute rise in number of T-suppressor/cytotoxic cells and to a concomitant reduction of the T-helper population; the depletion of helper cells is often less pronounced than in corresponding blood samples. Nodes with florid follicular hyperplasia may exhibit extreme follicular and interfollicular B-lymphocyte polyclonal activation, while in those with severe follicular involution and lymphocyte depletion, the lymphopenia results from decreased numbers of both T and B lymphocytes. Another important change revealed by immunostaining is the progressive disturbance of the DRC network.[2,3,29,151,152,217,264,278,394] This ranges from focal defects within hyperplastic follicles to more extensive disruption and loss of the DRC network in involuting follicles, while little trace of DRC may remain in AIDS cases showing generalized lymphocyte depletion.

Immunostaining for HIV core and envelope proteins points to a predominant localization of viral antigen within the hyperplastic follicles,[20,22,152,218,314,346,378] with apparent localization to the DRC network, to occasional blast-like lymphoid cells, and within extracellular immune complex deposits.[22,314,346] Some have also reported viral core antigen reactivity in nodal vascular endothelial cells.[20,22] In situ hybridization studies[22,28,346] aimed at localization of HIV viral RNA have similarly identified lymph node follicles as important sites of viral replication and trapping, but the precise cell types involved (whether lymphoid or dendritic) have not been clearly ascertained.

Of interest is the recent finding of multiple clonal B-cell expansions in nodes from a significant number of patients with the lymphadenopathy syndrome, in the absence of any morphological or immunophenotypic evidence of lymphoma.[260] This has obvious implications for the development of lymphoma in AIDS patients through expansion of B-cell clones under the influence of other factors such as immunosuppression and EBV infection.[260] Similar apparently discordant immunogenotypic and immunophenotypic findings have been described in other settings of immune dysfunction, for example multicentric Castleman's disease and AILD (see below).

Ultrastructure. Systematic EM of lymphoid tissue from PGL and AIDS patients has revealed a variety of unusual and characteristic ultrastructural changes. They can be divided into those which are novel and apparently pathognomonic of HIV infection,[10,11,45,73,185,187,267,278,345,379] and others which, although common in this infection, are also seen in other conditions,[8,175,176,246,321] and are therefore of more limited diagnostic value.

In the first category, and of particular significance, is a distinctive modification of follicular ultrastructure in the lymph nodes, tonsils, and splenic white pulp showing the histological patterns of follicular hyperplasia, or hyperplasia with commencing involution. The germinal centres and residual mantle zones are permeated by a pervasive labyrinth of cell processes of hypertrophied DRC,[10,11,185,187,267,345,379] inapparent in routine histological sections,[10] and extending between and around the germinal centre lymphocytes (Figs 29.10 and 29.11). Desmosomes linking DRC processes are larger and more conspicuous than those in unaffected follicles (Fig. 29.10, inset). Free lentivirus-like retroviral particles are sequestered extracellularly in the DRC labyrinths[10,11,185,187,267,345,379] (Fig 29.11), often associated with diffuse dense material which has been equated with immune complex deposits.[278] The virus particles, ranging from sparse to abundant in different germinal centres of the same lymph node, measure 90–120 nm in diameter. Each has a well-defined envelope with indistinct or absent spikes, and an asymmetrical dense core appearing rounded, conical or rod-like depending on the plane of section[45,186] (Fig. 29.11, left inset). In some cases, developmental particles have been found budding from the dendritic cells (Fig. 29.11, right inset), indicating that productive infection of DRC may occur in addition to surface trapping of virions.[11,45] Degeneration of affected DRC[267] and their

phagocytosis by tingible body macrophages may be observed,[45] particularly in lymph nodes showing follicular involution. Virtual loss of all DRC and their labyrinths may be found in lymphocyte-depleted nodes from advanced AIDS cases.[45]

With one exception,[310] EM studies have emphasized a predominant affinity of the retroviral particles for DRC rather than lymphocytes in tissue biopsy specimens, emphasizing viral tropism for non-lymphoid antigen-presenting cells as a significant factor in the pathogenesis of progressive HIV infection.[10,45,73,278] Cell-surface receptors involved in the tropism for dendritic-type cells are uncertain, but DRC are known to express class II MHC and CD4 antigens as well as the Fc and C3b complement receptors.[143,171,288,395]

The finding of typical, cored particles in germinal centres needs to be interpreted with caution, following the identification of virus-like particles, identical to those in seropositive PGL patients, in reactive nodes of patients not at risk for AIDS, and which fail to show any immunostaining for the HIV core protein p24.[243] It appears that particles similar to those found in PGL cases may occur outside the setting of HIV infection, and correct identification will depend on demonstrating viral antigens or viral RNA by other techniques.[243]

Other findings of interest but not specific for PGL and AIDS, include tubulo-reticular inclusions (TRI), cylindrical confronting cisternae (CCC) — also referred to as test-tube and ring-shaped forms (TRF) — and also crystalline or paracrystalline deposits (probably accumulated immunoglobulin) within the RER of plasmacytoid and plasma cells.[11,122]

TRI are frequently observed in a high percentage of cases. They comprise a system of coiled and branching tubules 20–28 nm in diameter containing electron-dense material. They occupy dilated segments of RER or the perinuclear space, and they are often seen in continuity with the cisternal membrane (Fig. 29.12). TRI are found in vascular endothelium, in paracortical and intrafollicular lymphocytes (particularly in T-cells),[113,114] and also in macrophages and plasma cells. Interestingly, they are infrequent in DRC. Indistinguishable TRI are commonly found in other conditions with immunological disturbances such as auto-immune diseases (especially SLE), in various viral infections, necrotizing lymphadenitis, and are occasional findings in a variety of malignant neoplasms (see ref. 191a for review). Their morphogenesis and pathogenetic or functional significance is not known, but there is some indication that elevated interferon levels may be at least partly concerned in their development.[113,114] We have noted a substantial increase in the numbers and prominence of TRI in sequential tissue biopsy specimens from two AIDS patients receiving interferon therapy.

CCC are found less frequently in the lymphocytes of PGL and AIDS patients, but they may be very numerous in individual patients. They have also been recorded in a case of Japanese adult T-cell leukaemia, in multiple sclerosis, and in experimental non-A, non-B hepatitis (see refs 32 and 191a for review). They are distinctive cytoplasmic cylindrical structures, appearing round on cross-section, consisting of intimately adherent, confronting cisternae of the endoplasmic reticulum (Fig. 29.13). A recent study employing serial sectioning[112] demonstrated these structures to be in fact open at both ends, and that the original 'test-tube' (closed-end) designation is erroneous, due to misinterpretation of obliquely-sectioned profiles. Observations of CCC and TRI in close proximity in the same cell,[112,176,247,248,278,320] and the recent demonstration that CCC can also be induced by interferon,[32] add support to the concept of a possibly common aetiology for these two RER-related entities. Orenstein et al[248] also describe the occurrence of another 'tubular' structure in some cases — from their illustrations we feel that these may be similar to filaments (rodlets) described in cases of necrotizing lymphadenitis (see below).

Clinico-pathological correlation. Some investigators have sought to correlate the clinical and serological status of patients with the nodal histopathology, immunohistology and ultrastructure in group and sequential studies of PGL and AIDS case material.[45,54a,152,278] Nodes from clinically-well PGL patients with high titres of circulating antibodies typically have hyperplastic follicles, with hypertrophied and intact DRC labyrinths, and a low to moderate load of germinal centre virus particles. In patients with lower, or declining, antibody levels, nodes commonly show onset of follicular involution; EM reveals maximal reservoirs of sequestered virions in the DRC labyrinths, together with some budding virus profiles and focal signs of DRC degeneration and ingestion by macrophages. The more advanced AIDS cases with severe follicle involution and lymphocyte depletion have shown extensive loss of DRC networks, and few or no virions remain demonstrable in the nodal tissue. As yet there is little information available relating to possible early ultrastructural lesions or virion localization in the lymphoid tissues of HIV-seropositive asymptomatic patients prior to onset of palpable lymphade-nopathy. Although time-consuming, it is increasingly evident that careful ultrastructural study of biopsied lymphoid tissue can be expected to make a useful contribution to the diagnosis, staging and prognostic assessment of individual PGL and AIDS cases, besides assisting in the exclusion of alternative or co-existing pathology.

Progressive transformation of germinal centers (PTGC)

This refers to a process of progressive enlargement of secondary follicles by small mantle lymphocytes infiltrating into germinal centres.[182] The boundary between the mantle and germinal centre is blurred, eventually resulting in a nodule of small lymphocytes whose origin from a secondary follicle can no longer be discerned. The pathogenesis is unknown, but it has been suggested that PTGC represents a transient phase in the formation of secondary follicles which manifests only when there is exaggerated follicle formation.[364] Of more practical importance is the possible association of PTGC with Hodgkin's disease, particularly the nodular lymphocyte and histiocyte predominant type,[40,273] but some discount any relationship.[249]

The small lymphocytes in the nodules are phenotypically mantle lymphocytes, and are clearly distinguishable from residual germinal centre cells.[330,364] Relatively large numbers of T-helper cells, very few T-suppressor cells, and moderate numbers of K- and NK cells are found in these nodules.[330,364] Some immunohistochemical studies have suggested that the DRC pattern in progressively transformed follicles is abnormal.[330,364] However, a recent comprehensive study of DRC in reactive lymph nodes revealed both abnormal and normal DRC networks in PTGC, in addition to disruption of the DRC pattern in ordinary follicles, suggesting that PTGC is part of a spectrum of continuous change within lymphoid follicles.[118] Comparative ultrastructural studies are needed to ascertain whether there are any consistent structural abnormalities of DRC in PTGC. Ultrastructural studies have thus far merely confirmed the presence of small lymphocytes within the abnormal follicles,[273] along with varying numbers of germinal centre lymphocytes and DRC.

Angio-follicular lymph node hyperplasia (Castleman's disease — CD)

Localized and multicentric forms of CD are recognized.

Localized CD. This form was initially described by Castleman et al[54] in 1956, and subsequently the hyaline-vascular (HV) and plasma-cell (PC) types were delineated;[166] a less well-defined 'intermediate' or 'mixed' form[90] was also described.

In the more common HV type (90%), patients typically have a mediastinal, intra-abdominal or peripheral (nodal or extranodal) mass without systemic symptoms or laboratory abnormalities. Histologically, the essential features are abnormal lymphoid follicles separated by hypervascular inter-follicular tissue. Small, vascular and hyaline germinal centres are surrounded by a prominent mantle of concentrically layered lymphocytes. Typically, one or more radially penetrating hyalinized or hypercellular vessels enter the germinal centres. The latter are characteristically composed chiefly of pale eosinophilic cells, often concentrically arranged, and contain few or no germinal centre lymphocytes. The interfollicular tissue is rich in hyalinized arborizing vessels and contains mainly small lymphocytes, with only a few plasma cells or immunoblasts.

Enzyme histochemical[48,155] and immunohistochemical[48,126,155,194,231,362,382] studies of the HV form of CD show that the cells constituting the abnormal germinal centres are mainly endothelial cells and DRC. This finding has been confirmed ultrastructurally (see below). The follicular mantle cells have the same phenotype as mantle cells of normal follicles.[155,194,362] B-cells are rare in the germinal centres, and reported proportions of T-cell subsets both in the follicular and interfollicular areas vary widely in the literature.[48,126,155,194,362] Clusters of plasmacytoid T-cells may also occur in the interfollicular areas.[127,376]

Most patients with the less common PC type of CD have a variety of systemic manifestations and laboratory abnormalities (reviewed by Frizzera[105]), and have masses located in the abdomen, mediastinum or peripheral nodes. Histologically, there are hyperplastic follicles of usual morphology without vascularization or hyalinization, and solid sheets of plasma cells are present in the interfollicular areas which usually do not show the prominent vascularity seen in the HV type. The diagnosis of CD, PC type, can be made only in the appropriate clinical setting, and after exclusion of other conditions which may also be associated with lymph node follicular hyperplasia and plasmacytosis.[105]

Multicentric CD. The multicentric form of CD (MCCD)[23,102,104,108,168,208,223,302,344,381] is typified by generalized adenopathy, hepatosplenomegaly, systemic symptoms, and various laboratory abnormalities which may include anaemia, high ESR, polyclonal hypergammaglobulinaemia, and bone marrow plasmacytosis. In contrast to localized CD, it occurs in older individuals, often has an aggressive clinical course, and patients are at risk of opportunisitic infections, Kaposi's sarcoma,[59,74,102,104,168,302,344,381] atypical lymphoproliferative disorders and malignant lymphoma[74,102,104,168,381] — all suggesting underlying disordered immune regulation. Morphologically, most cases show the PC-type histology, fewer show HV changes, and some have intermediate features.[381] Multiple biopsies may show variability in morphological patterns[102] possibly representing different phases of the same process.[105] Frizzera[105] believes the essential features of MCCD include plasmacytosis and abundant germinal centres of HV type. It is important to note that the morphological changes of MCCD are not specific, and have been described in other settings of immune disturbance, including AIDS.[103–105,178,190] The proliferating plasma cells are polyclonal in most instances.[72,74,168,205,208,216,223,344,382]

While the plasma cells in most cases of CD, PC type, are polyclonal, in some instances of localized CD or MCCD, the plasma cells are diffusely monoclonal and there may be a monoclonal peak in the serum.[35,58,126,131,231,399] In other cases, focal monoclonal mass lesions may be present.[64,177,231,311] The biological significance of this monoclonality is unclear, as many of the cases had benign clinical behaviour after limited follow-up, but it seems likely that CD with monoclonal plasma cells could be a precursor of plasmacytoma. This association is further strengthened by the occurrence of CD, PC type, changes in lymph nodes of patients with the POEMS syndrome (polyneuropathy; or-

ganomegaly; endocrinopathy; M protein; skin changes) in whom osteosclerotic myeloma is usually observed.[19,31] More recently, clonal B- and/or T-cell gene rearrangements have been described in a small number of patients with MCCD but not in patients with localized CD.[123] None of these had immunophenotypic evidence of monoclonality, and malignancy has not developed after limited follow-up. The biological significance of these clonal rearrangements remains to be determined. Frizzera[105] presents a plausible scheme which includes CD, PC type, as part of a wide spectrum of plasma cell disorders which range from reactive, through 'dysplastic', to frankly neoplastic states (myeloma).

Ultrastructural studies of solitary CD[96,124] and MCCD[72,216,223] are few, and vary in detail provided. The abnormal HV germinal centres contain large numbers of DRC and endothelial cells. The former are concentrically arranged and display labyrinthine cell processes coated with extracellular electron-dense material (Fig. 29.14).[124,223] DRC processes show desmosomal attachments and may contain many cytoplasmic microfilaments and dilated RER.[124] The vessels entering the follicles are lined by fenestrated, swollen endothelial cells surrounded by thickened, focally incomplete basement membrane; close contact between endothelial cells and DRC processes may occur (Fig. 29.15).[124] Germinal centre lymphocytes and macrophages vary in number. In the mantle, lymphocytes are arranged in rows between a concentric meshwork of fibroblasts and myofibroblasts.[72,124] Broad bands of collagen may be present around the cells in the germinal centres.

The interfollicular regions contain plasma cells, which may be bi- and tri-nucleate and have large Golgi fields, occasional immunoblasts, and small lymphocytes. Blood vessels are often of the HEV type, with voluminous organelle-rich cytoplasm and multilayering of basement membrane. Perivascular sclerosis with fibroblast and myofibroblast proliferation, haphazardly arranged coarse collagen which may be long-spacing, and granulofilamentous ground substance also occur.[72]

Sinus patterns of reaction

Sinus histiocytosis (SH)

Sinus histiocytes in SH show typical ultrastructural features[213,244] (Table 29.3 and Fig. 29.16) with varying degrees of phagocytic activity, and variable immunophenotypic profile.[363] In conditions such as dermatopathic lymphadenopathy they may contain large amounts of melanin within phagosomes, in addition to lipid.

'Monocytoid' B-cell proliferation — 'immature sinus histiocytosis'

Immature sinus histiocytes were first described by Lennert in Piringer's lymphadenitis. Their typical occurrence in toxoplasmosis has been described frequently,[75,200,316,331] but they occur in other reactive settings including infectious mononucleosis and in AIDS-associated lympha-denopathy.[41,146,203,324] Initially thought of as immature sinus histiocytes or monocytoid cells, enzyme histochemical, immunohistochemical and ultrastructural studies have revealed their lymphoid rather than histiocytic nature. The more recent designations of 'monocytoid' B-lymphocytes[316] or 'parafollicular-B-lymphocytes'[63] are therefore more appropriate.

Histologically they appear as clusters or sheets of medium-sized pale cells within trabecular or cortical sinuses, around HEV in the paracortex, or immediately juxtaposed to lymphoid follicles. They are often mingled with neutrophils, scattered small and larger lymphoid cells, histiocytes and plasma cells. They are quite distinct from epithelioid cell clusters which are also frequently seen in toxoplasmic lymphadenitis.

Immunohistochemical studies show that these cells are polyclonal B-lymphocytes with variable polyclonal expression of surface immunoglobulin heavy and light chains.[51,266,316,331,366] They are thought to be B-cells at an as yet undefined stage of differentiation and occuring only in certain conditions of lymphoid stimulation.[331] Because the cells often express surface IgG, it has been suggested that they may be post-antigen-stimulated B-cells, but their relationship to germinal centre development is not known.[51] On the basis of their similar morphology and phenotype to splenic marginal zone lymphocytes, it has been suggested that they represent proliferation of analogous marginal zone lymphocytes in lymph nodes[366] (a marginal zone analogous to that in the spleen has recently been suggested in reactive lymph nodes[328,368]). Differences in pan-B antigen and immunoglobulin expression reported by different workers may reflect different stages of differentiation of these B-cells into more mature mantle-zone, or antibody-forming cells.[366] Lymphomas of monocytoid B-cells have recently been described.[63,317]

The ultrastructural features of 'monocytoid' B-cells have been reported by several workers,[63,213,266,366] confirming the cells' intimate relationship to sinuses and walls of HEV.[266] They measure 10–16 μm in diameter. The nucleus is irregular and often indented, and it contains a moderately thick rim of heterochromatin. One or two inconspicuous nucleoli are present but occasionally one prominent nucleolus is seen. They have abundant cytoplasm with variable blunt cytoplasmic extensions. Organelles are generally few, and may be clustered near the nuclear indentation. Ribosomes may be numerous, while RER varies from little to moderate, with occasional long profiles. The Golgi apparatus is often well developed. There are some smooth vesicles, occasional dense granules, round or oval mitochondria, there may be focal glycogen deposits, and a lipid droplet is occasionally present (Fig. 29.17).

Sinus histiocytosis with massive lymphadenopathy (SHML)

This rare condition of unknown aetiology was defined as a clinico-pathological entity by Rosai & Dorfman.[294,295] The typical presentation is of bilateral, painless and often massive cervical lymphadenopathy occurring in the first or second decade of life, associated with fever, neutrophilic leucocytosis, elevated ESR and polyclonal hypergammaglobulinaemia. Other lymph node groups may be involved, and extra-nodal involvement occurs in about 30% of patients,[93] most commonly involving orbit and adnexa, upper respiratory tract, skin, bone and salivary glands.[307] Extranodal lesions may occur in the absence of adenopathy, eponymously referred to as 'Rosai–Dorfman disease'.[397] Although regarded as a benign disorder, it may cause severe morbidity, and, uncommonly death, as the result of involvement of vital organs,[94] or from infection and associated immunological abnormalities which are being increasingly recognized in this condition.[94,95]

Histologically, there is marked sinus distention by accumulation of large histiocytes containing numerous lymphocytes (emperipolesis), variable numbers of plasma cells, neutrophils, and less commonly erythrocytes, within the cytoplasm. The cell nuclei are large and vesicular with prominent nucleoli. Xanthoma cells may also be present. Mitoses are uncommon and there is no significant cytological atypia. The medullary cords often contain many plasma cells. Immunohistochemical studies reveal the cells to be S100$^+$, while variable results for the expression of other histiocytic markers have been reported.[9,34,57,148,201,239]

Apart from two series,[239,308] ultrastructural studies have been performed on single cases.[9,57,61,164,181,322] The most detailed reports[181,308] describe two types of large histiocytic cells in the sinuses, but with many cells showing overlapping features: (a) an epithelioid-like histiocyte possessing many mitochondria, moderate numbers of lysosomes, few residual bodies, and displaying interdigitating filopodic cell extensions which partially or completely envelop lymphocytes and plasma cells, and (b) very large histiocytes with smooth contours, prominent SER and Golgi complexes, fewer mitochondria, lipid vacuoles, and heterogenous residual bodies; there is prominent emperipolesis of lymphocytes chiefly, some plasma cells, and rarely neutrophil polymorphs and erythrocytes. The internalized cells are usually well preserved within their plasmalemma-bound vacuole, but various stages of degeneration may occur, finally resulting in electron-dense residual bodies. The lymphocytes may be large and activated, and plasma cells may also show signs of activation and protein synthesis, with accumulation of intracisternal secretory product. No microorganisms have ever been found. It has been suggested in one study that the S-100 positivity and elaborate filopodial processes indicate that the cells are phagocytic IDRC, but this remains to be confirmed.[9]

Diffuse patterns of reaction

T-zone reactions lead to a nodular or diffuse expansion of the paracortical area. For example, in dermatopathic lymphadenopathy very large tertiary nodules are formed, while in viral infections, following vaccinations, or in hypersensitivity to anticonvulsants, a more diffuse hyperplasia results. It has been suggested on the basis of immunohistochemical analysis of the cellular composition of reactive T-nodules that they undergo a series of maturational stages as part of the cellular immune response.[365]

Post-vaccinial, viral, and anticonvulsant-associated lymphadenopathy

A diffuse (and/or follicular) hyperplasia may result in these instances, characterized by proliferation of many immunoblasts, some with atypical morphology, which may mimic Hodgkin's or non-Hodgkin's lymphoma (Fig. 29.18).[128,306,398] Apart from anticonvulsants, some antibiotics, including cephalosporins, may produce identical changes.[12] Proliferation of IDRC and other histiocytic cells also occurs (Fig. 29.19).[163]

In most instances of paracortical hyperplasia of presumed viral aetiology, no infective agents are demonstrated. Occasionally viral particles may be seen in herpetic lymphadenitis. Necrotizing lymphadenitis with Warthin–Finkeldey giant cells has been described in an immunodeficient child with measles lymphadenopathy;[332] granular and coiled fibrillar membrane-bound intracytoplasmic inclusions were found, mainly in endothelial cells, and thought to be the ribonucleoprotein component of the measles virus.

Dermatopathic lymphadenopathy (DL)

In DL there is striking nodular paracortical expansion with accumulation of IDRC, LC, and macrophages which may contain melanin, haemosiderin, and lipid. In contrast to the diffuse postvaccinial or postviral reactions, mitoses and immunoblasts are few. This reaction typically accompanies chronic dermatoses and cutaneous T-cell lymphomas (CTCL); in the latter situation it may be difficult in routine sections to distinguish between DL and early nodal involvement by CTCL. Cerebriform lymphocytes occur in dermatopathic nodes from patients with or without mycosis fungoides (MF), without any difference in the quantity or distribution of these cells.[38] Despite the lack of obvious histological differences in DL nodes from MF as compared with non-MF patients,[38] at the ultrastructural level, it has been suggested that finding clusters of cerebriform lymphocytes is helpful in identifying involvement by MF.[117,296] Quantitative ultrastructural studies, similar to those which have proven useful in the early diagnosis of cutaneous MF,[389] should also prove useful. Some have suggested that, in DL occurring in MF patients, diffusely distributed sheets of S-100$^+$ cells occur, while in cases not associated with MF

the cells show a scattered distribution as seen in normal or reactive nodes.[130] Immunophenotypic analysis of T-cell subsets have provided conflicting results regarding their utility in identifying early nodal involvement by MF in DL,[39,384,388] while genotypic studies aimed at detecting clonal rearrangements of T-cell receptor genes are more sensitive in this regard.[383]

Immunohistochemical studies of the cellular composition in DL[323,360,365,384,385] show that the tertiary nodules are rich in S-100$^+$ IDRC, CD1a$^+$ LC, and T-helper cells with variable numbers of CD1a$^+$ dendritic cells in the sinuses. Weiss et al[385] found two subsets of nodal dendritic cells which were phenotypically and histochemically identical apart from their CD1a expression; in all likelihood the CD1a$^-$ dendritic cells are IDRC, while CD1a$^+$ cells are LC. It remains to be determined whether IDRC transform into LC locally,[360] whether there is an influx of LC from the skin, or whether both events occur. Interestingly, in dermatopathic nodes from patients with MF, but not in those from non-MF patients, C-type virus-like particles have been seen in Langerhans' cells and IDRC, and reverse transcriptase activity has been demonstrated.[323,370]

Ultrastructural studies[153,162,270,284,323,360] show that, in the tertiary nodules, IDRC predominate (see Table 29.3) and are present in much greater numbers than in normal nodes. Organelle-rich and organelle-poor variants are seen.[284,360] The former have well-developed Golgi complexes, many smooth vesicles and variable lysosomal granules (Fig. 29.9); rarely, heterophagic vacuoles containing melanin may be present. The RER may occasionally form Nebenkerne. Deep, slit-like cytoplasmic invaginations coated by electron-dense material form, and at points of cell-to-cell contact, condensation of cytoplasmic microfilaments results. IDRC are often surrounded by a 'rosette' of lymphocytes which may show deep and irregular invaginations and Golgi-related, localized aggregates of small lysosomes, typical of T-lymphocytes. Immunoblasts are rare. Ultrastructural differences of IDRC have been described in lymph nodes of patients with different cutaneous immunological disorders and may reflect functional differences in varying immunological settings.[173]

Langerhans' cells (Table 29.3) may also be numerous in DL, and are distinguishable from IDRC only by the presence of Birbeck granules which number from two to five per cell (Fig. 29.20).[284] Within the sinuses there are small and medium-sized lymphocytes, macrophages with pleomorphic phagosomes, many of which contain compound melanosomes, lipid or other heterogeneous contents. LC, some of which may be seen traversing the sinus walls, and other interdeterminate or veiled cells may also be found.

Necrotizing lymphadenitis (Kikuchi–Fujimoto disease)

This entity, which appears in the literature under various titles (the most recently suggested eponym being 'Kikuchi–

Fujimoto disease'[77]), was first described in Japan independently by Kikuchi and Fujimoto in 1972 (for review see refs 78 and 169), subsequently by other Japanese workers, and more recently outside Japan.[5,55,86,254,263,290,335,353,358] It is a subacute self-limiting disease most often involving lateral cervical nodes of young women; rarely there is generalized adenopathy and hepatosplenomegaly. The aetiology remains unknown, but it is generally considered to be a hyperimmune reaction possibly to viral, bacterial or other antigens. It has also been suggested that some cases may be related to SLE or an SLE-like auto-immune condition.[78,145] Histologically, there is focal or partial effacement of the node by paracortical collections of large cells comprising histiocytes and activated lymphocytes, admixed with lymphocytic karyorrhectic debris, and without significant numbers of neutrophils or plasma cells. Single-cell or more confluent necrosis occurs. The immunoblastic reaction may be florid and misinterpreted as lymphoma.

Immunohistochemical studies reveal the affected areas to be infiltrated by variable numbers of small lymphocytes, T-immunoblasts, macrophages and plasmacytoid T-cells, with only rare NK cells or B-cells, and occasional S-100$^+$ cells (presumed IDRC).[55,85a,86,169,290,353,358] The proportions of T-cell subsets vary, but cytotoxic T-cells usually predominate. The T-immunoblasts often express markers of activation and proliferation.[169,290]

Ultrastructural studies[5,82,145,169,377] have shown a mixture of histiocytes, large lymphoid cells including immunoblasts, occasional plasma cells and extremely rare neutrophils. Lymphocytic nuclear debris abounds and is recognizable within macrophages, which contain prominent heterophagic vacuoles and myelinoid figures. Vascular endothelial cells are swollen, and abundant fibrin and collagen fibrils may be discerned between cells (Fig. 29.21). Immunoblasts may show a range of morphological features. Some having irregular nuclei, clear cytoplasm with poorly developed RER, and focal clusters of lysosomal granules and mitochondria, may represent T-immunoblasts, consistent with the phenotypic findings. Others showing well-developed lamellae of RER, often localized to one part of the cytoplasm,[145] possibly correspond to plasmacytoid T-cells.[82,86]

Two characteristic but not diagnostic structures have been found by most workers. These are tubulo-reticular inclusions (TRI)[5,82,145,169] and intracytoplasmic rodlets.[82,169] The TRI are seen mainly in immunoblasts and endothelial cells, but may also occur in macrophages, small lymphocytes and plasma cells. They are identical to those seen in AIDS (see above) and in various hyperimmune lymphadenitides, such as SLE and related auto-immune diseases;[161] in the latter they are harder to find, and there are fewer inclusions per cell.[82] The intracytoplasmic rodlets are quasi-parallel, non-periodic aggregates of 12–20-nm diameter fibrils seen in immunoblasts and to a lesser extent in histiocytes in the affected areas (Fig. 29.21). Their nature is unknown. They

have not been seen in other reactive lymphadenitides studied so far,[82] and may be a useful marker of necrotizing lymphadenitis. Only very rarely have they been reported in cases of leukaemia[213] or lymphoma[82] (this has also been our experience). They are also remarkably similar to the 'tubular' structures (distinct from TRI) found in a small number of lymph nodal and thymic mononuclear cells from five AIDS patients, reported by Orenstein et al.[248] Further study is needed to ascertain whether these structures are indeed identical to those described in necrotizing lymphadenitis, and, if so, whether a common factor such as elevated interferon levels may be related to the development of both TRI and these unusual filaments.

Angio-immunoblastic lymphadenopathy with dysproteinaemia (AILD)

This is a systemic lymphoproliferative disease of uncertain aetiology usually affecting the elderly. It is characterized by marked constitutional symptoms, generalized lymphadenopathy, hepatosplenomegaly, skin rash, polyclonal hypergammaglobulinanaemia, and Coomb's-positive haemolytic anaemia, among other abnormal laboratory findings.[100,191] The immunological abnormalities present in these patients are similar to those evident in patients with AIDS.[269] Many cases have followed administration of a variety of drugs. Although there are some minor histological differences in the initial descriptions of angio-immunoblastic lymphadenopathy,[101] and immunoblastic lymphadenopathy (IBL),[191] the essential histological features are effacement of lymph node architecture, but often with marginal sinus preservation; proliferation of arborizing small blood vessels; infiltration of small mature lymphocytes, plasma cells, immunoblasts, and varying numbers of eosinophils, but often with an overall cell-depleted appearance; and the deposition of PAS-positive interstitial and perivascular amorphous material. There may be rare, atrophic 'burned-out' hypocellular follicles.[101]

Immunohistochemical studies have established the polyclonality of the plasma cells and other B-lymphocytes.[236,237,312] The immunoblasts may be of either B-cell or T-cell lineage.[154] In a high proportion of patients there is evolution into malignant lymphoma.[236] Certain histological features have been identified which suggest the presence of lymphoma,[236] but in difficult cases immunophenotypic or immunogenotypic analysis may be necessary to establish the diagnosis of lymphoma,[386] or at least to demonstrate underlying T-monoclonality which seems to be present in a high proportion of cases,[234,241] suggesting that many cases of AILD are neoplastic at the outset. When lymphoma supervenes, in most instances it appears to be of T-cell lineage,[236,318,380,386] and is often referred to as IBL-like T-cell lymphoma.[318,380] Recent data indicate that the pattern of clonal gene rearrangements in AILD may correlate with immunophenotype and clinical features.[87]

Table 29.6 Ultrastructural features of angio-immunoblastic lymphadenopathy*

Cytological features	Vascular changes	Interstitial changes
Polymorphous infiltrate which includes the following cells in varying proportions:	Proliferation of high endothelial venules	Granular, amorphous material (basement membrane-like) in which microfilaments (5–10 nm) may be seen
Small lymphocytes: round or polymorphic nuclei; condensed chromatin; focal clusters of lysosomal granules	Endothelial cells: hypertrophied and organelle-rich; TRI within endoplasmic reticulum may be found	Cell debris and cytoplasmic fragments from lymphoid cells and plasma cells
Immunoblasts: plasmablastic differentiation variable; TRI within endoplasmic reticulum; giant mitochondria in one case;[197] cytoplasmic blebbing or budding	Basal lamina and perivascular zone; three types of change may occur: (1) replacement of normal basal lamina by thick amorphous electron-dense layer (200–400 nm); (2) basal lamina splintered and multilayered, and of varying thickness (possibly a result of sequential synthesis by activated endothelium); (3) normally-structured basal lamina, surrounded by variably thick layer of amorphous granular material containing collagen fibres, often long-spacing; focally, re-duplicated thin strands of basal lamina may form beneath endothelial cells	Long-spacing (100–120 nm periodicity) collagen which may form thick tracts
Plasma cells and plasmacytoid lymphocytes: intracisternal accumulation of secretory product may occur, forming Russell bodies; intracisternal accumulation of TRI in one case ('macaroni cells')[14]		Normal collagen fibres and fibrils
		Amyloid fibrils (in one case) admixed with collagen and cytoplasmic fragments[192]
Clear cells: lymphocytes with abundant pale cytoplasm; small numbers of mono- and polyribosomes occurring in small clusters		Immunoglobulin deposition[312]
Phagocytic histiocytes: fragments of lymphocytes and plasma cells may be recognizable in phagosomes		*Comment.* Several of the above features have been thought to account for the PAS-positive interstitial material. In all likelihood, any or a combination of features are responsible. Some have found that the degree of PAS-positivity correlated with the type of interstitial change: pale staining in mainly collagenous cases, and stronger staining where abundant cell debris is present.[174] Long-spacing collagen is a useful finding, but we and others[209] have also observed it, albeit less frequently and in smaller amounts, in non-specific diffuse paracortical hyperplasia, dilantin-associated adenopathy, necrotizing lymphadenitis, dermatopathic lymphadenopathy, and angiofollicular lymph node hyperplasia
Epithelioid histiocytes; *eosinophils*; *interdigitating and fibroblastic reticulum cells*; *large granular lymphocytes*, possibly K–NK cells with many lysosomes, some having lamellar profiles (? parallel tubular arrays), described in one case[174]	Deposition of immunoglobulins has been shown in the perivascular zone	

Abbreviations: TRI = tubuloreticular inclusions; K–NK = killer–natural killer cells.
*References: 14, 27, 62, 174, 192, 197, 198, 226, 237, 251, 312, 359 and 380.

The ultrastructural changes in AILD are summarized in Table 29.6 (Fig. 29.22). Similar features have been found in other cases of hyperimmune reactions including hydantoin lymphadenopathy,[174] and also in the interfollicular areas and around blood vessels in Castleman's disease.[72] Hence, the changes are not diagnostic of AILD, but in the presence of cytoplasmic debris, abundant banded collagen and with small clusters of clear cells,[174] AILD may be reasonably diagnosed in the appropriate clinical setting. Features suggesting the possible evolution of lymphoma in AILD include zonal proliferation of medium-sized lymphoid cells with clear cytoplasm, or the occurrence of a polymorphic population of large, medium and small lymphocytes showing marked nuclear irregularities.[380]

Mixed patterns of reaction

Granulomatous disorders

Many granulomatous disorders, both infective and non-infective, may cause lymphadenopathy. The ultrastructure of the granulomas, apart from the presence or absence of necrosis, infectious agents or foreign material, is similar. Sarcoidosis may be used as an example to illustrate these conditions.

Sarcoid granulomata typically consist of collections of macrophages, epithelioid cells and multinucleate giant cells surrounded by lymphocytes and fibroblasts. Immunohistochemical studies of the cellular composition of the granulomata have yielded somewhat varying results.[361,372,375] The in vivo expression of the interleukin-2 receptor by the epithelioid and multinucleate cells and the localization of IL-2 and gamma interferon to the same cells has recently been demonstrated, and may prove to be of pathogenetic significance.[121]

There have been many ultrastructural studies of sarcoid granulomata.[52,53,107,149,158,159,211,220] Epithelioid cells arise from precursor phagocytic macrophages[255] but differ from activated macrophages by their absence of phagocytic activity, elaborate plasmalemmae, their enlarged Golgi apparatus, and extensive RER with many transport vesicles (Fig. 29.23). For further discussion of epithelioid cells the reader is referred to Chapter 13.

Asteroid and Schaumann inclusion bodies often occur in the granulomata, but may also be seen in other granulomatous conditions, albeit less frequently, including chronic berylliosis and tuberculosis,[157,158,160,309] and in silicone lymphadenopathy.[172] Schaumann bodies have a central crystalline nidus of calcium carbonate surrounded by a calcium-containing conchoidal body; the latter consists of concentrically laminated shells containing a mixture of carbohydrates, lipids, protein, RNA and minerals, thought to originate from aggregation of residual bodies formed by auto- or hetero-phagosomes.[156,157] They develop both in epithelioid cells and in giant cells, and after attaining a certain size may be extruded from the parent cell. The mechanism of their formation has been studied ultrastructurally in experimental tuberculous granulomata in hamsters.[80]

Asteroid bodies occur only in multinucleated giant cells. Varying theories as to their nature have been proposed.[15,42-44] Cain & Kraus[42-44] present compelling evidence that asteroids are derived from the cytosphere and that they are composed predominantly of densely packed vimentin filaments and of microtubules in smaller quantities; in the body of the asteroid occur many centrioles and procentrioles, and granular osmiophilic material. Others however, have not been able to demonstrate participation of the centriolar and microtubular systems in their formation.[172a] The tips of the asteroid arms are often related to elements of the Golgi apparatus, and to residual bodies (Fig. 29.24).

Progressive hyalinization occurs at the periphery of the granuloma. Capillaries here may show prominent reduplication of basal lamina, merging with a felt-like layer of fine filaments and collagen fibrils. Active fibroblasts are seen. The collagen fibrils may come into intimate contact with the epithelioid cells. Immuno-electron-microscopic studies reveal that the interstitial matrix of sarcoid granulomas contains collagen types I and III, and fibronectin, through all stages of the granulomas' evolution.[262]

The ultrastructural features of epithelioid cell granulomata in nodes draining cancer sites, in chronic berylliosis and in tuberculous lymphadenitis are similar.[158-160,337]

THE THYMUS GLAND

NORMAL STRUCTURE

Embryology

The two thymic lobes arise on either side of the neck during the sixth week of gestation. Human thymic epithelium is derived from both endoderm (the 3rd, and possibly 4th pharyngeal pouches), and ectoderm (the cervical vesicle from the 3rd branchial cleft), the latter completely enveloping the endodermal primordium.[511] It is postulated that the ectodermal cells give rise to cortical epithelial cells, while the medullary cells arise from pharyngeal pouch endoderm.[424,511] The ectodermal contribution to the thymus may account for the rare occurrence of sebaceous

glands within the thymus.[566] Bone marrow-derived lymphoid precursors populate the thymus at about the 9th gestational week. From the investing mesenchyme, septa carrying blood vessels divide each gland into pseudolobules. The paired anlage migrate into their definitive positions in the superior and anterior mediastinum, where the two lobes come together and appear as one gland invested by connective tissue. A comprehensive review of the ontogeny and cellular organization of the thymus is provided by von Gaudecker.[558]

Structure

By light microscopy the parenchyma is lobulated, with an outer dark-staining cortex containing densely packed lymphocytes, and a central, paler medulla possessing relatively fewer lymphocytes and containing distinctive Hassal's corpuscles. Connective tissue septa extend inward from the cortex, branch, and widen into broad perivascular spaces at the cortico-medullary junction. The subcapsular epithelial cells with their basal lamina form a continuous barrier between the true thymic parenchyma, and the capsule and perivascular space. Beginning early in life, the gland progressively involutes (see below) such that in older individuals it appears as a mass of adipose tissue containing scattered islands of thymic parenchyma.

A brief description of the various cell types occurring in the thymus gland follows.

Epithelial cells

These not only provide the structural framework of the thymus, but through their intimate contact with lymphoid cells and elaboration of various hormones they provide unique micro-environments needed for T-lymphocyte maturation. They exhibit considerable ultrastructural,[413,440,482,487,537,550,556,558] phenotypic[410,430,474,476,504,520,522,559] and functional (hormone production)[426,430,438,451] heterogeneity. Their essential ultrastructural features are their dendritic nature, intercellular desmosomes, tonofilament bundles in the cytoplasm, and basal lamina formation at parenchymal–mesenchymal interfaces (Figs 29.25 and 29.26). Dendritic cytoplasmic processes ramify throughout the cortex in particular, forming a three-dimensional mesh whose interstices are packed with lymphocytes in various stages of differentiation.

The fine-structural details of epithelial cells can vary considerably depending on their location in the thymus. Traditionally regarded as 'pale' (mainly cortical) or 'dark' (mainly medullary) cells,[413,537,555] more recent study has revealed even greater structural heterogeneity and compartmentalization of the various epithelial cell types. One may broadly distinguish between the flattened subcapsular epithelium, stellate cortical cells, medullary epithelial cells, and

Hassall's corpuscles, while some workers[487,550,559] identify as many as six epithelial cell subtypes on the basis of their morphology and location. The salient ultrastructural and immunophenotypic features of the thymic epithelium are presented in Tables 29.7 and 29.8 respectively.

Thymic nurse cells (TNC) are cortical epithelial cells, first described in thymic suspensions obtained from rats and mice, and are postulated to play a role in acquisition of T-lymphocyte MHC restriction and self-tolerance.[492,519,549,562,563] They contain up to 200 actively dividing thymocytes which are thought to enter the epithelial cell by emperipolesis. The caveolae containing the lymphocytes do not communicate with the extracellular space,[563] and intimate specialized contact sites between the epithelial cell membrane and lymphocyte plasmalemma occur.[562,563] The TNC express cortical epithelial antigens,[469,552] class I and II MHC antigens,[552,562,563] keratin filaments,[547] and seem capable of synthesizing thymic hormones.[492] It is debated whether TNC exist *in vivo* in the same form as in vitro. It has been suggested that, *in vivo*, TNC cytoplasmic processes incompletely envelope outer thymic lymphoblasts, whereas the appearance in vitro of the large lympho-epithelial complexes, with thymocytes fully contained within cytoplasmic vacuoles, results from the isolation procedures used.[491] We have rarely observed such lympho-epithelial complexes *in situ* (Fig. 29.27). From murine studies it appears that the TNC thymocytes are phenotypically heterogeneous, most being cortisone-sensitive and having an immature cortical phenotype, while a minority are cortisone-resistant, have a mature phenotype, and could be the reservoir from which the thymus is repopulated after exposure to cortisone.[431]

Some thymic epithelial cells are well equipped for protein synthesis by virtue of well-developed Golgi apparatus, abundant RER, secretory vesicles and granules and occasional intracytoplasmic lumens (Figs 29.28 and 29.29). In the medulla, distinctive Hassall's corpuscles are formed by concentrically arranged epithelial cells rich in tonofilaments, which may keratinize centrally or form a central lumen into which project microvilli coated with glycocalyx (Fig. 29.29). Immuno-electron microscopic studies have localized thymulin and thymosin alpha-1 within the cytoplasm of thymic epithelial cells.[401,402,527] Double-labelling immunohistological studies suggest that thymulin, thymopoietin and thymosin alpha-1 are present within the same epithelial cells, both in normal and pathological thymuses.[524] More recently, evidence that neurohypophyseal peptides may be produced by the thymus has been presented.[437]

Using monoclonal antibodies which detect various surface (and some cytoplasmic) antigens, the thymic micro-environment can be divided into four major regions showing particular phenotypic profiles. These are (i) mesenchymal capsule and septa (in early thymic ontogeny this mesodermal tissue induces epithelial maturation[495]), (ii) the subcapsular cortex, (iii) the inner cortex, and (iv) the medulla. These compartments provide the necessary 'milieu' for the various stages of T-cell ontogeny, acquisition of MHC restriction and elaboration of the various thymic hormone fractions (for reviews see refs 453 and 476).

Lymphocytes

Population of the fetal thymus by lymphoid precursors begins at about the 9th gestational week when large basophilic blast cells appear in the cortex.[556,557] These can still be seen in the adult thymus, principally in the outer subcapsular region. On the basis of fine structure, immunophenotype and in vitro functional properties, it is evident that lymphocytes are compartmentalized according to their different stages of maturation, with immature thymocytes occupying the cortex and more mature thymocytes occupying the medulla. The thymocytes can be divided into outer cortical large and medium-sized lymphocytes (Fig. 29.30), inner cortical small lymphocytes, and medullary medium-sized lymphocytes (see Table 29.9). Degenerating lymphocytes with pyknotic nuclei, often in large numbers, may be found mainly in the cortex but occur also in the medulla. They may be seen within macrophages and occasionally in Hassall's corpuscles. Most of the cortical lymphocytes arise intrathymically from subcapsular blast cells, are immuno-incompetent, short-lived, and die intrathymically, while a minority migrate into the medulla or to peripheral lymphoid organs. In contrast, medullary thymocytes are immunocompetent and express mature T-cell phenotypes.[453] While traditionally considered to be the domain of T-lymphocytes exclusively, recent evidence indicates that the normal thymus may in fact contain a distinct population of B-lymphocytes.[470,472]

The fine-structural features of thymic lymphocytes are presented in Table 29.9 (see Fig. 29.4 for a summary of T-cell differentiation).

Endocrine cells

Epithelial cells possessing dense-core secretory granules, 150–300 nm in diameter, have been described in the human thymic medulla.[413,537] These cells have well-developed abundant RER and Golgi apparatus, and are likely candidates for production of thymic hormones (Fig. 29.31). Similar secretory cells may be found among the cells constituting Hassall's corpuscles.[408,553] It is important not to mistake other intrathymic granulated cells as endocrine-like cells.[408]

Interdigitating reticulum cells

These cells, another component of the thymic micro-environment needed for differentiation of T-cells, are found mainly in the medulla and occasionally in the inner

Table 29.7 Ultrastructural characteristics of thymic epithelium*

	Subcapsular perivascular cells	Cortical epithelial cells (pale cells)	Medullary epithelial cells			Hassall's corpuscles (HC)
			Dark cells	'Undifferentiated' cells[550]	'Large-medullary' cells	
General features	Flat cells with long cell processes; small desmosomes; hemidesmosomes at basal laminal surface	Predominate in outer cortex, but also scattered in medulla; have electron-lucent cytoplasm; dendritic cytoplasmic processes ramify between lymphocytes	Mainly in medulla and around HC; some in deep cortex; electron-dense stellate cells; slender, dendritic processes between lymphocytes	Occur in clusters at cortico-medullary junction, or scattered in medulla; polyhedral, with blunt processes	Large, electron-lucent cells	Formed by concentric arrays of large medullary cells; may be *solid* (keratinize as in skin) or *cystic*.
Basal lamina	Continuous (50–60 nm wide) at mesenchymal and vascular interface	None	None	None	None	*Solid HC.* From the centre, and moving out, structure is as follows: central, dense amorphous, keratinized mass; concentric, flattened, anucleate epithelial lamellae, with homogenization of cytoplasm, packed with dense tonofilaments and keratohyaline; slit-like spaces between some lamellae into which project short microvilli; outer large, pale cells rich in tonofilaments. *Cystic HC.* Central cyst into which project microvilli. Cyst may contain macrophage, polymorph, or lymphocyte cell debris. Some of the cells at the periphery of both solid and cystic HC seem well equipped for secretory function; they are rich in RER, have a well developed Golgi, and contain secretory-granules, possibly thymic hormone-containing. (Figs 29.28, 29.29 and 29.31.)
Nucleus	Triangular or irregular; heterochromatinic; prominent nucleolus	Round or oval; occasionally multinucleate; euchromatinic; prominent nucleolus	Irregular; heterochromatinic; inconspicuous nucleolus	Round or oval, notched; marginated chromatin; prominent nucleolus	Large, round or ovoid; euchromatinic; prominent nucleolus	

Table 29.7 (continued)

Cytoplasm					
Filaments	Two types: intermediate and thin;[433] intermediate: 8–11 nm, as tonofilament bundles around nucleus and in processes; thin: 4–6 nm (actin), subplasmalemmal	Small tonofilament bundles	Many tonofilament bundles	Tonofilaments in small dispersed bundles	Prominent tonofilaments
Golgi	Well developed; smooth and coated vesicles prominent	Well developed; coated vesicles may be prominent	Poorly developed	Moderately developed	Well developed; many smooth vesicles
Granules	Some electron-dense granules	Small, 100–300 nm electron-dense granules, and larger lysosome-like granules	Vacuoles and residual bodies	Rare	Electron-dense secretion granules prominent
Ribosomes	Mainly single; few polyribosomes	Relatively sparse	Numerous, mainly single	Many polyribosomes	Prominent, including polyribosomes
RER	Long cisternae	Short profiles	Dilated	Few strands	Abundant; may be dilated with granular secretory material
Other features or comments	Pinocytotic vesicles along basal laminal aspect; nuclear bodies are commonly found in all epithelial cells and in non-epithelial cells as well	20 nm cytoplasmic tubules that may connect with cell membrane[550]	Mitochondria often swollen; dilated paranuclear cistern	Resemble fetal thymic epithelium[556]	20 nm tortuous cytoplasmic tubules as in pale cortical cells;[550] intracytoplasmic lumens containing microvilli, cilia, and mucin may occur (often at periphery of HC)

Comment
Up to six types of thymic epithelial cells are described[550,559] including 'pale' (mainly cortical) and 'dark' (mainly medullary) cells, and cells 'intermediate' in morphology. The relative proportion of these seems to vary with age; their varied structure may relate to the cells' functional states, the pale cells showing features of 'active' cells, while the dark cells may be degenerate.[550]
Thymic nurse cells: see text.
*References: 408, 413, 433, 457, 460, 462, 463, 467, 477, 486, 537, 550, 553–556, 558 and 559.

Table 29.8 Thymic epithelium — immunophenotype and hormone production*

	Cortex[a]		Medulla	
	Subcapsular epithelium	Cortical epithelium	Medullary epithelium	Hassall's corpuscles
Immunophenotype[b]				
HLA-DR	Variable: weak (+) or (−) except for strongly positive TE4$^+$ endocrine cells	(+) dendritic pattern	Variable; (+) confluent pattern described by some, but double-labelling studies suggest epithelium is (−), while IDRC are (+)[476]	(+)
HLA-A,B,C	(−) except for strongly positive TE4$^+$ endocrine cells			
Cytokeratin	(+)	(+)	(+)	(+)
Other MoAb[531] reactivities	Thy-1$^+$, p19$^+$ A2B5$^+$, RFD4$^+$ TE4$^+$, TE3$^-$ MR10$^+$, MR14$^+$, MR3$^-$, MR6$^-$ IP1$^+$, Ep-1$^+$ 21A62E$^-$, KiM3$^+$	Thy-1$^-$ (TNC are +), p19$^-$, A2B5$^-$, RFD4$^-$ TE4$^-$, TE3$^+$ MR10$^-$, MR14$^-$, MR3$^+$ MR6$^+$ IP1$^+$, IP2$^+$ (near medulla), Ep-1$^-$ 21 A62E$^+$, KiM3$^+$	Thy-1$^-$, p19$^+$ A2B5$^+$, RFD4$^+$ TE4$^+$, TE3$^-$ MR10$^+$, MR14$^+$ (a subpopulation only) IP1$^+$, Ep-1$^+$ 21A62E$^-$, KiM3$^+$	Thy-1$^-$, p19$^-$ TE4$^-$, TE8$^+$, TE16$^+$, TE15$^+$, TE19^{+c} MR14$^+$ IP3$^+$, IP4$^+$ KiM3$^+$
Hormone synthesis				
Thymosin	$\alpha 1^+$, $\alpha 7^-$, $\beta 3^+$, $\beta 4^+$	$\alpha 1^-$, $\alpha 7^-$, $\beta 4^-$	$\alpha 1^+$, $\alpha 7^-$, $\beta 4^-$	
Thymopoietin	(+)	(−)	(+)	
Thymulin (FTS)	(+)	(+)	(+)	
α-Metencephalin	(+)		(+)	

[a] See text for *thymic nurse cells*.

[b] Using antibodies of varying specificity for thymic epithelial antigens, several phenotypic subsets of thymic epithelium have been defined which most likely relate to different stages of T-cell differentiation. For example, antibodies A2B5, RFD4, TE4 and anti-p19 identify a peptide-secreting endocrine subset of thymic epithelium (subcapsular cortex and medulla), and reactivities correlate well with known localizations of various thymic hormones. It is not yet clear how the various antibody profiles relate to all of the structural subtypes of epithelial cells (Table 29.7) which have been identified. Analysis of a large panel of monoclonal antibodies reactive with thymic epithelium, at the Third International Workshop and Conference on Human Leucocyte Differentiation Antigens, has allowed a preliminary grouping of antibodies according to their distinctive reactivity.[531]

[c] The outermost layer of HC is TE4$^+$; the outer cells are TE8$^+$ and TE16$^+$ (these antibodies are markers of terminal stages of epidermal keratinization);[500] the entire HC is TE19$^+$.

* References: (*immunophenotype*)[531] HLA-DR: 410, 417, 454, 474, 476, 504, 519, 522, 559, 560; HLA-A,B,C: 474, 504, 522, 559, 560; keratin: 417, 430, 453, 476, 504, 530, 559; Thy-1: 476, 519; p19: 449; A2B5: 450, 452, 454, 504; RFD4: 417, 476; TE series: 452–454, 500, 504; MR and IP series: 430, 520; Ep-1, 21A62E, KiM3: 559.

(*thymic hormones*) Reviews: 403, 427, 438, 453, 512, 528, 529, 567; Specific: 401, 402, 426, 438, 450, 452, 468, 473, 524, 530, 559.

cortex.[481] Their precursors can be found as early as the twelfth gestational week, when they enter the thymus by diapedesis from the mesenchymal septa and perivascular spaces.[556] They have recently been studied and characterized in culture.[406,515] Ultrastructural and immunophenotypic details are provided in Table 29.9 (see also section on Lymph Node, above, Tables 29.3 and 29.4, and Fig. 29.9).

Myoid cells

These occur in thymus glands of all ages,[433,435,456–458,461,548,555] and appear as early as the eighth gestational week.[556] They react with anti-actin and anti-striated muscle myosin, but not with anti-smooth muscle myosin (cf. epithelial cells which react with anti-smooth muscle myosin but not with anti-striated muscle myosin).[433] They are unevenly distributed in the medulla, sometimes in clusters, and have also been described in the connective tissue of interlobular septa.[433] Their general structure resembles that

of degenerating skeletal muscle fibres. Rounded and spindle-shaped forms occur, often in excess of 40 μm in diameter. Cytoplasmic thick and thin filaments are present in varying numbers, often in a disorganized manner, but there may be sarcomere-like arrangements together with Z-band structures and triads (Fig. 29.32). Some workers have described cellular attachments between epithelial and myoid cells,[461,480] and transitional or hybrid cells (thought to arise by fusion) combining elements of both epithelial and myoid cells.[461,463] We and others have been unable to confirm this latter finding.[408,433,480]

Basal lamina surrounds these cells only at sites where they abut on connective tissue. There is no evidence that myoid cells are innervated.

Other cells

Macrophages containing phagocytozed nuclear debris are most numerous in the cortex and at the cortico-medullary

Table 29.9 Ultrastructural characteristics of thymic lymphocytes and interdigitating reticulum cells (IDRC)*

Lymphocytes	Size	Mitoses	Nuclei			Cytoplasm	
			Size and shape	Chromatin	Nucleoli	Amount	Organelles
Outer cortical[a]							
Large lymphocyte (blast)	12–15 μm	Frequent	7–9 μm; round or indented	Euchromatinic with thin rim peripheral heterochromatin	1–2, prominent, often on membrane	Moderate	Generally scant; many polyribosomes; scattered mitochondria; occasional single RER profiles; few small, dense granules
Medium lymphocyte	8–11 μm	Frequent	5–7 μm; round or indented	Small clumps throughout nucleoplasm and along nuclear membrane	1–2, may be prominent	Moderate	Similar to large cells; fewer polyribosomes, more monoribosomes
Inner cortical							
Small lymphocyte	5–8 μm	Infrequent	Round, ovoid or indented; occasional nuclear pockets	Heavily clumped along nuclear membrane and through nucleoplasm	Not prominent	Scant	Sparse; many free ribosomes; Golgi poorly developed; few mitochondria; aggregates of small dense granules near paired centrioles
Medullary							
Medium lymphocyte	5–8 μm	Infrequent	Irregular; multiple deep indentations	Clumped along nuclear membrane and through nucleoplasm	Not prominent	Moderate; interdigitations between adjacent lymphocytes and interdigitating reticulum cells	More abundant than small cortical lymphocytes; polyribosomes and free ribosomes; well-developed Golgi; prominent smooth vesicles; clustered small dense granules and mitochondria near Golgi and paired centrioles; single strands of RER; bundles of 7 nm thin filaments mainly in cell processes
Interdigitating reticulum cells[b]	Variable; often very large	Infrequent	Irregular and tortuous	Dispersed, with thin, marginated rim along nuclear membrane	One or more, central or peripheral	Voluminous; pale; complex interdigitating processes ramify between lymphocytes and epithelial cells	Well developed Golgi with associated vesicles and dense granules; occasional residual bodies and lysosomes; mitochondria dispersed; RER and SER variable, RER present as single strands or small groups of flat cisternae

[a] The large lymphoblasts and medium lymphocytes are found mainly in the outermost subcapsular and outer cortex respectively, but isolated cells can be seen elsewhere in the inner cortex and uncommonly in the medulla.

[b] IDRC strongly express HLA-DR;[276,474,543] are S-100+,[233,466] CD1a(T6)−,[233,466] 476 RFD-1+,[276,476] contain high levels of ATPase,[276,279] and show weak (Golgi-related), or no lysosomal enzyme activity.[276,476] This characteristic phenotype allows distinction from other dendritic cells, Langerhans' cells and macrophages. However, evidence has been presented that in culture IDRC do express CD1(T6).[406] See also Tables 29.3 and 29.4.

* References: 233, 276, 279, 406, 413, 463, 466, 473, 474, 476, 477, 543 and 555.

junction. Their numbers increase markedly in stress involution.[425] Multinucleated histiocytic cells may occur rarely (Fig. 29.33).[555] Mature eosinophils and eosinophil myelocytes,[408] mast cells and plasma cells[413,555] can be found in small numbers, principally in the medulla. Cells containing Birbeck granules, consistent with Langerhans' cells,[471] and plasmacytoid T-cells have also been described.[481] Very rare Leu 7+ (CD57) cells[319] in the medulla and, exceptionally, cortex of normal thymuses, and in the reactive follicles in thymuses of myasthenics[268,275] have also been described.

Blood vessels and perivascular space (PVS)

Blood vessels, nerves and efferent lymphatics are carried within the penetrating connective tissue septa. High-endothelial venules (analogous to the postcapillary venules of lymph nodes) are thought not to occur in the normal thymus.[538] Rather, wide venules with relatively thin endothelium are found, across which lymphocyte diapedesis may occur.[440,538] Surrounding the vessels there is a perivascular space (PVS) whose width is proportional to the size of the vessel it surrounds,[407] being widest around arteries in the septa and around venules at the cortico-medullary junction, but narrow around capillaries.[407] Various cells may be found in the PVS, chiefly lymphocytes, in addition to plasma cells, mast cells, eosinophils, neutrophils, polymorphs, macrophages and fibroblasts, along with collagen fibres.[408,413,486,555] Around the small capillaries, usually only collagen fibres, sometimes long-spacing, are seen.[407] In the normal thymus, lymphoid follicles with germinal centres may occur in the PVS with a wide range in reported incidence.[462] The PVS, bound by non-fenestrated endothelium[407,482] and endothelial basal lamina on one aspect, and thymic epithelium and epithelial basal lamina on the other, constitutes a 'blood–thymic' barrier separating the intrathymic parenchyma from the vascular compartment (Fig. 29.25).[482] This barrier may be incomplete in the inner cortex and medulla, where interruptions in the continuity of the epithelial basal lamina may occur (Fig. 29.26).[555]

NON-NEOPLASTIC ALTERATIONS OF THE THYMUS

Non-neoplastic changes in the thymus can be categorized as follows (based on Henry[462]):

1. Age-related (physiological) involution
2. Acute ('stress') involution
3. True thymic hyperplasia
4. Thymitis (follicular lymphoid hyperplasia) as seen in myasthaenia gravis and other auto-immune diseases (see Table 29.10)
5. Thymic dysplasia in congenital immunodeficiency syndromes
6. Graft-versus-host disease; AIDS.

Table 29.10 Conditions associated with thymic lymphoid follicular hyperplasia[405]

Myasthaenia gravis[441,446,498,542]
Systemic lupus erythematosus[439,440,446,501–503]
Rheumatoid arthritis[421,503]
Primary thyrotoxicosis[446,506,551]
Rheumatic heart disease[459]
Scleroderma[411]
Auto-immune haemolytic anaemia[446]
Behcet's syndrome[446]
Normal thymus

Comment.
Lymphoid follicles with germinal centres may occur in thymuses of normal individuals, with a wide range of reported incidence.[462,498] However, the number and size of germinal centres in myasthaenia gravis is greater than in the other conditions listed.[446,462]

Age-related (physiological) involution

Contrary to the classic belief that the human thymus grows to its maximum size until puberty, and then progressively involutes, recent studies suggest that the final size (volume and weight) of the thymus is reached during the first year of life, and that the overall size in healthy humans does not alter significantly with age.[541] There is marked variation in wet thymic weight at all ages, with a gradual decrease in wet weight with age and a small decrease in lean dry weight.[485,541] Physiological involution of cortex and medulla probably starts during the first year of life, is a continuous process, is not influenced by puberty-dependent endocrine changes, and is characterized by progressive accumulation of adipose tissue in an expanding perivascular space.[541] The decrease in thymic parenchymal volume is paralleled by changes in circulating hormone activity.[499] There are also decreased numbers of medullary thymosin alpha-1-positive cells.[468]

Results of frozen section immunohistological studies do not show any qualitative alterations of T-cell differentiation in the ageing thymus and suggest that the thymus is capable of generating T-cell clones and maintaining T-cell differentiation through life.[539,540] However, HLA-DR staining patterns of the cortex, as well as ultrastructural studies, reveal epithelial foci devoid of lymphocytes, and lymphocytic foci devoid of epithelial cells, together with ultrastructural evidence of lymphocytic apoptosis; this suggests a degenerative process with alteration of the cortical microenvironment.[541] As this phenomenon is also seen in the childhood thymus, it is in accord with the concept that involution begins very early in life.[541]

Apart from some minor alterations, the fine structural organization of the cortex and medulla in the adult parenchyma is similar to that in children.[507,555] Cortex and medulla may be physically separated in places; the medulla may be incompletely surrounded by cortex and, focally, may directly abut extra-thymic adipose tissue.[555] The cortex is still lymphocytopoietically and mitotically active,[555] but the overall number of lymphocytes is diminished.[507] The number of degenerating cortical lymphocytes and macrophages does not seem to be raised.[555] Cortical areas composed of epithelial cell complexes devoid of lymphocytes may occur,[507] but the ultrastructural features of cortical epithelial cells are not altered.[555] In the medulla, cystic Hassall's corpuscles are more frequent than in childen.[555] Apart from medullary foci composed entirely of tightly-packed epithelial cells with numerous desmosomes, the structure of the medulla is similar to that of the child.[555] Using anticytokeratin antibodies, it has been shown that, during involution, the epithelial cell framework remains intact, but that there is collapse of the structure as a result of lymphocyte depletion.[465] Interdigitating reticulum cells are present in undiminished numbers, and myoid cells may also be found.[555] Breaks in the continuity of the epithelial basal lamina at the epithelial–parenchymal interface around small capillaries in the inner cortex and medulla have been described, allowing direct contact between lymphocytes and the perivascular space (Fig. 29.26).[555] The presence of germinal centres in the perivascular space in aged thymuses of some individuals without any auto-immune disease has led to the suggestion that the lymphoid tissue here shows an arrangement similar to that in peripheral lymphoid organs.[507]

Acute ('stress') involution

Steroid-mediated rapid decrease in size and weight of the thymus occurs in many stressful situations; this may be temporary and reversible in physiological situations such as pregnancy, lactation, and weaning, or longer-lasting during steroid administration, malnutrition, severe infections, X-irradiation and chemotherapeutic treatment.[413,432,441] Both cortex and medulla show involutionary changes, but the cortex is affected more severely with profound loss of cortical lymphocytes. There is pyknosis and karyorrhexis of thymocytes, and marked increase in cortical lipid-rich macrophages leading to a picture of 'reversed lobulation' with the cortex now appearing clear, relative to a dense medulla. Hassall's corpuscles usually persist, become cystic, and accumulate keratin and necrotic debris.[432,464]

The ultrastructural changes in humans[413,414,432] are similar to those observed in experimental animals following injection of glucocorticoids.[425] Cortical lymphocytes show degenerative and apoptotic changes. Nuclear membranes become indistinct, nuclear chromatin condenses, and there is karyorrhexis. Macrophages are numerous and contain lipid vacuoles and many pleomorphic phagolysosomes. Epithelial cells also show degenerative changes; they accumulate vacuoles with electron–dense material, often develop intracellular cysts lined by microvilli, have increased numbers of lysosomes and lipid droplets, swollen mitochondria, and the presence of tonofilaments in concentrated dense bundles. Epithelial–mesenchymal boundaries are often irregular, and there is reduplication and tortuosity of the

epithelial basal lamina. The epithelial structural heterogeneity seen normally may be lacking.[414] Lipid-rich macrophages may also accumulate in connective tissue septa, and the mesenchymal cells often show residual bodies.[432] If there is recovery, increased mitotic activity of subcapsular stem cells is noted, repopulation of cortex by lymphocytes occurs within 8–10 days, and epithelial cells show increased RER and ribosomes, active Golgi zones and increased numbers of small, dense secretory granules.[413]

True thymic hyperplasia

True thymic hyperplasia, as distinct from thymic lymphoid hyperplasia, is defined as enlargement (increased size and weight) of a gland which is architecturally normal, beyond the normal range at any particular age.[498,521] Rarely, massive hyperplasia occurs which may cause respiratory distress.[404,480,484,493,513] Milder forms of thymic hyperplasia have also been described in patients after successful chemotherapy for various malignancies.[422,444,536] It has been postulated that the thymic hyperplasia in this setting may be an immunological rebound phenomenon following the immunosuppressive effects of the tumour and chemotherapy.[444,536] There are no ultrastructural details recorded in these situations.

Follicular lymphoid hyperplasia (thymitis) — myasthenia gravis (MG)

The thymus of myasthenics is histologically normal in 10% of patients, harbours a thymoma in 25% of cases, and shows lymphoid follicular hyperplasia without significant thymic enlargement in the remaining 65%.[498] Some prefer to describe the latter change as thymitis, arguing that the process is essentially chronic inflammatory in nature.[462,488] Histologically there are often numerous enlarged 'medullary' lymphoid follicles with prominent germinal centres.[462,463,521,526] The germinal centres are often polarized with their pale antigen-presenting dendritic cap regions close to medullary epithelium and epithelial–myoid cell complexes.[462,526] It should be noted that conditions other than MG may be associated with thymic lymphoid hyperplasia (Table 29.10).

The ultrastructural and immunopathological changes in the thymus occurring in MG are summarized in Table 29.11. Immunohistological studies have helped to place the structural alterations into some functional perspective. Using monoclonal antibodies with specificities for laminin and fibronectin, for the various thymic cellular constituents and for thymic hormone fractions, it has been possible to define distinct functional micro-environments in these hyperplastic glands[417,426,476,488,526,543] (see Table 29.11). Essentially these studies show three distinct micro-environmental regions: (i) reactive B-cell domains, surrounded by (ii) T-cell zones (similar to lymph nodal paracortex), located within an

Table 29.11 Thymic ultrastructural and immunopathological changes in myasthaenia gravis*

	Structural features	Immunopathological features
Lymphoid follicles with germinal centres		Immunohistology typical of reactive follicles in lymph nodes (see Table 29.2)
Structure	Similar to structure in peripheral lymphoid organs, with lymphocytes in various stages of activation, dendritic reticulum cells, macrophages and plasma cells	
Location	Exact location disputed; some consider them extrathymic and located in an expanded perivascular space,[497,498,542] while others maintain that they are truly intramedullary.[462,526] Our study of several thymuses suggests that the follicles are located in an expanded perivascular space, but there are focal disruptions of epithelium and basal lamina so that the extrathymic and intrathymic compartments merge at these points. This is supported by immunohistochemical studies.[417,488,514,543,546] Increased numbers of lymphocytes, some activated, immunoblasts and plasma cells surround the follicles, and together with high-endothelial venules (below) resemble the paracortical zone in lymph nodes	Perifollicular lymphoid tissue has phenotypic features of lymph node paracortical T-cell zones, with heavy fibronectin network;[417] T-cells have mature, peripheral phenotype with mixture of CD4[+] CD8[−] and CD4[−] CD8[+] cells; interdigitating reticulum cells in large numbers (see below); a continuous laminin-positive boundary separates the 'lymph nodal' zones (follicles and adjacent T-cell zones), from the thymic medulla proper, but this is focally disrupted or absent where germinal centres are closest to medullary epithelium and Hassall's corpuscles;[417] some germinal centres are entirely intramedullary, completely surrounded by medullary epithelium[488]
Perivascular space (PVS) and post-capillary venules	The perivascular space is expanded; high endothelial venules, absent in normal thymus, proliferate in the PVS, and display prominent lymphocyte diapedesis	
Plasma cells and other B-lymphocytes	Increased numbers in the medulla and perivascular space, including immature forms; RER cisternae may be distended by secretory product	Polyclonal plasma cell staining ($\kappa/\lambda = 2:1$); mainly IgG[+], some IgA[+], few IgM[+];[543] diffuse B-cell infiltration of PVS and medulla;[488] focal B-cell infiltration around Hassall's corpuscles
Medulla	Focal areas of epithelial hyperplasia with increased numbers of prominent desmosomes; degeneration of some epithelial cells at the perivascular interface; isolated cells contain membrane-bound secretory granules[462] (unrelated to Hassall's corpuscles where they are normally found);[553] increased numbers of cells containing cytoplasmic lumens; increased mucin secretion in these cells and in Hassall's corpuscles[463,526]	*Epithelium.* In most cases the medulla displays strong epithelial and thymocyte HLA-DR staining comparable to normal glands, but foci of compactly-organized RFD-4[+], HLA-DR[−] epithelial cells[417,564] paralleled by markedly increased numbers of, and strongly-staining thymosin $\alpha1^+$ epithelial cells[426] occur; islands of A2B5[+] endocrine epithelial cells isolated from thymocyte contact;[453] some epithelial cells express cytoplasmic ACh receptors, but not the main immunogenic region of the α-subunit[489]
		Lymphocytes. Increased numbers of medullary thymocytes,[453] but no differences in T-cell subsets[488,490,543,546]

expanded PVS; this 'peripheral' lymphoid tissue is separated from (iii) the thymic medullary parenchyma, by a continuous laminin boundary, which, however, becomes focally disrupted or absent where the B-follicles are in closest proximity to the medullary epithelium and Hassall's corpuscles. Recent studies suggest that B-cells and germinal centres first accumulate in the PVS and then extend into the medulla by virtue of the interrupted boundary between these two compartments.[488] This unique composite microenvironment, where hormone-producing medullary epithelium and myoid cells are in intimate contact with T- and B-lymphocytes and their antigen-presenting accessory cells, and perhaps with increased lymphocytic traffic across high endothelial venules, may facilitate sensitization to autoantigens, such as acetycholine receptor-like molecules.[417,476,514]

Thymic dysplasia in immunodeficiency states

Immunodeficiency states can occur as primary or acquired syndromes. A detailed discussion of the many types of immunodeficiency diseases is beyond the scope of this presentation (refer to refs 418, 442, 443, 494, 510 and 521); furthermore, ultrastructural accounts are very few.

The ultrastructural features of simple thymic dysplasia in a patient with the Swiss form of SCID were described by Bockman et al.[414] The epithelial framework was abnormal, with closely packed epithelial cells possessing numerous dense bundles of tonofilaments. Small lymphoid cells were rare and large thymocytes or blast cells absent. The epithelial–connective tissue interface was irregular and delimited by continuous but folded and reduplicated basal lamina. There were no Hassall's corpuscles. Scattered histio-

Table 29.11 (Continued)

	Structural features	Immunopathological features
Interdigitating reticulum cells (IDRC)	Increased numbers in medulla, and also present in perifollicular lymphoid tissue in the perivascular space; Birbeck granules described in IDRC in one report,[565] though we have not observed them	Increased numbers of RFD-1[+], HLA-DR[+], Ki-M1[+], Ki-M6[-] interdigitating reticulum cells, often closely associated with CD4[+] lymphocytes;[417,488,543] they are particularly prominent around Hassall's corpuscles and at the cortico-medullary junction;[488] a variable number, especially those clustered around Hassall's corpuscles, are said to express the CD1a(T6) antigen[488] and may in fact represent Langerhans' cells
Myoid cells	No difference in structure or number reported by some;[433] others report increased numbers;[463] some myoid cells may be degenerate or necrotic and phagocytized by macrophages; these cells are most numerous in medulla closely related to Hassall's corpuscles, but they are also seen in subcapsular cortex	Immunostaining has not revealed any increase in numbers of myoid cells;[433] they are most frequent in glands showing follicular hyperplasia, and less common in atrophic glands; express ACh receptors[483,561] including extracellular main immunogenic region of the α-subunit;[489] myoglobin staining in one study shows their close relationship to dendritic cap region of germinal centres[514] and may be concentrated around Hassall's corpuscles[488]
Cortex	Compressed and atrophic; yet to be adequately studied in order to correlate structure with variables such as age and concomitant therapy	Few studies done to date *Epithelium.* Normal HLA-DR and keratin patterns according to some;[490] others report abnormal epithelial framework (revealed by HLA-DR and keratin staining), with decreased numbers of thymic nurse cells, and focal areas completely devoid of epithelial cells;[488,508,564] the latter do occur in normal glands[507] but appear to be more extensive in MG[488] *Lymphocytes.* Decreased numbers of cortical thymocytes,[453,543] but of normal phenotype;[490] there is no B-cell infiltration Multinucleate cells, apparently of the macrophage system, and of unknown significance, occur at the cortico-medullary junction[488] (see Fig. 29.33)

Comments.
1. The changes tabulated are those seen in glands showing lymphoid follicular hyperplasia. In glands not containing hyperplastic follicles, or showing thymic atrophy, immunostaining reveals diffuse B-cell infiltration of medulla and PVS;[488] other structural changes are comparable to glands showing lymphoid follicular hyperplasia.
2. Nodular aggregates of histiocytes and eosinophils ('histio-eosinophilic granulomas') have been described in MG and non-MG patients who have undergone recent pneumomediastinoscopy. The histiocytic cells have many primary and secondary lysosomes but no Birbeck granules, and are S-100[-] and CD1 (T6)[-]. These infiltrates are similar to the reactive eosinophilic pleuritis seen in patients with spontaneous pneumothorax and may have the same (presumed iatrogenic) cause and pathogenesis.[447]
* References: (*structure*) 433, 440, 460, 462, 463, 497, 498, 526, 538, 542, 553, 564 and 565.
(*immunopathology*) 417, 426, 433, 453, 476, 483, 488–490, 507, 508, 514, 526, 543, 561 and 564.

cytes containing heterogeneous lysosomes and lipid droplets were present in the parenchyma. EM scrutiny of dysplasia with a pseudoglandular pattern in four cases of thymic alymphoplasia[412] showed pseudoglandular areas lined by tonofilament-rich polygonal epithelial cells resting on basal lamina. More centrally located cells were dendritic and had many cytoplasmic vacuoles. Complex epithelial–connective tissue interdigitations with fragments of basal lamina at epithelial cell margins are illustrated.

Using a variety of antibody probes of human thymic epithelium, heterogeneous abnormalities of surface marker expression have been found in patients with SCID and Nezelof syndrome, possibly indicating abnormal thymic epithelial maturation.[453,504] The endocrine thymic epithelium phenotypically appears arrested at an early stage of fetal development.[453] Thymus glands in SCID have been shown to contain thymopoietin and thymosin alpha-1, but the intrathymic content of thymosin alpha-1 is significantly decreased.[451]

Graft-versus-host disease (GVHD); AIDS

After allogeneic bone marrow transplantation, there is profound thymic involution, and, in addition, thymic epithelial damage occurs in patients with GVHD.[409,509,523,544] Damage to thymic medullary epithelium and Hassall's corpuscles in experimental and human GVHD results in a picture very similar to that seen in SCID.[532–534] Ultrastructural studies of GVHD in experimental animals[532,533] have shown, in addition to changes of acute involution, architectural effacement, epithelial cell injury, gradual disappearance of Hassall's corpuscles and macrophage accumulation (independent of adrenal corticosteroids), very similar to thymic dysplasia in SCID. Similar dysplasia-like changes were described in a human infant suffering GVHD after transfusion.[534] A recent study of a larger number of human allogeneic bone marrow transplant recipients reveals similar morphological changes, and furthermore furnishes evidence that the thymus may be capable of reconstituting its lympho-epithelial structure in some cases.[509]

Comparable changes have also been described in the thymus glands of AIDS patients.[429,434,445,478,479,535] In addition to severe involutionary changes and thymitis[479] there is progressive epithelial cell damage, with eventual reduction or total destruction of Hassall's corpuscles, changes resembling thymic dysplasia. Immunohistological analysis has shown loss of the normal reticular epithelial pattern, evidence of epithelial cell destruction, partial loss of thymic epithelial differentiation antigens, binding of antibodies and complement to epithelial cells, and decreased numbers of thymulin-positive cells.[525] These data support the histological impression that the thymic epithelium is a target of destruction in AIDS, and could account for the decreased thymic endocrine function in these patients.[428]

REFERENCES

Lymph node

1. Alavaikko M, Rinne A, Järvinen M, Jokinen K, Hopsu-Havu V K 1985 Acid cysteine–proteinase inhibitor, a new characteristic of reticulum cells in human lymphoid secondary follicles. Acta Histochemica 77: 1–6
2. Alavaikko M, Rinne A, Järvinen M, Hopsu-Havu V K, Meyer P R, Levine A M, Lukes R J 1985 Dendritic reticulum cells in AIDS-related lymphadenopathy. Experientia 41: 1173–1175
3. Alavaikko M, Rinne A, Järvinen M, Hopsu-Havu V K, Aine R, Levine A M, Meyer P R, Lukes R J 1986 Damage to secondary lymphoid follicles in AIDS-related persistent generalized lymphadenopathy, as revealed by the behaviour of dendritic reticulum cells possessing immunoreactive acid cysteine–proteinase inhibitor. Virchows Archiv B, Cell Pathology including Molecular Biology 50: 229–311
4. Alexander E, Sanders S, Braylan R 1976 Purported difference between human T- and B-cell surface morphology is an artefact. Nature 261: 239–241
5. Ali M H, Horton L W L 1985 Necrotising lymphadenitis without granulocytic infiltration (Kikuchi's disease). Journal of Clinical Pathology 38: 1252–1257
6. Anagnostou D, Harrison C V 1972 Angiofollicular lymph node hyperplasia (Castleman). Journal of Clinical Pathology 25: 306–311
7. Anderson K C, Bates M P, Slaughenhoupt B L, Pinkus G S, Schlossman S F, Nadler L M 1984 Expression of human B cell-associated antigens on leukemias and lymphomas: a model of human B cell differentiation. Blood 63: 1424–1433
8. Anderson M G, Key P, Tovey G, Murray-Lyon I M, Lawrence A, Byrom N, Dixey J, Ellis D S, McCaul T F, Gazzard B, Evans B, Zuckerman A J 1984 Persistent lymphadenopathy in homosexual men: a clinical and ultrastructural study. Lancet i: 880–882
9. Aoyama K, Terashima K, Imai Y, Katsushima N, Okuyama Y, Niikawa K, Mukada T, Takahashi K 1984 Sinus histiocytosis with massive lymphadenopathy. A histogenic analysis of histiocytes found in the fourth Japanese case. Acta Pathologica Japonica 34: 375–388
10. Armstrong J A, Horne R 1984 Follicular dendritic cells and virus-like particles in AIDS-related lymphadenopathy. Lancet ii: 370–372
11. Armstrong J A, Dawkins R L, Horne R 1985 Retroviral infection of accessory cells and the immunological paradox in AIDS. Immunology Today 6: 121–122
12. Asano S, Wakasa H 1985 Drug-induced lymphadenopathy — two biopsied cases treated with cephem-group antibiotics for a short time. Fukushima Journal of Medical Science 31: 71–78
13. Audouin J, Le Tourneau A, Marche C, Diebold J 1986 Etude immunopathologique des adénopathies persistantes liées à l'infection LAV-HTLV III. Annales de Pathologie (Paris) 6: 271–274
14. Averback P, Salama S S, Moinuddin M 1977 Hashimoto's thyroiditis with immunoblastic lymphadenopathy and unusual 'macaroni cells'. Canadian Medical Association Journal 117: 41–43
15. Azar H A, Lunardelli C 1969 Collagen nature of asteroid bodies of giant cells in sarcoidosis. American Journal of Pathology 57: 81–92
16. Babcock G F, Phillips J H 1983 Human NK cells: light and electron microscopic characteristics. Survey of Immunologic Research 2: 88–101
17. Balfour B M, Drexhage H A, Kamperdijk E W A, Hoefsmit E C M 1981 Antigen-presenting cells, including Langerhans cells, veiled cells and interdigitating cells. In: Porter R, Whelan J (eds) Micro-environments in haemopoietic and lymphoid differentiation. Ciba Foundation Symposium 84. Pitman Medical, London, pp 281–301
18. Banerjee D, Thibert R F 1983 Natural killer-like cells found in B-cell compartments of human lymphoid tissues. Nature 304: 270–272
19. Bardwick P A, Zvaifler N J, Gill G N, Newman D, Greenway G D, Resnick D L 1980 Plasma cell dyscrasia with polyneuropathy, organomegaly, endocrinopathy, and skin changes. Report on two cases and review of the literature. Medicine 59: 311–322
20. Baroni C D, Pezzella F, Mirolo M, Ruco L P, Rossi G B 1986 Immunohistochemical demonstration of p24 HTLV III major core protein in different cell types within lymph nodes from patients with lymphadenopathy syndrome (LAS). Histopathology 10: 5–13
21. Baroni C D, Vitolo D, Remotti D, Biondi A, Pezzella F, Ruco L P, Uccini S 1987 Immunohistochemical heterogeneity of macrophage subpopulations in human lymphoid tissues. Histopathology 11: 1029–1042
22. Baroni C D, Pezzella F, Pezzella M, Macchi B, Vitolo D, Uccini S, Ruco L P 1988 Expression of HIV in lymph node cells of LAS patients. Immunohistology, in situ hybridization, and identification of target cells. American Journal of Pathology 133: 498–506
23. Bartoli E, Massarelli G, Soggia G, Tanda F 1980 Multicentric giant lymph node hyperplasia. A hyperimmune syndrome with a rapidly progressive course. American Journal of Clinical Pathology 73: 423–426
24. Beckstead J H, Wood G S, Turner R R 1984 Histiocytosis X cells and Langerhans cells: enzyme histochemical and immunologic similarities. Human Pathology 15: 826–833
25. Beiske K, Langholm R, Godal T, Marton P F 1986 T-zone lymphoma with predominance of 'plasmacytoid T-cells' associated with myelomonocytic leukaemia — a distinct clinicopathological entity. Journal of Pathology 150: 247–255
26. Beiske K, Munthe-Kaas A, Davies C dL, Marton P F, Godal T 1987 Single cell studies on the immunological marker profile of plasmacytoid T-zone cells. Laboratory Investigation 56: 381–393
27. Bernuau D, Feldmann G, Brière J, Teillet F 1978 Angioimmunoblastic lymphadenopathy: demonstration of the ultrastructural site of immunoglobulin synthesis by immunoperoxidase method. Biomedicine 28: 232–237
28. Biberfeld P, Chayt K J, Marselle L M, Biberfeld G, Gallo R C, Harper M E 1986 HTLV-III expression in infected lymph nodes and relevance to pathogenesis of lymphadenopathy. American Journal of Pathology 125: 436–442
29. Biberfeld P, Öst A, Porwit A, Sandstedt B, Pallesen G, Böttiger B, Morfelt-Mänsson L, Biberfeld G 1987 Histopathology and immunohistology of HTLV-III/LAV related lymphadenopathy and AIDS. Acta Pathologica Microbiologica et Immunologica Scandinavica, Section A, Pathology 95: 47–65

30. Birbeck M S, Breathnach A S, Everall J D 1961 An electron microscope study of basal melanocytes and high-level clear cells (Langerhans cells) in vitiligo. Journal of Investigative Dermatology 37: 51–64

31. Bitter MA, Komaiko W, Franklin WA 1985 Giant lymph node hyperplasia with osteoblastic bone lesions and the POEMS (Takatsuki's) syndrome. Cancer 56: 188–194

32. Bockus D, Remington F, Luu JY, Bean M, Hammar S 1988 Induction of cylindrical confronting cisternae (AIDS inclusions) in Daudi lymphoblastoid cells by recombinant alpha-interferon. Human Pathology 19: 8–82

33. Boekstegers A, Grundmann E 1985 What's new in natural killer cells? Pathology, Research and Practice 180: 536–552

34. Bonetti F, Chilosi M, Menestrina F, Scarpa A, Pelicci P-G, Amorosi E, Fiore-Donati L, Knowles II D M 1987 Immunohistological analysis of Rosai-Dorfman histiocytosis. A disease of S-100 + CD1⁻ histiocytes. Virchows Archiv A, Pathological Anatomy and Histopathology 411: 129–135

35. Boniver J, Massart B, Tjean M, Van Lancker M A 1984 Monoclonal plasma cell populations in a case of Castleman's disease, plasma cell type. Pathology, Research and Practice 178: 155A (abs)

36. Boyd A W, Anderson K C, Freedman A S, Fisher D C, Slaughenhoupt B, Schlossman S F, Nadler L M 1985 Studies of in vitro activation and differentiation of human B lymphocytes. I. Phenotypic and functional characterization of the B cell population responding to anti-Ig antibody. Journal of Immunology 134: 1516–1523

37. Brynes R K, Chan W C, Spira T J, Ewing E P Jr, Chandler F W 1983 Value of lymph node biopsy in unexplained lymphadenopathy in homosexual men. Journal of the American Medical Association 250: 1313–1317

38. Burke J S, Colby T B 1981 Dermatopathic lymphadenopathy. Comparison of cases associated and unassociated with mycosis fungoides. American Journal of Surgical Pathology 5: 343–352

39. Burke J S, Sheibani K, Rappaport H 1986 Dermatopathic lymphadenopathy. An immunophenotypic comparison of cases associated and unassociated with mycosis fungoides. American Journal of Pathology 123: 256–263

40. Burns B F, Colby T V, Dorfman R F 1984 Differential diagnostic features of nodular L & H Hodgkin's disease, including progressive transformation of germinal centres. American Journal of Surgical Pathology 8: 253–261

41. Burns B F, Wood G S, Dorfman R F 1985 The varied histopathology of lymphadenopathy in the homosexual male. American Journal of Surgical Pathology 9: 287–297

42. Cain H, Kraus B 1977 Asteroid bodies: derivatives of the cytosphere. An electron microscopic contribution to the pathology of the cytocentre. Virchows Archiv B, Cell Pathology 26: 119–132

43. Cain H, Kraus B 1980 The ultrastructure and morphogenesis of asteroid bodies in sarcoidosis and other granulomatous disorders. In: Williams W J, Davies B H (eds) Eighth international conference on sarcoidosis and other granulomatous diseases. Alpha Omega Publishing, Cardiff, pp 30–37

44. Cain H, Kraus B 1983 Immunofluorescence microscopic demonstration of vimentin filaments in asteroid bodies of sarcoidosis. A comparison with electron microscopic findings. Virchows Archiv B, Cell Pathology including Molecular Biology 42: 23–226

45. Cameron P U, Dawkins R L, Armstrong J A, Bonifacio E 1987 Western blot profiles, lymph node ultrastructure and viral expression in HIV-infected patients: a correlative study. Clinical and Experimental Immunology 68: 465–478

46. Carbone A, Poletti A, Manconi R, Volpe R, Santi L 1985 Demonstration of S-100 protein distribution in human lymphoid tissues by the avidin–biotin complex immunostaining method. Human Pathology 16: 1157–1164

47. Carbone A, Manconi R, Poletti A, Volpe R, Santi L 1985 S-100 protein immunostaining in cells of dendritic morphology within reactive germinal centres by ABC immunoperoxidase method. Virchows Archiv A, Pathological Anatomy and Histopathology 406: 27–32

48. Carbone A, Manconi R, Volpe R, Poletti A, de Paoli P, Tirelli U, Santini G 1986 Immunohistochemical, enzyme histochemical, and immunologic features of giant lymph node hyperplasia of the hyaline-vascular type. Cancer 58: 908–916

49. Carbone A, Manconi R, Volpe R, Poletti A, Vaccher E, Tirelli U 1986 Multinucleated cells in the lymph nodes of HTLV-III seropositive intravenous drug abusers with generalized lymphadenopathy. Archives of Pathology and Laboratory Medicine 110: 871–872

50. Carbone A, Manconi R, Poletti A, Volpe R 1988 Heterogeneous immunostaining patterns of follicular dendritic reticulum cells in human lymphoid tissue with selected antibodies reactive with different cell lineages. Human Pathology 19: 51–56

51. Cardoso de Almeida P, Harris N L, Bhan A K 1984 Characterization of immature sinus histiocytes (monocytoid cells) in reactive lymph nodes by use of monoclonal antibodies. Human Pathology 15: 330–335

52. Carr I, Norris P 1977 The fine structure of human macrophage granules in sarcoidosis. Journal of Pathology 122: 29–33

53. Carr I 1980 Sarcoid macrophage giant cells. Ultrastructure and lysosyme content. Virchows Archiv B, Cell Pathology including Molecular Biology 32: 147–155

54. Castleman B, Iverson L, Menendez V P 1956 Localized mediastinal lymph-node hyperplasia resembling thymoma. Cancer 9: 822–830

54a. Chadburn A, Metroka C, Mouradian J 1989 Progressive lymph node histology and its prognostic value in patients with acquired immunodeficiency syndrome and AIDS-related complex. Human Pathology 20: 579–587

55. Chan J K C, Saw D 1986 Histiocytic necrotizing lymphadenitis (Kikuchi's disease). A clinicopathologic study of nine cases. Pathology 18: 22–28

56. Chan J K C, Ng C S 1987 Immunohistochemical studies on histiocytic necrotizing lymphadenitis. Pathology 19: 104

57. Chan K W, Chow Y Y N, Ghadially F N, Stansfeld A G, Woo C H 1985 Rosai–Dorfman disease presenting as spinal tumour. A case report with ultrastructural and immunohistochemical studies. Journal of Bone and Joint Surgery 67A: 1427–1431

58. Chan W C, Hargreaves H, Keller J 1984 Giant lymph node hyperplasia with unusual clinicopathologic features. Cancer 53: 2135–2139

59. Chen K T K 1984 Multicentric Castleman's disease and Kaposi's sarcoma. American Journal of Surgical Pathology 8: 287–293

60. Chu A, Eisinger M, Lee J S, Takezaki S, Kung P C, Edelson R L 1982 Immunoelectron microscopic identification of Langerhans cells using a new antigenic marker. Journal of Investigative Dermatology 78: 177–180

61. Codling B W, Soni K C, Barry D R, Martin-Walker W 1972 Histiocytosis presenting as swelling of orbit and eyelid. British Journal of Ophthalmology 56: 517–530

62. Cooperberg A A, Brisson de Champlain M, Siminovitch J, Rosenberg A, Schwartz J P 1977 Immunoblastic lymphadenopathy: case report and a literature review. Canadian Medical Association Journal 117: 53–57

63. Cousar J B, McGinn D L, Glick A D, List A F, Collins R D 1987 Report of an unusual lymphoma arising from parafollicular B-lymphocytes (PBLs) or so-called 'monocytoid' lymphocytes. American Journal of Clinical Pathology 87: 121–128

64. Cousineau S, Beauchamp G, Boileau J 1986 Extramedullary plasmacytoma associated with angiofollicular lymph node hyperplasia. Archives of Pathology and Laboratory Medicine 110: 157–158

65. Crocker J 1981 The enzyme histochemistry of lymphoid and non-lymphoid cells of the human palatine tonsil: a basis for the study of lymphomas. Journal of Pathology 134: 81–95

66. Crocker J, Jones E L, Curran R C 1983 Study of nuclear size in the centres of malignant and benign lymphoid follicles. Journal of Clinical Pathology 36: 1332–1334

67. Crocker J, Jones E L, Curran R C 1983 A comparative study of nuclear form factor, area and diameter in non-Hodgkin's lymphomas and reactive lymph nodes. Journal of Clinical Pathology 36: 298–302

68. Crocker J, Burnett D, Jones E L 1984 Immunohistochemical demonstration of cathepsin B in the macrophages of benign and malignant lymphoid tissues. Journal of Pathology 142: 87–94

69. Crocker J 1987 Reticulum cells and related structures in lymph nodes: their properties and roles in antigen processing. In: Thompson R A (ed) Recent advances in immunology, vol. 4. Churchill Livingstone, Edinburgh, pp 19–43

70. Dantchev D 1978 Scanning electron microscopy morphology of mononuclear leucocytes in normal subjects and in patients with lymphoid and monocytoid neoplasias. In: Mathé G, Seligmann M, Tubiana M (eds) Recent results in cancer research, vol. 64. Lymphoid neoplasias. I. Classification, categorization, natural history. Springer-Verlag, Berlin, pp 94–107

71. Dardick I, Sinnott N M, Hall R, Bajenko-Carr T A, Setterfield G 1983 Nuclear morphology and morphometry of B-lymphocyte transformation. Implications for follicular centre cell lymphomas. American Journal of Pathology 111: 35–49

72. Diebold J, Tulliez M, Bernadou A, Audouin J, Tricot G, Reynes M, Bilski-Pasquier G 1980 Angiofollicular and plasmacytic polyadenopathy: a pseudotumourous syndrome with dysimmunity. Journal of Clinical Pathology 33: 1068–1076

73. Diebold J, Marche C, Audouin J, Aubert J P, Le Tourneau A, Bouton C, Reynes M, Wizniak J, Capron F, Tricottet V 1985 Lymph node modification in patients with the acquired immunodeficiency syndrome (AIDS) or with AIDS-related complex (ARC). A histological, immuno-histopathological and ultrastructural study of 45 cases. Pathology, Research and Practice 180: 590–611

74. Dixon D, Ben-Ezra J M, Reed J, Flax H, Janis R 1985 Multicentric giant lymph node hyperplasia, Kaposi's sarcoma, and lymphoma. Archives of Pathology and Laboratory Medicine 109: 1013–1018

75. Dorfman R F, Remington J S 1973 Value of lymph-node biopsy in the diagnosis of acute acquired toxoplasmosis. New England Journal of Medicine 289: 878–881

76. Dorfman R F, Warnke R 1974 Lymphadenopathy simulating the malignant lymphomas. Human Pathology 5: 519–550

77. Dorfman R F 1987 Histiocytic necrotizing lymphadenitis of Kikuchi and Fujimoto. Archives of Pathology and Laboratory Medicine 111: 1026–1029

78. Dorfman R F, Berry G J 1988 Kikuchi's histiocytic necrotizing lymphadenitis: an analysis of 108 cases with emphasis on differential diagnosis. Seminars in Diagnostic Pathology 5: 329–345

79. Duijvestijn A, Horst E, Pals S T, Rouse B N, Steere A C, Picker L J, Meijer C J L M, Butcher E C 1988 High endothelial differentiation in human lymphoid and inflammatory tissues defined by monoclonal antibody HECA-452. American Journal of Pathology 130: 147–155

80. Dumont A, Sheldon H 1965 Changes in the fine structure of macrophages in experimentally produced tuberculous granulomas in hamsters. Laboratory Investigation 14: 2034–2055

81. Dvoretsky P, Wood G S, Levy R, Warnke R A 1982 T-lymphocyte subsets in follicular lymphomas compared with those in non-neoplastic lymph nodes and tonsils. Human Pathology 13: 618–625

82. Eimoto T, Kikuchi M, Mitsui T 1983 Histiocytic necrotizing lymphadenitis. An ultrastructural study in comparison with other types of lymphadenitis. Acta Pathologica Japonica 33: 863–879

83. Ewing E P, Chandler F W, Spira T J, Brynes R K, Chan W C 1985 Primary lymph node pathology in AIDS and AIDS-related lymphadenopathy. Archives of Pathology and Laboratory Medicine 109: 977–981

84. Facchetti F, de Wolf-Peeters C, van den Oord J J, Desmet V J 1987 Immunohistochemical visualization of plasmacytoid T cells in paraffin sections. Human Pathology 18: 1300

84a. Facchetti F, de Wolf-Peeters C, van den Oord J J, de Vos R, Desmet V J 1988 Plasmacytoid T cells: a cell population normally present in the reactive lymph node. An immunohistochemical and electronmicroscopic study. Human Pathology 19: 1085–1092

85. Facchetti F, de Wolf-Peeters C, Mason D Y, Pulford K, van den Oord J J, Desmet V 1988 Plasmacytoid T cells. Immunohistochemical evidence of their monocyte/macrophage origin. American Journal of Pathology 133: 15–21

85a. Facchetti F, de Wolf-Peeters C, van den Oord J J, de Vos R, Desmet V J 1989 Plasmacytoid monocytes (so-called plasmacytoid T-cells) in Kikuchi's lymphadenitis. An immunohistologic study. American Journal of Clinical Pathology 92: 42–50

86. Feller A C, Lennert K, Stein H, Bruhn H-D, Wuthe H-H 1983 Immunohistology and aetiology of histiocytic necrotizing lymphadenitis. Report of 3 instructive cases. Histopathology 7: 825–839

87. Feller A C, Griesser H, Schilling C V, Wacker H H, Dallenbach F, Bartels H, Kuse R, Mak T W, Lennert K 1988 Clonal gene rearrangement patterns correlate with immunophenotype and

clinical parameters in patients with angioimmunoblastic lymphadenopathy. American Journal of Pathology 133: 549–556

88. Fernandez R, Mouradian J, Metroka C, Davis J 1983 The prognostic value of histopathology in persistent generalized lymphadenopathy in homosexual men. New England Journal of Medicine 309: 185–186

89. Ferrarini M, Grossi C E 1984 Definition of the cell types within the 'null lymphocyte' population of human peripheral blood: an analysis of phenotypes and functions. Seminars in Hematology 4: 270–286

90. Flendrig J A 1970 Benign giant lymphoma. In: Clark R L, Cumley R W (eds) The year book of cancer. Year Book Medical Publishers, Chicago, pp 296–299

91. Forkert P-G, Thliveris J A, Bertalanffy F D 1977 Structure of sinuses in the human lymph node. Cell and Tissue Research 183: 115– 130

92. Fossum S, Ford W L 1985 The organization of cell populations within lymph nodes: their origin, life history and functional relationships. Histopathology 9: 469–499

93. Foucar E, Rosai J, Dorfman R F 1979 The ophthalmologic manifestations of sinus histiocytosis with massive lymphadenopathy. American Journal of Ophthalmology 87: 354–367

94. Foucar E, Rosai J, Dorfman R F 1984 Sinus histiocytosis with massive lymphadenopathy. An analysis of 14 deaths occurring in a patient registry. Cancer 54: 1834–1840

95. Foucar E, Rosai J, Dorfman R F, Eyman J M 1984 Immunologic abnormalities and their significance in sinus histiocytosis with massive lymphadenopathy. American Journal of Clinical Pathology 82: 515–525

96. Franco V, Aragona F, Rodolico V, Sangiorgi G B, Frada G, Campesi G 1984 Castleman's disease associated with hepatic amyloidosis. An immunohistochemical and ultrastructural study. Haematologica 69: 556–567

97. Freemont A J, Jones C J P 1983 Light microscopic, histochemical and ultrastructural studies of human lymph node paracortical venules. Journal of Anatomy 136: 349–362

98. Freemont A J, Matthews S, Stoddart R W, Jones C J P 1985 The distribution of cells of the monocytic-lineage in reactive lymph nodes and non-Hodgkin's lymphomata. Characterization using protein histochemistry, lectin binding and monoclonal antibodies. Journal of Pathology 146: 139–150

99. Freemont A J, Stoddart R W, Steven F, Jones C J P, Matthews S 1986 The structure of the basement membrane of human lymph node high endothelial venules: an ultrastructural, histochemical and immunocytochemical study. Histochemical Journal 18: 421–428

100. Frizzera G, Moran E M, Rappaport H 1974 Angio-immunoblastic lymphadenopathy with dysproteinaemia. Lancet i: 1070–1073

101. Frizzera G, Moran E M, Rappaport H 1975 Angio-immunoblastic lymphadenopathy. Diagnosis and clinical course. American Journal of Medicine 59: 803–817

102. Frizzera G, Banks P M, Massarelli G, Rosai J 1983 A systemic lymphoproliferative disorder with morphologic features of Castleman's disease. Pathological findings in 15 patients. American Journal of Surgical Pathology 7: 211–231

103. Frizzera G 1985 Castleman's disease: more questions than answers. Human Pathology 16: 202–205

104. Frizzera G, Peterson B A, Bayrd E D, Goldman A 1985 A systemic lymphoproliferative disorder with morphologic features of Castleman's disease: clinical findings and clinicopathologic correlations in 15 patients. Journal of Clinical Oncology 3: 1202–1216

105. Frizzera G 1988 Castleman's disease and related disorders. Seminars in Diagnostic Pathology 5: 346–364

106. Fujimori T, Shioda K, Sussman E B, Miura M, Katayama I 1981 Subacute necrotising lymphadenitis. A clinicopathologic study. Acta Pathologica Japonica 31: 791–797

107. Fuse Y, Hiraga Y 1974 The fine structures of sarcoidal and Kveim granulomas. In: Iwai K, Hosoda Y (eds) Proceedings of the VI international conference on sarcoidosis. University Park Press, Baltimore, pp 269–275

108. Gaba A R, Stein R S, Sweet D L, Variakojis D 1978 Multicentric giant lymph node hyperplasia. American Journal of Clinical Pathology 69: 86–90

109. Garcia C F, Lifson J D, Engleman E G, Schmidt D M, Warnke R

A, Wood G S 1986 The immunohistology of the persistent generalized lymphadenopathy syndrome (PGL). American Journal of Clinical Pathology 86: 706–715

110. Gerdes J, Stein H 1982 Complement (C3) receptors on dendritic reticulum cells of normal and malignant lymphoid tissue. Clinical and Experimental Immunology 48: 348–352

111. Gerdes J, Stein H, Mason D Y, Ziegler A 1983 Human dendritic reticulum cells of lymphoid follicles: their antigenic profile and their identification as multinucleated giant cells. Virchows Archiv B, Cell Pathology including Molecular Biology 42: 161–172

112. Ghadially F N, Senoo A, Fuse Y, Chan K W 1987 A serial section study of tubular confronting cisternae (so-called 'test tube and ring-shaped forms') in AIDS. Journal of Submicroscopic Cytology 19: 75–183

113. Grimley P M, Kang Y-H, Frederick W, Rook A H, Kostianowsky M, Sonnabend J A, Macher A M, Quinnan G V, Friedman R M, Masur H 1984 Interferon related leukocyte inclusions in acquired immune deficiency syndrome: localization in T-cells. American Journal of Clinical Pathology 81: 147–155

114. Grimley P M, Kang Y-H, Masur H, Frederick W, Hoofnagle J, Klippel J, Friedman R M 1984 Tubuloreticular inclusions in patients with AIDS: interferon-related effect in circulating T-cells and monocytes. In: Friedman-Kein A E, Laubenstein L J (eds) AIDS: the epidemic of Kaposi's sarcoma and opportunist infections. Masson, New York, pp 181–192

115. Grossi C E, Cadoni A, Zicca A, Leprini A, Ferrarini M 1982 Large granular lymphocytes in human peripheral blood: ultrastructural and cytochemical characterization of the granules. Blood 59: 277–283

116. Guarda L A, Butler J J, Mansell P, Hersh E M, Reuben J, Newell G R 1983 Lymphadenopathy in homosexual men. Morbid anatomy with clinical and immunologic correlations. American Journal of Clinical Pathology 79: 559–568

117. Guccion J G, Fischmann A B, Bunn P A Jr, Schechter G P, Patterson R H, Matthews M J 1979 Ultrastructural appearance of cutaneous T cell lymphomas in skin, lymph nodes, and peripheral blood. Cancer Treatment Reports 63: 565–570

118. Guettier C, Gatter K C, Heryet A, Mason D Y 1986 Dendritic reticulum cells in reactive lymph nodes and tonsils: an immunohistological study. Histopathology 10: 15–24

119. Haimoto H, Hosoda S, Kato K 1987 Differential distribution of immunoreactive S100-α and S100-β proteins in normal non-nervous human tissues. Laboratory Investigation 57: 489–498

120. Hammar S, Bockus D, Remington F, Bartha M 1986 The widespread distribution of Langerhans cells in pathologic tissues: an ultrastructural and immunohistochemical study. Human Pathology 17: 894–905

121. Hancock W W, Kobzik L, Colby A J, O'Hara C J, Cooper A G, Godleski J J 1986 Detection of lymphokines and lymphokine receptors in pulmonary sarcoidosis. Immunohistologic evidence that inflammatory macrophages express IL-2 receptors. American Journal of Pathology 123: 1–8

122. Hansmann M-L, Kaiserling E, Müller-Hermelink H K, Hui P-K 1987 Unusual crystalline inclusions in a case of AIDS-related complex. Ultrastructural Pathology 11: 389–395

123. Hanson C A , Frizzera G, Patton D F, Peterson B A, McLain K L, Gajl-Peczalska K J, Kersey J H 1988 Clonal rearrangements for immunoglobulin and T-cell receptor genes in systemic Castleman's disease. Association with Epstein–Barr virus. American Journal of Pathology 131: 84–91

124. Harigaya K, Mikata A, Kageyama K, Kameya T, Shimosato Y 1975 Histopathological study of 6 cases of Castleman's tumour. Acta Pathologica Japonica 25: 355–374

125. Harris N L 1984 Hypervascular follicular hyperplasia and Kaposi's sarcoma in patients at risk for AIDS. New England Journal of Medicine 310: 462–463

126. Harris N L, Bhan A K 1985 Immunohistology of Castleman's disease: a monoclonal antibody study. Laboratory Investigation 52: 28 (abs)

127. Harris N L, Bhan A K 1987 'Plasmacytoid T cells' in Castleman's disease. Immunohistologic phenotype. American Journal of Surgical Pathology 11: 109–113

128. Hartsock R J 1968 Postvaccinial lymphadenitis. Hyperplasia of lymphoid tissue that simulates malignant lymphomas. Cancer 21: 632–649

129. Herberman R B (ed) 1982 NK cells and other natural effector cells. Academic Press, New York

129a.Hercend T, Schmidt R E 1988 Characteristics and uses of natural killer cells. Immunology Today 9: 291–293

130. Herrera GA 1987 Light microscopic, S-100 immunostaining and ultrastructural analysis of dermatopathic lymphadenopathy with and without associated mycosis fungoides. American Journal of Clinical Pathology 87: 187–195

131. Hineman V L, Phyliky R L, Banks P M 1982 Angiofollicular lymph node hyperplasia and peripheral neuropathy. Association with monoclonal gammopathy. Mayo Clinic Proceedings 57: 379–382

132. Hoefsmit E C M, Duijvestijn A M, Kamperdijk E W A 1982 Relation between Langerhans cells, veiled cells and interdigitating cells. Immunobiology 161: 255–265

133. Hoffmann-Fezer G, Lohrs U, Rodt H V, Thierfelder S 1981 Immunohistochemical identification of T- and B-lymphocytes delineated by the unlabelled antibody enzyme method. III. Topographical and quantitative distribution of T- and B-cells in human palatine tonsils. Cell and Tissue Research 216: 361–375

134. Horny H-P, Fellar A C, Horst H-A, Lennert K 1986 Immunocytology of plasmacytoid T cells: marker analysis indicates a unique phenotype of this enigmatic cell. Human Pathology 18: 28–32

135. Howard D R, Batsakis J G 1982 Peanut agglutinin: a new marker for tissue histiocytes. American Journal of Clinical Pathology 77: 401–408

136. Hsu S-M, Cossman J, Jaffe E S 1983 Lymphocyte subsets in normal human lymphoid tissues. American Journal of Clinical Pathology 80: 21–30

137. Hsu S-M, Ree H J 1983 Histochemical studies on lectin binding in reactive lymphoid tissues. Journal of Histochemistry and Cytochemistry 31: 538–546

138. Hsu S-M, Jaffe E S 1984 Phenotypic expression of B-lymphocytes. I. Identification with monoclonal antibodies in normal lymphoid tissues. American Journal of Pathology 114: 387–395

139. Hsu S-M, Jaffe E S 1984 Phenotypic expression of B-lymphocytes. II. Immunoglobulin expression of germinal centre cells. American Journal of Pathology 114: 396–402

140. Hsu S-M, Jaffe E S 1985 Phenotypic expression of T lymphocytes in thymus and peripheral lymphoid tissues. American Journal of Pathology 121: 69–78

141. Hsu S-M 1987 Phenotypic expression of cells of stationary elements in human lymphoid tissues. A histochemical and immunohistochemical study. Hematologic Pathology 1: 45–56

142. Huhn D, Huber C, Gastl G 1982 Large granular lymphocytes: morphological studies. European Journal of Immunology 12: 985–988

143. Humphrey J H 1984 Virus-like particles in AIDS-related lymphadenopathy. Lancet ii: 643

144. Ide F, Iwase T, Saito I, Umemura S, Nakajima T 1984 Immunohistochemical and ultrastructural analysis of the proliferating cells in histiocytosis X. Cancer 53: 917–921

145. Imamura M, Ueno H, Matsuura A, Kamiya H, Suzuki T, Kikuchi K, Onoe T 1982 An ultrastructural study of subacute necrotizing lymphadenitis. American Journal of Pathology 107: 292–299

146. Ioachim H L, Lerner C W, Tapper M L 1983 The lymphoid lesions associated with the acquired immunodeficiency syndrome. American Journal of Surgical Pathology 7: 543–553

147. Isaacson P, Jones D B, Millward-Sadler G H, Judd M A, Payne S 1981 Alpha-1-antitrypsin in human macrophages. Journal of Clinical Pathology 34: 982–990

148. Jaffe E S 1988 Histiocytoses of lymph nodes: biology and differential diagnosis. Seminars in Diagnostic Pathology 5: 376–390

149. James E M V, Jones Williams W 1974 Fine structure and histochemistry of epithelioid cells in sarcoidosis. Thorax 29: 115–120

150. Janossy G, Tidman N, Selby W S, Thomas J A, Granger S, Kung P C, Goldstein G 1980 Human T lymphocytes of inducer and suppressor type occupy different microenvironments. Nature 288: 81–84

151. Janossy G, Pinching A J, Bofill M, Weber J, McLaughlin J E, Ornstein M, Ivory K, Harris J R W, Favrot M, MacDonald-Burns D C 1985 An immunohistological approach to persistent lymphadenopathy and its relevance to AIDS. Clinical and Experimental Immunology 59: 257–266

152. Janossy G, Racz P, Bofill M, Tenner-Racz K, Pinching A J, Foster S, Kernoff P 1987 Microenvironmental changes in lymph nodes of homosexual men with HIV infection. In: Gluckman J C, Vilmer E (eds) Acquired immunodeficiency syndrome — international conference on AIDS. Elsevier, Paris, pp 87–96

153. Jimbow K, Sato S, Kukita A 1969 Cells containing Langerhans granules in human lymph nodes of dermatopathic lymphadenopathy. Journal of Investigative Dermatology 53: 295–299

154. Jones D B, Castleden M, Smith J L, Mepham B L, Wright D H 1978 Immunopathology of angioimmunoblastic lymphadenopathy. British Journal of Cancer 37: 1053–1062

155. Jones E L, Crocker J, Gregory J, Guibarra M, Curran R C 1984 Angiofollicular lymph node hyperplasia (Castleman's disease): an immunohistochemical and enzyme-histochemical study of the hyaline-vascular form of lesion. Journal of Pathology 144: 131–147

156. Jones Williams W, Williams D 1967 'Residual bodies' in sarcoid and sarcoid-like granulomas. Journal of Clinical Pathology 20: 574–577

157. Jones Williams W, Williams D 1968 The properties and development of conchoidal bodies in sarcoid and sarcoid-like granulomas. Journal of Pathology and Bacteriology 96: 491–496

158. Jones Williams W, James E M V, Erasmus D A, Davies T 1970 The fine structure of sarcoid and tuberculous granulomas. Postgraduate Medical Journal 46: 496–500

159. Jones Williams W, Erasmus D A, Jenkins D, James E M V, Davies T 1971 A comparative study of the ultrastructure and histochemistry of sarcoid and tuberculous granulomas. In: Levinsky L, Macholda F (eds) Fifth international conference on sarcoidosis. Universita Karlova, Prague, pp 115–125

160. Jones Williams W, Fry E, James E M V 1972 The fine structure of beryllium granulomas. Acta Pathologica et Microbiologica Scandinavica. Section A, Pathology 80 (suppl 223): 195–202

161. Kaiserling E 1972 Intracytoplasmic undulating tubules in human lymph nodes. Beiträge zur Pathologie 147: 237–248

162. Kaiserling E, Lennert K 1974 Interdigitating reticulum cell in the human lymph node. A specific cell of the thymus dependent region. Virchows Archiv B, Cell Pathology 16: 51–61

163. Kamperdijk E W A, Raaymakers E M, de Leeuw J H S, Hoefsmit E C M 1978 Lymph node macrophages and reticulum cells in the immune response. I. The primary response to paratyphoid vaccine. Cell and Tissue Research 192: 1–23

164. Karpas A, Arno J, Cawley J 1973 Sinus histiocytosis with massive lymphadenopathy — properties of cultured histiocytes. European Journal of Cancer 9: 729–732

165. Karttunen T, Alavaikko M, Apaja-Sarkkinen M, Autio-Harmainen H 1986 Distribution of basement membrane laminin and type IV collagen in human reactive lymph nodes. Histopathology 10: 841–850

166. Keller A R, Hochholzer L, Castleman B 1972 Hyaline-vascular and plasma-cell types of giant lymph node hyperplasia of the mediastinum and other locations. Cancer 29: 670–683

167. Kelly R H, Balfour B M, Armstrong J A, Griffiths S 1978 Functional anatomy of lymph nodes. II. Peripheral lymph-borne mononuclear cells. Anatomical Record 190: 5–22

168. Kessler E 1985 Multicentric giant lymph node hyperplasia. A report of seven cases. Cancer 56: 2446–2451

169. Kikuchi M, Takeshita M, Tashiro K, Mitsui T, Eimoto T, Okamura S 1986 Immunohistological study of histiocytic necrotizing lymphadenitis. Virchows Archiv A, Pathological Anatomy and Histopathology 409: 299–311

170. Kim H, Pangalis G A, Payne B C, Kadin M E, Rappaport H 1982 Ultrastructural identification of neoplastic histiocytes — monocytes. An application of a newly developed cytochemical technique. American Journal of Pathology 106: 204–223

171. Kinet-Denoël C, Heinen E, Radoux D, Simar L 1984 Follicular dendritic cells isolated from human tonsils. Advances in Experimental Medicine and Biology 186: 985–991

172. Kircher T 1980 Silicone lymphadenopathy. A complication of silicone elastomer finger joint prostheses. Human Pathology 11: 240–244

172a. Kirkpatrick C J, Curry A, Bisset D L 1988 Light- and electron-microscopic studies on multinucleated giant cells in sarcoid granuloma: new aspects of asteroid and Schaumann bodies. Ultrastructural Pathology 12: 581–597

173. Klug H 1980 Ultrastructural differences of interdigitating cells in human lymph nodes. Virchows Archiv B, Cell Pathology including Molecular Biology 34: 291–298

173a. Knapp W, Rieber P, Dörken B, Schmidt R E, Stein H, v d Bore A E G 1989 Towards a better definition of human leucocyte surface molecules. Immunology Today 10: 253–258

174. Knecht H, Lennert K 1981 Ultrastructural findings in lymphogranulomatosis X ([angio-] immunoblastic lymphadenopathy). Virchows Archiv B, Cell Pathology including Molecular Biology 37: 29–47

175. Kostianovsky M, Kang Y-H, Grimley P M 1983 Disseminated tubuloreticular inclusions in acquired immunodeficiency syndrome (AIDS). Ultrastructural Pathology 4: 331–336

176. Kostianovsky M, Grimley P M 1985 Ultrastructural findings in the acquired immunodeficiency syndrome. Ultrastructural Pathology 8: 123–130

177. Kurihara K, Hashimoto N 1983 Extramedullary plasmacytoma associated with a Castleman's lesion of the cervical nodes. Journal of Oral Pathology 12: 131–138

178. Lachant N A, Sun N C J, Leong L A, Oseas R S, Prince H E 1985 Multicentric angiofollicular lymph node hyperplasia (Castleman's disease) followed by Kaposi's sarcoma in two homosexual males with the acquired immunodeficiency syndrome (AIDS). American Journal of Clinical Pathology 83: 27–33

179. Lauder I, Campbell A C 1986 The lymphadenopathy of human immunodeficiency virus infection. Histopathology 10: 1203–1207

180. Lennert K, Caesar R, Müller H K 1967 Electron microscopic studies of germinal centres in man. In: Cottier H, Odartchenko N, Schindler R, Congdon C C (eds) Germinal centres in immune responses. Springer-Verlag, Berlin, pp 49–59

181. Lennert K, Niedorf H R, Blumcke S, Hardmeier T 1972 Lymphadenitis with massive hemophagocytic sinus histiocytosis. Virchows Archiv Abteilung B, Zellpathologie 10: 14–29

182. Lennert K 1978 Malignant lymphomas other than Hodgkin's disease. Histology, cytology, ultrastructure, immunology. Springer-Verlag, Berlin, pp 1–71

183. Lennert K, Stein H 1982 The germinal centre: morphology, histochemistry, and immunohistology. In: Goos M, Christophers E (eds) Lymphoproliferative diseases of the skin. Springer-Verlag, Berlin, pp 3–15

184. Lennert K, Stein H, Müller-Hermelink H K, Vollenweider R 1984 T-cells with plasmacytoid features. In: Bernard A, Boumsell L, Dausett J, Millstein C, Schlossmann S F (eds) Leucocyte typing. Human leucocyte differentiation antigens detected by monoclonal antibodies. Specification, classification, nomenclature. Springer-Verlag, Berlin, Heidelberg, New York, Tokyo, p 711

185. Le Tourneau A, Audouin J, Aubert J P, Denis J, Baufine-Ducrocq H, Duterque M, Diebold J 1985 Mise en évidence de particules de type viral dans les centres germinatifs au cours d'un syndrome lymphadénopathique relié au SIDA. Annales de Pathologie (Paris) 5: 137–142

186. Le Tourneau A, Audouin J, Diebold J 1986 Etude ultrastructurale des ganglions chez les sujets à risque pour la SIDA. Annales de Pathologie (Paris) 6: 275–277

187. Le Tourneau A, Audouin J, Diebold J, Marche C, Tricottet V, Reynes M 1986 LAV-like viral particles in lymph node germinal centres in patients with the persistent lymphadenopathy syndrome and the acquired immunodeficiency syndrome-related complex: an ultrastructural study of 30 cases. Human Pathology 17: 1047–1053

188. Levine G D, Dorfman R F 1975 Nodular lymphoma: an ultrastructural study of its relationship to germinal centres and a correlation of light and electron microscopic findings. Cancer 35: 148–164

189. Ling N R, Maclennan I C M, Mason D Y 1987 B-cell and plasma cell antigens: new and previously defined clusters. In: McMichael A J (ed) Leucocyte typing III. White cell differentiation antigens. Oxford University Press, Oxford, pp 302–335

190. Lowenthal D A, Filippa D A, Richardson M E, Bertoni M, Straus D J 1987 Generalized lymphadenopathy with morphologic features of Castleman's disease in an HIV-positive man. Cancer 60: 2454–2458

191. Lukes R J, Tindle B H 1975 Immunoblastic lymphadenopathy. A hyperimmune entity resembling Hodgkin's disease. New England Journal of Medicine 292: 1–8

191a. Luu J, Bockus D, Remington F, Bean M A, Hammar S P 1989 Tubuloreticular structures and cylindrical confronting cisternae: a review. Human Pathology 20: 617–627

192. Madri J A, Fromowitz F 1978 Amyloid deposition in immunoblastic lymphadenopathy. Human Pathology 9: 157–162

193. Mangkornkanok-Mark M, Mark A S, Dong J 1984 Immunoperoxidase evaluation of lymph nodes from acquired immune deficiency patients. Clinical and Experimental Immunology 55: 581–586

194. Martin J M E, Bell B, Ruether D A 1985 Giant lymph node hyperplasia (Castleman's disease) of hyaline vascular type. Clinical heterogeneity with immunohistologic uniformity. American Journal of Clinical Pathology 84: 439–446

195. Mason D Y, Taylor C R 1975 The distribution of muramidase (lysosyme) in human tissues. Journal of Clinical Pathology 28: 124–132

196. Mason D Y, Ladyman H, Gatter K C 1986 Immunohistochemical analysis of monoclonal anti-B cell antibodies. In: Reinherz E L, Haynes B F, Nadler L M, Bernstein I D (eds) Leukocyte typing II, vol. 2. Human B lymphocytes. Springer-Verlag, Berlin, pp 245–255

197. Matsumoto N, Ishihara T, Fujii H, Shiomura T, Yamauchi K, Yamashita Y, Uchino F, Miwa S 1977 Ultrastructural study of immunoblastic lymphadenopathy. Tohoku Journal of Experimental Medicine 122: 129–141

198. Matz L R, Papadimitriou J M, Carrol J R, Barr A L, Dawkins R L, Jackson J M, Herrmann R P, Armstrong B K 1977 Angioimmunoblastic lymphadenopathy with dysproteinaemia. Cancer 40: 2152–2160

199. Metroka C E, Cunningham-Rundles S, Pollack M S, Sonnabend J A, Davis J M, Gordon B, Fernandez R D, Mouradian J 1983 Generalized lymphadenopathy in homosexual men. Annals of Internal Medicine 99: 585–591

200. Miettinen M 1981 Histological differential diagnosis between lymph node toxoplasmosis and other benign lymph node hyperplasias. Histopathology 5: 205–216

201. Miettinen M, Paljakka P, Haveri P, Saxén E 1987 Sinus histiocytosis with massive lymphadenopathy. A nodal and extranodal proliferation of S-100 positive histiocytes? American Journal of Clinical Pathology 88: 270–277

202. Mildvan D, Mathur U, Enlow R, Armstrong D, Gold J, Sears C, Wong B et al 1982 Persistent, generalized lymphadenopathy among homosexual males. Morbidity and Mortality Weekly Report 31: 249–251

203. Millard P R 1984 AIDS: histopathological aspects. Journal of Pathology 143: 223–239

204. Miller M L, Tubbs R R, Fishleder A J, Savage R A, Sebek B A, Weick J K 1984 Immunoregulatory Leu-7[+] and T8[+] lymphocytes in B-cell follicular lymphomas. Human Pathology 15: 810–817

205. Miller R T, Mukai K, Banks P M, Frizzera G 1984 Systemic lymphoproliferative disorder with morphologic features of Castleman's disease. Immunoperoxidase study of cytoplasmic immunoglobulins. Archives of Pathology and Laboratory Medicine 108: 626–630

206. Mirchandani I, Palutke M, Tabaczka P, Goldfarb S, Eisenberg L, Pak M S Y 1985 B-cell lymphomas morphologically resembling T-cell lymphomas. Cancer 56: 1578–1583

207. Modlin R L, Meyer P R, Ammon A J, Rea T H, Hofman F M, Vaccaro S A, Conant M A, Taylor C R 1983 Altered distribution of B and T lymphocytes in lymph nodes from homosexual men with Kaposi's sarcoma. Lancet ii: 768–771

208. Moir D H, Choy T, Dalton W R 1982 Giant lymph node hyperplasia: persistence of symptoms for 15 years. Cancer 49: 748–750

209. Mollo F, Monga G 1971 Banded structures in the connective tissue of lymphomas, lymphadenitis, and thymomas. Virchows Archiv Abteilung B, Zellpathologie 7: 356–366

210. Monda L, Warnke R, Rosai J 1986 A primary lymph node malignancy with features suggestive of dendritic reticulum cell differentiation. A report of 4 cases. American Journal of Pathology 122: 562–572

211. Morgenroth K, Fasske E 1974 Examination of mediastinal lymph node sarcoidosis by electron microscope. Beiträge zur Pathologie 153: 51–64

212. Mori S, Mohri N, Morita H, Yamaguchi K, Shimamine T 1983 The distribution of cells expressing a natural killer cell marker (HNK-1) in normal human lymphoid organs and malignant lymphomas. Virchows Archiv B, Cell Pathology including Molecular Biology 43: 253–263

213. Mori Y, Lennert K 1969 Electron microscopic atlas of lymph node cytology and pathology. Springer-Verlag, Berlin

214. Morris H B, Mason D Y, Stein H, Lennert K 1983 An immunohistological study of reactive lymphoid tissue. Histopathology 7: 809–823

215. Motoi M, Stein H, Lennert K 1980 Demonstration of lysozyme, alpha-1-antichymotrypsin, alpha-1-antitrypsin, albumin, and transferrin with the immunoperoxidase method in lymph node cells. Virchows Archiv B, Cell Pathology including Molecular Biology 35: 73–82

216. Mufarrij A, Fazzini E, Feiner H D 1982 Giant lymph node hyperplasia. An immunopathologic and ultrastructural study of a case of the multicentric plasma cell variant. Archives of Pathology and Laboratory Medicine 106: 92–95

217. Müller H, Falk S, Stutte H J 1985 Lymph nodes, accessory cells and the staging of AIDS. Immunology Today 6: 257

218. Müller H, Falk S, Stutte H J 1986 Accessory cells as primary target of human immunodeficiency virus HIV infection. Journal of Clinical Pathology 39: 1161

219. Müller-Hermelink H K 1974 Characterization of the B-cell and T-cell regions of human lymphatic-tissue through enzyme histochemical demonstration of ATPase and 5′-nucleotidase activities. Virchows Archiv B, Cell Pathology 16: 371–378

220. Müller-Hermelink H K, Kamiyama R, Kaiserling E, Lennert K 1980 In: Jones Williams W, Davies B H (eds) Eighth international conference on sarcoidosis and other granulomatous diseases. Alpha Omega Publishing, Cardiff, pp 23–29

221. Müller-Hermelink H K, Von Gaudecker B, Drenckhahn D, Jaworsky K, Feldmann C 1981 Fibroblastic and dendritic reticulum cells of lymphoid tissue. Ultrastructural, histochemical, and ³H-thymidine labelling studies. Journal of Cancer Research and Clinical Oncology 101: 149–164

222. Müller-Hermelink H K, Stein H, Steinmann G, Lennert K 1983 Malignant lymphoma of plasmacytoid T-cells. Morphologic and immunologic studies characterising a special type of T-cell. American Journal of Surgical Pathology 7: 849–862

223. Muretto P, Cinti S, Staccioli M P 1985 Multicentric giant lymph-node hyperplasia: immunohistochemical and ultrastructural study of 2 cases. Haematologica 70: 120–131

224. Murphy G F, Bhan A K, Sato S, Harrist T J, Mihm M C Jr 1981 Characterization of Langerhans cells by the use of monoclonal antibodies. Laboratory Investigation 45: 465–468

225. Muse K E, Koren H S 1982 The uropod as an integral and specialised structure of large granular lymphocytes. In: Herberman R B (ed) NK cells and other natural effector cells. Academic Press, New York, pp 1035–1040

226. Myers T J, Cole S R, Pastuszak W T 1978 Angioimmunoblastic lymphadenopathy: pleural-pulmonary disease. Cancer 40: 266–271

227. Nadler L M, Korsmeyer S J, Anderson K C, Boyd A W, Slaughenhoupt B, Park E et al 1984 B-cell origin of non-T cell acute lymphoblastic leukaemia. A model for discrete stages of neoplastic and normal pre-B cell differentiation. Journal of Clinical Investigation 74: 332–340

228. Nadler L M, Anderson K C, Bates M, Park E, Slaughenhoupt B, Schlossman S F 1984 Human B cell-associated antigens: expression on normal and malignant B lymphocytes. In: Bernard A, Boumsell L, Dausset J, Milstein C, Schlossman S F (eds) Leucocyte typing. Human leucocyte differentiation antigens detected by monoclonal antibodies. Specification, classification, nomenclature. Springer-Verlag, Berlin, pp 354–363

229. Nadler L M, Anderson K C, Marti G, Bates M, Park E, Daley J F,

Schlossman S F 1983 B4, a human B lymphocyte–associated antigen expressed on normal, mitogen-activated, and malignant B lymphocytes. Journal of Immunology 131: 244–250

230. Nadler L M 1986 B cell/leukemia panel workshop: summary and comments. 1986. In: Reinherz E L, Haynes B F, Nadler L M, Bernstein I D (eds) Leucocyte typing II, vol. 2. Human B lymphocytes. Springer-Verlag, Berlin, pp 3–43

231. Nagai K, Sato I, Shimoyama N 1986 Pathohistological and immunohistochemical studies on Castleman's disease of the lymph node. Virchows Archiv A, Pathological Anatomy and Histopathology 409: 287–297

232. Naiem M, Gerdes J, Abdulaziz Z, Stein H, Mason D Y 1983 Production of a monoclonal antibody reactive with human dendritic reticulum cells and its use in the immunohistological analysis of lymphoid tissue. Journal of Clinical Pathology 36: 167–175

233. Nakajima T, Watanabe S, Sato Y, Shimosato Y, Motoi M, Lennert K 1982 S-100 protein in Langerhans cells, interdigitating reticulum cells and histiocytosis X cells. Gann 73: 429–432

234. Namikawa R, Suchi T, Ueda R, Itoh G, Koike K, Ota K, Takahashi T 1987 Phenotyping of proliferating lymphocytes in angioimmunoblastic lymphadenopathy and related lesions by the double immunoenzymatic staining technique. American Journal of Pathology 127: 279–287

235. Nathwani B N, Sheibani K, Winberg C D, Burke J S, Rappaport H 1985 Neoplastic B cells with cerebriform nuclei in follicular lymphomas. Human Pathology 16: 173–180

236. Nathwani B N, Winberg C D, Bearman R M 1985 Angioimmunoblastic lymphadenopathy with dysproteinaemia and its progression to malignant lymphoma. In: Jaffe E S (ed) Major problems in pathology, vol. 16. Surgical pathology of the lymph nodes and related organs. Saunders, Philadelphia, pp 57–85

237. Neiman R S, Dervan P, Haudenschild C, Jaffe R 1978 Angioimmunoblastic lymphadenopathy. An ultrastructural and immunologic study with review of the literature. Cancer 41: 507–518

238. Newell D G, Roath S, Smith J L 1976 The scanning electron microscopy of normal human peripheral blood lymphocytes. British Journal of Haematology 32: 309–316

239. Ngendahayo P, Roels H, Quatacker J, Boddaert J, Ntabomuvra V, Mbonyingabo P 1983 Sinus histiocytosis with massive lymphadenopathy in Rwanda: report of 8 cases with immunohistochemical and ultrastructural studies. Histopathology 7: 49–63

240. Nieuwenhuis P, Opstelten D 1984 Functional anatomy of germinal centres. American Journal of Anatomy 170: 421–435

241. O'Connor N T J, Crick J A, Wainscoat J S, Gatter K C, Stein H, Falini B, Mason D Y 1986 Evidence for monoclonal T lymphocyte proliferation in angioimmunoblastic lymphadenopathy. Journal of Clinical Pathology 39: 1229–1232

242. O'Hara C J, Said J W, Pinkus G S 1986 Non-Hodgkin's lymphoma, multilobated B-cell type: report of 9 cases with immunohistochemical and immunoultrastructural evidence for a follicular centre cell derivation. Human Pathology 17: 593–599

243. O'Hara C J, Groopman J E, Federman M 1988 The ultrastructural and immunohistochemical demonstration of viral particles in lymph nodes from human immunodeficiency virus-related and non-human immunodeficiency virus-related lymphadenopathy syndromes. Human Pathology 19: 545–549

244. Oláh I, Röhlich P, Törö I 1975 Ultrastructure of lymphoid organs. An electron-microscopic atlas. Lippincott, Philadelphia

245. O'Murchadha M T, Wolf B C, Neiman R S 1987 The histologic features of hyperplastic lymphadenopathy in AIDS-related complex are non-specific. American Journal of Surgical Pathology 11: 94–99

246. Onerheim R M, Wang N-S, Gilmore N, Jothy S 1984 Ultrastructural markers of lymph nodes in patients with acquired immune deficiency syndrome and in homosexual males with unexplained persistent lymphadenopathy. A quantitative study. American Journal of Clinical Pathology 82: 280–288

247. Orenstein J M 1983 Ultrastructural markers in AIDS. Lancet ii: 284–285

248. Orenstein J M, Schulof R S, Simon G L 1984 Ultrastructural markers in acquired immune deficiency syndrome. Archives of Pathology and Laboratory Medicine 108: 857–859

249. Osborne B M, Butler J J 1984 Clinical implications of progressive transformation of germinal centres. American Journal of Surgical Pathology 8: 725–733

250. Palestro G, Valente G, Micca F B, Novero D, Godio L, Stramignoni A 1982 Histochemical study on human germinal centre, mantle-zone and extra-follicular area lymphoid cell subpopulations. Immunological and cytochemical correlations with lymphomatous cells, peripheral normal and leukaemic lymphocytes. Virchows Archiv B, Cell Pathology including Molecular Biology 41: 253–265

251. Palutke M, Khilanani P, Weise R 1976 Immunologic and electron microscopic characteristics of a case of immunoblastic lymphadenopathy. American Journal of Clinical Pathology 65: 929–941

252. Papadimitriou C S, Stein H, Papacharalampous N X 1980 Presence of alpha-1-antichymotrypsin and alpha-1-antitrypsin in haematopoietic and lymphoid tissue cells as revealed by the immunoperoxidase method. Pathology, Research and Practice 169: 287–297

253. Papadimitriou C S, Stephanaki-Nikou S N, Malamou-Mitsi V D 1983 Comparative immunostaining of T-associated plasma cells and other lymph-node cells in paraffin sections. Virchows Archiv B, Cell Pathology including Molecular Biology 43: 31–36

254. Papadimitriou C S, Papacharalampous N X 1985 Histiocytic necrotizing lymphadenitis without granulocytic infiltration. Archives of Pathology and Laboratory Medicine 109: 107–108

255. Papadimitriou J M, Spector W G 1971 The origin, properties and fate of epithelioid cells. Journal of Pathology 105: 187–203

256. Parwaresch M R, Radzun H J, Hansmann M-L, Peters K-P 1983 Monoclonal antibody Ki-M4 specifically recognises human dendritic reticulum cells (follicular dendritic cells) and their possible precursor in blood. Blood 62: 585–590

257. Parwaresch M R, Radzun H J, Kreipe H, Hansmann M-L, Barth J 1986 Monocyte/macrophage-reactive monoclonal antibody Ki-M6 recognizes an intracytoplasmic antigen. American Journal of Pathology 124: 141–151

258. Payne B C, Kim H, Pangalis G A, Rothman A, Rappaport H 1980 A method for the ultrastructural demonstration of non-specific esterase in human blood and lymphoid tissue. Histochemical Journal 12: 71–86

259. Payne C M, Glasser L, Fiederlein R, Lindberg R 1983 New ultrastructural observations: parallel tubular arrays in human T lymphoid cells. Journal of Immunological Methods 65: 307–317

260. Pelicci P-G, Knowles II D M, Arlin Z A, Wieczorek R, Luciw P, Dina D, Basilico C, Dalla-Favera R 1986 Multiple monoclonal B cell expansions and c-myc oncogene rearrangements in acquired immune deficiency syndrome-related lymphoproliferative disorders. Implications for lymphomagenesis. Journal of Experimental Medicine 164: 2049–2060

261. Peters J P J, Rademakers L H P M, Roelofs J M M, de Jong D, Van Unnik J A M 1984 Distribution of dendritic reticulum cells in follicular lymphoma and reactive hyperplasia. Light microscopic identification and general morphology. Virchows Archiv B, Cell Pathology including Molecular Biology 46: 215–228

262. Peyrol S, Takiya C, Cordier J-F, Grimaud J-A 1986 Organization of the connective matrix of the sarcoid granuloma. Evolution and cell–matrix interactions. In: Johns C J (ed) Tenth international conference on sarcoidosis and other granulomatous disorders. Annals of the New York Academy of Sciences 465: 268–285

263. Pileri S, Kikuchi M, Helbron D, Lennert K 1982 Histiocytic necrotizing lymphadenitis without granulocytic infiltration. Virchows Archiv A, Pathological Anatomy and Histopathology 395: 257–271

264. Pileri S, Rivano M T, Raise E, Gualandi G, Gobbi M, Martuzzi M, Gritti F M, Gerdes J, Stein H 1986 The value of lymph node biopsy in patients with the acquired immunodeficiency syndrome (AIDS) and the AIDS-related complex (ARC): a morphological and immunohistochemical study of 90 cases. Histopathology 10: 1107–1129

265. Pinkus G S, Warhol M J, O'Connor E M, Etheridge C L, Fujiwara K 1986 Immunohistochemical localization of smooth muscle myosin in human spleen, lymph node, and other lymphoid tissues. Unique staining patterns in splenic white pulp and sinuses,

lymphoid follicles, and certain vasculature, with ultrastructural correlations. American Journal of Pathology 123: 440–453

266. Piris M A, Rivas C, Morente M, Oliva H, Rubio C 1986 Immature sinus histiocytosis. A monocytoid B-lymphoid reaction. Journal of Pathology 148: 159–167

267. Piris M A, Rivas C, Morente M, Rubio C, Martin C, Olivia H 1987 Persistent and generalized lymphadenopathy: a lesion of follicular dendritic cells? American Journal of Clinical Pathology 87: 716–724

268. Pizzolo G, Semenzato G, Chilosi M, Morittu L, Ambrosetti A, Warner N, Bofill M, Janossy G 1984 Distribution and heterogeneity of cells detected by HNK-1 monoclonal antibody in blood and tissues in normal, reactive and neoplastic conditions. Clinical and Experimental Immunology 57: 195–206

269. Pizzolo G, Vinante F, Agostini C, Zambello R, Trentin L, Masciarelli M et al 1987 Immunologic abnormalities in angioimmunoblastic lymphadenopathy. Cancer 60: 2412–2418

270. Poblete M T, Figueroa C D, Caorsi I 1987 Ultrastructural characteristics of the interdigitating dendritic cell in dermatopathic lymphadenopathy of mycosis fungoides patients. Journal of Pathology 151: 263–269

271. Polliak A 1977 Normal, transformed and leukemic leukocytes. A scanning electron microscopy atlas. Springer-Verlag, Berlin

272. Polliak A 1978 Surface morphology of lymphoreticular cells: review of data obtained from scanning electron microscopy. In: Mathé G, Seligmann M, Tubiana M (eds) Recent results in cancer research, vol. 64. Lymphoid neoplasias I. classification, categorization, natural history. Springer-Verlag, Berlin, pp 66–93

273. Poppema S, Kaiserling E, Lennert K 1979 Nodular paragranuloma and progressively transformed germinal centres. Ultrastructural and immunohistologic findings. Virchows Archiv B, Cell Pathology including Molecular Biology 31: 211–225

274. Poppema S, Bhan A K, Reinherz E L, McCluskey R T, Schlossmann S F 1981 Distribution of T cell subsets in human lymph nodes. Journal of Experimental Medicine 153: 30–41

275. Porwit-Ksiazek A, Ksiazek T, Biberfeld P 1983 Leu7⁺(HNK-1⁺) cells. I. Selective compartmentalization of Leu7⁺ cells with different immunophenotypes in lymphatic tissues and blood. Scandinavian Journal of Immunology 18: 485–493

276. Poulter L W, Janossy G 1985 The involvement of dendritic cells in chronic inflammatory disease. Scandinavian Journal of Immunology 21: 401–407

277. Prasthofer E F, Grizzle W E, Prchal J T, Grossl C E 1985 Plasmacytoid T cell lymphoma associated with chronic myeloproliferative disorder. American Journal of Surgical Pathology 9: 380–387

278. Rácz P, Tenner-Rácz K, Kahl C, Feller A C, Kern P, Dietrich M 1986 Spectrum of morphologic changes of lymph nodes from patients with AIDS or AIDS-related complexes. Progress in Allergy 37: 81–181

279. Rademakers L H P M, Peters J P J, Van Unnik J A M 1983 Histiocytic and dendritic reticulum cells in follicular structures of follicular lymphoma and reactive hyperplasia. Virchows Archiv B, Cell Pathology including Molecular Biology 44: 85–98

280. Radzun H J, Parwaresch M R 1983 Differential immunohistochemical resolution of the human mononuclear phagocyte system. Cellular Immunology 82: 174–183

281. Radzun H J, Parwaresch M R, Feller A C, Hansmann M-L 1984 Monocyte/macrophage-specific monoclonal antibody Ki-M1 recognizes interdigitating reticulum cells. American Journal of Pathology 117: 441–450

282. Ralfkiaer E, Plesner T, Wantzin G L, Thomsen K, Nissen N I, Hou-Jensen K 1984 Immunohistochemical identification of lymphocyte subsets and accessory cells in human hyperplastic lymph nodes. The functional significance of the compartmentalization of lymphoid tissue. Scandinavian Journal of Haematology 32: 536–543

283. Ralfkiaer E, Stein H, Plesner T, Hou-Jensen K, Mason D 1984 In situ immunological characterisation of Langerhans' cells with monoclonal antibodies: comparison with other dendritic cells in skin and lymph nodes. Virchows Archiv A, Pathological Anatomy and Histopathology 403: 401–412

284. Rausch E, Kaiserling E, Goos M 1977 Langerhans cells and interdigitating reticulum cells in the thymus-dependent region in

285. Ree H J, Kadin M E 1985 Macrophage-histiocytes in Hodgkin's disease. The relation of peanut-agglutinin-binding macrophage-histiocytes to clinicopathologic presentation and course of disease. Cancer 56: 333–338

286. Ree H J, Kadin M E 1986 Peanut agglutinin. A useful marker for histiocytosis X and interdigitating reticulum cells. Cancer 57: 282–287

287. Reyes B F, Lejonc J L, Gourdin M F, Mannoni P, Dreyfus B 1975 The surface morphology of human B lymphocytes as revealed by immunoelectron microscopy. Journal of Experimental Medicine 141: 392–410

288. Reynes M, Aubert J P, Cohen J H M, Audouin J, Tricottet V, Diebold J, Kazatchkine M D 1985 Human follicular dendritic cells express CR1, CR2 and CR3 complement receptor antigens. Journal of Immunology 135: 2687–2694

289. Rinne A, Alavaikko M, Järvinen M, Martikainen J, Karttunen T, Hopsu-Havu V 1983 Demonstration of immunoreactive acid cysteine-proteinase inhibitor in reticulum cells of lymph node germinal centres. Virchows Archiv B, Cell Pathology including Molecular Biology 43: 121–126

290. Rivano M T, Falini B, Stein H, Canino S, Ciani C, Gerdes J, Ribacchi R, Gobbi M, Pileri S 1987 Histiocytic necrotizing lymphadenitis without granulocytic infiltration (Kikuchi's lymphadenitis). Morphological and immunohistochemical study of eight cases. Histopathology 11: 1013–1027

291. Rodriguez E M, Caorsi I 1978 A second look at the ultrastructure of the Langerhans cell of the human epidermis. Journal of Ultrastructure Research 65: 279–295

292. Roholl P J M, Kleyne J, Pijpers H W, Van Unnik J A M 1985 Comparative immunohistochemical investigation of markers for malignant histiocytes. Human Pathology 16: 763–771

293. Roholl P J M, Kleyne J, Prins M E F, Hooijkass H, Vroom T M, Van Unnik J A M 1988 Immunologic marker analysis of normal and malignant histiocytes. A comparative study of monoclonal antibodies for diagnostic purposes. American Journal of Clinical Pathology 89: 187–194

294. Rosai J, Dorfman R F 1969 Sinus histiocytosis with massive lymphadenopathy. A newly recognised benign clinicopathological entity. Archives of Pathology 87: 63–70

295. Rosai J, Dorfman R F 1972 Sinus histiocytosis with massive lymphadenopathy: a pseudolymphomatous benign disorder. Analysis of 34 cases. Cancer 30: 1174–1188

296. Rosas-Uribe A, Variakojis D, Molnar Z, Rappaport H 1974 Mycosis fungoides: an ultrastructural study. Cancer 34: 634–645

297. Rouse R V, Ledbetter J A, Weissman I L 1982 Mouse lymph node germinal centres contain a selected subset of T cells — the helper phenotype. Journal of Immunology 128: 2243–2246

298. Rouse R V, Weissman I L, Ledbetter J A, Warnke R A 1982 Expression of T cell antigens by cells in mouse and human primary and secondary follicles. Advances in Experimental Medicine and Biology 149: 751–756

299. Rouse R V, Reichert R A, Gallatin W M, Weissman I L, Butcher E C 1984 Localisation of lymphocyte subpopulations in peripheral lymphoid organs: directed lymphocyte migration and segregation into specific micro-environments. American Journal of Anatomy 170: 391–405

300. Rowden G, Lewis M G, Sullivan A K 1977 Ia antigen expression on human epidermal Langerhans cells. Nature 268: 247–248

301. Rowden G 1981 The Langerhans cell. Critical Reviews in Immunology 3: 95–180

302. Rywlin A M, Rosen L, Cabello B 1983 Coexistence of Castleman's disease and Kaposi's sarcoma. Report of a case and a speculation. American Journal of Dermatopathology 5: 277–281

303. Said J W, Shintaku P, Teitelbaum A, Chien K, Sassoon A F 1984 Distribution of T-cell phenotypic subsets and surface immunoglobulin-bearing lymphocytes in lymph nodes from male homosexuals with persistent generalized lymphadenopathy. Human Pathology 15: 785–790

304. Said J W, Sassoon A F, Chien K, Shintaku B, Pinkus G S 1986 Immunoultrastructural and morphometric analysis of B lymphocytes in human germinal centres. Evidence for alternate pathways of

follicular transformation. American Journal of Pathology 123: 390–397

305. Sakuma H, Asana S, Kojima M 1981 An ultrastructural study of the primary follicle in the lymph node. Acta Pathologica Japonica 31: 473–493

306. Saltzstein S L, Ackerman L V 1959 Lymphadenopathy induced by anticonvulsant drugs and mimicking clinically and pathologically malignant lymphomas. Cancer 12: 164–182

307. Sanchez R, Rosai J, Dorfman R F 1977 Sinus histiocytosis with massive lymphadenopathy: an analysis of 113 cases with special emphasis on extra-nodal manifestations. Laboratory Investigation 36: 349–350

308. Sanchez R, Sibley R K, Rosai J, Dorfman R F 1981 The electron microscopic features of sinus histiocytosis with massive lymphadenopathy: a study of 11 cases. Ultrastructural Pathology 2: 101–119

309. Scadding J G 1967 Sarcoidosis. Eyre & Spottiswoode, London

310. Schiaffino E, Bestetti-Bosisio M, Toia G, Onida L, Riboli P, Schmid C 1986 Ultrastructural alterations and virus-like particles in lymph nodes of drug addicts with lymphadenopathy syndrome (LAS). Pathology, Research and Practice 181: 755–760

311. Schlosnagle D C, Chan W C, Hargreaves H K, Nolting S F, Brynes R K 1982 Plasmacytoma arising in giant lymph node hyperplasia. American Journal of Clinical Pathology 78: 541–544

312. Schnaidt U, Thiele J, Georgeii A 1980 Angioimmunoblastic lymphadenopathy. Fine structure of the lymph nodes by correlation of light and electron microscopical findings. Virchows Archiv A, Pathological Anatomy and Histology 389: 381–395

313. Schuurman H-J, Kluin P M, Gmelig Meijling F H J, Van Unnik J A M, Kater L 1985 Lymphocyte status of lymph node and blood in acquired immunodeficiency syndrome (AIDS) and AIDS-related complex disease. Journal of Pathology 147: 269–280

314. Schuurman H-J, Krone W J A, Broekhuizen R, Goudsmit J 1988 Expression of RNA and antigens of human immunodeficiency virus type-1 (HIV-1) in lymph nodes from HIV-1 infected individuals. American Journal of Pathology 133: 516–524

315. Shamoto M, Kaplan C, Katoh A K 1971 Langerhans cell granules in human hyperplastic lymph nodes. Archives of Pathology 92: 46–52

316. Sheibani K, Fritz R M, Winberg C D, Burke J S, Rappaport H 1984 'Monocytoid' cells in reactive follicular hyperplasia with and without multifocal histiocytic reactions: an immunohistochemical study of 21 cases including suspected cases of toxoplasmic lymphadenitis. American Journal of Clinical Pathology 81: 453–458

317. Sheibani K, Sohn C C, Burke J S, Winberg C D, Wu A M, Rappaport H 1986 Monocytoid B-cell lymphoma. A novel B-cell neoplasm. American Journal of Pathology 124: 310–318

318. Shimoyama M, Minato K, Saito H, Takenaka T, Watanabe S, Nagatani T, Naruto M 1979 Immunoblastic lymphadenopathy (IBL)-like T-cell lymphoma. Japanese Journal of Clinical Oncology 9 (suppl): 347–356

319. Si L, Whiteside T L 1983 Tissue distribution of human NK cells studied with anti-Leu-7 monoclonal antibody. Journal of Immunology 130: 2149–2155

320. Sidhu G S, Stahl R E, el-Sadr W, Zolla-Pazner S 1983 Ultrastructural markers of AIDS. Lancet i: 990–991

321. Sidhu G S, Stahl R E, el-Sadr W, Cassai N D, Forrester E M, Zolla-Pazner S 1985 The acquired immunodeficiency syndrome. An ultrastructural study. Human Pathology 16: 377–386

322. Sinclair-Smith C C, Kahn L B, Uys C J 1974 Sinus histiocytosis with massive lymphadenopathy. Report of 2 additional cases with ultrastructural observations. South African Medical Journal 48: 451–454

323. Slater D N, Rooney N, Bleehen S, Hamed A 1985 The lymph node in mycosis fungoides: a light and electron microscopy and immunohistological study supporting the Langerhans cell–retrovirus hypothesis. Histopathology 9: 587–621

324. Sohn C C, Sheibani K, Winberg C D, Rappaport H 1985 Monocytoid B lymphocytes: their relation to the patterns of the acquired immunodeficiency syndrome (AIDS) and AIDS-related lymphadenopathy. Human Pathology 16: 979–985

325. Soler P, Chollet S, Jacque C, Fukuda Y, Ferrans V J, Basset F 1985 Immunocytochemical characterization of pulmonary histiocytosis X cells in lung biopsies. American Journal of Pathology 118: 439–451

326. Spry C J F, Pflug A J, Janossy G, Humphrey J H 1980 Large mononuclear (veiled) cells with 'Ia-like' membrane antigens in human afferent lymph. Clinical and Experimental Immunology 39: 750–755

327. Stanley M W, Frizzera G 1986 Diagnostic specificity of histologic features in lymph node biopsy specimens from patients at risk for the acquired immunodeficiency syndrome. Human Pathology 17: 1231–1239

328. Stein H, Bonk A, Tolksdorf G, Lennert K, Rodt H, Gerdes J 1980 Immunohistologic analysis of the organization of normal lymphoid tissue and non-Hodgkin's lymphomas. Journal of Histochemistry and Cytochemistry 28: 746–760

329. Stein H, Gerdes J, Tolksdorf G, Klatt U 1981 Human membrane-bound C3 receptors. Serological and immunohistological demonstration of C3 receptors. Scandinavian Journal of Immunology 13: 67–76

330. Stein H, Gerdes J, Mason D Y 1982 The normal and malignant germinal centre. Clinics in Haematology 11: 531–559

331. Stein H, Lennert K, Mason D Y, Liangru S, Ziegler A 1984 Immature sinus histiocytes. Their identification as a novel B-cell population. American Journal of Pathology 117: 44–52

332. Stejskal J 1980 Measles lymphadenopathy. Ultrastructural Pathology 1: 243–247

333. Stingl G, Wolff-Schreiner E C, Pichler W J, Gschnait F, Knapp W, Wolff K 1977 Epidermal Langerhans cells bear Fc and C3 receptors. Nature 268: 245–246

334. Strauchen J A 1984 Lectin receptors as markers of lymphoid cells. 1. Demonstration in tissue section by peroxidase technique. American Journal of Pathology 116: 297–304

335. Suseelan A V, Augusty T S, Harilal K R 1984 Necrotizing lymphadenitis. An analysis of seventeen cases. Indian Journal of Pathology and Microbiology 27: 331–334

336. Swerdlow S H, Murray L J 1984 Natural killer (Leu7 +) cells in reactive lymphoid tissues and malignant lymphomas. American Journal of Clinical Pathology 81: 459–463

337. Syrjanen K J 1981 Epithelial cell granulomas in the lymph nodes draining human cancer: ultrastructural findings of a breast cancer case. Diagnostic Histopathology 4: 291–294

338. Szakal A K, Gieringer R L, Kosco M H, Tew J G 1985 Isolated follicular dendritic cells: cytochemical antigen localization, Nomarski, SEM, and TEM morphology. Journal of Immunology 134: 1349–1359

339. Takahashi K, Yamaguchi Y, Ishizeki J, Nakajima T, Nakazato Y 1981 Immunohistochemical and immunoelectron microscopic localization of S-100 protein in the interdigitating reticulum cells of the human lymph node. Virchows Archiv B, Cell Pathology including Molecular Biology 37: 125–135

340. Takahashi K, Eto K, Takeya M, Naito M, Yaginuma Y, Ichihara A 1983 Long-term polyvinylpyrrolidone storage. Histochemical and ultrastructural observations in 2 biopsy cases. Acta Pathologica Japonica 33: 985–997

341. Takahashi K, Isobe T, Ohtsuki Y, Akagi T, Sonobe H, Okuyama T 1984 Immunohistochemical study on the distribution of α and β subunits of S-100 protein in human neoplasm and normal tissues. Virchows Archiv B, Cell Pathology including Molecular Biology 45: 385–396

342. Takahashi K, Yoshino T, Hayashi K, Sonobe H, Ohtsuki Y 1987 S-100 beta positive human T lymphocytes: their characteristics and behaviour under normal and pathologic conditions. Blood 70: 214–220

343 Tanaka Y 1986 Immunocytochemical study of human lymphoid tissue with monoclonal antibodies against S-100 protein subunits. Virchows Archiv A, Pathological Anatomy and Histopathology 410: 125–132

344 Tanda F, Massarelli G, Costanzi G 1983 Multicentric giant lymph node hyperplasia: an immunohistochemical study. Human Pathology 14: 1053–1058

345. Tenner-Rácz K, Rácz P, Dietrich M, Kern P 1985 Altered follicular dendritic cells and virus-like particles in AIDS and AIDS-related lymphadenopathy. Lancet i: 105–106

346. Tenner-Rácz K, Rácz P, Bofill M, Schulz-Meyer A, Dietrich M, Kern P, Weber J, Pinching A J, Veronese-Dimarzo F, Popovic M,

Klatzmann D, Gluckman J C, Janossy G 1986 HTLV-III/LAV viral antigens in lymph nodes of homosexual men with persistent generalized lymphadenopathy and AIDS. American Journal of Pathology 123: 9–15

347. Tew J G, Thorbecke J, Steinman R M 1982 Dendritic cells in the immune response: characteristics and recommended nomenclature (a report from the Reticuloendothelial Society Committee on Nomenclature). RES: Journal of the Reticuloendothelial Society 31: 371–380

348. Toccanier-Pelte M-F, Skalli O, Kapanci Y, Gabbiani G 1987 Characterization of stromal cells with myoid features in lymph nodes and spleen in normal and pathological conditions. American Journal of Pathology 129: 109–118

349. Tosi P, Leoncini L, Spina D, Del Vecchio M T 1984 Morphometric nuclear analysis of lymphoid cells in center cell lymphomas and in reactive germinal centers. American Journal of Pathology 117: 12–17

350. Travis W D, Balogh K, Abraham J L 1985 Silicone granulomas: report of 3 cases and review of the literature. Human Pathology 16: 19–27

351. Trinchieri G, Perussia B 1984 Human natural killer cells: biologic and pathologic aspects. Laboratory Investigation 50: 489–513

352. Turk J L, Narayanan R B 1982 The origin, morphology, and function of epithelioid cells. Immunobiology 161: 274–282

353. Turner R R, Martin J, Dorfman R F 1983 Necrotizing lymphadenitis. A study of 30 cases. American Journal of Surgical Pathology 7: 115–123

354. Turner R R, Levine A M, Gill P S, Parker J W, Meyer P R 1987 Progressive histopathologic abnormalities in the persistent generalized lymphadenopathy syndrome. American Journal of Surgical Pathology 11: 625–632

355. Turner R R, Meyer P R, Taylor C R, Gill P S, Hofman F H, Nichols P, Rasheed S, Levine A M 1987 Immunohistology of persistent generalized lymphadenopathy. Evidence for progressive lymph node abnormalities in some patients. American Journal of Clinical Pathology 88: 10–19

356. Tykocinski M, Schinella R A, Greco M A 1983 Fibroblastic reticulum cells in human lymph nodes. An ultrastructural study. Archives of Pathology and Laboratory Medicine 107: 418–422

357. Uccini S, Vitolo D, Stoppacciaro A, Paliotta D, Cassano A M, Barsotti P, Ruco L P, Baroni C D 1986 Immunoreactivity for S-100 protein in dendritic and lymphocyte-like cells in human lymphoid tissues. Virchows Archiv B, Cell Pathology including Molecular Biology 52: 129–141

358. Unger P D, Rappaport K M, Strauchen J A 1987 Necrotizing lymphadenitis (Kikuchi's disease). Report of four cases of an unusual pseudolymphomatous lesion and immunologic marker studies. Archives of Pathology and Laboratory Medicine 111: 1031–1034

359. Valdes A J, Blair O M 1976 Angioimmunoblastic lymphadenopathy with dysproteinaemia. Immunohistologic and ultrastructural studies. American Journal of Clinical Pathology 66: 551–559

360. van den Oord J J, de Wolf-Peeters C, de Vos R, Desmet V J 1984 The paracortical area in dermatopathic lymphadenitis and other reactive conditions of the lymph node. Virchows Archiv B, Cell Pathology including Molecular Biology 45: 289–299

361. van den Oord J J, de Wolf-Peeters C, Facchetti F, Desmet V J 1984 Cellular composition of hypersensitivity-type granulomas: immunohistochemical analysis of tuberculous and sarcoidal lymphadenitis. Human Pathology 15: 559–565

362. van den Oord J J, de Wolf-Peeters C, Tricot G, Desmet V J 1984 Distribution of lymphocyte subsets in a case of angiofollicular lymph node hyperplasia. American Journal of Clinical Pathology 82: 491–495

363. van den Oord J J, de Wolf-Peeters C, Desmet V J 1985 The paracortical area in reactive lymph nodes demonstrating sinus histiocytosis. An enzyme- and immunohistochemical study. Virchows Archiv B, Cell Pathology including Molecular Biology 48: 77– 85

364. van den Oord J J, de Wolf-Peeters C, Desmet V J 1985 Immunohistochemical analysis of progressively transformed follicular centres. American Journal of Clinical Pathology 83: 560–564

365. van den Oord J J, de Wolf-Peeters C, Desmet V J, Takahashi K, Ohtsuki Y, Akagi T 1985 Alteration of the paracortical area. An in situ immunohistochemical analysis of primary, secondary, and tertiary T-nodules. American Journal of Pathology 120: 55–66

366. van den Oord J J, de Wolf-Peeters C, de Vos R, Desmet V J 1985 Immature sinus histiocytosis. Light- and electron-microscopic features, immunologic phenotype, and relationship with marginal zone lymphocytes. American Journal of Pathology 118: 266–277

367. van den Oord J J, de Wolf-Peeters C, Desmet V J 1986 The composite nodule. A structural and functional unit of the reactive human lymph node. American Journal of Pathology 122: 83–91

368. van den Oord J J, de Wolf-Peeters C, Desmet V J 1986 The marginal zone in the human reactive lymph node. American Journal of Clinical Pathology 86: 475–479

369. van den Oord J J, de Wolf-Peeters C, de Vos R, Thomas J, Desmet V J 1986 Sarcoma arising from interdigitating reticulum cells: report of a case, studied with light and electron microscopy, and enzyme- and immunohistochemistry. Histopathology 10: 509–523

370. van der Loo E M, van Muijen G N P, van Vloten W A, Beens W, Scheffer E, Meijer C J L M 1979 C-type virus-like particles specifically localised in Langerhans cells and related cells of skin and lymph nodes of patients with mycosis fungoides and Sezary's syndrome. A morphological and biochemical study. Virchows Archiv B, Cell Pathology including Molecular Biology 31: 193–203

371. van der Valk P, van der Loo E M, Jansen J, Daha M R, Meijer C J L M 1984 Analysis of lymphoid and dendritic cells in human lymph node, tonsil and spleen. A study using monoclonal and heterologous antibodies. Virchows Archiv B, Cell Pathology including Molecular Biology 45: 169–185

371a. van Krieken J H J M, von Schilling C, Kluin M, Lennert K 1989 Splenic marginal zone lymphocytes and related cells in the lymph node: a morphologic and immunohistochemical study. Human Pathology 20: 320–325

372. van Maarsseven A C M T, Mullink H, Alons C L, Stam J 1986 Distribution of T-lymphocyte subsets in different portions of sarcoid granulomas: immunologic analysis with monoclonal antibodies. Human Pathology 17: 493–500

373. Velardi A, Tilden A B, Millo R, Grossi C E 1986 Isolation and characterization of Leu7[+] germinal-center cells with the T helper-cell phenotype and granular lymphocyte morphology. Journal of Clinical Immunology 6: 205–215

374. Vernon M L, Fountain L, Krebs H M, Horta-Barbosa L, Fuccillo D A, Sever J L 1973 Birbeck granules (Langerhans cell granules) in human lymph nodes. American Journal of Clinical Pathology 60: 771–779

375. Viale G, Codecasa L, Bulgheroni P, Giobbi A, Madonini E, Dell'Orto P, Coggi G 1986 T-cell subsets in sarcoidosis: an immunocytochemical investigation of blood, bronchoalveolar lavage fluid, and prescalenic lymph nodes from eight patients. Human Pathology 17: 476–481

376. Vollenweider R, Lennert K 1983 Plasmacytoid T-cell clusters in non-specific lymphadenitis. Virchows Archiv B, Cell Pathology including Molecular Biology 44: 1–14

377. Wakasa H, Takahashi H, Kimura N 1978 Necrotizing lymphadenitis. Recent Advances in RES Research 18: 85–95

378. Ward J M, O'Leary T J, Baskin G B, Benveniste R, Harris C A, Nara P L, Rhodes R H 1987 Immunohistochemical localization of human and simian immunodeficiency viral antigens in fixed tissue sections. American Journal of Pathology 127: 199–205

379. Warner T F C S, Uno H, Gabel C, Tsai C-C 1984 A comparative ultrastructural study of virions in human pre-AIDS and simian AIDS. Ultrastructural Pathology 7: 251–259

380. Watanabe S, Shimosato Y, Shimoyama M, Minato K, Suzuki M, Abe M, Nagatani T 1980 Adult T-Cell lymphoma with hypergammaglobulinaemia. Cancer 46: 2472–2483

381. Weisenburger D D, Nathwani B N, Winberg C D, Rappaport H 1985 Multicentric angiofollicular lymph node hyperplasia: a clinicopathologic study of 16 cases. Human Pathology 16: 162–172

382. Weisenburger D, Grierson H L, Purtilo D 1986 Immunologic studies of multicentric (M) and unicentric (U) angiofollicular

lymphoid hyperplasia (AFH). Laboratory Investigation 54: 68A (abs)

383. Weiss L M, Hu E, Wood G S, Moulds C, Cleary M L, Warnke R, Sklar J 1985 Clonal rearrangements of T-cell receptor genes in mycosis fungoides and dermatopathic lymphadenopathy. New England Journal of Medicine 313: 539–544

384. Weiss L M, Wood G S, Warnke, R A 1985 Immunophenotypic differences between dermatopathic lymphadenopathy and lymph node involvement in mycosis fungoides. American Journal of Pathology 120: 179–185

385. Weiss L M, Beckstead J H, Warnke, R A, Wood G S 1986 Leu-6-expressing cells in lymph nodes. Dendritic cells phenotypically similar to interdigitating cells. Human Pathology 17: 179–184

386. Weiss L M, Strickler J G, Dorfman R F, Horning S J, Warnke R A, Sklar J 1986 Clonal T-cell populations in angioimmunoblastic lymphadenopathy and angioimmunoblastic lymphadenopathy-like lymphoma. American Journal of Pathology 122: 392–397

387. Weiss R L, Kjeldsberg C R, Colby T V, Marty J 1985 Multilobated B cell lymphomas. A study of 7 cases. Hematological Oncology 3: 79–86

388. Willemze R, Scheffer E, Meijer C J L M 1985 Immunohistochemical studies using monoclonal antibodies on lymph nodes from patients with mycosis fungoides and Sezary's syndrome. American Journal of Pathology 120: 46–54

389. Willemze R, Cornelisse C J, Hermans J, Pardoel V P A M, van Vloten W A, Meijer C J L M 1986 Quantitative electron microscopy in the early diagnosis of cutaneous T-cell lymphomas. A long-term follow-up study of 77 patients. American Journal of Pathology 123: 166–173

390. Wolff K 1967 The fine structure of the Langerhans cell granule. Journal of Cell Biology 35: 468–473

391. Wolff K 1972 The Langerhans cell. Current Problems in Dermatology 4: 79–145

392. Wolff K, Stingl G 1983 The Langerhans cell. Journal of Investigative Dermatology 80: 17s–21s

393. Wood G S, Morhenn V B, Butcher E C, Kosek J 1984 Langerhans cells react with pan-leucocyte monoclonal antibody: ultrastructural documentation using a live cell suspension immunoperoxidase technique. Journal of Investigative Dermatology 82: 322–325

394. Wood G S, Burns B F, Dorfman R F, Warnke R A 1985 The immunohistology of non-T cells in the acquired immunodeficiency syndrome. American Journal of Pathology 120: 371–379

395. Wood G S, Turner R R, Shiurba R A, Eng L, Warnke R A 1985 Human dendritic cells and macrophages. In-situ immunophenotypic definition of subsets that exhibit specific morphologic and microenvironmental characteristics. American Journal of Pathology 119: 73–82

396. Wood G S, Burns B F, Dorfman R F, Warnke R A 1986 In-situ quantitation of lymph node helper, suppressor and cytotoxic T cell subsets in AIDS. Blood 67: 596–603

397. Wright D H, Richards D B 1981 Sinus histiocytosis with massive lymphadenopathy (Rosai–Dorfman disease): report of a case with widespread nodal and extranodal dissemination. Histopathology 5: 697–709 .

398. Yates P, Stockdill G, Mcintyre M 1986 Hypersensitivity to carbamazepine presenting as pseudolymphoma. Journal of Clinical Pathology 39: 1224–1228

399. York G C, Taylor C R, Lukes R J 1981 Monoclonality in giant lymph node hyperplasia. Laboratory Investigation 44: 77A (abs)

400. Ziegler T, Tubbs R, Alanis A, Calabrese L, Petras R, Weinstein A, Ahmad M, Bergfeld W 1983 Lymph node immunohistology in homosexual males with acquired immunodeficiency. Laboratory Investigation 48: 97A (abs)

Thymus gland

401. Auger C, Monier J C, Dardenne M, Pleau J M, Bach J F 1982 Identification of FTS (Facteur Thymique Sérique) on thymus ultrathin sections using monoclonal antibodies. Immunology Letters 5: 213–216

402. Auger C, Stahli C, Fabien N, Monier J-C 1987 Intracellular localization of thymosin alpha 1 by immunoelectron microscopy using a monoclonal antibody. Journal of Histochemistry and Cytochemistry 35: 181–187

403. Bach J F (ed) 1983 Thymic hormones. Clinics in immunology and allergy, vol 3, no. 1. Saunders, London

404. Balcolm R J, Hakanson D O, Werner A, Gordon L P 1985 Massive thymic hyperplasia in an infant with Beckwith-Wiedemann syndrome. Archives of Pathology and Laboratory Medicine 109: 153–155

405. Barnes E W, Irvine W J 1973 Clinical syndromes associated with thymic disorders. Proceedings of the Royal Society of Medicine 66: 151–154

406. Barthélémy H, Pelletier M, Landry D, Lafontaine M, Perreault C, Tautu C, Montplaisir S 1986 Demonstration of OKT6 antigen on human thymic dendritic cells in culture. Laboratory Investigation 55: 540–545

407. Bearman R M, Bensch K G, Levine G D 1975 The normal human thymic vasculature: an ultrastructural study. Anatomical Record 183: 485–498

408. Bearman R M, Levine G D, Bensch K G 1978 The ultrastructure of the normal human thymus: a study of 36 cases. Anatomical Record 190: 755–782

409. Beschorner W E, Hutchins G M, Elfenbein G J, Santos G W 1978 The thymus in patients with allogeneic bone marrow transplants. American Journal of Pathology 92: 173–186

410. Bhan A K, Reinherz E L, Poppema S, McCluskey R T, Schlossman S F 1980 Location of T cell and major histocompatibility complex antigens in the human thymus. Journal of Experimental Medicine 152: 771–782

411. Biggart J D, Nevin N C 1967 Hyperplasia of the thymus in progressive systemic sclerosis. Journal of Pathology and Bacteriology 93: 334–337

412. Blackburn W R, Gordon D S 1967 The thymic remnant in thymic alymphoplasia. Light and electron microscopic studies. Archives of Pathology 84: 363–375

413. Bloodworth J M B Jr, Hiratsuka H, Hickey R C, Wu J 1975 Ultrastructure of the human thymus, thymic tumours and myasthenia gravis. In: Sommers S C (ed) Pathology annual, vol. 10. Appleton–Century–Crofts, New York, pp 329–391

414. Bockman D E, Lawton A R, Cooper M D 1972 Fine structure of thymus after bone marrow transplantation in an infant with severe combined immunodeficiency. Laboratory Investigation 26: 227–239

415. Bodger M P, Francis G E, Delia D, Granger S M, Janossy G 1981 A monoclonal antibody specific for immature human hemopoietic cells and T lineage cells. Journal of Immunology 127: 2269–2274

416. Bofill M, Janossy G, Janossa M, Burford G D, Seymour G J, Wernet P, Kelemen E 1985 Human B cell development. II. Subpopulations in the human fetus. Journal of Immunology 134: 1531–1538

417. Bofill M, Janossy G, Willcox N, Chilosi M, Trejdosiewicz L K, Newsom-Davis J 1985 Microenvironments in the normal thymus and the thymus in myasthenia gravis. American Journal of Pathology 119: 462–473

418. Borzy M S, Schulte-Wissermann H, Gilbert E, Horowitz S D, Pellett J, Hong R 1979 Thymic morphology in immunodeficiency diseases: results of thymic biopsies. Clinical Immunology and Immunopathology 12: 31–51

419. Boyd A W 1987 Human leukocyte antigens: an update on structure, function and nomenclature. Pathology 19: 329–337

420. Bradstock K F, Janossy G, Pizzolo G, Hoffbrand A V, McMichael A, Pilch J R, Milstein C, Beverley P, Bollum F J 1980 Subpopulations of normal and leukemic human thymocytes: an analysis with the use of monoclonal antibodies. Journal of the National Cancer Institute 65: 33–42

421. Burnet F M, MacKay I R 1962 Lymphoepithelial structures and autoimmune disease. Lancet ii: 1030–1033

422. Carmosino L, DiBenedetto A, Feffer S 1985 Thymic hyperplasia following successful chemotherapy. Cancer 56: 1526–1528

423. Ceredig R, Lopez-Botet M, Moretta L 1984 Phenotypic and functional properties of mouse and human thymocytes. Seminars in Hematology 21: 244–256

424. Cordier A C, Haumont S M 1980 Development of thymus, parathyroids, and ultimo-branchial bodies in NMRI and nude mice. American Journal of Anatomy 157: 227–263

425. Cowan W K, Sorenson G D 1964 Electron microscopic observations of acute thymic involution produced by hydrocortisone. Laboratory Investigation 13: 353–370

426. Dalakas M C, Engel W K, McClure J E, Goldstein A L, Askanas V 1981 Immunocytochemical localization of thymosin alpha-1 in thymic epithelial cells of normal and myasthenia gravis patients and in thymic cultures. Journal of the Neurological Sciences 50: 239–247

427. Dardenne M, Bach J-F 1981 Thymic hormones. In: Kendall M D (ed) The thymus gland. Academic Press, London, pp 113–131

428. Dardenne M, Bach J-F, Safai B 1983 Low serum thymic hormone levels in patients with acquired immunodeficiency syndrome. New England Journal of Medicine 309: 48–49

429. Davis A E Jr 1984 The histopathological changes in the thymus gland in the acquired immune deficiency syndrome. Annals of the New York Academy of Sciences 437: 493–502

430. De Maagd R A, Mackenzie W A, Schuurman H-J, Ritter M A, Price K M, Broekhuizen R, Kater L 1985 The human thymus microenvironment: heterogeneity detected by monoclonal anti-epithelial cell antibodies. Immunology 54: 745–754

431. de Waal Malefijt R, Leene W, Roholl P J M, Wormmeester J, Hoeben K A 1986 T cell differentiation within thymic nurse cells. Laboratory Investigation 55: 25–34

432. Dourov N 1986 Thymic atrophy and immune deficiency in malnutrition. Current Topics in Pathology. 75: 127–150

433. Drenckhahn D, von Gaudecker B, Müller-Heimelink H K, Unsicker K, Groschel-Stewart U 1979 Myosin and actin containing cells in the human postnatal thymus. Ultrastructural and immunohistochemical findings in normal thymus and in myasthenia gravis. Virchows Archiv B, Cell Pathology including Molecular Biology 32: 33–45

434. Elie R, Laroche A C, Arnoux E, Guerin J-M, Pierre G, Malebranche R 1983 Thymic dysplasia in acquired immunodeficiency syndrome. New England Journal of Medicine 308: 841–842

435. Feltkamp-Vroom T 1966 Myoid cells in human thymus. Lancet i: 1320–1321

436. Foon K A, Todd R F III 1986 Immunologic classification of leukaemia and lymphoma. Blood 68: 1–31

437. Geenen V, Legros J-J, Franchimont P, Baudrihaye M, Defresne M-P, Boniver J 1986 The neuroendocrine thymus: co-existence of oxytocin and neurophysin in the human thymus. Science 232: 508–511

438. Goldstein A L, Low T L K, Thurman G B, Zatz M M, Hall N, Chen J, Hu S-K, Naylor P B, McClure J E 1981 Current status of thymosin and other hormones of the thymus gland. Recent Progress in Hormone Research 37: 369–415

439. Goldstein G, Mackay I R 1967 The thymus in systemic lupus erythematosus: a quantitative histopathological analysis and comparison with stress involution. British Medical Journal 2: 475–478

440. Goldstein G, Abbot A, Mackay I R 1968 An electron-microscope study of the human thymus: normal appearances and findings in myasthenia gravis and systemic lupus erythematosus. Journal of Pathology and Bacteriology 95: 211–215

441. Goldstein G, Mackay I R 1969 The human thymus. University Press, Glasgow

442. Gosseye S, Nezelof C 1981 T system immunodeficiencies in infancy and childhood. Pathology, Research and Practice 171: 142–158

443. Gosseye S, Diebold N, Griscelli C, Nezelof C 1983 Severe combined immunodeficiency disease: a pathological analysis of 26 cases. Clinical Immunology and Immunopathology 29: 58–77

444. Grissom J R, Durant J R, Whitley R J, Flint A 1983 Thymic hyperplasia in a case of Hodgkin's disease. Southern Medical Journal 76: 1189–1192

445. Grody W W, Fligiel S, Naeim F 1985 Thymus involution in the acquired immunodeficiency syndrome. American Journal of Clinical Pathology 84: 85–95

446. Habu S, Kameya T, Tamaoki N 1971 Thymic lymphoid follicles in autoimmune diseases. 1. Quantitative studies with special reference to myasthenia gravis. Keio Journal of Medicine 20: 45–56

447. Halicek F, Rosai J 1984 Histioeosinophilic granulomas in the thymuses of 29 myasthenic patients: a complication of pneumomediastinum. Human Pathology 15: 1137–1144

448. Haynes B F 1981 Human T-lymphocyte antigens as defined by monoclonal antibodies. Immunological Reviews 57: 127–161

449. Haynes B F, Robert-Guroff M, Metzgar R S, Franchini G, Kalyanaraman V S, Palker T J, Gallo R C 1983 Monoclonal antibody against human T-cell leukaemia virus p19 defines a human thymic epithelial antigen acquired during ontogeny. Journal of Experimental Medicine 157: 907–920

450. Haynes B F, Shimizu K, Eisenbarth G S 1983 Identification of human and rodent thymic epithelium using tetanus toxin and monoclonal antibody A2B5. Journal of Clinical Investigation 71: 9–14

451. Haynes B F, Warren R W, Buckley R H, McClure J E, Goldstein A L, Henderson F W, Hensley L L, Eisenbarth G S 1983 Demonstration of abnormalities in expression of thymic epithelial surface antigens in severe cellular immunodeficiency diseases. Journal of Immunology 130: 1182–1188

452. Haynes B F 1984 Phenotypic characterization and ontogeny of components of the human thymic microenvironment. Clinical Research 32: 500–507

453. Haynes B F 1984 The human thymic microenvironment. Advances in Immunology 36: 87–142

454. Haynes B F, Scearce R M, Lobach D F, Hensley L L 1984 Phenotypic characterization and ontogeny of mesodermal-derived and endocrine epithelial components of the human thymic microenvironment. Journal of Experimental Medicine 159: 1149–1168

455. Haynes B F 1986 Summary of T cell studies performed during the Second International Workshop and Conference on Human Leukocyte Differentiation Antigens. In: Reinherz E L, Haynes B F, Nadler L M, Bernstein I D (eds) Leukocyte typing II, vol. 1. Human T-lymphocytes. Springer-Verlag, Berlin, pp 3–30

456. Hayward A R 1972 Myoid cells in the human foetal thymus. Journal of Pathology 106: 45–49

457. Henry K 1966 Mucin secretion and striated muscle in the human thymus. Lancet i: 183–185

458. Henry K 1968 Striated muscle in human thymus. Lancet i: 638–639

459. Henry K 1968 The thymus in rheumatic heart disease. Clinical and Experimental Immunology 3: 509–523

460. Henry K, Petts V 1969 Nuclear bodies in human thymus. Journal of Ultrastructure Research 27: 330–343

461. Henry K 1972 An unusual thymic tumour with a striated muscle (myoid) component (with a brief review of the literature on myoid cells). British Journal of Diseases of the Chest 66: 291–299

462. Henry K 1981 The human thymus in disease with particular emphasis on thymitis and thymoma. In: Kendall M D (ed) The thymus gland. Academic Press, London, pp 85–111

463. Henry K, Farrer-Brown G 1981 A colour atlas of thymus and lymph node histopathology with ultrastructure. Wolfe Medical Publications, London

464. Henry L 1968 'Accidental' involution of the human thymus. Journal of Pathology and Bacteriology 96: 337–343

465. Henry L, Anderson G 1987 Epithelial-cell architecture during involution of the human thymus. Journal of Pathology 152: 149–155

466. Higley H R, Rowden G 1984 Thymic interdigitating reticulum cells demonstrated by immunocytochemistry. Thymus 6: 243–253

467. Hirokawa K 1969 Electron microscopic observation of the human thymus of the fetus and the newborn. Acta Pathologica Japonica 19: 1–13

468. Hirokawa K, McClure J E, Goldstein A L 1982 Age-related changes in localization of thymosin in the human thymus. Thymus 4: 19–29

469. Hirokawa K, Utsuyama M, Moriizumi E, Handa S 1986 Analysis of the thymic microenvironment by monoclonal antibodies with special reference to thymic nurse cells. Thymus 8: 349–360

470. Hofmann W J, Momburg F, Möller P 1988 Thymic medullary cells expressing B lymphocyte antigens. Human Pathology 19: 1280–1287

471. Hoshino T, Kukita A, Sato S 1970 Cells containing Birbeck granules (Langerhans cell granules) in the human thymus. Journal of Electron Microscopy 19: 271–276

472. Isaacson P G, Norton A J, Addis B J 1987 The human thymus contains a normal population of B lymphocytes. Lancet ii: 1488–1491

473. Jambon B, Montagne P, Bene M-C, Brayer M-P, Faure G, Duheille J 1981 Immunohistologic localization of 'facteur thymique sérique' (FTS) in human thymic epithelium. Journal of Immunology 127: 2055–2059

474. Janossy G, Thomas J A, Bollum F J, Granger S, Pizzolo G, Bradstock K F, Wong L, McMichael A, Ganeshaguru K, Hoffbrand A V 1980 The human thymic microenvironment: an immunohistologic study. Journal of Immunology 125: 202–212

475. Janossy G, Tidman N, Papageorgiou E S, Kung P C, Goldstein G 1981 Distribution of T lymphocyte subsets in the human bone marrow and thymus: an analysis with monoclonal antibodies. Journal of Immunology 126: 1608–1613

476. Janossy G, Bofill M, Trejdosiewicz L K, Willcox H N A, Chilosi M 1986 Cellular differentiation of lymphoid subpopulations and their microenvironments in the human thymus. Current Topics in Pathology 75: 89–125

477. Jones D L, Thomas K, Williams W J 1975 A fine structure study of human thymus. Beiträge zur Pathologie 156: 387–400

478. Joshi V V, Oleske M M 1985 Pathologic appraisal of the thymus gland in acquired immune deficiency syndrome in children. Archives of Pathology and Laboratory Medicine 109: 142–146

479. Joshi V V, Oleske J M, Saad S, Gadol C, Connor E, Bobila R, Minnefor A B 1986 Thymus biopsy in children with acquired immunodeficiency syndrome. Archives of Pathology and Laboratory Medicine 110: 837–842

480. Judd R L 1987 Massive thymic hyperplasia with myoid cell differentiation. Human Pathology 18: 1180–1183

481. Kaiserling K, Stein H, Müller-Hermelink H K 1974 Interdigitating reticulum cells in the human thymus. Cell and Tissue Research 155: 47–55

482. Kameya T, Watanabe Y 1965 Electron microscopic observations on human thymus and thymoma. Acta Pathologica Japonica 15: 223–246

483. Kao I, Drachman D B 1977 Thymic muscle cells bear acetylcholine receptors: possible relation to myasthenia gravis. Science 19: 74–75

484. Katz S M, Chatten J, Bishop H C, Rosenblum H 1977 Massive thymic enlargement. Report of a case of gross thymic hyperplasia in a child. American Journal of Clinical Pathology 68: 786–790

485. Kendall M D, Johnson H R M, Singh J 1980 The weight of the human thymus gland at necropsy. Journal of Anatomy 131: 485–499

486. Kendall M D 1981 The cells of the thymus. In: Kendall M D (ed) The thymus gland. Academic Press, London, pp 63–83

487. Kendall M D, van de Wijngaert F P, Schuurman H-J, Rademakers L H P M, Kater L 1985 Heterogeneity of the human thymus epithelial microenvironment at the ultrastructural level. Advances in Experimental Medicine and Biology 186: 289–297

488. Kirchner T, Schalke B, Melms A, von Kugelgen, Müller-Hermelink H K 1986 Immunohistological patterns of non-neoplastic changes in the thymus in myasthenia gravis. Virchows Archiv B, Cell Pathology including Molecular Biology 52: 237–257

489. Kirchner T, Tzartos S, Hoppe F, Schalke B, Wekerle H, Müller-Hermelink H K 1988 Pathogenesis of myasthenia gravis. Acetylcholine receptor-related antigenic determinants in tumor-free thymuses and thymic epithelial tumours. American Journal of Pathology 130: 268–280

490. Kornstein M J, Brooks J J, Anderson A O, Levinson A I, Lisak R P, Zweiman B 1984 The immunohistology of the thymus in myasthenia gravis. American Journal of Pathology 117: 184–194

491. Kyewski B A, Kaplan H S 1982 Lymphoepithelial interactions in the mouse thymus: phenotypic and kinetic studies on thymic nurse cells. Journal of Immunology 128: 2287–2294

492. Kyewski B A 1986 Thymic nurse cells: possible sites of T-cell selection. Immunology Today 7: 374–379

493. Lack E E 1981 Thymic hyperplasia with massive enlargement: report of two cases with review of diagnostic criteria. Journal of Thoracic and Cardiovascular Surgery 81: 741–746

494. Landing B H, Yutuc I L, Swanson V L 1978 Clinicopathologic correlations in immunologic deficiency diseases of children, with emphasis on thymic histologic patterns. In: Kobayashi N (ed) Immunodeficiency: its nature and etiological significance in human diseases. University Park Press, Baltimore, pp 3–35

495. Le Douarin N M, Jotereau F V 1975 Tracing of cells of the avian thymus through embryonic life in interspecific chimeras. Journal of Experimental Medicine 142: 17–40

496. Le Douarin N M, Jotereau F V 1981 The ontogeny of the thymus. In: Kendall M D (ed) The thymus gland. Academic Press, London, pp 37–62

497. Levine G D, Rice D D F 1977 A revised concept of the location of thymic germinal centers in myasthenia gravis: an ultrastructural and immunologic study. Laboratory Investigation 36: 345A (abs)

498. Levine G D, Rosai J 1978 Thymic hyperplasia and neoplasia: a review of current concepts. Human Pathology 9: 495–515

499. Lewis V M, Twomey J J, Bealmear P, Goldstein G, Good R A 1978 Age, thymic involution, and circulating thymic hormone activity. Journal of Clinical Endocrinology and Metabolism 47: 145–150

500. Lobach D F, Scearce R M, Haynes B F 1985 The human thymic microenvironment. Phenotypic characterization of Hassall's bodies with the use of monoclonal antibodies. Journal of Immunology 134: 250–257

501. Mackay I R, de Gail P 1963 Thymic 'germinal centres' and plasma cells in systemic lupus erythematosus. Lancet ii: 667

502. Mackay I R, Masel M, Burnet F M 1964 Thymic abnormality in systemic lupus erythematosus. Australasian Annals of Medicine 13: 5–14

503. MacSween R N M, Anderson J R, Milne J A 1967 Histological appearances of the thymus in systemic lupus erythematosus and rheumatoid arthritis. Journal of Pathology and Bacteriology 93: 611–619

504. McFarland E J, Scearce R M, Haynes B F 1984 The human thymic microenvironment: cortical thymic epithelium is an antigenically distinct region of the thymic microenvironment. Journal of Immunology 133: 1241–1249

505. McMichael A J, Gotch F M 1987 T-cell antigens: new and previously defined clusters. In: McMichael A J (ed) Leucocyte typing III. White cell differentiation antigens. Oxford University Press, Oxford, pp 31–62

506. Michie W, Swanson Beck J S, Mahaffey R G, Honein E F, Fowler G B 1967 Quantitative radiological and histological studies of the thymus in thyroid disease. Lancet i: 691–695

507. Müller-Hermelink H K, Steinman G, Stein H 1982 Structural and functional alterations of the aging human thymus. Advances in Experimental Medicine and Biology 149: 303–312

508. Müller-Hermelink H K, Steinmann G G 1984 Age-related alterations of intrathymic micro-environments. In: de Weck A I (ed) Lymphoid cell functions in aging. Topics in aging research in Europe, vol. 3. Eurage, Rijswijk, pp 75–82

509. Müller-Hermelink H K, Sale G, Borisch B, Storb R 1987 Pathology of the thymus after allogeneic bone marrow transplantation in man. A histologic immunohistochemical study of 36 patients. American Journal of Pathology 129: 242–256

510. Nezelof C 1986 Pathology of the thymus in immunodeficiency states. Current Topics in Pathology 75: 151–177

511. Norris E H 1938 The morphogenesis and histogenesis of the thymus gland in man: in which the origin of the Hassall's corpuscles of the human thymus is discovered. Contributions to Embryology 27: 191–207

512. Oates K K, Goldstein A L 1984 Thymosins: hormones of the thymus gland. Trends in Pharmacological Sciences 5: 347–352

513. O'Shea P A, Pansatiankul B, Farnes P 1978 Giant thymic hyperplasia in infancy: immunologic, histologic, and ultrastructural observations. Laboratory Investigation 38: 39IA (abs)

514. Palestro G, Tridente G, Micca F B, Novero D, Valente G, Godio L 1983 Immunohistochemical and enzyme histochemical contributions to the problem concerning the role of the thymus in the pathogenesis of myasthenia gravis. Virchows Archiv B, Cell Pathology including Molecular Biology 44: 173–186

515. Pelletier M, Tautu C, Landry D, Montplaisir S, Chartrand C, Perreault C 1986 Characterization of human thymic dendritic cells in culture. Immunology 58: 263–270

516. Puchtler H, Meloan S N, Branch B W, Gropp S 1975 Myoepithelial cells in human thymus: staining, polarization and fluorescence microscopic studies. Histochemistry 45: 163–176

517. Reinherz E L, Schlossman S F 1980 The differentiation and function of human T lymphocytes. Cell 19: 821–827

518. Reinherz E L, Kung P C, Goldstein G, Levey R H, Schlossman S F 1980 Discrete stages of human intrathymic differentiation: analysis of normal thymocytes and leukemic lymphoblasts of T-cell lineage. Proceedings of the National Academy of Sciences of the USA 77: 1588–1592

519. Ritter M A, Sauvage C A, Cotmore S F 1981 The human thymus microenvironment: in vivo identification of thymic nurse cells and other antigenically-distinct subpopulations of epithelial cells. Immunology 44: 439–446

520. Ritter M A, Schuurmann H-J, MacKenzie W A, deMaagd R A, Price K M, Brockhuizan R, Kater L 1985 Heterogeneity of human thymus epithelial cells revealed by monoclonal anti-epithelial cell antibodies. Advances in Experimental Medicine and Biology 186: 283–288

521. Rosai J, Levine G D 1976 Tumours of the thymus. Atlas of tumour pathology, second series, fascicle 13. Armed Forces Institute of Pathology, Washington, DC

522. Rouse R V, Parkam P, Grumet F C, Weissman I L 1982 Expression of HLA antigens by human thymic epithelial cells. Human Immunology 5: 21–34

523. Sale G E 1984 Pathology of the lymphoreticular system. In: Sale G E, Shulman H M (eds) The pathology of bone marrow transplantation. Masson, New York, pp 171–191

524. Savino W, Dardenne M 1984 Thymic hormone-containing cells. VI. Immunohistologic evidence for the simultaneous presence of thymulin, thymopoietin and thymosin alpha-1 in normal and pathological human thymuses. European Journal of Immunology 14: 987–991

525. Savino W, Dardenne M, Marche C, Trophilme D, Dupuy J-M, Pekovic D, Lapointe M, Bach J-F 1986 Thymic epithelium in AIDS. An immunohistologic study. American Journal of Pathology 122: 302–307

526. Scadding G K, Vincent A, Newsom-Davis J, Henry K 1981 Acetylcholine receptor antibody synthesis by thymic lymphocytes: correlation with thymic histology. Neurology 31: 935–943

527. Schmitt D, Monier J C, Dardenne M, Pleau J M, Deschaux P, Bach J F 1980 Cytoplasmic localization of FTS (facteur thymique sérique) in thymic epithelial cells. An immunoelectronmicroscopical study. Thymus 2: 177–186

528. Schulof R S, Low T L K, Thurman G B, Goldstein A L 1981 Thymosins and other hormones of the thymus gland. Progress in Clinical and Biological Research 58: 191–215

529. Schulof R S 1985 Thymic peptide hormones: basic properties and clinical applications in cancer. Critical Reviews In Oncology/Haematology 3: 309–376

530. Schuurman H J, Van de Wijngaert F P, Delvoye L, Broekhuizen R, McClure J E, Goldstein A L, Kater L 1985 Heterogeneity and age dependency of human thymus reticuloepithelium in production of thymosin components. Thymus 7: 13–23

531. Schuurman H J, Ritter M A, Broekhuizen R, Ladyman H, Larche M 1987 The thymic epithelium panel of antibodies: immunohistologic analysis of human tissues. In: McMichael A J (ed) Leucocyte typing III. White cell differentiation antigens. Oxford University Press, Oxford, pp 259–262

532. Seemayer T A, Lapp W S, Bolande R P 1977 Thymic involution in murine graft-versus-host reaction. Epithelial injury mimicking human thymic dysplasia. American Journal of Pathology 88: 119–134

533. Seemayer T A, Lapp W S, Bolande R P 1978 Thymic epithelial injury in graft-versus-host reactions following adrenalectomy. American Journal of Pathology 93: 325–338

534. Seemayer T A, Bolande R P 1980 Thymic involution mimicking thymic dysplasia. A consequence of transfusion-induced graft versus host disease in a premature infant. Archives of Pathology and Laboratory Medicine 104: 141–144

535. Seemayer T A, Laroche A C, Russo P, Malebranche R, Arnoux E, Guerin J-M, Pierre G, Dupuy J-M, Gartner J G, Lapp W S, Spira

536. Shin M S, Ho K-J 1983 Diffuse thymic hyperplasia following chemotherapy for nodular sclerosing Hodgkin's disease. An immunologic rebound phenomenon? Cancer 51: 30–33

537. Singh J 1981 The ultrastructure of epithelial reticular cells. In: Kendall M D (ed) The thymus gland. Academic Press, London, pp 133–149

538. Söderström N, Axelsson J-A, Hagelqvist E 1970 Postcapillary venules of the lymph node type in the thymus in myasthenia. Laboratory Investigation 23: 451–458

539. Steinmann G G, Müller-Hermelink H K 1984 Immunohistological demonstration of terminal transferase (TdT) in the age-involuted human thymus. Immunobiology 166: 45–52

540. Steinmann G G, Müller-Hermelink H K 1984 Lymphocyte differentiation and its microenvironment in the human thymus during aging. Monographs in Developmental Biology 17: 142–155

541. Steinmann G G 1986 Changes in the human thymus during aging. Current Topics in Pathology 75: 43–87

542. Tamaoki N, Habu S, Kameya T 1971 Thymic lymphoid follicles in autoimmune diseases. II. Histological, histochemical and electron microscopic studies. Keio Journal of Medicine 20: 57–68

543. Thomas J A, Willcox H N A, Newsom-Davis J 1982 Immunohistological studies of the thymus in myasthenia gravis. Correlation with clinical state and thymocyte culture responses. Journal of Neuroimmunology 3: 319–335

544. Thomas J A, Sloane J P, Imrie S F, Ritter M A, Schuurman H-J, Huber J 1986 Immunohistology of the thymus in bone marrow transplant recipients. American Journal of Pathology 122: 531–540

545. Tidman N, Janossy G, Bodger M, Granger S, Kung P C, Goldstein G 1981 Delineation of human thymocyte differentiation pathways utilizing double-staining techniques with monoclonal antibodies. Clinical and Experimental Immunology 45: 457–467

546. Tridente G 1985 Immunopathology of the human thymus. Seminars in Haematology 22: 55–67

547. Vakharia D D, Mitchison N A 1984 Thymic epithelial cells derived from the cultures of thymic nurse cells. Immunology Letters 7: 261–266

548. Van de Velde R L, Friedman N B 1970 Thymic myoid cells and myasthenia gravis. American Journal of Pathology 59: 347–368

549. Van de Wijngaert F P, Rademakers L H P M, Schuurman H-J, De Weger R A, Kater L 1983 Identification and in-situ localization of the 'thymic nurse cell' in man. Journal of Immunology 130: 2348–2351

550. Van de Wijngaert F P, Kendall M D, Schuurman H-J, Rademakers L H P M, Kater L 1984 Heterogeneity of epithelial cells in the human thymus. An ultrastructural study. Cell and Tissue Research 237: 227–237

551. Van Herle A J, Chopra I J 1971 Thymic hyperplasia in Graves' disease. Journal of Clinical Endocrinology and Metabolism 32: 140–146

552. Van Vliet E, Melis M, van Ewijk 1984 Immunohistology of thymic nurse cells. Cellular Immunology 87: 101–109

553. Vetters J M, MacAdam R F 1973 Fine structural evidence for hormone secretion by the human thymus. Journal of Clinical Pathology 26: 194–197

554. von Gaudecker B, Schmale E-M 1974 Similarities between Hassal's corpuscles of the human thymus and the epidermis. An investigation by electron microscopy and histochemistry. Cell and Tissue Research 151: 347–368

555. von Gaudecker B 1978 Ultrastructure of the age-involuted adult human thymus. Cell and Tissue Research 186: 507–525

556. von Gaudecker B, Müller-Hermelink H-K 1980 Ontogeny and organization of the stationary non-lymphoid cells in the human thymus. Cell and Tissue Research 207: 287–306

557. von Gaudecker B, Müller-Hermelink H-K 1982 Ultrastructural investigation of the lympho-epithelial and the lympho-mesenchymal interactions in the ontogeny of the human thymus. In: Fabris N (ed) Immunology and aging. Developments in hematology and immunology, vol. 3. Nijhoff, The Hague, pp 51–58

558. von Gaudecker B 1986 The development of the human thymus microenvironment. Current Topics in Pathology 75: 1–41

T J, ElIe R 1984 Precocious thymic involution manifest by epithelial injury in the acquired immune deficiency syndrome. Human Pathology 15: 469–474

559. von Gaudecker B, Steinmann G G, Hansmann M-L, Harpprecht J, Milicevic N M, Müller-Hermelink H-K 1986 Immunohistochemical characterization of the thymic microenvironment. A light-microscopic and ultrastructural immunocytochemical study. Cell and Tissue Research 244: 403–412

560. Weissman I L, Rouse R V, Kyewski B A, Lepault F, Butcher E C, Kaplan H S, Scollay R G 1982 Thymic lymphocyte maturation in the thymic micro-environment. Behring Institute Mitteilungen 70: 242–251

561. Wekerle H, Ketelson U P, Zurn A D, Fulpius B W 1978 Intrathymic pathogenesis of myasthenia gravis: transient expression of acetylcholine receptors on thymus-derived myogenic cells. European Journal of Immunology 8: 579–582

562. Wekerle H, Ketelsen U-P 1980 Thymic nurse cells — Ia-bearing epithelium involved in T-lymphocyte differentiation? Nature 283: 402–404

563. Wekerle H, Ketelsen U-P, Ernst M 1980 Thymic nurse cells. Lymphoepithelial cell complexes in murine thymuses: morphological and serological characterization. Journal of Experimental Medicine 151: 925–944

564. Wekerle H, Müller-Hermelink H-K 1986 The thymus in myasthenia gravis. Current Topics in Pathology 75: 179–206

565. Wiersbowsky-Schmeel A, Helpap B, Totovic V, Grouls V 1984 Thymus in myasthenia gravis: a light and electron microscopic study of a case with thymic follicular hyperplasia. Pathology, Research and Practice 178: 323–331

566. Wolff M, Rosai J, Wright D H 1984 Sebaceous glands within the thymus: report of three cases. Human Pathology 15: 341–343

567. Zatz M M, Goldstein A L 1985 Thymosins, lymphokines, and the immunology of aging. Gerontology 31: 263–277

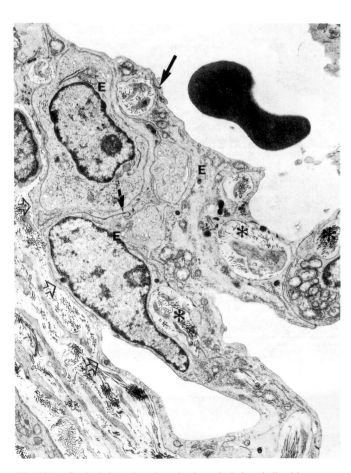

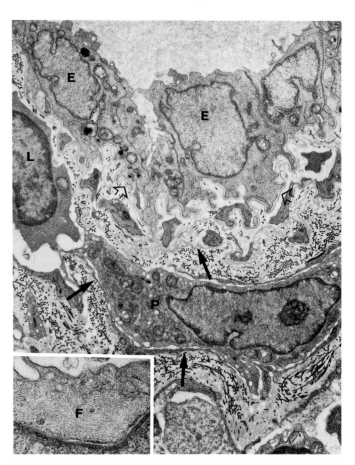

Fig. 29.1 Cortical sinus: lymph node. A cortical sinus is lined by endothelial cells (E) resting on a continuous basal lamina (open arrows), and is invested by collagen and stromal cell processes. Tight junctions (arrows) are evident between endothelial cells. Projections of the sinus wall extend across the lumen, where pockets of stroma are seen surrounded by endothelium (asterisks). (× 39 300)

The endothelial lining and basal lamina of the marginal sinus outer wall, and trabecular side of the deep cortical sinuses is continuous, whereas endothelial gaps are evident along the inner wall of the marginal sinus, the parenchymal aspect of intermediate sinuses, and in the medullary sinus walls.[91] Here the endothelium may rest directly on collagen fibres or ground substance.[182] Organelles are most abundant in endothelial cells of intermediate and medullary sinuses and may include well-developed Golgi zones, endoplasmic reticulum and numerous vesicles. References: 91, 165, 182 and 213.

Fig. 29.2 High endothelial venule: lymph node. This HEV is lined by distinctive plump, tall endothelial cells (E) having pale cytoplasm due to the high content of cytoplasmic intermediate filaments (see inset). A basal lamina (open arrows) invests the endothelium and also surrounds a pericytic cell (P) and pericytic processes (arrows) on their abluminal aspects. A migrating lymphocyte (L) is present in the space between the pericytic layer and endothelial basal lamina. (× 13 860) *Inset* This details the cytoplasmic aspect of an endothelial cell, displaying a rich network of vimentin intermediate filaments (IF) and prominent pinocytotic vesicles. (× 25 800)

The endothelial cells typically have well-developed tight junctions and complex cytoplasmic interdigitations. The Golgi zone, smooth vesicles and tubular elements of the SER, and RER are all well-developed, and Weibel–Palade bodies may be prominent. The basal lamina has a distinctive complex structure[99] and is associated with a network of collagen fibrils and pericytic processes rich in myofilaments and mitochondria.

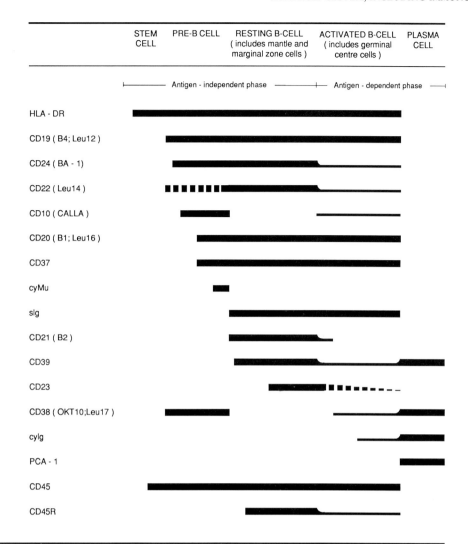

Abbreviations: cy = cytoplasmic; s = surface. In parentheses are some prototype antibodies recognising leucocyte associated antigens defined by the CD nomenclature system.

Comments: CD22 antibodies bind strongly to follicular mantle and marginal zone B cells, and weakly to germinal centre cells, but the antigen is present in the cytoplasm of almost all B cells, and appears at approximately the same time as the CD19 antigen in B-progenitor cells. In resting B cells, the CD22 antigen is expressed on the cell surface, and disappears with activation. CD10, while strongly expressed on centroblastic/centrocytic lymphoma cells, shows only limited distribution on normal germinal centre cells.
CD23 appears to be a low affinity receptor for Fc of IgE. It is variably expressed on follicular mantle cells, but while some resting B cells increase their CD23 expression upon activation, those in germinal centres do not express surface CD23.

References: 7,36,133,136,138,139,173a,183,189,196,227-230,240,282,328-330,371.

Fig. 29.3 B-cell differentiation.

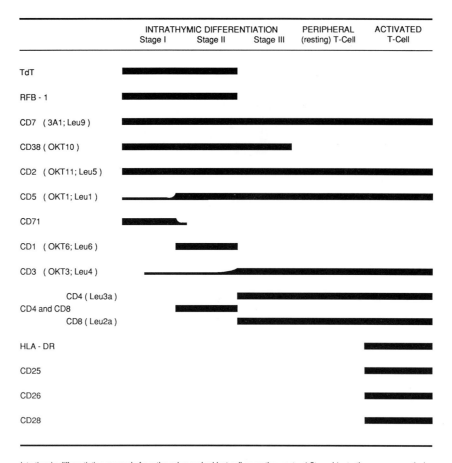

Intrathymic differentiation proceeds from the subcapsular blast cell or prothymocyte (Stage I), to the common cortical thymocyte (Stage II), to the mature medullary thymocyte (Stage III).

In parentheses are some prototype antibodies recognising leucocyte associated antigens defined by the CD nomenclature system.

References: 81, 136, 140, 150, 173a, 274, 282, 371, 410, 415, 419, 420, 423, 436, 448, 452, 455, 474-476, 505, 517, 518, 545.

Fig. 29.4 T-cell differentiation.

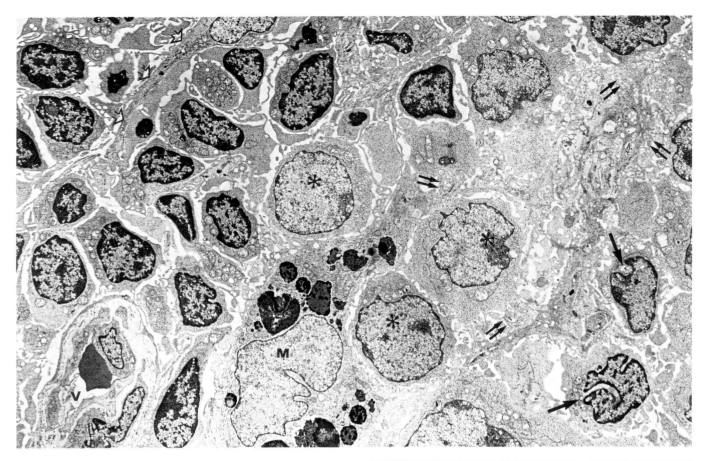

Fig. 29.5 (Above) Reactive lymphoid follicle: lymph node. Portion of a reactive lymphoid follicle is illustrated, whose mantle zone (left) is composed of small lymphocytes having little cytoplasm and heterochromatinic nuclei. A long tapering myofibroblastic cell process (open arrows) courses between mantle lymphocytes, and a vessel (V) can be seen entering the follicle. Within the germinal centre can be found several large non-cleaved lymphocytes (asterisks), small cleaved lymphocytes (arrows), and a tingible body macrophage (M) replete with dense heterophagosomes. A network of delicate cytoplasmic processes originating from dendritic reticulum cells occupies the cellular interstices (double arrows). (× 3700) See Table 29.1.

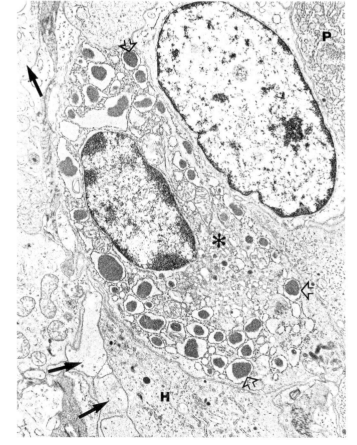

Fig. 29.6 (Right) Plasma cell: lymph node paracortex. The nucleus of this plasma cell shows the characteristic marginal masses of heterochromatin. The RER cisternae are distended by electron-dense secretory material (open arrows) consistent with immunoglobulin. Such intracisternal accumulation of secretions may be very large, resulting in the Russell bodies seen histologically. A well-developed Golgi zone with associated vesicles (asterisk) would appear as a paranuclear *hof* light-microscopically. Portions of a histiocyte (H), another plasma cell (P) and processes of IDRC (arrows) are also evident in this micrograph. (× 69 700)

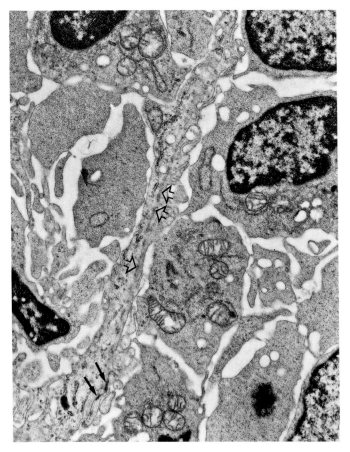

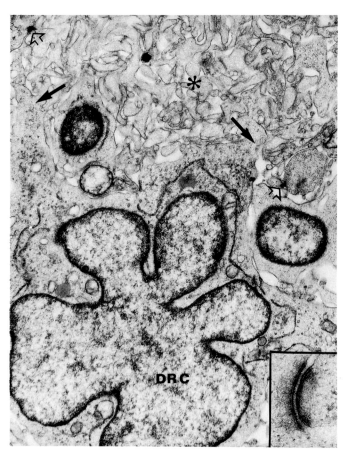

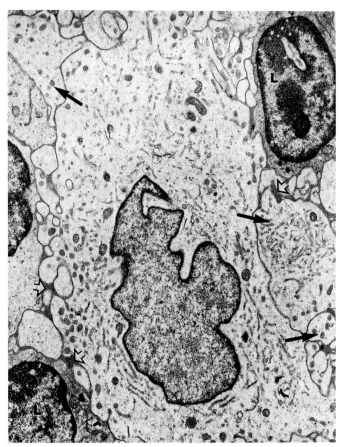

Fig. 29.7 (Above) Fibroblastic reticulum cell: lymph node. Coursing through the mantle zone of a lymphoid follicle is a long cytoplasmic process of a fibroblastic reticulum cell. Fascicles of ill-defined thin filaments with focal densities (open arrows) are seen in the cytoplasm along with short profiles of RER. Intermediate junctions (arrows) are formed with other processes. (× 7700) See Table 29.3.

Fig. 29.8 (Above right) Follicular dendritic reticulum cell: lymph node. A follicular dendritic reticulum cell (DRC) and a labyrinth of DRC cytoplasmic processes (asterisk) separate two small lymphocytes. Broad cytoplasmic extensions emanate from the DRC (arrows) and ramify into smaller processes. Desmosomes between some of the DRC processes are evident (open arrows) (× 11 300). *Inset* A desmosome between DRC processes. (× 42 400) See Table 29.3.

Fig. 29.9 (Right) Interdigitating reticulum cell: lymph node paracortex. This IDRC in the paracortex of a reactive lymph node possesses abundant pale cytoplasm, and has a characteristically irregular nucleus. Many broad cytoplasmic processes arise from the cell (arrows), interdigitate with those of other IDRC and come into intimate contact with paracortical lymphocytes (L). Electron-dense granular material coats the cytoplasmic processes (open arrows). Note that lysosomes are few, the smooth ER is well-developed and phagocytic activity is absent. (× 6000)

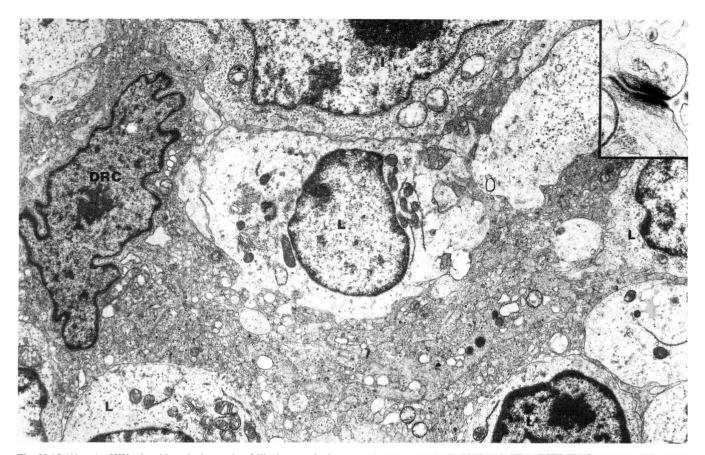

Fig. 29.10 (Above)   HIV-related lymphadenopathy: follicular germinal centre. This low-power micrograph illustrates a portion of a follicular germinal centre in a patient with HIV-related PGL. The lymph node histology revealed florid follicular hyperplasia. A hypertrophied dendritic reticulum cell (DRC) with its characteristically serrated nucleus, gives rise to a complex labyrinth of cytoplasmic processes separating and partly surrounding several large lymphoid cells (L) and an immunoblast (I). In the interstices of the labyrinth there are myriads of small dense, rounded particles, not further resolved at this magnification. (× 4950) *Inset* Detail of a desmosome between DRC cytoplasmic processes which contain prominent cytoplasmic microfilaments. On the surface of one of the processes can be seen a round membrane-bound particle, 95 nm in diameter, containing a somewhat conical dense core, consistent with an HIV virion. (× 23 100)

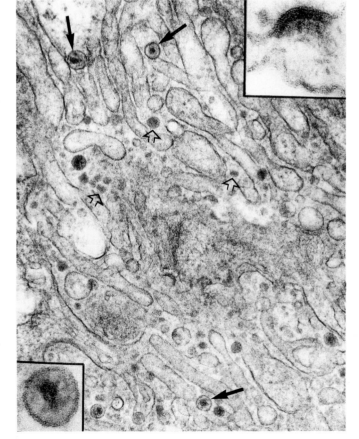

Fig. 29.11 (Right)   Germinal centre DRC labyrinth: HIV-related lymphadenopathy. Detail of a DRC labyrinth with numerous swollen cytoplasmic processes is illustrated. In the interstices there are numerous rounded particles of varying morphology. Some (arrows), as detailed in the *left inset*, have a distinct membrane, and a well-defined, often eccentric, dense core. In the setting of HIV-seropositivity in this case, these particles are consistent with human immunodeficiency virus. The true nature of the other amorphous rounded particles (open arrows) cannot be ascertained. (× 45 540) *Right inset* A developmental viral particle budding from the surface of a swollen DRC process. (Left inset, × 132 000; right inset, × 138 600)

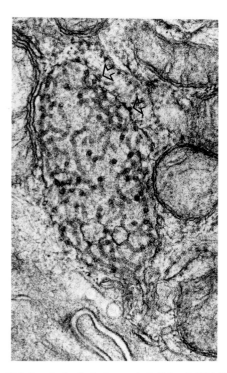

Fig. 29.12 Tubuloreticular inclusion: endothelial cell. This TRI in an endothelial cell from a patient with PGL displays typical branching tubules containing electron-dense material, located within a dilated segment of the RER. Ribosomal particles (open arrows) can be seen attached to the cisternal membrane. (× 75 900)

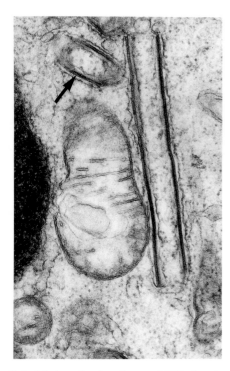

Fig. 29.13 Cylindrical confronting cisternae (CCC): lymphocyte. Cylindrical confronting cisternae of the RER have given rise to this inclusion in the cytoplasm of a lymphocyte from a patient with HIV infection. A second, obliquely-sectioned, ellipsoid CCC is also present (arrow). (× 36 000)

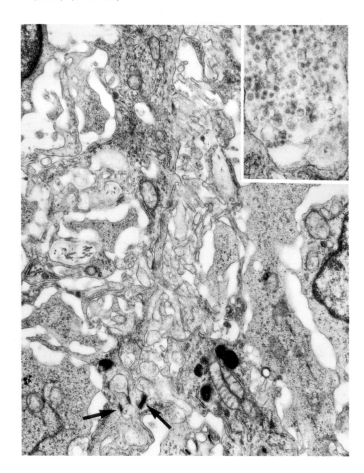

Fig. 29.14 (Right) Localized Castleman's disease, hyaline-vascular type: germinal centre. An abnormal germinal centre from a patient with CD, HV type, is illustrated. An elaborate network of DRC cytoplasmic processes is evident, with desmosomal attachments present between some processes (arrows). In some of the HV germinal centres amorphous granular material, sometimes spherular in outline, and occasional vesicular structures, were present in the interstices of the DRC processes (*inset*). This material possibly represents antigen–antibody complexes, and is not to be confused with viral particles. (× 12 200; inset, × 36 000)

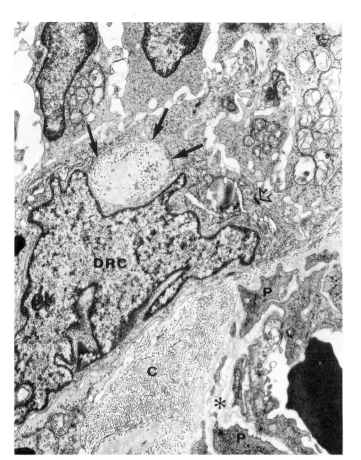

Fig. 29.15 (Left)   Localized Castleman's disease, HV type: germinal centre. A vessel entering an HV germinal centre is surrounded by several pericytic cell processes (P), reduplicated layers of external lamina (asterisk) and a mantle of collagen (C). Focal collections of fine filamentous material are present within this collagen, and also entrapped by processes (arrows) of a dendritic reticulum cell (DRC); the latter has a markedly irregular nucleus, and a small desmosome is evident between two cytoplasmic processes (open arrow). Two small lymphocytes, consistent with mantle lymphocytes are present in the upper left of the field. (× 7550)

Fig. 29.16 (Below)   Sinus histiocytosis: lymph node. This is a panoramic view of a deep cortical sinus in a lymph node showing prominent sinus histiocytosis histologically. The outline of one of the sinus walls is indicated by the dashed line. The sinus endothelium (S) often rests directly on collagen fibres, without any intervening external lamina. Projections of endothelium investing cores of stroma (arrows) extend across the sinus lumen (L) which is all but obliterated by the masses of reactive histiocytes. The histiocytes possess indented nuclei, and their cytoplasm is replete with heterophagosomes including myelinoid bodies (open arrows) and electron-dense erythrocyte fragments (asterisks). Some of the histiocytes display elaborate filopodia (double arrows). In the lower right of the field are small lymphocytes, and a stromal myofibroblast (mf) with a long cytoplasmic process. (× 3450)

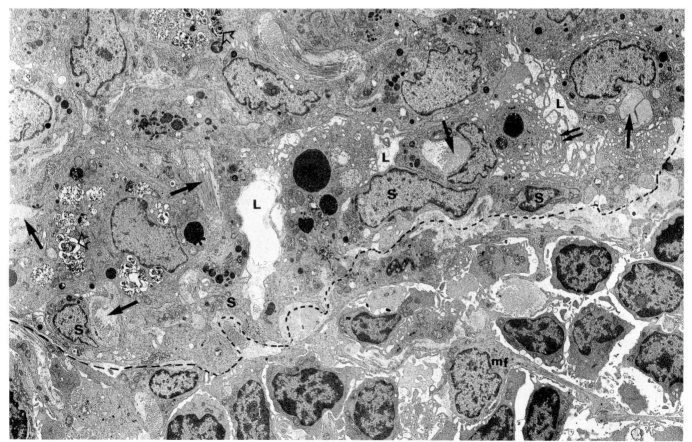

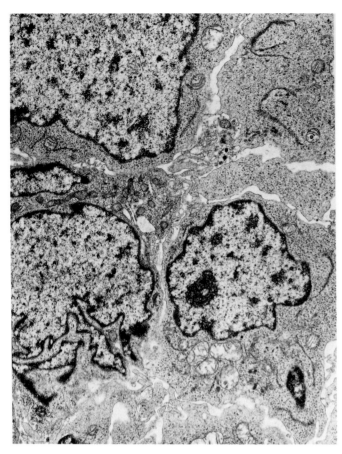

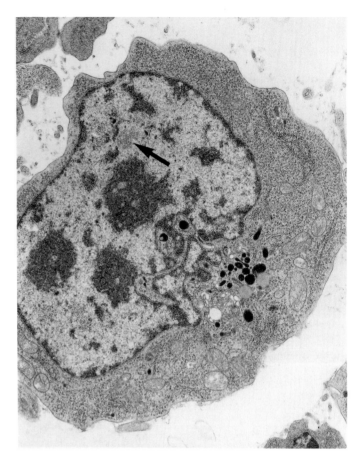

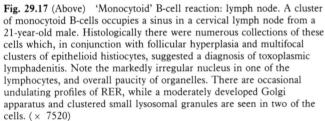

Fig. 29.17 (Above) 'Monocytoid' B-cell reaction: lymph node. A cluster of monocytoid B-cells occupies a sinus in a cervical lymph node from a 21-year-old male. Histologically there were numerous collections of these cells which, in conjunction with follicular hyperplasia and multifocal clusters of epithelioid histiocytes, suggested a diagnosis of toxoplasmic lymphadenitis. Note the markedly irregular nucleus in one of the lymphocytes, and overall paucity of organelles. There are occasional undulating profiles of RER, while a moderately developed Golgi apparatus and clustered small lysosomal granules are seen in two of the cells. (× 7520)

Fig. 29.18 (Above right) Dilantin lymphadenopathy: immunoblast. A paracortical immunoblast from the node of a patient with dilantin lymphadenopathy is shown. Histologically there was florid paracortical hyperplasia, with proliferation of numerous immunoblasts including atypical forms. This immunoblast has an irregular nucleus containing three very large nucleoli and a nuclear body (arrow). The clustering of dense lysosomal granules and Golgi apparatus in the centriolar region indicates that it may be a T-immunoblast. The cytoplasm contains many polyribosomes, large mitochondria and relatively little RER. (× 8600)

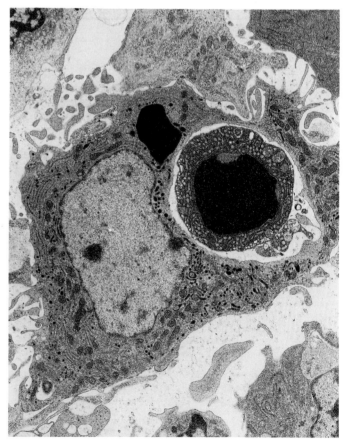

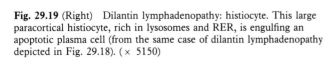

Fig. 29.19 (Right) Dilantin lymphadenopathy: histiocyte. This large paracortical histiocyte, rich in lysosomes and RER, is engulfing an apoptotic plasma cell (from the same case of dilantin lymphadenopathy depicted in Fig. 29.18). (× 5150)

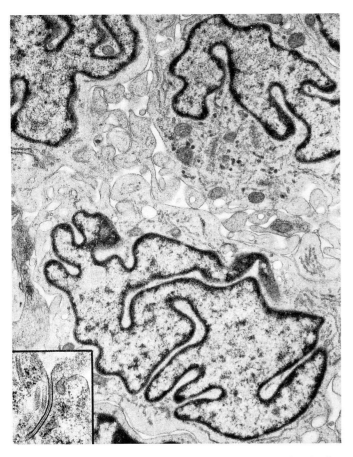

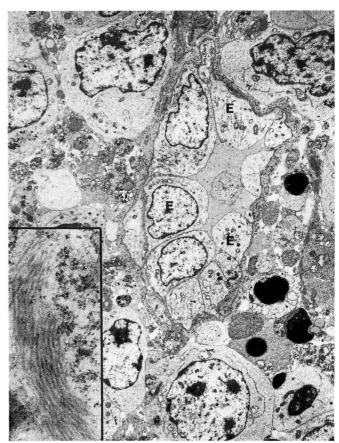

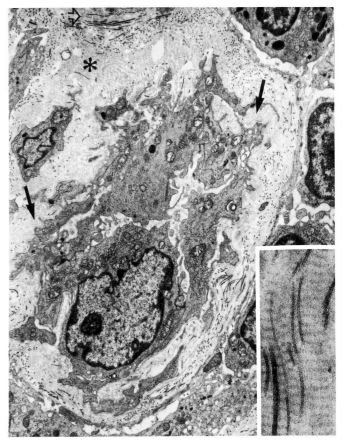

Fig. 29.20 (Above)   Dermatopathic lymphadenopathy: Langerhans' cells. This cluster of Langerhans' cells occurred in a lymph node showing DL. Note the characteristic, markedly irregular, nuclear contours with deep, serpiginous clefts, and the pale dendritic cytoplasmic processes. Golgi fields and elements of the SER are well-developed. Ill-defined small Birbeck granules are evident, related to the Golgi apparatus. Elsewhere, the granules are present near the cell surface, fused with the cell membrane (*inset*). (× 11 300; inset, × 30 100)

Fig. 29.21 (Above right)   Necrotizing lymphadenitis. This micrograph is from the paracortex of a cervical lymph node from a 17-year-old female who had the typical clinicopathological features of necrotizing lymphadenitis. The central paracortical venule is lined by swollen endothelial cells (E). Surrounding it are transformed large lymphoid cells, and abundant lymphocytic nuclear and cytoplasmic debris. Endothelial cells and some lymphoid cells contained TRI (not illustrated). (× 3700) *Inset* Aggregates of filaments approximately 20-nm thick found in the cytoplasm of an immunoblast. These filaments were quite easily found in the lymphoid cells of this case. (× 35 700)

Fig. 29.22 (Right)   Angioimmunoblastic lymphadenopathy with dysproteinaemia. A paracortical venule is surrounded by a wide 'mantle' of reduplicated basal lamina (arrows) and amorphous granular material (asterisk), within which are some pericytic processes. Portion of an eosinophil is seen at upper right. Long-spacing collagen is evident in the surrounding interstitium (open arrow). (× 47 500) *Inset* Detail of long-spacing collagen in the stroma, with periodic banding of approximately 96 nm. (× 26 100)

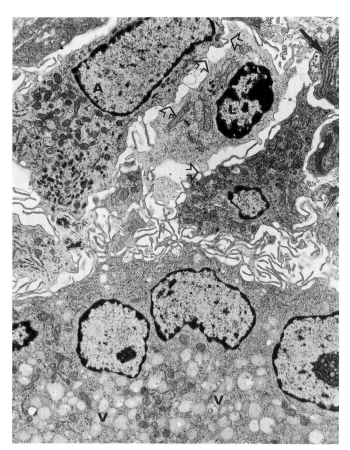

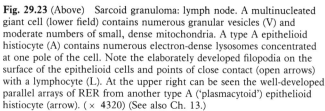

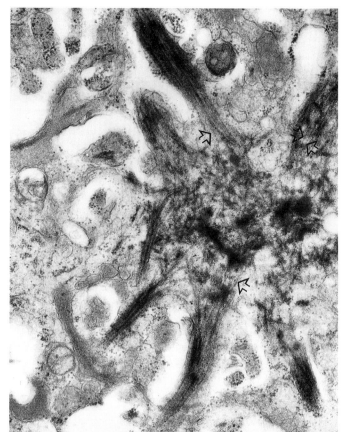

Fig. 29.23 (Above)   Sarcoid granuloma: lymph node. A multinucleated giant cell (lower field) contains numerous granular vesicles (V) and moderate numbers of small, dense mitochondria. A type A epithelioid histiocyte (A) contains numerous electron-dense lysosomes concentrated at one pole of the cell. Note the elaborately developed filopodia on the surface of the epithelioid cells and points of close contact (open arrows) with a lymphocyte (L). At the upper right can be seen the well-developed parallel arrays of RER from another type A ('plasmacytoid') epithelioid histiocyte (arrow). (× 4320) (See also Ch. 13.)

Fig. 29.24 (Above right)   Asteroid body: sarcoid granuloma. Detail of a 'mature' asteroid body within a multinucleated giant cell. The radiating arms appear electron-dense as a result of lateral aggregation of individual intermediate filaments, which can occasionally be discerned closer to the body of the asteroid (open arrows). The latter displays criss-crossing filaments of varying thickness, and condensations of amorphous electron-dense material. Centrioles are not evident in this plane of section. Note that the asteroid is not enclosed by a membrane, and that the arms are surrounded by optically clear spaces; these are said to occur around fully developed asteroids.[44] (× 26 750)

Fig. 29.25 (Right)   Epithelial cells: thymus gland. The thymus gland from this 52-year-old female harboured a histologically benign thymoma, while the residual non-neoplastic thymus showed pronounced lymphoid follicular hyperplasia in the absence of MG or other auto-immune disease. The micrograph is from the non-neoplastic thymus, and includes portions of two subcapsular epithelial cells (Ep). One of the these possesses prominent paranuclear tonofilament bundles (arrow), and, in addition, there are subplasmalemmal thin filaments with fusiform densities (curved arrows); the latter are rarely discerned in epithelial cells elsewhere in the thymus. Continuous basal lamina surrounds the subcapsular epithelium. At the lower left is the edge of a septal vessel including a portion of an endothelial cell (E) and a pericyte (P), surrounded by basal lamina. The perivascular space (asterisk) contains collagen fibres, some amorphous ground substance, and cytoplasmic processes of stromal cells. (× 12 300) **Inset** Detail of a desmosome between processes of two epithelial cells. (× 15 000)

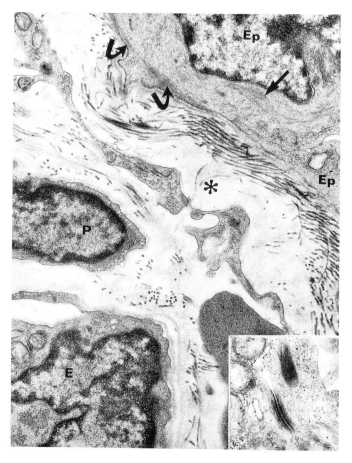

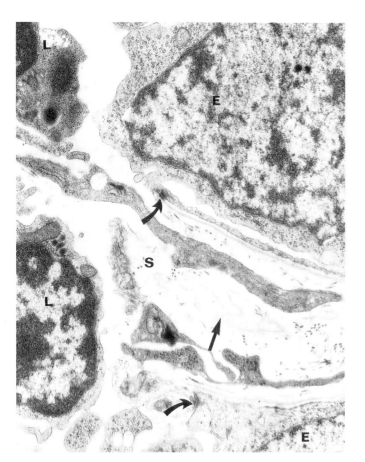

Fig. 29.26 (Left) Interruption of 'blood-thymic' barrier: thymus gland in MG. This thymus gland from a 31-year-old female with MG histologically revealed pronounced lymphoid follicular hyperplasia. The micrograph is from an area deep in the medulla showing focal discontinuity of the parenchymal–mesenchymal interface. Epithelial cells (E) with their basal lamina flank a delicate invaginating septum (S) containing scant collagen fibres, some redundant loops of basal lamina (arrow), and processes of stromal fibroblasts. The basal laminal integrity is interrupted in the region of small desmosomes between epithelial cell processes (curved arrows). Here, the extra-thymic space is in intimate contact with medullary lymphocytes (L). Such gaps have also been demonstrated immunohistochemically, and may be found in the ageing thymus, but more commonly in MG (see text). (× 13 250)

Fig. 29.27 (Below) Lymphoepithelial complex: thymus gland in MG. The micrograph depicts a lymphoepithelial complex, one of several found in the outer cortex of this gland from a 16-year-old female with MG. Cytoplasmic processes from a large putative thymic nurse cell (TNC) completely or partially encircle several lymphocytes. The lymphocytes do not show any degenerative changes; their plasmalemmae are intact and they establish close contact with the cell membrane of the epithelial cell. The TNC displays multiple, well-developed Golgi fields (arrows), and several small, dense secretory granules are present (open arrows). Occasional autophagic vacuoles (asterisks) can be seen. Small desmosomes are formed with processes of other epithelial cells (curved arrows). (× 8000)

Care must be taken not to mistake cortical macrophages for possible TNC. The latter, in our experience are difficult to find in vivo, whereas macrophages are relatively frequently found: lymphocytes or fragments thereof contained within them are often degenerate and lie within phagocytic vacuoles; broad ramifying cytoplasmic processes typically are not formed, and desmosomal attachments to other cells never form.

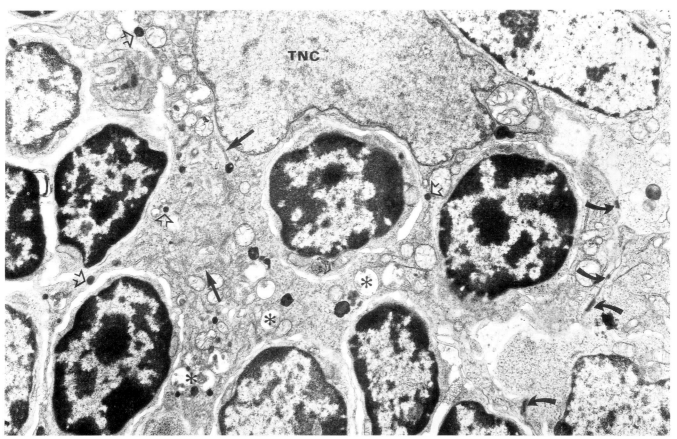

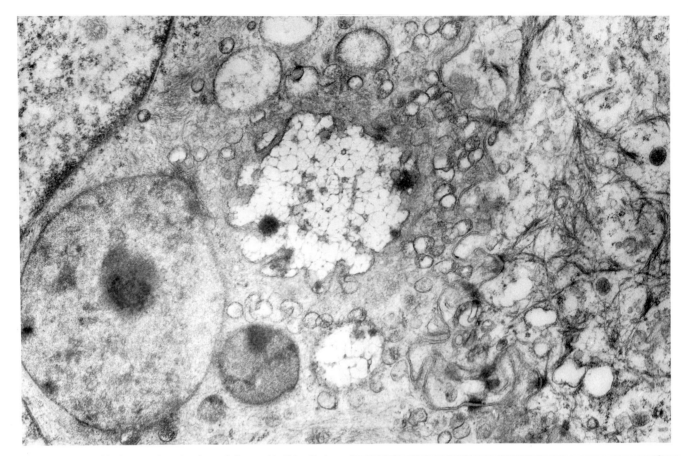

Fig. 29.28 (Above)   Mucin secretion: thymic medullary epithelial cell. A medullary thymic epithelial cell from a 34-year-old female with MG shows intracytoplasmic lumen formation, with accumulation of mucin granules in the surrounding cytoplasm. The neighbouring epithelial cell on the right contains prominent tonofilament bundles in the cytoplasm in addition to occasional similar secretory granules. (× 19 400)

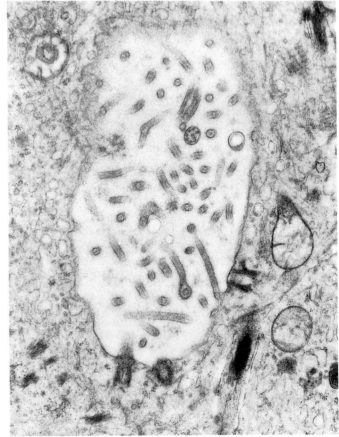

Fig. 29.29 (Right)   Intracytoplasmic lumen: Hassall's corpuscle. An intracytoplasmic lumen in an epithelial cell from the outer part of a Hassall's corpuscle is illustrated. Microvilli and cilia project into the lumen, which is surrounded by clear secretory vesicles. (× 19 400)

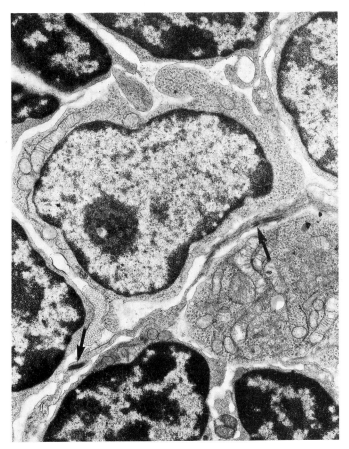

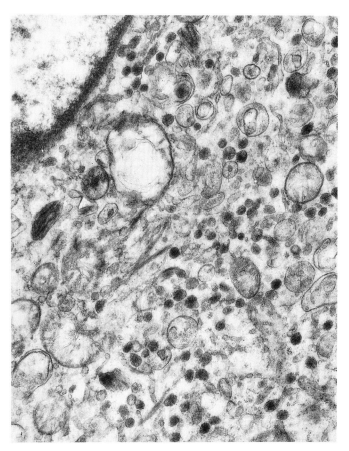

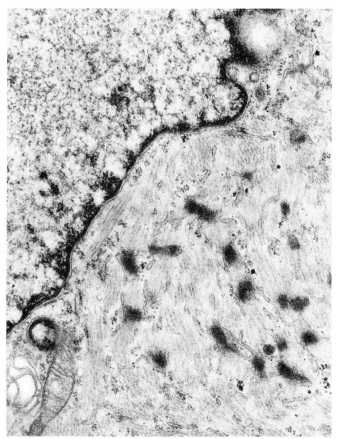

Fig. 29.30 (Above)   Cortical lymphoblast: thymus gland. A cortical blast cell is surrounded by small cortical lymphocytes. Slender, dendritic processes of epithelial cells joined by desmosomes (arrows), course between the thymocytes. The blast cell nucleus has relatively smooth contours, displays only a thin marginated rim of heterochromatin and much euchromatin, and possesses a prominent nucleolus. The cytoplasm has scanty organelles consisting mainly of polyribosomes, few mitochondria and rare cisternae of RER. The nuclear characteristics contrast sharply with the more densely heterochromatinic nuclei lacking distinct nucleoli, of the small cortical thymocytes. (× 8200)

Fig. 29.31 (Above right)   Secretory granules: thymic epithelium. Occasional epithelial cells, as depicted in this micrograph, from the thymus of a 14-year-old female with MG, contained numerous randomly-distributed electron-dense secretory granules ranging from approximately 130 nm to 190 nm in diameter. (× 19 400)

Fig. 29.32 (Right)   Myoid cells: thymic medulla. The same case as Fig. 29.31. Readily found in the medulla of this thymus, and often concentrated near Hassall's corpuscles, were spindle- or epithelioid-shaped myoid cells possessing many cytoplasmic thin and thick filaments, often forming disorganized, sarcomere-like arrangements with dense Z-lines. (× 5600)

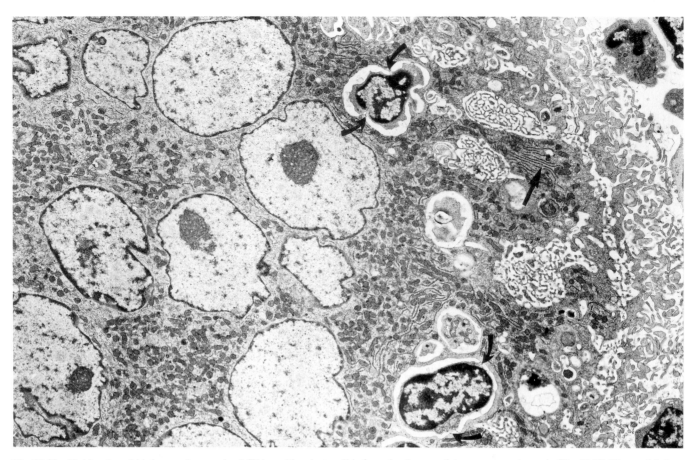

Fig. 29.33   Multinucleated histiocyte: thymus gland. This multinucleate cell is from the thymus of the same case shown in Fig. 29.27. The nuclei show features of 'activation', possessing abundant euchromatin, large nucleoli, and multiple sphaeridia. The cytoplasm contains numerous mitochondria, and well-developed cisternae of RER sometimes arranged in parallel arrays (arrow). There are no tonofilaments, and no cell attachments were found after careful scrutiny. There is striking development of labyrinthine cytoplasmic processes along the cell surface and within otherwise empty spaces enclosed by cell cytoplasm. Occasional well-preserved lymphocytes are contained within caveolar spaces, and points of close contact (curved arrows) with the caveolar membranes are evident. The overall features are in keeping with a multinucleated histiocytic cell, possibly actively secreting, as evidenced by the paucity of lysosomes. The lack of cell junctions and tonofilaments, and the elaborate surface development argue against this being a TNC, with which it might be confused. (× 4300)

30. Blood and bone marrow

Janine Breton-Gorius   Elisabeth Cramer

INTRODUCTION

In a few uncommon genetic defects of red cells, platelets and granulocytes, ultrastructural techniques in conjunction with cytochemistry and immunogold methods are desirable for confirmation of the diagnosis. Consequently electron microscopy (EM), although not crucial in the diagnosis of congenital dyserythropoietic anaemia (CDA), sideroblastic anaemia (SA), the haemoglobinopathies, the grey platelet syndrome (GPS), the Hermansky-Pudlak syndrome (HPS), the Chèdiak-Higashi syndrome (CHS) or lactoferrin deficiency has, nevertheless made significant contributions to our knowledge of these various disorders. The aim of this general review is to focus upon and to illustrate the characteristic ultrastructural changes in each of these syndromes.

TECHNIQUES

Preparation of bone marrow cells and peripheral blood cells in suspension for ultrastructural examination has previously been described in detail.[17] Methods for detection of the different peroxidases have been similarly described.[14,17,18,32] Table 30.1 summarizes the localization of peroxidatic activities in various haematopoietic cells. This cytochemical method can also be combined with immunolabelling of various glycoproteins on the cell membrane of red cell, platelet and granulocyte precursors.[18] Monoclonal antibodies raised against different normal or leukaemic cell lineages bind to the specific antigens, and such immunoreactive sites may be visualized either by anti-immunoglobulin coupled to colloidal gold or to colloidal gold conjugated to protein A which binds to the Fc-portion of several immunoglobulin subclasses.[30]

Intracytoplasmic proteins can also be visualized by the immunogold technique. However, in order to facilitate penetration of the antibody into the cytoplasm, several procedures can be employed: a detergent (saponin) added to fixative enhances permeability of the cells and permits entry of antibody.[24] This pre-embedding immunolabelling technique preserves the immunoreactivity of intragranular proteins but the ultrastructure is poor, despite careful adjustment of saponin concentration to ensure membrane permeability and granule preservation. The immune reaction may also be applied to thin sections of tissue fixed and embedded in water-soluble embedding media such as glycol methacrylate;[24,25] this avoids the use of organic solvents and allows polymerization at 4°C. A further procedure consists of performing the immune reaction on thin frozen sections.[66,68]

CONGENITAL DYSERYTHROPOIETIC ANAEMIA

The term congenital dyserythropoietic anaemia (CDA) was introduced by Crookston et al[28] and Wendt & Heimpel[76] to designate hereditary anaemia characterized by the presence of erythroid hyperplasia in the bone marrow as well as various morphological abnormalities of erythroblasts. Intramedullary cell death, which is characteristic of CDA, is responsible for the ineffective erythropoiesis and secondary haemochromatosis.

CDA can be classified into three types, I, II and III, according to the various morphological abnormalities of erythroblasts and serological differences in the red cells.[49] In addition, variants of CDA not conforming to one of the classical types have been reported.[6,12,29] Table 30.2 summarizes the differential diagnosis of the three CDA types.

The defect responsible for CDA I and III remains unknown, but a defect in glycosylation of erythrocyte membrane proteins was recently reported in CDA II.[38]

Since *in vitro* culture of committed erythroid progenitors permits the growth of erythroid colonies, this method was employed to determine whether the burst-forming cells (BFU-E) — the earliest committed erythroid progenitors — are defective in CDA I, II and III.[65,70-72] Ultrastructural investigations of individual mature colonies derived from CDA I, II and III BFU-E show a mixture of normal and abnormal erythroblasts which exhibit the typical aberrations found *in vivo*. These results suggest that all BFU-E are abnormal, but the severity of the defect in their progeny is

Table 30.1 Comparative localization of peroxidatic activities*

	Myeloperoxidase Eosinophil peroxidase Basophil peroxidase		Platelet peroxidase		Pseudoperoxidatic activity of haemoglobin	
	Bone marrow promyelocytes and promonocytes	Peripheral blood granulocytes and monocytes	Immature megakaryocytes	Mature megakaryocytes and platelets	Pro-erythroblasts	Mature erythroblastic cells
Endoplasmic reticulum	+ + +	−	+ + +	+ + +	−	−
Golgi apparatus	+ + +	−	−	−	−	−
Granules	+ + +	+ + +	−	−	−	−
Diffuse cytoplasmic reactivity	−	−	−	−	±	+ + +

*Reference: 16.

Table 30.2 Comparative features of congenital dyserythropoietic anaemias (CDA)*

CDA type	Inheritance	Frequency	Serology	Clinical and light microscopic findings	Electron microscopy features	Remarks
I	Autosomal recessive	Rare	No anomaly	Macrocytic anaemia, increased unconjugated bilirubin and plasma iron turnover; exclusion of haemoglobin anomaly and red cell enzymopathies; presence of internuclear chromatin bridges connecting two erythroblasts, with megaloblastoid changes	Widening of nuclear pores; chromatin with spongy appearance; invasion of the nucleus by cytoplasmic organelles; intramitochondrial iron	Aberration not specific, and may be present in: thalassaemia; CDA III; acquired dyserythropoietic states in preleukaemia
II (HEMPAS) Hereditary erythroblastic multinuclearity associated with a positive acidified serum test	Autosomal recessive	The most frequent CDA	Haemolysis in acidified serum; increased agglutination of red cells by anti-i antibody	Anaemia; jaundice of variable intensity; increased unconjugated bilirubin; haemosiderosis, increased serum iron levels; binucleation of late erythroblasts, and karyorrhexis	Excess of endoplasmic reticulum cisternae close to the cell membrane of erythroblasts and red cells	
III	Autosomal dominant?	Very rare	Increased agglutination and lysis by anti-i antibody	Minimal anaemia; giant and multinucleated erythroblasts	Nuclear clefts and disrupted nuclear membranes; asynchrony of mitosis in all nuclei in multinucleated erythroblasts; few of them also exhibit CDA I anomaly; intramitochondrial iron	Aberration not specific

*References: 7, 11, 15, 22, 41, 42, 50 and 74.

expressed variably. Figures 30.1 to 30.7 illustrate the abnormalities found *in vivo* and reproduced in *in vitro* cultures.

SIDEROBLASTIC ANAEMIA

Sideroblastic anaemia (SA) represents a heterogeneous group of disorders[58] characterized by a diversity of clinical and biochemical abnormalities.[51,64] However, in all cases, erythroblasts exhibit abnormal ring sideroblasts (see, in Table 30.3, the comparison between normal and ring sideroblasts) and macrophages contain an excess of iron stores. There is also ineffective erythropoiesis, and hyper-ferraemia. These conditions may be acquired, or they may be congenital. Refractory primary SA[55] may be an acquired condition. A variable number of such patients develop acute myelogeneous leukaemia. It is, however, not clear whether the leukaemia evolves as a separate disorder or whether the refractory SA represents a preleukaemic state.[73] Acquired SA may also be secondary (and reversible) to certain drugs, including ethanol and lead;[51] pyridoxine-responsive anaemia is classified separately and represents about 20% of all reported cases of SA.[48]

Hereditary forms of SA have also been described.[19,56] As in acquired SA, some of these forms are pyridoxine-responsive and some are not. The most common varieties appear to be transmitted as an X-linked recessive trait and all affected males have severe manifestations. A few mildly affected females appear to be heterozygous carriers; however, in a small number of female patients the anaemia is more severe[19,23,59,67] and possibly the transmission here is auto-somal. In both acquired and congenital SA, defects in the erythroid haem-synthesis pathway have been observed[13] (especially a defect in 5-aminolevulinic acid synthesis).

In all types of SA abnormal accumulation of iron is observed in the matrix between the cristae of mitochondria from normoblasts. The iron present in mitochondria and examined by EM has an appearance distinct from ferritin molecules (Fig. 30.8). For this reason, the term 'iron micelles' is sometimes employed to distinguish such intra-mitochondrial iron from ferritin. Electron-probe X-ray analysis confirms that the mitochondrial iron deposits have an elemental composition different from that of ferritin or haemosiderin.[40,46]

The abnormal iron accumulation occurs primarily in late normoblasts in congenital SA (Figs 30.9 and 30.10), in contrast to patients showing acquired primary refractory anaemia in whom mitochondrial iron overload is seen in early proliferating erythroid cells.[5,51] The abnormal presence of glycogen also varies according to the type of sideroblastic anaemia (Table 30.4).

Iron-laden mitochondria are not specific for sideroblastic anaemia and may also be observed in various congenital and acquired disorders (Table 30.5). In all varieties of SA, in addition to iron-loaded mitochondria, many ferritin mole-

Table 30.3 Characteristics of normal and ring sideroblasts*

	Light microscopy	Electron microscopy
Normal sideroblast	One or several Prussian blue-positive granules	Cluster of ferritin particles in the cytoplasm
Ring sideroblast	Perinuclear distribution of Prussian blue-positive granules	Ferruginous micelles in mitochondria and clusters of ferritin particles in the cytoplasm

*References: 2–4, 20, 31, 46, 47, 57 and 61.

Table 30.4 Comparison of ultrastructural features of erythroblasts in different types of sideroblastic anaemia*

	Mitochondrial iron overload in early proliferating erythroid cells	Glycogen particles
Primary refractory sideroblastic anaemia	+ + +	+
Alcoholic sideroblastic anaemia	±	–
Pyridoxine-responsive anaemia	±	–
Congenital sideroblastic anaemia	–	+

*References: 5, 43 and 51.

cules are deposited between adjacent erythroblastic membranes.[36,39]

HAEMOGLOBINOPATHIES

These disorders represent heterogeneous congenital abnormalities of the production or structure of the globin chains. A brief summary and the characteristics of the different varieties of haemoglobinopathies are given in Table 30.6.

EM has been employed to study the structure of fibres formed by deoxygenated haemoglobin S[27,33–35,39] as well as the organization of fibres of polymerized haemoglobin in sickled red cells.[1,26,77] The irregular and rigid membrane contours which characterize the sickling process appear to be caused by bundles of closely-packed fibres.[1] EM has also been used to study the structure of erythrocytes and reticulocytes in the bone marrow of homozygous patients with sickle cell anaemia,[44] and marked phagocytosis of sickled reticulocytes and red cells was observed. Under conditions of deoxygenation in bone marrow aspirates, haemoglobin polymers can also be observed in the nucleus and cytoplasm of polychromatophilic and orthochromatic

Table 30.5   Differential diagnosis between sideroblastic anaemia and other diseases with iron-loaded mitochondria in erythroblasts*

Disease	Characteristics
Thalassaemia minor	Ringed sideroblasts few in number Moderate degree of anaemia present only in periods of stress Increased haemoglobin A_2 level
Beta thalassaemia major	Ringed sideroblasts but presence of Heinz bodies Defect in synthesis of the beta globin chain Increased level of fetal haemoglobin
Sickle-cell anaemia	Iron-loaded mitochondria predominantly in late normoblasts and reticulocytes Haemoglobin S detectable by electrophoresis
CDA I and III	Ringed sideroblasts Nuclear abnormalities of erythroblasts
Sideroblastic anaemia associated with preleukaemia	Abundant sideroblasts in all stages of erythroid maturation Abnormal myeloid and megakaryocyte precursors

*References: 5, 10, 44 and 63.

Table 30.6   Classification and main characteristics of the various haemoglobinopathies*

Type	Defect	Geographic distribution	Clinical course	Laboratory features
Sickle cell anaemia	Structural alteration in one of the globin chains (haemoglobin S and variants C, D, E)	Tropical Africa	Normochromic anaemia Various types of crisis due to obstruction of blood vessels by rigid, sickled red cells in homozygous subjects	Transformation to sickled forms in an oxygen-poor environment
Thalassaemia	Total/partial absence of beta or alpha globin chain production	Mediterranean countries, Middle East, Southeast Asia and East Asia	Severe hypochromic anaemia with ineffective erythropoiesis and marked iron overload in homozygous subjects	Formation of Heinz bodies resulting from imbalanced chain production
Unstable haemoglobins	Changes of the amino acid sequence of one chain of globin which weakens the stability of haemoglobin (about 75 variants are recognized)	No preferential distribution	Haemolytic anaemia due to loss of deformability because of attachment of Heinz bodies to the cell membrane	Formation of Heinz bodies

*References: 8, 9, 60 and 75.

normoblasts, but are absent in more immature erythroblasts. This suggests that the aggregation and polymerization of haemoglobin occurs when the haemoglobin concentration is sufficiently high.[45]

In beta thalassaemia, ultrastructural studies have shown that the alpha chains precipitate in the cytoplasm and in the nucleus in late polychromatic erythroblasts. All aggregates of denatured haemoglobin are collectively termed Heinz bodies.[10,63,78,81] Frequently, there is also an accumulation of glycogen particles (Fig. 30.11). The precipitates constituting Heinz bodies are sometimes grouped in a cytoplasmic zone isolated from the other parts of the cell. These inclusions seem to have a different appearance from those found in non-Asian patients with haemoglobin H disease in whom

abnormal formation of tetramers of beta chains occurs.[79] In this situation, the inclusions appear as irregular branching masses.

All Heinz bodies — including those present in erythrocytes of patients with unstable haemoglobin — are often fixed to the cell membrane, the membrane attachment being well seen by scanning electron microscopy.[54] It has been proposed that disulphide bonding may account for the attachment of certain unstable haemoglobins to membrane,[53] but more recently it was suggested that the formation of hydrophobic bonds appears to be a more likely mechanism of membrane attachment.[21,80] In reticulocytes or erythroblasts the denatured haemoglobin may co-precipitate with ribosomes, ferritin and iron-containing mitochondria[37,52,62,69] (Fig. 30.12) — while in erythrocytes fixation of Heinz bodies to the cell membrane produces regional membrane alterations (Fig. 30.12) leading to premature destruction.

HERMANSKY–PUDLAK SYNDROME (HPS)

Four distinct classes of granules which differ in both their contents and their ultrastructural appearances have been recognized in normal platelets:

1. Alpha-granules represent the largest class of granules and contain various proteins which can be demonstrated by immunogold methods, namely fibrinogen, beta-thromboglobulin, platelet factor 4, thrombospondin, fibronectin, von Willebrand factor and immunoglobulins.[86,87,93,101,107,111,115,118]

2. Small lysosomal granules can be recognized by the ultrastructural cytochemical demonstration of acid phosphatase and aryl sulphatase,[83] and by the immunogold localization of cathepsin D.[112,113]

3. Catalase-containing granules (microperoxisomes) can be distinguished from other granule classes by the cytochemical demonstration of catalase.[84]

4. Dense bodies. EM techniques — including autoradiography and analytical EM — and biochemistry have been employed to demonstrate that the last category, the dense bodies (DB), are the storage sites for serotonin, the non-metabolic pool of adenine nucleotides and calcium.[88,91,102,116,120] These organelles appear as a vacuole with highly opaque core. In the rabbit, DB cannot be detected in megakaryocytes by conventional EM. However, the administration of 5-hydroxytryptamine (5-HT) induces the appearance of characteristic DB in megakaryocytes, suggesting that megakaryocytes store exogenous 5-HT in organelles which represent the precursors of DB.[117] In man, their visualization requires either the addition of calcium to the fixative[121] or the use of the uranaffin reaction[110] — which probably localizes the phosphonucleotides of adenine nucleotides. Mepacrine (a fluorescent acridine derivative) can be used to visualize dense bodies as fluorescent dots in platelets and megakaryocytes on ultraviolet irradiation.[89,100,114] All of the substances sequestered in DB are secreted to the exterior when platelets are stimulated by agonists which trigger the release reaction.[92] Thus, it is expected that defects in DB or their secretion will be associated with abnormal aggregation and will cause a bleeding tendency; HPS is an example.

In 1959, Hermansky & Pudlak[96] described several patients with a mild bleeding tendency and a prolonged bleeding time; these patients also had oculocutaneous albinism and a ceroid-like pigment was found in macrophages, including those in the bone marrow.[82,123,124] Subsequent studies on similar patients revealed that the platelets, which were normal in number, had very low levels of serotonin and a marked reduction in the non-metabolic pool of adenine nucleotides.[95,119] In addition, HPS platelets were shown to contain significantly less calcium than normal platelets,[98] and by EM, either the absence or a severe reduction of DB was observed.[90,103,104,109,122] Of the megakaryocytes incubated with mepacrine, 74% contained no granules and only 4.5% had a normal granule concentration; platelets contained only 33% of the normal value.[97] HPS appears to be an inherited autosomal recessive disease; to date about 50 cases have been reported in the literature. In addition, variants of HPS have been described.[109,123]

Figures 30.20 and 30.21 compare the distribution of DB in normal and HPS platelets, and Fig. 30.22 illustrates the ceroid-like pigment in bone marrow macrophages.

GREY PLATELET SYNDROME

The grey platelet syndrome (GPS) is a rare congenital platelet disorder, autosomal and recessive,[106] in which the platelets lack normal alpha granules (and therefore appear grey with the Romanovsky stain, allowing diagnosis by light microscopy). The syndrome was first described in 1971 by Raccuglia[108] as an association of a bleeding tendency with morphological abnormalities of platelets which were shown by EM to correspond to a deficiency of alpha-granules. Otherwise, these platelets have a normal number of dense bodies, peroxisomes, lysosomes and mitochondria.[99,125] Although the primary defect giving rise to the selective deficiency of alpha-granules in grey platelets has not yet been elucidated, EM has been of great value in understanding the disorder.

By EM, grey platelets are pleomorphic; their size is irregular, mostly enlarged, and sometimes assume giant proportions. Vacuolization is a striking but inconstant feature, some platelets appearing to be devoid of organelles and filled with vacuoles of variable size (Fig. 30.13).[99,105,108,125] Other abnormalities can occasionally be encountered, including the following: masses of dense tubular systems or surface-connected canalicular system (SCCS) disposed in stacks or in circular areas; sequestration of cytoplasmic organelles by an enclosing membrane; and the presence of numerous vacuoles unrelated to the exterior and distinct from the SCCS. The main morphological abnormality detected by EM is the almost complete lack of normal alpha-granules in the majority of platelets. The other types of granule, including dense bodies (Fig. 30.14), and the catalase-containing granules[84] (Fig. 30.15), are present in either normal or increased numbers.

The absence of normal alpha-granules has been confirmed by biochemical studies showing that the concentrations of proteins normally present in the alpha-granules such as thrombospondin, fibrinogen and beta-thromboglobulin are severely decreased[94,105] but are not completely absent. Indeed, we have recently shown by immunogold detection of fibrinogen (Fg) and von Willebrand factor (vWF) — two components normally present in the alpha-granules (Fig. 30.16) — that two types of abnormal alpha-granules could be identified (Fig. 30.17). The first type consisted of granules which were normal in size but which lacked nucleoids, and were partially empty; the scant material remaining in their matrices labelled with vWF and Fg. The second type comprised very small granules (less than 0.1 μm in diameter), and these were either spherical or elongated. Because they are considerably smaller than normal alpha-granules, this type may resemble other platelet granules, such as lysosomes or microperoxisomes; therefore, they can be identified as abnormal alpha-granules only by immunoelectron microscopy.[86]

In the bone marrow, typical mature alpha-granules are absent from the megakaryocytes of patients with GPS.[85] Smaller granules, less than 0.1 μm in diameter are present; these frequently appear elongated, often possessing a light grey periphery and an electron-dense core. They are especially present in the Golgi zone. White,[125] from his observation of one patient's bone marrow, raised the hypothesis that Golgi complexes were abnormal in GPS; however, the two patients described by Breton-Gorius et al[85] had normal Golgi complexes. Generally, large areas of cytoplasm lacked granules but contained membrane complexes which were associated with the demarcation membrane system and smooth endoplasmic reticulum. The lumina of the demarcating membranes were often dilated and contained dense material (Fig. 30.19). Immunolabelling for vWF stained small vesicles in the vicinity of the Golgi complex and some small granules, identical to those found in platelets. Although vWF is eccentrically located in normal platelet alpha-granules, and coincides with tubular structures which may represent the vWF molecule itself,[87] in GPS, immunolabelling shows it to be distributed randomly in the matrices, and an underlying abnormality of the platelet vWF molecule may be present. The dense material deposited in the SCCS of megakaryocytes was also found within blood platelet SCCS and was identified as having been lost from the alpha-granules (Fig. 30.18).

Finally, EM study of GPS is extremely useful in the diagnosis and understanding of the disease:

1. It allows recognition of the absence or marked reduction of normal alpha-granules and the concomitant presence of the other types of granules.

2. It has permitted the observation of normal synthesis of alpha-granule proteins, the formation of immature alpha-granules, and the loss of alpha-granule proteins into the extracellular space before the formation of mature alpha-granules.

THE CHEDIAK–HIGASHI SYNDROME

The Chèdiak–Higashi syndrome (CHS) is a rare autosomal recessive disease characterized by partial oculo-cutaneous albinism, frequent pyogenic infections, neutropenia and characteristic giant lysosomes. It was first described in man in 1943 by Bèguez-Cèsar.[127] Further studies on the affected family were then reported by Chèdiak in 1952 and an additional patient was described by Steinbrick in 1948 and later by Higashi in 1954. In 1955 Sato recognized the similarities between the patients described by Chèdiak and Higashi and proposed the eponym of CHS for the disease. Detailed references of these early reports together with descriptions of CHS in man and in animal homologues (mink, cattle, mice, killer whales, cats) can be found in the extensive review by Windhorts and Padgett.[156] In man the susceptibility to infection is associated with granulocytopenia, an abnormality of leukocyte chemotaxis, delayed killing of phagocytozed bacteria, and abnormal distribution of leukocyte lysozymes.[128,133,148] Abnormal microtubule assembly and cyclic nucleotide metabolism have been implicated in the pathophysiology of the leukocyte dysfunction, and ascorbic acid — a known stimulant of leukocyte cyclic GMP — was reported to induce partial correction of the leukocyte function *in vitro* and *in vivo*.[130,135,141,154] However, recent appraisal of microtubule number and length by high-voltage stereo EM in neutrophils from patients with CHS has shown that these were identical to normal polymorphonuclear leukocytes (PMN), but that the responsiveness to stimulation of microtubule polymerization was irregular.[145]

Microscopy is essential to establish the diagnosis of the disease, and EM is a valuable means of defining the various abnormalities. The main observation allowing diagnosis of CHS is the presence of abnormal giant granules in the cytoplasm of all granule-containing cells, and these are related to the occurrence of the other features of the syndrome — namely, albinism and an abnormal propensity to infection. Although present in non-haemopoietic tissues like renal tubular epithelial cells, gastric mucosa, thyroid and melanocytes, the massive intracellular inclusions are more easily demonstrated in leukocytes. We describe here the abnormal features which can be observed in CHS blood cells by electron microscopy, their mode of formation during cell maturation, their nature and morphology in mature neutrophils (PMN), and their particular morphology in each cell type.

The formation of CHS granules in myeloid precursors has been most extensively studied in animals, but some ultrastructural studies of human bone marrow cells have appeared. Most authors have concluded that the giant granules develop by fusion of granules of normal size, with changes in internal granule structure taking place subsequently (Fig. 30.23). The fusion can also occur between granules of normal size and between giant granules and nearby normal granules. The giant inclusions with complex internal structure are present as early as the promyelocyte stage (Fig. 30.24). The subsequent appearance of specific granules is normal.

While the lysosomal nature of the giant PMN granules has been generally accepted on the basis of earlier histochemical studies, White[151] was the first to demonstrate this fact by the ultrastructural demonstration of acid phosphatase within the giant inclusions. Some authors have indicated that the azurophilic or primary granules are exclusively involved and that the process of giant granule formation is complete before the PMN leaves the bone marrow. This hypothesis is supported by data illustrated in Fig. 30.26, which shows a giant inclusion containing myeloperoxidase (the specific marker of primary granules), the virtual absence of primary granules of normal size, and the presence in normal number of specific granules of normal morphology without apparent fusion with the giant granules. The alternative hypothesis has been supported by immunocytochemical identification of both primary and secondary granule markers in the giant organelles of CHS neutrophils.[156] However, the light microscopy techniques have limited resolution and cannot reveal the exclusive presence of normal secondary granules in the cytoplasm of these PMN as does EM. Apart from these giant granules resembling normal granules with a surrounding unit membrane and generally homogeneous internal structures, some internal reticular membranous and myelin-like figures are seen (Fig. 30.25). They were interpreted by White[152] as cytoplasmic sequestration, corresponding to a peculiar form of autophagy, initiated by a leakage of acid hydrolase from giant granules.[152,155] Degranulation induced by phagocytosis of foreign particles is impaired, the appearance of myeloperoxidase (MPO) within the phagosomes is delayed, and the giant inclusions do not participate in early degranulation. The administration of ascorbic acid either in vivo or in vitro corrects to some extent (under certain conditions) the morphological and functional abnormalities of neutrophils in human and animal disease: the polymerization of microtubules is increased, and in maturing CHS neutrophils the formation of giant granules is prevented.

Other blood cells also display giant cytoplasmic granules, including eosinophils and basophils (Fig. 30.27), this abnormality also being found in tissue mast cells. Monocytes have been shown to contain ring-shaped organelles due to the fusion of the cytoplasmic granules; however, numerous normal azurophilic granules remain in the cytoplasm.[153] These structures are also found infrequently in neutrophils, eosinophils and lymphocytes. Lymphocyte subpopulations are variably abnormal: natural killer cells display giant lysosomes, B-cells are structurally abnormal, but T-cells are morphologically intact.[138] Finally, it has also been shown by EM that platelets in CHS are deficient in serotonin-storage granules or dense bodies,[147] and although other granule constituents are normal, this dense granule defect has an influence on the release mechanism of other normal granules.

CONGENITAL LACTOFERRIN DEFICIENCY

Human blood neutrophils contain two main populations of cytoplasmic granules that are formed in the bone marrow at different stages of maturation.[126,144] The azurophil granules are packaged in promyelocytes and are identified by LM and EM by their peroxidase activity; specific granules are formed later, during the myelocyte stage, and have been categorized by electron microscopy by an absence of peroxidase activity (Fig. 30.31), and more recently by their lactoferrin content as demonstrated by immunocytochemistry[134] (Fig. 30.32). There have been reports of five cases of patients with susceptibility to bacterial infections and neutrophil dysfunction associated with a congenital absence of secondary or specific granules and abnormal nuclear lobulation (Table 30.7). This abnormality was detected by the absence of immunocytochemical reactivity for lactoferrin[132,136,150] and/ or myeloperoxidase-negative granules at the EM level.[132,137,142,149,150]

Since the work of Masson et al[140] which demonstrated the presence of lactoferrin in neutrophils, biochemical studies using subcellular fractionation and light microscopic immunocytochemical studies[139,144] have shown lactoferrin to be associated with the secondary granules. More recently, an ultrastructural immunogold technique confirmed this localization.[134] The identification of patients with a deficiency of specific granules provides an important model to assess their function. The specific granules are involved in exocytosis and contain a number of substances capable of regulating inflammation. These include factors that generate the chemotactically active fragments of the fifth complement component and the glycoprotein lactoferrin which plays an important role in neutrophil adherence and aggregation as well as regulation of myelopoiesis and modulation of hydroxyl radical production. The specific granules may also provide a source for renewal of the plasma membrane during neutrophil locomotion.[136]

Lactoferrin-deficient neutrophils have been shown to contain less than 10% of this protein, but it is not completely absent. The other components of specific granules are also decreased in proportion to lactoferrin (for example, vitamin B12 binding protein and lysozyme, half of which is normally located in the secondary granule).[131,149] The cytochemical activity of alkaline phosphatase, the localization of which is still controversial (plasma membrane or secondary granules), is generally low or negative. Cytochrome B-245 — a key component of the oxidative burst of neutrophils and normally located in the specific granule membrane — is found in association with the plasma membrane.[129] One hypothesis raised was that specific granules had fused with the plasma membrane because of a possible pre-activated state of the cells.[129,131] The functional consequences of this absence of specific granule abnormality have been studied; in vivo mobilization and in vitro chemotaxis are impaired, bactericidal activity is decreased and oxidative metabolism following stimulation displays several abnormalities.[129,131,136] The neutrophil homogenates do not have the usual chemotactic activity on monocytes; when stimulated by specific degranulants, such as phorbol myristate acetate, there is no increase in PMN surface area and a subnormal increase in surface chemotactic receptors.

Lactoferrin-deficient PMN display several types of morphological abnormality (Fig. 30.29). Apart from the absence

Table 30.7 Analysis of five cases of lactoferrin deficiency reported in the literature

Reference	Sex and age	Infections	Neutrophils					
			Blood count	Nuclei	Primary granules	Alkaline phosphatase cytochemistry	Chemotaxis	Microbicidal capacity
129, 131, 143, 150	M, 14	Staphylococcal and respiratory infections	Normal	Bilobed nuclei	Abnormal complex carbohydrate content	Absent	Reduced	*Candida*: normal *Staphylococcus*: decreased
137	F, 7	Abscesses, otitis, mastoiditis, eczema, due to *Staphylococcus* A, *Pseudomonas* A	Normal	Bilobed nuclei with nuclear blebs, clefts, pockets	Normal	Present in less than 3% of PMN	Reduced	*Staphylococcus*: decreased
137	M, 43	Recurrent bacterial infections	?	No abnormality mentioned	Normal	Normal	No data	*E. coli* and *alpha-streptococci* A: decreased
			Neutrophils					
142	F, 5½	Ear and throat infections, diarrhoea, oral lesions due to *Pseudomonas*, *Klebsiella* and *E. coli*	Severe neutropenia	Multiple small nuclear lobes, or notched nuclei	Presence of electron-lucent MPO-deficient granules, and myelin figures	Decreased	Decreased	No data
132	M, 6	Staphylococcal skin infections; infections by *pneumococcus* and *Candida albicans*	Normal	Bilobed nuclei	Presence of electron-lucent, MPO-deficient granules	Decreased	Normal	*Staphylococcus aureus*: normal *Serratia marcescens*: normal

of detectable peroxidase-negative granules (Fig. 30.33), they also display abnormal nuclear segmentation (generally bilobulation resembling the Pelger–Huet anomaly), microlobes, nuclear clefts and pockets (Fig. 30.30).[132,137,142,150] Abnormalities involving primary granules are also present; their number may be increased, as observed on spread PMN from one patient, and their morphology may be abnormal, appearing to be partially extracted but with a dense nucleoid.[132,137,141] Their complex carbohydrate content — demonstrated ultrastructurally by the periodic acid–thiocarbohydrazide–silver proteinate staining method — was normal in immature primary granules, but masking of this carbohydrate reactivity did not occur in mature primary granules, as seen in normal neutrophils.[143] In addition, some small flattened vesicles are found in the cytoplasm of PMN.

In the bone marrow, macrophages loaded with phagocytozed abnormal neutrophils can be observed. Granulocyte maturation at the myeloblast and promyelocyte stage is mainly normal, apart from rare abnormal nuclear segmentation and the presence of some azurophilic granules with a dense core and a lack of myeloperoxidase (MPO) (Fig. 30.30). At the myelocyte stage, the cell organelles generally appear normal, including the nuclear chromatin, and the rough and smooth endoplasmic reticulum. The primary granules are abundant, and they may appear either normal or abnormally electron-lucent with a dense core; the defective granules do not contain MPO (Fig. 30.28). The Golgi apparatus is prominent, but only minute and flattened vesicles are present in the vicinity of its convex surface where specific granules would arise under normal circumstances. However, flattened elongated granules are also seen scattered in the cytoplasm,[132,142] and these have been interpreted as abnormal specific granules (Fig. 30.33). Indeed they appear at the myelocyte stage and disappear after treatment with phorphol myristate acetate (a selective degranulant of normal secondary granules).

It would be worth studying the ultrastructural distribution of lactoferrin in these PMN in order to demonstrate whether the remaining lactoferrin is located in these vesicles and that they indeed correspond to abnormal specific granules. Alternatively, the specific granules may be completely missing because they were not formed, or — less likely — because they were redistributed during a possible preactivation.

REFERENCES

Techniques, dyserythropoietic and sideroblastic anaemias and haemoglobinopathies

1. Bertles J F, Dobler J 1969 Reversible and irreversible sickling: a distinction by electron microscopy. Blood 33: 884–898
2. Bessis M C, Breton-Gorius J 1959 Ferritin and ferruginous micelles in normal erythroblasts and hypochromic hypersideremic anemias. Blood 14: 423–432
3. Bessis M C, Breton-Gorius J 1962 Iron metabolism in the bone marrow as seen by electron microscopy: a critical review. Blood 19: 635–663
4. Bessis M C, Jensen W N 1965 Sideroblastic anaemia, mitochondria and erythroblastic iron. British Journal of Haematology 11: 49–51
5. Bessis M C, Dreyfus B, Breton-Gorius J, Sultan C 1969 Etude au microscope électronique de onze cas d'anémies réfractaires avec enzymopathies multiples. Nouvelle Revue Française d'Hématologie 9: 87–104
6. Bethlenfalvay N C, Hadnagy C S, Heimpel H 1985 Unclassified type of congenital dyserythropoietic anaemia (CDA) with prominent peripheral erythroblastosis. British Journal of Haematology 60: 541–550
7. Bethlenfalvay N C, Phaure T A J, Phyliky R L, Bowman R P 1986 Nuclear bridging of erythroblasts in acquired dyserythropoiesis: an early and transient preleukemic marker. American Journal of Hematology 21: 315–322
8. Beutler E 1983 The sickle cell diseases and related disorders. In: Williams W J, Beutler E, Erslev A, Lichtman M A (eds) Hematology, 3rd edn. McGraw-Hill, New York, pp 583–609
9. Beutler E 1983 Hemoglobinopathies associated with unstable hemoglobin. In: Williams W J, Beutler E, Erslev A, Lichtman M A (eds) Hematology, 3rd edn. McGraw-Hill, New York, pp 609–617
10. Beuzard Y, Tulliez M, Breton-Gorius J, Griscelli C, Cosson A, Schaison G 1978 Beta thalassemia with reticulocytopenia. Clinical biochemical and ultrastructural studies. Blood Cells 4: 269–286
11. Björkstén B, Holmgren G, Roos G, Stenling R 1978 Congenital dyserythropoietic anaemia, type III: an electron microscopic study. British Journal of Haematology 38: 37–42
12. Boogaerts M A, Verwilghen R L 1982 Variants of congenital dyserythropoietic anaemia: an update. Haematologia 15: 211–219
13. Bottomley S S 1977 Porphyrin and iron metabolism in sideroblastic anemia. Seminars in Hematology 14: 169–185
14. Breton-Gorius J 1970 Utilisation de la diaminobenzidine pour la mise en évidence au microscope électronique, de l'hémoglobine intracellulaire. La réactivité des différents organelles des érythroblastes. Nouvelle Revue Française d'Hématologie 10: 243–256
15. Breton-Gorius J, Daniel M T, Clauvel J P, Dreyfus B 1973 Anomalies ultrastructurales des érythroblastes et des érythrocytes dans six cas de dysérythropoïèse congénitale. Nouvelle Revue Française d'Hématologie 13: 23–50
16. Breton-Gorius J, Reyes F 1976 Ultrastructure of human bone marrow cell maturation. International Review of Cytology 46: 251–321
17. Breton-Gorius J, Gourdin M F, Reyes F 1981 Ultrastructure of the leukemic cell. In: Catovsky D (ed) Methods in hematology. The leukemic cell. Churchill Livingstone, Edinburgh, pp 87–128
18. Breton-Gorius J, Vanhaeke D, Pryzwansky K B, Guichard J, Tabilio A, Vainchenker W, Carmel R 1984 Simultaneous detection of membrane markers with monoclonal antibodies and peroxidase activities in leukaemia: ultrastructural analysis using a new method of fixation preserving the platelet peroxidase. British Journal of Haematology 58: 447–458
19. Buchanan G R, Bottomley S, Nitschke A 1980 Bone marrow delta-amino laevulinate synthetase deficiency in a female with congenital sideroblastic anemia. Blood 55: 509–515
20. Cartwright G E, Deiss A 1975 Sideroblasts, siderocytes and sideroblastic anemia. New England Journal of Medicine 292: 185–193
21. Chan E, Desforges J F 1976 The role of disulfide bonds in Heinz body attachment to membranes. British Journal of Haematology 33: 371–378
22. Clauvel J P, Cosson A, Breton-Gorius J, Flandrin G, Faille A, Bonnet-Gajdos, Turpin F, Bernard J 1972 Dyserythropoïèse congénitale (étude de 6 observations). Nouvelle Revue Française d'Hématologie 12: 653–672
23. Cotton H B, Harris J W 1962 Familial pyridoxine-responsive anemia. Journal of Clinical Investigation 31: 1352 (abstr)
24. Cramer E, Pryzwansky K B, Villeval J L, Testa U, Breton-Gorius J 1985 Ultrastructural localization of lactoferrin and myeloperoxidase in human neutrophils by immunogold. Blood 65: 423–432
25. Cramer E, Meyer D, Le Menn R, Breton-Gorius J 1985 Eccentric localization of von Willebrand factor in an internal structure of platelet α-granule resembling that of Weibel–Palade bodies. Blood 66: 710–713
26. Crepeau R H, Dykes G, Garrell R, Edelstein S J 1978 Diameter of hemoglobin S fibres in sickled cells. Nature 274: 616–617
27. Crepeau R H, Edelstein S J 1984 Polarity of the 14 strand fibres of hemoglobin determined by cross-correlation methods. Ultramicroscopy 13: 11–18
28. Crookston J H, Godwin T F, Wightman K J R, Dacie J V, Lewis S M, Patterson M J L 1966 Congenital dyserythropoietic anaemia. XIth Congress of the International Society Hematology, Sydney. AB8 p 18 (abs)
29. David G, van Dorpe A 1977 Aberrant congenital dyserythropoietic anaemias. In: Lewis S M, Verwilghen R L (eds) Dyserythropoiesis. Academic Press, London, pp 93–100
30. De Mey J 1983 A critical review of light and electron microscopy immunocytochemical techniques used in neurobiology. Journal of Neuroscience Methods 7: 1–18
31. Douglas A S, Dacie J V 1953 The incidence and significance of iron-containing granules in human erythrocytes and their precursors. Journal of Clinical Pathology 6: 307–313
32. Dvorak A M, Dvorak H F, Karnovsky M J 1972 Cytochemical localization of peroxidase activity in the developing erythrocyte. American Journal of Pathology 67: 303–326
33. Dykes G, Crepeau R J, Edelstein S J 1979 Three-dimensional reconstruction of the 14-filaments fibers of hemoglobin S. Journal of Molecular Biology 130: 451–472
34. Edelstein S J 1981 Molecular topology in crystals and fibers of hemoglobin S. Journal of Molecular Biology 150: 557–575
35. Finch J T, Peruta M F, Bertles J F, Dobler J 1973 Structure of sickled erythrocytes and of a sickle cell hemoglobin fiber. Proceedings of the National Academy of Sciences of the United States of America 70: 719–722
36. Flandrin G, Daniel M T, Breton-Gorius J, Brouet J C, Bernard J 1974 Ilot erythroblastique anormal dû au développement de jonctions intercellulaires (synarthèse érythroblastique). Un nouveau mécanisme d'anémie. Problèmes posés par le diagnostic. Nouvelle Revue d'Hématologie 14: 161–180
37. Frisch B, Lewis S M, Sherman D, White J M, Gordon-Smith E C 1974 The ultrastructure of erythropoiesis in two haemoglobinopathies. British Journal of Haematology 28: 109–117
38. Fukuda M, Papayannopoulou T, Gordon-Smith E C, Rochant H, Testa U 1984 Defect in glycosylation of erythrocyte membrane proteins in congenital dyserythropoietic anemia type II (HEMPAS). British Journal of Haematology 56: 55–68
39. Garrell R L, Crepeau R H, Edelstein S J 1979 Cross-sectional views of hemoglobin S fibers by electron microscopy and computer modeling. Proceedings of the National Academy of Sciences of the USA 76: 1140–1144
40. Ghadially F N, Lalonde J M A, Mukherjee T M 1979 Electron probe X-ray analysis of intramitochondrial iron deposits in sideroblastic anaemia. Journal of Submicróscopical Cytology 11: 503–510
41. Goudsmit R, Beckers D, De Bruisne J I, Engelfriet C P, James J, Morselt A F W, Reynierse E 1972 Congenital dyserythropoietic anaemia, type III. British Journal of Haematology 23: 97–105
42. Goudsmit R 1977 Congenital dyserythropoietic anaemia, type III. In:

Lewis S M, Verwilghen R L (eds) Dyserythropoiesis. Academic Press, London, pp 83–92

43. Grasso J A, Hines J D 1969 A comparative electron microscopic study of refractory and alcoholic sideroblastic anaemia. British Journal of Haematology 17: 35–44

44. Grasso J A, Sullivan A L, Sullivan L W 1975 Ultrastructural studies of the bone marrow in sickle cell anaemia. I. The structure of sickled erythrocytes and reticulocytes and their phagocytic destruction. British Journal of Haematology 31: 135–148

45. Grasso J A, Sullivan A L, Sullivan L W 1975 Ultrastructural studies of the bone marrow in sickle cell anaemia. II. The morphology of erythropoietic cells and their response to deoxygenation in vitro. British Journal of Haematology 31: 381–389

46. Grasso J A, Myers T J, Hines J D, Sullivan A L 1980 Energy-dispersive X-ray analysis of mitochondria of sideroblastic anaemia. British Journal of Haematology 46: 57–72

47. Gruneberg H 1941 Siderocytes: a new kind of erythrocyte. Nature 148: 114–115

48. Harris J W, Whittington R M, Weisman R, Horrigan D L 1956 Pyridoxine-responsive anemia in the human adult. Proceedings of the Society for Experimental Biology and Medicine 91: 427–432

49. Heimpel H, Wendt F 1968 Congenital dyserythropoietic anemia with karyorrhexis and multinuclearity of erythroblasts. Helvetica Medica Acta 34: 103–115

50. Heimpel H 1976 Congenital dyserythropoietic anaemia type I: clinical and experimental aspects. In: Congenital disorders of erythropoiesis. Ciba Foundation Symposium 37. Elsevier, North-Holland, Amsterdam, pp 135–149

51. Hines J D, Grasso J A 1970 The sideroblastic anemias. Seminars in Hematology 7: 86–106

52. Hollan S R, Szelenyi J G, Lelkes G, Berzy H, Farago S, Rappay G 1968 Ultrastructural and microspectrophotometric studies of the red cell inclusion bodies in unstable haemoglobin disease. Haematologia 2: 291–312

53. Jacob H S 1970 Mechanisms of Heinz body formation and attachment to red cell membrane. Seminars in Hematology 7: 341–354

54. Jensen W, Lessin L S 1970 Membrane alterations associated with hemoglobinopathies. Seminars in Hematology 7: 409–426

55. Kushner J P, Lee G R, Wintrobe M M, Cartwright G E 1971 Idiopathic refractory sideroblastic anemia. Clinical and laboratory investigation of seventeen patients and review of the literature. Medicine 50: 139–159

56. Lee G R, MacDiarmid W D, Cartwright G E, Wintrobe M M 1968 Hereditary, X-linked, sideroachrestic anemia. The isolation of two erythrocyte populations differing in Xg^a blood type and porphyrin content. Blood 32: 59–69

57. MacFadzean A J S, Davis L J 1947 Iron staining erythrocyte inclusions with special reference to acquired haemolytic anemia. Glasgow Medical Journal 28: 237–279

58. MacGibbon B H, Mollin D L 1965 Sideroblastic anemia in man: observations on seventy cases. British Journal of Haematology 11: 59–69

59. Manabe Y, Seto S, Furusho K, Aoki Y 1982 A study of a female with congenital sideroblastic anemia. American Journal of Hematology 12: 63–67

60. Mohandas N, Phillips W M, Bessis M 1979 Red cell deformability and hemolytic anemias. Seminars in Hematology 16: 95–114

61. Mollin D L 1965 Introduction: sideroblasts and sideroblastic anaemia. British Journal of Haematology 11: 41–48

62. Najman A, Breton-Gorius J, Turpin F, Duhamel G, Andre R 1972 Double population érythrocytaire au cours d'une érythro-leucémie avec hémoglobine H. Etude au microscope électronique et en microspectrophotométrie. Nouvelle Revue Française d'Hématologie 12: 43–64

63. Polliack A, Yataganas X, Thorell B, Rachmilewitz E A 1974 An electron microscopic study of the nuclear abnormalites in erythroblasts in beta-thalassaemia major. British Journal of Haematology 26: 201–204

64. Prasad A S, Tranchida L, Konno E T, Berman L, Albert S, Sing C F, Brewer G J 1968 Hereditary sideroblastic anemia and glucose-6-phosphate-dehydrogenase deficiency in a negro family. Journal of Clinical Investigation 47: 1415–1422

65. Roodman G D, Clare C N, Mills G 1982 Congenital dyserythropoietic anaemia type II (CDA II): chromosomal banding studies and adherent cell effects on erythroid colony (CFU-E) and burst (BFU-E) formation. British Journal of Haematology 50: 499–507

66. Sander H J, Slot J W, Bouma B N, Bolhuis P A, Pepper D S, Sixma J J 1983 Immunocytochemical localization of fibrinogen, platelet factor 4 and beta-thromboglobulin in thin frozen sections of human blood platelets. Journal of Clinical Investigation 72: 1277–1287

67. Seip M, Gjessing L R, Lie S O 1971 Congenital sideroblastic anaemia in a girl. Scandinavian Journal of Haematology 8: 501–512

68. Stenberg P E, Shuman M A, Levin S P, Bainton D F 1984 Optimal techniques for the immunocytochemical demonstration of beta-thromboglobulin, platelet factor 4 and fibrinogen in the alpha granules of unstimulated platelets. Histochemical Journal 16: 983–1002

69. Tanaka Y, Goodman J R 1972 Electron microscopy of human blood cells. Harper & Row, New York, p 75

70. Vainchenker W, Guichard J, Breton-Gorius J 1979 Morphological abnormalities in cultured erythroid colonies (BFU-E) from the blood of two patients with HEMPAS. British Journal of Haematology 42: 363–369

71. Vainchenker W, Guichard J, Bouguet J, Breton-Gorius J 1980 Congenital dyserythropoietic anemia I: absence of clonal expression in the nuclear abnormalities of cultured erythroblasts. British Journal of Haematology 46: 33–37

72. Vainchenker W, Breton-Gorius J, Guichard J, Bouguet J, Henri A, Rochant H, Goudsmit R 1980 Congenital dyserythropoietic anemia type III. Studies on erythroid differentiation of blood erythroid progenitor cells (BFU-E) in vitro. Experimental Hematology 8: 1057–1062

73. Valentine W N 1973 Sideroblastic anemias. In: Williams W J, Beutler E, Erslev A J, Lichtman M A (eds) Hematology, 3rd edn. McGraw-Hill, New York, pp 537–546

74. Verwilghen R L 1976 Congenital dyserythropoietic anaemia, type II (HEMPAS). In: Congenital disorders of erythropoiesis. Ciba Foundation Symposium 37. Elsevier, North-Holland, Amsterdam, pp 151–170

75. Weatherall D J 1983 The thalassemias. In: Williams W J, Beutler E, Erslev A, Lichtman M A (eds) Hematology, 3rd edn. McGraw-Hill, New York, pp 493–521

76. Wendt F, Heimpel H 1967 Kongenitale dyserythropoietische Anämie bei Eeinem zweieiigen Zwillingspaar. Medizinische Klinik 62: 172–177

77. White J G 1968 The fine structure of sickled hemoglobin in situ. Blood 31: 561–579

78. Wickramasinghe S N, Bush V 1975 Observations on the ultrastructure of erythropoietic cells and reticulum cells in the bone marrow of patients with homozygous β thalassaemia. British Journal of Haematology 30: 395–399

79. Wickramasinghe S N, Hugues M, Hollan S R, Horanyi M, Szelenyi J 1980 Electron microscope and high resolution autoradiographic studies of the erythroblasts in haemoglobin H disease. British Journal of Haematology 45: 401–404

80. Winterbourn C C, Carrell R W 1973 The attachment of Heinz bodies to the red cell membrane. British Journal of Haematology 25: 585–592

81. Yataganas X, Gahrton G, Thorell B O 1974 Intranuclear hemoglobin in erythroblasts of β thalassemia. Blood 43: 243–250

The Hermansky–Pudlak and grey platelet syndromes

82. Brednar B, Hermansky F, Lojdas 1964 Vascular pseudohemophilia associated with ceroid pigmentophagia in albinos. American Journal of Pathology 45: 283–294

83. Bentfeld-Barker M E, Bainton D F 1982 Identification of primary lysosomes in human megakaryocytes and platelets. Blood 59: 472–481

84. Breton-Gorius J, Guichard J 1975 Two different types of granules in megakaryocytes and platelets as revealed by the diaminobenzidine method. Journal de Microscopie et de Biologie Cellulaire 23: 197–202

85. Breton-Gorius J, Vainchenker W, Nurden A, Levy-Toledano S, Caen J 1981 Defective α-granule production in megakaryocytes from gray platelet syndrome. Ultrastructural studies of bone marrow cells and megakaryocytes growing in culture from blood precursors. American Journal of Pathology 102: 10–19

86. Cramer E M, Vainchenker W, Vinci G, Guichard J, Breton-Gorius J 1985 Gray platelet syndrome: immunoelectron microscopic localization of fibrinogen and von Willebrand factor in platelets and megakaryocytes. Blood 66: 1309–1316

87. Cramer E M, Meyer D, Lemen R, Breton-Gorius J 1985 Eccentric localization of von Willebrand factor in an internal structure of platelet α-granule resembling that of Weibel–Palade bodies. Blood 66: 710–713

88. Da Prada M, Pletscher A, Tranzer J P, Knuche L H 1967 Subcellular localization of 5-hydroxytryptamine and histamine in blood platelets. Nature 216: 1315–1317

89. Da Prada M, Pletscher A 1975 Accumulation of basic drugs in 5-hydroxytryptamine storage organelles of rabbit blood platelets. European Journal of Pharmacology 32: 179–185

90. Da Prada M, Richards J G, Kettler R 1981 Amine storage organelles in platelets. In: Gordon A S (ed) Platelets in biology and pathology. Elsevier, Amsterdam, pp 107–145

91. Davis R B, White J G 1968 Localization of 5-hydroxytryptamine in blood platelets: an ultrastructural and autoradiographic study. British Journal of Haematology 15: 93–99

92. Day H J, Holmsen H 1971 Concepts of the blood platelet release reaction. Series of Hematology 4: 3–27

93. George J N, Saucerman S, Levine S P, Knieriem L K, Bainton D F 1985 Immunoglobulin G is an alpha-granule secreted protein. Journal of Clinical Investigation 76: 2020–2025

94. Gerrard J M, Phillips D R, Rao G H, Plow L F, Walz D, Ross R, Harker L A, White J G 1980 Biochemical studies of two patients with the gray platelet syndrome. Selective deficiency of platelet α-granules. Journal of Clinical Investigation 66: 102–109

95. Hardisty R M, Mills D B C, Ketsa-Ard K 1972 The platelet defect associated with albinism. British Journal of Haematology 23: 679–692

96. Hermansky F, Pudlak P 1959 Albinism associated with hemorrhagic diathesis and unusual pigmented reticular cells in the bone marrow: report of two cases with histochemical studies. Blood 14: 162–169

97. Hourdille P, Fialon P, Belloc F, Boisseau M R, Andrieu J M 1982 Mepacrine labelling test and uranaffin cytochemical reaction in human megakaryocytes. Thrombosis and Haemostasis 47: 232–235

98. Lages B, Scrutton M C, Holmsen H, Day H J, Weiss J H 1975 Metal ion contents of gel-filtered platelets from patients with storage pool disease. Blood 46: 119–130

99. Levy-Toledano S, Caen J P, Breton-Gorius J, Rendu F, Cywiner-Golenzer C, Dupuy E, Legrand Y, Maclouf J 1981 Gray platelet syndrome: α-granule deficiency. Its influence on platelet function. Journal of Laboratory and Clinical Medicine 98: 831–848

100. Lorez H P, Da Prada M, Rendu F, Pletscher A 1977 Mepacrine, a tool for investigation for 5-hydroxytryptamine organelles of blood platelets by fluorescence microscopy. Journal of Laboratory and Clinical Medicine 89: 200–206

101. MacLaren K M, Pepper D 1982 Immunological localization of β thromboglobulin and platelet factor 4 in human megakaryocytes and platelets. Journal of Clinical Pathology 35: 1227–1231

102. Martin J H, Carson F L, Race G J 1974 Calcium containing platelet granules. Journal of Cell Biology 60: 775–777

103. Maurer H M, Buckingham S, McGilvray E, Spielvogel A R, Wolff J A 1968 Prolonged bleeding time, abnormal binding of platelet serotonin (5-HT), absent platelet 'dark body', defective platelet factor 3 activation, bone marrow inclusions and chromosome breaks in albinism. In: Jaffe E R (ed) XII Congress of the International Society of Hematology, New York, p 198

104. Maurer H M, Wolff J A, Buckingham S, Spielvogel A R 1977 'Impotent' platelets in albinos with prolonged bleeding times. Blood 39: 490–499

105. Mouri K, Suzuki S, Sugai K 1984 Electron microscopic and functional studies of patients with gray platelet syndrome. Tohoku Journal of Experimental Medicine 143: 262–287

106. Nurden A T, Kunicki T J, Dupuis D, Soria C, Caen J P 1982 Specific protein and glycoprotein deficiencies in platelets isolated from two patients with the gray platelet syndrome. Blood 59: 709–718

107. Pham T D, Kaplan K L, Butler V P 1983 Immunoelectron microscopic localization of platelet factor 4 and fibrinogen in the granules of human platelets. Journal of Histochemistry and Cytochemistry 31: 905–910

108. Racuglia G 1971 Gray platelet syndrome. A variety of qualitative platelet disorder. American Journal of Medicine 51: 818–828

109. Rendu F, Breton-Gorius J, Trugnan G, Castro-Malaspina H, Andrieu J M, Bereziat G, Lebret M, Caen J P 1978 Studies on a new variant of the Hermansky–Pudlak syndrome: qualitative, ultrastructural and functional abnormalities of the platelet dense bodies associated with a phospholipase A defect. American Journal of Hematology 4: 387–399

110. Richards J G, Da Prada M 1977 Uranaffin reaction: a new cytochemical technique for the localization of adenine nucleotides in organelles storing biogenic amine. Journal of Histochemistry and Cytochemistry 25: 1322–1336

111. Sander H J, Slot J W, Bouma B N, Bolhuis P A, Pepper D S, Sixma J J 1983 Immunocytochemical localization of fibrinogen, platelet factor 4 and beta-thromboglobulin in thin sections of human blood platelets. Journal of Clinical Investigation 72: 1277–1287

112. Sixma J J, van den Berg A, Geuze H J, Hasilik A, von Figura K, Nieuwenhuis H K, van Iwaarden F, Bouma B N 1985 Localization of various proteins, granule secretion in platelets and megakaryocytes by immunoelectron microscopy. Nouvelle Revue Française d'Hématologie 27: 47 (abs)

113. Sixma J J, van den Berg A, Hasilik A, von Figura K, Geuze H J 1985 Immuno-electron microscopical demonstration of lysosomes in human blood platelets and megakaryocytes using anti-cathepsin D. Blood 65: 1287–1291

114. Skaer R J, Flemans R J, McQuilkan S 1981 Mepacrine stains the dense bodies of human platelets and not platelet lysosomes. British Journal of Haematology 49: 435–438

115. Stenberg P E, Shuman M A, Levine S P, Bainton D F 1984 Optimal techniques for the immunocytochemical demonstration of beta-thromboglobulin, platelet factor 4 and fibrinogen in the alpha-granules of unstimulated platelets. Histochemical Journal 16: 983–1002

116. Tranzer J P, Da Prada M, Pletscher A 1966 Ultrastructural localization of 5-hydroxytryptamine in blood platelets. Nature 212: 1574–1575

117. Tranzer J P, Da Prada M, Pletscher A 1972 Storage of 5-hydroxytryptamine in megakaryocytes. Journal of Cell Biology 52: 191–197

118. Wencel-Drake J D, Printer R G, Zimmerman T S, Ginsberg M H 1985 Ultrastructural localization of human platelet thrombospondin, fibrinogen, fibronectin and von Willibrand factor in frozen thin section. Blood 65: 929–938

119. Weiss H J, Tschopp T B, Roger S J, Brand H 1974 Studies of platelet 5-hydroxytryptamine (serotonin) in storage pool disease and albinism. Journal of Clinical Investigation 54: 421–432

120. White J G 1969 The dense bodies of human platelets: inherent electron opacity of serotonin storage particles. Blood 33: 598–606

121. White J G 1971 Serotonin storage organelles in human megakaryocytes. American Journal of Pathology 63: 403–408

122. White J G, Gerrard J M 1976 Ultrastructural features of abnormal blood platelets. A review. American Journal of Pathology 83: 590–614

123. White J G, Edson J R, Desnick S J, Witkop C J 1971 Studies of platelets in a variant of the Hermansky–Pudlak syndrome. American Journal of Pathology 63: 319–330

124. White J G, Witkop C J, Gerritsen S M 1972 The Hermansky–Pudlak syndrome. Ultrastructure of bone marrow macrophages. American Journal of Pathology 70: 329–344

125. White J G 1979 Ultrastructural studies of the gray platelet syndrome. American Journal of Pathology 95: 445–462

The Chediak–Higashi syndrome and congenital lactoferrin deficiency

126. Bainton D F, Ullyot J L, Farquhar M G 1971 The development of neutrophilic polymorphonuclear leukocytes in human bone marrow.

Origin and content of azurophil and specific granules. Journal of Experimental Medicine 134: 907–934

127. Bèguez-Cèsar A 1943 Neutropenia cronica maligna familiar con granulaciones atipicas de los leucocitos. Sociedad Cubana de Pediatrica. Boletin 15: 900–922

128. Blume R S, Wolff S M 1972 The Chèdiak–Higashi syndrome: studies of host defenses. Annals of Internal Medicine 76: 293–306

129. Borregard N, Boxer L A, Smolen J E, Tauber A I 1985 Anomalous neutrophil granule distribution in a patient with lactoferrin deficiency: pertinence to the respiratory burst. American Journal of Hematology 18: 255–260

130. Boxer L A, Albertini D F, Baehner R L, Oliver J M 1979 Impaired microtubule assembly and polymorphonuclear leucocyte function in the Chèdiak–Higashi syndrome correctable by ascorbic acid. British Journal of Haematology 43: 207–213

131. Boxer L A, Coates T D, Haak R A, Baruch Wolach J, Hoffstein S, Baehner R L 1982 Lactoferrin deficiency associated with altered granulocyte function. New England Journal of Medicine 307: 404–410

132. Breton-Gorius J, Mason D Y, Buriot D, Vilde J L, Griscelli C 1980 Lactoferrin deficiency as a consequence of a lack of specific granules in neutrophils from a patient with recurrent infections. American Journal of Pathology 99: 413–428

133. Clawson C C, Repine J E, White J G 1979 The Chèdiak–Higashi syndrome: quantitation of a deficiency in maximal bactericidal capacity. American Journal of Pathology 94: 539–548

134. Cramer E, Pryzwansky K B, Villeval J L, Testa U, Breton-Gorius J 1985 Ultrastructural localization of lactoferrin and myeloperoxidase in human neutrophils by immunogold. Blood 65: 423–432

135. Gallin J I, Elin R J, Hubert R T, Fauci A S, Kaliner M A, Wolff S M 1979 Efficacy of ascorbic acid in Chèdiak–Higashi syndrome (CHS): studies in humans and mice. Blood 53: 226–231

136. Gallin J I, Fletcher M P, Seligmann B E, Hoffstein S, Cehrs K, Mounessa N 1982 Human neutrophil-specific granule deficiency: a model to assess the role of neutrophil-specific granules in the evolution of the inflammatory response. Blood 59: 1317–1329

137. Komiyama A, Morosawa H, Nakahata T, Miyagawa Y, Akabane T 1979 Abnormal neutrophil maturation in a neutrophil defect with morphologic abnormality and impaired function. Journal of Pediatrics 94: 19–25

138. Grossi C E, Crist W H, Abo T, Velardi A, Cooper M D 1985 Expression of the Chèdiak Higashi lysosomal abnormality in human peripheral blood lymphocyte subpopulations. Blood 65: 937–944

139. Mason D Y, Farrell C, Taylor C R 1975 The detection of intracellular antigens in human leukocytes by immunoperoxidase staining. British Journal of Haematology 31: 361–370

140. Masson P L, Heremans J F, Schowne E 1969 Lactoferrin, an iron-binding protein in neutrophil leukocytes. Journal of Experimental Medicine 130: 643–658

141. Oliver J M, Zurier R B 1976 Correction of the characteristic abnormalities of microtubule function and granule morphology in Chèdiak–Higashi syndrome with cholinergic agonists: studies in vitro in man and in vivo in the beige mouse. Journal of Clinical Investigation 57: 1239–1247

142. Parmley R T, Ogawa M, Darby C P Jr, Spicer S S 1975 Congenital neutropenia: neutrophil proliferation with abnormal maturation. Blood 46: 723–734

143. Parmley R T, Tzeng D, Baehner R L, Boxer L A 1983 Abnormal distribution of complex carbohydrates in neutrophils of a patient with lactoferrin deficiency. Blood 62: 538–548

144. Pryzwansky K B, Rausch P G, Spitznagel J K, Nerion J C 1979 Immunocytochemical distinction between primary and specific granule formation in developing human neutrophils: correlations with Romanovsky stains. Blood 53: 179–185

145. Pryzwansky K B, Schilwa M, Boxer L A 1985 Microtubule organization of unstimulated and stimulated adherent neutrophils in Chèdiak–Higashi syndrome. Blood 66: 1393–1403

146. Rausch P G, Pryzwansky K B, Spitznagel J K 1978 Immunocytochemical identification of azurophilic and specific granule markers in the giant granules of Chèdiak–Higashi neutrophils. New England Journal of Medicine 298: 693–698

147. Rendu F, Breton-Gorius J, Lebret M, Klebanoff C, Buriot D, Griscelli C, Levy-Toledano S, Caen J P 1983 Evidence that abnormal platelet functions in human Chèdiak–Higashi syndrome are the result of a lack of dense bodies. American Journal of Pathology 111: 307–314

148. Root R K, Rosenthal A S, Balestra D J 1972 Abnormal bactericidal, metabolic and lysosomal functions of Chèdiak–Higashi syndrome leukocytes. Journal of Clinical Investigation 51: 649–665

149. Spitznagel J K, Cooper M R, McCall A E, DeChatelet L R, Welsh I R H 1972 Selective deficiency of granules associated with lysozyme and lactoferrin in human polymorphonuclear leukocytes with reduced microbicidal capacity. Journal of Clinical Investigation 51: 93a

150. Strauss R G, Boue K E, Jones J F, Mauer A M, Fulginiti V A 1974 An anomaly of neutrophil morphology with impaired function. New England Journal of Medicine 290: 478–484

151. White J G 1966 The Chèdiak–Higashi syndrome: a possible lysosomal disease. Blood 28: 143–156

152. White J G 1967 The Chèdiak–Higashi syndrome: cytoplasmic sequestration in circulating leukocytes. Blood 29: 435–450

153. White J G, Clawson C C 1979 The Chèdiak–Higashi syndrome: ring-shaped lysosomes in circulating monocytes. American Journal of Pathology 96: 781–798

154. White J G, Clawson C C 1979 The Chèdiak–Higashi syndrome: microtubules in monocytes and lymphocytes. American Journal of Hematology 7: 349–356

155. White J G, Clawson C C 1980 The Chèdiak–Higashi syndrome: the nature of the giant neutrophil granules and their interactions with cytoplasm and foreign particulates. American Journal of Pathology 98: 151–196

156. Windhorts D B, Padgett G 1973 The Chèdiak–Higashi syndrome and the homologous trait in animals. Journal of Investigative Dermatology 60: 529–537

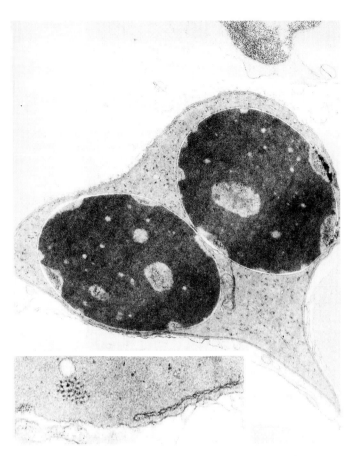

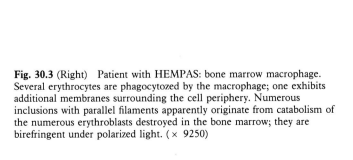

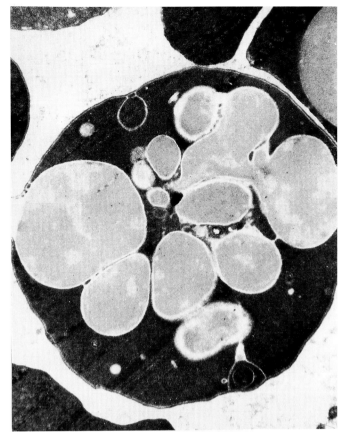

Fig. 30.1 (Above) Type II congenital dyserythropoietic anaemia (HEMPAS): bone marrow binucleated normoblast. A continuous cisterna surrounds the cell periphery at a constant distance from the cell membrane. Note the pyknotic appearance of the nucleus and the presence of some polyribosomes in the cytoplasm. (× 13 500) *Inset* Enlargement of the cell periphery. No ribosomes are attached to the cisterna beneath the plasma membrane (× 40 300)

Fig. 30.2 (Above right) Patient with HEMPAS: normoblast from bone marrow incubated in the diaminobenzidine medium to stain haemoglobin. The dark staining of the cytoplasm, identical to that of erythrocytes, indicates a fully mature cell. The additional cisterna which appears to be continuous beneath the cell membrane is visualized as a white line because the cisterna does not contain haemoglobin: two loops are seen in continuity with the cisterna. Note the extreme multilobulation of the nucleus. (× 9200) From Breton-Gorius et al.[15]

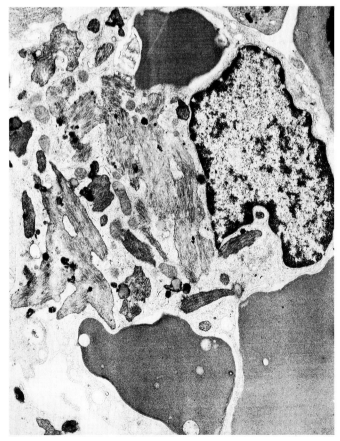

Fig. 30.3 (Right) Patient with HEMPAS: bone marrow macrophage. Several erythrocytes are phagocytozed by the macrophage; one exhibits additional membranes surrounding the cell periphery. Numerous inclusions with parallel filaments apparently originate from catabolism of the numerous erythroblasts destroyed in the bone marrow; they are birefringent under polarized light. (× 9250)

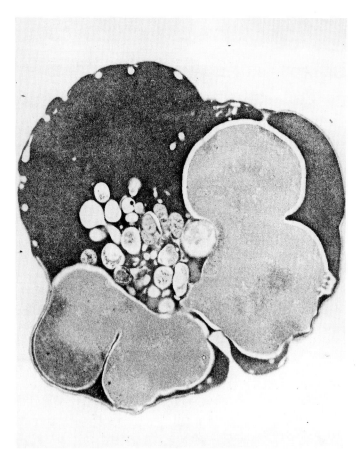

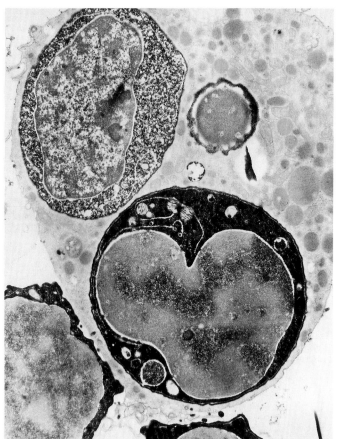

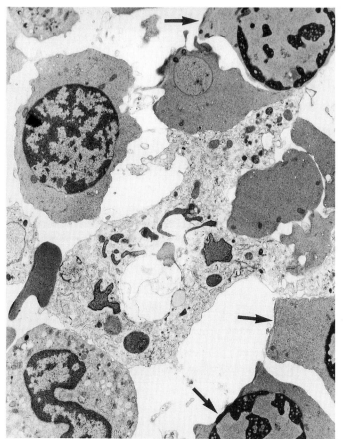

Fig. 30.4 (Above)   Patient with HEMPAS: a multilobulated erythroblast growing in plasma clot medium from a BFU-E in a patient with HEMPAS. The abnormalities of the nucleus are similar to those seen in vivo, as well as the presence of the additional membrane beneath the cell membrane. This finding indicates that the defect is present at the level of the erythroid stem cells. (× 9000)

Fig. 30.5 (Above right)   Patient with HEMPAS: phagocytosis of the abnormal erythroblasts maturing in vitro. After the lysis of the clot, macrophages present in the culture rapidly engulf several erythroblasts, containing variable amounts of haemoglobin as detected by the oxidized DAB. Under normal conditions only the expelled nuclei are phagocytozed. (× 7500) From Vainchenker et al.[70]

Fig. 30.6 (Right)   Patient with congenital dyserythropoietic anaemia (CDA) type I: erythroblastic island in the bone marrow. Several normoblast nuclei exhibit the spongy appearance of the chromatin (arrows) and dilated nuclear pores. (× 5720) From Vainchenker et al.[71]

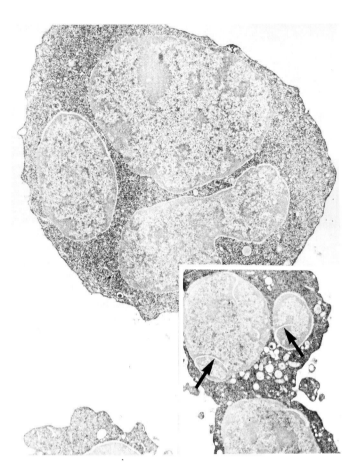

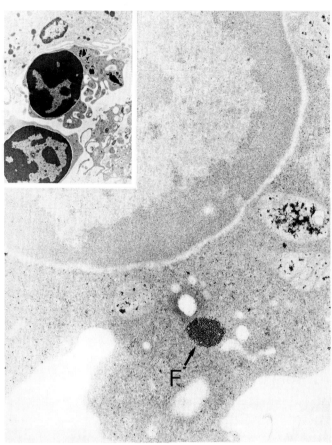

Fig. 30.7 Patient with CDA type III: giant and multilobulated or multinucleated erythroblast in the bone marrow. The density of the cytoplasm, due to the oxidized DAB, indicates normal haemoglobin formation. (× 5060) *Inset* Similar giant erythroblast obtained in culture. Note the nuclear clefts (arrows) which can also be observed in the erythroblasts in vivo (× 4180) From Vainchenker et al.[71]

Fig. 30.8 Congenital severe sideroblastic anaemia due to ALA-synthetase deficiency: normoblast. A cluster of ferritin molecules (F) and intramitochondrial iron deposit with a distinct appearance can be seen. (× 29 500) *Inset* A mature normoblast from the same patient showing intense iron deposit between the mitochondrial cristae. In addition, clumps of glycogen particles are present in the cytoplasm. (× 4500)

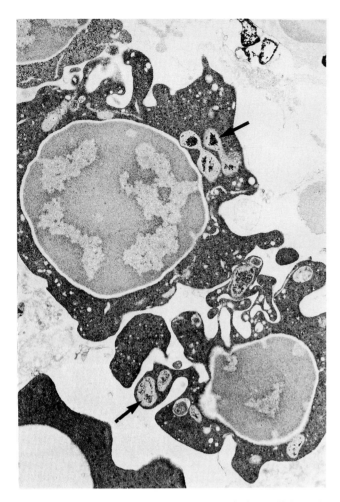

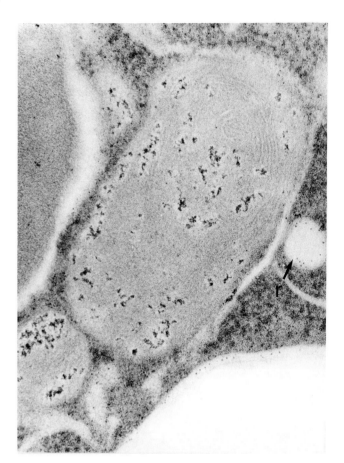

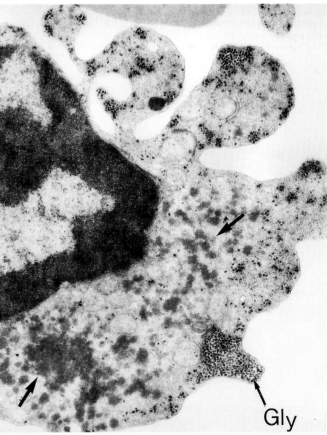

Fig. 30.9 (Above)   Congenital sideroblastic anaemia due to ALA-synthetase deficiency: normoblasts after incubation in DAB medium to detect pseudo-peroxidatic activity of haemoglobin. The same patient as in Fig. 30.8. The density of the cytoplasm is proportional to the amount of haemoglobin. Mitochondria (arrows), which are somewhat swollen, show a variable deposit of iron between the cristae. ($\times$ 10 360)

Fig. 30.10 (Above right)   Congenital sideroblastic anaemia due to ALA-synthetase deficiency: mitochondria in a polychromatophilic erythroblast. The same patient as in Figs 30.8 and 30.9. At the early phase of iron deposition in the mitochondria it is easier to see the filamentous appearance compared to that of individual ferritin molecules seen in rhopheocytotic vesicle (r) and at the surface of the cell membrane. Note the concentric arrangement of the cristae in the mitochondria. ($\times$ 62 300)

Fig. 30.11 (Right)   Homozygous beta thalassaemia: bone marrow erythroblast. Abundant masses of denatured alpha globin chain precipitate within the cytoplasm (arrows). Aggregates of glycogen (Gly) particles are located at the cell periphery. ($\times$ 20 300) From Beuzard et al.[10]

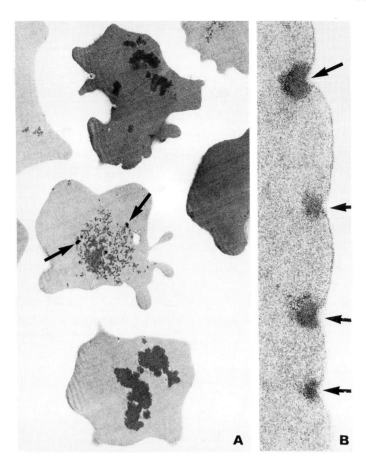

Fig. 30.12 Patient with unstable haemoglobin: cytoplasmic inclusions. **A** Large irregular masses and aggregates of small dense inclusions predominate in the middle of the reticulocytes and red cells. Note the presence of mitochondrial iron in a reticulocyte (arrows). ($\times$ 7600) **B** The cell membrane appears to be modified on each side where it meets the dense inclusions or Heinz bodies (arrows). ($\times$ 66 500)

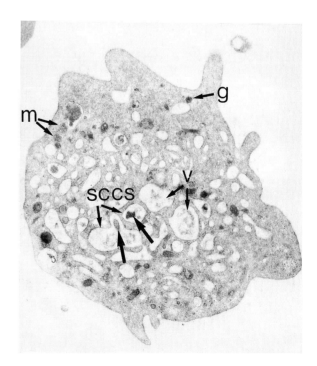

Fig. 30.13 (Right) Grey platelet: virtual absence of alpha-granules. In addition to profoundly reduced alpha-granules, this platelet is characterized by marked vacuolization (v) of the cytoplasm and dilated cisternae of the SCCS with deposits of dense material (arrow). Some small granules (g) and mitochondria (m) are present. ($\times$ 34 020) From Levy-Toledano et al[99]

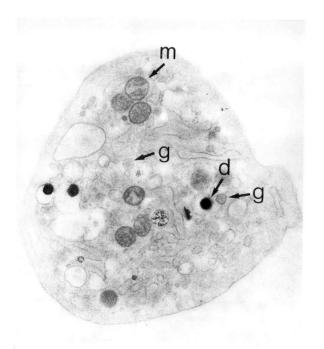

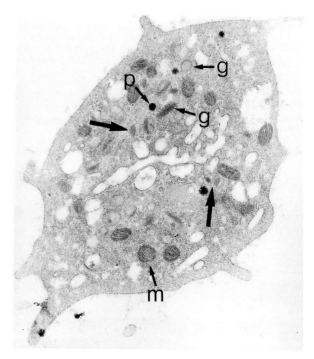

Fig. 30.14 Grey platelet fixed in the presence of calcium: dense bodies. The dense bodies are easily identified by their dense content (d). Numerous mitochondria (m) can be seen, but there are no normal alpha-granules. Some unidentified small granules (g) are scattered in the cytoplasm. (× 21 580)

Fig. 30.15 Grey platelet: cytochemical demonstration of catalase. Four small granules (p) are identified as microperoxisomes. Small granules (g) of other types are present also, and some exhibit a dense core (arrow). There are numerous mitochondria (m). (× 18 900) From Levy-Toledano et al[99]

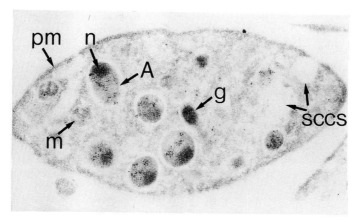

Fig. 30.16 Normal platelet treated with an anti-Fg antibody and immunogold: topographical distribution. Gold particles are localized on the matrix of the α granules (A), with the exception of the dense nucleoids (n). Small granules of other types (g), mitochondria (m), the plasma membrane (pm) and SCCS are not labelled. (× 30 160) From Cramer et al[86]

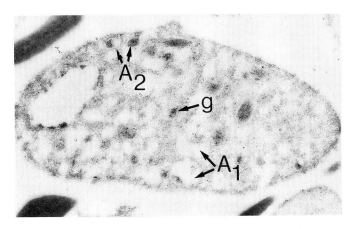

Fig. 30.17 Grey platelet treated with an anti-vWF antibody and immunogold: topographical distribution. Two populations of abnormal granules are identified: some are normal in size but with little internal structure (A₁), while others are of small size (A₂), resembling small granules of other types (g). (× 28 440) From Cramer et al[86]

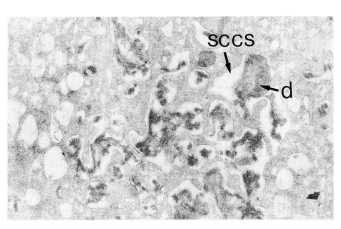

Fig. 30.18 Grey platelet syndrome: megakaryocyte. Part of a bone marrow megakaryocyte displaying dense material (d) within the dilated cisternae of its demarcation membranes (SCCS). (× 16 200)

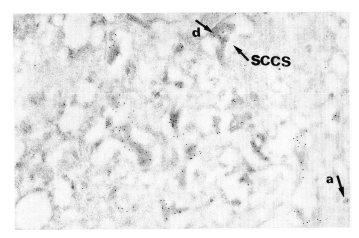

Fig. 30.19 Grey platelet syndrome: dilatation of SCCS. Grey platelet displaying a dilated SCCS containing dense material (d) identical to that found in megakaryocytes. This material is specifically labelled for Fg and thus indicates release of normal alpha-granule content into the SCCS. Small abnormal alpha-granules (a) are also visible in this section. (× 19 440) From Cramer et al[86]

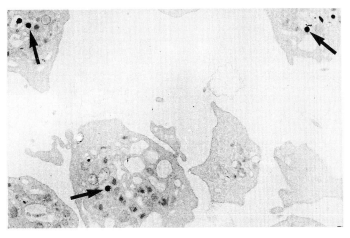

Fig. 30.20 General view of normal platelets showing dense bodies. Dense cores of variable size are located in a vacuole (arrows). They are distinguished from α granules by their opacity, with a nucleoid which is less dense. (× 8800)

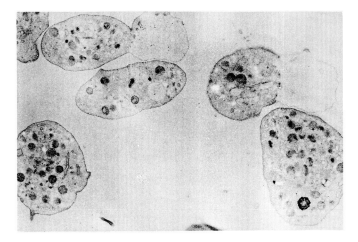

Fig. 30.21 (Above)   General view of Hermansky–Pudlak syndrome (HPS) platelets. Only one abnormal DB is seen in a single platelet. (× 7500)

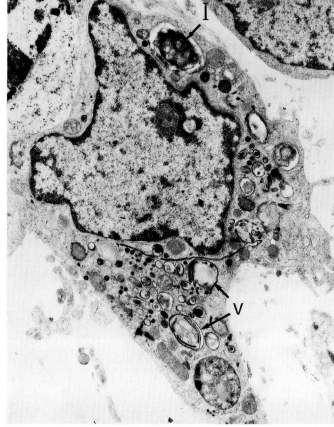

Fig. 30.22 (Above right)   Patient with HPS: bone marrow macrophage. Numerous heterogeneous inclusions (I) and vacuoles (V) containing a few membranous residues and material of low electron-density. (× 10 800)

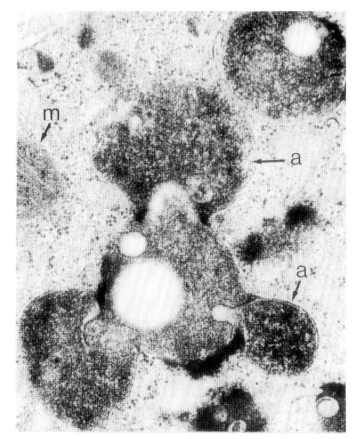

Fig. 30.23 (Right)   Chèdiak–Higashi syndrome (CHS): promyelocyte. Part of a bone marrow promyelocyte from a CHS patient. Four azurophilic granules (a) are fusing to form a typical giant granule. m = mitochondrion. (× 38 800)

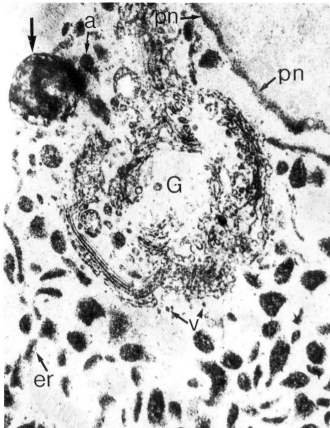

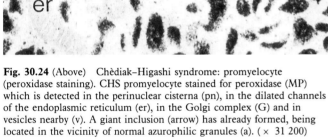

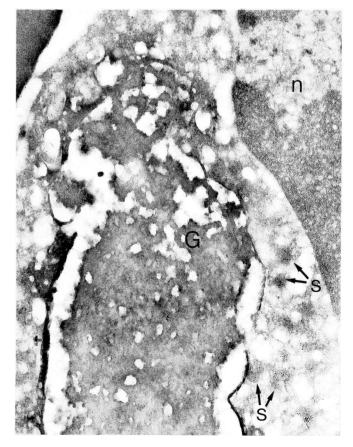

Fig. 30.24 (Above) Chèdiak–Higashi syndrome: promyelocyte (peroxidase staining). CHS promyelocyte stained for peroxidase (MP) which is detected in the perinuclear cisterna (pn), in the dilated channels of the endoplasmic reticulum (er), in the Golgi complex (G) and in vesicles nearby (v). A giant inclusion (arrow) has already formed, being located in the vicinity of normal azurophilic granules (a). (× 31 200)

Fig. 30.25 (Above right) Chèdiak-Higashi syndrome: polymorphonuclear leukocyte. Part of a CHS PMN stained for peroxidase, displaying giant inclusions and granules (G), myelin figures (m), rare normal azurophilic granules (a) and an apparently normal number of specific granules (s). n = nucleus. (× 25 200)

Fig. 30.26 (Right) Chèdiak–Higashi syndrome: peroxidase and lactoferrin in a neutrophil. Peroxidase cytochemistry and immunogold localization of lactoferrin in a CHS PMN: the giant inclusion (G) is MPO-positive, but contains virtually no gold labelling for lactoferrin, which is still evident in the cytoplasm within the specific granules (s). No normal azurophilic granules remain in the cell. n = nucleus. (× 52 000)

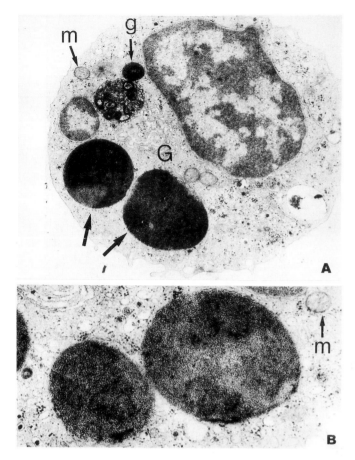

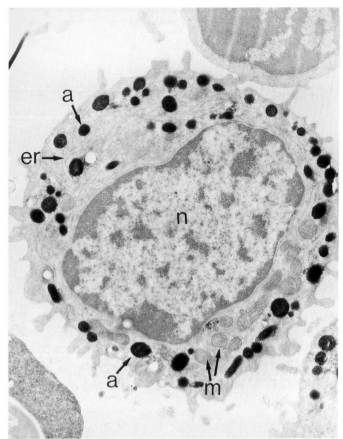

Fig. 30.27 (Above)   Chèdiak–Higashi syndrome: basophil myelocyte. **A** In CHS bone marrow, basophil myelocytes contain giant granules (arrows) as well as granules of intermediate and normal size (g) in the vicinity of the Golgi complex (G), whose cisternae are dilated. m = mitochondria. (× 11 760) **B** In the giant granules of CHS basophils, the structure of normal basophil granules is still present and identifiable. m = mitochondria. (× 21 400)

Fig. 30.28 (Above right)   Lactoferrin deficiency: myelocyte (peroxidase cytochemistry). Bone marrow myelocyte from a patient with lactoferrin deficiency. Endoplasmic reticulum (er) is negative for MPO, showing that the synthesis of MPO has ceased. However, no specific granules are found in the cytoplasm, only azurophilic MPO positive granules (a) being present. n = nucleus; m = mitochondria. (× 11 250)

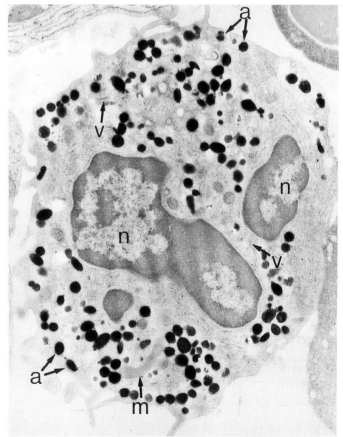

Fig. 30.29 (Right)   Lactoferrin deficiency: neutrophil (peroxidase cytochemistry). Mature PMN from a lactoferrin-deficient patient. Numerous azurophilic MPO- positive granules (a) are present in the cytoplasm, but no typical specific granules can be seen. Some rare elongated flat vesicles (v) — previously interpreted as abnormal specific granules — are also present. m = mitochondria; n = nucleus. (× 13 500) From Breton-Gorius et al[132]

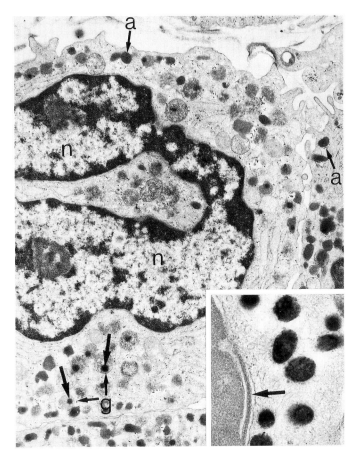

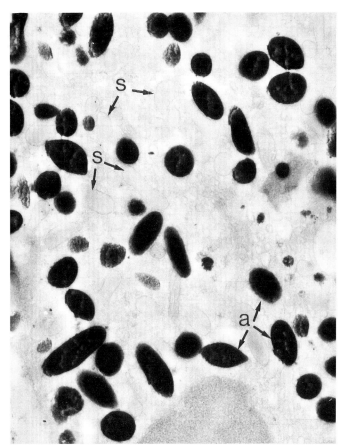

Fig. 30.30 Lactoferrin deficiency: promyelocyte. Abnormal promyelocyte from a lactoferrin-deficient patient's bone marrow. The nucleus (n) is abnormally segmented. Some azurophilic granules (a) are normal but others are abnormal (g), being partially extracted with a dense core (arrow). (× 10 800) *Inset* Several nuclear abnormalities are found in lactoferrin-deficient neutrophils, among them nuclear clefts (arrow). (× 25 740)

Fig. 30.31 Normal polymorphonuclear leukocyte: peroxidase cytochemistry. Large MPO-positive azurophilic granules (a), and numerous smaller electron-lucent specific granules (s) can be seen. (× 22 440)

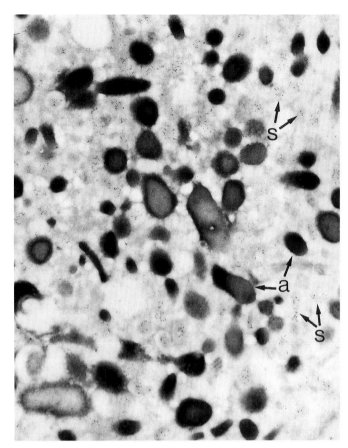

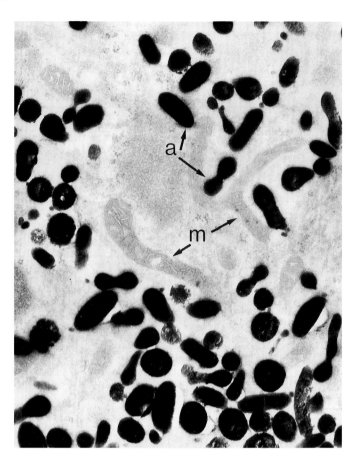

Fig. 30.32 Normal polymorphonuclear leukocyte: peroxidase cytochemistry and immunogold demonstration of lactoferrin. Beside dense MPO-positive azurophilic granules (a), the specific granules (s) are labelled by gold particles due to their lactoferrin content. (× 18 480) From Cramer et al.[134]

Fig. 30.33 Lactoferrin deficiency: detail of polymorphonuclear leukocyte. Only MPO-positive azurophilic granules (a) are present in the cytoplasm. No specific granules are observed. m = mitochondria. (× 22 440) From Breton-Gorius et al.[134]

Index